FAUST'S
ANESTHESIOLOGY REVIEW
Fourth Edition

FAUST'S ANESTHESIOLOGY REVIEW

Fourth Edition

Edited by

Michael J. Murray, MD, PhD
Consultant, Department of Anesthesiology
Mayo Clinic, Phoenix, Arizona
Professor of Anesthesiology
Mayo Clinic College of Medicine

Associate Editors

Barry A. Harrison, MD
Consultant, Department of Anesthesiology
Mayo Clinic, Jacksonville, Florida
Assistant Professor of Anesthesiology
Mayo Clinic College of Medicine

Jeff T. Mueller, MD
Consultant, Department of Anesthesiology
Mayo Clinic, Phoenix, Arizona
Assistant Professor of Anesthesiology
Mayo Clinic College of Medicine

Steven H. Rose, MD
Consultant, Department of Anesthesiology
Mayo Clinic, Rochester, Minnesota
Professor of Anesthesiology
Mayo Clinic College of Medicine

C. Thomas Wass, MD
Consultant, Department of Anesthesiology
Mayo Clinic, Rochester, Minnesota
Associate Professor of Anesthesiology
Mayo Clinic College of Medicine

Denise J. Wedel, MD
Consultant, Department of Anesthesiology
Mayo Clinic, Rochester, Minnesota
Professor of Anesthesiology
Mayo Clinic College of Medicine

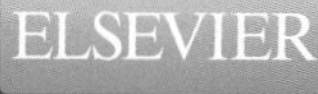

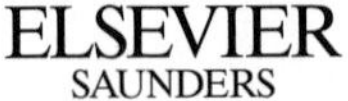
ELSEVIER
SAUNDERS

1600 John F. Kennedy Blvd.
Ste 1800
Philadelphia, PA 19103-2899

FAUST'S ANESTHESIOLOGY REVIEW,
FOURTH EDITION

ISBN: 978-1-4377-1369-5

Notices

Knowledge and best practice in this field are constantly changing. As new research and experience broaden our understanding, changes in research methods, professional practices, or medical treatment may become necessary.

Practitioners and researchers must always rely on their own experience and knowledge in evaluating and using any information, methods, compounds, or experiments described herein. In using such information or methods they should be mindful of their own safety and the safety of others, including parties for whom they have a professional responsibility.

With respect to any drug or pharmaceutical products identified, readers are advised to check the most current information provided (i) on procedures featured or (ii) by the manufacturer of each product to be administered, to verify the recommended dose or formula, the method and duration of administration, and contraindications. It is the responsibility of practitioners, relying on their own experience and knowledge of their patients, to make diagnoses, to determine dosages and the best treatment for each individual patient, and to take all appropriate safety precautions.

To the fullest extent of the law, neither the Publisher nor the authors, contributors, or editors, assume any liability for any injury and/or damage to persons or property as a matter of products liability, negligence or otherwise, or from any use or operation of any methods, products, instructions, or ideas contained in the material herein.

Library of Congress Cataloging-in-Publication Data

Anesthesiology review (Faust)
Faust's anesthesiology review / edited by Michael J. Murray ; associate editors, Steven H. Rose, Denise J. Wedel, C. Thomas Wass, Barry A. Harrison, Jeff T. Mueller. -- Fourth edition.
p. ; cm.
Preceded by: Anesthesiology review / edited by Ronald J. Faust. 3rd ed. 2002.
Includes bibliographical references and index.
ISBN 978-1-4377-1369-5 (hardcover : alk. paper)
I. Murray, Michael J. (Michael James), 1949- editor of compilation. II. Rose, Steven H., editor of compilation. III. Wedel, Denise J., editor of compilation. IV. Wass, C. Thomas, editor of compilation. V. Harrison, Barry A., editor of compilation. VI. Mueller, Jeff T., editor of compilation. VII. Title.
[DNLM: 1. Anesthesiology. 2. Anesthesia. WO 200]
RD82.3
617.9'6076--dc23
2014001771

Executive Content Strategist: William Schmitt
Senior Content Development Specialist: Deidre Simpson
Publishing Services Manager: Catherine Jackson
Senior Project Manager: Mary Pohlman
Design Direction: Louis Forgione

Printed in Canada

Last digit is the print number: 9 8 7 6 5 4 3 2

Dedication

Catherine Friederich Murray - who provided phenomenal writing and editing skills for the entire edition.

Contributors

Martin D. Abel, MD
Consultant, Department of Anesthesiology, Mayo Clinic, Rochester, Minnesota
Professor of Anesthesiology, Mayo Clinic College of Medicine

Adebola Adesanya, MD, MPH
Medical Director, Critical Care Services, Medical City Dallas Hospital, Dallas, Texas

Brooke E. Albright, MD, Major USAF
Adjunct Assistant Professor, Department of Anesthesiology, USUHS
Department of Anesthesiology and Pain Medicine, Landstuhl Regional Medical Center, Landstuhl, Germany

Bradley Anderson, MD
Resident, Department of Anesthesiology, Baylor College of Medicine, Houston, Texas

Richard L. Applegate II, MD
Professor and Vice Chair, Department of Anesthesiology, Loma Linda University School of Medicine, Loma Linda, California

Katherine W. Arendt, MD
Consultant, Department of Anesthesiology, Mayo Clinic, Rochester, Minnesota
Assistant Professor of Anesthesiology, Mayo Clinic College of Medicine

Anna E. Bartunek, MD
Associate Professor, Medical Doctor, Department of Cardiothoracic and Vascular Anesthesia and Intensive Care, Medical University of Vienna, Vienna, Austria

Keith H. Berge, MD
Consultant, Department of Anesthesiology, Mayo Clinic, Rochester, Minnesota
Assistant Professor of Anesthesiology, Mayo Clinic College of Medicine

Michael L. Bishop, MD
Professor, Department of Anesthesiology, University of California San Diego, San Diego, California

Susan Black, MD
Professor and Vice Chair, Department of Anesthesiology, University of Alabama School of Medicine, Birmingham, Alabama

Gilbert A. Blaise, MD
Professeur Titulaire, Département d'anesthésiologie, Université de Montréal, Montréal, Québec, Canada

Eric L. Bloomfield, MD, MS, MMI, FCCM
Consultant, Department of Anesthesiology and the Division of Critical Care Medicine, Mayo Clinic, Rochester, Minnesota
Associate Professor of Anesthesiology, Mayo Clinic College of Medicine

Caridad Bravo-Fernandez, MD
Anesthesiologist, Froedtert Health-Froedtert Hospital, Milwaukee, Wisconsin

Daniel R. Brown, MD, PhD, FCCM
Director, Critical Care Multidisciplinary Practice, Department of Anesthesiology, Mayo Clinic, Rochester, Minnesota
Associate Professor of Anesthesiology, Mayo Clinic College of Medicine

David L. Brown, MD
Anesthesiology Institute Chair, Cleveland Clinic, Cleveland, Ohio

Sorin J. Brull, MD, FCARCSI (Hon)
Consultant, Department of Anesthesiology, Mayo Clinic, Jacksonville, Florida
Professor of Anesthesiology, Mayo Clinic College of Medicine

Daniel R. Bustamante, MD
Assistant Professor, Department of Anesthesiology, University of Tennessee Graduate School of Medicine, Knoxville, Tennessee

Paul E. Carns, MD
Consultant, Department of Anesthesiology, Mayo Clinic, Rochester, Minnesota
Assistant Professor of Anesthesiology, Mayo Clinic College of Medicine

Edmund Carton, MD
Department of Critical Care Medicine, Mater Misericordiae University Hospital, Dublin, Ireland

Renee E. Caswell, MD
Consultant, Department of Anesthesiology, Mayo Clinic, Phoenix, Arizona
Assistant Professor of Anesthesiology, Mayo Clinic College of Medicine

Steven R. Clendenen, MD
Consultant, Department of Anesthesiology, Mayo Clinic, Jacksonville, Florida
Assistant Professor of Anesthesiology, Mayo Clinic College of Medicine

Norman A. Cohen, MD
Associate Professor, Department of Anesthesiology and Perioperative Medicine, Oregon Health & Science University, Portland, Oregon

Daniel J. Cole, MD
Consultant, Department of Anesthesiology, Mayo Clinic, Phoenix, Arizona
Professor of Anesthesiology and Vice Dean for Continuous Professional Development, Mayo Clinic College of Medicine

Craig M. Combs, MD
Assistant Professor, Department of Anesthesiology, University of Tennessee Medical Center, Knoxville, Tennessee

James P. Conterato, MD
Assistant Clinical Professor,
Department of Anesthesiology,
Medical College of Wisconsin, Milwaukee, Wisconsin

David J. Cook, MD
Consultant, Department of Anesthesiology, Mayo Clinic, Rochester, Minnesota
Professor of Anesthesiology, Mayo Clinic College of Medicine

Eric G. Cornidez, MD
Interventional Pain Physician, Pain Management, The Pain Institute of Southern Arizona, Tucson, Arizona

Douglas B. Coursin, MD
Professor, Department of Anesthesiology and Medicine, University of Wisconsin School of Medicine and Public Health, Madison, Wisconsin

Robert M. Craft, MD
Professor, Department of Anesthesiology, University of Tennessee Graduate School of Medicine, Knoxville, Tennessee

Claudia C. Crawford, MD
Consultant, Department of Anesthesiology, Mayo Clinic, Jacksonville, Florida
Assistant Professor of Anesthesiology, Mayo Clinic College of Medicine

Frank D. Crowl, MD
Anesthesiology & Pain Management, Atlantic Pain Management Center, Wilmington, North Carolina

Efrain Israel Cubillo, IV, MD
Fellow in Anesthesiology, Mayo School of Graduate Medical Education, Phoenix, Arizona

Roy F. Cucchiara, MD
Consultant, Department of Anesthesiology, Mayo Clinic, Jacksonville, Florida
Professor of Anesthesiology, Mayo Clinic College of Medicine

Nancy J. Cummings, Esq.
Senior Legal Council, Legal Department, Mayo Clinic, Scottsdale, Arizona

David R. Danielson, MD
Consultant, Department of Anesthesiology, Mayo Clinic, Rochester, Minnesota
Assistant Professor of Anesthesiology, Mayo Clinic College of Medicine

Nicole M. Dawson, MD
Anesthesiologist, Portland, Oregon

Marie L. De Ruyter, MD
Consultant, Department of Anesthesiology, Mayo Clinic, Jacksonville, Florida
Assistant Professor of Anesthesiology, Mayo Clinic College of Medicine

Martin L. De Ruyter, MD
Professor, Department of Anesthesiology, University of Kansas Medical Center, Kansas City, Kansas

Peter A. DeSocio, DO
Associate Professor-Clinical, Department of Anesthesiology, The Ohio State University Wexner Medical Center, Columbus, Ohio

Daniel A. Diedrich, MD
Consultant, Department of Anesthesiology, Division of Critical Care Medicine, Mayo Clinic, Rochester, Minnesota
Assistant Professor of Anesthesiology, Mayo Clinic College of Medicine

Niki M. Dietz, MD
Consultant, Department of Anesthesiology, Mayo Clinic, Rochester, Minnesota
Professor of Anesthesiology, Mayo Clinic College of Medicine

John A. Dilger, MD
Consultant, Department of Anesthesiology, Mayo Clinic, Rochester, Minnesota
Associate Professor of Anesthesiology, Mayo Clinic College of Medicine

Gavin D. Divertie, MD
Chair, Department of Critical Care Medicine, Mayo Clinic, Jacksonville, Florida
Assistant Professor of Anesthesiology, Mayo Clinic College of Medicine

Karen B. Domino, MD, MPH
Professor, Department of Anesthesiology & Pain Medicine, University of Washington School of Medicine, Seattle, Washington

Brian S. Donahue, MD, PhD
Associate Professor, Department of Anesthesiology, Vanderbilt University, Nashville, Tennessee

Carla L. Dormer, MD
Supplemental Consultant, Department of Anesthesiology, Mayo Clinic, Phoenix, Arizona

Jerry A. Dorsch, MD
Emeritus Associate Professor of Anesthesiology, Mayo Clinic College of Medicine

Douglas A. Dubbink, MD
Surgery Medical Director, Department of Anesthesiology, Woodwinds Hospital, Woodbury, Minnesota

Andrea P. Dutoit, MD
Assistant Professor, Department of Anesthesiology, University of Oklahoma Health Sciences Center, Oklahoma City, Oklahoma

Beth A. Elliott, MD
Consultant, Department of Anesthesiology, Mayo Clinic, Rochester, Minnesota
Assistant Professor of Anesthesiology, Mayo Clinic College of Medicine

Brian Emerson, MD
Assistant Professor, Department of Pediatric Anesthesiology, Monroe Carrel Jr. Children's Hospital at Vanderbilt, Nashville, Tennessee

Jerry L. Epps, MD
Associate Professor, Department of Anesthesiology, University of Tennessee Graduate School of Medicine, Knoxville, Tennessee

Kirstin M. Erickson, MD
Consultant, Department of Anesthesiology, Mayo Clinic, Rochester, Minnesota
Assistant Professor of Anesthesiology, Mayo Clinic College of Medicine

Scott A. Eskuri, MD
Medical Director of Perioperative Services, Department of Anesthesiology, Essentia Health, Duluth, Minnesota

Jonathan A. Faust, MD
Anesthesiologist, Mercy Hospital, Minneapolis, Minnesota

Neil G. Feinglass, MD, FASE, FCCP
Director, Intra-operative Echocardiography; Consultant, Department of Anesthesiology, Mayo Clinic, Jacksonville, Florida
Assistant Professor of Anesthesiology, Mayo Clinic College of Medicine

James Y. Findlay, MB, ChB, FRCA
Consultant, Department of Anesthesiology, Mayo Clinic, Rochester, Minnesota
Assistant Professor of Anesthesiology, Mayo Clinic College of Medicine

Randall P. Flick, MD, MPH
Consultant, Department of Anesthesiology, Mayo Clinic, Rochester, Minnesota
Associate Professor of Anesthesiology and Pediatrics, Mayo Clinic College of Medicine

William David Freeman, MD
Director, Neurosciences ICU, Departments of Neurology, Neurosurgery, and Critical Care, Mayo Clinic, Jacksonville, Florida
Associate Professor of Neurology, Mayo Clinic College of Medicine

Robert J. Friedhoff, MD
Consultant, Department of Anesthesiology, Mayo Clinic, Rochester, Minnesota
Assistant Professor of Anesthesiology, Mayo Clinic College of Medicine

Brantley Dollar Gaitan, MD
Consultant, Department of Anesthesiology, Mayo Clinic, Phoenix, Arizona
Assistant Professor of Anesthesiology, Mayo Clinic College of Medicine

Scott A. Gammel, MD
Medical Director, Park Place Surgical Hospital, Lafayette, Louisiana

Carol B. Garrison, CPMSM
CPCS Manager, Medical Staff Services, Mayo Clinic, Scottsdale Arizona

Halena M. Gazelka, MD
Consultant, Department of Anesthesiology, Mayo Clinic, Rochester, Minnesota
Instructor in Anesthesiology, Mayo Clinic College of Medicine

Adrian Gelb, MB, ChB
Professor, Department of Anesthesia & Perioperative Care, University of California, San Francisco, California

Salim Michel Ghazi, MD
Chair, Department of Pain Medicine, Mayo Clinic, Jacksonville, Florida
Assistant Professor of Anesthesiology, Mayo Clinic College of Medicine

James A. Giacalone, BS, MEd
Adjunct Faculty, Department of Biology, Lebanon Valley College, Annville, Pennsylvania

R. Scott Gorman, MD
Consultant, Department of Internal Medicine, Mayo Clinic, Scottsdale, Arizona
Assistant Professor of Medicine, Mayo Clinic College of Medicine

Robert E. Grady, MD
Anesthesiologist, Sanford Hospital, Sioux Falls, South Dakota

Roy A. Greengrass, MD
Consultant, Department of Anesthesiology, Mayo Clinic, Jacksonville, Florida
Professor of Anesthesiology, Mayo Clinic College of Medicine

Alina M. Grigore, MD, MHS, FASE
Associate Professor, Department of Anesthesiology, Director, Division of Cardiothoracic Anesthesiology University of Maryland School of Medicine, Baltimore, Maryland

Cornelius B. Groenewald, MB, ChB
Acting Assistant Professor, Anesthesiology and Pain Medicine, Seattle Children's Hospital, Seattle, Washington

Heidi A. Hadley, MD
Resident Physician, Department of Anesthesiology, University of Arizona Medical Center, Tucson, Arizona

Dawit T. Haile, MD
Consultant, Department of Anesthesiology, Mayo Clinic, Rochester, Minnesota
Assistant Professor of Anesthesiology, Mayo Clinic College of Medicine

Robert G. Hale, DDS
Commander, Dental and Trauma Research Detachment, U.S. Army Institute of Surgical Research, Oral & Maxillofacial Surgeon, San Antonio, Texas

Brian A. Hall, MD
Consultant, Department of Anesthesiology, Mayo Clinic, Rochester, Minnesota
Professor of Anesthesiology, Mayo Clinic College of Medicine

James D. Hannon, MD
Consultant, Department of Anesthesiology, Mayo Clinic, Rochester, Minnesota
Assistant Professor of Anesthesiology, Mayo Clinic College of Medicine

Kenneth C. Harris, MD
Anesthesiologist, San Antonio, Texas

Barry A. Harrison, MD
Consultant, Department of Anesthesiology, Mayo Clinic, Jacksonville, Florida
Assistant Professor of Anesthesiology, Mayo Clinic College of Medicine

Terese T. Horlocker, MD
Consultant, Department of Anesthesiology, Mayo Clinic, Rochester, Minnesota
Professor of Anesthesiology and Orthopedics, Mayo Clinic College of Medicine

Joshua Horowitz, DO
Anesthesiology Resident, Department of Anesthesiology and Critical Care Medicine, Johns Hopkins Hospital, Baltimore, Maryland

Michael P. Hosking, MD
Associate Professor, Department of Anesthesiology, University of Tennessee Medical Center, Knoxville, Tennessee

Srikanth Hosur, MD
Assistant Professor, Department of Anesthesia and Pain Management, University of Texas Southwestern Medical Center, Dallas, Texas

Clint Grant Humpherys, MD
Anesthesiologist, Providence Anchorage Medical Center, Anchorage, Alaska

Michael G. Ivancic, MD
Anesthesiologist, Liberty Hospital, Liberty, Missouri

Daniel J. Janik, MD
Associate Professor, Department of Anesthesiology, University of Colorado School of Medicine, Aurora, Colorado

Aaron M. Joffe, DO
Associate Professor, Anesthesiology and Pain Medicine, University of Washington, Harborview Medical Center, Seattle, Washington

Michael Egon Johnson, MD, PhD
Consultant, Department of Anesthesiology, Mayo Clinic, Rochester Minnesota
Assistant Professor of Anesthesiology, Mayo Clinic College of Medicine

Keith A. Jones, MD
Alfred Habeeb Professor and Chair, Department of Anesthesiology, The University of Alabama at Birmingham, Birmingham, Alabama

Mark T. Keegan, MB, MRCPI, MSc
Consultant, Department of Anesthesiology, Division of Critical Care, Mayo Clinic, Rochester, Minnesota
Professor of Anesthesiology, Mayo Clinic College of Medicine

James D. Kindscher, MD
Professor, Department of Anesthesiology, Kansas University, Kansas City, Kansas

Melinda A. King, MD
Volunteer Professor, Department of Anesthesiology and Critical Care, University of New Mexico School of Medicine, Albuquerque, New Mexico

Michelle A. O. Kinney, MD
Consultant, Department of Anesthesiology, Mayo Clinic, Rochester, Minnesota
Assistant Professor of Anesthesiology, Mayo Clinic College of Medicine

Suneerat Kongsayreepong, MD
Professor, Head of the General Surgical Intensive Care Unit, Department of Anesthesiology, Siriraj Hospital, Mahidol University, Bangkok, Thailand

Sandra L. Kopp, MD
Consultant, Department of Anesthesiology, Mayo Clinic, Rochester, Minnesota
Associate Professor of Anesthesiology, Mayo Clinic College of Medicine

Sarang S. Koushik, MD
Fellow in Anesthesiology, Mayo School of Graduate Medical Education, Phoenix, Arizona

Beth L. Ladlie, MD, MPH
Consultant, Department of Anesthesiology, Mayo Clinic, Jacksonville, Florida
Assistant Professor of Anesthesiology, Mayo Clinic College of Medicine

Tim J. Lamer, MD
Consultant, Division of Pain Medicine, Mayo Clinic, Rochester, Minnesota
Associate Professor of Anesthesiology, Mayo Clinic College of Medicine

David Layer, DO
Anesthesiologist, Madigan Healthcare System, Tacoma, Washington

Alaric C. LeBaron, MD
Staff Anesthesiologist, Master Clinician, Department of Anesthesia, David Grant Medical Center, Travis AFB, California

Sten Lindahl, MD, PhD, FRCA
Professor, Karolinska Institutet, Director of Research and Education, Karolinska University Hospital, Stockholm, Sweden

Timothy R. Long, MD
Consultant, Department of Anesthesiology, Mayo Clinic, Rochester, Minnesota
Assistant Professor of Anesthesiology, Mayo Clinic College of Medicine

Jeffrey J. Lunn, MD
Director of Anesthesiology and Perioperative Services, Kingman Regional Medical Center, Kingman, Arizona

Christopher V. Maani, MD
Chief of Anesthesia & PeriOperative Services,
U.S. Army Institute of Surgical Research & Army Burn Center,
San Antonio Military Medical Center,
Fort Sam Houston, Texas

Ian MacVeigh, MD
Consultant Anesthesiologist, Department Head, Clínica Cemtro, Madrid, Spain

Aaron J. Mancuso, MD
Adult Cardiothoracic Fellow, Department of Anesthesia, Critical Care and Pain Medicine, Beth Israel Deaconess Medical Center, Boston, Massachusetts

Carlos B. Mantilla, MD, PhD
Consultant, Department of Anesthesiology, Mayo Clinic, Rochester, Minnesota
Professor of Anesthesiology and Physiology, Mayo Clinic College of Medicine

H. Michael Marsh, MB, BS
Professor, Department of Anesthesiology, Wayne State University School of Medicine, Detroit, Michigan

David P. Martin, MD, PhD
Consultant, Department of Anesthesiology, Mayo Clinic, Rochester, Minnesota
Associate Professor of Anesthesiology, Mayo Clinic College of Medicine

William J. Mauermann, MD
Consultant, Department of Anesthesiology, Mayo Clinic, Rochester, Minnesota
Assistant Professor of Anesthesiology, Mayo Clinic College of Medicine

Patrick O. McConville, MD
Assistant Professor of Anesthesiology, University of Tennessee Graduate School of Medicine, Knoxville, Tennessee

Craig C. McFarland, MD
Assistant Professor, Department of Anesthesiology, Uniformed Services University of the Health Sciences, Bethesda, Maryland

Brian P. McGlinch, MD
Consultant, Department of Anesthesiology, Mayo Clinic, Rochester, Minnesota
Assistant Professor of Anesthesiology, Mayo Clinic College of Medicine

K. A. Kelly McQueen, MD, MPH
Associate Professor, Department of Anesthesiology, Vanderbilt Institute for Global Health, Vanderbilt University Medical Center, Nashville, Tennessee

Sharon K. Merrick, MS, CCS-P
Director, Payment and Practice Management, American Society of Anesthesiologists, Washington, DC

Colin George Merridew, MBBS, FANCZA
Clinical Senior Lecturer, School of Medicine, University of Tasmania, Tasmania, Australia

Julia I. Metzner, MD
Associate Professor, Department of Anesthesiology & Pain Medicine, University of Washington School of Medicine, Seattle, Washington

Lopa Misra, DO
Consultant, Department of Anesthesiology, Mayo Clinic, Phoenix, Arizona
Instructor in Anesthesiology, Mayo Clinic College of Medicine

Susan M. Moeschler, MD
Consultant, Department of Anesthesiology, Mayo Clinic, Rochester, Minnesota
Instructor in Anesthesiology, Mayo Clinic College of Medicine

Steven T. Morozowich, DO, FASE
Supplemental Consultant, Department of Anesthesiology, Mayo Clinic, Phoenix, Arizona
Instructor in Anesthesiology, Mayo Clinic College of Medicine

Jeff T. Mueller, MD
Consultant, Department of Anesthesiology, Mayo Clinic, Phoenix, Arizona
Assistant Professor of Anesthesiology, Mayo Clinic College of Medicine

David R. Mumme, MD
Anesthesiologist, Anesthesia Consultants, Indianapolis, Indiana

Michael J. Murray, MD, PhD
Consultant, Department of Anesthesiology, Mayo Clinic, Phoenix, Arizona
Professor of Anesthesiology, Mayo Clinic College of Medicine

Teresa M. Murray
Medical Student, Pritzker School of Medicine, University of Chicago, Chicago, Illinois

Bradly J. Narr, MD
Chair, Department of Anesthesiology, Mayo Clinic, Rochester, Minnesota
Associate Professor of Anesthesiology, Mayo Clinic College of Medicine

Heather L. Naumann, MD
Acting Assistant Professor, Department of Pediatric Anesthesiology, University of Washington, Seattle, Washington

Stephanie A. Neuman, MD
Pain Medicine, Gundersen Health System, La Crosse, Wisconsin

Doris B.M. Ockert, MD
Associate Professor, Department of Anesthesiology, University of Wisconsin School of Medicine and Public Health, Madison, Wisconsin

William C. Oliver, Jr., MD
Consultant, Department of Anesthesiology, Mayo Clinic, Rochester, Minnesota
Professor of Anesthesiology, Mayo Clinic College of Medicine

Jeffrey J. Pasternak, MS, MD
Consultant, Department of Anesthesiology, Mayo Clinic, Rochester, Minnesota
Associate Professor of Anesthesiology, Mayo Clinic College of Medicine

Prith Peiris, MD
Consultant, Department of Anesthesiology, Mayo Clinic, Jacksonville, Florida
Instructor in Anesthesiology, Mayo Clinic College of Medicine

Nicole W. Pelly, MD
Assistant Clinical Professor, Department of Anesthesiology & Pain Medicine, University of Washington/Seattle Children's Hospital, Seattle, Washington

Steven G. Peters, MD
Consultant, Department of Pulmonary and Critical Care Medicine, Mayo Clinic, Rochester, Minnesota
Professor of Medicine, Mayo Clinic College of Medicine

Roxann D. Barnes Pike, MD
Consultant, Department of Anesthesiology, Mayo Clinic, Rochester, Minnesota
Assistant Professor of Anesthesiology, Mayo Clinic College of Medicine

Karl A. Poterack, MD
Consultant, Department of Anesthesiology, Mayo Clinic, Phoenix, Arizona
Assistant Professor of Anesthesiology, Mayo Clinic College of Medicine

Jennifer A. Rabbitts, MB, ChB
Anesthesiology and Pain Medicine, Seattle Children's Hospital, Seattle, Washington

Peter Radell, MD, PhD
Associate Professor, Department of Pediatric Anesthesia and Intensive Care, Karolinska University Hospital, Astrid Lindgren Children's Hospital, Stockholm, Sweden

Mary M. Rajala, MS, MD
Staff Anesthesiologist, Winona Health, Winona, Minnesota

Harish Ramakrishna, MD, FASE
Consultant, Department of Anesthesiology and Chair, Division of Cardiovascular and Thoracic Anesthesiology, Mayo Clinic, Phoenix, Arizona
Assistant Professor of Anesthesiology, Mayo Clinic College of Medicine

Manoch Rattanasompattikul, MD
Nephrology and Internal Medicine, Renal Unit, Golden Jubilee Medical Center, Mahidol University, Nakhon Pathom, Thailand

Guy S. Reeder, MD
Consultant, Department of Cardiovascular Diseases, Mayo Clinic, Rochester, Minnesota
Professor of Medicine, Mayo Clinic College of Medicine,

Kent H. Rehfeldt, MD, FASE
Consultant, Department of Anesthesiology, Mayo Clinic, Rochester, Minnesota
Assistant Professor of Anesthesiology, Mayo Clinic College of Medicine

Edwin H. Rho, MD
Consultant, Department of Anesthesiology, Mayo Clinic, Rochester, Minnesota
Assistant Professor of Anesthesiology, Mayo Clinic College of Medicine

Richard H. Rho, MD
Consultant, Department of Anesthesiology, Mayo Clinic, Rochester, Minnesota
Assistant Professor of Anesthesiology, Mayo Clinic College of Medicine

Christopher B. Robards, MD
Consultant, Department of Anesthesiology, Mayo Clinic, Jacksonville, Florida
Assistant Professor of Anesthesiology, Mayo Clinic College of Medicine

Kip D. Robinson, MD
Assistant Professor and Associate Program Director, Department of Anesthesiology, University of Tennessee College of Medicine, Knoxville, Tennessee

Eduardo S. Rodrigues, MD
Consultant, Department of Anesthesiology, Mayo Clinic, Jacksonville, Florida
Instructor in Anesthesiology, Mayo Clinic College of Medicine

Steven H. Rose, MD
Consultant, Department of Anesthesiology, Mayo Clinic, Rochester, Minnesota
Professor of Anesthesiology, Mayo Clinic College of Medicine

David M. Rosenfeld, MD
Consultant, Department of Anesthesiology, Mayo Clinic, Phoenix, Arizona
Assistant Professor of Anesthesiology, Mayo Clinic College of Medicine

Joseph J. Sandor, MD
Valley Anesthesiology & Pain Consultants Ltd., Phoenix/Scottsdale, Arizona

Wolfgang Schramm, MD
Associate Professor, Medical Doctor, Department of Anesthesiology and General Intensive Care, Medical University of Vienna, Vienna, Austria

David P. Seamans, MD
Consultant, Department of Anesthesiology, Mayo Clinic, Phoenix, Arizona
Assistant Professor of Anesthesiology, Mayo Clinic College of Medicine

Lisa S. Seip, MD
Supplemental Anesthesiologist, Mayo Clinic, Phoenix Arizona

Deepesh M. Shah, MD
Interventional Pain Physician-Partner, Atlantis Medical Specialists, Phoenix, Arizona

William Shakespeare, MD
Anesthesiologist, Intermountain Healthcare, Murray, Utah

David P. Shapiro, MD
Anesthesiologist, Jacksonville, Florida

Yu Shi, MD, MPH
Resident in Anesthesiology, Medical College of Wisconsin, Milwaukee, Wisconsin

Timothy S.J. Shine, MD
Consultant, Department of Anesthesiology, Mayo Clinic, Jacksonville, Florida
Assistant Professor of Anesthesiology, Mayo Clinic College of Medicine

Allen Brian Shoham, MD
Anesthesiologist, Interventional Pain Management, Tri-City Orthopaedics, Richland, Washington

Jeffrey W. Simmons, MD
Assistant Professor, Department of Anesthesiology, Trauma Section, University of Alabama at Birmingham, Birmingham, Alabama

Daniel V. Simula, MD
Consultant, Department of Anesthesiology, Mayo Clinic, Phoenix, Arizona
Instructor in Anesthesiology, Mayo Clinic College of Medicine

Molly Solorzano, MD
Supplemental Consultant, Department of Anesthesiology, Mayo Clinic, Phoenix, Arizona

J. Robert Sonne, JD
Legal Counsel, Legal Department, Mayo Clinic, Scottsdale Arizona

Thomas N. Spackman, MD, MS
Chair, Department of Anesthesiology, Mayo Clinic, Jacksonville, Florida
Assistant Professor of Anesthesiology, Mayo Clinic College of Medicine

Wolf H. Stapelfeldt, MD
Professor & Chairman, Department of Anesthesiology & Critical Care Medicine, Saint Louis University Medical Center, St. Louis, Missouri

Joshua D. Stearns, MD
Consultant, Department of Anesthesiology, Mayo Clinic, Phoenix, Arizona
Assistant Professor of Anesthesiology, Mayo Clinic College of Medicine

Petter Andreas Steen, MD, PhD, FERC
Professor, Department of Emergency Medicine, Institute of Clinical Medicine, University of Oslo, Oslo, Norway

Robert A. Strickland, MD
Associate Professor, Department of Ambulatory and Outpatient Anesthesiology, Wake Forest Baptist Health, Winston-Salem, North Carolina

Kjetil Sunde, MD, PhD
Professor, Institute of Clinical Medicine, Faculty of Medicine, University of Oslo, Oslo, Norway

Barbara E. Switzer, MD
Pediatric Resident, Medical Education Miami Children's Hospital, Miami, Florida

Kamthorn Tantivitayatan, MD
Assistant Professor, Mahidol University, Thailand

Brian J. Thomas, JD
Director of Risk Management, Preferred Physicians Medical, Shawnee Mission, Kansas

Christopher A. Thunberg, MD
Consultant, Department of Anesthesiology, Mayo Clinic, Phoenix, Arizona
Instructor in Anesthesiology, Mayo Clinic College of Medicine

Klaus D. Torp, MD
Consultant, Department of Anesthesiology, Mayo Clinic, Jacksonville, Florida
Assistant Professor of Anesthesiology, Mayo Clinic College of Medicine

Nichole T. Townsend, RN, MD
Fellow in Anesthesiology, Mayo School of Graduate Medical Education, Phoenix, Arizona

Robert J. Trainer, DO, MBA
Anesthesiologist, Stony Brook Medical Center, Islandia, New York

Terrence L. Trentman, MD
Chair, Department of Anesthesiology, Mayo Clinic, Phoenix, Arizona
Associate Professor of Anesthesiology, Mayo Clinic College of Medicine

MAJ Ali Akber Turabi, MD
Assistant Adjunct Professor, Department of Anesthesiology, Uniformed Services University of the Health Sciences, Bethesda, Maryland

Inge Falk van Rooyen, MD
Anesthesiologist, Harborview Medical Center, Seattle, Washington

John M. VanErdewyk, MD
Medical Director of Anesthesia, Queen of Peace Hospital, Mitchell, South Dakota

Gurinder M. S. Vasdev, MD, MBBS
Consultant, Department of Anesthesiology, Mayo Clinic, Rochester, Minnesota
Assistant Professor of Anesthesiology, Mayo Clinic College of Medicine

Jörg H. Vetterman, MD
Anesthesiology and Intensive Care, Evangelisches Krankenhaus, Mulheim/ Ruhr, Germany

Amorn Vijitpavan, MD
Anesthesiologist, Samitivej Hospital, Bangkok, Thailand

Amy G. Voet, DO, MS
Resident, Department of Anesthesiology, Penn State University, Hershey Medical Center, Hershey, Pennsylvania

Wayne H. Wallender, DO
Anesthesiologist, Ozark Anesthesia Associates, Springfield, Missouri

R. Doris Wang, MD
Consultant, Department of Anesthesiology, Mayo Clinic, Jacksonville, Florida
Assistant Professor of Anesthesiology, Mayo Clinic College of Medicine

David O. Warner, MD
Consultant, Department of Anesthesiology, Mayo Clinic, Rochester, Minnesota
Professor of Anesthesiology, Mayo Clinic College of Medicine

Mary Ellen Warner, MD
Consultant, Department of Anesthesiology, Mayo Clinic, Rochester, Minnesota
Associate Professor of Anesthesiology, Mayo Clinic College of Medicine

C. Thomas Wass, MD
Consultant, Department of Anesthesiology, Mayo Clinic, Rochester, Minnesota
Associate Professor of Anesthesiology, Mayo Clinic College of Medicine

Mary B. Weber, MD
Anesthesiologist, Wyoming Medical Center, Casper, Wyoming

Denise J. Wedel, MD
Consultant, Department of Anesthesiology, Mayo Clinic, Rochester, Minnesota
Professor of Anesthesiology, Mayo Clinic College of Medicine

Toby N. Weingarten, MD
Consultant, Department of Anesthesiology, Mayo Clinic, Rochester, Minnesota
Associate Professor of Anesthesiology, Mayo Clinic College of Medicine

Eric Werner, MD
Clinical Anesthesiologist, Department of Anesthesiology, Central DuPage Hospital, Winfield, Illinois

Jack L. Wilson, MD
Consultant, Department of Anesthesiology, Mayo Clinic, Rochester, Minnesota
Assistant Professor of Anesthesiology, Mayo Clinic College of Medicine

Gilbert Y. Wong, MD
Anesthesiologist/Pain Medicine, Palo Alto, California

Glenn E. Woodworth, MD
Assistant Professor, Department of Anesthesiology and Perioperative Medicine, Oregon Health & Science University, Portland, Oregon

Qinghao Xu, PhD
Department of Anesthesiology, University of California-San Diego, La Jolla, California

Tony L. Yaksh, PhD
Department of Anesthesiology, University of California-San Diego, La Jolla, California

Avishai Ziser, MD
Anesthesiologist, Rambam Medical Center, Haifa, Israel

Preface

Dear Readers,

This fourth edition of *Faust's Anesthesiology Review* is different from its predecessors in a number of ways, not the least of which is that Ron Faust has retired from clinical practice, requiring a new editor-in-chief and several new associate editors for this edition. Ron's foresight and tenacity in bringing his eponymous text to completion will be missed, but hopefully the new editors have continued the tradition that he established.

With Ron's retirement, a subsequent edition of his widely used textbook might never have come to fruition; however, because his colleagues at Mayo continually received inquiries about when a fourth edition would be published, we realized that this book met a need among anesthesia residents and faculty in preparing didactic lectures for daily residency conferences. With a lapse of more than a decade since the third edition was published, the need for an update was clear.

The book has changed in other ways. Previous editions were meant to serve as a Board review, but, with that as a goal, we are tempted to "teach to the test." When writing a Board review, authors tend to write what the American Board of Anesthesiologists believes to be the correct approach to a clinical problem and not necessarily the physiologically and scientifically correct approach (e.g., see the chapter on one-lung ventilation). This new edition is, instead, a comprehensive review of anesthesiology in general, covering 254 concepts of importance to anesthesia care providers so that they might provide the best care to their patients. Because of this approach, we made no attempt to use keywords, the American Board of Anesthesiologists content outline, or information provided to program chairs by the American Board of Anesthesiologists.

We either deleted several chapters from previous editions or included the information covered in those chapters in others with a similar focus, a process that freed up space so that the editors could include new topics that reflect recent advances in the practice of anesthesiology. We also reorganized the book. The previous editions had three major sections—the physiologic sciences, the physical sciences, and the clinical sciences—whereas this edition has 13 sections, with the specialty section further divided into 8 subsections covering most of the major subspecialties in our field.

The authors of this edition either have had training or experience with the Mayo Clinic and the Mayo Clinic Health System or are current members of the United States military and were recommended by Mayo faculty who knew of their reputation (e.g., Chris Maani and colleagues, who work in the burn unit at the San Antonio Military Medical Center, who wrote the chapter on burn injury). Of more importance, several of the previous authors are now on faculty at other academic institutions, and several have gone on to leadership positions within those institutions as program directors, department chairs, deans, etc., and within organized medicine, both in the United States and overseas. While maintaining the tradition of excellence of the all-Mayo faculty that Dr. Faust established in previous editions, these new authors bring insights and approaches to clinical problems that greatly enhance the educational value of the material covered in this textbook.

However such diversity of opinion enhances the final product, diversity of style can be distracting in a multi-authored textbook. With more than 250 chapters, writing styles, chapter lengths, and content can vary widely. In this edition, we attempted to edit chapters to a standard length and style and undertook extensive reviews of the literature to ensure that the content was similar and as up to date as possible across all chapters.

The publisher, Elsevier, has also made significant changes. The introduction of color definitely enhances the interpretation and understanding of tables and figures. Furthermore, both the Mayo Foundation and Elsevier allowed us full access to their extensive collection of artwork to select material that facilitates interpretation of concepts. The use of Netter's well-known collection of medical graphics is an invaluable addition to the book.

We hope that you will find that the improvements in the textbook have continued the tradition that Ron Faust established and that the textbook will serve as an easily accessible reference for maintaining your knowledge of what we consider to be the most important topics in anesthesiology. As authors and editors, our most fervent hope is that the information contained in this book will improve the care that we provide to our patients.

Michael J. Murray, MD, PhD
Barry A. Harrison, MD
Jeff T. Mueller, MD
Steven H. Rose, MD
C. Thomas Wass, MD
Denise J. Wedel, MD

Contents

B. NEUROANESTHESIA

C. CARDIAC ANESTHESIA

D. THORACIC ANESTHESIA

E. GENERAL/UROLOGIC/ENT

F. ANESTHESIA FOR UNIQUE SITUATIONS OR FOR SPECIFIC PATIENT POPULATIONS

SECTION XI CRITICAL CARE MEDICINE

SECTION XII RISK MANAGEMENT

SECTION XIII PRACTICE MANAGEMENT

SECTION I Operating Room

CHAPTER 1

Medical Gas Supply

Martin L. De Ruyter, MD

Medical gases most common to anesthesia include oxygen (O_2), nitrous oxide (N_2O), and air. Historically the less frequently used medical gases include helium (He), nitrogen (N_2), and carbon dioxide (CO_2), but there has been a recent surge in the use of CO_2 secondary to the advancement of laparoscopic and robotic procedures. Several governing bodies regulate medical gases, but the containment and delivery of these gases via a medical gas cylinder system is controlled via standards set by the United States Department of Transportation. Medical gas cylinders are the foundation for central pipeline supply of gases to the operating room (OR) and hospital. Additionally, a cylinder system (typically the smaller E cylinders) exists in the OR as a backup for unanticipated failure of the central pipeline supply (Figures 1-1 to 1-3).

Medical gas cylinders store compressed gas. Cylinder sizes vary and are designated by letters, with A being the smallest and H being the largest. H cylinders are large-capacity storage containers that typically provide the central pipeline supply of medical gas that is piped into the OR. E cylinders are smaller and are the most commonly encountered cylinders in the OR. A typical anesthesia machine will have an attachment for two (O_2 and N_2O) or three (two O_2 and one N_2O) E cylinders. E cylinders are also commonly used to supply O_2 to patients during transport. Cylinders are color coded according to the gas they contain. Unfortunately, there is no global agreement, and the colors in the United States are not the same as those accepted internationally. Table 1-1 lists the common medical gases, the cylinder capacity, the color of the cylinders, and the form under which medical gases are stored.

At ambient temperature, when gases are compressed and stored in cylinders, gases will either liquefy or remain in a gas state. When stored in medical cylinders, compressed O_2, He, and air remain as gases at ambient temperature. In contrast, N_2O, when compressed and stored in medical cylinders, becomes a liquid at ambient temperature. Knowledge of nonliquefied gases and liquefied gases allows one to estimate the amount of gas that remains in a cylinder as the gas is being consumed. As gas is consumed, the pressure gauge will decrease in a linear proportion to the cylinder's remaining content. For example, an E cylinder filled with O_2 contains approximately 660 L of nonliquefied O_2 at a pressure of approximately 2000 pounds per square inch (psi). When the gauge reads 1000 psi, approximately 330 L of O_2 remain. One can, therefore, estimate how long before a cylinder will empty when delivering gas at a certain flow rate. An equation to estimate the time remaining in a cylinder is as follows:

$$\text{Approximate remaining time (h)} = \frac{O_2 \text{ cylinder pressure (psi)}}{200 \times O_2 \text{ flow rate (L/min)}}$$

The volume remaining in a cylinder of liquefied gases, such as N_2O, cannot be estimated in the same manner. The pressure gauge of the N_2O cylinder reads the pressure of the small amount of vapor above the liquid. As gas is consumed, more gas moves from the liquid phase to the gas phase, maintaining the vapor pressure and, hence, the reading of the pressure gauge. Only when nearly all of the liquid N_2O is vaporized does the pressure start to fall. For example, a full E cylinder of N_2O contains 1590 L and reads 745 psi; this pressure will remain constant until nearly all of the N_2O is vaporized, at which point the pressure starts to drop. At this point, approximately 400 L of N_2O remain in the cylinder. The only reliable way to estimate the volume of N_2O remaining in a cylinder is to weigh the cylinder. Each cylinder is stamped with a tare weight (empty weight), and the difference between the measured weight and tare weight represents the amount of liquefied gas present.

E cylinders attach directly to the anesthesia machine via a hanger-yoke assembly. This assembly orients and supports the cylinder, provides a gas-tight seal, and ensures unidirectional flow of gases into the machine. As a safety measure, to prevent connecting the wrong gas cylinder to the machine

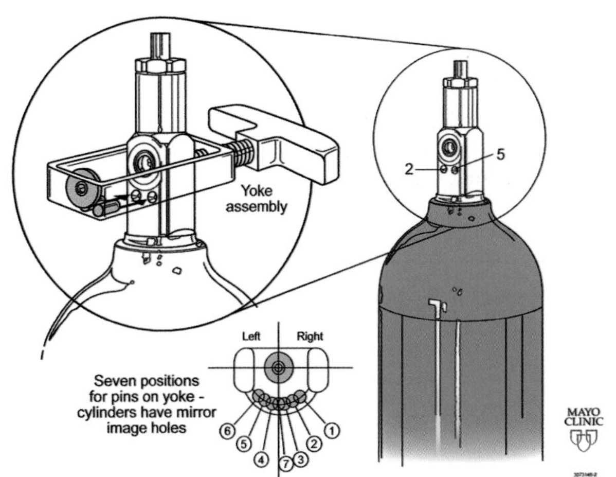

Figure 1-1 The index safety system is one of several features of medical gas cylinders that is in place to ensure that the correct cylinder is attached to the correct gas inlet in the back of the anesthesia machine. Cylinders are color coded; each cylinder has a label identifying which gas it contains, and the cylinders attach to the back of the anesthesia machine using the pin-index safety system. Two pins incorporated into the yoke of the machine, just below the gas inlet, line up with two holes on the gas cylinder, allowing only the correct cylinder to be connected to the correct inlet. (© Mayo Foundation for Medical Education and Research. All rights reserved.)

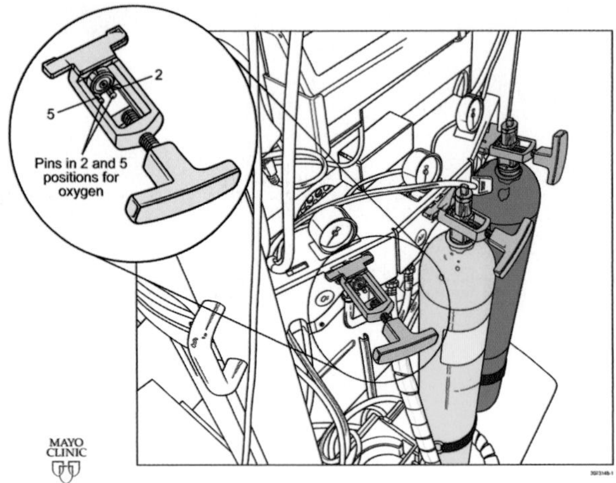

Figure 1-2 A close-up view of the yoke assembly in the back of the anesthesia machine. The two pins that are immediately below the gas inlet on the anesthesia machine occupy one of seven possible standardized positions. For O_2, the pins are in the 2 and 5 position and line up with the corresponding inlet on the O_2 cylinder. As the clamp on the yoke assembly is tightened, the cylinder is secured up against the gas inlet for O_2. If the pins line up correctly, when the valve on the cylinder is open, the correct gas will flow into the correct inlet. If the pins are *not* lined up correctly, the cylinder will not be able to be tightened into the yoke, no contact will be made between the gas inlet and cylinder, and, therefore, the gas won't flow into the inlet. (© Mayo Foundation for Medical Education and Research. All rights reserved.)

(and thus potentially delivering a hypoxic mixture), a pin index safety system is in use. Each gas cylinder has two holes in its cylinder valve that interface with corresponding pins in the yoke of the anesthesia machine. The positioning of the holes on the cylinder valve and the pins on the yoke are unique for each gas. This safety measure is designed to prevent the wrong gas cylinder from being attached to the anesthesia machine. This safety mechanism can be breached if the yoke pins are broken or missing or intentionally instrumented in some way.

Today's ORs commonly have a pipeline supply of medical gases. Large-capacity tanks, such as liquid O_2 storage tanks or H cylinders connected in series by a manifold, use pipes to deliver O_2 throughout the hospital. In the OR, these pipes connect to one of three common systems: gas columns, hose drops, or articulating arms. Color-coded hoses with a quick-coupling mechanism connect to one of these systems, and, in turn, the hoses then interface with the anesthesia machine via a diameter index system.

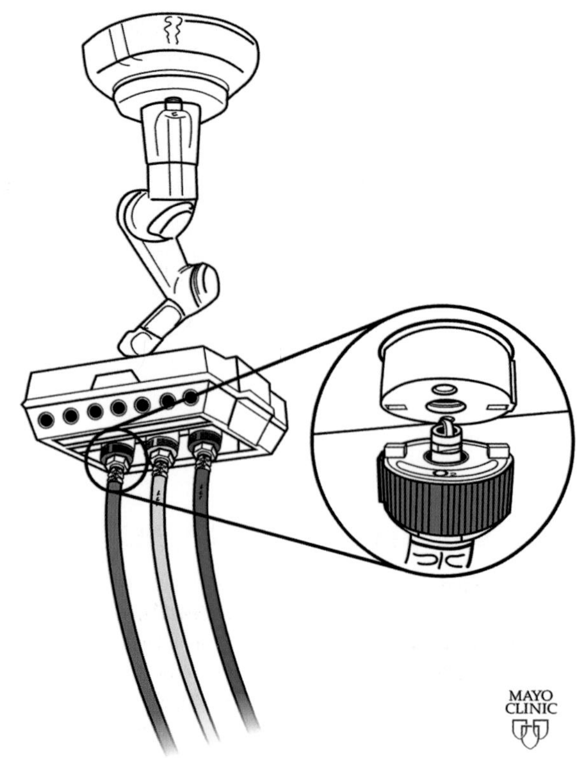

Figure 1-3 Hoses, color coded for each gas, can be connected to the appropriate gas outlet with an adaptor that has a disc-index system unique to the gas for that outlet. The system comprises a central tube, through which the gas flows, and two small metal rectangles placed on the surface of the adaptor that are, again, unique to each gas, such that an O_2 hose can only be connected to an O_2 outlet. (© Mayo Foundation for Medical Education and Research. All rights reserved.)

Suggested Readings

Dorsch JA, Dorsch SE. Medical gas cylinders and containers. In: Dorsch, JA, Dorsch SE, eds. *Understanding Anesthesia Equipment*. 5th ed. Philadelphia: Wolters Kluwer/Lippincott Williams & Wilkins; 2007:1-24.

Dorsch JA, Dorsch SE. Medical gas pipeline systems. In: Dorsch, JA, Dorsch SE, eds. *Understanding Anesthesia Equipment*. 5th ed. Philadelphia: Wolters Kluwer/Lippincott Williams & Wilkins; 2007:25-50.

Table 1-1 Medical Gas Cylinders

	Cylinder Capacity (L)*			Color		
Gas	**E**	**H**	**Pressure (psi) at 20° C**	**U.S.**	**Non-U.S.**	**Form**
O_2	625-700	6000-8000	1800-2200	Green	White Blue[†]	Gas
Air	625-700	6000-8000	1800-2200	Yellow	White and black	Gas
N_2O	1590	15,900	745	Blue	Blue	Liquid

*Cylinder sizes are designated by letters, with A being the smallest and H the largest.
[†]China.
psi, Pounds per square inch.

CHAPTER 2

Electrical Supply

Brian A. Hall, MD

Electrical Safety in the Operating Room

Efforts to reduce the risk of explosions and to improve electrical safety in operating rooms (ORs) were first instituted when flammable inhalation agents were in use. These endeavors have continued because, even though explosions are unlikely to occur today, the amount of electrical equipment used throughout health care facilities and in the OR, in particular, has dramatically increased. Any electrical equipment has the potential to create macroshock, an electric shock on the order of 5 mA to 1000 mA or more that can burn a patient or fibrillate the patient's heart. Patients in the OR are at particular risk for incurring a macroshock because the normal resistance of dry skin (~ 100 kΩ) is reduced if the skin is wet or abraded (~ 1 kΩ).

Power Systems

The two types of power systems used in health care facilities include a grounded power system (GPS) and an isolated power system (IPS). Which system is used in a specific area depends upon the patient care provided at that location as well as the characteristics of the electrical system that supplies the patient care area.

Grounded Power Systems

The main wiring in an OR is similar to that of a typical home in the United States—a GPS—comprised of a live (hot, positive) wire carrying alternating current at 120 V (120 VAC), a neutral (cold, negative) wire that completes the circuit by transmitting the current from the house back to the power-generating station, and an earth wire, or ground wire. If a person is grounded and comes in contact with the hot limb of a GPS, an electric shock will be delivered.

In a home, ground-fault circuit interrupters (GFCIs) are installed in a GPS that is used in wet locations (e.g., bathrooms and kitchens). Likewise, in the OR, GFCIs can be placed on each circuit of a GPS to minimize the likelihood of a macroshock occurring. The circuit will "trip" in milliseconds if a current greater than 4 to 6 mA begins to flow between the live wire and any other pathway other than the neutral wire. The concern with using GFCIs in an OR, however, is that, if the circuit trips, every electrical device plugged into that circuit will lose power.

In a "dry" OR with a GPS, the live (hot) wire is connected to the narrower of the two parallel prongs of an electrical plug and can be inserted only into the wider of the two parallel holes in the outlet. The neutral wire has the same potential difference from ground as the ground wire itself (i.e., 0 V). The single pole switches used in a GPS disconnect only the "hot" wire. If a person or a patient standing or lying in water comes in contact with the neutral or ground wire, no current flows. However, if the person contacts the hot wire, possible electrocution could occur unless protected by a GFCI.

Isolated Power Systems

Electricity in IPS is supplied by a transformer that is separate from the power-station electrical supply. The term *isolated* means precisely that—isolated from earth ground; the electrons in the circuit are not seeking the path of least resistance back to the power-generating station.

Electrical plugs and receptacles in an IPS look exactly like those in a GPS (i.e., one prong is wider than the other). The difference is that, in an IPS, both wires are "hot," and the voltage between either of the lines and ground is zero. (It is one way to differentiate IPS from GPS; in a GPS, the difference between the hot wire and ground is 120 VAC.)

Circuit breakers in the electrical panel of an IPS are double-pole breakers that disconnect both wires of the circuit when tripped. Because neither wire in an IPS circuit is connected to an earth ground, a person could stand in a pool of water while holding either of the wires of the circuit without macroshock occurring because no circuit is completed. Touching both wires simultaneously, of course, would deliver a macroshock.

Line Isolation Monitors

Any piece of equipment that has a power supply will have a small amount of current that reaches the earth ground without a physical connection to that ground. The phenomenon is termed *capacitance coupling*. With the amount of electrical equipment in a modern OR, it should not be a surprise that the net potential current of this capacitance coupling can be 2 to 5 mA or higher.

In an OR with an IPS, a line isolation monitor (LIM) must be used to continually monitor the leakage current from both lines or wires to ground to ensure that the system remains "isolated" from the earth ground. This device measures how much current could "leak" to earth ground (in milliamperes)—a quantitative assessment of how well the IPS is isolated. The LIM must be installed so that the green (status OK) lamp and the red (hazard leakage current) lamp are visible to personnel in the care areas where the IPS is used (Figure 2-1).

The LIM helps to protect against macroshock but not microshock. Currents up to 5 mA can pass to ground without triggering an LIM alarm. An activated LIM alarm does not indicate that the patient is receiving an electric shock; instead, the audible warning signal indicates that the impedance (to ground) within the circuit has decreased to the point that a current greater than 5 mA (macroshock threshold) could flow (leakage current). If no intervention is made and a circuit is completed (e.g., the patient is lying on a wet metal OR table), the patient may receive a macroshock. With higher currents (~70-100 mA), fibrillation of the heart through intact skin may occur.

When an audible warning signal from an LIM is triggered, OR personnel should expediently search for the cause. Violations usually occur when wires become frayed and are exposed to the metal casing of the plug. The third prong in both isolated and nonisolated circuits is always grounded, as are the metal face plates and housings of equipment; these parts serve as the

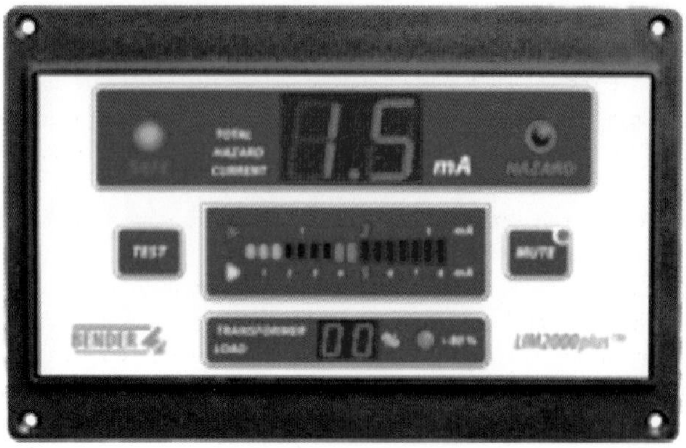

Figure 2-1 Example of a line isolation monitor, the LIM2000plus. (Courtesy of Isotrol, Inc., Coatesville, PA.)

violation points where IPSs most frequently become grounded. If the LIM sounds, OR personnel should unplug the last device connected, then the one before that, and so on, until the offending device is identified.

Electrical Requirements in the Operating Room

From 1948 to 1988, IPS and LIMs were required at all anesthetizing locations in the United States to reduce the risk of macroshock. As originally developed, LIMs alarmed if the current that could flow were greater than 2 mA; with the elimination of ether from ORs and the decreased concern about an electric spark triggering an explosion or fire, the Occupational Health and Safety Administration raised the threshold for the LIM to alarm at 5 mA.

In 1988, the national standards for electrical safety in health care institutions changed again; an IPS or a GPS with GFCI was required only if the OR was considered to be "wet." Many hospitals and health care systems (e.g., the Department of Defense and the Veterans Administration) have objected to installing the more expensive IPS or GFCIs and have declared the majority of their ORs, including cystoscopy rooms, to be "dry." A person who is in such a room and is standing or lying on a wet surface becomes grounded. If that person comes into contact with faulty electrical equipment, he or she will receive a macroshock, with the potential for serious harm occurring. In 2012, the National Fire Protection Association deemed all ORs to be wet procedure locations unless the health care governing body had conducted a risk assessment and determined otherwise. Therefore, all ORs should be provided with special protection against electric shock unless a risk assessment proves otherwise.

Electrical cords should not traverse the OR floor because they create a tripping hazard. Articulated booms or ceiling outlets should be used to bring the power supply close to the OR table. No multiple-plug outlet boxes that could become grounded if they come in contact with body fluids or liquids should be on the floor. Containers or liquids should not be placed on electrical equipment. Equipment operated by surgeons (e.g., lasers or electrosurgical [cautery] units) should be plugged into circuits separate from circuits used for anesthesia monitoring equipment; plugging these devices into the same circuit can increase the likelihood of 60-cycle electrical interference creating artifacts on the monitors. The use of lasers increases the risk of a fire occurring in a high-oxygen environment and, though electrosurgical units, especially modern bipolar units, do not cause macroshocks because they use very high frequency and low-voltage current, they can trigger cardiac defibrillators and interfere with cardiac pacemakers.

Suggested Readings

Barker SJ, Doyle DJ. Electrical safety in the operating room: Dry versus wet. *Anesth Analg*. 2010;110(6):1517-1518.

Day FJ. Electrical safety revisited: a new wrinkle. *Anesthesiology*. 1994;80(1):220-221.

Electrical safety Q&A. A reference guide for the clinical engineer. *Health Devices*. 2005;34:57-75.

Hull CJ. Electrocution hazards in the operating theatre. *Br J Anaesth*. 1978;50:647-657.

Wills JH, Ehrenwerth J, Rogers D. Electrical injury to a nurse due to conductive fluid in an operating room designated as a dry location. *Anesth Analg*. 2010;110:1647-1649.

CHAPTER 3 Microshock Hazards

Brian A. Hall, MD

Electricity is ubiquitous in the operating room environment; its use poses inherent risks to health care workers and special risks to patients. Isolated power systems were developed several decades ago when ether was used in operating rooms. Line-isolation monitors (LIMs) were originally set to trigger at 2 mA, to decrease the chances of a spark occurring, which, in an ether-enriched environment, could create an explosion or fire. With the elimination of ether in operating rooms, in the late 1980s, the Occupational Health and Safety Administration increased the alarm threshold to 5 mA for LIMs used in operating rooms that had isolated power transformers to decrease the possibility of macroshocks occurring.

The 5-mA level was selected because (1) this level was thought to be potentially injurious to a grounded patient, depending on the site at which the current would contact the patient, thereby creating a path through which current might flow, and (2) the resistance (impedance) to current flow is estimated by convention to be 500 Ω.

A potential current leak to ground can occur and will go undetected by the LIM if the leak is well below the detection threshold. For this reason, the American National Standards Institute mandates that the maximum 60-Hz current leakage from an indwelling device not exceed 10 μA. This level is well below the ventricular fibrillation threshold (~100 μA).

Independent of which system exists in an operating room, it is always prudent to ensure that, to the extent possible, a patient is never grounded. However, patients are connected to many electrical devices (e.g., via electrodes and electrical leads to monitoring devices). The chassis of the device is grounded, and such devices must be checked by a biomedical engineer no less frequently than every 3 months. All electrical devices have some leakage of current; extracorporeal electrical devices that are connected to patients cannot have more than 300 μA of leakage of current. The goal of isolated power transformers, ground-fault circuit interrupters (GFCIs), and even grounded circuits is to prevent macroshocks (i.e., patients exposed to electrical current flows of >5 mA).

With the advent of intracorporeal placement of electrical devices in or on the heart (e.g., pacemakers, defibrillators, oximetric and pacing pulmonary artery catheters, and cardiac output devices), the concept of *microshock* was born. The hazard associated with microshock is the low current threshold that may cause serious arrhythmias. A current as low as 100 μA can produce ventricular fibrillation. The threshold for the microshock is therefore in stark contrast with that of macroshock, which is the aforementioned 5 mA (i.e., 5000 μA). The difference in the magnitude of current needed to produce a macroshock versus a microshock is related to current density. When an electrical conductor is in direct contact with the myocardium, current density is several orders of magnitude higher than the current density produced when the conducting electrode is in contact with the outside of the body, such as with the hand.

It is blatantly obvious how a pacemaker with leads embedded in the myocardium could cause patient harm if electricity were conducted through those leads; however, anesthesia providers must also be aware that any catheter they insert into a patient, such as an internal jugular catheter or pulmonary catheter that is filled with conducting solution (e.g., saline or, especially, total parenteral nutrition), has the potential to conduct electricity directly to the heart. Manufacturers of devices used to monitor pressures from a central line go to great efforts to ensure that these devices are well grounded with maximum impedances everywhere possible. However, an anesthesia provider could overcome these safety measures by placing an electrical device with a relatively large leakage current in close proximity to, or touching, one of these central cannulas or catheters.

Care must be taken to avoid this scenario, and care must be used when handling wires that are in direct contact with the heart, such as intravascular guidewires or pacemaker leads. When procedures are performed in which these wires will be manipulated, the health care professional must ensure immediate availabiliy of equipment for direct-current cardioversion should a life-threatening arrhythmia occur. All personnel working in an operating room must be aware of the potential for the occurrence of microshock. Of equal importance is having a skilled biomedical engineer as part of the operating room staff.

Suggested Readings

Aggarwal A, Farber NE, Kotter GS, Dhamee MS. Electrosurgery-induced ventricular fibrillation during pacemaker replacement—A unique mechanism. *J Clin Monit*. 1996;12:339-342.

Amicucci GL, Di Lollo L, Fiamingo F, et al. Electrical safety during transplantation. *Transplant Proc*. 2010;42:2175-2180.

Baas LS, Beery TA, Hickey CS. Care and safety of pacemaker electrodes in intensive care and telemetry nursing units. *Am J Crit Care*. 1997;6:302-311.

Fish RM, Geddes LA. Conduction of electrical current to and through the human body: A review. *Eplasty*. 2009;9:e44.

Leeming MN. Protection of the "electrically susceptible patient": A discussion of systems and methods. *Anesthesiology*. 1973;38:370-383.

Monies-Chass I, Vilensky A, Mordechowitz B, Birkhahn J. Hidden risk in operating room. Micro-shock. *Acta Anaesthesiol Belg*. 1986;37:39-44.

Ruppen W, Enderlin M, Schüpfer G, Urwyler A. Electrical shock in the operating theatre: What to do? *Acta Anaesthesiol Scand*. 2006;50:641-642.

Tooley M. Electrical hazards: Their causes and prevention. *Anesth Intensive Care Med*. 2004;5:366-368.

CHAPTER 4
Operating Room Fires

Daniel A. Diedrich, MD

With the movement away from the use of flammable anesthetic gases, the incidence of fires in the operating room (OR) has decreased. However, with the increased use of disposable drapes and alcohol-based prepping solutions, there is concern that the incidence may increase. Although the precise incidence of OR fires is difficult to determine because of a lack of a structured reporting system, it is estimated that 50 to 200 fires occur in the OR annually in the United States.

Fire Triangle

For a fire to occur, three elements must come together: (1) an oxidizer, (2) fuel, and (3) an ignition source. These three elements are commonly called the "fire triad" and can be represented as a "fire triangle" (Figure 4-1). An OR fire can be prevented by removing any one element of the triangle.

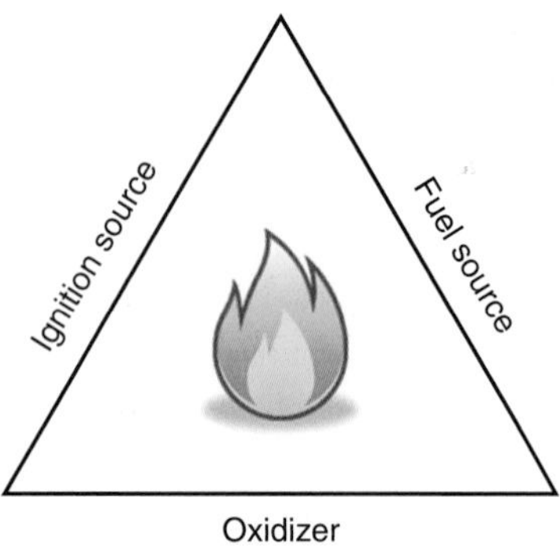

Figure 4-1 The fire triangle.

The two oxidizing agents most prevalent in the OR are oxygen (O_2) and nitrous oxide (N_2O). In the OR, many potential fuel sources are present (Box 4-1). The most common ignition source is diathermy or electrocautery with other ignition sources listed in Box 4-1.

Prevention

General OR fire prevention strategies are summarized in Box 4-2 and involve minimizing or avoiding oxidizer-enriched atmospheres, fuels or ignition sources. A useful strategy for prevention of an OR fire is the identification of a high risk procedure, (i.e., a procedure in which an ignition source will be used in proximity to an oxidizer-enriched environment). The presence of an oxidizer (O_2 and N_2O) lowers the combustion threshold and increases the intensity of a fire. This oxidizer-enriched atmosphere exists in (and around) the patient's breathing circuit and the risk of fire is increased in these areas. The risk of ignition is magnified when certain procedures (e.g., electrosurgery during tracheostomy, cauterization of airway lesions) are performed in close proximity to this environment. A number of techniques can be employed to reduce the fire risk during these high-risk procedures (Box 4-3).

Box 4-1 Components of the Fire Triangle

Oxidizers	Ignition source
Oxygen (O_2) Nitrous oxide (N_2O)	Malfunctioning electrical devices Electrosurgical devices Electrocautery devices Lasers Heated probes Fiberoptic scopes Defibrillators Static electricity
Fuel	
Patient Intestinal gases Drapes Blankets Gauze Sponges Dressings Gloves Gowns Alcohol-containing solutions Ointment Tracheal tubes Ventilator circuits O_2 masks	

Box 4-2 General Operating Room Fire Prevention Strategies

- Allow sufficient drying time of flammable skin-prepping solution
- Avoid using ignition sources close to an oxidizer-enriched environment
- Configure surgical drapes to avoid trapping oxidizer-enriched gases
- Minimize oxidizer concentration (e.g., minimize inspired O_2 concentration)
- Moisten sponges and gauze that are placed near an O_2-enriched environment

Box 4-3 Techniques to Minimize the Risk of Fires in the Operating Room During High-Risk Procedures

- The inspired oxygen concentration should be decreased to as low as physiologically acceptable as guided by pulse oximetry. By doing so, this lowers the amount of available oxidizer.
- A cuffed tracheal tube (TT) should be used and will minimize leak of oxygen.
- A laser-resistant TT should be used for laser procedures. Additionally the cuffs should be filled with colored saline to allow detection of a perforation.
- Communication should be optimized between the surgeon and the anesthesia provider. Although communication is important at all times, it is critically important in high-risk situations to minimize the risk of airway fires. Entry of the airway with an ignition source such as an electrosurgery device should be avoided, but, if such a device is required, the surgeon needs to alert the anesthesia provider so that risks can be minimized.

Preparation

The development of a multidisciplinary fire prevention and management plan is an important strategy that can minimize the severity of an OR fire. It involves good communication among all personnel and should begin with a team meeting prior to the patient entering the OR. The meeting should focus on (1) determining whether the procedure has a high risk with regard to fire, and (2) assignment of a specific fire management task that should be performed if a fire did occur.

Management of an Operating Room Fire

An overall strategy for management of an OR fire has been developed by the American Society of Anesthesiologists (Figure 4-2). Once a fire is detected, the surgical procedure should be immediately halted and all OR personnel and appropriate external resources should be notified.

If the fire involves an airway device, ventilation and gas flows should be stopped and the airway device or any burning material should be removed immediately. Saline should be used to extinguish the fire. Once extinguished, a patent airway should be reestablished and ventilation resumed. Reassessment of the patient and situation should occur. Retained intraluminal fragments should be removed by bronchoscopy.

For a non-airway fire, ventilation and gas flows should be stopped. Patient drapes and all burning material should be immediately removed from the patient and saline used to extinguish the fire. Once all burning material has been extinguished, ventilation should be resumed and reassessment of the patient and situation should occur.

Following any fire, the involved personnel should be appropriately debriefed. A review of procedural techniques, including the fire response, should also be conducted.

Suggested Readings

Airway fires during surgery. *PA-PSRS Patient Saf Advis*. 2007;4:1-4.

Apfedbaum JL, Caplan RA, Barker SJ, et al. Practice Advisory for the Prevention and Management of Operating Room Fires. *Anesthesiology*. 2013;118:271-290.

Bayley G, McIndoe AK. Fires and explosions. *Anesth Intensive Care Med*. 2004;5:364-366.

Lypson ML, Stephens S, Colletti L. Preventing surgical fires: Who needs to be educated. *Jt Comm J Qual Patient Saf*. 2005;31:522-527.

Prasad R, Quezado Z, St. Andre A. Fires in the operating room and intensive care unit: Awareness is the key to prevention. *Anesth Analg*. 2006;102:172-174.

Rinder CS. Fire safety in the operation room. *Curr Opin Anesth*. 2008;21: 790-795.

OPERATING ROOM FIRES ALGORITHM

Fire Prevention:

- Avoid using ignition sources [1] in proximity to an oxidizer-enriched atmosphere [2]
- Configure surgical drapes to minimize the accumulation of oxidizers
- Allow sufficient drying time for flammable skin prepping solutions
- Moisten sponges and gauze when used in proximity to ignition sources

Is this a High-Risk Procedure?
An ignition source will be used in proximity to an oxidizer-enriched atmosphere

No → Early Warning Signs of Fire

YES

- Agree upon a team plan and team roles for preventing and managing a fire
- Notify the surgeon of the presence of, or an increase in, an oxidizer-enriched atmosphere
- Use cuffed tracheal tubes for surgery in the airway; appropriately prepare laser-resistant tracheal tubes
- Consider a tracheal tube or laryngeal mask for monitored anesthesia care (MAC) with moderate to deep sedation and/or oxygen-dependent patients who undergo surgery of the head, neck, or face.
- *Before* an ignition source is activated:
  - o *Announce* the intent to use an ignition source
  - o *Reduce* the oxygen concentration to the minimum required to avoid hypoxia[3]
  - o *Stop* the use of nitrous oxide[4]

Fire Management:

Early Warning Signs of Fire[5]

HALT PROCEDURE
Call for Evaluation

Fire is not present; Continue procedure

FIRE IS PRESENT

AIRWAY[6] ***Fire:***

IMMEDIATELY, without waiting

- Remove tracheal tube
- Stop the flow of all airway gases
- Remove sponges and any other flammable material from airway
- Pour saline into airway

NON-AIRWAY Fire:

IMMEDIATELY, without waiting

- Stop the flow of all airway gases
- Remove drapes and all burning and flammable materials
- Extinguish burning materials by pouring saline or other means

If Fire is Not Extinguished on First Attempt
Use a CO_2 fire extinguisher [7]
If fire persists: activate fire alarm, evacuate patient, close OR door, and turn off gas supply to room

Fire out (airway fire):

- Re-establish ventilation
- Avoid oxidizer-enriched atmosphere if clinically appropriate
- Examine tracheal tube to see if fragments may be left behind in airway
- Consider bronchoscopy

Fire out (non-airway fire):

- Maintain ventilation
- Assess for inhalation injury if the patient is not intubated

Assess patient status and devise plan for management

[1] Ignition sources include but are not limited to electrosurgery or electrocautery units and lasers.
[2] An oxidizer-enriched atmosphere occurs when there is any increase in oxygen concentration above room air level, and/or the presence of any concentration of nitrous oxide.
[3] After minimizing delivered oxygen, wait a period of time (*e.g.*, 1-3 min) before using an ignition source. For oxygen dependent patients, *reduce* supplemental oxygen delivery to the minimum required to avoid hypoxia. Monitor oxygenation with pulse oximetry, and if feasible, inspired, exhaled, and/or delivered oxygen concentration.
[4] After stopping the delivery of nitrous oxide, wait a period of time (*e.g.*, 1-3 min) before using an ignition source.
[5] Unexpected flash, flame, smoke or heat, unusual sounds (*e.g.*, a "pop," snap or "foomp") or odors, unexpected movement of drapes, discoloration of drapes or breathing circuit, unexpected patient movement or complaint.
[6] In this algorithm, airway fire refers to a fire in the airway or breathing circuit.
[7] A CO_2 fire extinguisher may be used on the patient if necessary.

Figure 4-2 The American Society of Anesthesiologists operating room fire algorithm. (Copyright © 2013, the American Society of Anesthesiologists, Inc. Lippincott Williams & Wilkins. Anesthesiology 2013;118:271-90.)

CHAPTER 5

Operating Room Management

James D. Kindscher, MD

The operating room (OR) is a complex and dynamic part of a health care system. Although many centers expect the OR to produce strong profit margins, it is also well recognized that this unit is very expensive to run. The OR relies on coordinated activities among medical specialties, nursing, and support staff to function at an optimal level. The subject of OR management is broad and can be found in more detail in the literature. This chapter will describe aspects of OR management that are important to the anesthesiologist.

Operating Room Governance

Most hospitals have an OR committee that is active in directing the function of this unit. This committee usually consists of leaders in the different sections of surgery, anesthesiology, and hospital management. The scope and authority of the OR committee depend upon local facility and medical practice governance structures. Often this committee will review performance standards, develop policies, offer budgetary guidance, and allocate OR time to surgeons or divisions.

The OR committee is not designed to meet the day-to-day needs of the OR, nor is it able to personally intervene when a challenge occurs in this unit. Therefore, many hospitals have created the position of medical director of the OR. This person is charged with leading improvements in the OR and ensuring compliance with the directives of the OR committee and hospital leadership. The medical director must balance the needs of physicians, nurses, hospital, and patients to maximize OR performance. Anesthesiologists frequently serve in the role of medical director because they are present in the OR on a daily basis, understand the different aspects of OR throughput, and can balance the needs of the different groups working in this area. The medical director position may require significant time and energy from the physician and should be supported by both the physician's group and the hospital. The expectations for this position must be clearly defined. Responsibilities may include policy development, conflict resolution, regulatory compliance, participation on committees related to OR function, and daily supervision of the unit.

Operating Room Efficiency

Surgeons, anesthesiologists, nurses, and hospital leadership all have different views on what OR efficiency means. Surgeons want convenient and readily available OR access, anesthesiologists want smooth-running schedules, nurses desire predictable shifts, and hospitals seek maximal profit margins for this costly unit. The medical director can help bridge these different interests to help the OR achieve its best function. Some of the key areas of focus for OR efficiency are scheduling, first-case starts, turnovers, and daily schedule management. Agreement on the definitions of these terms is essential.

Scheduling may be the single most important step in making an OR function well. Accuracy of the data is paramount; the procedure description and case length should realistically match what is to be performed. Errors in scheduling will inevitably lead to delays, lack of proper equipment, and dissatisfaction among the OR team. OR time may be granted to surgeons at regular intervals, called blocks. Surgeons are given a set time to schedule cases in an OR, based on their previous usage of OR time. This block time may be held for this surgeon up to several days prior to the anticipated date of surgery. If the block is not filled, then it may be released so that another surgeon can post a case in the unused time. Most ORs have a combination of block time and open (unblocked) time. The percentage of block versus open time is dependent on the surgery makeup in each hospital.

First-case on-time starts set the emotional tone for an OR. Usually an OR that has a high percentage of on-time starts will also be efficient in other areas of OR throughput. Delays in starting the first case may be related to the surgeon, anesthesiologist, nurse, patient, or hospital support. An objective analysis of delays may help to direct resources in the best way to improve on-time starts.

Perhaps the biggest area of focus by OR committees is turnover time. An immense amount of activity is required by the OR team to prepare an OR from one case to the next. Despite this fact, many members of the OR committee believe turnover times can be reduced to unreasonably short intervals. The OR may set goals for turnover time based on case complexity and personnel. Reasonable turnover times of 15 to 30 minutes are often achievable with commitment of the entire OR team.

Daily schedule management is an essential part of a well-run OR. Because there are frequent changes in the surgery list of cases, with add-ons and cancellations, it is important that the OR be adaptable to applying resources where they can best be utilized. Delays or complications in a surgical procedure may necessitate moving patients into different rooms. Communication between the OR medical director and OR nursing leadership is a key step in making this process work smoothly. It is also important to plan ahead and to anticipate potential roadblocks to the progress of the surgical schedule.

Operating Room Utilization

A common method of measuring the function of an OR is calculating the amount of time that this resource is used in actually performing surgical cases. There are different ways to define OR utilization. Perhaps the most commonly used calculation of OR utilization is the amount of time devoted to a case (room set-up time plus OR time for the case plus OR cleanup time) divided by the amount of time the OR is staffed and available. OR utilization goals are dependent on the types of operations performed in a hospital, the need for open time to manage emergencies, and the percentage of trauma or transplant cases that require short schedule-to-incision intervals. A utilization of 80% or more is most often necessary to balance the costs of staffing this unit.

One misunderstood aspect of OR utilization is the concept that utilization equates to OR productivity. Utilization is only a measure of consumption of a resource; it does not account for how well that resource is managed. As an example, if one surgeon spends twice as long to do a common procedure as a different surgeon, then the first surgeon may have greater utilization than the faster surgeon. Likewise, surgeons who perform long, complex procedures often have greater utilization than do surgeons who are efficient in performing short cases. When an analysis is made of the cost effectiveness of an OR, a better picture of value may be obtained. Subtracting the cost per minute of a case from the revenue per minute of the case allows a better measure of OR value for a procedure or surgeon. This information is important to a hospital in determining allocation of resources or expansion of services.

Cost Management

Because the majority of hospital revenue is derived from a bundled payment (diagnosis-related group, or DRG) structure, it is essential that costs for delivery of a service are well controlled. The OR represents one of the most expensive units in a hospital. Most surgeons perform cases that can be profitable to a hospital (contribute a positive margin); however, the range of profitability between surgeons is broad and important to understand before expanding service lines. Infrastructure support, such as capital equipment and intensive care unit availability, are also considerations during surgical services planning

Anesthesia management is also an important area of hospital cost management. When anesthesia personnel are not performing procedures, they are not generating revenue. When the hospital requires availability of an anesthesia service but has lower utilization of that service, then gaps in that support must be accounted for. Examples of areas in which these gaps occur include low utilization of elective OR times and specialty-call coverage (e.g., cardiac, obstetric, pediatric, transplant, and trauma). Because of these issues, hospitals will often contract with the anesthesia group to provide this service coverage in exchange for a fixed level of support.

Anesthesia pharmaceutical costs average 6% of the total costs for a surgical patient's hospitalization. Although cost differences between various agents used by anesthesiologists may seem like a potential area for cost reduction, many of these drug costs are fixed, and switching to a less expensive agent is unlikely to reduce overall expense. Regularly reviewing anesthesia drug costs and seeking best pricing in acquisition are the best strategies to employ when addressing this aspect of OR costs.

Conclusion

OR management is an important and necessary discipline; anesthesiologists are frequently leaders in improving OR performance. An integrated understanding of surgical, nursing, hospital, and patient needs uniquely qualifies anesthesiologists to serve in OR leadership roles.

Suggested Readings

Dexter F, Abouleish AE, Epstein RH, et al. Use of operating room information system data to predict the impact of reducing turnover times on staffing costs. *Anesth Analg*. 2003;97:1119-1126.

Macario A. Are your hospital operating rooms "efficient"? *Anesthesiology*. 2006; 105:237-240.

Marjamaa R, Vakkuri A, Kirvelä O. Operating room management: why, how and by whom? *Acta Anaesthesiol Scand*. 2008;52:596-600.

McIntosh C, Dexter F, Epstein RH. Impact of service-specific staffing, case scheduling, turnovers, and first-case starts on anesthesia group and operating room productivity: Tutorial using data from an Australian hospital. *Anesth Analg*. 2006;103:1499-1516.

SECTION II Equipment

CHAPTER 6

Vaporizers

Jerry A. Dorsch, MD

The vapor pressures of most modern inhalation anesthetic agents at room temperature are much greater than the partial pressure required to produce anesthesia (Table 6-1). To produce clinically useful concentrations, a vaporizer must bring about dilution of the saturated vapor. The total gas flow from the flowmeters goes through the vaporizer, picks up a predictable amount of vapor, and then flows to the common gas outlet. A single calibrated knob or dial is used to control the concentration of the agent.

Concentration-Calibrated Vaporizers

All vaporizers in common use today in developed countries are calibrated by the output concentration, expressed in volume percent. This is known as a concentration-calibrated (variable bypass, direct-reading) vaporizer. The American Society for Testing and Materials anesthesia workstation standard requires that all vaporizers on the anesthesia workstation be concentration calibrated. In addition, all vaporizer control dials must turn counterclockwise to increase the output concentration. These vaporizers must be placed between the flowmeters and the outlet on the anesthesia machine.

Concentration calibration may be accomplished by splitting the flow of gas that passes through the vaporizer. Some gas passes through the vaporizing chamber (the part of the vaporizer containing the liquid anesthetic agent), and the remainder goes through a bypass to the vaporizer outlet (Figure 6-1). The ratio of bypass gas to the gas flowing to the vaporizing chamber is called the *splitting ratio* and depends on the resistances in the two pathways. It also depends on the setting of the concentration dial that allows more gas to pass through the vaporizing chamber as higher output concentrations are set. The splitting ratio may also depend on the total gas flow through the vaporizer. Another method of controlling the outlet concentration is to direct enough carrier gas to flow through the vaporizing chamber to achieve the concentration set on the vaporizer. This is determined by a computer.

In many concentration-calibrated vaporizers, the composition of the carrier gas affects vaporizer output (vaporizer aberrance). Most vaporizers are calibrated using O_2 as the carrier gas. Usually, little change in output occurs if air is substituted for O_2. Addition of N_2O to the carrier gas typically results in both temporary and long-lasting effects on vaporizer output. The temporary effect is usually reduced vapor concentration. The duration depends on the gas flow rate and on the volume of liquid in the vaporizer. The longer-term effect may be increased or decreased output concentration, depending on the construction of the vaporizer.

At low barometric pressure (higher altitudes), variable-bypass concentration-calibrated vaporizers will deliver approximately the same anesthetic partial pressure but increased concentrations measured in volume percent. At high barometric pressure (as in a hyperbaric chamber), these vaporizers deliver decreased output measured in volume percent because the vapor pressure of the agent is affected only by temperature

Table 6-1 Vapor Pressure of Inhaled Anesthetic Agents at 20° C

Anesthetic Agent	Vapor Pressure, mm Hg
Isoflurane	239
Sevoflurane	160
Desflurane	664

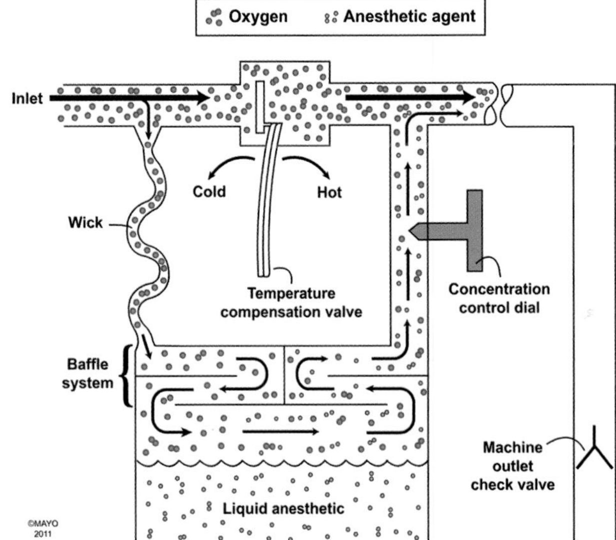

Figure 6-1 A schematic of a variable bypass vaporizer. Oxygen, air, or both O_2 and air flow into the inlet, and a small amount is diverted into the vaporizing chamber—the concentration valve and a temperature compensation valve control the amount that is diverted. As the gas flowing through the vaporizing chamber absorbs the inhalation agent, the temperature of the liquid drops. To maintain a constant output of the inhalation agent, the temperature compensation valve diverts more gas into the vaporizing chamber. Conversely, if the room temperature were to rise—and, therefore, the temperature of the entire vaporizer, the valve would move to the left, and less gas would be diverted into the vaporizing chamber.

and not by ambient pressure. The partial pressure and clinical effects remain relatively unchanged.

Vaporization Methods

Flow Over

In a flow-over vaporizer, carrier gas passes over the surface of the liquid. Increasing the area of the carrier gas-liquid interface can enhance the efficiency of vaporization. This can be done using baffles or spiral tracks to lengthen the pathway of the gas exposed to the liquid. Another method is to use wicks with their bases in the liquid. The liquid moves up the wicks by capillary action.

Bubble Through

Another way to increase contact between the carrier gas and the volatile liquid is to bubble the gas through the liquid. The gas may break up into small bubbles, further increasing the gas-liquid interface.

Injection

Some vaporizers control the vapor concentration by injecting a known amount of liquid anesthetic agent (from a reservoir in the vaporizer or from the bottle of agent) into a known volume of gas.

Temperature Compensation

When a liquid is vaporized, energy, in the form of heat, is lost. The vapor pressure decreases as the temperature of the liquid drops. Three methods have been employed to maintain a constant vapor output with fluctuations in liquid anesthetic temperature.

Thermostatic Compensation

Most concentration-calibrated vaporizers compensate for changes in vapor pressure with temperature by altering the flow of carrier gas through the vaporizing chamber. This is accomplished by changing the splitting ratio. In mechanical vaporizers, a thermostatic element performs this function by increasing resistance to the bypass gas flow, allowing more gas to flow through the vaporizing chamber when the vaporizer cools.

Computer Controlled

In electronic vaporizers, gas flow is controlled by a computer that alters the flow of carrier gas through the vaporizing chamber to maintain the set output concentration.

Supplied Heat

An electric heater can be used to supply heat to a vaporizer and maintain it at a constant temperature. Desflurane vaporizers (Tec 6, Datex-Ohmeda, GE Healthcare, Helsinki, Finland; Dräger Vapor-D, Telford, PA; and Penlon Sigma Alpha, Abingdon, UK) present unique problems for vaporizer design. The low boiling point (22.8° C) of desflurane makes the volume of gas delivered by either a measured-flow or a variable-bypass vaporizer unpredictable. The Ohmeda Tec 6 vaporizer pressurizes the liquid desflurane to 1500 mm Hg and warms it to around 40° C. It delivers a flow of pure saturated gas to the bypass gas. The amount of vapor that is delivered to the bypass gas will depend on the concentration selected on the concentration dial and the fresh gas flow.

Suggested Readings

Andrews JJ. Delivery systems for inhaled anesthetics. In: Barash PG, Cullen BF, Stoelting RK, eds. *Clinical Anesthesia*. 3rd ed. Philadelphia: Lippincott-Raven; 1997:535-572.

Dorsch JA, Dorsch SE. Vaporizers (anesthetic agent delivery devices). In: Dorsch JA, Dorsch SE, eds. *Understanding Anesthesia Equipment*. 5th ed. Baltimore: Williams & Wilkins; 2008:121-190.

Sezdi M, Akan A, Tank F. Anesthetic gas concentration changes related to the temperature and humidity in high and low flow anesthesia. *Conf Proc IEEE Eng Med Biol Soc*. 2009;2009:877-880.

CHAPTER 7

Flowmeters and the Physics of Gas Flow

Mary M. Rajala, MS, MD

A flowmeter assembly is a device that measures, controls, and indicates the flow of gas passing through it. Originally, flowmeters on anesthesia machines were mechanical devices, and, on many machines, they still are; however, newer machines control the flow of gases electronically.

Traditional flowmeters, known as variable orifice or Thorpe flowmeters, are vertically placed, tempered-glass, tapered tubes that have the smallest diameter at the bottom (Figure 7-1). Flow into the tube is controlled by a needle valve at the base of the glass tube. As the needle valve is opened, gas enters the base of the tube, where it encounters an indicator float or bobbin that, through the force of gravity, lies at the base of the tube. The pressure of the gas exerts a force that moves the float in the tapered tube to a point of equilibrium, the point at which the downward force of gravity on the float is equal to the upward force of the gas flow. The float is prevented from leaving the tube by a stop at the top. A scale calibrated specifically for each gas is marked along the side of the tube, indicating the gas flow. The higher the float rises in the tube, the greater is the gas flow around it. Likewise, when gas flow is decreased, gravity causes the float to settle at a lower level in the tube.

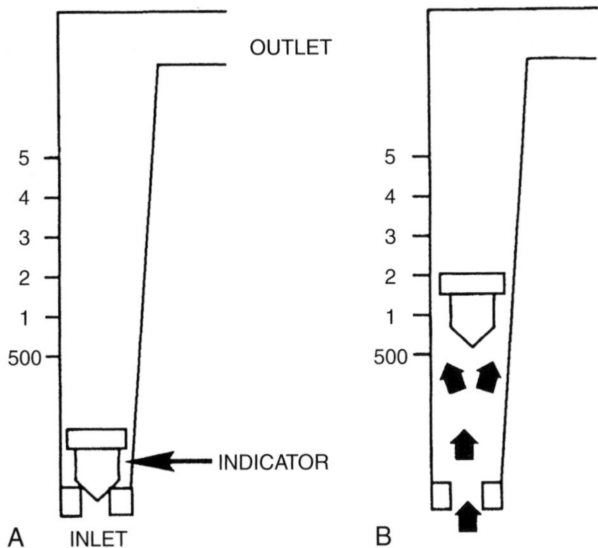

Figure 7-1 Variable orifice flowmeter. Gas enters at the base and flows through the tube, causing the float to rise. The gas passes through the annular opening around the float. The area of this annular space increases with the height of the indicator. Thus, the height of the indicator is a measure of gas flow. (Reprinted, with permission, from Dorsch JA, Dorsch SE. Understanding Anesthesia Equipment. 5th ed. Philadelphia: Lippincott, Williams & Wilkins; 2008:103-109, 114-117, 405-407, 933, 940-941.)

Physical Principles

Pressure Change Across the Constriction

Any liquid or gas flowing through a tube obeys Poiseuille's law: $Q = \Delta P \pi r^4/(8\eta L)$. This law states that the flow (Q) in a tube is directly proportional to the pressure drop (ΔP) along the length of the tube, and to the fourth power of the radius (r) of the tube, and is inversely proportional to the length (L) of the tube and the viscosity (η) of the fluid or gas.

The Bernoulli principle can be used to describe what happens when the gas encounters, and then flows around, the float. The float, in essence, creates a stricture such that flow around the float is more rapid than that below the float. The rate of gas flow through the flowmeter is proportional to this pressure change around the float; this change, in turn, is related to the radius of the float in relationship to the radius of the glass tube and the physical properties of the gas.

As the needle valve is opened, gas enters the tube, increasing the pressure at the base of the tube and forcing the float to rise. The change in pressure around the float is constant for all positions of the float within the tube. As the needle valve is opened and flow around the float increases, the pressure above the float decreases, and the float rises higher in the tube to a position at which the pressure around the float is the same as it was at the previous position of the float. Increased flow does not change the pressure around the float at the new position because the change in pressure is proportional to the weight of the float and to the flow and is inversely proportional to the cross-sectional area of the float.

Physical Properties of the Gas

Flowmeters are calibrated for use with a specific gas density and viscosity and, thus, cannot be interchanged. At low flows, the gap around the float will be narrow and the float will hover near the bottom of the tube. When the tube is narrow, gas flow is laminar and varies according to the viscosity of the gas.

With increasing flow, the opening enlarges as the float rises. At high flows, the tube is wider and flow becomes turbulent and becomes a function of the density of the gas.

Effects of Temperature and Pressure

Changes in temperature and pressure alter both the viscosity and density of gases, thereby affecting the accuracy of the indicator on the flowmeters, which are calibrated at atmospheric pressure (760 mm Hg) and room temperature (20° C). Practically speaking, temperature changes are slight and are not responsible for significant changes. Large fluctuations in temperature, however, will make calibrations inaccurate.

As altitude increases, barometric pressure decreases, potentially resulting in a flow that is greater than indicated. At low flow rates, flow is laminar and dependent on gas viscosity, a property independent of altitude. However, at high flow rates, flow becomes turbulent, and flow becomes a function of density, a property that is influenced by altitude. The resulting decrease in density will increase the actual flow rate, so the flowmeter will read lower than the actual flow rate. At pressures below 630 mm Hg, the delivered flow rate will exceed the set flow rate by 9% to 20%.

At increased pressure, as in a hyperbaric chamber, the reverse is seen, with the delivered flow rate slightly less than indicated.

Types of Indicators

The indicator float is generally made of aluminum, nickel, sapphire, or glass. Numerous styles are in use, including the free-spinning float, rotameter ball float, nonrotating float, and H float (Figure 7-2). These floats are designed so that gas flowing through the tube keeps the float in the center

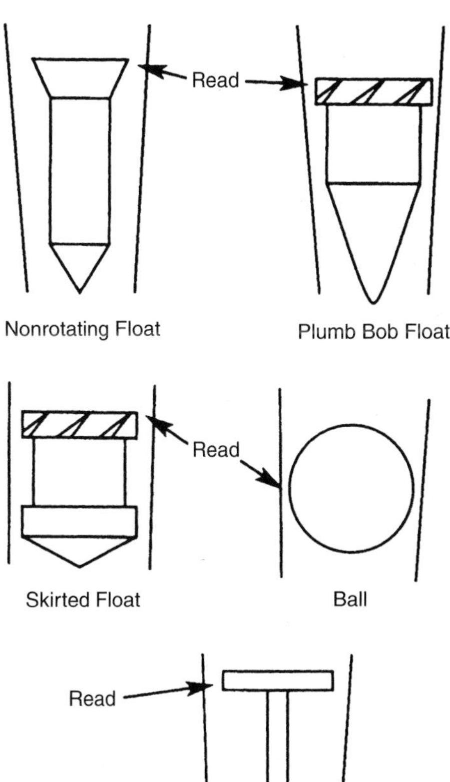

Figure 7-2 Flowmeter indicators. The plumb bob and skirted floats are examples of rotameters, which are kept centered in the tube by constant rotation; the reading is taken at the top. The ball indicator is held centered by rib guides; the reading is taken at the center. The nonrotating float and H float do not rotate and are kept centered by gas flow. (Reprinted, with permission, from Dorsch JA, Dorsch SE. Understanding Anesthesia Equipment. 5th ed. Philadelphia: Lippincott, Williams & Wilkins; 2008:103-109, 114-117, 405-407, 933, 940-941.)

of the tube and allows the float to spin freely (for types that rotate), maintaining the central position, reducing friction, and improving accuracy. Deviations of the tube from a vertical position cause the float to strike the side of the tube.

Arrangement of Flowmeters

Two flowmeter tubes for the same gas may be arranged in series or in parallel for finer control of gas flow at low rates. Modern machines have a series arrangement, using only one valve for each gas. Normal flow is from bottom to top and from left to right. One tube is for low flow (less than 1 L/min) and one is for high flow (1-10 L/min) and the greatest accuracy is in the middle half of the tube. An O_2 analyzer must be used to determine whether a hypoxic mixture exists. Different manufacturers have created different designs for regulating O_2 pressure. The practitioner needs to be familiar with the equipment and should attempt to create a hypoxic mixture by adjusting O_2, as well as N_2O, in performing routine machine checkout to ensure that the O_2 analyzer is functioning properly.

A hypoxic gas mixture can result from unsafe sequencing of flowmeters (Figure 7-3). When the O_2 flowmeter is upstream, a leak in the system will cause O_2 to leak out before being added to other gases, a potentially dangerous situation. It is safer to have O_2 as the most downstream gas. In the United States and Canada, the standard is for the O_2 flowmeter to occupy the right-hand location nearest the normal outlet and downstream from all other gases. Some machines are manufactured with pin indexing of the flowmeter module as a safety feature. Often flowmeters are serviced as a unit, preventing transposition of the rotameter tubes. Some newer models have incorporated identical flowmeter tubes that are entirely interchangeable, relying instead on exterior scales that are etched. Other new trends include electronic flow controls. To avoid problems, only qualified personnel should service flowmeters or dissemble the anesthesia machine.

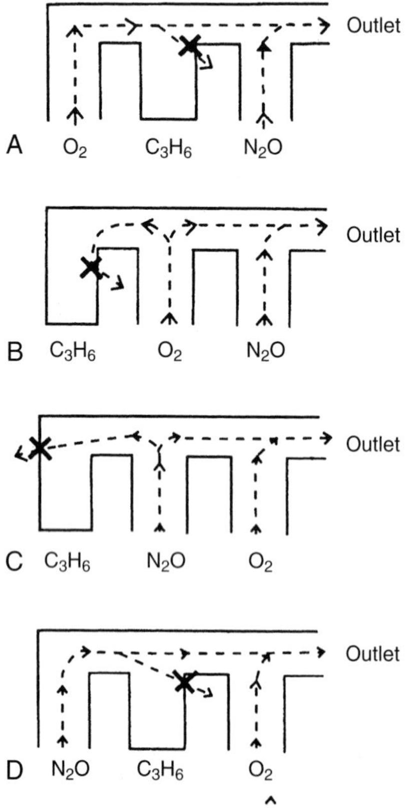

Figure 7-3 Flowmeter sequence. **A** and **B**—With the O_2 flowmeter upstream, a potentially dangerous situation arises if a leak should occur. **C** and **D**—With the O_2 entering downstream from the other gases, a safer situation is achieved. (Reprinted, with permission, from Eger EI, Hylton RR, Irwin RH, Guadagni N. Anesthetic flow meter sequence: A cause for hypoxia. Anesthesiology. 1963;24:396-397.)

Hypoxic gas mixtures can also result from human error on older machines. To prevent this, modern machines have mandatory minimum O_2 flows, mechanical or pneumatic linkages between O_2 and N_2O flow control valves, and alarms to prevent administration of hypoxic mixtures. The anesthesia provider should refer to the American Society of Anesthesiologists Guidelines for Determining Anesthesia Machine Obsolescence to assist in the decision as to when to retire equipment that is outdated and perhaps unsafe.

Problems

Flowmeters are more likely to malfunction when there has been a repair or installation, if mechanical damage has occurred, or when turning on the gas supply. To prevent this problem, the anesthesia provider should always turn the flowmeters to the off position before turning off the gas supply, connecting pipeline hoses, or opening cylinders to the machine. Compressed gas may contain particles that cause floats to become stuck. For this reason, preanesthesia checks and required routine maintenance should be performed.

Inaccuracy

Flowmeters are calibrated to the lowest point on the scale. Therefore, on a 1 L/min to a 10 L/min flowmeter at flows of greater than 1 L/min, the actual flow is ± 5% of the flow denoted by the float. Error increases inversely with the rate of flow and may become clinically significant (up to 70%) at flows below 1 L/min. Flows extrapolated below the first mark on the scale are not accurate. Low-flow tubes arranged in series allow greater accuracy when low gas flow is desired. It is important to measure O_2 concentration (F_{IO_2}) during low flow to avoid a hypoxic mixture caused by flowmeter inaccuracy. When there is a discrepancy between low-flow and high-flow meters, the low-flow tube is more likely to be accurate.

Back Pressure

If pressure at the common outlet increases, then the gas above the float is compressed and the pressure above the indicator rises, forcing the float down and causing the flowmeter to read lower than the actual gas flow rate.

Improper Alignment

Inaccuracy may result from improper alignment of the floats in the flowmeter tube, leading to an asymmetric circumference of the channel around the float.

Improper Sequence

A 1998 report by Walmsley and Holloway describes a case in which rotameter tubes for CO_2 and N_2O were transposed after servicing. The anesthesiologist recognized the problem after the gas flows were turned on—when the calibration for N_2O was incorrect in scale, color, and labeling; the anesthesiologist was able to compensate by using 100% O_2 and an inhalation agent.

Static Electricity

Inaccuracy may result from static electricity causing the float to stick to the side of the tube. The electrostatic charges are negligible as long as the float rotates freely. Moisture or antistatic spray applied to the outside of the tube will successfully remove charges. More technical approaches are required to remove charges from within the tube.

Hidden Floats

The float may adhere to the stop at the top of the tube even if no gas is flowing. If the stops are broken or are not replaced after cleaning, the float may disappear from view. Dirt particles, frequent components of compressed air, can cause a float to stick and create inaccurate gas flow readings; excessive pressure buildup inside the tube can lead to explosion.

Erratic Movement of the Float

The float may exhibit jumping or up-and-down movement from dirt in the tube. This can result in incorrect and potentially hypoxic gas mixtures, a reason for FIO_2 monitoring. If this is observed, the sealed unit containing the tube needs cleaning or replacement.

Suggested Readings

American Society of Anesthesiologists. *Guidelines for Determining Anesthesia Machine Obsolescence*. Available at: http://www.psanes.org/Portals/0/docs/ASAGuidelines.pdf. Accessed on: January 13, 2011.

Dorsch JA, Dorsch SE. *Understanding Anesthesia Equipment*. 5th ed. Philadelphia: Lippincott, Williams & Wilkins; 2008:103-109, 114-117, 405-407, 933, 940-941.

Eger EI, Hylton RR, Irwin RH, Guadagni N. Anesthetic flow meter sequence: A cause for hypoxia. *Anesthesiology*. 1963;24:396-397.

Walmsley AJ, Holloway J. Transposition of rotameter tubes. *Br J Anesth*. 1998; 80:124-125.

CHAPTER 8

Carbon Dioxide Absorption

John M. VanErdewyk, MD

Scientists first began experimenting with substances capable of absorbing carbon dioxide (CO_2) in the early 1900s. Progress was made during World War I, when chemical warfare stimulated research to eliminate CO_2 from the closed breathing system of the gas mask. Today, CO_2 absorption is used daily to remove CO_2 from semiclosed or closed anesthetic circuits.

CO_2 Absorbers

An ideal CO_2 absorber would have the following characteristics: efficiency, ease of handling, low resistance to airflow, low cost, lack of toxicity, and lack of reactivity when used with common anesthetics.

The amount of CO_2 that can be absorbed varies depending upon the absorbent. In practical use, the maximum amount is rarely achieved because of factors such as channeling of gas flow around the granules of absorbent. Channeling refers to the preferential passage of exhaled gases through the canister via the pathways of least resistance. Excessive channeling will bypass much of the granule bulk and decrease efficiency. Proper canister design—with screens and baffles plus proper packing—helps decrease channeling (Figure 8-1).

A dual-chamber canister is more efficient than a single-chambered canister, and an ideal water content of the absorbent is needed for optimal CO_2 absorption. For the greatest efficiency of absorption, the patient's entire tidal volume should be accommodated within the void space of the container. Therefore, a properly packed canister should contain approximately one half of its volume in granules and one half as intergranular space.

The greater the surface area available for CO_2 absorption, the greater the absorptive ability. However, as granule size decreases (surface area increases), the resistance to airflow through the canister increases. A compromise has been reached in a granule size of 4 to 8 mesh, which allows good CO_2 absorption with an acceptable resistance to flow.

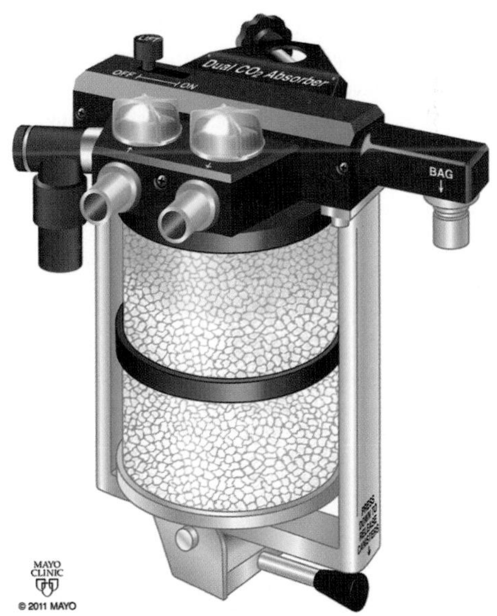

Figure 8-1 The dual-chamber absorber is now the most commonly used type of absorber for containing CO_2 absorbent. This device is permanently mounted, with a vertical gas-flow axis. This positioning eliminates dusting, channeling, and packing problems. Because condensation may collect at the bottom of the chamber, forming a caustic lye solution with the dust, it is important that the unit contains a drain valve. Each absorber design has unique opening, closing, and sealing components; however, most have a single-action clamp mechanism.

Benefits

CO_2 absorption is cost effective because it allows lower gas flows and use of less inhalation agent when using a semiclosed or closed circuit to deliver a general anesthetic. The use of lower gas flows decreases pollution in the operating room. In addition, the CO_2 absorber generates both heat and water, which help warm and humidify inspired gases.

Degradation of Inhaled Anesthetic Agents

All CO_2 absorbers utilize $Ca(OH)_2$ as the primary component. Some absorbents contain various amounts of NaOH and KOH (e.g., sodalime) to serve as catalysts. Unfortunately inhalation anesthetic agents can interact with these catalysts to produce toxic byproducts (compound A, carbon monoxide [CO], methanol, and formaldehyde) and thermal injuries.

Compound A is a vinyl ether degradation product formed from the interaction of sevoflurane (only) with the bases KOH and NaOH (KOH > NaOH). Compound A is produced with either a moist or desiccated CO_2 absorber and is present in any rebreathing circuit utilizing sevoflurane and sodalime. Despite the initial concern of possible renal toxicity, extensive evaluation has found no clinically significant adverse effect on renal function in humans.

Thermal Injuries and CO Production

All modern inhalation anesthetic agents interacting with a desiccated CO_2 absorber containing KOH or NaOH cause an exothermic reaction and production of CO. CO production is increased with increasing temperature. Desflurane is more likely to result in CO production, as compared with isoflurane, with sevoflurane being the least likely. Other factors related to CO production include the dryness of absorbent and the concentration of the anesthetic agent.

Desiccation of the absorber can occur after a prolonged period of high fresh-gas flow rates, such as occurs when an anesthesia machine is inadvertently left on over a weekend. When an inhalation agent is introduced during the first case on Monday morning, the reaction can occur. Effects of CO can range from subclinical to severe, with carboxyhemoglobin concentrations greater than 30% described in case reports. Signs and symptoms of subclinical CO toxicity are nonspecific, or masked under anesthesia, making diagnosis difficult without a high degree of suspicion; the measurement of arterial blood-gas concentrations with a co-oximeter will document the concentration of carboxyhemoglobin.

Despite the lesser quantity of CO produced, sevoflurane has been proved to generate the most heat. Case reports have described explosions and fire in the CO_2 absorbers secondary to the interaction of sevoflurane with desiccated Baralyme. In experimental settings, sevoflurane has been shown to produce canister temperatures of 400°C, with associated smoldering, melting of plastic, explosion, and fire. Cases of severe heat associated with the use of sodalime have also been reported.

New Absorbents

As a result of the reported dangerous reactions, Baralyme was withdrawn from the market in 2004. New CO_2 absorbents (e.g., Amsorb Plus, LoFloSorb, and Dragersorb 800 PLUS) without NaOH or KOH have been introduced. Composed of $Ca(OH)_2$ with small amounts of $CaCl_2$ and $CaSO_4$, they are not known to react with inhalation anesthetic agents or to produce compound A or CO. Thermal injuries should also be markedly reduced or eliminated.

An Anesthesia Patient Safety Foundation conference report recommends the use of a CO_2 absorbent that does not significantly degrade inhalation anesthetic agents or, if conventional CO_2 absorbents are used, that specific policies be instituted to prevent their desiccation.

Suggested Readings

Fatheree R, Leighton B. Acute respiratory distress syndrome after an exothermic baralyme-sevoflurane reaction. *Anesthesiology*. 2004;101:531-533.

Hirabayashi G, Uchino H, Nakajima T, et al. Effects of temperature gradient reduction in three different carbon dioxide absorbents. *Eur J Anaesthesiol*. 2009;26:469-474.

Junzheng W, Previte J, Adler E, et al. Spontaneous ignition, explosion, and fire with sevoflurane and barium hydroxide lime. *Anesthesiology*. 2004;101:534-537.

Keijzer C, Perez RS, de Lange JJ. Compound A and carbon monoxide production from sevoflurane and seven different types of carbon dioxide absorbent in a patient model. *Acta Anaesthesiol Scand*. 2007;51:31-37.

Olympio MA. Carbon dioxide absorbent desiccation safety conference convened by APSF. *APSF Newsletter*. 2005;20:25-29.

Waters RM. Carbon dioxide absorption technic in anesthesia. *Ann Surg*. 1936;103(1):38-45.

Wissing H, Kuhn I, Warnken U, Dudziak R. Carbon monoxide production from desflurane, enflurane, halothane, isoflurane, and sevoflurane with dry soda lime. *Anesthesiology*. 2001;95:1205-1212.

Yamakage M, Takahashi K, Takahashi M, et al. Performance of four carbon dioxide absorbents in experimental and clinical settings. *Anaesthesia*. 2009;64:287-292.

CHAPTER 9

Carbon Dioxide Retention and Capnography

Michael G. Ivancic, MD

The monitoring of CO_2, the most abundant gas produced by the human body during anesthesia, has become a standard of practice strongly encouraged by the American Society of Anesthesiologists. CO_2 is a by-product of cellular metabolism, transported to the lungs by the systemic venous system and eliminated from the alveoli during ventilation (see Chapter 22).

CO_2 Retention

Rebreathing of CO_2 is undesirable, although, during mechanical ventilation, allowing the patient to rebreathe CO_2 is infrequently used to achieve normocarbia in those patients who are being hyperventilated (i.e., when large tidal volumes may be desirable for other reasons). A leak or obstruction in the anesthesia machine circuit, common gas outlet, or fresh gas supply line may also cause an increase in CO_2 concentration.

When Mapleson systems are used, inadequate fresh gas flow is the primary cause of an increase in CO_2 because these systems do not contain unidirectional valves or absorbent canisters. Specifically, systems with inner tubes, such as the Bain system, can cause rebreathing if there is any dysfunction (kink) in that tube. The Mapelson D (Bain circuit) is the most efficient for controlled ventilation with regard to a relatively low flow of fresh gas, whereas the Mapleson A is most suitable for patients who are spontaneously breathing (see Chapter 193). Specific minimum fresh gas flow rates for the various Mapleson apparatuses are recommended for spontaneous ventilation as well as controlled ventilation (Box 9-1).

Increased dead space, whether mechanical or physiologic, can increase rebreathing and CO_2 retention if the dead space is particularly large, especially in smaller patients. A heat and moisture exchanger in the breathing circuit may also be a source of dead space, with the larger the volume of the heat and moisture exchanger, the larger the dead space.

In the closed-circle systems used in modern anesthesia machines, minimal rebreathing of CO_2, if any, should occur; however, malfunction of either of the unidirectional valves may lead to CO_2 rebreathing. If an inspiratory valve is stuck open, rebreathing can occur because, during expiration, alveolar gas can backfill the inspiratory limb of the circle. A malfunctioning expiratory valve can lead to CO_2 rebreathing in a spontaneously breathing patient because, during inspiration, the negative pressure generated by the patient can entrain alveolar gas from the expiratory limb of the circuit.

Other causes of inadvertent CO_2 rebreathing usually involve the CO_2 absorber. If the absorbent color indicator malfunctions—and, therefore, is not reflecting the true level of CO_2 in the system—rebreathing can occur without the anesthesia provider being aware of the problem. In older anesthesia machines, the CO_2 absorber could be bypassed. Older absorbent canisters had a rebreathing valve on them that, if engaged, would lead to CO_2 rebreathing. Channeling of gas through the canister without contacting any active absorbent can also lead to CO_2 rebreathing. Independent of the cause, absorbent malfunction is best corrected immediately by increasing the fresh gas flow and then troubleshooting the underlying cause.

Box 9-1 Circumstances in Which Rebreathing of CO_2 May Occur with the Use of a Closed-Circle Anesthesia System

- Absorbent-related situations
  - Malfunction of the color indicator
  - Intentional or unintentional bypass of the absorber*
  - Unintentional engagement of the rebreathing valve*
  - Channeling of the gas through the canister without contacting any active absorbent
- Unidirectional-valve malfunction during spontaneous or mechanical ventilation
  - Inspiratory valve
  - Expiratory valve

*In an older machine.

Capnography

During induction of and emergence from anesthesia, rebreathing of CO_2 will lengthen each process because of alterations in alveolar tensions associated with rebreathing of exhaled alveolar anesthetic gases. Capnography can help troubleshoot malfunctioning equipment, such as the problems noted above. The classic rebreathing pattern on the capnogram will show an elevation of the waveform baseline that does not return to 0, as well as a higher end-tidal CO_2 (P_{ETCO_2}) reading, although the $Paco_2$ value may be normal, depending on the degree of alveolar ventilation.

Terminology

Capnometry is the measurement and numeric display of the partial pressure or gas concentration of CO_2. A capnometer is the device that measures and displays the concentration of CO_2. Capnography is the graphic record of CO_2 concentration, and the capnograph is the device that generates the waveform, with the capnogram being the actual waveform.

Sidestream Versus Mainstream Sampling

The CO_2 may be measured from a mainstream or sidestream device. Mainstream sampling uses a device that is placed close to the tracheal tube, with all the inhaled and exhaled gas flowing through the device. One benefit to the use of mainstream sampling is that the response time is faster, so no uncertainty exists regarding the rate of gas sampling. Drawbacks include the bulkiness of the device and the need for it to be heated to 40° C, therefore increasing the risk of burning the patient's skin.

Sidestream sampling is the method most commonly used in today's operating rooms. Sampling flow rate is an important aspect of this system and is usually in the range of 150 to 250 mL/min, with a mean of approximately 200 mL/min. If the sampling flow is less than 150 mL/min, the sampling time is too slow; if the flow is greater than 250 mL/min, the likelihood increases of fresh-gas contamination occurring. Water condensation can also be a problem as expired air condenses within the sampling tube walls. Various water-trap systems have been devised but may fail. Changing or flushing of the CO_2 sampling tube with an air-filled syringe may alleviate some moisture and the sampling error, but a new filter is often required.

CO_2 Measurement Methods

Infrared spectrometry is the most commonly used method of measuring gas concentration. Other methods include mass spectrometry, Raman scattering, and chemical colorimetric analysis.

Infrared spectrometry systems work by analyzing infrared light absorption from gas samples and comparing them with a known reference to determine the type and concentration of that particular gas. The advantages associated with the infrared system include the ability of the system to accurately analyze multiple gases—from CO_2 to N_2O and all the potent inhalation agents—as well as the fact that the unit is relatively small, lightweight, and inexpensive. The greatest disadvantage is that water vapor can interfere with measurements, resulting in falsely elevated readings of CO_2 and inhalation agents.

Mass spectrometry can measure nearly every gas pertinent to anesthesia by separating gases and vapors according to differences in their mass-to-charge ratios, including O_2 and N_2, which cannot be measured by infrared. Mass spectrometry also has a relatively fast response time. The disadvantages to this system include the relatively large size of the unit, the need for warm-up time, and the cost.

Raman spectroscopy relies on the inelastic, or Raman, scattering of monochromatic light (e.g., a laser) by different gases, thereby providing information about the phonon modes (an excitation state, a quantum mechanical description of a special type of vibrational motion of molecules) in a system. The advantages to the use of Raman spectroscopy include the fact that multiple gases can be analyzed simultaneously, the system is very accurate, and the response time is rapid. However, this system is relatively large and expensive.

Colorimetric detection consists of a pH-sensitive paper within a chamber placed between the tracheal tube and ventilation device. The color change is reversible and can change from breath to breath. Several brands are marketed, but most use a color scale that is similar (i.e., purple: $ETCO_2$ <4 mm Hg [<0.5% CO_2]; tan: $ETCO_2$ 4-15 mm Hg [0.5% to 2% CO_2]; yellow: $ETCO_2$ >15 mm Hg [>2% CO_2]). Advantages are portability, low cost, and no need for other equipment. The use of colorimetric detection is most applicable outside of the operating room to confirm tracheal-tube placement. The disadvantages are that the results are only semiquantitative.

Capnograms

Capnograms rely on time or volume to assess CO_2 concentrations. Time capnograms are further divided into slow and fast tracings. All have their advantages, but the time capnogram is the most commonly used system (fast speed for trends and slow speed for detailed waveform analysis). Volume capnograms are unique in that a breath-by-breath measurement of CO_2 concentration can be made, dead space can be divided into components, and significant changes in the morphology of the expired waveform can be detected as they relate to ventilation and perfusion. Normal CO_2 waveforms and several abnormal capnograms are shown in Figures 9-1 and 9-2. Pa_{CO_2} and P_{ETCO_2} trends of metabolism, circulation, ventilation, and various equipment failures are summarized in Table 9-1. Changes in P_{ETCO_2} and the capnogram may indicate one of a number of potential changes in the patient's condition, requiring the clinician to act appropriately.

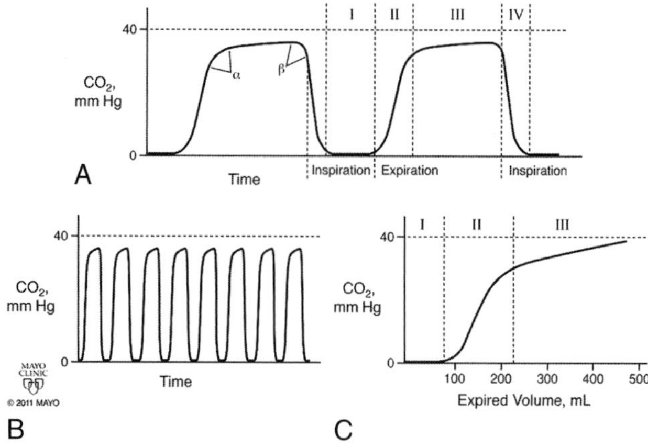

Figure 9-1 Normal capnograph waveforms. **A,** Phase I—Inspiration; CO_2 should be 0. Phase II—Beginning of expiration; CO_2 rises rapidly as dead space gas containing no CO_2 is exhaled. Phase III contains almost all alveolar gas, and, in a healthy individual, the plateau should be relatively flat. Phase IV—Beginning of inhalation. The α angle, the angle between phase II and III, should be between 100 and 110 degrees; patients with obstructive lung disease will have an angle greater than 110 degrees. The β angle, the angle between phase III and IV, is less than 100 degrees but will increase if there is any rebreathing because the gas being inhaled will contain some of the previously exhaled CO_2. **B,** Normal capnogram tracing over time—The end-tidal CO_2 should be relatively constant. **C,** Capnogram of a patient with obstructive lung disease. Such patients require a longer expiratory time; the capnogram has a more rounded appearance during the initial phase of expiration, a more obtuse α angle, and an upward slope to the alveolar plateau.

Table 9-1 Causes of Altered End-Tidal CO_2 during Anesthesia*

Cause	P_{ETCO_2}	P_{ETCO_2}-to-Pa_{CO_2} Gradient
CO_2 insufflation	Increased	Normal
Increased CO_2 production†	Increased	Normal
Right-to-left shunt	Increased	Widened
Increased physiologic or anatomic dead space, or both	Decreased	Widened
Increased apparatus dead space	Increased	Normal
Hyperventilation	Decreased	Normal
Hypoventilation	Increased	Normal
Leak in sampling line	Decreased	Widened
Poor seal around tracheal tube	Decreased	Widened
High sampling rate	Decreased	Widened
Low sampling rate	Decreased	Widened
Rebreathing due to malfunctioning breathing valve	Increased	Decreased
Rebreathing with low fresh gas in the Mapleson system	Increased	Decreased
Rebreathing with circle system (absorbent problem)	Increased	Normal

*Normal pressure of end-tidal CO_2 (P_{ETCO_2}) is 38 mm Hg (5%). The Pa_{CO_2}-to-P_{ETCO_2} gradient is normally <5 mm Hg.

†From hyperthermia, malignant hyperthermia, convulsions, pain, or bicarbonate administration.

Adapted, with permission, from Dorsch JA, Dorsch SE. Gas monitoring. In: Dorsch JA, Dorsch SE, eds. Understanding Anesthesia Equipment, 5th ed. Philadelphia: Lippincott, Williams & Wilkins; 2007:706-707.

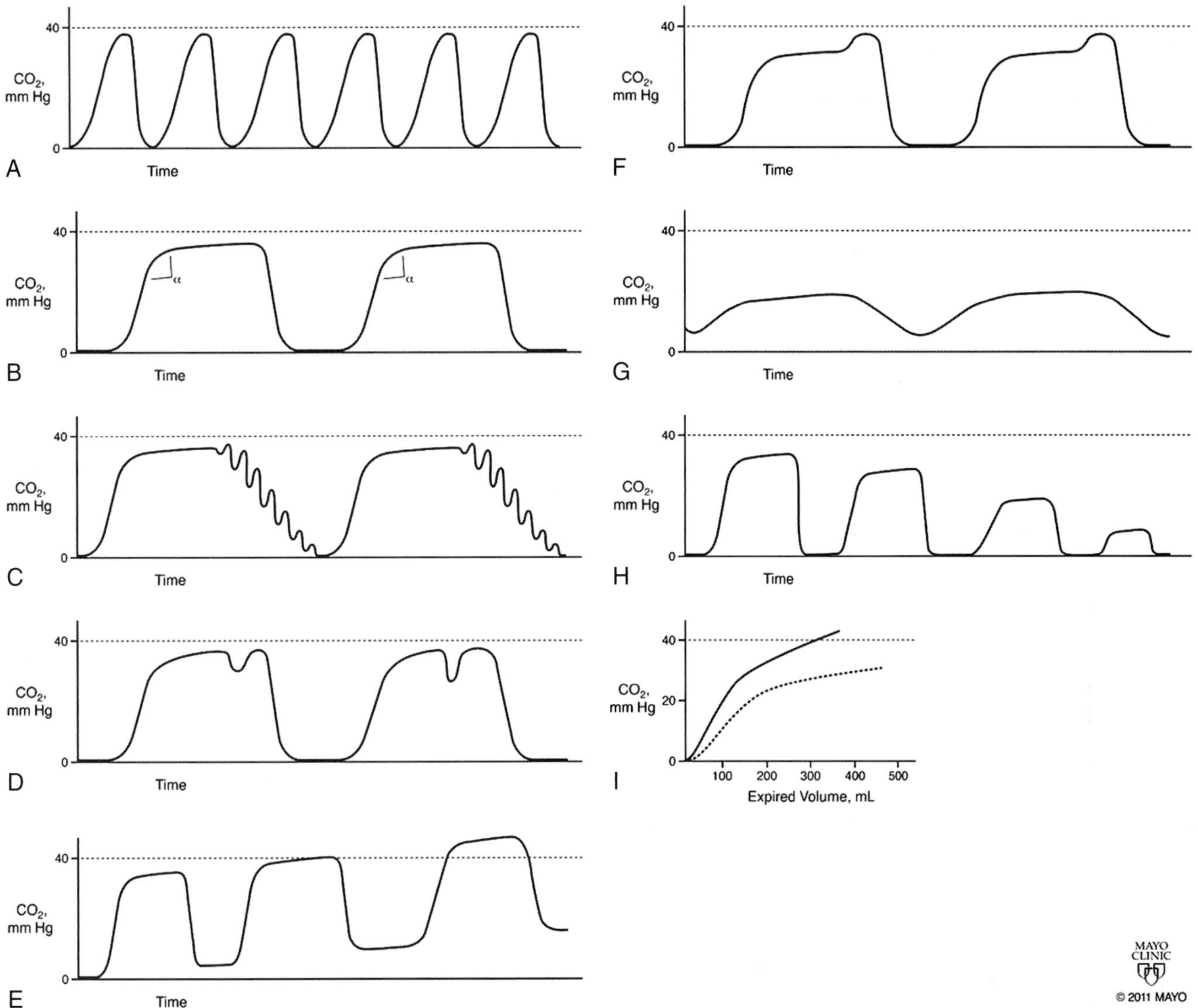

Figure 9-2 Examples of various capnograph waveforms and their interpretation. **A,** Normal spontaneous breathing. **B,** Normal mechanical ventilation. **C.** Cardiogenic oscillations seen during the terminal portion of exhalation. **D,** "Curare" cleft—seen normally in the last part of phase III caused by a lack of synchrony between diaphragm and intercostal muscles in a patient who has received neuromuscular-blocking agents and in whom muscle strength is returning. **E,** Patient rebreathing CO_2 due either to exhausted absorbent or incompetent inspiratory valve. The figure overdramatizes the increase in inspired CO_2 that will occur over time if the underlying problem is not corrected. **F,** Dual-plateau waveform because of a break in the sample line—early during exhalation, room air is entrained, lowering the CO_2; toward the end of exhalation, as pressure in the tubing increases, less air is entrained—hence, a second "tail." **G,** Patient with severe obstructive lung disease (forced expiratory volume at 1 second 20% or less of predicted. **H,** Obstruction in the sampling line as less air is withdrawn. **I,** Shift right (*dotted line*) to left (*solid line*) as would occur in a patient with obstructive lung disease whose disease worsened (e.g., bronchospasm in a patient with chronic obstructive pulmonary disease).

Suggested Readings

Bhende MS, LaCovey DC. End-tidal carbon dioxide monitoring in the prehospital setting. *Prehosp Emerg Care*. 2001;5:208-213.

Dorsch JA, Dorsch SE. Gas monitoring. In: Dorsch JA, Dorsch SE. *Understanding Anesthesia Equipment*. 5th ed. Philadelphia: Lippincott, Williams & Wilkins; 2007:685–727.

Kodali BS. Capnography: A comprehensive educational web site. Available at: www.capnography.com. Accessed on: May 28, 2011.

Nagler J, Krauss B. Capnography: A valuable tool for airway management. *Emerg Med Clin North Am*. 2008;26:881-897.

Thompson JE, Jaffe MB. Capnographic waveforms in the mechanically ventilated patient. *Respir Care*. 2005;50:100-109.

CHAPTER 10
Tracheal Tubes

Molly Solorzano, MD

Magill first developed a tracheal tube in response to the need to deliver anesthetic gases to patients in the United Kingdom who incurred facial injuries in World War I. The original tubes, subsequently manufactured and sold by Portex, were cut from a roll of red rubber tubing, resulting in a natural curve. Because these devices were not cuffed, swabs of cotton were placed at the side of the tube once the tube was in place in the patient's trachea.

Contemporary tracheal tubes have circular walls, which help prevent kinking. The proximal portion (the machine end) attaches through a standardized connector to the anesthetic circuit. The distal portion (the patient end) typically includes a slanted portion, called the bevel, and a Murphy eye (Figure 10-1), which provides an alternative conduit for gas flow should the tip of the tube obstruct if pressed against the carina or wall of the trachea. Tracheal tubes also commonly have a radiopaque marker that runs the length of the tube and can be used radiographically to determine tube position within the trachea.

Most adults are intubated with cuffed tubes, whereas the practice of using cuffed versus uncuffed tubes varies in children (Figure 10-2). The cuff acts as a seal between the tube and the trachea, the purpose of which is threefold: to prevent aspiration of pharyngeal, gastric, or foreign objects into the trachea; to prevent gas leak; and to center the tube in the trachea. If the tracheal tube includes a cuff, it will also have an inflation valve, a pilot balloon, and an inflation tube at the proximal end. Several different cuff systems are in use (Table 10-1).

Because a variety of factors may lead to changes in cuff pressure, some authorities recommend that cuff pressures be measured at end expiration in operations that last longer than 4 to 6 hours (Box 10-1). Pressure measurements can be obtained by connecting the inflation tube to a manometer or to the pressure channel of a monitor by using an air-filled transducer. Using the "feel" of the pilot balloon as a measurement of intracuff pressure has not been shown to be reliable. Pressures should be maintained between 25 and 34 cm H_2O (18-25 mm Hg) in normotensive adults. N_2O can diffuse into the cuff, leading to increased intracuff volume and pressure if the cuff is filled with air. When N_2O use is discontinued, the intracuff pressure decreases rapidly; therefore, if the tracheal tube is to be left in postoperatively, the cuff should be deflated and reinflated with air to prevent a leak.

Tracheal tubes contribute to airway resistance and increase the work of breathing. The internal diameter (ID) correlates with the tube size and is the main determinant of the resistance to flow. The length of the tube also contributes to resistance. The smaller and longer the tracheal tube, the greater the resistance. There is no dedicated method for determining the appropriate tube size for a given patient. A 7.0-mm ID tube is adequate for most women and an 8.0-mm ID tube is appropriate for most men. Age is the most reliable indicator of tube size for children. A tracheal tube should be inserted until the cuff is 2.25 to 2.5 cm past the vocal cords. Typically, this correlates with an insertion distance of 23 cm at the incisors for a man and 21 cm for a woman.

Tracheal tubes have many desirable features, such as providing a secure protected airway; decreasing pollution in the operating room by inhibiting escape of anesthetic gases; and allowing for accurate monitoring of end-tidal gases, tidal volume, and pulmonary compliance. However, their use is

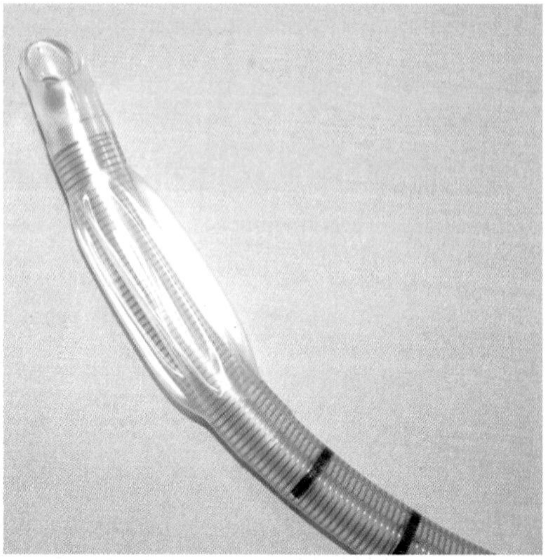

Figure 10-1 A wire-spiral or reinforced tube has a metal or nylon spiral-wound reinforcing wire incorporated into the wall of the lumen.

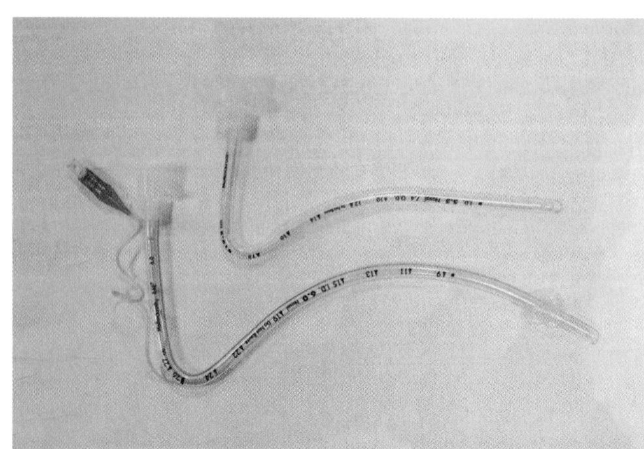

Figure 10-2 Preformed tubes are commonly used during oral surgery and for operations involving the head and neck.

Table 10-1 Characteristics of Various Types of Airway Cuffs

Type of Cuff	Description	Advantages	Disadvantages
Low-volume, high-pressure	Standard cuffed tracheal tube	Provides better protection against aspiration Use is associated with a lower incidence of sore throat	Can lead to ischemia of the tracheal wall
High-volume, low-pressure	Standard cuffed tracheal tube Thin and compliant and does not stretch the tracheal wall	Better for prolonged use owing to a decreased ischemic risk	May be more difficult to insert Can tear during intubation Is more easily dislodged Its use may be associated with an increased incidence of postoperative sore throat May not as effectively protect the lower airway from aspiration
Foam cuff *	—	Less likely to cause mucosal ischemia with resultant ulceration and cartilage damage	—
Lanz cuff *	Controlled-pressure device with a latex reservoir balloon	—	—

*Alternative systems that do not require cuff pressure measurements.

Box 10-1 Factors That May Lead to Changes in Cuff Pressure

↑ Pressure	↓ Pressure
Hypothermic cardiopulmonary bypass	Pressure from nearby surgical procedures Increased altitude Change in head position Diffusion of O_2 into the cuff Coughing, straining, and changes in muscle tone The use of certain topical anesthetic agents

associated with a variety of complications (Box 10-2). Trauma from multiple attempts to intubate the trachea, excessive force, or a stylet through the Murphy eye can cause hematomas, lacerations, vocal cord avulsions and fractures, and even tracheal perforations. Obstruction from kinking, external compression, displacement, change in the patient's body position, material in the lumen, or the patient biting the tube can occur.

A variety of tracheal tubes are marketed. Typically, tracheal tubes are made of polyvinylchloride or silicone or, less commonly, red rubber. They can be cuffed, uncuffed, nasal, oral, reinforced (wire, see Figure 10-1), preformed (see Figure 10-2), laser-resistant (Figure 10-3), flexed (to aid with difficult intubations), reusable, disposable, and single-lumen or multilumen. Tracheal tubes with electrodes imbedded in their outer wall are being marketed for intraoperative monitoring of the recurrent laryngeal nerves during thyroid or parathyroid operations (Figure 10-4).

Reinforced tubes, also known as wire spirals, usually have a metal-wound or nylon-wound spiral reinforcing wire incorporated into the wall of the lumen, which makes them relatively resistant to bending, compression, and kinking and, therefore, well suited for use in tracheal operations (see Figure 10-1). However, these tubes may be difficult to pass nasally without a stylet or orally through an intubating laryngeal mask airway (LMA). Perhaps most disadvantageous is that a patient may bite through the tube.

Box 10-2 Complications That May Occur with the Placement of Tracheal Tubes

- Airway edema
- Emergence phenomena (coughing, bucking, tachycardia, etc.)
- Hoarseness
- Infection
- Macroglossia
- Nerve injuries
- Postoperative sore throat
- Tracheal stenosis
- Ulcerations
- Vocal cord dysfunction

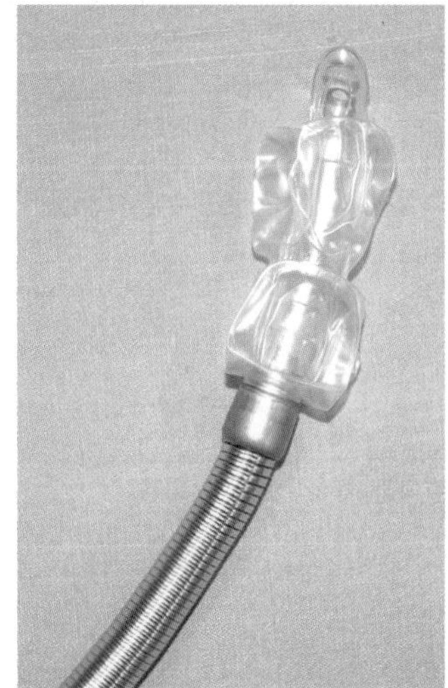

Figure 10-3 A metal laser-resistant tube with a double cuff at the tip. Laser-resistant tubes can be made of malleable metal and have two cuffs at their tip. Each cuff is typically filled with 1 to 3 mL of saline, with the more proximal or cephalad tube sometimes containing blue dye, though many surgeons prefer that no dye be added. Surgeons know if they perforate the proximal cuff with the laser beam because they will see the saline well up in the trachea. If the saline contains dye, the dye stains tissue, making continued surgical excision difficult. If the proximal cuff is compromised, the distal cuff will continue to secure the airway. Because metal tubes reflect the laser beam, many companies have developed tubes made of either noncombustible material or polyvinylchloride wrapped in noncombustible material that will not reflect the laser beam.

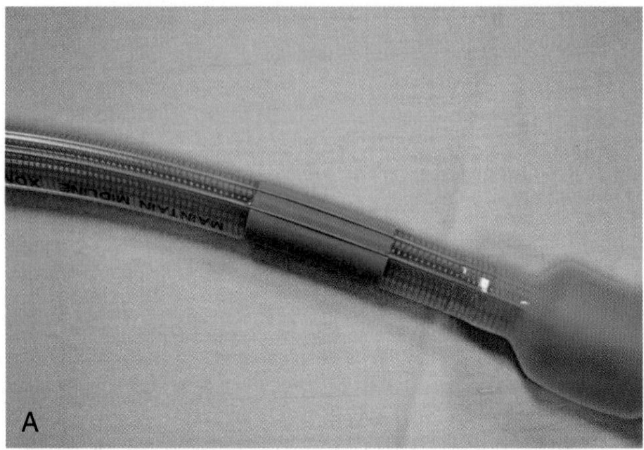

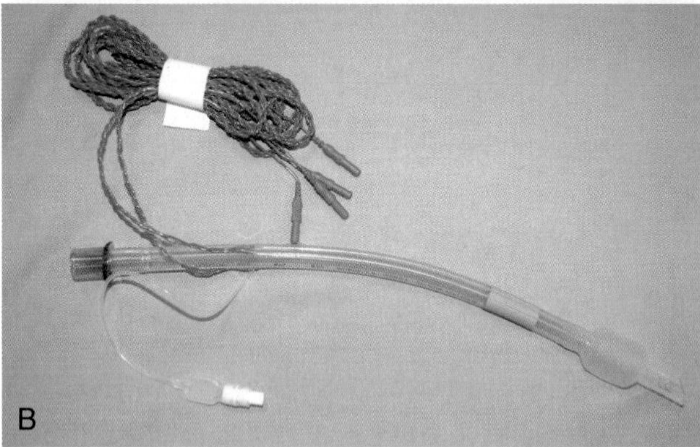

Figure 10-4 Intraoperative monitoring of the recurrent laryngeal nerve or vagus nerve during thyroid and parathyroid operations is possible with the use of a tracheal tube with two electrodes embedded in its side. The blue portion of the tracheal tube is placed between the vocal cords (**A**), and the electrodes are connected to an appropriate monitoring system (**B**).

Preformed tubes, also known as Ring-Adair-Elwin (RAE) tubes, are useful during oral surgery and for head and neck operations (see Figure 10-2). They have a preformed bend that directs the tube away from the surgical field. An oral RAE tube rests on the patient's chin and is directed toward the chest. A nasal RAE is longer and directs the proximal end of the tube toward the patient's forehead.

Laser-resistant tubes (see Figure 10-3) were designed to be nonflammable for use during operations in which a laser is used; however, airway fires may still occur if the laser power is great enough or if the duration of application of the laser is too long. Different laser-resistant tubes vary in their compatibility with various laser types; compatibility should always be checked prior to use. The most common lasers are CO_2, potassium titanyl phosphate (KTP), neodymium:yttrium-aluminum-garnet (Nd:YAG), and argon. Cuffs are not laser resistant and, therefore, should be filled with water or saline. Some tubes have two cuffs so that if one cuff is damaged, the other can be inflated to provide a seal and prevent a leak.

Multilumen tubes are used for gas sampling, suctioning, airway pressure monitoring, fluid and drug injection, jet ventilation, and lung isolation. The double-lumen tube (DLT) is commonly used for lung isolation and can be right- or left-sided (Figure 10-5). The tracheal lumen is placed above the carina, and the bronchial lumen is angled to fit into either the right or left mainstem bronchus. DLTs are sized according to the external diameter of the tracheal segment. The margin of safety is greater for a left-sided tube, and therefore, it is often the tube of choice even for left-lung operations. A right-sided DLT is necessary in specific circumstances (Box 10-3). The tracheal cuff should be inflated in the same manner in which a regular tracheal tube is inflated. The bronchial cuff should be inflated incrementally until a seal is achieved. Volumes in the bronchial cuff should be less than 3 mL. Complications associated with the use of the DLT include difficulty with insertion and positioning, hypoxemia, obstructed ventilation, trauma, poor seal, and cuff rupture.

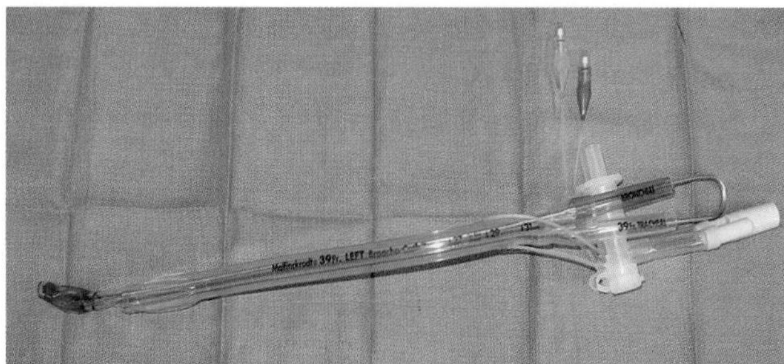

Figure 10-5 Left-sided double-lumen tracheal tube. The bronchial tube and its pilot balloon are color-coded blue; the tracheal tube and its pilot balloon are made of clear polyvinylchloride.

Supraglottic Airways

The most commonly used supraglottic airway, the LMA, is less invasive than a tracheal tube and creates a hands-free seal. The LMA is a curved tube (shaft) that is connected to an elliptical spoon-shaped mask (cup). The two flexible bars where the tube attaches to the mask prevent obstruction by the epiglottis (Figure 10-6). The LMA also comes with an inflatable cuff, inflation tube, and self-sealing pilot balloon. When placed correctly, the mask

Box 10-3 Indications for the Use of a Right-Sided Double-Lumen Tube

- When manipulation or intubation of the left main bronchus is contraindicated
- When the left main bronchus is narrowed or positioned too cephalad
- If a left main bronchus stent is present
- If there is left tracheobronchial disruption

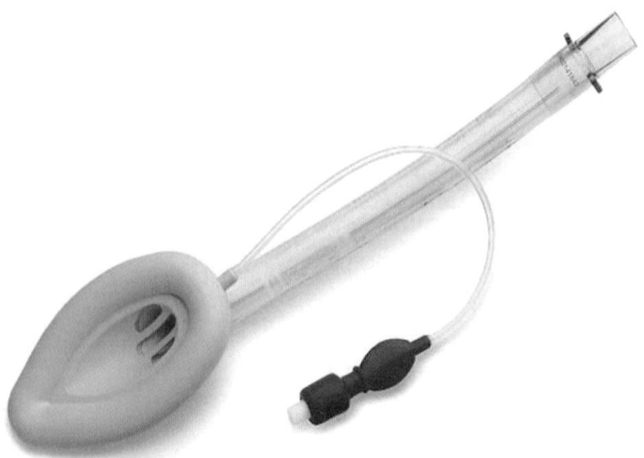

Figure 10-6 A laryngeal mask airway has a curved shaft connected to an elliptical cup with a pilot balloon and inflatable cuff. The two bars at the orifice of the shaft (or tube) that connects to the cup (or mask) prevent obstruction of the mask by the epiglottis.

Box 10-4 Contraindications to the Use of Laryngeal Mask Airways

- Increased aspiration risk
- Bleeding disorder
- Cervical trauma or disease
- Hiatal hernia
- Laparoscopic surgery
- Restricted airway access
- Supraglottic trauma or disease
- Tracheomalacia
- Unusual oropharyngeal axis

should rest on the hypopharyngeal floor, the sides should face the piriform fossae, and the upper portion of the cuff should sit behind the tongue base. Although weight-based formulas can be used for sizing, a man or larger adult will typically require a size 5, and a woman or smaller adult, a size 4. For pediatric sizing, matching the widest part of the mask to the width of the second to fourth fingers works well.

The cuff on an LMA should be inflated to a pressure of 40 cm H_2O, and pressures can be monitored periodically. CO_2 and N_2O can diffuse into the cuff, leading to increased intracuff pressures. The leak pressure should be greater than 20 cm H_2O if using positive pressure or greater than 10 cm H_2O with spontaneous ventilation. The LMA can be used with mechanical ventilation, but the peak inspiratory pressure should not exceed 20 cm H_2O to prevent leak, gastric distention, and pollution in the operating room.

The LMA can be useful for a patient in whom mask ventilation is difficult; the use of an LMA is included in the American Society of Anesthesiologists' algorithm to facilitate tracheal intubation for management of the patient with a difficult airway. LMAs are typically easy to insert and use, are cost effective, and provide for a smooth awakening. However, they do not protect against aspiration, can lead to gastric distention, can cause airway trauma, and have relative contraindications to their use; therefore, their use is contraindicated in specific situations (Box 10-4).

Facemasks

Facemasks can be made of black rubber, clear plastic, elastomeric material, or a combination thereof. They include a body, seal, and connector (Figure 10-7) and can be used to ventilate with positive pressure and to administer inhaled anesthetic gases. Advantages include a decreased incidence of postoperative sore throat, cost effectiveness, and decreased anesthetic requirement. Facemask anesthesia, however, is demanding of the anesthesia provider, requires higher fresh-gas flows, leads to increased pollution in the operating room, causes more O_2 desaturation, increases the work of breathing, and can cause pressure necrosis, dermatitis, nerve injury, jaw pain, and increased movement of the cervical spine.

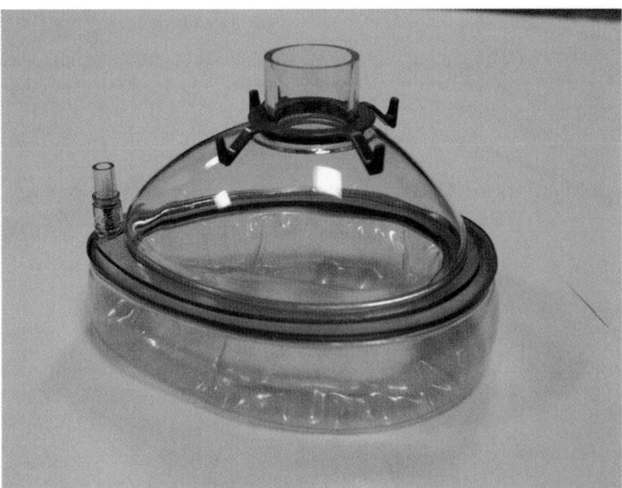

Figure 10-7 Facemasks include a body, seal, and connector and can be used to ventilate with positive pressure and to administer inhaled anesthetic gases.

Pharyngeal Airways

Pharyngeal airways are typically made of plastic or elastomeric material (Figure 10-8) and help prevent obstruction of the laryngeal space by the tongue or epiglottis without the anesthesia provider having to manipulate the patient's cervical spine. They can also reduce the work of breathing, as compared with a facemask. Oropharyngeal airways (Figure 10-8, *A*) are made up of a flange, bite portion, and air channel and are useful for maintaining an open airway, preventing biting, facilitating suctioning, and providing a pathway for inserting devices, such as a fiberscope or endoscope,

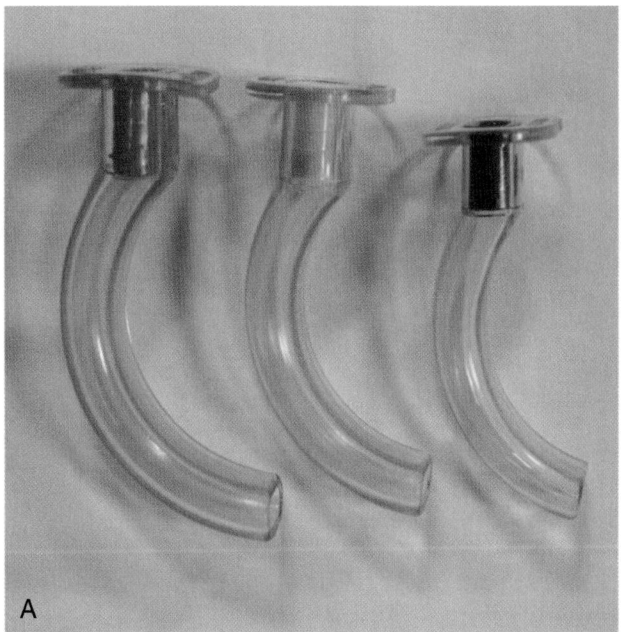

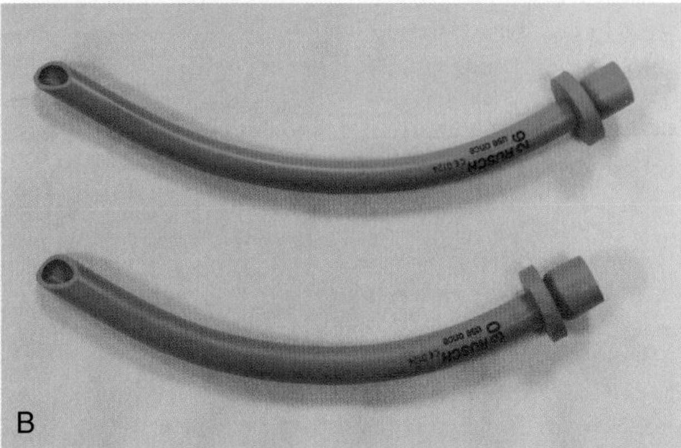

Figure 10-8 Pharyngeal airways. **A,** Oropharyngeal airways are available in different sizes and are frequently color-coded for rapid identification of an appropriate-sized airway. **B,** Nasopharyngeal airways also come in various sizes. They also can be color-coded, but more commonly, the clinician inserting the device will size the nasopharyngeal airway, choosing one that extends from the tip of the patient's nose to the lobe of the ear, and will then lubricate and insert the device.

into the pharynx. Oropharyngeal airways can stimulate pharyngeal and laryngeal reflexes, leading to coughing or laryngospasm. Nasopharyngeal airways (Figure 10-8, *B*) are better tolerated in a patient with intact airway reflexes and can be used for many of the same purposes as the oral airway. In addition, they can be used to administer continuous positive airway pressure, treat hiccoughs, and dilate the nasal passages for nasotracheal intubation. The use of a nasopharyngeal airway should be avoided when the patient is anticoagulated or has a basilar skull fracture, nasal deformity, nasal infection, or history of nosebleeds requiring treatment. A vasoconstrictor can be applied topically to the patient's nasopharynx before the airway is inserted to decrease the risk of bleeding and to facilitate passage—vasoconstriction decreases mucosal thickness, enlarging the nasal passageway.

Suggested Readings

Chee WK. Orotracheal intubation with a nasal Ring-Adair-Elwyn tube provides an unobstructed view in otolaryngologic procedures. *Anesthesiology*. 1995; 83:1369.

Dimitriou VK, Zogogiannis ID, Douma AK, et al. Comparison of standard polyvinyl chloride tracheal tubes and straight reinforced tracheal tubes for tracheal intubation through different sizes of the Airtraq laryngoscope in anesthetized and paralyzed patients: A randomized prospective study. *Anesthesiology*. 2009;111:1265-1270.

El-Orbany M, Woehlck HJ. Difficult mask ventilation. *Anesth Analg*. 2009; 109:1870-1880.

Hameed AA, Mohamed H, Al-Mansoori M. Acquired tracheoesophageal fistula due to high intracuff pressure. *Ann Thorac Med*. 2008;3:23-25.

Hooshangi H, Wong DT. Brief review: The Cobra Perilaryngeal Airway (CobraPLA and the Streamlined Liner of Pharyngeal Airway (SLIPA) supraglottic airways. *Can J Anaesth*. 2008;55:177-185.

Morris LG, Zoumalan RA, Roccaforte JD, Amin MR. Monitoring tracheal tube cuff pressures in the intensive care unit: A comparison of digital palpation and manometry. *Ann Otol Rhinol Laryngol*. 2007;116:639-642.

Rinder CS. Fire safety in the operating room. *Curr Opin Anaesthesiol*. 2008;21: 790-795.

Weiss M, Dullenkopf A, Fischer JE, et al. European Paediatric Endotracheal Intubation Study Group. Prospective randomized controlled multi-centre trial of cuffed or uncuffed endotracheal tubes in small children. *Br J Anaesth*. 2009; 103:867-873.

Williams DL, Wong SM, Pemberton EJ, et al. A randomised, single-blind, controlled trial of silicone disposable laryngeal masks during anaesthesia in spontaneously breathing adult patients. *Anaesth Intensive Care*. 2009;37: 992-997.

CHAPTER 11
Complications of Tracheal Intubation

Scott A. Eskuri, MD

Standards for tracheal tube (TT) design, testing, and manufacturing were established decades ago by the American National Standards Institute and the American Society for Testing and Materials. Polyvinyl chloride is currently the most commonly used TT material because of its ability to soften at body temperature, which decreases pressure on laryngotracheal mucosa; however, this device is still a poor substitute for the human larynx. Complications of TT intubation can be divided into those that occur during intubation, those that occur while the TT is in place, and those that occur after extubation.

Complications That Occur During Intubation

Eye and Facial Soft Tissue Injury

Contusions or lacerations of the upper and lower lip can occur secondary to trauma from the laryngoscope blade or TT. Trauma to the hard and soft palate has been reported when anesthesia providers use a video laryngoscope and watch the video monitor without directly observing the passage of the blade into the hypopharynx. Corneal abrasions may also occur when an instrument (e.g., wristwatch) or the arm or sleeve of the anesthesia provider who is performing the intubation brushes the patient's eye.

Tooth Trauma

Dental injuries are the most common reasons for anesthesia-related malpractice claims (30%-40%). The incidence of perioperative dental injury ranges from 1 in 150 to 1 in 1500, with 75% of injuries occurring during intubation (25% with emergence). Care must be taken to recover all pieces of a broken tooth to prevent aspiration. If an entire tooth is dislodged, it should be promptly reimplanted, and dental consultation should be obtained.

Cervical Spine Injury

Patients with trauma, osteogenesis imperfecta, severe osteoporosis, rheumatoid arthritis, Down syndrome, Morquio's syndrome, or lytic bone lesions are at increased risk of experiencing a cervical spine and spinal cord injury during intubation, a time during which the anesthesia provider manipulates the patient's jaw and head, often leading to considerable movement of the cervical spine.

Laryngeal and Pharyngeal Trauma

Minor trauma—including lacerations, vocal cord injury with subsequent paralysis, subluxation of the arytenoids, and vocal cord hematoma—occurs in up to 6% of intubations. Long-term sequelae are unusual.

Stimulation of Airway Reflexes

Stimulation of pharyngeal or laryngeal mucosa results in laryngovagal-mediated reflexes, such as laryngospasm, bronchospasm, bradycardia, and arrhythmias. Sympathetic activation can cause hypertension and tachycardia.

In addition, tactile stimulation can cause cough, straining, or vomiting, which, in turn, can increase intraocular and intracranial pressure. Aspiration can occur before the trachea is intubated.

Esophageal Intubation

Unrecognized esophageal intubation is the most disastrous complication associated with intubation. Many methods are used to assess correct position; however, the "gold standard" is to confirm the presence of expired CO_2.

Bronchial Intubation

Bronchial intubation may be difficult to detect, but monitoring of flow-volume loops, as is possible on newer anesthesia machines, allows the anesthesia provider to more readily recognize this complication. The sequelae of bronchial intubation may be minor if the patient's underlying pulmonary function is good. A simple rule of thumb that results in correct positioning in nearly 100% of adults is to place the tube 23 cm from the teeth in men and 21 cm in women. In children, the tip should be advanced 2 to 3 cm beyond the cords or the following formula should be used:

Premature: 6 to 7 cm
Full term: 8 to 10 cm
1 year: 11 cm
2 year: 12 cm
Age 3 to 18: 12 + (age/2)

Tracheal or Bronchial Rupture

The risk factors that are associated with the anesthesia provider causing a tracheal or bronchial rupture include stylets protruding from the end of the TT, the use of excessive force during intubation, and multiple attempts at intubation. Chest drainage and open surgical repair may be required to treat a tracheal or bronchial rupture.

Complications That Occur with the Tracheal Tube in Place

Excessive Leak or Resistance

The selection of a properly sized tube is necessary in adults and critically important in children. In children older than 1 year, tube diameter can be determined by the following formula:

$$\text{TT size, in mm} = 4 + (\text{age, in years}/4)$$

Obstruction

TT obstruction is caused by external force (most commonly, the patient biting down), internal obstruction, or tube abnormalities. Kinking or herniation of the cuff over the tip of the TT can externally obstruct the tube; however, lumen obstruction (with, e.g., secretions, blood, tumor, foreign body) is more common. Clearing with irrigation and suction is indicated, and replacing the TT may be necessary.

Migration

Head flexion and extension can advance and withdraw (respectively) the TT by 2 cm to 5 cm from full flexion to full extension. This movement can lead to bronchial intubation or tracheal extubation. (When long-term intubation is anticipated, a chest radiograph should be obtained to verify that the tip of the TT is 3 to 6 cm above the carina.)

Mucosal Ulceration or Necrosis

Mucosal ulceration can occur anteriorly on the trachea where the tip of the TT lies. Necrosis can be induced if mucosal blood flow is impeded (cuff pressures >25 mm Hg).

Ignition

The TT can ignite during operations in which a laser is employed.

Dehydration/Hypothermia

Dehydration or hypothermia may occur with the use of nonhumidified, nonwarmed gas-delivery systems. Dehydration causes thickened secretions and decreased ciliary function, increasing the risk of the patient developing postoperative pulmonary complications.

Nasal Alar Necrosis

Nasal alar necrosis can occur in patients who have had a nasotracheal tube in place for an extended period of time.

Sinusitis

The incidence of clinically significant sinusitis is 2% to 20% in patients who are nasotracheally intubated for more than 5 days.

Miscellaneous

Airway reflexes, unintentional extubation, tracheal perforation (with subsequent tracheal esophageal fistula), aspiration, and nasal or oral excoriation may occur.

Complications That Occur Immediately After Extubation

Supraglottic, Glottic, or Subglottic Edema

Edema is the most significant complication in the early postextubation period, especially in pediatric patients; however, adults with an allergic response to lubricant or plastic may develop stridor. In pediatric patients, the strongest predictor of postextubation stridor is the absence of an air leak if 30 cm H_2O pressure is applied to the TT. The use of intravenously administered steroids, racemic epinephrine nebulizers, or a combination thereof has been advocated, but proof of their efficacy is not conclusive.

Laryngeal Dysfunction

Immediately after extubation, patients frequently have difficulty protecting their airway. Risk factors associated with laryngeal injury include prolonged intubation, traumatic intubation, and large TT size (>8 mm in men and >7 mm in women). The incidence of aspiration is highest after prolonged intubation; the risk declines with time after extubation.

Sore Throat

A high prevalence of sore throat has been reported (up to 90%). Risk factors for postextubation sore throat or hoarseness include large TT size, female sex, and use of lubricant.

Vocal Cord Paralysis

Vocal cord paralysis may be secondary to surgical trauma of the vagus or recurrent laryngeal nerve. However, it has also been postulated that pressure from the TT cuff could compress the recurrent laryngeal nerve against the thyroid lamina.

Miscellaneous

Laryngospasm, bronchospasm, acute sialadenopathy ("surgical mumps"), sore jaw, dysphonia, and tracheal collapse may occur.

Delayed Complications

Mucosal Lesions

In patients intubated for more than 1 week, up to 67% have been reported to have vocal cord ulcerations. Most lesions resolve within 8 weeks. Laryngeal ulcers may develop as quickly as 6 hours after intubation occurs, but most heal without sequelae. Laryngeal granulomas and polyps occur in 1 in 150 to 1 in 250 cases of prolonged intubation and usually require surgical excision.

Laryngeal or Tracheal Stenosis

The risk of laryngeal or tracheal stenosis is lowered by the use of a TT with a high-volume, low-pressure cuff. If laryngeal or tracheal stenosis does occur, surgical correction is usually required.

Cricoid Abscess

Cricoid abscess is an extremely rare complication that develops in the retrocricoid region after mucosal injury from the TT and secondary bacterial infection.

Vocal Cord Paralysis

The cause of vocal cord paralysis is unknown. However, direct trauma or pressure or a local reaction to an ethylene-oxide sterilized TT may contribute to the occurrence of this complication.

Suggested Readings

Liu J, Zhang X, Gong W, et al. Correlations between controlled endotracheal tube cuff pressure and postprocedural complications: A multicenter study. *Anesth Analg*. 2010;111:1133-1137.

McCulloch TM, Bishop MJ. Complications of translaryngeal intubation. *Clin Chest Med*. 1991;12:507-521.

Gaudio RM, Feltracco P, Barbieri S, et al. Traumatic dental injuries during anaesthesia: Part I: Clinical evaluation. *Dent Traumatol*. 2010;26:459-465.

Santos PM, Afrassiabi A, Weymuller EA Jr. Risk factors associated with prolonged intubation and laryngeal injury. *Otolaryngol Head Neck Surg*. 1994;111:453.

Scuderi PE. Postoperative sore throat: More answers than questions. *Anesth Analg*. 2010;111:831-832.

Sitzwohl C, Langheinrich A, Schober A, et al. Endobronchial intubation detected by insertion depth of endotracheal tube, bilateral auscultation, or observation of chest movements: Randomised trial. *BMJ*. 2010;341:c5943.

CHAPTER 12
Disconnect Monitors

Glenn E. Woodworth, MD

A review of studies looking at closed-claims databases indicates that the percentage of total claims related to the gas-delivery system has been steadily decreasing over the past few decades—from 3% in the 1970s to 2% in the 1980s, and representing only 1% of total claims in the 1990s. In the most recent closed claims update on patient injuries from anesthesia gas delivery equipment from 2000 through 2011, there were no claims for breathing circuit disconnects. In addition, the morbidity rate from these claims appears to be decreasing as well. However, major anesthesia-related morbidity and mortality risk is still often related to problems with the patient's airway and ventilation, including problems with the breathing circuit and, in particular, disconnections of the circuit. Therefore, anesthesia providers must be ever vigilant to prevent and detect breathing-circuit problems. One closed-claims analysis indicated that 78% of breathing-circuit problems were deemed preventable by appropriate monitoring.

One of the most common critical incidents with gas-delivery systems is disconnection of the breathing circuit during mechanical ventilation—the most common disconnection sites are between the breathing circuit and the tracheal tube connection and between the breathing circuit and the heat-moisture exchanger, if one is used. Of note, cost-containment measures often advocate reusing breathing-circuit components; however, sterilization procedures may degrade conical plastic fittings, making them more likely to disconnect.

Risk-reduction measures have focused on three general areas: (1) secure locking of mated components (several devices are available; however, their use increases cost, may inhibit quick disconnection if an emergency disconnection is warranted, and may be undesirable if their use leads to an increased risk of an accidental extubation or barotrauma), (2) education, and (3) the use of disconnect monitors and alarms for detection of disconnects.

Disconnects cannot be completely prevented; therefore, monitoring for such an event is essential. Disconnect alarms can be classified into four categories (Box 12-1).

Low Airway Pressure Alarms

The American Society of Anesthesiologists and the American Association of Nurse Anesthetists recommend that patients being mechanically ventilated have a monitor in the expiratory line of their breathing circuit that is activated if the airway pressure falls below a set value. Called a low-pressure (or disconnect) alarm, the device triggers if the maximum inspiratory pressure does not exceed a set threshold within a predetermined time (usually 15 seconds). This aspect of the pressure monitor is not enabled during spontaneous respiration.

Certain conditions can cause a disconnection, yet can fail to trigger the low-pressure monitor. One potential circumstance that is especially likely is a disconnection of the tracheal tube itself from the 15-mm connector

Box 12-1 Types of Disconnect Alarms

Pressure monitors
Respiratory volume monitors
CO_2 monitors
Miscellaneous monitors

(a site of high resistance). A similar situation occurs if the disconnection is partially obstructed and generates a resistance, for example, if the circuit is disconnected at the Y-piece and is obstructed by bed sheets. The high resistance in these situations creates upstream pressure that may fall above the alarm threshold.

Factors that influence pressure-alarm effectiveness include the disconnection site, pressure-sensor site, threshold alarm limits, inspiratory flow rate, and resistance within the disconnected circuit. Once the ventilator has been activated, the airway pressures should be verified to be within expected limits. The low-pressure alarm should be activated (most modern ventilators activate the low-pressure monitor when the ventilator is turned on and deactivate the monitor when the ventilator is turned off, whereas the high-pressure alarm is always on).

Most modern ventilators set the low-pressure threshold to a factory default or to the last setting entered by the user. It is absolutely essential that the low-threshold pressure and high-pressure alarm be set approximately 5 cm of H_2O below and 5 cm of H_2O above the peak inspiratory pressure, respectively. If the low-pressure alarm threshold is set too low, the alarm may fail to detect a disconnection. Finally, the anesthesia provider must make sure that the audible alarm can be heard over ambient room noise.

In addition to disconnections of the breathing circuit, a low-pressure alarm may signify other problems in the breathing circuit or anesthesia machine that can lead to problems with ventilation (e.g., subatmospheric, high, or continuing pressure conditions). The optimal location of the pressure monitor is at the Y-piece; however, condensation of water vapor may interfere with the monitor, and many systems place the sensor just proximal to the inspiratory valve to minimize moisture within the sensing line and to provide ready access.

Respiratory Volume Monitors

The respiratory volume monitor is normally located in the expiratory limb of the breathing circuit. Its function is to measure the exhaled tidal volume, respiratory rate, minute volume, and flow direction. Several different types of volume meters are available. Many include electronic analysis and alarms under conditions of low rate, low volume, or reverse flow and provide a graphic display of flow and volumes during the respiratory cycle. These monitors are useful during spontaneous respiration as well as mechanical ventilation.

Like pressure alarms, volume alarms can fail to signal during a disconnect. Failure to signal is most likely to occur when using a ventilator with bellows that descend during exhalation (e.g., descending or hanging bellows). During expiration, in the presence of a disconnect, descent of the bellows due to gravity may entrain room air and generate a flow within the circuit. A false-negative alarm may also occur even if the breathing circuit is totally obstructed. The compliance of the breathing circuit and compression of gas during an inspiratory cycle may yield an "exhaled volume" that can exceed alarm limits. In addition, during spontaneous respiration, a disconnect on the machine side of either directional valve will go undetected, depending on the location of the volume meter. A frequent criticism of these monitors is that flow in the expiratory limb does not guarantee gas exchange.

CO_2 Monitors

CO_2 monitors not only allow titration of ventilation, but also can serve as disconnect monitors. CO_2 is monitored by mass spectrometry, infrared absorption, or Raman scattering. A change in CO_2 concentration or absence of CO_2 in the exhaled gas can implicate various ventilatory problems, including a disconnect. The CO_2 monitor is probably the best monitor for evaluating the adequacy of ventilation. Capnography is discussed in Chapter 9.

Miscellaneous Monitors

The esophageal stethoscope, with which breath sounds should be monitored continuously, is an excellent monitor for detecting disconnects. A disconnect can be picked up immediately. Observation of chest wall excursion may also be helpful.

Ascending bellows will often fail to refill completely when there is a disconnect because they utilize expired gas to help refill the bellows (this would usually trigger the low-pressure or volume alarm because ensuing breaths with an inadequately filled bellows would not deliver a complete tidal volume).

Pulse oximeters offer a late warning of disconnections that lead to hypoxemia. Blood pressure and heart rate changes may indicate a disconnection. Hypoxemia typically produces increases in heart rate and blood pressure as hypoxemia sets in. When the hypoxemia becomes severe, the initial "pressor response" is followed by bradycardia and hypotension. Occasionally, an oxygen analyzer will detect oxygen concentrations within the breathing circuit that are lower than expected in the presence of a disconnect.

In summary, alarm monitors with properly set threshold limits should be enabled and functioning. Many experts would testify that it is essential to do this. Finally, even with all of the currently available monitors in use, under certain circumstances, a disconnect or partial disconnect may be missed.

Suggested Readings

Adams AP. Breathing system disconnections. *Br J Anaesth.* 1994;73:46-54.

Caplan RA, Vistica MF, Posner KL, et al. Adverse anesthesia outcomes arising from gas delivery equipment: A closed claims analysis. *Anesthesiology.* 1997; 87:741-748.

Dorsch JA, Dorsch SE, eds. *Understanding Anesthesia Equipment.* Philadelphia: Lippincott, Williams & Wilkins; 2008:410,704-705,731-744.

Eichorn JH. Risk management. In: Benumoff JL, Saidman LJ, eds. *Anesthesia and Perioperative Complications.* St. Louis: Mosby; 1992:648.

Eisenkraft J. Hazards of anesthesia gas delivery systems. *Can J Anesth.* 2004;51:R7.

Metha SP, Eisenkraft JB, Posner KL, Domino KB. Patient injuries from anesthesia gas delivery equipment: A closed claims update. *Anesthesiology.* 2013; 119:788–785.

CHAPTER 13

Closed-Circuit Anesthesia

Allen B. Shoham, MD

Closed-circuit anesthesia refers to a technique in which, during the delivery of an inhalation anesthetic agent using an anesthesia work station (machine) with a circle system, the adjustable pressure relief valve is closed and the fresh gas inflow is adjusted such that it is just sufficient to match the amount of inhaled anesthetic gas and O_2 that is taken up by the patient and the amount of gas removed by any side-stream monitors (for measurement of anesthetic gas concentration, CO_2, and O_2) (Box 13-1). To prevent hypercapnia, a CO_2 absorber must be used; all exhaled gases except CO_2 are rebreathed when this technique is used. One must ensure that the circuit is free of any leaks (more than 20 potential sites exist for gases to leak from the circuit/system) (Box 13-2).

Whereas, during administration of most inhalation anesthetics, one monitors only the fractional inspired O_2 concentration (FIO_2), when using a closed-circuit anesthetic technique, one should monitor both the FIO_2 and the expired oxygen concentration (FEO_2). Normally, the FEO_2 is not significantly different from the FIO_2; however, during closed-circuit anesthesia, the FEO_2 may be significantly less if the amount of O_2 delivered in the fresh-gas inflow is inadequate to meet the patient's O_2 consumption. Oxygen consumption determines the amount of O_2 one must deliver through the fresh-gas inflow. Anesthetic uptake, on the other hand, is proportional to blood/gas solubility and the alveolar-venous inhalation anesthetic concentration gradient and cardiac output.

During the use of a closed-circuit anesthetic, it is important that flowmeters and vaporizers have been calibrated to be accurate at low flows and varying circuit pressures. It may be difficult to deliver the required amount of inhalation anesthetic using this technique with certain vaporizers that are inaccurate at low flow rates (see Box 13-2). If this is the case, one can inject the inhalation anesthetic directly into the expiratory limb of the circle system, but this is rarely done.

Some major obstacles must be overcome if anesthesia is induced using a closed-circuit anesthesia system (see Box 13-2). Before tissue uptake of the anesthetic can occur, an adequate amount of the inhalation anesthetic must be in the breathing circuit, the patient's alveoli, and the arterial circulation. During conventional inhalation anesthetic induction, uptake of the inhalation anesthetic agent is greatest during the initial phases of induction; uptake decreases as venous concentration approaches alveolar concentration of the inhalation anesthetic. During induction with a closed-circuit anesthetic, it is difficult to denitrogenate the patient; the N_2 that the patient exhales dilutes the breathing circuit, thereby slowing induction and increasing the risk for awareness and, possibly, resulting in delivery of a hypoxic gas mixture.

During closed-circuit anesthesia, O_2 is the preferred carrier gas because its uptake is relatively constant. The administration of N_2O makes induction more complicated because its uptake follows a power function and requires constant titration during induction and further increases the risk of delivery of a hypoxic gas mixture. To avoid these difficulties, most clinicians use high flows on induction to denitrogenate the breathing circuit and the patient's functional residual capacity and to establish adequate anesthetic concentrations prior to switching to a closed system (Figure 13-1).

Box 13-1 Advantages of Closed-Circuit Anesthesia

- Allows for economic use of inhalation and medical gases
- Minimizes anesthetic gas contamination of operating room and atmosphere
- Maintains airway temperature and humidity
- Allows continuous monitoring of O_2 consumption, which may signal early symptoms of malignant hyperthermia, inadequate depth of anesthesia, or decreased O_2 consumption, indicating circulatory depression
- Provides less danger of barotraumas, as elevated pressures take longer to develop with very low flows

Box 13-2 Disadvantages of Closed-Circuit Anesthesia

- Depends on operator vigilance and safety devices; failure in any of these may result in delivery of a hypoxic gas mixture or inadequate inhalation anesthetic gas mixture.
- Has many potential sites for gas leaks, including the tracheal tube cuff; any leaks or negative pressure applied to the circuit may entrain room air, thereby decreasing O_2 concentration.
- May increase risk for awareness when inhalation anesthetic gas concentrations decrease during intermittent high-flow flushing or dilution of gases in the circuit.
- N_2O, carbon monoxide, compound A, acetone, ethanol, methane, and acrylic monomer accumulate when using surgically cemented joint prostheses.
- Inability to quickly titrate inspired inhalation anesthetic concentration.
- CO_2 absorbent will be consumed more quickly, creating an exothermic reaction, significantly elevating the temperature of inspired gases as well as a hypercarbic inspired gas mixture when absorbent is saturated.

Maintenance of Anesthesia

If N_2O is used as one of the carrier gases for the maintenance of anesthesia using a closed-circuit system, one must be particularly vigilant in monitoring O_2 concentration. As N_2O uptake by the patient decreases, alveolar N_2O concentration increases, thereby displacing O_2 with a subsequent decrease in O_2 concentration within the alveolus; therefore, constant titration of O_2 and N_2O inflow is essential. Once the inhalation anesthetic gas concentration is at a steady state, the requirement for additional inhalation anesthetic decreases, remaining relatively constant.

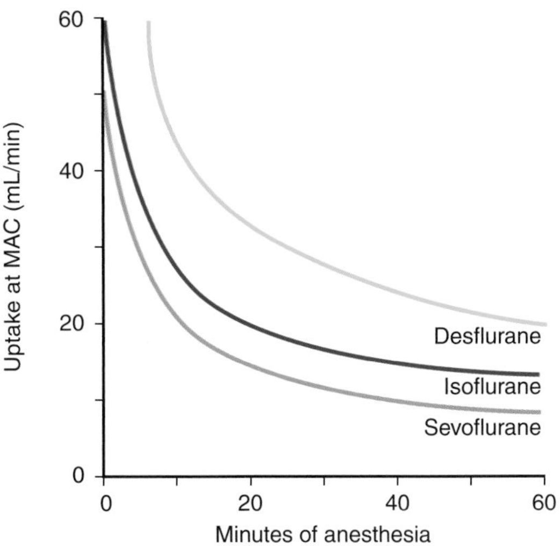

Figure 13-1 Uptake of inhalation anesthetic is dependent on alveolar-venous gradient, solubility, and cardiac output. The vessel-rich group equilibrates after approximately 5 minutes and uptake slows. After approximately 10 minutes, uptake slows further as the reservoir within the muscle groups equilibrates. Therefore, many practitioners induce anesthesia with high gas flows for approximately 5 to 10 minutes before switching to a closed circuit. MAC, Minimum alveolar concentration. (Modified, with permission, from Yasuda IV, Lockhart SH, Eger EI 2nd, et al. Kinetics of desflurane, isoflurane, and halothane in humans. Anesthesiology. 1991;74:489-498.)

Each milliliter of liquid inhalation anesthetic (isoflurane, sevoflurane, desflurane) produces approximately 200 mL of vapor (±10%). Closed-circuit anesthesia can be maintained with a vaporizer or by intermittent injections of inhalation anesthetic at appropriate time intervals.

During the maintenance phase, a constant circuit volume must be maintained by (1) adjusting flows to maintain a constant reservoir-bag size; (2) with ascending bellows, adjusting the flow to be just below the top of the housing of the bellows at end exhalation; and (3) with descending bellows, adjusting the fresh-gas flow to allow the bellows to just reach the bottom of its housing at end exhalation. It is crucial that there are no gas leaks in the circuit or a negative pressure transmitted to the bellows at any time, as this may entrain room air and decrease O_2 and the concentration of inhalation anesthetic gas.

Nitrogen accumulates in the breathing circuit over time; therefore, the system should be flushed for a few minutes every hour to denitrogenate the system and prevent production of a hypoxic gas mixture. Accumulation of carbon monoxide, compound A, methane, ethanol, and acetone are other reasons for flushing the system. The clinical consequences of these compounds are unknown; however, they have been proposed to cause an increased incidence of postoperative nausea and vomiting. The clinical significance of compound A is still controversial; therefore, it is not recommended to use sevoflurane in closed-circuit anesthesia.

Emergence from Anesthesia

Emergence is prolonged when using closed-circuit anesthesia, even with the newer low-solubility inhalation anesthetics. Therefore, most clinicians increase fresh-gas flow at the end of the procedure so that the patient will emerge more quickly from anesthesia. Since the inhalation anesthetic is discontinued at the end of the procedure, nothing is gained by continuing low flows for emergence.

Suggested Readings

Dorsch JA, Dorsch SE, eds. *Understanding Anesthesia Equipment*. 5th ed. Philadelphia: Lippincott Williams & Wilkins; 2008.

Morgan GE, Mikhail MS, Murray MJ. *Clinical Anesthesiology*. 4th ed. New York: McGraw-Hill Medical Publishing Division; 2006:174-178.

Schober P, Loer SA. Closed system anaesthesia—Historical aspects and recent developments. *Eur J Anaesthesiol*. 2006;23:914-920.

SECTION III Monitoring

CHAPTER 14

Pulse Oximetry

Klaus D. Torp, MD

Technology

Oximetry involves the measurement of oxyhemoglobin (HbO_2) concentration based on the Lambert-Beer law. Fractional oximetry, which measures arterial O_2 saturation (SaO_2), is defined as HbO_2 divided by total hemoglobin (Hb). Total Hb is calculated as the sum of HbO_2, reduced or deoxyhemoglobin (HHb), methemoglobin (metHB), and carboxyhemoglobin (COHb). In contrast, functional oximetry, which measures O_2 saturation using pulse oximetry (SpO_2), is defined as HbO_2 divided by the sum of HbO_2 and HHb. In clinical practice, SpO_2 is measured using a pulse oximeter to estimate SaO_2.

$$SaO_2 = HbO_2/(HbO_2 + HHb + metHb + COHb)$$

$$SpO_2 = (HbO_2/HbO_2 + HHb)$$

HHb absorbs more light in the red band (600 to 750 nm) than does HbO_2, whereas HbO_2 absorbs more light in the infrared band (850 to 1000 nm) than does HHb. The conventional pulse oximeter probe contains two light-emitting diodes (LEDs) that emit light at specific wavelengths: one in the red band and one in the infrared band. Typical wavelengths are 660 nm and 940 nm. When the probe is placed on the patient, the light emitted from the LEDs is transmitted or reflected (depending on the site of the sensor) through the intervening blood and tissue and is detected by sensors built into the probe. The amount of transmitted light is sensed several hundred times per second to allow precise estimation of the peak and trough of each pulse waveform. At the pressure trough—during diastole—light is absorbed by the intervening arterial, capillary, and venous blood, as well as by the intervening tissue. At the pressure peak—during systole—additional light is absorbed in both the red and infrared bands by an additional quantity of purely arterial blood, the pulse volume. The typical pulse amplitude accounts for 1% to 5% of the total signal. Pulse oximeters isolate the pulsatile components from the blood volume signal (photoplethysmogram) and calculate the red over infrared red ratio, which is then used to calculate SpO_2 by using an algorithm, based on a nomogram, built into the software of the pulse oximeter. Isolation and measurement of the pulsatile component allows individuals to act as their own controls and, thus, eliminates potential problems with interindividual differences in baseline light absorbance. The "calibration curve" used to calculate SpO_2 was derived from studies of healthy volunteers.

The process to identify the pulse, which is initiated with application of the probe to the subject, includes sequential trials of various intensities of light to find those strong enough to transmit through the tissue without overloading the sensors.

Accuracy

Pulse oximeters have generally been found to be accurate to within 5% of in vitro oximeters, in the range of 70% to 100%. The most widely used "gold standard" for comparison is the IL282 co-oximeter. Sensors are calibrated to the site of application (digit, ear, forehead, etc.). Applying them to a different site may give false SpO_2 readings even when showing an acceptable plethysmographic waveform. In discussing the accuracy of pulse oximeters, the terms *bias* and *precision* are used. Bias is the mean value of SaO_2 minus SpO_2. Precision is the standard deviation of the bias.

There are two potential problems with the accuracy of pulse oximetry below values of 70%. First, as stated previously, pulse oximeters have been calibrated using studies of healthy volunteers (an Olympic athlete, in one case). Therefore, it is unlikely that much data have been collected for calibration at low saturation levels. Second, the absorption spectrum of HHb is maximally steep at 600 nm. Therefore, any slight variance in the light emitted from the 660-nm LED has significant potential to introduce measurement error into the system. Because decreasing levels of SpO_2 lead to an increasing proportion of HHb, there is the potential for increasing inaccuracy as SpO_2 decreases. These potential problems are unlikely to be of much clinical significance. For example, it is unlikely that a treatment decision would be based on whether an SpO_2 is 50% versus 60% at a given time. Some studies have reported poor accuracy of pulse oximeters at SpO_2 values of less than 70%.

Response Time

Most pulse oximeters average pulse data over 5 to 8 seconds before displaying a value. Some oximeters allow for an override of this lag by providing for a shortened averaging interval or allowing a beat-by-beat display. Response time is also related to probe location and perfusion. Desaturation response times range from 7.2 to 19.8 seconds for ear probes, from 19.5 to 35.1 seconds for finger probes, and from 41.0 to 72.6 seconds for toe probes.

Low-Amplitude States

Pulse oximeters depend on a pulsatile waveform to calculate SpO_2. Therefore, under conditions of low or absent pulse amplitude, the pulse oximeter may not accurately reflect SaO_2 or may not provide a reading at all (e.g., during cardiac arrest, proximal blood pressure cuff inflation, tourniquet application, hypovolemia, hypothermia, vasoconstriction, or cardiac bypass). In addition, pulse oximeters are more sensitive to movement artifact during low-pulse–amplitude states.

The earlobe and forehead appear to be areas that are least sensitive to a decreased pulse. If the SpO_2 decreases without an obvious physiologic cause (e.g., asystole) and changing the site of the sensor does not produce the desired result, changing to a different brand of pulse oximeter, with a different signal-processing algorithm, may provide a reading. There has been some question of the accuracy of pulse oximeter readings in the face of an arrhythmia in which not all electrocardiographic complexes produce a sufficient stroke volume, creating a pulse deficit. However, a relationship between pulse deficit and bias has not been identified.

Dyshemoglobins

Conventional pulse oximeters use only two wavelengths of light; therefore, conventional pulse oximeters can accurately measure only HbO_2 and HHb. The presence of a third or fourth species of hemoglobin (e.g., metHb or COHb) can interfere with accurate measurement by causing changes in the absorbance of light in the critical red and infrared regions.

The COHb is interpreted by the pulse oximeter as a mixture of approximately 90% HbO_2 and 10% HHb. Thus, at high levels of COHb, the pulse oximeter will overestimate true SaO_2, as may occur in patients with recent CO exposure (e.g., house fire, combustion engine exhaust, or cigarette smoking).

metHb is formed when the heme iron is oxidized from the ferrous (Fe^{2+}) to the ferric (Fe^{3+}) state. metHb is very dark and tends to absorb equal amounts of red and infrared light, resulting in a red:infrared ratio of 1. When extrapolated on the calibration curve, a ratio of 1 corresponds with a saturation of 85%. Thus, as metHb increases, SpO_2 approaches 85% regardless of the true level of HbO_2. Drugs capable of causing methemoglobinemia (defined as greater than 1% metHb) include nitrates, nitrites, chlorates, nitrobenzenes, antimalarial agents, amyl nitrate, nitroglycerin, sodium nitroprusside, and local anesthetic agents. High levels of metHb create mitochondrial hypoxia caused by the diminished O_2-carrying capacity of blood and a leftward shift in the HbO_2 dissociation curve. Recent advances in pulse oximetry, some of which use more than seven wavelengths (Rainbow SET Technology, Masimo Corp., Irvine, CA) allow approximate measure of levels of COHb and metHb, but these newer pulse oximeters do not correct for COHb and metHb in the SpO_2 readings.

Pulse oximeters underestimate the SaO_2, especially at low saturation values, in patients with anemia; however this finding has little clinical significance because an intervention would likely take place before the SaO_2 would fall to a low level. Some new pulse oximeters have the capability of measuring total hemoglobin either continuously or as a spot check device.

Dyes and Pigments

Injections of methylene blue produce a large and consistent spurious decrease in SpO_2, with readings remaining below baseline for 1 to 2 minutes. Injection of indocyanine green decreases SpO_2 to approximately 80% to 90%, which lasts for a minute or less. Injection of indigo carmine decreases the SpO_2 the least, with the decrease lasting approximately 30 seconds.

Elevated serum bilirubin concentrations, per se, do not affect the accuracy of the pulse oximeter.

Ambient Light

Inaccurate SpO_2 readings have been reported to occur because of interference by the light of surgical lamps, fluorescent lights, infrared-light–emitting devices, and fiberoptic light sources.

Skin Pigment

Obtaining an accurate pulse oximetry reading may not be possible in deeply pigmented individuals because of a failure of LED light transmission.

Electrocautery

Electrocautery results in decreased SpO_2 readings caused by interference from the wide-spectrum radiofrequency emissions, which affect the pulse oximeter probe. Interference is usually of little clinical significance unless electrocautery is used for a lengthy time in patients who have decreased or unstable O_2 saturation. Some manufacturers have attenuated this problem by improving the electrical shielding of sensors and cables.

Motion Artifact

Repetitive and persistent motion artifact of any kind tends to cause the SpO_2 to display the local venous SaO_2 level. The susceptibility to motion artifacts may also depend on the signal-processing algorithm of the pulse oximeter brand.

Fingernail Polish

The presence of fingernail polish may cause a low of SpO_2 value, although this effect is not constant and may be related to the number of layers and the color of the polish. Acrylic nails usually have no significant effect, but depending on the color may also result in a lower SpO_2 reading. Placing the sensor sideways on the finger may produce a reading, but the preferred action would be to remove the nail polish or choose another site.

Other Useful Data

While some pulse oximeters measure COHb and met Hb, In addition to measuring SpO_2, COHb, and metHb, most pulse oximeters also provide plethysmography, which can provide useful information regarding the patient's volume status by assessing the respiratory variation, where the plethysmographic amplitude changes during the respiratory cycle. Plethysmographic waveforms however are highly processed and filtered so that a visual estimate of the extent of the respiratory variation of the pulse amplitude may not be correct. However some devices now provide a numeric index of that variability, which correlates with change in intravascular volume status and fluid responsiveness in hypotensive patients during positive pressure ventilation. Some pulse oximeters also provide measurements of perfusion in a digit, which can be used to assess a change in sympathetic tone during general and regional anesthesia.

Complications of Pulse Oximetry

Complications are very rare and generally minor, including mild skin erosions and blistering, tanning of the skin with prolonged continuous use, and ischemic skin necrosis.

Suggested Readings

Ginosar Y, Weiniger CF, Meroz Y, et al. Pulse oximeter perfusion index as an early indicator of sympathectomy after epidural anesthesia. *Acta Anaesthesiol Scand.* 2009; 53:1018-1026.

Cannesson M, Desebbe O, Rosamel P, et al. Pleth variability index to monitor the respiratory variations in the pulse oximeter plethysmographic waveform amplitude and predict fluid responsiveness in the operating theatre. *Br J Anaesth.* 2008;101:200-206.

Mannheimer PD. The light-tissue interaction of pulse oximetry. *Anesth Analg.* 2007;105: S10-S17.

CHAPTER 15

The Pulmonary Artery Catheter

Avishai Ziser, MD

The pulmonary artery catheter (PAC), an invasive monitor of cardiac function, provides not only cardiac but also respiratory information. Hemodynamic and respiratory parameters, which can be calculated from PAC-derived data, are combined with an assessment of the patient's clinical status, with resultant therapy based on the interpretation of this combined information. PACs can be placed with ease, are simple to use, and allow for continuous or intermittent data monitoring. In addition, atrial and right ventricular (RV) wires can be placed through the PAC to enable cardiac pacing. Although the PAC provides substantial and unique hemodynamic information, it is unclear if its use is associated with improved patient outcome.

Indications for the Use of Pulmonary Artery Catheter

PACs may be inserted in patients undergoing high-risk surgical procedures and in patients who are critically ill and in the intensive care unit. Patient comorbid conditions, elective versus emergency operations, and local practice settings should all be considered before placing a PAC. Many cardiac anesthesiologists place a PAC in patients undergoing cardiac operations or ascending aorta and aortic arch procedures, in patients with poor left ventricular (LV) or RV function who are undergoing any open heart or major noncardiac procedure, and for patients undergoing redo cardiac operations. The most recent comprehensive list of indications can be found in the 2003 American Society of Anesthesiologists practice guidelines on PAC.

Insertion and Complications of Pulmonary Artery Catheter

The PAC can be inserted from any central or femoral vein, with the pressure waveform recorded from the distal pulmonary artery port guiding the clinician in advancing and placing the catheter. The highest success rate is typically achieved using the right internal jugular vein approach. Ultrasound guidance is strongly recommended. Fluoroscopy is rarely required for placement, and few centers require a chest radiograph before the PAC is used clinically. Complications may occur during catheter insertion or while the catheter is in place long term (Box 15-1).

Box 15-1 Potential Complications with the Use of a Pulmonary Artery Catheter

During Insertion

Arrhythmias
Arterial puncture
Balloon rupture
Catheter knotting
Conduction block
Hematoma
Hemorrhage
Hemothorax
Pneumothorax
Pulmonary artery rupture
Venous air embolism

After Insertion, Long Term

Infection
Pulmonary embolism
Pulmonary infarction
Valve injury

Data and Interpretation

Central venous pressure, pulmonary artery pressure, pulmonary artery occlusion pressure (PAOP), cardiac output (CO), mixed venous oxygen saturation ($S\bar{v}O_2$), and RV ejection fraction can all be measured with a PAC. In addition, several hemodynamic and oxygenation parameters can be calculated based on the PAC data. To avoid misinterpretation of the data, it is critical that the pressure transducers be leveled with the right atrium and calibrated. Mechanical ventilation, positive end-expiratory pressure, catheter location, artifacts, and cardiac diseases may affect the results of the various measurements. Incorrect measurements and misinterpretation of data can be minimized by implementation of an education program targeting physicians, nurses, and therapists.

The Cardiac Output

RV output can be measured using thermodilution. If no intracardiac shunts are present, the RV output reflects the LV output, or the CO. The CO provides a global evaluation of cardiovascular function. To obtain the CO measurement, a 10-mL bolus of saline (either iced or at room temperature) is injected via the proximal port of the PAC. The change in blood temperature is detected by a thermistor, located 4 cm proximal to the PAC tip. The temperature change is recorded, and the data are integrated to calculate the CO (modified Stewart-Hamilton equation). The thermodilution CO technique has become the gold standard for measuring CO.

To obtain an accurate CO measurement, the use of repeated indicator injections is recommended. Usually, three sequential CO measurements, the results of which are within 10% of one another, can be considered to be an accurate CO reading. In a supine patient under general anesthesia, misreadings rarely occur.

Several factors may affect this measurement (Box 15-2) and may, therefore, influence the reliability of the CO value that is measured. A 0.5-mL

Box 15-2 Factors That May Impact Measurements Obtained via a Pulmonary Artery Catheter

Patient-Related Factors

Arrhythmia
Change in position
Deep spontaneous respirations
Movement
Valsalva maneuver

Catheter-Related Factors

Improper tip location
Long injection time (longer than 4 sec)

change in injectate volume will cause a 5% to 10% change in CO results; conversely, a lower volume will result in a higher CO reading. Injectate temperature also affects the reading, with an increase of 1° C in the injectate temperature reading causing a 3% overestimation of the CO.

Right-sided valve regurgitation and intracardiac shunt render the CO measurement unreliable. The value of measuring CO in these conditions is questionable, and the procedure should be used with caution, if at all, when the patient has right-sided valve regurgitation or an intracardiac shunt.

The Pulmonary Artery Occlusion Pressure

Accurate measurement of PAOP mandates that the catheter tip rest in West lung zone 3, where there is a continuous column of blood between the catheter tip and the left atrium and the effect of alveolar pressure is minimal. The pulmonary artery diastolic pressure and PAOP are indexes of LV preload and usually correlate closely with the LV end-diastolic pressure (LVEDP) and volume. However, in many clinical situations (Box 15-3), the pulmonary artery diastolic pressure and the PAOP either underestimate or overestimate the LVEDP.

Box 15-3 Situations in Which the Underestimation or Overestimation of Left Ventricular End-Diastolic Pressure by Pulmonary Artery Diastolic or Occlusion Pressure Occur

Overestimation

Positive end-expiratory pressure
Increased intrathoracic pressure
Pulmonary artery hypertension
Mitral stenosis and regurgitation
Ventricular septal defect
Tachycardia
Tip position outside West lung zone 3
Chronic obstructive pulmonary disease
Left atrial myxoma

Underestimation

Diastolic dysfunction
Aortic stenosis and regurgitation
Pulmonary regurgitation
Right bundle branch block
Postpneumonectomy
Hypertension
Left atrial pressure >25 mm Hg

The Mixed Venous Oxygen Saturation

The $S\bar{v}O_2$ is a global index of the balance of oxygen delivery ($\dot{D}O_2$), consumption ($\dot{V}O_2$), and extraction. It can be obtained by aspirating blood from the distal port of the PAC and subsequently analyzing the gases in this venous blood or by continuous measurement with an oximetric PAC. The normal value of $S\bar{v}O_2$ is 70% to 75%. In the presence of stable arterial oxygen saturation, oxygen consumption, and hemoglobin concentration, the $S\bar{v}O_2$ is a sensitive indicator of change in CO. A change in CO may reflect a hemodynamic change or a compensation for the change in other parameters. A high $S\bar{v}O_2$ reading may be caused by a wedged PAC, low oxygen consumption, cyanide or carbon monoxide toxicity, hypothermia, high CO states (e.g., sepsis, burns, and pancreatitis), left-to-right intracardiac shunts, and the use of inotropic drugs. A low $S\bar{v}O_2$ usually reflects inadequate oxygen delivery and an imbalance between the $\dot{D}O_2$ and the $\dot{V}O_2$. Low CO is the most common cause of a low $S\bar{v}O_2$ reading, but anemia, hypoxemia, and high $\dot{V}O_2$ should also be considered as potential causes.

Right Ventricular Function

Originally, central venous pressure and CO were the main parameters for assessing RV function by the PAC. The measurements of central venous pressure and RV pressure have a limited value in estimating RV preload. Currently, a PAC with faster thermistor response is available to calculate RV ejection fraction, which can also be used to calculate stroke volume, RV end-diastolic volume, and end-systolic volume. The placement of a PAC that can measure RV ejection fraction is indicated primarily in patients with RV failure, pulmonary hypertension, intrinsic lung disease, sepsis, acute respiratory distress syndrome, and heart failure following acute myocardial infarction and in patients who have received a heart transplant whose condition is rapidly deteriorating. No study has demonstrated improved outcome using this type of PAC, or any type of PAC, for that matter.

The Pulmonary Artery Catheter Controversy

For many years, the PAC provided valuable information and was considered to be the gold standard for hemodynamic monitoring and therapy, but a great deal of controversy exists as to whether the use of a PAC improves patient outcome. Several studies and meta-analyses have shown improvement, no change, or worse outcome with the use of a PAC. Experienced clinicians may choose different therapies based on a review of the same clinical data, emphasizing the point that there is no "standard" or "best" practice when it comes to the use of PACs. Several less invasive monitoring instruments that have the capability of measuring CO and calculating hemodynamic parameters are currently on the market. The PAC should be used by experienced clinicians who base their management decision on physiologic and hemodynamic principles, modified to reflect their local practice settings. Selected patient populations may benefit from the use of PACs.

Suggested Readings

American Society of Anesthesiologists Task Force on Pulmonary Artery Catheterization. Practice guidelines for pulmonary artery catheterization: An updated report by the American Society of Anesthesiologists Task Force on Pulmonary Artery Catheterization. *Anesthesiology*. 2003;99:988-1014.

Greenberg SB, Murphy GS, Vender JS. Current use of the pulmonary artery catheter. *Curr Opin Crit Care*. 2009;15:249-253.

Leibowitz AB, Oropello JM. The pulmonary artery catheter in anesthesia practice in 2007: An historical overview with emphasis on the last 6 years. *Semin Cardiothorac Vasc Anesth*. 2007;11:162-176.

Vincent JL, Pinsky MR, Sprung CL, et al. The pulmonary artery catheter: In medio virtus. *Crit Care Med*. 2008;36:3093-3096.

CHAPTER 16
The Arterial Waveform

Avishai Ziser, MD

The use of arterial catheters is classically indicated for continuous hemodynamic monitoring and for obtaining blood for laboratory determinations in critically ill patients and those undergoing major operations. The beat-to-beat visual arterial pressure wave and numerical pressure display enable prompt identification of trends or changes in blood pressure that could potentially be missed with noninvasive blood pressure monitoring. The systolic pressure variation (SPV), the pulse pressure variation (PPV), and the stroke volume variation (SVV) based on the arterial waveform may provide an indication of the patient's volume status and prediction of fluid responsiveness. Accurate measurement of cardiac output (CO) can be performed based on the arterial waveform. Several monitoring instruments apply this technology at the patient's bedside.

Equipment and Cannulation

The arterial catheter is placed in a peripheral artery or the femoral artery, with the radial artery being the most commonly used cannulation site. Arterial spasm and thrombosis, local infection and hematoma, distal ischemia, hemorrhage, and air embolism are the main complications. A 20G cannula is appropriate for the cannulation of a small artery, and an 18G for a larger one. Aseptic technique should always be applied. The arterial cannula is connected to a pressure transducer via high-pressure tubing. The pressure transducer should usually be located at the level of the right atrium, or at the level of the external auditory meatus for the sitting patient who is undergoing a neurosurgical procedure. Air should be thoroughly evacuated from the entire system. Zeroing to atmospheric pressure is done before first use and as needed afterward. The continuous flash device is connected to a bag of normal saline under a pressure of 300 mm Hg that brings a continuous flash of 1 to 3 mL/h to prevent clot formation at the tip of the arterial cannula. Heparin (1-2 μ/mL or 10-20 μgr/mL) can be added to the flush solution, but this is not mandatory, and the risk of heparin-induced thrombocytopenia should be kept in mind.

Waveform Interpretation

The arterial waveform provides valuable and continuous hemodynamic information. It changes as the measuring catheter is located more distally from the heart. The pulse pressure increases, and the dicrotic notch is delayed and then disappears. The systolic pressure is higher in a peripheral artery, compared with the ascending aorta, but the mean pressure is minimally affected or slightly reduced. The heart rate and rhythm can be determined from the arterial tracing. The effect of ectopic beats on arterial pressure and waveform can be evaluated. The pulse pressure may help to evaluate the patient's hemodynamic status. High pulse pressure can be seen after exercise and in patients with hyperthyroidism, aortic insufficiency, peripheral vasodilatation, arteriovenous malformation, increased stiffness of the aorta (most common in older patients), and mild hypovolemia. Narrow pulse pressure can be seen in patients with hypovolemia, pericardial tamponade, congestive heart failure, aortic stenosis, and shock states. The area under the arterial curve, from the onset of systole to the dicrotic notch, can estimate the stroke volume (SV), and the systolic rise may reflect myocardial contractility. However, the arterial curve changes as the location of the arterial cannula insertion moves distally from the ascending aorta.

Dynamic Indexes of Fluid Responsiveness

The SPV and PPV derived from the arterial waveform during a mechanical breath (Figure 16-1) are more pronounced during hypovolemia because the left ventricle operates on the steep portion of the Frank-Starling curve. Changes in right and left ventricular preload, which are highly sensitive to changes in intrathoracic pressure induced by a mechanical breath, cause the variation in the left ventricular SV. Observing the various components of SPV and PPV can establish the presence and cause of hypovolemia, with dynamic changes in the arterial waveform predicting the response to fluid challenge. SPV, PPV, and SVV (measured by pulse contour analysis) are currently the most accurate indicators for fluid responsiveness in patients in the intensive care unit and in many surgical patients. Given that only 50% of patients in the intensive care unit respond to fluid loading, this measurement may provide valuable data for determining which patients should be first treated with fluids and which may benefit from inotropic support as the first intervention to increase CO. Although simply viewing the arterial waveform on the arterial pressure tracing can provide information about the presence of respiratory variation, an accurate electronic measurement can quantify the pressure variation and its components, allowing the effect of fluid loading to be continually assessed.

Measurements of SPV, SVV, and PPV are currently limited to the sedated mechanically ventilated patient who is in normal sinus rhythm. Spontaneous breathing, frequent arrhythmia, high positive end-expiratory pressure, high airway pressure, high and low tidal volumes, low chest wall compliance, increased intra-abdominal pressure, and the use of vasodilators may all cause inaccurate representations of the dynamic indexes on tracings from arterial catheters.

Many studies have demonstrated the superiority of the dynamic indexes—as compared with the static indexes (central venous pressure, pulmonary capillary occlusion pressure, left ventricular end-diastolic area, and global end-diastolic volume)—in predicting patient response to fluid loading. The dynamic indexes of fluid responsiveness should be evaluated as a component of the entire clinical scenario related to a given patient. They should not be used as a single "best" index for clinical decisions but, rather, should be used in the context of the other clinical parameters.

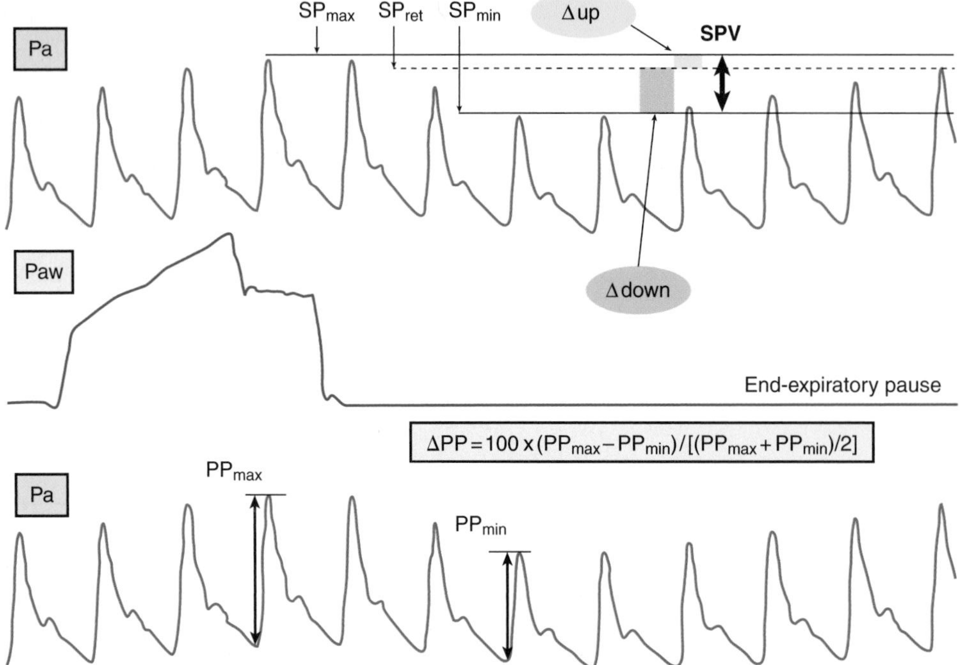

Figure 16-1 Analytical description of respiratory changes in arterial pressure during mechanical ventilation. The systolic pressure and pulse pressure (systolic – diastolic pressure) are maximum (SP_{max} and PP_{max}, respectively) a few heartbeats later (i.e., during the expiratory period). The systolic pressure variation (SPV) is the difference between SP_{max} and SP_{min}). The assessment of a reference systolic pressure (SP_{ref}) during an end-expiratory pause allows the discrimination between the inspiratory increase (Δup) and the expiratory decrease (Δdown) in systolic pressure. Pa, Arterial pressure; Paw, airway pressure; PP, pulse pressure. (Adapted from Michard F. Changes in arterial pressure during mechanical ventilation. Anesthesiology 2005;103:419-428.)

Cardiac Output Derived from the Arterial Pressure Waveform

Arterial pressure waveform analysis is now used in clinical practice with several commercially available devices that can be used to continuously measure CO, based on the arterial pressure waveform. These devices provide a CO value derived from pulse-contour measurements that correlates well with the value derived from the pulmonary artery catheter thermodilution technique (a bias of 0.03-0.3 L/min), but, under various clinical conditions and therapies, this correlation might be disrupted. Compared with the thermodilution technique, these devices are less invasive and their use is associated with potentially fewer complications. Examples of commercially available devices include the PiCCO (Pulsion Medical Systems, Munich, Germany) and LiDCO (LiDCO, Ltd, Cambridge, UK), and the EV1000 Clinical Platform (Edwards Lifesciences, Irvine, CA) which require an invasive calibration and recalibration, and the FloTrac/Vigileo (Edwards Lifesciences) device, which uses individual demographic data to estimate arterial compliance and, therefore, does not require invasive calibration. These devices use pulse-contour analysis with various algorithms to estimate SV from the arterial waveform. The SV is calculated by a mathematical computation of the area under the systolic portion of the arterial pressure waveform. The algorithm incorporates parameters such as aortic impedance, arterial compliance, and peripheral vascular resistance. These devices can also calculate other hemodynamic variables (e.g., static preload parameters, peripheral resistance, oxygen delivery, and the dynamic indexes of fluid responsiveness [see earlier]). The hemodynamic profile is continuously displayed, with the option to follow trends and changes during patient care (Figure 16-2).

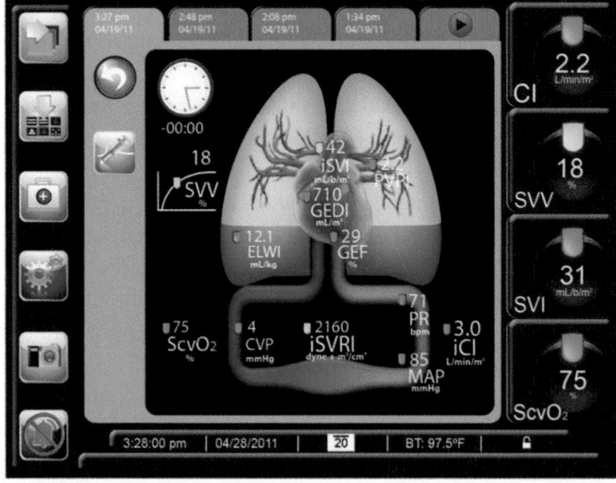

Figure 16-2 EV1000 Clinical Platform. Several and continuous hemodynamic parameters. (Courtesy Edwards Lifesciences Corporation, Irvine, CA.)

Suggested Readings

Bendjelid K, Marx G, Kiefer N, et al. Performance of a new pulse contour method for continuous cardiac output monitoring: Validation in critically ill patients. *Br J Anaesth*. 2013;111(4):573–579.

Cannesson M, de Backer D, Hofer CK. Using arterial pressure waveform analysis for the assessment of fluid responsiveness. *Expert Rev Med Devices*. 2011;8:635-646.

Chew MS, Aneman A. Haemodynamic monitoring using arterial waveform analysis. *Curr Opin Crit Care*. 2013;19:234-241.

Funk DJ, Moretti EW, Gan TJ. Minimally invasive cardiac output monitoring in the perioperative setting. *Anesth Analg*. 2009;108:887-807.

Marik PE, Cavallazzi R, Vasu T, Hirani A. Dynamic changes in arterial waveform derived variables and fluid responsiveness in mechanically ventilated patients: A systemic review of the literature. *Crit Care Med*. 2009;37:1-6.

Mathews L, Singh KRK. Cardiac output monitoring. *Ann Card Anaesth*. 2008;11:56-68.

Michard F. Changes in arterial pressure during mechanical ventilation. *Anesthesiology*. 2005;103:419-428.

Su BC, Tsai YF, Chen CY, et al. Cardiac output derived from arterial pressure waveform analysis in patients undergoing liver transplantation: Validity of a third-generation device. *Transplant Proc*. 2012;44:424-428.

CHAPTER 17

Intermittent Noninvasive Blood Pressure Monitoring

Clint Grant Humpherys, MD, and Michael J. Murray, MD, PhD

Obtaining frequent blood pressure (BP) measurements is an essential component to delivering a safe anesthetic. The American Society of Anesthesiologists (ASA) Standards for Basic Anesthetic Monitoring states that "every patient receiving anesthesia shall have arterial blood pressure and heart rate determined and evaluated at least every five minutes." A variety of ways exist by which to noninvasively measure BP, such as palpation, auscultation, Doppler, finger plethysmography with pulse oximetry, tonometry, and oscillometry.

Methods of Obtaining Blood Pressure

Palpation

Systolic BP, but not diastolic BP, can be measured by palpating a peripheral pulse while inflating a BP cuff until flow is occluded and then slowly releasing the cuff pressure until a pulse is palpable. A similar technique can be used by substituting a pulse oximeter for palpation and placing it on one digit of the extremity, noting the pressure at which the Spo_2 measurement returns.

Auscultation

When measuring BP by auscultation, the BP cuff is connected to a sphygmomanometer, the cuff is inflated above the systolic pressure, and the cuff pressure is then gradually released while simultaneously auscultating with a stethoscope in the antecubital fossa for Korotkoff sounds. The first and last audible Korotkoff sounds represent the systolic and diastolic BPs, respectively.

Doppler

When utilizing the Doppler technique to ascertain BP, a small probe that emits ultrasound waves is placed above a peripheral artery. A BP cuff is inflated above systolic pressure and then slowly deflated. When blood begins to flow, it causes the characteristic Doppler shift in the ultrasound wave, which is created by the difference in the transmitted and received frequencies; this shift is recorded as the systolic pressure. Following the now-continuous blood flow in the artery, another shift in frequency occurs; this second shift is recorded as diastole.

Finger Plethysmography

With finger plethysmography, a probe that emits infrared light is placed on the patient's finger. With the probe in place, the cuff pressure is increased to above the systolic BP and the volume of blood in the finger decreases, which is measured as a change in the waveform of the light transmitted across the finger. As the cuff is subsequently deflated and systolic BP is reached, the volume of blood changes again. The subsequent change in wavelength is an indication of systolic BP, until the volume of blood in the finger is stable (i.e., diastolic pressure).

Tonometry

With tonometry, a pressure transducer is applied to the skin above a peripheral artery. The transducer measures the contact stress between the transducer over the artery and the skin, reflecting the intraluminal pressure. Tonometry provides the capability of measuring beat-to-beat arterial BP.

Oscillometry

Oscillometry has become the most common method to measure arterial BP in the operating room.

Equipment for Oscillometric Blood Pressure Monitoring

Intermittent noninvasive BP monitoring with oscillometry requires several pieces of equipment: an inflatable cuff, pressure tubing, a cuff-inflation pump, and a bleed valve. Inflatable cuffs are available in varying sizes and are marked to indicate an appropriate limb circumference for the cuff size. Oscillometric devices have either one or two tubes that permit inflation and deflation of the cuff while simultaneously allowing measurement of the oscillations of the pressure in the cuff secondary to the impact of the pulse pressure in the underlying artery.

The cuff-inflation pump and bleed valve incorporate a sensing mechanism, a timing circuit, a control circuit, and alarms. The sensing mechanism is a pressure transducer containing a piezoelectric crystal that is distorted by the oscillations in the pressure of the cuff; this mechanical energy is converted to a measureable electric current that is amplified and recorded as the systolic, diastolic, and mean arterial pressures by the amplifier in the recording device. The timing circuit determines the frequency of BP measurement to be taken. A manual cycling option is also often available. The control circuit regulates the maximum pressure in the cuff, artifact rejection, deflation rate, and automatic cutoff. All monitors should be capable of triggering alarms when sensing abnormal BP measurements.

Oscillometry Operation and Function

Most intermittent noninvasive BP monitors use oscillometry to measure BP. In most situations, a BP cuff is applied above the patient's elbow of either the left or right upper extremity. The cycle begins with the cuff inflating to a pressure above the measurable arterial systolic BP. The cuff is then deflated slowly in a stepwise or linear manner until oscillations (arterial pressure pulsations) begin to be detected. The oscillations initially increase to a maximum and then decrease to an immeasurable level. After the final oscillation is detected, the cuff quickly bleeds out the remaining air. The point of maximum amplitude of the oscillations corresponds with the mean arterial pressure (Figure 17-1). The device then calculates the systolic and diastolic BP by an empirically derived algorithm; because the algorithms are proprietary, the systolic and diastolic BP measurements may vary from one device to another, depending on the manufacturer's algorithm. In contrast,

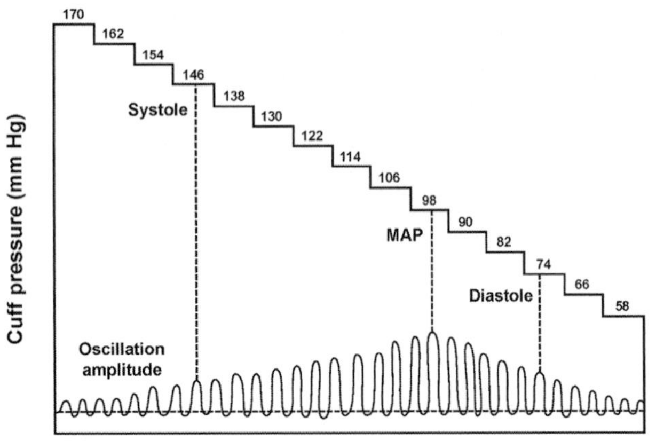

Figure 17-1 An oscillometer measures the oscillations in the pressure within the blood pressure cuff. The point at which the oscillations have a maximum amplitude is the mean arterial pressure (MAP). Once oscillations are barely perceptible, the device releases the air remaining in the cuff and then calculates the systolic and diastolic blood pressure, using an algorithm unique to each manufacturer.

direct arterial BP monitoring via arterial catheter measures both the systolic and diastolic pressures and calculates the mean.

Factors Affecting the Accuracy of Oscillometric Blood Pressure Monitoring

Relationship Between the Size of the Cuff and the Size of the Arm It is recommended that the width of the cuff be 40% to 50% of the arm's circumference (or 125% to 150% of the arm's diameter). The bladder should encircle the arm's circumference by 50% or more. If the upper arm is too large or conically shaped, it may be better to place the cuff at the forearm, ankle, or thigh. Placing the cuff over superficial nerves, bony prominences, or joints should be avoided. A cuff that is too loose or too large may underestimate the BP; conversely, a cuff that is too tight or too small may overestimate the BP.

Site of Monitoring As the cuff moves more peripherally, the systolic pressure increases, whereas the diastolic pressure decreases secondary to changes in the amplitude of the pulse of blood being conducted down the underlying artery. Vascular disease and peripheral vasoconstriction may reduce pressure values at distal locations. As a general rule, venous engorgement has little effect on accuracy.

Arm Positioning The cuff should remain at the level of the patient's heart. If the cuff is placed 10 cm above or below heart level, a correction of 7.4 mm Hg needs to be added or subtracted from the measured BP.

Arrhythmias Oscillometric noninvasive BP monitoring is often inaccurate in patients with arrhythmias. If the patient has a history of an arrhythmia, the provider should consider placing an arterial line catheter for direct BP monitoring.

Potential Adverse Events During Oscillometric Blood Pressure Monitoring

Artifacts from intrinsic and extrinsic motion of the patient and staff, mechanical problems, and equipment failure may occur during oscillometric monitoring and may lead to inaccurate measurement of the patient's BP. Several complications may arise during oscillometric monitoring of BP. Damage to the skin and underlying tissue may occur when the cuff is placed improperly. The patient may also develop neuropathies of the median, ulnar, or radial nerves, or a combination thereof. Compartment syndrome is most likely to develop in patients in whom the use of oscillometric monitoring of BP is prolonged or if the device malfunctions and the malfunction is undetected if the patient's extremity is covered.

Suggested Readings

Committee of Standards and Practice Parameters. *Standards for Basic Anesthetic Monitoring*. San Francisco, CA: American Society of Anesthesiologists House of Delegates; October 21, 1986, Amended October 20, 2010. Effective July 1, 2011.

Dorsch JA, Dorsch SE. In: ed. *Understanding Anesthesia Equipment*. 5th ed. Philadelphia: Lippincott Williams & Wilkins; 2008:837-842.

CHAPTER 18

Depth of Anesthesia

Daniel J. Cole, MD, and Karen B. Domino, MD, MPH

A fundamental component of general anesthesia is unconsciousness. Patients consenting to general anesthesia do so with the expectation that they will not see, hear, feel, or remember intraoperative events. Recently, there has been increased public concern regarding intraoperative awareness, and studies show that a large percentage of patients who undergo general anesthesia report preoperative fears of awareness or recall. In the past, conventional monitoring of anesthetic depth (i.e., risk for awareness) has included rudimentary signs such as patient movement, autonomic changes, and subjective clinical instinct. A considerable effort has been devoted to establishing a monitor that will reliably determine a patient's depth of anesthesia. Several different methods have been evaluated, yet none are 100% effective. At present there are at least three inherent obstacles in the development of a "foolproof" monitor of anesthetic depth, and the ability of that monitor to prevent intraoperative awareness. The first is that we have an

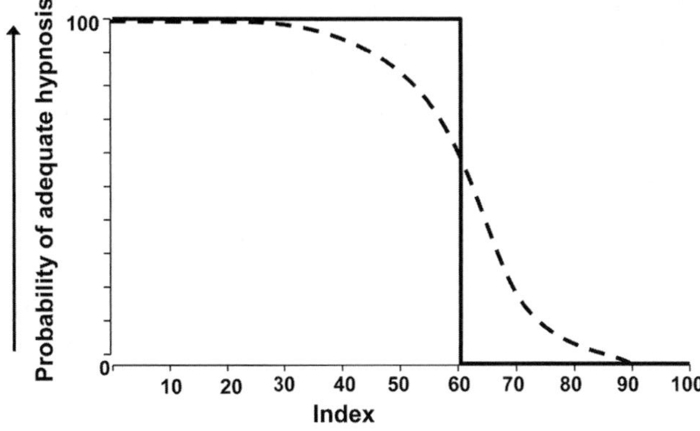

Figure 18-1 The probability of adequate hypnosis based upon brain function monitoring index. The solid line is the ideal probability curve with 100% sensitivity and specificity. The dashed line is a more realistic expectation of monitoring in which a progressive decrease of the monitored index value correlates with increased probability of adequate hypnosis.

Table 18-1 Reported Incidence of Intraoperative Awareness

Incidence (%)	No. of Patients	Prospective Methodology	Study
0.6	4001	Yes	Errando et al., 2008
0.41	11,101	Yes	Xu et al., 2009
0.2	1000	Yes	Nordstrom et al., 1997
0.15	11,785	Yes	Sandin et al., 2000
0.13	19,575	Yes	Sebel et al., 2004
0.1	10,811	No	Myles et al., 2000
0.023	44,006	No	Mashour et al., 2009
0.0068	211,842	No	Pollard et al, 2007

incomplete understanding of the mechanism of general anesthesia. The second is that general anesthesia occurs on a continuum without a quantitative dimension, and there is considerable interpatient and interanesthetic variability. Attempting to translate a conscious or unconscious state into a quantitative number can, at best, be limited to the practice of probability (Figure 18-1). Finally, the sensitivity and specificity of measured cortical electrical activity may not be related to a general anesthesia-induced biochemical event within subcortical structures.

Incidence of Intraoperative Awareness

The incidence of awareness is greater than most practitioners believe because the incidence is best estimated by formally interviewing patients postoperatively. Patients may not voluntarily report awareness if they were not disturbed by it. In addition, memory for awareness may be delayed. A minority of cases are identified in the immediate postanesthetic period. A structured interview is therefore used to evaluate the incidence of awareness. Although the data are variable and controversial (Table 18-1), in prospective studies in which a structured interview has been used, it was found that intraoperative awareness occurs with surprising frequency. A prospective evaluation of awareness in nearly 12,000 patients undergoing general anesthesia conducted in Sweden revealed an incidence of awareness of 0.18% in cases in which neuromuscular blocking agents were used and 0.10% in the absence of such agents. A similar incidence has been observed in tertiary care centers in the United States, with a higher proportion among patients with coexisting morbidity. Studies in Spain and China have reported a higher incidence (0.4% to 0.6%). Studies showing a lower incidence (see Table 18-1) have relied upon quality-improvement data rather than the structured interview. The incidence of awareness is higher when light anesthesia is used, such as with patients undergoing obstetric or cardiac surgical procedures or patients undergoing surgery to treat the sequelae of traumatic injury. The incidence of awareness is higher in children (0.5% to 1%), but psychological sequelae are fewer.

Risk Factors for Intraoperative Awareness

The most common causes of intraoperative awareness include light anesthesia, increased anesthetic requirement, or malfunction or misuse of the anesthetic delivery system. Light anesthesia may be necessary for physiologic stability in hypovolemic patients or those with limited cardiovascular reserve. Patients with an American Society of Anesthesiologists physical class of 3 or greater, who undergo emergency surgery or cesarean section, or who have a history of intraoperative awareness have a higher likelihood of experiencing awareness. Neuromuscular blockade prevents the most common sign of light anesthesia, patient movement. An inadequately anesthetized nonparalyzed patient usually moves first, as lower anesthetic concentrations are needed to prevent awareness than to render immobility. Some patients, such as those using alcohol, opiates, amphetamines, and cocaine may require an increase in anesthetic dose. In addition, equipment problems with the vaporizer or intravenous infusion devices may lead to awareness, although these are less common causes of awareness, especially with use of end-tidal anesthetic gas analysis.

Prevention of Awareness

Suggestions for the prevention of awareness include premedicating the patient with an amnesic agent, giving adequate doses of induction agents, avoiding muscle paralysis unless necessary, and administering at least a 0.7 minimum alveolar concentration of an inhalation agent with monitoring of end-tidal levels to ensure delivery of adequate levels of inhalation anesthetic gases. Hypertension and tachycardia do not reliably predict awareness.

Brain-Function Monitoring

In general, devices that monitor brain electrical activity for the purpose of assessing depth of anesthesia record electroencephalographic (EEG) activity. Some process spontaneous EEG and electromyographic activity, and others measure evoked responses to auditory stimuli. Most of the research concerning depth of anesthesia and all of the research concerning awareness have been performed on the Bispectral Index (BIS, Aspect Medical Systems, Norwood, Mass; BIS now marketed by Covidien, Mansfield, Mass) monitor.

The BIS uses a proprietary algorithm to convert a single channel of frontal EEG activity into an index of hypnotic level, ranging from 100 (awake) to 0 (isoelectric EEG). Specific ranges (40-60) reflect a low probability of consciousness during general anesthesia. A number of other events (cerebral ischemia or hypoperfusion), other drugs (neuromuscular blocking agents or ephedrine), or conditions (elderly with low-amplitude EEG) may affect BIS level.

Evidence in support of a reduction in awareness under general anesthesia with BIS monitoring is derived from two sources: a randomized controlled trial in high-risk patients and a nonrandomized cohort comparison with historical control subjects. Myles and associates performed a randomized controlled trial of BIS monitoring in 2500 patients at high risk for intraoperative awareness (e.g., high-risk cardiac surgery, impaired cardiovascular status, trauma, cesarean section, chronic benzodiazepine or opiate use, heavy alcohol intake, history of awareness). Explicit recall occurred in 0.17% (2 patients) when BIS monitors were used to guide anesthesia and in 0.91% (11 patients) managed by routine clinical practice (P <0.02). Although these results are promising, it is important to realize that if only one additional patient had reported awareness, the difference in the two groups would have not been statistically significant. This is particularly relevant because the end point "awareness" has no "gold standard," unlike death, myocardial infarction, or stroke. Unresolved issues in this study included difficulties in determining "possible" compared with "definite" awareness and the optimal time to interview a patient for possible awareness.

Ekman and colleagues compared the incidence of awareness in a prospective cohort of 5057 patients in whom BIS was used to guide anesthetic administration with the incidence in a historical control group of 7826 patients. Explicit recall occurred in 0.04% of the BIS-monitored patients versus 0.18% of the historical control subjects ($P < 0.038$). Again, if one additional patient had been classified with awareness in the BIS-monitored cohort and one fewer in the historical cohort, the difference would not have been statistically significant. In addition, anesthetic practice may have been changed unrelated to BIS monitoring, as well as affected by the "Hawthorne effect" (people perform better when they know they are being studied). Another prospective nonrandomized cohort study ($n = 19{,}575$) in which BIS was monitored but values were not used to guide anesthetic depth found no difference in the incidence of awareness in the BIS-monitored group.

In 2008, Avidan and colleagues reported the effect of BIS and end-tidal anesthetic gas monitoring on the incidence of intraoperative awareness. Patients were randomly assigned to either BIS-guided therapy ($n = 967$), in which the intent was to maintain the BIS level between 40 and 60, or end-tidal anesthetic gas therapy ($n = 974$), in which the intent was to maintain the end-tidal anesthetic gas concentration between 0.7 and 1.3 minimum alveolar concentration. There was no difference in the incidence of definite awareness between the two groups (two for each group). It is important to note in this study that there was no control group of standard anesthetic practice in allowing lower levels of inhaled anesthetic gases. More recently, Avidan performed a similar prospective randomized study in a population that was at high risk for experiencing intraoperative awareness ($n = 5713$) comparing the two methods and came to similar conclusions: monitoring BIS was not superior to monitoring end-tidal anesthetic gas concentration. However, using a post hoc analysis, Mashour and associates found BIS monitoring may decrease intraoperative awareness compared to routine anesthetic care.

Finally, Whitlock and associates examined data from 1100 patients and concluded that BIS monitoring does not correlate well with end-tidal anesthetic gas concentration, is not sensitive to clinical correlates of changes in end-tidal anesthetic gas concentration, and has high interindividual variability and is not, therefore, amenable for use in finely titrating maintenance of anesthesia.

Summary

Depth of anesthesia is an important factor in the anesthetic management of patients. When considering depth of anesthesia as it relates to the risk of intraoperative awareness, the following points are key:

- The incidence of intraoperative awareness is 1 to 2 per 1000 inhalation anesthetic procedures, and the incidence is higher with light anesthesia and in children.
- The potential exists for serious psychological or medicolegal sequelae to occur.
- Ensuring the functionality of equipment to be used to deliver general anesthesia is paramount in the prevention of intraoperative awareness.
- The clinician may consider administering an amnestic agent as a premedicant in patients who are at risk for developing intraoperative awareness or as a treatment when patients are lightly anesthetized.
- Readministering hypnotic agents may be suitable in clinical situations that place patients at increased risk for developing intraoperative awareness (e.g., difficult airway).
- Hemodynamic measures are unreliable predictors of inadequate anesthesia.
- No monitor has proved to be 100% sensitive and specific for detecting awareness.
- The end-tidal anesthetic gas concentration should be monitored.
- Consider administering at least a 0.7 minimum alveolar concentration of a inhalation anesthetic agent.
- Neuromuscular blocking agents will mask an important indicator of inadequate anesthesia—movement.
- Consider monitoring brain function as an adjunct to other available indicators of anesthetic depth.

Suggested Readings

Apfelbaum JL, Arens JF, Cole DJ, et al. Practice advisory for intraoperative awareness and brain function monitoring: A report by the American Society of Anesthesiologists Task Force on Intraoperative Awareness. *Anesthesiology.* 2006;104:847-864.

Avidan MS, Jacobsohn E, Glick D, et al. BAG-RECALL Research Group. Prevention of intraoperative awareness in a high-risk surgical population. *N Engl J Med.* 2011;365:591-600.

Avidan MS, Mashour GA. Prevention of intraoperative awareness with explicit recall: making sense of the evidence. *Anesthesiology.* 2013:118(2):449-456.

Avidan MS, Zhang L, Burnside BA, et al. Anesthesia awareness and the bispectral index. *N Engl J Med.* 2008;358:1097-1108.

Davidson AJ, Huang GH, Czarnecki C, et al. Awareness during anesthesia in children: a prospective cohort study. *Anesth Analg.* 2005;100(3):653-661.

Ekman A, Lindholm ML, Lennmarken C, Sandin R. Reduction in the incidence of awareness using BIS monitoring. *Acta Anaesthesiol Scand.* 2004;48:20-26.

Errando CL, Perez-Caballero P, Gelb AW, Sigl JC. Methodology, human factors, and incidence of intraoperative awareness. *Acta Anaesthesiol Scand.* 2010; 54(6):781-783.

Errando CL, Sigl JC, Robles M, et al. Awareness with recall during general anaesthesia: A prospective observational evaluation of 4001 patients. *Br J Anaesth.* 2008;101(2):178-185.

Ghoneim MM. Awareness during anesthesia. *Anesthesiology.* 2000;92:597-602.

Malviya S, Galinkin JL, Bannister CF. The incidence of intraoperative awareness in children: childhood awareness and recall evaluation. *Anesth Analg.* 2009; 109(5):1421-1427.

Mashour GA, Shanks A, Tremper KK, et al. Prevention of intraoperative awareness with explicit recall in an unselected surgical population: a randomized comparative effectiveness trial. *Anesthesiology.* 2012;117(4):717-725.

Mashour GA, Wang LY, Turner CR, et al. A retrospective study of intraoperative awareness with methodological implications. *Anesth Analg.* 2009;108(2): 521-526.

Myles PS, Leslie K, McNeil J, et al. Bispectral index monitoring to prevent awareness during anaesthesia: The B-Aware randomised controlled trial. *Lancet.* 2004;363(9423):1757-1763.

Nordström O, Engström AM, Persson S, Sandin R. Incidence of awareness in total I.V. anesthesia based on propofol, alfentanil, and neuromuscular blockade. *Acta Anaesthesiol Scand.* 1997;41(8):978-984.

Pollard RJ, Coyle JP, Gilbert RL, Beck JE. Intraoperative awareness in a regional medical system: A review of 3 years data. *Anesthesiology.* 2007;106(2): 269-274.

Sandin RH, Enlund G, Samuelsson P, Lennmarken C. Awareness during anaesthesia: A prospective case study. *Lancet.* 2000;355(9205):707-711.

Sebel PS, Bowdle TA, Ghoneim MM, et al. The incidence of awareness during anesthesia: A multicenter United States study. *Anesth Analg.* 2004;99(3): 833-839.

Whitlock EL, Villafranca AJ, Lin N, et al. Relationship between bispectral index values and volatile anesthetic concentrations during the maintenance phase of anesthesia in the B-Unaware trial. *Anesthesiology.* 2011;115(6):1209-1218.

Xu L, Wu A-S, Yue Y. The incidence of intra-operative awareness during general anesthesia in China: a multi-center observational study. *Acta Anaesthesiol Scand.* 2009;53(7):873-882.

CHAPTER 19

Monitoring Integrity of the Neuromuscular Junction

Jeffrey J. Lunn, MD

Neuromuscular Transmissions

When a nerve impulse arrives at the neuromuscular junction, voltage-gated ion channels open, leading to an influx of calcium within the terminal that causes several hundreds of vesicles of acetylcholine to fuse with the nerve membrane (Figure 19-1). The acetylcholine within these vesicles is released into the synaptic cleft, combining with and activating nicotinic receptors on the motor endplate, the activation of which opens ion channels on the muscle membrane and depolarizes the membrane. The release of calcium from intracellular stores stimulates an interaction between actin and myosin, resulting in muscle contraction.

To facilitate tracheal intubation and many surgical procedures, neuromuscular blocking agents (NMBAs) are often administered to inhibit the nicotinic receptor. A multitude of factors affect patients' responses to NMBAs, therefore making it essential to monitor the extent of blockade of the nicotinic receptor.

Clinical Indicators of Neuromuscular Blockade

Clinically, it is most important that patients are able to maintain adequate ventilation and protect their airway at the end of a surgical procedure; however, patients may have a normal tidal volume and yet 80% of nicotinic receptors may still be blocked. If such patients are extubated, they may have impaired swallowing, and if they also have a weak or absent cough, these patients may aspirate if gastric contents are in the oropharynx.

Sustained ability to raise the head (headlift) is a much more sensitive indicator of return of neuromuscular function; sustained headlift indicates that at least 70% of function has returned and is the best clinical indicator of return of adequate muscle function.

Neuromuscular Monitoring

Generally, the degree of neuromuscular blockade induced by an NMBA is evaluated by the response induced by a supramaximal electrical stimulus delivered to a peripheral nerve with measurement of a mechanical response of the muscle to the stimulus. When a peripheral nerve is stimulated with a supramaximal stimulus, each muscle fiber enervated by that nerve responds in an all-or-none fashion, and the aggregate response of the whole muscle is dependent upon the number of individual fibers that respond. Muscle fibers with nicotinic receptors still inhibited by NMBAs do not respond to a stimulus.

Nerve Stimulators

To test the degree of neuromuscular blockade—either to ensure muscle paralysis for tracheal intubation or a surgical procedure or to assess the adequacy of muscle strength at the end of an anesthetic—it is important to deliver a supramaximal stimulus, one that is at least 10% to 20% greater than the current necessary to produce a maximum response and 200% to 300% greater than the threshold stimulus. The ability to generate a supramaximal response requires that at least 50 to 80 mA of current be applied to the peripheral nerve. So that a constant current is applied throughout the entire impulse, the stimulus must be monophasic and delivered as a rectangular square wave with a duration of 0.2 to 0.3 ms. Pulses exceeding 0.5 ms may stimulate muscle directly or cause repetitive firing of nerves.

The resistance to current flow increases as skin temperature decreases; conversely, removing hair or degreasing the skin decreases resistance. Modern nerve stimulators deliver a constant current, despite the resistance, by varying voltage to ensure that the amount of current selected is equal to the amount of current delivered.

Nerve stimulators should be able to deliver several different types of stimuli, such as a single twitch, train of four (TOF), continuous (tetanic) stimulation, posttetanic stimulation, and double-burst stimulation (DBS). Nerve stimulators should also have polarity indicators, and most have a display indicating the amount of current applied.

Nerve stimulators have two cables, one with a positive and one with a negative polarity, that are attached to pregelled silver or silver chloride electrodes, each having a minimum of about an 8-mm diameter conducting area, that attach to the skin with a self-contained adhesive. Subcutaneous needle electrodes are rarely, if ever, used for routine neuromuscular monitoring.

Sites for Monitoring

Stimulation of the ulnar nerve at the wrist—with measurement of the response in the adductor pollicis muscle—remains the most popular site for monitoring the degree of neuromuscular blockade. If the arm is not available, the facial nerve or the posterior tibial or the common peroneal nerve is stimulated, with monitoring of their respective muscle groups. The facial nerve can be stimulated with the electrodes placed on the mandible-maxilla; overlying the facial nerve. Placement of the electrodes behind and in front of the ear provides very good sensitivity and specificity, with little chance of direct nerve stimulation.

There are differences when these sites are stimulated because the muscles themselves have different sensitivity to NMBAs. The diaphragm itself is the most resistant muscle, requiring up to two times the dose of NMBAs required to block the adductor pollicis. The muscles of the face enervated by the facial nerve are less resistant to blockade than is the diaphragm but are more resistant than the adductor pollicis.

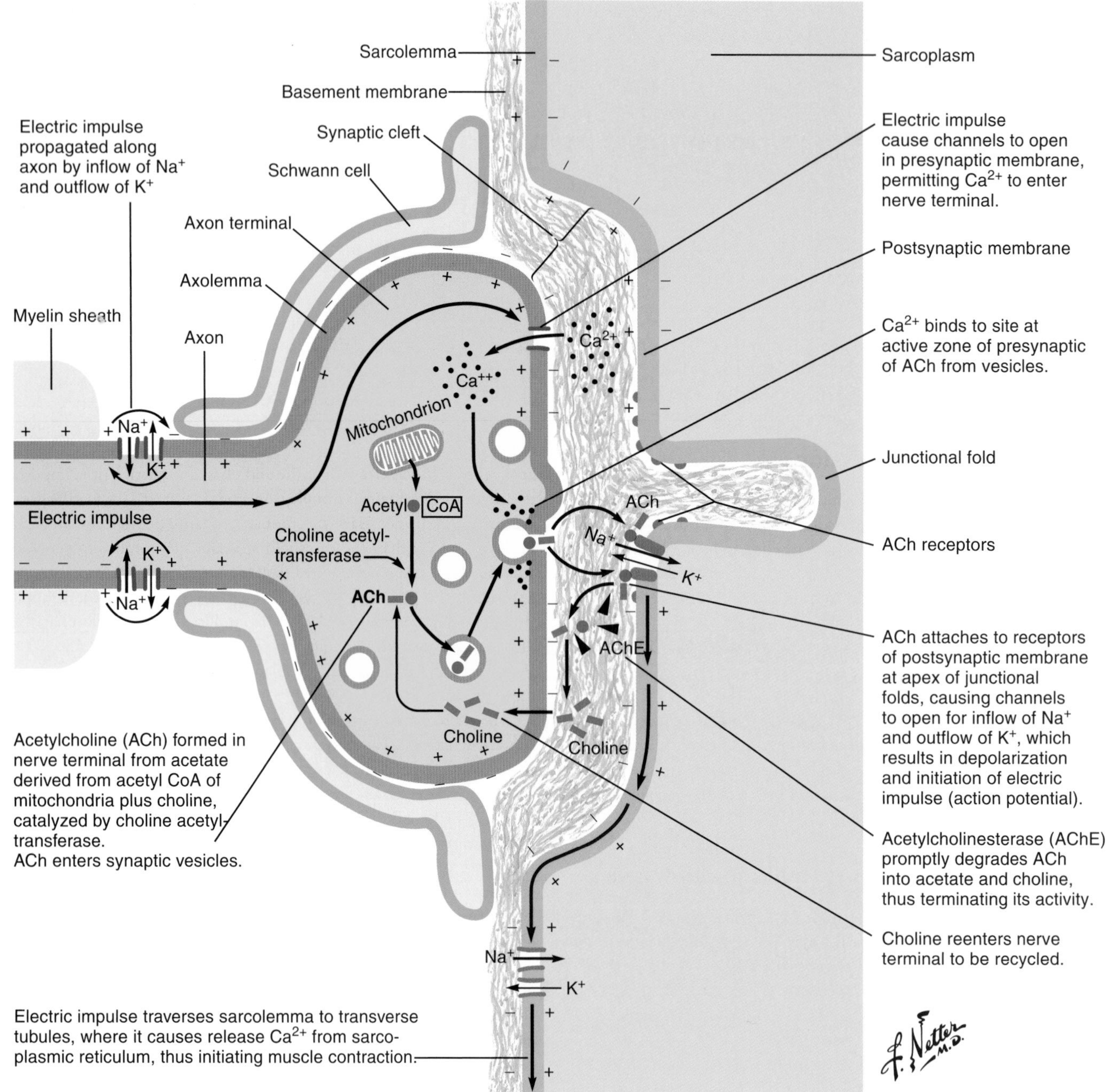

Figure 19-1 Physiology of the neuromuscular junction. (Netter illustration from www.netterimages.com. © Elsevier Inc. All rights reserved.)

Modes of Stimulation

Single Twitch

Single twitches are supramaximal stimuli delivered at between 0.1 and 1 Hz. The response to the stimulus is measured by visual or tactile means and will remain static until approximately 75% of nicotinic receptors are blocked. A linear decrease occurs in response until no twitch can be observed, which occurs at about 95% of nicotinic receptor blockade.

Train of Four

TOF comprises four supramaximal stimuli at 2 Hz that are delivered and may be repeated at a minimum of every 10 sec. Each stimulus can produce a motor response; the degree of receptor blockade is based upon the fade of the individual responses, the presence of subsequent responses, or both. All four responses are identical when no neuromuscular blockade is present. When the fourth stimulus produces no response (3-4), approximately 75% to 80% of receptors are blocked. When the third response is lost (2-4), approximately 85% of receptors are blocked. When the second response is lost (1-4), approximately 90% of receptors are blocked. If there are no responses to any stimuli (0-4), more than 95% of receptors are inhibited.

If there are four responses, the ratio of the strength of the fourth to the first twitch also can be used to assess the degree of neuromuscular function.

At the end of a procedure, a T4/T1 of 0.9 is the gold standard, indicating that a sufficient degree of neuromuscular strength has returned so that clinicians can assure themselves that patients will be able to maintain adequate ventilation and can protect their airways. The advantage of a TOF is that no baseline control twitch is required. When measuring the ratio of T4/T1, an objective measure of the mechanical response is performed using a device that objectively quantifies the strength of the muscle contraction.

Though it is uncommon to use TOF monitoring in patients who have received a depolarizing NMBA, such as succinylcholine, for those patients who have prolonged weakness associated with depolarizing blockade, the TOF may be helpful. Normally, depolarizing blockade decreases the twitch height of all four responses equally. If fade occurs, and the first twitch is greater than subsequent twitches, a phase II block should be considered.

Tetanus

Tetanus is obtained by the delivery of repetitive stimuli, usually at 50 to 100 Hz. In the absence of an NMBA, a tetanic contraction results. If fade is observed with a nondepolarizing neuromuscular blocker and a decrease occurs in the amplitude of force over the duration of the stimulus, neuromuscular block (or phase II block) is present. If a single twitch is administered shortly following tetanic stimulation, posttetanic facilitation should be observed, indicating that not all nicotinic receptors are blocked.

Posttetanic Facilitation

Not commonly used clinically, posttetanic facilitation can be used to assess the degree of neuromuscular blockade if there is no response to TOF stimulation or single-twitch stimulation. As noted earlier, a 50-Hz tetanic stimulation for 5 sec followed 3 sec later by a 1-Hz single stimulus should result in posttetanic stimulation, indicating that 0% to 5% of receptors are unoccupied.

Double-Burst Stimulation

DBS can be used in detecting small degrees of neuromuscular blockade by tactile means when recording devices are not available. DBS involves the delivery of two short 50-Hz stimuli separated by 750 ms, in which three impulses are delivered in each burst (DBS 3, 3). The response of the second burst is decreased if there is any degree of neuromuscular blockade present, and the ratio of the second burst to the first burst correlates well with a T4/T1 ratio but is readily perceptible to touch.

Techniques to Monitor Muscular Response

As mentioned previously, response to stimulation is most frequently measured visually; however, tactile evaluation of the twitches is recommended. For research and for assessing degrees of neuromuscular blockade at either end of the spectrum, an objective measurement of response is desired.

Electromyography

Electromyography is sensitive but has problems inherent in electrical interference, inconvenience, expense, direct muscle stimulation, and other issues.

Mechanomyography

Mechanomyography is the gold standard of monitoring neuromuscular blockade because it measures the actual force of isometric contraction using a force transducer. It is typically used on the hand (adductor pollicis) with ulnar stimulation.

Acceleromyography

Using a piezoelectric transducer, acceleromyography measures isotonic acceleration. It can be used on a variety of muscle sites and has good correlation with mechanomyography.

Phonomyography

Phonomyography measures the low-frequency sounds of muscle contraction. It correlates well with mechanomyography and can be applied to any muscles.

Suggested Readings

Hemmerling TM. Neuromuscular monitoring: An update for the clinician. *Can J Anesth.* 2007;54:58-72.

Trager G, Michand G, Deschamps S, Hemmerling T. Comparison of phonomyography, linemyography, and mechanomyography for neuromuscular monitoring. *Can J Anesth.* 2006;53:130-135.

Viby-Morgensen J. Neuromuscular monitoring. *Curr Opin Anesth.* 2001;14:655-659.

CHAPTER 20

Evoked Potential Monitoring

Jeffrey J. Pasternak, MS, MD

Recording of evoked potentials (EPs) is used to assess the integrity of select neuronal pathways within the central and peripheral nervous systems. EP monitoring is especially useful intraoperatively when general anesthesia otherwise limits or prevents performance of a clinical neurologic examination. Evaluation of four major neuronal systems can be accomplished via four EP measurements: somatosensory (SSEP), brainstem auditory evoked responses (BAER), visual (VEP), and motor (MEP). BAERs are the most resistant to the effects of anesthetic agents, and VEPs are the most sensitive; SSEP and MEP responses are intermediate in sensitivity to the effects of anesthetic agents.

The Evoked Potential Waveform

All four EP techniques involve the application of a stimulus that generates a neuronal response with measurement of that response. Typical recordings are expressed as a graph of time (in milliseconds) on the abscissa (i.e., *x*-axis) and voltage (mV) as the ordinate (i.e., *y*-axis) (Figure 20-1). The responses are very low voltage and require signal averaging to enhance their quality, that is, recorded waveforms are a composite of 50 to 100 or more measurements following multiple stimulation measurement cycles that serve to "subtract out" higher-voltage interference (e.g., electrocardiogram, electroencephalogram, and electrical noise within the operative suite). Peak voltages in the measured waveform refer to positive or negative deflections, designated by a *P* or *N*, respectively.

Two major characteristics of the measured waveform are usually described: amplitude and latency. Amplitude refers to the voltage difference between either a successive peak or a designated reference voltage. Latency refers to the length of time following stimulation for a specific peak to appear and is usually designated as a subscript of the positively or negatively deflected peak (e.g., N_{20} is a negatively deflected peak occurring 20 ms after stimulation). Interpeak latency refers to the time difference (in ms) between two different peaks.

Many factors influence the recorded waveform. Monitoring variables may include displacement of monitoring leads or electrical impedance, and improper patient positioning may compress a nerve, which can then interfere with conduction, even if the surgical site is remote (e.g., ulnar nerve compression in the prone position during spine operations).

Anesthetic agents have variable effects, depending on the EP modality and the anesthetic drug. Surgical factors (e.g., injury to a neural pathway from compression, reduced perfusion, or transection) are the reasons to intraoperatively monitor EPs. Physiologic variables include decreased O_2 delivery to the neural pathway being monitored, which can occur with hypotension, anemia, and hypoxia. Hypothermia can also reduce the rate of neural conduction and impact recordings.

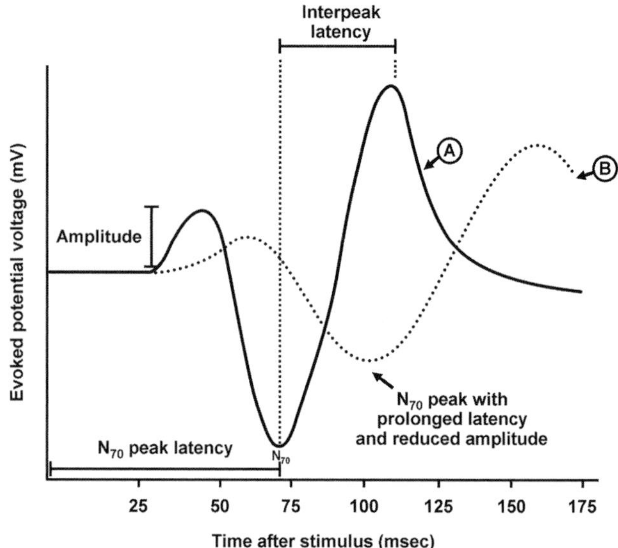

Figure 20-1 The solid line (A) represents a typical evoked potential waveform described in terms of latency (time from delivery of stimulus to onset of response) and amplitude (size in microvolts). Interpeak latency refers to the time difference between two peaks on the tracing. Waveform B represents a decrease in amplitude and an increase in latency compared to waveform A. This change can occur due to neuronal ischemia or injury, effects of various anesthetic agents, or changes in physiologic variables leading to reduced neuronal perfusion. (Modified, with permission, from Mahla ME. Neurologic monitoring. In: Cucchiara RF, Black S, Michenfelder JD, eds. Clinical Neuroanesthesia. 2nd ed. New York, Churchill Livingstone, 1998.)

Brainstem Auditory Evoked Responses

BAERs allow monitoring of the integrity of the auditory pathway both peripherally and centrally. Stimuli are loud, repetitive clicks produced by a device placed over or in the auditory canal or canals. Measurement of the response is from electrodes placed on the scalp or external ears to record contralateral and ipsilateral signals that have and have not decussated, respectively. BAER monitoring allows assessment of the acoustic transduction system of the middle and inner ear, the cochlear nerve (i.e., cranial nerve VIII), and the entire central auditory pathway rostrally to the primary auditory cortex located in the temporal lobe of the brain (Figure 20-2). Some anesthetic agents may cause minor changes in amplitude or latency of recorded waveforms; however, these changes are usually very small, even with large changes in anesthetic dose. Therefore, significant intraoperative BAER changes are usually indicative of a surgical trespass.

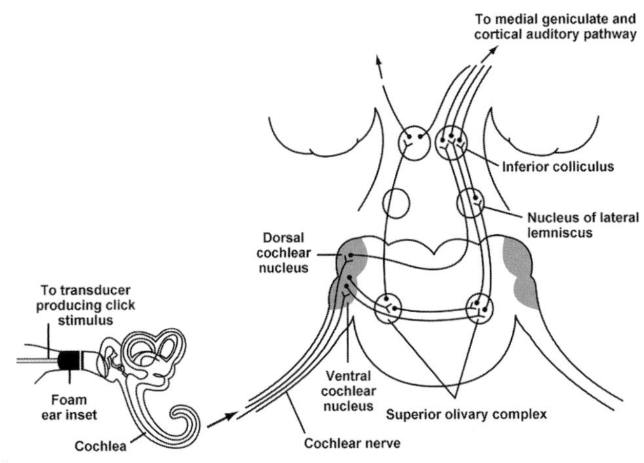

Figure 20-2 Brainstem auditory evoked potentials involve stimulation via the transducer placed within the external auditory canal. Neuronal impulses travel from the cochlea via the cochlear nerve (cranial nerve VIII) to the auditory cortex in the temporal lobes. (Reprinted, with permission, from Mahla ME. Neurologic monitoring. In: Cucchiara RF, Black S, Michenfelder JD, eds. Clinical Neuroanesthesia. 2nd ed. New York, Churchill Livingstone, 1998.)

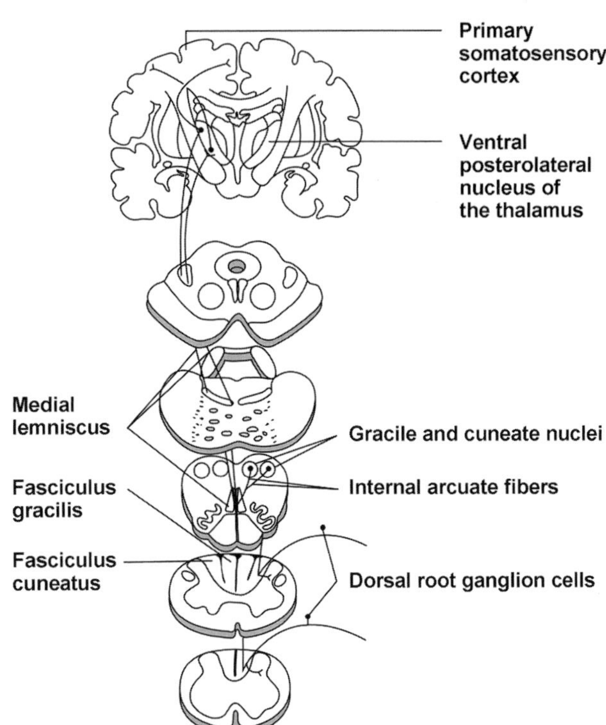

Figure 20-3 The dorsal column medial lemniscus pathway is the primary afferent pathway impulses from touch, vibration, and proprioception receptors. (Reprinted, with permission, from Burt AM. Textbook of Neuroanatomy. Philadelphia, WB Saunders; 1993:202-221.)

Potential indications for intraoperative BAERs include monitoring for microvascular decompression of cranial nerve V or VII, resection of tumors in the cerebellopontine angle, or resection of brainstem lesions, and in the intensive care unit BAERs may help in the declaration of brain death.

Placement of the cerebellar retractor during microvascular decompression of cranial nerve V or VII can stretch cranial nerve VIII and increase the risk of subsequent postoperative hearing impairment. Brainstem compression, direct trauma to cranial nerve VIII or its blood supply, or cerebellar retraction during resection of tumors in the cerebellopontine angle, such as acoustic neuromas, may result in injury to the auditory pathway.

Somatosensory Evoked Potentials

Monitoring of SSEPs permit assessment of major sensory pathways (within the dorsal column medial lemniscus) responsible for transmission of touch, vibration, and proprioception (Figure 20-3). These sensory pathways consist of first-order neurons originating at peripheral sensory receptors and entering the spinal cord to travel rostrally within the ipsilateral posterior column to synapse on the second-order neurons located within the gracile and cuneate nuclei at the cervicomedullary junction. These neurons then decussate and proceed rostrally through the brainstem as the medial lemniscus to reach the ventral posterolateral nucleus of the thalamus. The second-order neurons synapse here with third-order neurons that then travel rostrally to the primary somatosensory cortex located on the postcentral gyrus.

Stimulation and monitoring of SSEPs from the median, posterior tibial, or peroneal nerve are commonly performed. Measurement of the response can be accomplished by recording more proximally along the same nerve, over the spine, or from the contralateral scalp. Maintenance of adequate blood supply to the central portions of the pathway within the spinal cord is of critical importance when interpreting the results. Specifically, the dorsal columns within the spinal cord are supplied by the posterior spinal arteries. Accordingly, SSEP measurements are generally not reliable for the detection of ischemia in regions of the cord supplied by the anterior spinal artery (e.g., motor pathways).

SSEP monitoring can be used for procedures involving the spine (e.g., scoliosis surgery, spinal cord tumor resection, laminectomy with fusion, vertebral fractures with instability), posterior fossa operations (e.g., tumor resection), and vascular operations (e.g., carotid endarterectomy, aneurysm clipping). Anesthetic agents have variable effects on recordings of SSEPs. Stimulation and measurement of potentials from peripheral nerves and subcortical regions are often minimally affected by anesthetic agents. However, anesthetic agents can have a significant modulatory effect on the waveforms recorded from the cortex. In general, agents that cause increased latency and decreased amplitude include inhalation anesthetic agents (e.g., isoflurane, sevoflurane, desflurane), N_2O, propofol, benzodiazepines, and opioids. The magnitude of the effect on either latency or amplitude varies among these agents. For example, inhalation anesthetic agents and benzodiazepines have a much greater suppressant effect of EPs than do opioids. Therefore, moderate to high doses of inhalation anesthetic agents or benzodiazepines may obliterate SSEP waveforms. On the other hand, reliable signal recording can often be accomplished even with high-dose opioid technique. Increased latency or decreased amplitude can also occur with ischemia or injury to the sensory pathway. Conversely, ketamine and etomidate increase the amplitude of SSEP waveforms. As such, these agents can actually be used to enhance signals due to their effect on amplitude. Neuromuscular blocking agents (NMBAs) have no significant effect on SSEPs.

Motor Evoked Potentials

Unlike SSEP techniques that assess the integrity of afferent neural pathways, MEPs assess the efferent motor pathway: the corticospinal tract (Figure 20-4). Cell bodies of first-order motor neurons exist in the precentral gyrus of the frontal lobe. Axons extend via the internal capsule into the crux cerebri of the midbrain, basal pons, and pyramidal tracts of the medulla. In the caudal region of the medulla, these axons decussate and travel in the lateral region of the spinal cord (i.e., the lateral corticospinal tract) to synapse on secondary motor neurons. These secondary motor neurons then leave the ventral spinal cord, combine to form nerves and plexuses, and proceed to innervate muscles. Blood to the primary motor pathway comes from branches of the middle and anterior cerebral arteries in the cerebrum, the vertebrobasilar system in the brainstem, and the anterior spinal artery in the spinal cord.

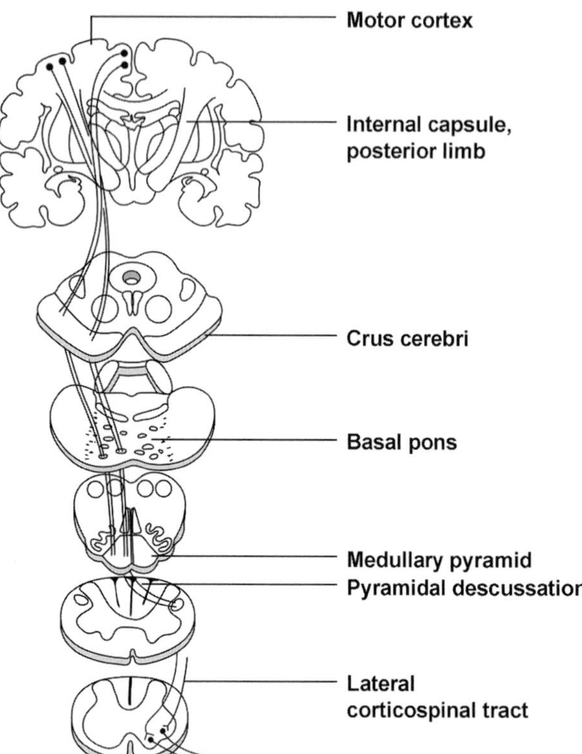

Figure 20-4 The corticospinal tract is the primary efferent motor pathway. (Reprinted, with permission, from Burt AM. Textbook of Neuroanatomy. Philadelphia, WB Saunders; 1993:202-221.)

Stimulation of MEPs can be accomplished from the cerebral cortex or spinal cord by applying either an electric or magnetic stimulus. Recording can be accomplished anywhere caudal to the site stimulated; however, recording within the muscle is most commonly used.

Intraoperative recording of MEPs can be used during spine operations (e.g., scoliosis correction, spinal tumor resection) or operations involving peripheral nerves (e.g., brachial plexus or peripheral nerve reconstruction/transposition). Intraoperative MEP recording may also provide valuable information during repair of thoracoabdominal aortic aneurysms. The artery of Adamkiewicz, a branch of the aorta, often has a variable location and supplies the lower two thirds of the anterior spinal cord; occlusion of the artery of Adamkiewicz either directly or via occlusion of the aorta at a site proximal to the artery's origin places a large portion of the spinal cord at risk. MEP recording may also be used during cerebral aneurysm clipping, especially for aneurysms located within the middle cerebral, anterior cerebral, or vertebrobasilar systems because these vascular territories supply different parts of the motor pathway, and also for resection of tumors in the posterior fossa.

As with sensory EPs, MEPs are also subject to interference by anesthetic agents and physiologic variables. Electrically induced MEPs are less sensitive to anesthetic effects than are magnetically induced MEP signals. Utilization of multipulse (versus single-pulse) electrical stimulation will further reduce the sensitivity of MEPs to the effects of anesthetic agents and will improve signal quality because of summation and recruitment of a greater number of axons to transmit the stimulus. MEPs that do not involve cerebral cortical stimulation (i.e., stimulation at the level of the spinal cord or peripheral nerve) are less sensitive to the effects of anesthetic agents than are those involving cortical stimulation.

The use of NMBAs is not absolutely contraindicated when MEPS are used. In fact, low-dose infusions of NMBAs can be helpful to reduce noise within the MEP signal; however, complete neuromuscular blockade will result in loss of myogenically recorded MEPs. If NMBAs are used, compound motor action potentials can be recorded from a peripheral nerve with care taken to retain 5% to 10% of the original compound motor action potential. Inhalation anesthetic agents, N_2O, propofol, barbiturates, and benzodiazepines produce decreased signal amplitude and increased signal latency, especially when given in high doses. The use of a continuous propofol infusion or low-dose inhalation anesthesia agents is typically compatible with successful MEP monitoring. Ketamine, etomidate, dexmedetomidine, and opioids have minimal effects on MEPs such that these agents can be used at moderate doses during MEP monitoring.

Visual Evoked Potentials

VEPs allow for assessment of the integrity of the entire visual system, including the ophthalmic globe, optic nerve, optic chiasm, optic tracts and radiations, and visual cortex of the occipital lobe. Measurement of VEPs involves delivery of repetitive bright flashes of light through goggles or placement of contact lenses containing light-emitting diodes. Traditionally, intraoperative recording of VEPs has been attempted for resection of tumors near the optic nerve (i.e., skull base meningioma) or optic chiasm (i.e., pituitary tumors); however, the exquisite sensitivity of VEPs to the depressant effects of anesthetic agents make them impractical for intraoperative use.

Intraoperative Changes in Evoked Potential Signals

If EPs are being recorded intraoperatively, the clinician should have a very systematic approach to assess the reason for changes in signals. Ischemia, injury, or transection of a neural pathway will generally result in either a decrease in signal amplitude with an increase in signal latency or a complete loss of signal (i.e., isoelectricity). The following should be considered to rule out anesthetic and monitoring-based causes:

- Was a drug recently administered or was the dose of a drug recently changed?
- Was an NMBA given during MEP monitoring?
- Is there a physiologic reason for neural ischemia or hypoxia (e.g., hypotension, hypoxia, anemia)? An increase in blood pressure, the O_2 content of blood, and hemoglobin concentration may all be helpful in improving O_2 delivery to compromised neural tissue even in the event of a surgical cause of signal decrease or loss.
- Is there significant hypothermia?
- Is there a positioning problem that may result in peripheral nerve compression?
- Is there a problem with the monitoring equipment (e.g., displacement of a monitoring lead)?

Once anesthetic, physiologic, and monitoring-based causes have been ruled out or corrected and the signal amplitude and latency still do not improve, surgical causes for neural compromise should be sought and corrected, if possible.

Suggested Readings

Bhalodia VM, Sestokas AK, Tomak PR, Schwartz DM. Transcranial electric motor evoked potential detection of compressional peroneal nerve injury in the lateral decubitus position. *J Clin Monitor Comp*. 2008;22:319-326.

Burt AM. *Textbook of Neuroanatomy*. Philadelphia: WB Saunders; 1993:202-221.

Lotto M, Banoub M, Schubert A. Effects of anesthetic agents and physiologic changes on intraoperative motor evoked potentials. *J Neurosurg Anesth*. 2004;16:32-42.

Mahla ME. Neurologic monitoring. In: Cucchiara RF, Black S, Michenfelder JD, eds. *Clinical Neuroanesthesia*. 2nd ed. New York: Churchill Livingstone; 1998.

CHAPTER 21

Oxygen Transport

David R. Mumme, MD

The amount of O_2 delivered to tissues is equal to the amount contained in the blood (the arterial O_2 content) times the cardiac output (CO): CO = stroke volume × the heart rate (Figure 21-1). The arterial O_2 content is a product of the hemoglobin (Hb) concentration in grams per deciliter times the amount of O_2 in each gram of Hb times the O_2 saturation, expressed as a fraction, usually given as 1.39 mL of O_2 for every gram of Hb. The affinity of Hb for O_2 (Figure 21-1) determines the characteristics of the oxyhemoglobin (Hbo_2) dissociation curve, with pH, temperature, and concentration of 2,3-diphosphoglycerate (2,3-DPG) having the greatest impact on the affinity of Hb for O_2. Five variables affect O_2 delivery: (1) Hb concentration, (2) Hb affinity for O_2 (P_{50}), (3) percent O_2 saturation of Hb (Sao_2), (4) CO, and (5) the amount of O_2 dissolved in blood (usually trivial amounts).

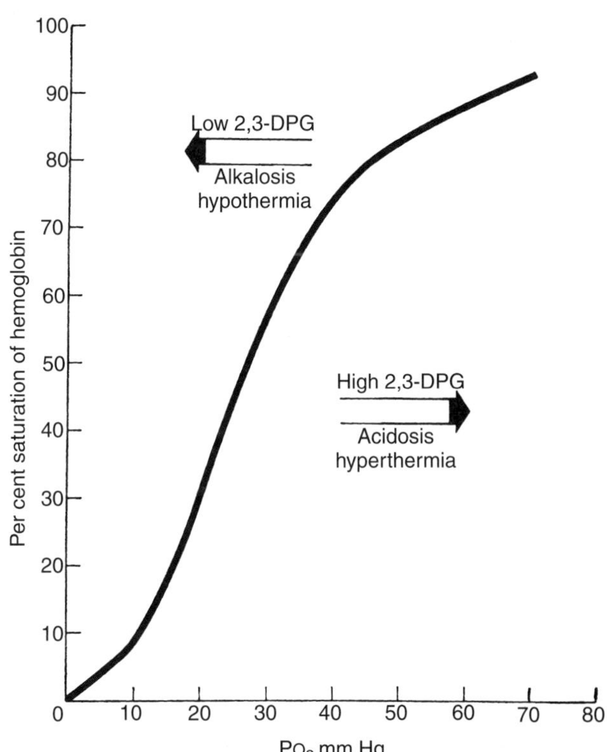

Figure 21-1 The oxyhemoglobin dissociation curve plots hemoglobin saturation (ordinate) at varying O_2 tensions (abscissa). Note that hemoglobin is approximately 80% saturated at a Pao_2 of 50 mm Hg (P_{50}), 75% saturated at a Pao_2 of 40 mm Hg (venous), and 30% saturated at a Pao_2 of 20 mm Hg. The normal P_{50} of adult humans is 26.7 mm Hg. 2,3-DPG = 2,3-Diphosphoglycerate. (Reprinted, with permission, from Miller RD, ed. Anesthesia. 6th ed. Philadelphia, Elsevier Churchill Livingstone, 2005:1799-1827.)

The arterial O_2 content (Cao_2) is calculated as the sum of the O_2 bound by Hb and the O_2 dissolved in the plasma.

$$Cao_2 = (Hb \times 1.39 \times Sao_2/100) + (Pao_2 \times 0.003)$$

For example, if Hb is 15 g/dL, Sao_2 is 100%, and Pao_2 is 100 mm Hg, then

$$\begin{aligned} Cao_2 &= (15 \times 1.39 \times 1) + (100 \times 0.003) \\ &= 20.85 + 0.3 \\ &= 21.15 \text{ mL/dL (or 211.5 mL/L)} \end{aligned}$$

Note that dissolved O_2 ($Pao_2 \times 0.003$) typically has little impact on Cao_2. Notable exceptions occur when O_2 carried by Hb is severely diminished, such as in severe anemia or carbon monoxide intoxication or if the Pao_2 is very high.

The O_2 content of mixed venous blood is usually 25% less than that of arterial blood due to O_2 extraction by the tissues. At a mixed venous O_2 saturation of 75% and mixed venous O_2 tension of 40 mm Hg, mixed venous O_2 content ($C\bar{v}o_2$) is

$$\begin{aligned} C\bar{v}o_2 &= (15 \times 1.39 \times 0.75) + (40 \times 0.003) \\ &= 15.64 + .12 \\ &= 15.76 \text{ mL/dL} \end{aligned}$$

Oxygen delivery ($\dot{D}o_2$) to the tissues is the product of CO and Cao_2. For example, if the CO is 5.0 L/min in the first example, then the $\dot{D}o_2$ is

$$\begin{aligned} \dot{D}o_2 &= 21.15 \text{ dL/L} \times 50 \text{ dL/min} \\ &= 1057 \text{ mL/min (approximately 1 L/min)} \end{aligned}$$

Oxygen consumption ($\dot{V}o_2$), approximately 250 mL/min for an adult, is the CO multiplied by the difference between arterial and venous O_2 content (assuming no shunt). This calculation uses the Fick principle:

$$\dot{V}o_2 = CO \times C(a - \bar{v})O_2$$

Thus, for a constant $\dot{V}o_2$, a decrease in the CO requires a proportionate increase in the $C(a - \bar{v})O_2$, usually achieved by increasing ti- extraction. Conversely, if $\dot{V}o_2$ increases, CO, C(a - … $C(a - \bar{v})O_2$ must increase.

The Oxyhemoglobin Dissociatic

The Hbo_2 dissociation curve is the measured relat So_2 (see Figure 21-1). The position of this curve position at which Hb is 50% saturated, which is normally 26.7 mm Hg in adult humans. Shifting this curve to the left or right has little effect on So_2 greater than 90%, at which point the curve is relatively horizontal; a much greater effect is seen for values in the steeper parts of the curve ($So_2 < 90\%$).

Variables shifting the Hbo_2 dissociation curve are listed in Table 21-1. A left-shifted Hbo_2 dissociation curve indicates a higher affinity of Hb for O_2 and, thus, a higher saturation at a given Pao_2 (e.g., fetal hemoglobin). This increased affinity of Hb for O_2 may require higher tissue perfusion to produce the same O_2 unloading. Note that banked blood is markedly depleted of 2,3-DPG within 1 to 2 weeks, which can affect O_2 delivery after massive transfusion.

Table 21-1 Variables That Shift the Oxyhemoglobin Dissociation Curve

Left	Right
Alkalosis	Acidosis
Hypothermia	Hyperthermia
Decreased 2,3-diphosphoglycerate	Increased 2,3-diphosphoglycerate
Abnormal hemoglobin (fetal)	Abnormal hemoglobin
Carboxyhemoglobin	Increased CO_2
Methemoglobin	

A right-shifted Hbo_2 dissociation curve implies lower affinity and, thus, lower saturation at a given Pao_2, but may permit lower tissue perfusion because the lower affinity in effect allows easier unloading of O_2 to the tissues. Adding hydrogen ions, 2,3-DPG, and heat causes a rightward shift of the curve.

Chronic acid-base changes will cause a compensatory change in 2,3-DPG within 24 to 48 hours and restore the Hbo_2 dissociation curve back toward normal.

Suggested Readings

Rutter TW, Tremper KK. The physiology of oxygen transport and red cell transfusion. In: Healy TEJ, Knight PR, eds. *A Practice of Anesthesia*. 7th ed. London: Arnold; 2003:167-183.

CHAPTER 22

Carbon Dioxide Transport

Michael J. Murray, MD, PhD, and Jörg H. Vetterman, MD

CO_2, one of the end products of metabolism, is produced in mitochondria and follows a concentration gradient through the cytoplasm, extracellular fluid, venous blood, and alveolar gas and then, by way of exhalation, disperses in ambient air. The elimination of CO_2 is dependent on blood flow and alveolar ventilation:

$$CHO + O_2 = H_2O + CO_2$$

CO_2 Transport

Because more CO_2 is produced than can be dissolved and transported in blood, a number of mechanisms have developed over time to enable the body to eliminate CO_2. When CO_2 enters plasma from cells, 5% to 10% of the gas remains dissolved in plasma; some combines with H_2O to form carbonic acid, which dissociates into bicarbonate and hydrogen ion; and some combines with plasma proteins, but 90% to 95% of the CO_2 is taken up by red blood cells (RBCs) (Figure 22-1).

O_2 in Plasma

CO₂ that does not enter RBCs, some, as mentioned, remains dissolved a and is transported to the lungs (the solubility coefficient of CO_2 is 0.03 mmol·L-1·mm Hg-1 at 37° C). One in 700 molecules of the dissolved CO_2 reacts with plasma water and, through hydrolysis, forms carbonic acid:

$$CO_2 + H_2O \leftrightarrow H_2CO_3$$

Because of the lack of carbonic anhydrase in plasma, this reaction is very slow. In fact, the concentration of CO_2 in plasma is nearly 1000 times greater than that of carbonic acid. The small amount of carbonic acid that is formed in plasma dissociates into hydrogen and bicarbonate ions:

$$H_2CO_3 \rightarrow H^+ + HCO_3^-$$

Finally, a negligible amount of CO_2 combines with the amino groups of plasma proteins to form carbamino compounds according to the equation:

$$R{-}NH_2 + CO_2 \leftrightarrow R{-}NH{-}COOH$$

Role of Red Blood Cells

Most of the CO_2 that dissolves in plasma passes into the erythrocytes where three processes can occur: (1) A negligible amount of this CO_2 remains in solution within the RBC. (2) A much larger amount of CO_2 (5% to 10% of the total amount of CO_2 carried in the blood) combines with hemoglobin to form carbaminohemoglobin, a reaction that is facilitated by the release of

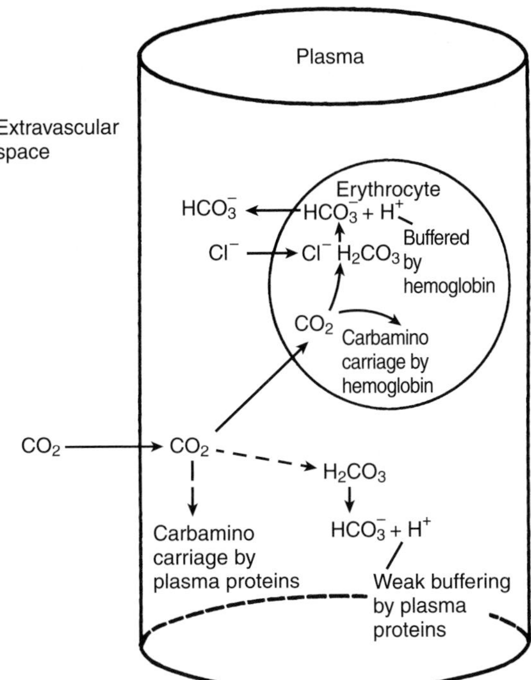

Figure 22-1 Diagrammatic representation of CO_2 transport in plasma and in the erythrocyte. (From Lumb AB. Nunn's Applied Respiratory Physiology. 5th ed. Boston, Butterworth-Heinemann, 2000.)

O_2 from hemoglobin. The release of hydrogen ions when carbonic acid dissociates (more acidic environment) shifts the O_2 dissociation curve to the right; O_2 is given up more readily by hemoglobin. The deoxygenated hemoglobin has a greater ability than oxygenated hemoglobin to form carbaminohemoglobin. This is known as the Haldane effect (Figure 22-2). The opposite occurs in the lungs, where blood is more alkalotic: CO_2 is released from hemoglobin more readily—the reduced hemoglobin more readily carries O_2 (the Bohr effect). Finally, (3) the greatest fraction of CO_2 in RBCs is hydrated by carbonic anhydrase to form carbonic acid, almost 99.9% of which dissociates into bicarbonate and hydrogen ions. The negatively charged bicarbonate ion produced from the dissociation of carbonic acid diffuses out of the RBCs into plasma. To maintain electrical neutrality within the RBCs, chloride ions diffuse from plasma into the RBC in a process called the Hamburger phenomenon, or chloride shift.

CO_2 Dissociation Curve

The CO_2 dissociation curve defines the relationship between the total CO_2 content of blood and the partial pressure of CO_2. Two important differences exist between the oxyhemoglobin dissociation curve and the CO_2 dissociation curve. First, the CO_2 dissociation curve is much more linear than the O_2 dissociation curve. Second, the CO_2 dissociation curve has a steeper slope, meaning that, for a given change in partial pressure, significantly more CO_2 than O_2 can be carried in blood (Figure 22-3). The degree of hemoglobin oxygenation affects the position of the CO_2 dissociation curve. The lower the saturation of hemoglobin with O_2, the higher the CO_2 content for a given P_{CO_2}.

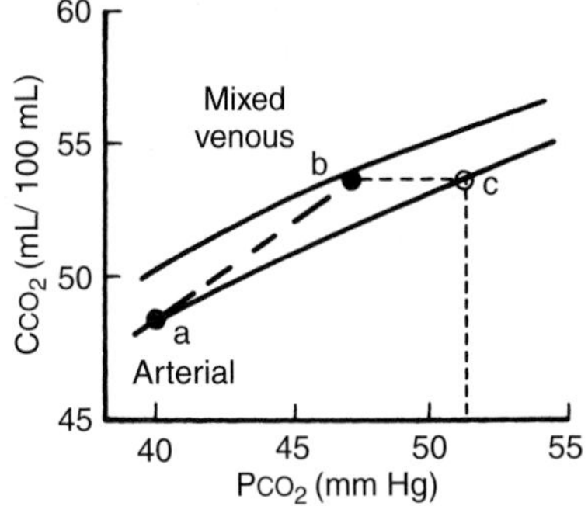

Figure 22-2 The Haldane effect, as illustrated here, is of physiologic importance in CO_2 transport. Deoxygenated (mixed venous) blood has a greater capacity to carry CO_2 than does oxygenated (arterial) blood. In the absence of this shift in the CO_2 dissociation curve, tissue P_{CO_2} would need to increase considerably to load the same amount of CO_2.

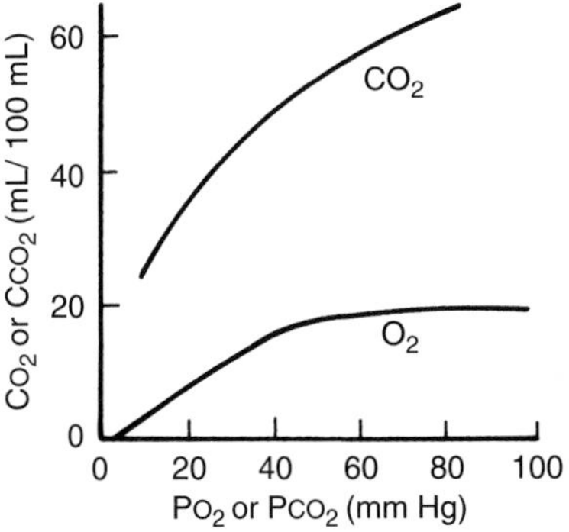

Figure 22-3 Comparison of the shape of the oxyhemoglobin and CO_2 dissociation curves. The slope of the CO_2 dissociation curve is approximately three times steeper than that of the oxyhemoglobin dissociation curve. C_{CO_2}, CO_2 content of blood; C_{O_2}, O_2 content of blood; P_{CO_2} and P_{O_2}, partial pressures of CO_2 and O_2 in blood, respectively. (From Taylor AE, Rehder K, Hyatt RE, et al. Clinical Respiratory Physiology. Philadelphia, WB Saunders, 1989.)

Suggested Readings

Lumb AB. *Nunn's Applied Respiratory Physiology*. 5th ed. Boston: Butterworth-Heinemann; 2000.

Taylor AE, Rehder K, Hyatt RE, et al. *Clinical Respiratory Physiology*. Philadelphia: WB Saunders; 1989.

CHAPTER 23

Interpretation of Arterial Blood Gases

Bradly J. Narr, MD, and Steven G. Peters, MD

The clinical utility of arterial blood gas (ABG) measurements includes assessment of oxygenation (arterial O_2 tension [$Pa{O_2}$]), ventilation (arterial CO_2 tension [$Pa{CO_2}$]), and acid-base status (pH). The bicarbonate (HCO_3^-) value in an ABG measurement is calculated from the CO_2 tension and pH, as opposed to the bicarbonate value on an electrolyte panel, which is actually measured. Modern blood gas machines also have a means to measure hemoglobin concentration and a co-oximeter to measure hemoglobin O_2 saturation. These measurements allow quantitative assessment of the functions of the cardiorespiratory system. Recognition of abnormal measurements permits specific diagnostic and therapeutic interventions in the operating room, postanesthesia care unit, and intensive care unit. Specific clinical situations for which ABG analysis can guide patient care include management of hypoxia or hypercarbia, weaning from mechanical ventilation, use of permissive hypercapnia as a component of lung-protective ventilation strategies, and diagnosis and management of acid-base disorders.

Acid-Base Disturbances

Intracellular pH is tightly regulated; several buffering systems minimize the changes in pH that are associated with the addition of acid or base. In humans, the major extracellular buffer pair is bicarbonate/carbonic acid. The Henderson-Hasselbalch equation describes the effect of the dissociation of carbonic acid to hydrogen ion and bicarbonate:

$$pH = pK + \log\frac{HCO_3^-}{H_2CO_3^-}$$

Using 6.1 as the pK for carbonic acid, and expressing the concentration of carbonic acid as dissolved CO_2 ($0.03 \times P{CO_2}$), the pH determined by the Henderson-Hasselbalch equation becomes:

$$pH = 6.1 + \frac{\log(HCO_3^-)}{0.03 \times Pa{CO_2}}$$

The physiologic response to an acid-base disturbance is threefold. Initially, the acid or base is buffered immediately in that body-fluid compartment. In plasma and interstitial fluid, bicarbonate is the major buffer, with proteins and phosphate compounds contributing to a lesser extent. In erythrocytes, hemoglobin is the major buffer, with bicarbonate contributing approximately 30% and phosphate 10% of the buffering capacity. Secondary and tertiary compensation for the underlying acid-base abnormality occurs via the lungs and kidneys. Elimination of CO_2 by hyperventilation is the initial compensatory mechanism for metabolic acidemia. The kidneys eliminate organic acids and [H^+] as ammonium ions and reabsorb bicarbonate from tubular fluids, with formation of titratable acid. Ultimately, however, to restore true homeostasis, the underlying pathophysiologic process must be corrected (e.g., administration of fluids and insulin for diabetic ketoacidosis or antibiotics for pneumonia in a patient with chronic obstructive lung disease).

Acid-base abnormalities are the result of pathophysiologic processes and are not unique disease entities. The differential diagnosis of any specific acid-base pattern begins with obtaining the patient's history and performing a physical examination. Common conditions and disease states associated with acid-base disturbances include metabolic acidosis (septic or cardiogenic shock, renal failure, diabetic ketoacidosis), metabolic alkalosis (diuretics, nasogastric suction, vomiting), respiratory acidosis (narcosis, neuromuscular blockade or profound weakness of respiratory muscles, chronic obstructive pulmonary disease), and respiratory alkalosis (hyperventilation).

Ventilation

Normal $Pa{CO_2}$ values range between 36 and 44 mm Hg. Production of CO_2 is relatively constant in most clinical settings, so the elimination of CO_2 is proportional to alveolar ventilation. As diagrammed in Figure 23-1, a $Pa{CO_2}$ below 36 mm Hg implies hyperventilation and a $Pa{CO_2}$ above 44 mm Hg implies hypoventilation, unless these situations occur as respiratory compensation for metabolic acid-base abnormalities.

When interpreting $Pa{CO_2}$, the initial question that the clinician should answer is whether this change in $Pa{CO_2}$ (from 40 mm Hg) accounts for the change in pH from 7.40. This effect can be estimated by employing the "golden rule" of ABG interpretation: For every 10-mm Hg change in $Pa{CO_2}$, the pH will change 0.08 unit in the opposite direction.

If the change in pH can be accounted for by the change in $Pa{CO_2}$, then the abnormality causing the change in $Pa{CO_2}$ is a primary respiratory disturbance.

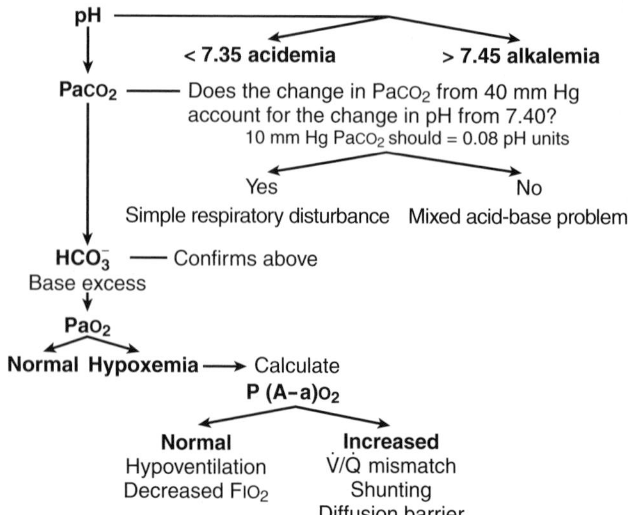

Figure 23-1 An algorithm for blood gas interpretation. $F{IO_2}$, Fractional content of inspired O_2; $\dot{V}/\dot{Q}$, ventilation/perfusion.

If not, then a metabolic acid-base disturbance or, more commonly, a mixed metabolic-respiratory acid-base abnormality accounts for the change.

Oxygenation

The PaO_2 depends on inspired O_2 concentration, alveolar ventilation, mixed venous O_2 saturation, and ventilation/perfusion matching ($\dot{V}/\dot{Q}$). The lung is not a perfect gas-exchange unit, and, to the extent that ventilation and perfusion are not matched, a gradient between the alveolar and the arterial PO_2 exists [$P(A-a)O_2$]. Abnormalities in lung function increase this gradient and produce hypoxemia.

When interpreting the PaO_2, the clinician's first step is to determine if hypoxemia is present. In most patients, hypoxemia would be considered to be a PaO_2 below 60 mm Hg because, below this level, the oxyhemoglobin dissociation curve is steep and the O_2 content of the blood drops rapidly with small decreases in the PaO_2. If hypoxemia is present, then knowing the [$P(A-a)O_2$] helps the clinician determine the severity of the disturbance. The PaO_2 is measured and the PAO_2 is calculated as:

$$PAO_2 = FIO_2\ (PB - PH_2O) - \frac{PaCO_2}{R}$$

Simplified for clinical use, this equation reads as follows:

$$PAO_2 = (FIO_2 \times 713) - (PaCO_2 \times 1.25)$$

where FIO_2 is the fractional content of inspired O_2; PB, the barometric pressure; PH_2O, the vapor pressure of water in alveoli at 37° C (47 mm Hg); and R, the respiratory quotient (CO_2 production/O_2 consumption = 0.8). PaO_2 and $PaCO_2$ are determined from ABG analysis.

If the $P(A-a)O_2$ gradient is normal, (i.e., ≤ 20), then the hypoxemia must be the result of hypoventilation or decreased FIO_2 concentration. If the $P(A-a)O_2$ gradient is increased, then the hypoxemia is the results of a $\dot{V}/\dot{Q}$ mismatch, shunting, or, rarely, a diffusion barrier (see Figure 23-1).

Finally, O_2 saturation should be assessed relative to the PaO_2 expected for a normal oxyhemoglobin dissociation curve. If the measured O_2 saturation is less than expected for the PaO_2, then other hemoglobin abnormalities (such as carboxyhemoglobin, methemoglobin, or sulfhemoglobin) must be present. Modern co-oximeters are designed to measure all of these values.

Case Examples

Acute Respiratory Acidosis—Buffering

A 38-year-old woman comes to the operating room for repair of perineal lacerations sustained during a recent vaginal delivery. A spinal anesthetic is placed, and 10 min later, the patient complains of respiratory difficulty and arm weakness. An ABG analysis obtained with the patient receiving supplemental O_2 via nasal cannula reveals the following: PaO_2, 98 mm Hg; $PaCO_2$, 70 mm Hg; pH, 7.16; and HCO_3^-, 26 mmol/L.

Interpretation Algorithm

The pH is in the acidemic range. The $PaCO_2$ varies from normal $PaCO_2$ (40 mm Hg) by 30. An estimate of the respiratory component to acidosis can be calculated as the variance from normal $PaCO_2$ (i.e., 30) divided by 10 and then multiplied by 0.08 pH units (remember the golden rule). The result of this calculation is a pH that is 0.24 below normal. The measured pH of 7.16 corresponds exactly with this calculation, indicating a simple acute respiratory acidosis. The interpretation of this ABG is acute respiratory acidosis due to impaired ventilation, most likely the result of a high spinal anesthetic. The process is so acute that no compensation by retention of bicarbonate could occur and only buffering has taken place. The $P(A-a)O_2$ gradient is calculated by estimating the FIO_2 to be 27% with an O_2 flow of 2 L/min. The PAO_2 equals (0.27 × 713) minus 70/0.8, or 193 – 88, or 105 mm Hg, which calculates to a $P(a-a)O_2$ gradient of 7 mm Hg. The measured PaO_2 of 98 mm Hg implies normal oxygenation in the setting of significant CO_2 retention due to hypoventilation.

Chronic Metabolic Acidosis—Compensation

A woman on chronic hemodialysis sustains a femur fracture in a motor vehicle crash but has no other apparent injuries. Her extremity is dusky below the fracture. The patient is brought to the operating room immediately for open reduction and fixation. She appears to be breathing deeply during induction of anesthesia. After the patient is draped, an ABG sample obtained while she is breathing 50% O_2 reveals a PaO_2 of 266 mm Hg; $PaCO_2$, 32 mm Hg; pH, 7.17; and HCO_3^-, 12 mmol/L.

Interpretation Algorithm

The pH is in the acidemic range. The $PaCO_2$ is below normal, so this is a metabolic acidosis and probably a mixed disorder, based on the history. According to Winters formula defining the confidence interval for expected respiratory compensation for chronic metabolic acidosis ($PaCO_2 = [1.5 \times HCO_3^-] + 8 \pm 2$), the expected $PaCO_2$ is 1.5 + 12 + 8, or 26, whereas the measured $PaCO_2$ is 32, so we have a mixed metabolic-respiratory acidosis due to chronic renal failure and less-than-expected respiratory compensation due to general anesthesia. The $P(A-a)O_2$ gradient is calculated as PAO_2 = (0.5 × 713) – 32/0.8 (356 – 40), or 316 mm Hg. The measured PaO_2 is 266 mm Hg, implying $\dot{V}/\dot{Q}$ mismatch in the setting of chronic renal failure, recent trauma, and general anesthesia.

Carbon Monoxide Exposure—Correction

The first patient anesthetized in an operating room on a Monday morning is preoxygenated for 2 min, anesthesia is induced with intravenously administered medications and then maintained on desflurane and a mixture of N_2O and O_2. Fifteen minutes into the case, the patient's pulse has increased by 40 beats/min, and respirations have increased by 10/min. Pulse oximetry reveals an SpO_2 of 88%. An ABG measurement shows a $PaCO_2$ of 155 mm Hg; PCO_2, 33 mm Hg; pH, 7.25; HCO_3^-, 20 mmol/L; O_2 saturation, 55%; and carboxyhemoglobin concentration, 45%. A presumptive diagnosis is made of carbon monoxide poisoning due to production of carbon monoxide by exposure of dry sodalime to desflurane. The operation is canceled, and the patient is transferred to the intensive care unit breathing 95% O_2. Four hours later, an ABG analysis reveals PaO_2, 550 mm Hg; PCO_2, 39 mm Hg; pH, 7.38; HCO_3^-, 24 mmol/L; and carboxyhemoglobin concentration, 3.2%.

Interpretation Algorithm

Carbon monoxide avidly binds to hemoglobin, interfering with O_2 binding and delivery, and thereby interfering with aerobic cellular metabolism. A rare cause of this problem is the interaction of several inhalation anesthetic agents with desiccated sodalime.

The initial ABG sample shows a significant metabolic acidosis and normal PaO_2, with a critically elevated carboxyhemoglobin level consistent with severe carbon monoxide poisoning. The elimination half-life of carbon monoxide in a person breathing 100% O_2 is approximately 1 hour and results in complete correction of the acid-base disorder with normalization of O_2-carrying capacity.

Suggested Readings

Hemmila MR, Napolitano LM. Severe respiratory failure: Advanced treatment options. *Crit Care Med.* 2006;34:S278-290.

Keijzer C, Perez RS, De Lange JJ. Carbon monoxide production from five volatile anesthetics in dry sodalime in a patient model: Halothane and sevoflurane do produce carbon monoxide; temperature is a poor predictor of carbon monoxide production. *BMC Anesthesiol.* 2005;5:6.

Khamiees M, Raju P, DeGirolamo A, et al. Predictors of extubation outcome in patients who have successfully completed a spontaneous breathing trial. *Chest.* 2001;120:1262-1270.

Morris CG, Low J. Metabolic acidosis in the critically ill: Part 2. Causes and treatment. *Anaesthesia.* 2008;63:396-411.

CHAPTER 24

Blood Gas Temperature Correction

John M. VanErdewyk, MD

The values of arterial CO_2 tension ($Paco_2$), arterial O_2 tension (Pao_2), and pH are highly dependent on temperature. Most blood gas analysis machines are calibrated to 37° C and, thus, run samples at 37° C. If the patient's actual temperature is near 37° C, then the machine values are approximately the same as those of the patient in vivo. However, the further the patient's temperature is from 37° C, the greater the difference between the numbers reported by the machine and the patient's actual values.

When the sample is analyzed, it is heated to 37° C, which causes a decrease in the solubility and falsely elevates partial-pressure values. Conversely, if the temperature of the blood decreases, the solubility of O_2 and CO_2 increases, which consequently lowers the partial pressures of these gases (i.e., decreases Po_2 and Pco_2). Pco_2 decreases by approximately 4.5% for each 1° C temperature decrease (Table 24-1). Therefore, temperature correction—the process of correcting the machine values to the patient values in vivo at the patient's actual temperature—is needed to determine the patient's actual partial pressures of Po_2 and Pco_2. Changes in temperature also affect pH. As temperature decreases, less water is dissociated into OH^- and H^+, and, thus, pH will rise, as will the pOH. The pH rises approximately 0.015 unit for each 1° C decrease in temperature. If the patient's temperature is less than 37° C, but the blood sample is subsequently heated to 37° C in the analyzer, then elevated levels of H^+ (and OH^-) will be recorded, leading to a falsely decreased pH value compared with the patient's actual pH.

pH-Stat Versus α-Stat Method

Two major approaches have been proposed to handle the management of blood gases during cardiopulmonary bypass–induced hypothermia.

The pH-Stat Method

In the pH-stat approach, which was used almost exclusively for the first several decades of cardiopulmonary bypass, CO_2 is added to the inspired gases in an attempt to keep the temperature-corrected $Paco_2$ normal at 40 mm Hg and the pH normal at 7.4 or greater. The goal of this method is to maintain a constant pH despite varying patient temperatures. Because, during cardiopulmonary bypass using hypothermia, the patient's temperature is much lower than 37° C, a temperature-corrected system would produce a decreased $Paco_2$ and an elevated pH in vivo.

The α-Stat Method

In the early 1980s, many physicians began using the α-stat system to manage patient care because of its potential theoretic benefits, despite a lack of randomized trials or clinical outcome studies. The goal of this approach is to keep a constant ionic charge on amino acids in proteins, principally the α-imidazole ring of histidine, which functions as an important pH buffer in hemoglobin and other body proteins. The ratio (α) of dissociated to undissociated imidazole groups stays constant (α-stat) with cooling because of changes of blood pH when CO_2 content is held constant. Constant imidazole ionization makes optimal enzyme function possible. As the patient cools, pH must rise because less H^+ is dissociated. However, equally less OH^- is available, and, therefore, electrochemical neutrality is maintained. Proponents argue that the α-stat method keeps a patient's uncorrected $Paco_2$ and pH at normal levels, as this method preserves more physiologic values by maintaining electrochemical neutrality despite varying body temperature. Temperature correction of blood gases is therefore unnecessary.

Comparison of the Two Systems

Patients managed by the pH-stat approach would be considered hypercarbic and have a lower pH (i.e., a respiratory acidosis) by the α-stat approach, and α-stat management would be considered a relative respiratory alkalosis by the pH-stat system (Table 24-2). The blood of cold-blooded animals (ectotherms) undergoes pH changes during cooling, parallel to the changes that water undergoes (α-stat). On the other hand, homeothermic mammals, in effect, have "corrected" blood gases during hibernation, and their decreased metabolic function produces anesthetic effects.

Some controversy exists as to whether the α-stat or the pH-stat method yields better patient outcomes. Concerns exist with either system as to how the fluctuating pH and Pco_2 levels affect cerebral and cardiac function. Very few outcome studies exist in the literature, however, and those that do exist have failed to demonstrate any important differences in outcome of these regimens.

Table 24-1 Effects of Hypothermia on Pco_2, Po_2, and pH

Parameter	Effect of Hypothermia	Effect/Change in Temperature
Pco_2	↓	4.5%/° C
Po_2	↓	4.5%/° C
pH	↑	0.015 unit/° C

Table 24-2 Effects of Temperature Correction

Parameter	pH-Stat as Viewed by α-Stat	α-Stat as Viewed by pH-Stat
CO_2	↑	↓
pH	↓	↑
Condition	Respiratory acidosis	Respiratory alkalosis

Suggested Readings

Griffin DA. Blood gas strategies and management during pediatric cardiopulmonary bypass. *ASAIO J*. 2005;51:657-658.

Hoover LR, Dinavahi R, Cheng WP, et al. Jugular venous oxygenation during hypothermic cardiopulmonary bypass in patients at risk for abnormal cerebral autoregulation: Influence of alpha-stat versus pH-stat blood gas management. *Anesth Analg*. 2009;108:1389-1393.

Kiziltan HT, Baltali M, Bilen A, et al. Comparison of alpha-stat and pH-stat cardiopulmonary bypass in relation to jugular venous oxygen saturation and cerebral glucose-oxygen utilization. *Anesth Analg*. 2003;96:644-650.

Kollmar R, Georgiadis D, Schwab S. Alpha-stat versus pH-stat guided ventilation in patients with large ischemic stroke treated by hypothermia. *Neurocrit Care*. 2009;10:173-180.

Murkin JM. Cerebral autoregulation: The role of CO_2 in metabolic homeostasis. *Semin Cardiothorac Vasc Anesth*. 2007;11:269-273.

CHAPTER 25

Central Regulation of Ventilation

Michael P. Hosking, MD

Ventilation is regulated to maintain optimal and unchanging levels of pH, CO_2, and O_2 in the blood. This regulation is provided via the respiratory center, which receives afferent input from chemical stimuli and peripheral chemoreceptors. The respiratory center is composed of a group of nuclei in four major areas within the medulla and pons (Table 25-1).

Neural Control

Inspiratory Center

The inspiratory center, the site of basic respiratory drive, located dorsally in the medulla, extends the full length of the medulla (Figure 25-1). The neurons within the inspiratory center are located near the termination sites of afferent fibers from the glossopharyngeal (IX) and vagus (X) nerves. These neurons have intrinsic automaticity and normally fire for 2 sec, with a ramp effect of increasing efferent activity to the diaphragm until it abruptly ceases with a 3-sec pause before initiating a new cycle.

Pneumotaxic Center

Located in the pons, the pneumotaxic center continually communicates signals to the inspiratory center to turn off inspiration (see Figure 25-1). A strong signal results in a short (0.5-sec to 1-sec) inspiratory cycle and, consequently, a more rapid respiratory rate.

Expiratory Center

The expiratory center extends the full length of the ventral medulla and stimulates the muscles of expiration (see Figure 25-1) but is normally quiescent because expiration is a passive process. With increased demand, the expiratory center sends efferent signals and stimulates the muscles of expiration (see Figure 25-1).

Apneustic Center

The apneustic center is located in the lower pons. Its role is to antagonize the effects of the pneumotaxic center, and it plays no role in normal respiration.

Table 25-1 Neurons within the Medulla and Pons That Constitute the Respiratory Center

Center	Location	Nuclei	Function
Dorsal respiratory (inspiratory center)	Dorsal portion of the medulla	Nucleus tractus solitarius	Results in inspiration when stimulated
Pneumotaxic center	Upper portion of the pons	Nucleus parabrachialis	Controls rate and pattern of breathing; limits inspiration
Ventral respiratory group (expiratory center)	Anterolateral portion of the medulla (~5 mm anterior and lateral to dorsal respiratory group)	Nucleus ambiguus and nucleus retroambiguus	Primarily causes expiration; depending upon which neurons are stimulated, can cause expiration or inspiration; transmits inhibitory impulses to the apneustic center
Apneustic center	Lower portion of the pons		Discharges stimulatory impulses to the inspiratory center, resulting in inspiration; receives inhibitory impulses from the pneumotaxic center and from stretch receptors of lung; discharges inhibitory impulses to the expiratory center

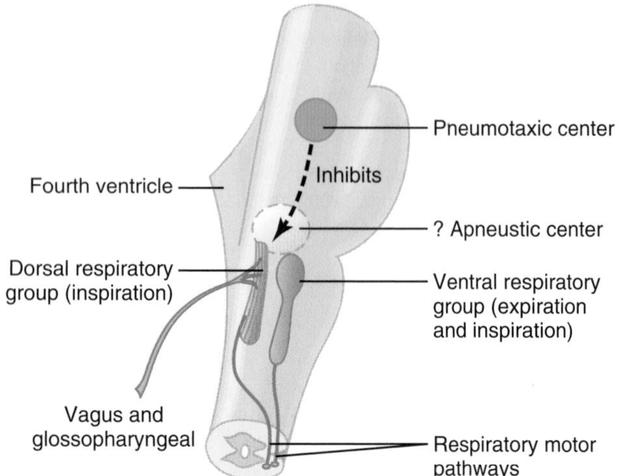

Figure 25-1 Organization of the respiratory center. (From Guyton AC, Hall JE. Textbook of Medical Physiology. 11th ed. Philadelphia: Elsevier Saunders; 2005:515, F41-1.)

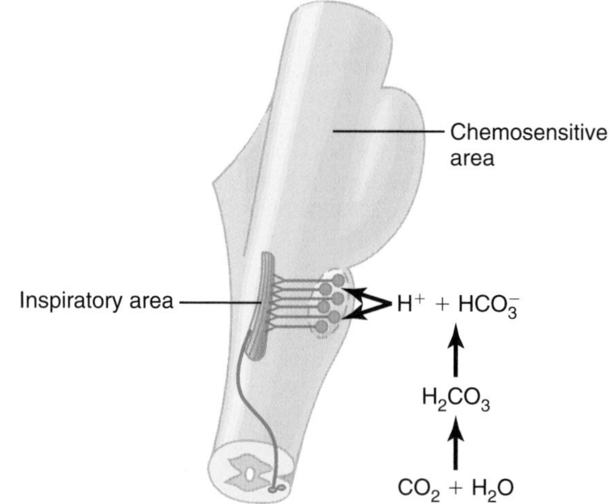

Figure 25-3 Stimulation of the inspiratory area by the chemosensitive area located bilaterally in the medulla, only a few microns beneath the ventral medullary surface. Note also that H^+ ions stimulate the chemosensitive area, whereas mainly CO_2 in the fluid gives rise to the H^+ ions. (From Guyton AC, Hall JE. Textbook of Medical Physiology. 11th ed. Philadelphia: Elsevier Saunders; 2005:516, F41-2.)

In the Hering-Breuer reflex, bronchiolar stretch receptors feed back to the inspiratory center via the vagus nerve to limit lung overexpansion. This reflex plays a minimal role in normal ventilation but becomes active when tidal volume exceeds 1.5 L (Figure 25-2).

Chemical Control

Central

The chemosensitive area is located bilaterally in the medulla several microns beneath the ventral surface (Figure 25-3). This area is extremely sensitive to hydrogen ions (H^+). However, H^+ cross the blood-brain barrier poorly, and thus, CO_2 indirectly controls this region through formation of carbonic acid with dissociation to H^+. When stimulated, this chemosensitive area then stimulates the inspiratory center to increase the rate of rise of the ramp effect and, thus, increases the rate of respiration.

$$CO_2 + H_2O \rightarrow H_2CO_3 \rightarrow H^+ + HCO_3^-$$

Therefore, $Paco_2$ indirectly influences the level of H^+ in cerebrospinal fluid and controls respiratory drive. Peak effect is reached within 1 min. The effect begins to wane over the next several hours, and, by 48 h, is only one eighth the peak effect. Compensation is secondary to increased active transport of HCO_3^- into the cerebrospinal fluid to neutralize the increased H^+.

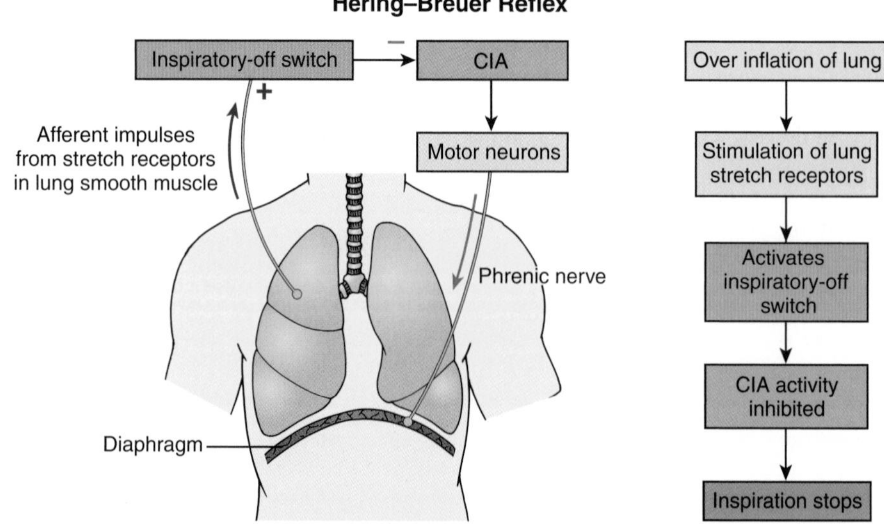

Figure 25-2 The Hering-Breuer inflation reflex is triggered to prevent overinflation of the lungs. Stretch receptors present in airway smooth muscle respond to excessive stretching of the lung during large inspirations. When these receptors are activated, they send action potentials through the vagus nerves to the inspiratory and apneustic areas, directly inhibiting the inspiratory area and inhibiting the apneustic area via activation of the inspiratory area, thus stopping inspiration and allowing expiration to occur. CIA, Central inspiratory activity.

Peripheral

Peripheral chemoreceptors are located in the carotid bodies (cranial nerve IX) and aortic bodies (cranial nerve X). These areas of high blood flow are sensitive to changes in O_2, CO_2, and pH. They stimulate the inspiratory center when Pao_2 decreases; the effect is greatest between 30 and 60 mm Hg (Figure 25-4).

If the mean arterial blood pressure drops below 70 mm Hg, respiratory drive increases. The effect of peripheral chemoreceptors in response to hypoxia is eliminated by as little as 0.1 minimum alveolar concentration of a volatile anesthetic agent, which may be critical in patients with chronic obstructive lung disease who are dependent on hypoxic respiratory drive. Loss of the carotid body, as may occur with carotid endarterectomy, decreases response to hypoxia, a 30% decrease in responsiveness to changes in $Paco_2$, and no change in the resting level of respiration.

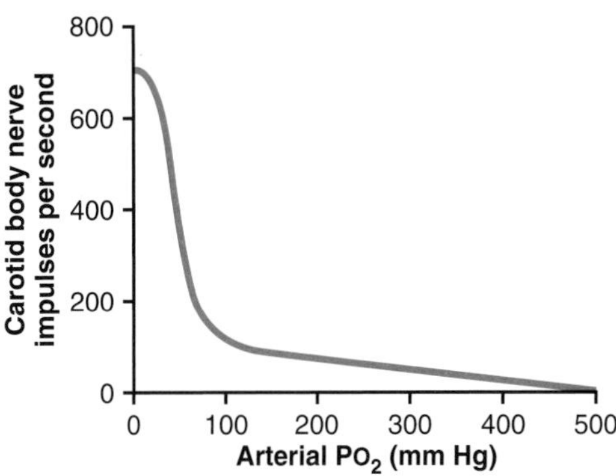

Figure 25-4 The effect of arterial Po_2 on impulse rate from the carotid body of a cat. (From Guyton AC, Hall JE. Textbook of Medical Physiology. 11th ed. Philadelphia, Elsevier Saunders, 2005:518, F41-5.)

Suggested Readings

Guyton AC, Hall JE. *Textbook of Medical Physiology*. 11th ed. Philadelphia: Elsevier Saunders; 2005.

West JB. *Respiratory Physiology: The Essentials*. 8th ed. Philadelphia: Lippincott, Williams & Wilkins; 2008.

CHAPTER 26

Physiologic Effects of Hypercarbia and Hypocarbia

Douglas A. Dubbink, MD

Hypercarbia exists when the $Paco_2$ exceeds 45 mm Hg; hypocarbia is present when the $Paco_2$ is below 35 mm Hg.

CO_2 Transport

CO_2 is transported in blood from the cells, where it is produced, to the lungs, where it is excreted through an ingenious transport system. Between 70% and 90% of total CO_2 is in plasma in the form of bicarbonate. Bicarbonate is synthesized primarily in erythrocytes in peripheral tissue beds through the following reaction:

$$CO_2 + H_2O \xleftrightarrow[\text{anhydrase}]{\text{carbonic}} H_2CO_3 \leftrightarrow H^+ + HCO_3^-$$

Between 5% and 10% of CO_2 is bound to the terminal amino groups of blood proteins and transported by these carbamino compounds. The remaining 5% to 10% of CO_2 is physically dissolved in the plasma and is delivered to the lungs for excretion.

Effects of CO_2 Changes on Various Organ Systems

Central Nervous System

Within the $Paco_2$ range of 20 to 80 mm Hg, for each 1-mm Hg increase of CO_2, cerebral blood flow (CBF) increases 1.8 $mL \cdot 100g^{-1} \cdot min^{-1}$ and cerebral blood volume increases 0.04 mL/100 g (Figure 26-1). CO_2 vasoactivity occurs in response to changes in local H^+ concentration in the smooth muscle

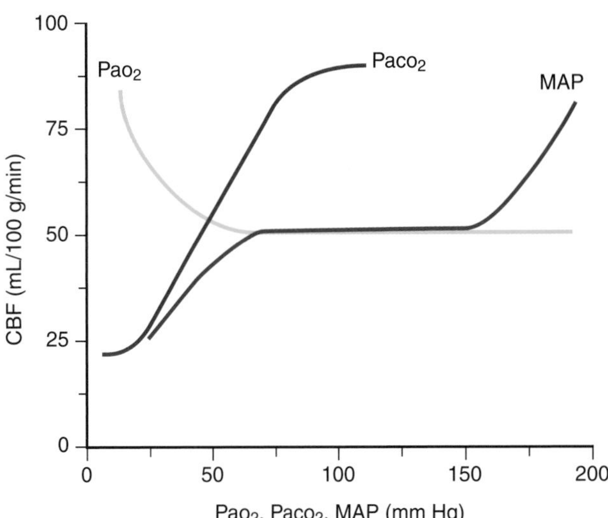

Figure 26-1 Changes in cerebral blood flow (CBF) caused by independent alterations in $Paco_2$, Pao_2, and mean arterial pressure (MAP). (Reprinted from Patel PM, Drummond JA. Cerebral physiology and the effects of anesthetic drugs. In: Miller RD, Eriksson LI, Fleisher LA, et al, eds. Miller's Anesthesia. 7th ed. Philadelphia: Churchill Livingstone; 2009.)

cells of the arteriolar walls on the brain side of the blood-brain barrier (BBB). HCO_3^- does not cross the BBB, but CO_2 does; when CO_2 crosses the BBB, carbonic acid (H_2CO_3) is formed, which dissociates to HCO_3^- and H^+, resulting in a decreased pH of the periarteriolar cerebrospinal fluid. Nitric oxide and prostaglandins (PGI_2) are the primary mediators of CO_2-induced vasodilation. Vasodilation occurs within 20 to 30 sec of a change in $Paco_2$. The pH of cerebrospinal fluid normalizes over about 6 to 8 h through active changes in HCO_3^- concentration, limiting the utility of hyperventilation in treating increased intracranial pressure. The CO_2 response in gray matter exceeds that in white matter because of the greater vascular density in gray matter. Hypercarbia has the greatest effect on vessels less than 100 μm in diameter.

Pathologic states may decrease the response to CO_2; for example, 12 min of global ischemia, BBB disruption (e.g., due to trauma), and severe transient focal ischemia abolish CO_2 responsiveness for approximately 24 h. Narcosis occurs in humans when the $Paco_2$ exceeds 90 mm Hg, but the set point is lowered by the use of opioids, benzodiazepines, and other drugs.

If the $Paco_2$ drops below 20 to 30 mm Hg, vasoconstriction leads to ischemia, manifested by confusion and electroencephalographic slowing. Hypocarbia secondary to hyperventilation can lead to lightheadedness, dizziness, visual disturbances, and, possibly, hypocalcemia due to increased calcium binding by albumin because of respiratory alkalosis (see Chapter 70, Effects of pKa, pH, and Protein Binding).

Respiratory System

The maximal stimulation of minute ventilation occurs at a $Paco_2$ of about 100 mm Hg. Any further increase in $Paco_2$ results in ventilatory depression. Hypercarbia increases pulmonary vascular resistance, and the resulting respiratory acidosis augments hypoxic pulmonary vasoconstriction. Hypocarbia inhibits hypoxic pulmonary vasoconstriction and causes bronchoconstriction and decreased lung compliance. Many anesthetic agents depress the response of the respiratory center to CO_2.

Cardiovascular System

The effects of hypercarbia on the cardiovascular system result from alterations in the balance between the direct depressant effects of CO_2 and increased sympathetic nervous system (SNS) activity. As CO_2 rises, blood pressure and cardiac output usually increase in awake and in anesthetized patients. At very high levels (80-90 mm Hg), however, hypercarbia causes a reduction in cardiac output, blood pressure, and heart rate, with resultant cardiovascular collapse.

Arrhythmias may be associated with hypercarbia, especially during administration of halothane because halothane sensitizes the myocardium to the effects of epinephrine, which will be increased through activation of the SNS by the hypercarbia.

Hypocarbia can cause decreased cardiac output by several mechanisms. During positive pressure ventilation, if minute ventilation is increased by increasing tidal volume to at least 10 to 20 mL/kg, venous return may be decreased. Vasoconstriction in the central nervous system depresses SNS activity, which leads to a decreased inotropic state. Respiratory alkalosis secondary to hypocarbia reduces ionized calcium, which also decreases the inotropic state.

Gastrointestinal System

In awake patients, hypercarbia (respiratory acidosis) increases hepatic and portal venous blood flow; conversely, hypocarbia (respiratory alkalosis) decreases hepatic and portal venous blood flow. If the SNS is not completely suppressed during general anesthesia, increasing $Paco_2$ levels will lead to splanchnic vasoconstriction and decreased hepatic blood flow. With significant SNS suppression, as would occur during deep anesthesia, increased $Paco_2$ levels result in increased hepatic blood flow because of vasodilation.

Renal System

Chronic hypercarbia results in renal retention of HCO_3^- and a compensatory metabolic alkalosis. Chronic hypocarbia results in HCO_3^- wasting by the kidney and a compensatory metabolic acidosis.

Box 26-1 Signs That May Be Present in Patients with Hypercarbia

Cardiac arrhythmias, especially ventricular extrasystoles or tachycardia
Coma
Flushed skin
Hypertension*
↓ Respiratory rate
↓ Tidal volume

*When hypertension is unexplained, increased $Paco_2$ should always be considered.

Metabolic

As $Paco_2$ rises, plasma levels of epinephrine and norepinephrine increase. Hypercarbia and respiratory acidosis result in an increased transfer of K^+ from cells into the plasma. Reuptake of K^+ by cells is slow, and repeated episodes of hypercarbia can cause a stepwise increase in plasma K^+.

Pharmacologic Effects of CO_2 Changes

Hypercarbia and respiratory acidosis can affect the pharmacokinetics of many anesthetic agents. For example, it is the nonionized form of local anesthetic agents that readily cross cell membranes. Because local anesthetic agents are weak bases, in the presence of acidemia, the relative amount of nonionized drug will decrease, resulting in less transport across cell membranes and decreased activity. An increased $Paco_2$ level shifts the O_2 dissociation curve to the right, resulting in less O_2 availability in the periphery. A decreased $Paco_2$ has the opposite effect.

Effects of CO_2 Changes on Minimum Alveolar Concentration

There is no difference in the MAC (minimum alveolar concentration) for any of the inhalation anesthetic agents between $Paco_2$ levels of 20 and 100 mm Hg. Anesthesia can be achieved with very high levels of CO_2. A $Paco_2$ of 245 mm Hg produces about 1.0 MAC anesthesia.

Signs and Symptoms

There are no absolute diagnostic signs of hypercarbia, but several clues may be present (Box 26-1). Clinical signs are not consistently present; therefore, arterial blood gas analysis or respiratory gas monitoring is often required to make the diagnosis.

Suggested Readings

Adrogué HJ, Madias NE. Secondary responses to altered acid-base status: The rules of engagement. *J Am Soc Nephrol*. 2010;21:920-923.

Azzam ZS, Sharabi K, Guetta J, et al. The physiological and molecular effects of elevated CO_2 levels. *Cell Cycle*. 2010;9(8):1528-1532.

Brian, JE. Carbon dioxide and the cerebral circulation. *Anesthesiology*. 1998;88: 1365-1386.

Curley G, Laffey JG, Kavanagh BP. Bench-to-bedside review: Carbon dioxide. *Crit Care*. 2010;14:220.

Dorrington KL, Balanos GM, Talbot NP, Robbins PA. Extent to which pulmonary vascular responses to Pco_2 and Po_2 play a functional role within the healthy human lung. *J Appl Physiol*. 2010;108:1084-1096.

Fencl V, Jabor A, Kazda A, Figge J. Diagnosis of metabolic acid-base disturbances in critically ill patients. *Am J Respir Crit Care Med*. 2000;162:2246-2251.

Lumb AB, ed. *Nunn's Applied Respiratory Physiology*. 6th ed. Philadelphia: Elsevier/ Butterworth Heinemann; 2005.

Michenfelder JD. *Anesthesia and the Brain*. New York: Churchill Livingstone; 1988.

O'Croinin D, Ni Chonghaile M, Higgins B, Laffey JG. Bench-to-bedside review: Permissive hypercapnia. *Crit Care*. 2005;9:51-59.

Ogoh S, Nakahara H, Ainslie PN, Miyamoto T. The effect of oxygen on dynamic cerebral autoregulation: Critical role of hypocapnia. *J Appl Physiol*. 2010;108: 538-543.

CHAPTER 27

Surfactant and Lung Mechanics in Health and Disease

James P. Conterato, MD

Surfactant Production and Composition

Pulmonary surfactant is a phospholipid-protein mixture secreted by type II pneumocytes that acts to stabilize alveolar structure via reducing the surface tension inherent at air-water interfaces, thus preventing alveolar and distal airway collapse during end expiration. Additionally, this compound functions to incite immune responses to inhaled pathogens.

Production of Surfactant

Lung tissue first develops in the fetus off the esophagus during the first trimester to give rise to conducting airways, with the canalicular stage occurring between 16 and 34 weeks. As this process progresses under the influence of the hypothalamic-pituitary-adrenal axis (cortisol, thyroxine, and retinoic acid), type II pneumocytes develop and initiate secretion of surfactant by 34 weeks. This process can be accelerated by the administration of steroids. Numerous insults, such as inflammatory atelectasis, toxin exposure, infection, and oxygen toxicity, can all markedly diminish surfactant production, impairing alveolar and airway stability and pulmonary gas exchange, and can, over the long term, lead to restrictive lung disease.

Composition of Surfactant

Surfactant is produced within organelles of type II pneumocytes that are known as lamellar bodies. These bodies consist of whorls of phospholipids, specialized surfactant proteins (SP-A, SP-B, SP-C, SP-D), and calcium (as a cofactor). The phospholipid is mainly dipalmitoylphosphatidylcholine (DPPC). It is an amphipathic molecule that orients at air-water interfaces (e.g., the alveolar surface) with the hydrophobic (lipid) ends exposed to air and the hydrophilic (phosphate) ends immersed in water. Aided by SP-B and SP-C proteins, which are also amphipathic, a phospholipid monolayer forms spontaneously along the alveolar surface at the air-water interface. Congenital deficiency of SP-B results in fatal postnatal respiratory distress, whereas congenital SP-C deficiency is associated with familial interstitial pulmonary fibrosis. SP-A and SP-D are hydrophilic proteins belonging to the collectin family of host-defense proteins. They bind microorganisms and modulate leukocyte chemotaxis, cytokine function, and phagocytosis.

The lamellar bodies are secreted by type II pneumocytes into the alveolar space by exocytosis. Initially, the extrusions are in the form of bundles of tubular myelin, which then reorient into the phospholipid monolayer film. Under normal circumstances, some of the phospholipid-surfactant protein complex undergoes reuptake by these cells and is recycled under the influence of SP-D.

Physics of Surfactant

Under normal circumstances, water molecules exert strong interattractive forces. (This is what holds a raindrop together.) The effect of an air-water interface on a sphere that it covers (alveolus) is described by the law of Laplace, which states:

$$P \sim 2T/r$$

where P equals the net pressure exerted on the sphere; T, the surface tension; and r, the radius of the sphere.

In simple terms, the strong attraction that water molecules lining the alveolus exert on one another (surface tension) produces a positive pressure on the alveolus that is inversely proportional to its radius. So, as its radius decreases (exhalation), the alveolus experiences an increasingly positive pressure that will cause complete collapse unless the surface tension acting on the alveolus decreases, which is what surfactant achieves via the properties of the phospholipid membrane. Alveolar fluid devoid of surfactant exerts a surface tension of approximately 50 dynes/cm^2. Alveolar fluid with normal surfactant content has a decreased surface tension, varying between 5 and 30 dynes/cm^2. Under normal conditions, the positive pressure exerted on an alveolus is approximately 3 mm Hg, which is easily resisted by the negative intrapleural pressure. However, without surfactant, this pressure can increase to over 18 mm Hg, leading to alveolar collapse and resistance to reexpansion (not enough negative suction to counteract the pressure developed by the air-water interface).

A similar mechanism exists for terminal airway patency (e.g., asthma). These distal airways are cylinders, and their correlation with the law of Laplace is:

$$P = T/r$$

As long as surface tension decreases more than the radius, the pressure will decrease and the surrounding airway and alveolar fluids will not be sucked into the narrowest part of the airway (terminal bronchioles). If surfactant is inadequate in supply or if inflammation is too great, the surface tension will not decrease, and surrounding surface fluids will redistribute from the wider airways into the narrowest, dropping the radius there further. This mechanism may be an integral component of airway collapse with an inflammatory process, such as asthma. Additionally, both β-adrenergic receptor agonists and glucocorticoids enhance secretion of surfactant, which may partially explain the benefit that these agents exert in reactive airway diseases.

Therapeutic Applications of Surfactant

Exogenous aerosolized preparations of surfactant have been employed therapeutically for certain acute lung diseases, some with more success than others. The sources of surfactant are both natural (animal-lung homogenates) and synthetic (DPPC mixed with chemicals that enhance adsorption and spreading but that are devoid of surfactant proteins).

Established roles have been demonstrated for surfactant in both neonatal respiratory distress syndrome (prophylactic and selective applications) and meconium aspiration. Less dramatic benefits have been observed with pediatric and adult forms of respiratory distress syndrome, but trials are ongoing.

Suggested Readings

Nkadi PO, Merritt TA, Pillers DA. An overview of pulmonary surfactant in the neonate: Genetics, metabolism, and the role of surfactant in health and disease. *Mol Genet Metab.* 2009;97:95-101.

Ochs M. The closer we look the more we see. Quantitative microscopic analysis of the pulmonary surfactant system. *Cell Physiol Biochem.* 2010;25:27-40.

Pfister RH, Soll R, Wiswell TE. Protein-containing synthetic surfactant versus protein-free synthetic surfactant for the prevention and treatment of respiratory distress syndrome. *Cochrane Database Syst Rev.* 2009:CD006180.

CHAPTER 28

Factors Affecting Pulmonary Compliance and Airway Resistance

H. Michael Marsh, MB, BS, and Michael L. Bishop, MD

In an open thorax, an isolated lung contracts, because of its elastic recoil, until, over time, all contained gas is expelled; conversely, the thoracic cage, freed from contact with the lung, expands, assuming a volume that, in the adult, reaches approximately 1 L more than functional residual capacity (FRC). In a closed thorax, the lung and thorax, which are now in contact, come to rest at FRC, as their resting shapes dictate. FRC is thus determined by the opposing elastic recoil of lung and chest wall and the resting tone of the respiratory muscles.

When at FRC, respiratory muscle activity is required to either increase or decrease the thoracic cage, with the lung itself passively following the changes in thoracic wall (to include the diaphragm) shape so engendered. However, (1) elastic forces in lung tissue and chest wall, (2) surface tension at the alveolar gas/liquid alveolar lining interface (3) frictional resistance to airway gas flow, (4) viscoelastic tissue resistance from deformation of thoracic tissues, and (5) inertia of gas and tissue movement combine to resist or impede and, thus, limit changes in chest wall shape and volume in response to muscle force. These five factors contributing to respiratory system impedance can be grouped as "elastic" resistance (factors 1 and 2) and "nonelastic" resistance (factors 3, 4, and 5).

Elastic Resistance and Pulmonary and Chest Wall Compliance

Elasticity is that passive property of tissue that causes a return to resting shape after deformation by an external force. Perfectly elastic tissues obey the Hooke law, such that 1 unit of applied force will result in 1 unit of stretch, 2 units of force, 2 units of stretch, and so on up to the elastic limit of the tissue. The slope of the line that results from plotting length (unit of stretch, volume) against force (unit of force, pressure) indicates the elasticity (stretchiness, compliance) of that tissue.

Thus, for the respiratory system, elastic recoil, or compliance after deformation, is defined as change in volume divided by change in pressure (L/cm H_2O). The system comprises the lung and the chest wall (thoracic wall and diaphragm), which both have about twice the compliance of the combined system. Thus, the normal value for lung compliance (C_L) is 0.2 L/cm H_2O, for chest wall compliance (C_{CW}) is 0.2 L/cm H_2O, and for respiratory system compliance (C_{RS}) is 0.1 L/cm H_2O.

Elastance is the reciprocal of compliance, and elastances of components can be summed.

Thus,

$$\frac{1}{C_{RS}} = \frac{1}{C_L} + \frac{1}{C_{CW}}$$

where the total respiratory system elastance equals the sum of the component lung and chest wall elastances.

Lung elastance and compliance are also influenced by the surface tension at the alveolar gas/liquid alveolar lining interface. Thus, the lung is *not* a perfectly elastic tissue and demonstrates both significant hysteresis (time-dependent elastic behavior) and volume-dependent changes in compliance. Lung hysteresis may be due to a variety of factors (Box 28-1).

Experiments have demonstrated that compliance varies with lung volume. Thus, compliance measurements must be interpreted with knowledge of the

Box 28-1 Factors That May Lead to Lung Hysteresis

Change in surfactant activity*
Stress relaxation
Gas redistribution between slow-filling and fast-filling alveoli
Alveolar recruitment, as closed alveoli open
Displacement of pulmonary blood volume

*The Laplace law may operate (see Chapter 27, Surfactant and Lung Mechanics in Health and Disease).

starting lung volume (usually FRC). For example, a lung compliance of 60% of normal does not indicate that the lungs are stiffer than normal unless the lung volume (FRC) is known to be normal. To address this problem, some investigators report specific compliance (compliance related to FRC).

Major Factors Affecting Pulmonary Compliance

The pressure in a bubble (or alveolus) is inversely proportional to the radius (Laplace's law). That is, a small bubble would empty into a larger one. Pulmonary surfactant increases compliance by altering surface tension relationships in the alveoli; surfactant decreases surface tension as alveoli decrease in size, allowing small alveoli to exist at the same pressure as larger alveoli. Pulmonary edema decreases compliance, perhaps by altering surfactant concentration or by changing alveolar geometry.

When pulmonary surfactant is damaged or removed, increased surface tension in smaller alveoli causes them to collapse. High pressure is needed to open and reexpand ("recruit") them.

Ascites, pleural effusion, pericardial effusion, and cardiomegaly all decrease compliance by decreasing FRC, among other mechanisms. Pleural, interstitial, and alveolar fibrosis all decrease compliance by decreasing the elastic properties of the lung tissue and decreasing FRC. Atelectasis and pneumonia decrease compliance secondary to decreased FRC and decreased surfactant.

Poliomyelitis and kyphoscoliosis decrease compliance secondary to decreased FRC. Pulmonary artery obstruction decreases compliance by decreasing FRC and pulmonary surfactant. General anesthesia decreases compliance by decreasing FRC.

Emphysema increases compliance secondary to loss of normal elastic recoil of the lungs. (Normal transpulmonary pressure results in an elevated FRC.) Normal to moderate obstructive or reactive airway disease increases compliance because FRC increases.

Major Factors Affecting Thoracic Cage Compliance

Kyphoscoliosis, pectus excavatum, arthritic spondylitis, skeletal muscle diseases resulting in rigidity or spasticity, abdominal disorders with marked diaphragmatic elevation, and marked obesity all decrease thoracic cage compliance.

Major Effects of Decreased Compliance

Decreased compliance results in increased work of breathing because higher pressures are needed to increase lung volume. Compensatory mechanisms to decrease the work of breathing include increased respiratory rate, decreased tidal volume, and breathing with pursed lips. Because the bronchi behave as Starling resistors, pursing the lips moves the equal pressure point away from the mouth toward the bronchi maintaining airway patency. However, no matter the effort, depending on how much C_{RS} is decreased, areas of the lung will collapse, leading to an increase in pulmonary shunt. And even in those areas in which patency is maintained, the compliance is not uniform throughout the lung, and thus alveolar ventilation is not distributed equally within the lung, leading to an increased ventilation/perfusion mismatch.

Nonelastic Resistance, Including Airway Resistance

The majority of nonelastic impedance to respiratory system motion is provided by frictional resistance to airway gas flow and by viscoelastic tissue resistance to deformation, with very small contributions from inertia of gas to change in flow and from tissue to change in shape. Inertia really becomes a factor only with very high frequency ventilation, whereas "airway resistance" and "tissue resistance" usually contribute about 50% each to "respiratory system" resistance, as usually measured. Airway resistance is the major modifiable factor in clinical situations; thus, viscoelastic "tissue resistance" will not be further discussed here.

Airway Resistance

Driving pressure is that pressure necessary to move air through the airways during inspiration and expiration. Driving pressure equals atmospheric pressure minus alveolar pressure during inspiration and alveolar pressure minus atmospheric pressure during expiration. Because pressure equals flow times resistance (Ohm's law), resistance equals driving pressure divided by flow. Airway resistance is created by friction between molecules of flowing gas and the airway walls; it is expressed in units of cm $H_2O \cdot L^{-1} \cdot sec^{-1}$.

For laminar gas flow, by Poiseuille's law, resistance equals $8\,l\eta/\pi r^4$, where l equals the length of the airway; η, the viscosity of the gas in poise; and r, the radius of the airway. Thus, resistance to flow is affected most significantly by the radius of the airway. Reducing the radius by 50% increases resistance sixteenfold (i.e., 2^4). Anesthesia may directly affect the size of small airways.

Resistance is also dependent on the nature of the gas flow. With laminar flow, pressure is proportional to the volume of gas flow times a constant related to gas viscosity. However, with turbulent flow, pressure is proportional to the volume of the gas flow squared times a constant related to gas density. Assuming constant flow, according to Ohm's law, resistance with turbulent flow exceeds that during laminar flow. Turbulence occurs at airway branch points and with irregularities in the walls of the airways (e.g., mucus, exudates, tumor, foreign body, and partial glottic closure). In normal lungs, most airway resistance occurs in the large lobar bronchi and diminishes progressively as gas moves peripherally because of progressively increased total airway area with resultant decreased flow velocity. Resistance is minimal in peripheral respiratory bronchioles. Thus, large changes can occur in the diameter of peripheral bronchioles before changes occur in measured airway resistance. Normal adult airway resistance is 0.5 to 1.5 cm $H_2O \cdot L^{-1} \cdot sec^{-1}$.

Major Factors Affecting Airway Resistance

Airway resistance decreases with increased lung volume as the elastic tissues of the lung increase airway diameter. Bronchospasm and airway secretions associated with asthma result in increased airway resistance, thereby facilitating turbulent flow. Emphysema causes increased resistance because airways tend to collapse. In addition, as patients with emphysema attempt to overcome the increased resistance with forced expiration, the positive intrapleural pressure developed tends to collapse airways further.

Airway resistance is increased by other causes of decreased airway lumen size, including mucosal congestion, edema, inflammation, pneumothorax, presence of exudates or foreign bodies, compression, and fibrosis. Iatrogenic causes of increased resistance include long narrow tracheal tubes.

Major Effects of Increased Airway Resistance

Increased resistance increases the time needed to complete exhalation. This results in increased FRC (gas trapping) if the respiratory rate is kept constant. To compensate, patients may depend on active exhalation, which increases the work of breathing. In chemically paralyzed patients who are unable to actively exhale, gas trapping may severely decrease cardiac output by both decreasing preload to both ventricles and increasing afterload in both ventricles.

In an attempt to decrease airway resistance, patients may decrease their rate of breathing to allow decreased flow velocity. They may also exhale against pursed lips to decrease the pressure gradient within the tracheobronchial tree. Pursing the lips, as mentioned previously, moves the equal pressure point proximally in the airways, thus keeping them slightly more open.

Suggested Readings

Lumb AB, ed. *Nunn's Applied Respiratory Physiology*. 5th ed. Boston: Heinemann-Butterworth; 2000.

Rehder K, Marsh HM. Respiratory mechanics during anesthesia and mechanical ventilation. In: Geiger SR, ed. *Handbook of Physiology—The Respiratory System III*. Bethesda, MD, The American Physiological Society. 1986:737-752.

Satoh J-I, Yamakage M, Kobayashi T, et al. Desflurane but not sevoflurane can increase lung resistance via tachykinin pathways. *Br J Anaesth*. 2009;102:704.

CHAPTER 29

Pulmonary Ventilation and Perfusion

H. Michael Marsh, MB, BS

This chapter examines gas exchange in the normal lung and in the lung under general anesthesia. Maximal gas-exchange efficiency for O_2 and CO_2 in an ideal single-lung unit has a ventilation/perfusion ($\dot{V}/\dot{Q}$) ratio of 1 in a situation of continuous countercurrent flow of gas to blood, with a blood-to-gas exposure of 0.75 sec. Human lung, by contrast, is only relatively efficient, showing a range of $\dot{V}/\dot{Q}$ ratios for its many alveoli, determined by the distribution of $\dot{V}$ and $\dot{Q}$ throughout the lungs.

Ventilation

Inspired gas flows into the lungs influenced by pulmonary compliance and airway resistance. Gravity, interacting with posture, and regional alveolar time constants for filling and emptying of lung regions, interacting with the frequency of respiration, are the other two major factors determining the distribution of $\dot{V}$ within the lungs. The right lung is larger than the left lung, receiving approximately 52% to 53% of a tidal breath in the supine position, during both spontaneous breathing and with mechanical ventilation. These percentages change under the influence of gravity with change in posture. Anesthesia, paralysis, and mechanical ventilation introduce further changes.

At functional reserve capacity, in each slice of lung, from nondependent (apex in sitting position, anterior lung in supine, up lung in lateral decubitus position) to most dependent portion, the alveolar volume decreases. Basal alveoli are one quarter the volume of apical alveoli at end expiration. This puts the basal alveolar characteristics on a steeper portion of their pressure-volume (P-V) curve (Figure 29-1); although the basal alveoli are smaller than apical alveoli at functional reserve capacity, the basal alveoli expand more than do the apical alveoli during inspiration. Therefore, in an awake, spontaneously breathing patient, in all positions, ventilation per unit of lung volume is smallest at the highest portion (e.g., the apex in an upright patient) and increases with vertical distance down the lung.

In the supine patient, general anesthesia with paralysis and mechanical ventilation decreases the difference between the ventilation of the dependent and nondependent alveoli, causing nearly uniform distribution of ventilation throughout the lung. This is attributed to a decreased functional reserve capacity, shifting alveolar characteristics downward on their P-V curves (see Figure 29-1). When the patient is in the lateral decubitus position, anesthesia reverses the distribution of ventilation so that the nondependent (upper) part of the lung receives more ventilation than does the dependent (lower) part of the lung. This arrangement holds for both spontaneous and mechanical ventilation and is clinically significant because the dependent lung has greater perfusion, which causes increased $\dot{V}/\dot{Q}$ mismatch. The change in distribution of $\dot{V}$ to lung regions in the lateral decubitus position is attributed to (1) decreased functional reserve capacity, causing a shift along the P-V curve (which can be partially reversed by positive end-expiratory pressure); (2) more compression of the dependent lung by the mediastinum and abdominal contents; and (3) increased compliance of the nondependent hemithorax.

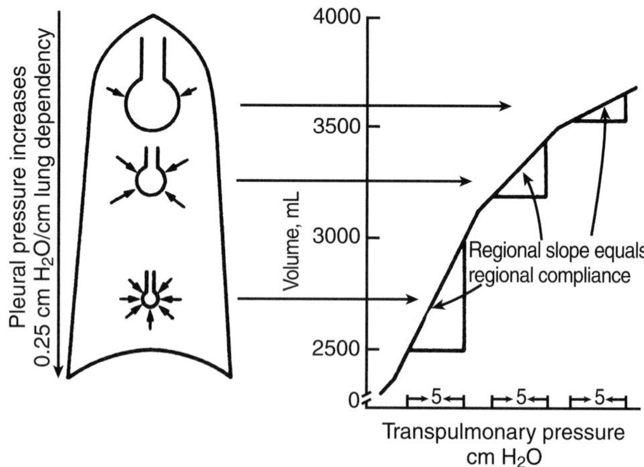

Figure 29-1 Pleural pressure increases 0.25 cm H_2O every centimeter down the lung. The increase in pleural pressure causes a fourfold decrease in alveolar volume. The caliber of the air passages also decreases as lung volume decreases. When regional alveolar volume is translated over to a regional transpulmonary pressure–alveolar volume curve, small alveoli are on a steep (large slope) portion of the curve, and large alveoli are on a flat (small slope) portion of the curve. The regional slope equals regional compliance. Over the normal tidal volume range (2500 to 3000 mL), the pressure-volume relationship is linear. Lung volume values in this diagram relate to the upright position. (From Benumof JL. Respiratory physiology and respiratory function during anesthesia. In: Miller RD, ed. Anesthesia. 5th ed. Philadelphia: Churchill Livingstone; 2000:578-618.)

The time constant for filling and emptying of a lung region is determined by the product of compliance and resistance of the region. If respiratory frequency is such that complete emptying of a region does not occur before the next inspiratory effort is applied, gas trapping will occur. This is a concern when obstructive airways disease is present. Incomplete filling or emptying of lung regions may also increase $\dot{V}/\dot{Q}$ mismatching. Anesthesia may reverse bronchoconstriction and favorably impact this factor.

Pulmonary Blood Flow

The two major determinants of distribution of pulmonary blood flow ($\dot{Q}$) within the lung are (1) gravity and (2) hypoxic pulmonary vasoconstriction (HPV). Pulmonary artery pressure (Ppa) decreases by 1 mm Hg or 1.35 cm H_2O for every cm of vertical distance up the lung. Because the pulmonary circulation is a low-pressure system, this causes significant differences in $\dot{Q}$ between the lower and higher regions of the lung, with greater $\dot{Q}$ going to the lower lung regions. The actual $\dot{Q}$ to an alveolus also depends on the alveolar pressure (Palv), which opposes the Ppa and pulmonary venous pressure (Ppv). This interaction is summarized in Figure 29-2.

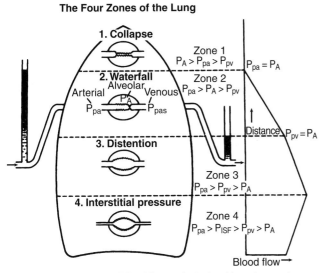

Figure 29-2 Distribution of blood flow in the isolated lung. In zone 1, alveolar pressure (PA) exceeds pulmonary artery pressure (Ppa) and no flow occurs, presumably because collapsible vessels are directly exposed to alveolar pressure. In zone 2, arterial pressure exceeds alveolar pressure, but alveolar pressure exceeds venous pressure (Ppv). Flow in zone 2 is determined by the arterial-alveolar pressure difference, which steadily increases down the zone. In zone 3, pulmonary venous pressure now exceeds alveolar pressure and flow is determined by the arterial-venous pressure difference (Ppa – Ppv), which is constant down the lung. However, the pressure across the walls of the vessels increases down zone 3, so that their caliber increases, as does flow. In zone 4, flow is determined by the arterial pressure–interstitial flow (ISF) pressure difference (Ppa – PISF), because interstitial pressure exceeds both Ppv and PA. (From Benumof JL. Respiratory physiology and respiratory function during anesthesia. In: Miller RD, ed. Anesthesia. 5th ed. Philadelphia: Churchill Livingstone; 2000:578-618.)

All of these relationships are dynamic, varying throughout the cardiac and respiratory cycles. There are four defined zones of blood flow in the lung. In zone 1, at the apex of an upright lung, PALV is greater than PPA, preventing any blood flow and thereby creating alveolar dead space. Zone 1 is negligible in healthy lungs. In zone 2, PPA is greater than PALV, which is greater than PPV, so that $\dot{Q}$ depends only on PPA minus PALV. In zone 3, PPA is greater than PPV, which is greater than PALV, and $\dot{Q}$ is a function of PPA minus PPV independent of PALV. In zone 4 flow is determined by the difference between PPA and PISF. In general, decreases in PPA (e.g., hemorrhagic shock) will increase the size of the upper zones (1 and 2) at the expense of the lower zones (2 and 3), whereas increases in PPA have the opposite effect. Increases in PALV (e.g., with positive end-expiratory pressure) may recruit alveoli from lower zones into higher zones (i.e., increase the volumes of zones 1 and 2).

HPV is a local response of pulmonary arterial smooth muscle to a decreased regional alveolar Po_2. It acts to decrease $\dot{Q}$ to underventilated regions of lung and maintain normal $\dot{V}/\dot{Q}$. HPV is effective only when there is a significant section of normally ventilated and oxygenated lung to which flow can be diverted (e.g., one-lung ventilation during thoracic operations). Intravenously administered anesthetic agents do not inhibit HPV, whereas the inhaled anesthetic agents and potent vasodilators do. Therapeutically inhaled NO is a unique pulmonary-specific vasodilator that may attenuate HPV and often improves oxygenation because it is delivered only to alveoli that are already being ventilated.

Ventilation/Perfusion Ratio

Both $\dot{V}$ and $\dot{Q}$ increase toward the dependent part of the lung, but at different rates (Figure 29-3). Therefore, $\dot{V}/\dot{Q}$ is greater than 1 at the top, $\dot{V}/\dot{Q}$ equals 1.0 at the third rib in upright lungs, and $\dot{V}/\dot{Q}$ is less than 1 below the third rib. $\dot{V}/\dot{Q}$ is, of course, also affected by the factors that affect $\dot{V}$ or $\dot{Q}$ separately.

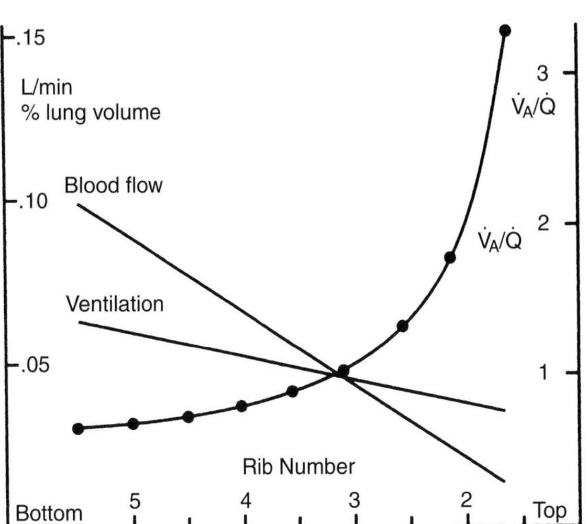

Figure 29-3 Distribution of ventilation and perfusion (left vertical axis) and the ventilation/perfusion ratio (right vertical axis) in normal upright lung. Both ventilation and perfusion are expressed in L/min/percent alveolar volume and have been drawn as smoothed-out linear functions of vertical height. The closed circles mark the ventilation/perfusion ratios of horizontal lung slices. A cardiac output of 6 L/min and a total minute ventilation of 5.1 L/min were assumed. $\dot{V}_A/\dot{Q}$, alveolar ventilation-perfusion ratio. (From West JB. Respiratory Physiology. 2nd ed. Baltimore: Williams & Wilkins; 1970.)

Dead Space

Dead space (VD) is the volume of a breath that does not participate in gas exchange, VT is the total tidal volume, and VD/VT is the fraction of the tidal volume composed of dead space volume. Anatomic dead space, VD(AN), is that volume of gas that ventilates only the conducting airways. Alveolar dead space, VD(ALV), is that volume of gas not taking part in effective gas exchange at the alveolar level, that is, ventilated but unperfused alveoli. Total (or physiologic) VD equals VD(AN) plus VD(ALV). Normally, the ratio of the physiologic dead space to the tidal volume (VD/VT) equals one third, and VD(AN) equals 0.5 mL/kg of body weight. In awake, healthy, supine patients, the VD(ALV) is negligible. One mechanism contributing to this is a bronchiolar constrictive reflex that constricts airways to alveoli that are unperfused.

VD/VT may be measured by the Bohr method, based on the fact that all expired CO_2 comes from perfused alveoli and none from dead space:

$$V_D/V_T = \frac{P_{ACO_2} - \text{mixed expired } P_{CO_2}}{P_{ACO_2}}$$

Clinically, we assume that arterial Pco_2 equals alveolar Pco_2. Mixed expired Pco_2 is the average Pco_2 in an expired gas sample; this is *not* the same as end-tidal Pco_2.

Factors Affecting Dead Space and Dead Space/Tidal Volume

VD and VD/VT are affected by $\dot{V}/\dot{Q}$ and the anatomy of the conducting airways. Decreased PPA (e.g., hemorrhage, drug effects) causes increased VD(ALV) owing to an increase in zone 1.

Loss of perfusion to ventilated alveoli despite normal or high PPAS causes increased VD(ALV) and, therefore, an increase in VD/VT. These conditions may result from pulmonary emboli (including venous air embolism), pulmonary arterial thrombosis, surgical manipulation of the pulmonary arterial tree, or emphysema with loss of alveolar septa and vasculature.

Increased airway pressure (e.g., positive-pressure ventilation) causes increased VD(AN) from radial traction on conducting airways by surrounding lung parenchyma and increased VD(ALV) from increased zone 1. When the patient's neck is extended and jaw is protruded, the VD(AN) increases twofold, compared with a flexed neck and depressed chin. Compared with supine posture, erect posture causes increased VD(ALV) because decreased perfusion to the uppermost alveoli causes an increased volume of zone 1.

The dead space of anesthesia apparatus increases the VD/VT ratio from the normal 0.3 to values of 0.4 to 0.5 with tracheal intubation and Y-piece connectors or 0.64 with facemask ventilation. Tracheostomy or intubation decreases the VD(AN) by roughly half unless anesthesia apparatus is added to the breathing circuit.

General anesthesia, with spontaneous or controlled ventilation, increases VD and VD/VT. The etiology is multifactorial and incompletely understood; it may be partially due to moderate pulmonary hypotension, loss of skeletal muscle tone, or loss of bronchoconstrictor tone. Rapid short inspirations increase VD by ventilating a greater fraction of noncompliant and badly perfused alveoli, as compared with slower deeper inspirations.

Increasing age increases both anatomic and alveolar dead space due to decreased elasticity of lung tissues. Additionally, closing volume and closing capacity increase with aging.

Shunt

Shunt ($\dot{Q}S$) is that portion of blood flow that does not participate in gas exchange. $\dot{Q}S/\dot{Q}T$ is that fraction of pulmonary blood flow (total cardiac output) that is shunt. There are anatomic contributions to shunt from thebesian veins, bronchial veins, and any other anatomic right-to left shunt paths directly emptying into the left side of the heart beyond the lungs. These shunts may deflect up to 5% to 7% of $\dot{Q}T$. $\dot{V}/\dot{Q}$ mismatching may contribute about a further 1% to 3% such that total shunt may be 6% to 10% of cardiac output in normal lungs (Box 29-1). $\dot{Q}S/\dot{Q}T$ may be estimated using the Fick principle embodied in the shunt equation:

$$\dot{Q}S/\dot{Q}T = \frac{Cc'O_2 - CaO_2}{Cc'O_2 - C\bar{v}O_2}$$

where $Cc'O_2$ is end-capillary O_2 content, CaO_2 is arterial O_2 content, and $C\bar{v}O_2$ is mixed venous O_2 content.

Box 29-1 Factors Affecting Shunt

- Thebesian veins drain blood directly from left ventricular muscle wall into the left ventricle; this blood has a very low O_2 content but is only 0.3% of $\dot{Q}T$.
- Flow in the bronchial veins may be large in patients with bronchial disease and up to 7% to 10% of $\dot{Q}T$ in patients with a coarctation.
- Congenital right-to-left cardiac shunt
- Pulmonary edema increases $\dot{Q}S$ in dependent and flooded alveoli.
- Pulmonary diseases may increase diffusion block and create regions of low $\dot{V}/\dot{Q}$.
- Any airway closure will increase $\dot{Q}S$; thus, use of PEEP and alveolar-recruitment maneuvers may decrease $\dot{Q}S$ and improve oxygenation.

PEEP, Positive end-expiratory pressure; $\dot{Q}S$, shunt; $\dot{Q}T$, total cardiac output; $\dot{V}/\dot{Q}$, ventilation/perfusion.

Acknowledgment

The author wishes to thank Michael E. Johnson, MD, PhD, for his work in previous editions.

Suggested Readings

Gattinoni L, Carlesso E, Brazzi L, Caironi P. Positive end-expiratory pressure. *Curr Opin Crit Care*. 2010;16:39-44.

Lumb AB, ed. *Nunn's Applied Respiratory Physiology*. 6th ed. Oxford: Butterworth-Heinemann; 2005.

CHAPTER 30

Pulmonary Function Test Interpretation

H. Michael Marsh, MB, BS, and David O. Warner, MD

Basic pulmonary function tests measure three sets of data: (1) gas flow rates, to assess airway narrowing; (2) lung volumes, to assess lung tissue loss or change induced by chest wall muscle disease; and (3) arterial blood gases or diffusing capacity (DLCO) for carbon monoxide, to assess gas exchange efficiency of the blood-gas interface within the lung.

More complex testing can also be done. For example, data used to assess cardiopulmonary interactions and metabolism can be obtained using cardiopulmonary exercise stress testing, measuring $\dot{V}O_2$ max (maximal O_2 consumption) and metabolic rate at rest. Respiratory muscle strength and endurance can be assessed separately using resistive or elastance loading, measuring power and fatigability of these muscles, whereas central respiratory control can be assessed further using CO_2 and hypoxic response estimates and sleep polysomnography studies.

This range of pulmonary function tests has been conveniently divided into levels of increasing sophistication and complexity, as shown in Box 30-1. The usual tests comprise levels 1 and 2. Normal values for these usual tests vary with age, body size, and sex. Values for an average 40-year-old man and woman are shown in Table 30-1. The highest prevalence of respiratory disease in surgical patients in the United States is seen in two major groups: patients with obstructive diseases, including asthma, bronchitis, bronchiectasis, and emphysema; and those with restrictive diseases, including morbid obesity with obstructive sleep apnea and kyphoscoliosis. Patterns of change in lung function, as seen in level 1 and 2 testing, typical of obstructive and restrictive disease are shown in Table 30-2. The anesthesiologist must be familiar with these diseases and the risks they pose in the perioperative period. However, we should also be aware that, although pulmonary function tests may confirm clinical diagnoses and show response to therapy, allowing assessment of severity of these diseases, no single test or combination of tests is necessarily predictive for pulmonary perioperative complications. However, one can use predicted postoperative changes in gas flow (FEV_1%), DLCO, and baseline exercise tolerance to predict risks for lung resection (Figure 30-1).

The individual level 1 and 2 pulmonary function tests are discussed here, and a conservative recommendation for choice of testing is provided.

Table 30-1 Normal Values for a 40-Year-Old Man and Woman

Measurement	Man*	Woman†
VC or FVC, L	5	3.5
RV, L	1.8	1.7
TLC, L	6.8	5.2
FRC, L	3.4	2.6
FEV_1, L	4.1	2.9
FEV_1%, %	82	83
FEF_{25-75}, L/sec	4.3	3.3
MVV, L/min	168	112
DLCO, $mL \cdot min^{-1} \cdot mm\ Hg^{-1}$	33	24

*Height, 178 cm.
†Height, 165 cm.
DLCO, Diffusing capacity of lung for carbon monoxide; *FEF_{25-75}*, the forced expiratory flow, i.e., the flow (or speed) of air coming out of the lung during the middle portion of a forced expiration; *FEV_1*, forced expiratory volume in the first second of the experiment; *FEV_1%*, the ratio of *FEV_1* to forced vital capacity; *FRC*, functional residual capacity; *FVC*, forced vital capacity; *MVV*, maximum voluntary ventilation; *RV*, residual volume; *TLC*, total lung capacity; *VC*, vital capacity.
Adapted from Taylor AE, Rehder K, Hyatt RE. Clinical Respiratory Physiology. Philadelphia: WB Saunders; 1989.

Box 30-1 Pulmonary Function Tests

Level 1 Tests

- Spirometry/spirography
  - FEV_1
  - FEV_1%
  - FEF_{25-75}
  - MVV
- Response to bronchodilator
- Pulse oximetry on room air or O_2 supplementation

Level 2 Tests

- Arterial blood gases
  - PaO_2/FIO_2 ratio
- Lung volumes
  - TLC
  - FRC
  - RV
- DLCO

Level 3 Tests

- Flow-volume loops
- Pressure-volume loops
  - C_{RS}
  - Pst
- Respiratory muscle strength
  - PImax
  - PEmax
- Hypoxic and hypercapnic responsiveness
- Exercise tests
- Sleep studies

C_{RS}, Compliance of the entire respiratory system; *DLCO*, diffusing capacity of lung for carbon monoxide, the carbon monoxide uptake from a single inspiration in a standard time, usually 10 sec; *FEV_1*, *the forced expiratory volume*, i.e., the volume of air that can be forcibly blown out in 1 sec, after full inspiration; *FEV_1%*, *the ratio of FEV_1 to forced vital capacity (FVC)*, the volume of air that can forcibly be blown out in 1 sec, after full inspiration; *FEF_{25-75}*, *the forced expiratory flow*, i.e., the flow (or speed) of air coming out of the lung during the middle portion of a forced expiration; *FIO_2*, fraction of inspired O_2; *FRC*, functional residual capacity; *MVV*, maximum voluntary ventilation, i.e., the maximum amount of air that can be inhaled and exhaled within 1 min, usually extrapolated from a 15-sec testing period; *PEmax*, maximum expiratory pressure; *PImax*, maximum inspiratory pressure; *Pst*, static lung recoil pressure; *RV*, residual volume; *TLC*, total lung capacity, the maximum volume of air present in the lungs.

Table 30-2 Patterns of Lung Disease

	Restriction		Obstruction		
Parameter	Chest Wall	Parenchyma	Asthma	Bronchitis	Emphysema
TLC	↓	↓	↑	– or ↑	↑
VC	↓	↓	– or ↓	– or ↓	– or ↓
RV	– or ↑	↓	↑	↑	↑
FRC	↓	↓	↑	↑	↑
MVV	– or ↓	– or ↓	↓	↓	↓
DL_{CO}	–	↓	– or ↑	– or ↓	↓
FEV_1	↓	↓	↓	↓	↓
FEV_1%	–	–	↓	↓	↓

DLCO, Diffusing capacity of lung for carbon monoxide; *FEV_1*, forced expiratory volume in the first second of the experiment; *FEV_1%*, the ratio of FEV_1 to forced vital capacity; *FRC*, functional residual capacity; *MVV*, maximum voluntary ventilation; *RV*, residual volume; *TLC*, total lung capacity; *VC*, vital capacity; ↓, decreased; ↑, increased; –, normal.
Adapted from Taylor AE, Rehder K, Hyatt RE. Clinical Respiratory Physiology. Philadelphia: WB Saunders; 1989.

Tests of Gas Flow

Forced Expiratory Spirography

In this test, the subject exhales as forcefully as possible from a maximal inhalation, and expiratory flow and volume are measured using a spirometer or pneumotachograph (Figures 30-2 and 30-3). In any individual, the maximal forced expiratory flow (FEF_{max}) obviously depends on effort. Flow during continued expiration—typically measured as forced flow from 75% to 25% of forced vital capacity (FVC) (FEF_{25-75}), depends only on lung volume and lung characteristics and less on the effort. In fact, these tests are considered to be effort independent. Because the airways behave as Starling "variable" resistors, no matter how forcefully the individual exhales, as the intrathoracic pressure increases, the airways constrict, and resistance increases, with the changes counterbalancing one another; maximum flow does not change.

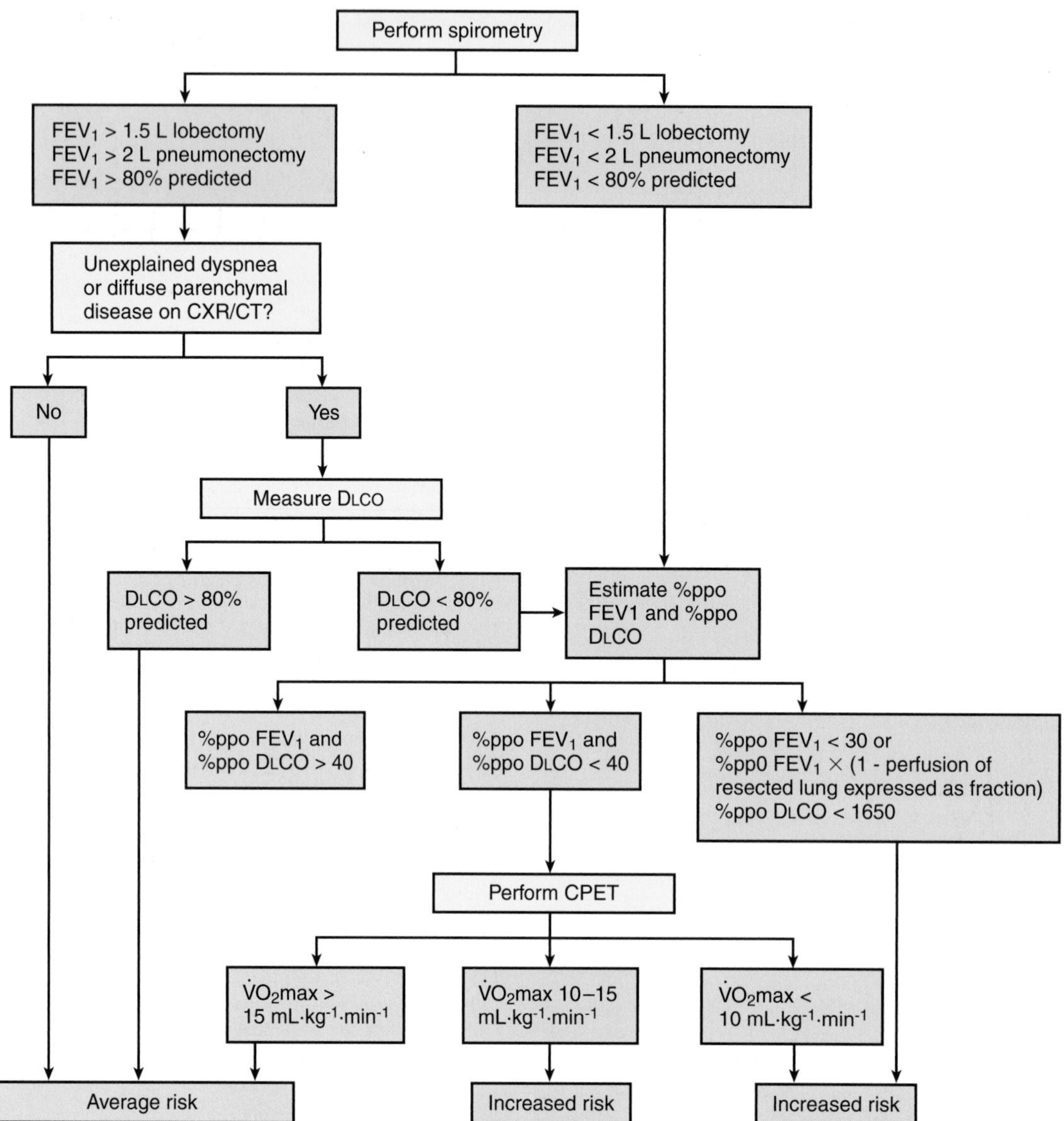

Figure 30-1 Evidence-based guidelines for resection operation of lung: Physiologic assessment. CPET, Cardiopulmonary exercise testing; CT, computed tomography; CXR, radiograph of the chest; DLCO, diffusing capacity of lung for carbon monoxide; FEV_1, the forced expiratory volume in the first second of the experiment; %ppo, predicted postoperative values, calculated by estimating the percentage of lung to be removed and reducing measured FEV_1% (the ratio of FEV_1 to forced vital capacity) or DLCO, accordingly; $\dot{V}O_2$ max, maximum O_2 consumption. (Adapted from Colice GL, Shafazand S, Griffin JP, et al. Physiologic evaluation of the patient with lung cancer being considered for resectional surgery: ACCP Evidence-Based Practice Guidelines. 2nd ed. Chest. 2007;132:35, 161.)

The most useful parameters obtained from forced expiratory spirography are FVC and forced expiratory volume in 1 sec (FEV_1). The ratio of FEV_1 to FVC (FEV_1%) normalizes FEV_1 measurements for each individual's lung volume. For example, a patient with restrictive lung disease will have a low FEV_1 because of low lung volume, not airway obstruction. FEV_1% is the hallmark of obstructive lung disease. FEV_1% values of 60% to 70% indicate mild obstruction; 40% to 60%, moderate obstruction; and less than 40%, severe obstruction. These measurements are not valid if the patient does not perform at maximum effort. In the laboratory, $FEF_{25\text{-}75}$ of vital capacity (VC) is another spirography measurement that may be less effort dependent. If maximal inspiratory flows are also measured, then the flow-volume loops can be useful in identifying the source of airway obstruction (Figure 30-4).

In patients with obstructive lung disease, forced expiratory spirography may be done before and after the inhalation of a bronchodilator to assess the reversibility of airway obstruction. (A greater than 10% improvement in FEV_1 indicates reversibility.) Analogously, the inhalation of methacholine, which causes bronchoconstriction, is used to diagnose asthma. Patients with asthma will exhibit abnormally decreased flow parameters (a greater than 15% decrease in FEV_1) in response to methacholine.

Maximal Voluntary Ventilation

In this test, the subject breathes as quickly and deeply as possible through a pneumotachograph for 12 sec. The exhaled volume is measured and multiplied by 5 to yield the maximal ventilation during 1 min. Because this test measures patient motivation and effort as well as lung and thorax properties, it may be a particularly useful screening test before surgery.

Tests to Measure Lung Volumes

Spirometry

Spirometry measures the volume of gas passing through the airway opening. During spirometry, the patient first breathes normally, then is asked to inhale maximally and exhale maximally, as discussed earlier (see Figure 30-1).

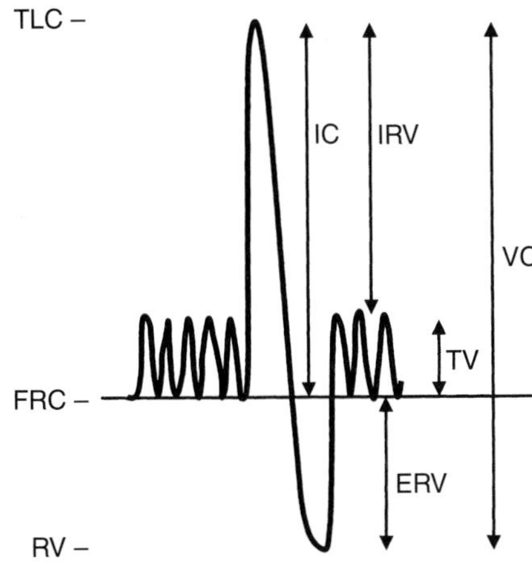

Figure 30-2 Changes in lung volume over time during spirometry. ERV, Expiratory reserve volume; FRC, functional residual capacity; IC, inspiratory capacity; IRV, inspiratory reserve volume; RV, residual volume; TLC, total lung capacity; TV, tidal volume; VC, vital capacity. (Adapted from Conrad SA, George RB. Clinical pulmonary function testing. In: George RB, Light RW, Mathay RA, eds. Chest Medicine. New York: Churchill Livingstone; 1984:161.)

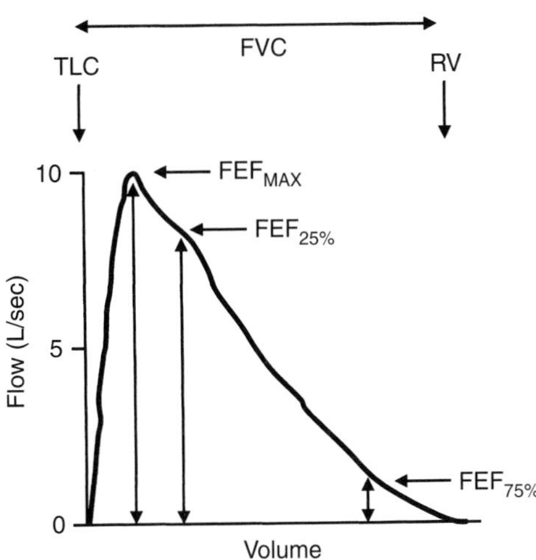

Figure 30-3 Maximal expiratory flow-volume curve. FEF$_{MAX}$, Maximal forced expiratory flow; FEF$_{25\%}$, 25% of forced expiratory flow (FEF); FEF$_{75\%}$, 75% of FEF; FVC, forced vital capacity; RV, residual volume; TLC, total lung capacity. (Adapted from Conrad SA, George RB. Clinical pulmonary function testing. In: George RB, Light RW, Mathay RA, eds. Chest Medicine. New York: Churchill Livingstone; 1984:161.)

Measurements obtained by spirometry include inspiratory capacity (IC), inspiratory reserve volume (IRV), expiratory reserve volume (ERV), and VC. One can also measure total lung capacity (TLC) and deduce residual volume (RV) by measuring functional residual capacity (FRC).

Measurements of Functional Residual Capacity

FRC measures the amount of gas in the lungs at the end of expiration during tidal breathing. Three types of methods are available: (1) equilibration methods, in which FRC is calculated from the concentration of a tracer gas (usually helium) in a closed system in equilibrium with the patient's lungs; (2) washout methods, in which FRC is calculated from the lung washout of a tracer gas (usually nitrogen); and (3) plethysmographic methods, in which the total thoracic gas volume is measured by a technique based on Boyle's law (subjects attempt to breathe against a closed airway while sitting in an airtight chamber; a body box—pressure and volume change can be assessed). This method measures the total amount of gas in the thorax, whereas the other two methods measure the amount of gas in communication with the

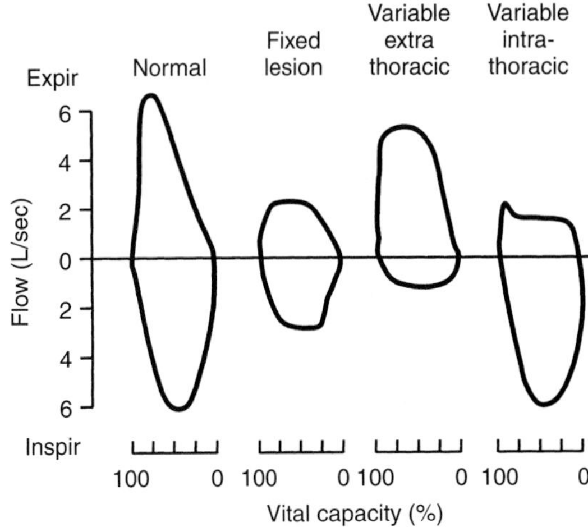

Figure 30-4 Maximal inspiratory and expiratory flow-volume curves used to diagnose airway obstruction. (Adapted from Taylor AE, Rehder K, Hyatt RE. Clinical Respiratory Physiology. Philadelphia: WB Saunders; 1989.)

airway opening. When combined with spirometry, FRC measurements allow calculation of TLC and RV. Decreased TLC and decreased RV are the hallmark of restrictive lung disease.

Closing Volume Measurement

Closing volume is the volume above RV at which airway closure, in the dependent parts of the lung, can be detected using a tracer gas. This gas may be nitrogen in a single-breath nitrogen washout after a maximal breath from RV of O_2, or He, or Xe. The test is based on the differing concentrations of tracer gas in nondependent and dependent alveoli achieved during a single maximal inspiration. This test assesses dynamic airway closure in small airways, and the closing volume, if above FRC, will determine gas trapping and some ventilation/perfusion inequality leading to gas exchange inefficiency. Measurement of closing volume is a level 3 test, and though this test is not commonly performed, anesthesiologists must understand the importance of the measurement.

Tests of Gas Exchange Efficiency

Arterial blood gas and co-oximeter sampling are used to assess oxygenation and to measure CO_2 values and establish acid-base parameters. One can measure O_2 uptake and CO_2 clearance during rest or during exercise. A ventilatory ratio for CO_2 clearance has recently been suggested as a simple bedside estimate of ventilatory gas exchange efficiency. Its widespread utility has not yet been tested.

Diffusing Capacity

Several methods are available to measure diffusing capacity, all of which measure the diffusion of CO across the alveolar-capillary membrane. DLCO decreases with the loss of parenchyma (e.g., in emphysema) or thickening of the alveolar-capillary membrane (e.g., in fibrosis).

Choosing Pulmonary Function Tests

Perhaps the most critical decisions resting on pulmonary function testing for anesthesiologists center upon preoperative assessment of perioperative risk for lung resection. The American College of Chest Physicians, in 2007, published an algorithm for this purpose (see Figure 30-1). Poor results on spirometry, symptoms of dyspnea, or diffuse chest radiographic changes indicate the need for DLCO measurement. Estimation of predicted postoperative values for FEV_1 and DLCO indicate risk and the possible need for cardiopulmonary exercise testing as a final level of assessment. The anesthesiologist must be aware of this algorithm and the risks entailed by poor performance.

Detection of the usual obstructive airway diseases can be made from history, physical examination, and bedside observation. Pulmonary function testing can then be reserved for severity assessment or adjustment of bronchodilator therapy but is not usually indicated prior to routine surgery.

Increasingly, obstructive sleep apnea and the restrictive changes associated with morbid obesity are seen in anesthetic practice. In this case, an anesthesiologist may be the first physician to detect the problem and should then refer and follow these patients up in promoting aftercare. Again, detection of these conditions is usually relatively easy, using history, physical examination, and bedside observation. Thus, although close postoperative monitoring and supportive care are mandatory, definitive pulmonary function testing can await specialist referral.

Suggested Readings

Bernstein WK. Pulmonary function testing. *Curr Opin Anesthesiol*. 2012;25:11-16.

Colice GL, Shafazand S, Griffin JP, et al. Physiologic evaluation of the patient with lung cancer being considered for resectional surgery. ACCP Evidence-Based Practice Guidelines. 2nd ed. *Chest*. 2007;132:35, 161.

Gross JB, Bachenberg KL, Benumof JL, et al. Practice guidelines for the perioperative management of patients with obstructive sleep apnea: A report by the American Society of Anesthesiologists Task Force on Perioperative Management of patients with obstructive sleep apnea. *Anesthesiology*. 2006;104:1081-1093.

Ridgway ZA, Howell SJ. Cardiopulmonary exercise testing: A review of methods and applications in surgical patients. *Eur J Anesthesiol*. 2012;27:858-865.

Siuha P, Farwel NJ, Singh S, Soni N. Ventilatory ratio: A simple bedside test of ventilation. *Br J Anaesth*. 2009;102:692.

Taylor AE, Rehder K, Hyatt RE. *Clinical Respiratory Physiology*. Philadelphia: WB Saunders; 1989.

CHAPTER 31

Chronic Obstructive Pulmonary Disease and Restrictive Lung Disease

Kamthorn Tantivitayatan, MD

Chronic Obstructive Pulmonary Disease

The Global Initiative for Obstructive Lung Disease defines *chronic obstructive lung (pulmonary) disease* (COPD) as "a common preventable and treatable disease, is characterized by persistent airflow limitation that is usually progressive and associated with an enhanced chronic inflammatory response in the airways and the lung to noxious particles or gases. Exacerbations and comorbidities contribute to the overall severity in individual patients." The definition does not include the pathologic term *emphysema* and the clinical and epidemiologic term *chronic bronchitis*.

Patients with COPD frequently have a combination of obstructive bronchiolitis or small-airway disease and parenchymal destruction or emphysema (Figure 31-1). A ratio of forced expiratory volume in 1 sec (FEV_1) to functional vital capacity (FVC) of less than 0.7 is essential to make the diagnosis of COPD. Total lung capacity, residual volume, and functional residual capacity are all increased in COPD, which is different from the pattern seen with restrictive lung disease.

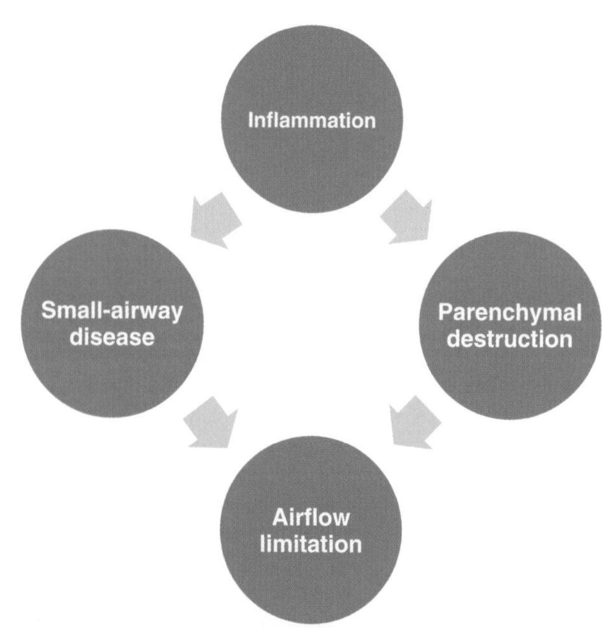

Figure 31-1 Patients with chronic obstructive pulmonary disease often have a combination of small-airway disease and parenchymal destruction or emphysema.

Clinical Features

The Global Initiative for Obstructive Lung Disease has calculated the prevalence of COPD to be 6.1% and 13.5%, respectively, after 9-year and 10-year cumulative studies. In young adults, the prevalence was found to be 2.2%, and in patients 40 to 44 years of age, it was 4.4%. The primary cause of COPD is cigarette smoking (with α_1-antitrypsin deficiency as another cause in the young). Approximately half of patients older than 60 years of age who have a smoking history of at least 20 pack-years have a spirometry result consistent with COPD. Lung parenchymal destruction leads to loss of diffusing capacity and loss of the radial traction force on the airways. Airway inflammation produces increased mucus secretions and mucosal thickening, resulting in ventilation-perfusion mismatch and, finally, hypoxemia and CO_2 retention. Airway collapse on expiration results in air trapping, leading to dynamic hyperinflation because of auto-positive end-expiratory pressure (Figure 31-2).

Signs and symptoms of COPD vary from asymptomatic to overt disease, depending on the severity of the disease (Table 31-1). Extrapulmonary symptoms include diaphragmatic dysfunction, right-sided heart failure, anxiety, depression, and weight loss with evidence of malnutrition.

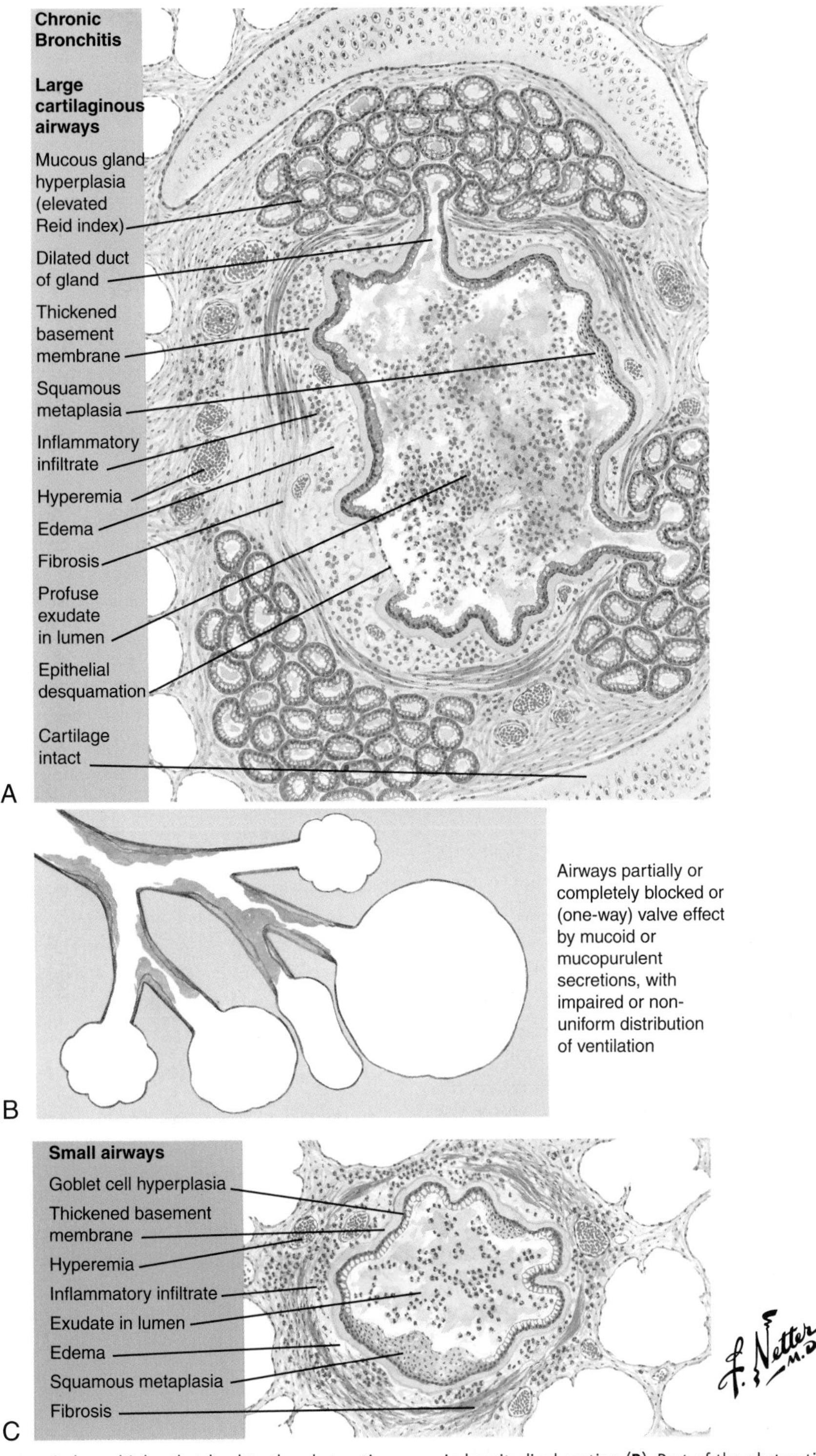

Figure 31-2 **A,** Pathologic changes in bronchioles that lead to the obstruction, seen in longitudinal section (**B**). Part of the obstruction is due to collapse of small airways caused by loss of elastic recoil (**C**). (Netter illustration from www.netterimages.com.)

Table 31-1 GOLD Classification of COPD Severity

Severity	Spirometry Results	
	FEV_1/FVC	FEV_1 % of predicted value
Mild	< 0.7	≥ 80
Moderate	< 0.7	≥ 50 and < 80
Severe	< 0.7	≥ 30 and <50
Very severe	< 0.7	< 30 or < 50 plus signs of respiratory or right-sided heart failure

COPD, Chronic obstructive pulmonary disease; FEV_1, forced expiratory volume in 1 sec; FEV_1/FVC, the ratio of FEV_1 to FVC; FVC, forced vital capacity; GOLD, Global Initiative for Obstructive Lung Diseases.

Management

Smoking cessation can halt the decline of pulmonary function, and although it produces only a small improvement in FEV_1, smoking cessation results in a subsequent rate of decline that eventually becomes equivalent to that of a nonsmoker. The use of short-acting β_2-adrenergic receptor agonists and anticholinergic agents as combined bronchodilators is superior to the use of either agent alone. Long-acting bronchodilators provide sustained symptomatic relief. The use of inhaled corticosteroids is indicated for severe and repeated exacerbations but is not recommended as monotherapy. Theophylline may be tried in patients with severe COPD that is unresponsive to other regimens; blood levels of theophylline must be monitored to minimize potential side effects.

The Global Initiative for Obstructive Lung Disease defines an acute exacerbation of COPD as "an event in the natural course of the disease characterized by a change in the patient's baseline dyspnea, cough, and/or sputum that is beyond normal day-to-day variations, is acute in onset, and may warrant a change in regular medications in a patient with underlying COPD." Exacerbations are commonly caused by infection and air pollution and are treated with antibiotics. Bronchodilator therapy should be reviewed and changed if appropriate. Mechanical ventilation is sometimes required for acute exacerbations of COPD; noninvasive mechanical ventilation without tracheal intubation can be tried. Lung volume reduction surgery and lung transplantation have a limited role in the treatment of patients with COPD.

Perioperative Considerations

Perioperative morbidity and mortality rates are not influenced by the use of general versus regional anesthetic techniques in patients with COPD. The main goal is to avoid excessive airway manipulation, thus lessening reflex-induced bronchospasm. Surgery should be postponed for symptomatic patients with severe dyspnea or acute exacerbations of symptoms who are scheduled to undergo elective operations.

Preoperative optimization of pulmonary function focuses on cessation of smoking, optimization of bronchodilator therapy, control of infections, and provision of chest physiotherapy, such as incentive spirometry, breathing exercises, and postural drainage techniques. Appropriate investigations such as arterial blood gas analysis, electrocardiography, echocardiography, and chest radiography provide information that is often helpful in determining gas exchange efficiency, right ventricular function, and the presence of asymptomatic bullae.

Intraoperative monitoring of airway pressure, O_2 saturation, and end-tidal CO_2 provides useful information about the degree of airflow obstruction. Anesthetics of choice include short-acting agents, such as propofol and remifentanyl, and drugs that do not stimulate histamine release. The respiratory rate of the ventilator should be lower than normal to allow for prolonged expiration and to minimize the chance of dynamic hyperinflation occurring. Postoperatively, the use of noninvasive positive-pressure ventilation is an attractive alternative to tracheal intubation and mechanical ventilation.

Restrictive Lung Disease

Clinical Features

Limited lung expansion or restrictive lung disease may result from any of several pulmonary and extrapulmonary causes—pulmonary fibrosis, sarcoidosis, obesity, pleural effusion, scoliosis, or respiratory muscle weakness. Interstitial edema and acute lung injury/acute respiratory distress syndrome (ALI/ARDS) are classified as acute restrictive lung diseases. Spirometry can help differentiate between obstructive and restrictive patterns: in the latter, total lung capacity is reduced, airway resistance is normal, and airflow is preserved. Reduced FEV_1 with a normal or increased FEV_1/FVC suggests the presence of restrictive lung disease, but the diagnosis and severity grading are based on measurement of decreased total lung capacity (Figure 31-3). In patients who have restrictive lung disease with an intrinsic cause, reduced gas transfer is manifest as desaturation after exercise.

The prevalence rates of the mortality and morbidity associated with restrictive lung disease vary based on the underlying cause: idiopathic pulmonary fibrosis is found in 27 to 29 cases per 100,000 persons and has a median survival time of less than 3 years.

Management

The treatment of restrictive lung disease is dependent upon the specific diagnosis; for example, the mainstay of treatment in many interstitial lung diseases includes corticosteroids plus immunosuppressive and cytotoxic agents. Supplemental O_2 therapy alleviates exercise-induced hypoxemia and improves performance.

Perioperative Considerations

For patients who have pulmonary lesions, preoperative spirometry, arterial blood gas analysis, and measurements of lung volume and gas transfer should be performed within 8 weeks before surgery to identify disease severity. Supplemental doses of corticosteroids and postoperative O_2 therapy may be required; respiratory infections should be treated immediately. Patients who have extrapulmonary causes of their restrictive lung disease usually breathe rapidly and shallowly, which is not effective in clearing sputum, particularly after thoracic or upper abdominal operations. Providing vigorous chest physiotherapy and adequate analgesia are important. Patients who are mechanically ventilated during the operative and postoperative periods typically tolerate relatively low tidal volumes and high breathing rates.

Conclusion

In summary, spirometry is used to differentiate obstructive from restrictive pulmonary dysfunction patterns. The treatment and prognoses of these conditions vary according to the cause. Perioperative concerns include bronchospasm, air trapping, chest physiotherapy, and postoperative pain control in patients with COPD, whereas gas exchange, supplementary doses of steroids, and ventilatory management should be considered in patients with restrictive lung disease.

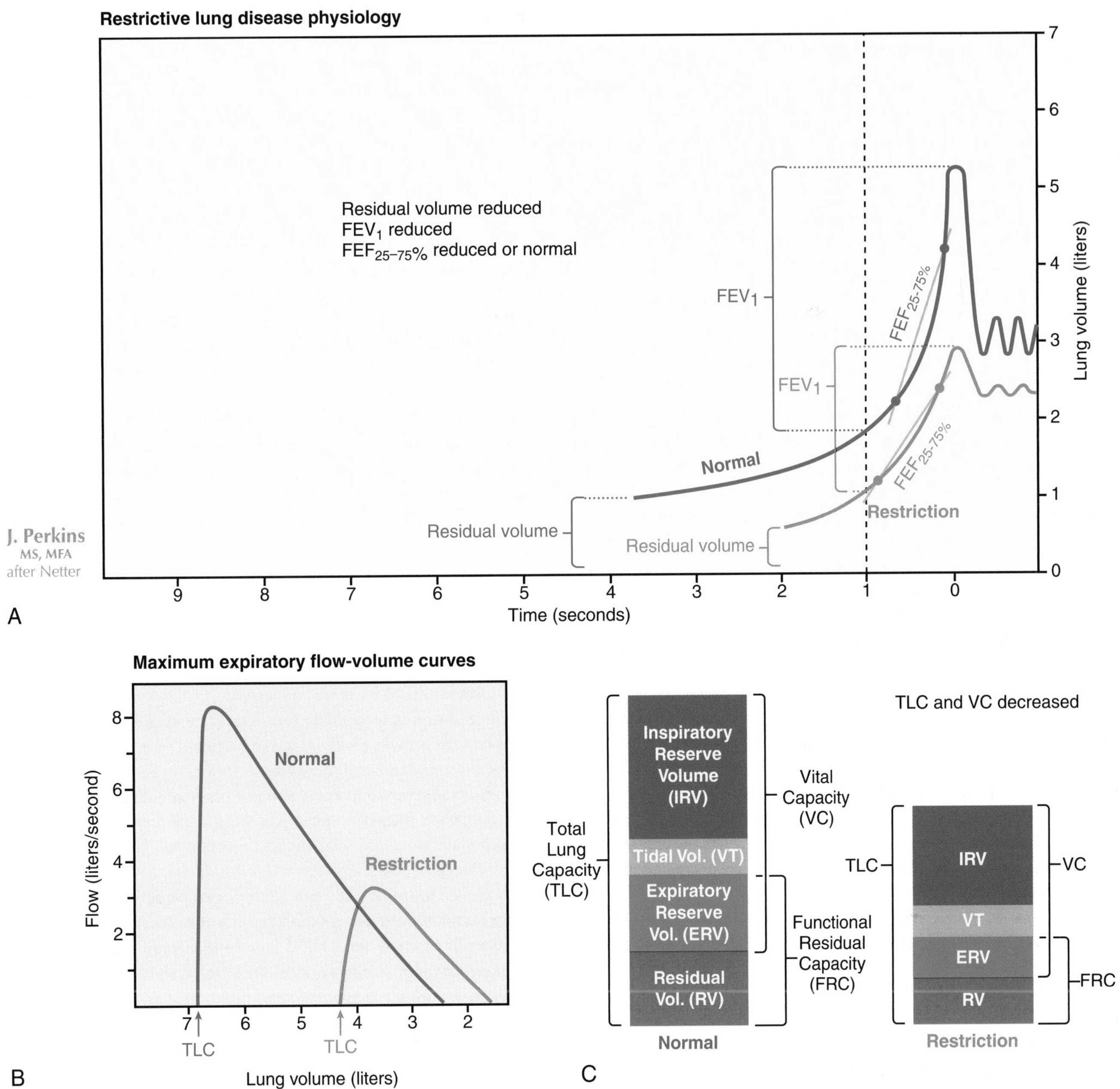

Figure 31-3 Physiology of restrictive lung disease. **A,** Normal forced vital capacity maneuver in green; in orange, a similar maneuver in an individual with restrictive lung disease showing a reduced forced expiratory volume in 1 second (FEV_1), and forced vital capacity. **B,** Maximum expiratory flow volume curve in a normal individual (*green*) and in someone with restricted lung disease (*orange*). **C,** Comparison of lung volumes and lung capacities in a normal lung and in an individual with restrictive lung disease. (Netter illustration from www.netterimages.com. © Elsevier Inc. All rights reserved.)

Suggested Readings

Cazzola M, Donner CF, Hanania NA. One hundred years of chronic obstructive pulmonary disease (COPD). *Respir Med*. 2007;101:1049-1065.

Global Initiative for Chronic Obstructive Lung Disease. *Global strategy for the diagnosis, management, and prevention of chronic obstructive pulmonary disease*. 2013. http://www.goldcopd.com. Accessed December 6, 2013.

Tamul PC, Peruzzi WT. Assessment and management of patients with pulmonary disease. *Crit Care Med*. 2004;32:S137-145.

Ward NS, Dushay KM. Clinical concise review: Mechanical ventilation of patients with chronic obstructive pulmonary disease. *Crit Care Med*. 2008; 36;5:1614-1619.

CHAPTER 32

Measurement and Implications of the $\dot{Q}s/\dot{Q}t$

Robert A. Strickland, MD

Hypoxemia can be caused by a variety of factors (Box 32-1). This chapter will focus on the primary cause of hypoxemia—shunting, which may, at times, be due to ventilation/perfusion ($\dot{V}/\dot{Q}$) mismatch.

Ventilation/Perfusion Mismatch

Ideally, pulmonary perfusion ($\dot{Q}$) evenly matches alveolar ventilation at all levels of the lung; however, perfect matching does not occur because the distribution of ventilation and perfusion and the $\dot{V}/\dot{Q}$ ratio vary throughout the lung. A normal lung has a $\dot{V}/\dot{Q}$ ratio of approximately 0.8. A $\dot{V}/\dot{Q}$ ratio of 0 (i.e., a shunt) exists when perfused alveoli have no ventilation and the values for Po_2 and Pco_2 of the trapped air are the same as those of mixed venous blood (Po_2 = 40 mm Hg and Pco_2 = 47 mm Hg). Conversely, a $\dot{V}/\dot{Q}$ ratio of ∞ exists when ventilated alveoli have no perfusion and, at sea level, the Po_2 and Pco_2 equal approximately 150 and 0 mm Hg, respectively. Nonperfused alveoli (i.e., alveolar dead space) is approximately 25 to 50 mL in a healthy 70-kg person. Figure 32-1 depicts the progression of a $\dot{V}/\dot{Q}$ ratio from 0 to ∞; the normal, idealized, alveolar-capillary unit is shown as example A.

Box 32-1 Causes of Hypoxemia

- An O_2-deficient environment, such as occurs at high altitude
- Hypoventilation, which can be caused by the use of opioid or sedative agents
- Diffusion abnormalities at the alveolar-capillary membrane
- Shunting

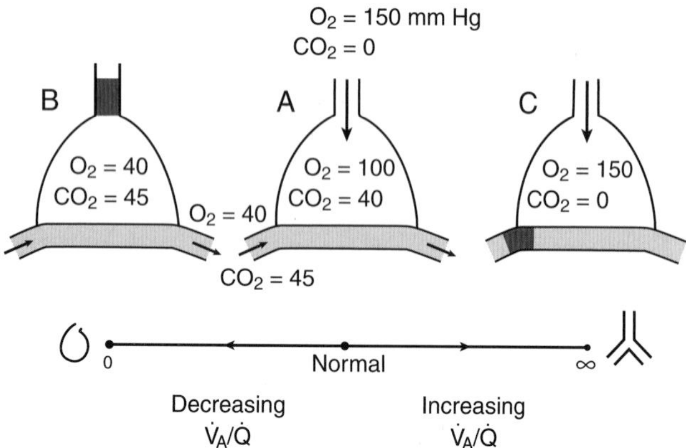

Figure 32-1 Effect of altering the ventilation-perfusion ratio on the Po_2 and Pco_2 in a lung unit from 0 (**B**) to normal (**A**) to ∞ (**C**). (From West JB. Respiratory physiology: the essentials. 9th ed. Philadelphia: Lippincott Williams & Wilkins; 2012:64.)

In contrast with blood vessels in all other tissues, which dilate in response to hypoxemia, the blood vessels of intact lung constrict in response to hypoxia (termed *hypoxic pulmonary vasoconstriction* [HPV]). Blood flow is directed away from poorly ventilated regions of a lung to better ventilated lung fields. Thus, the overall $\dot{V}/\dot{Q}$ ratio improves, better oxygenating blood. A low Po_2 in the pulmonary arteries and pulmonary capillaries is the predominant stimulus that produces HPV, although a low mixed venous O_2 pressure ($P\bar{v}o_2$) also plays a role. A Po_2 below 100 mm Hg will initiate HPV; marked vasoconstriction occurs with a Po_2 less than 70 mm Hg, becoming progressively more severe as Po_2 levels continue to decrease. The mechanism for HPV is not well understood, but it appears that pulmonary vascular endothelium responds to a low O_2 tension, with endothelium-derived vasoconstrictor biochemicals (e.g., leukotrienes and prostaglandins) constricting arteriolar smooth muscle.

A variety of physiologic alterations and pharmacologic interventions alter HPV. Respiratory acidosis and metabolic acidosis increase HPV, whereas respiratory alkalosis and metabolic alkalosis decrease HPV. In vitro studies have shown that inhaled anesthetic agents uniformly inhibit HPV, but the results of in vivo studies have not often yielded clinically significant effects. Systemically administered vasodilators, such as nitroprusside and nitroglycerin, generally adversely affect HPV, which may be of consequence in patients with significant obstructive lung disease or during one-lung ventilation.

Shunting Due to Other Causes

A small fraction of blood in the cardiac output, normally 2% to 5%, enters the arterial circulation without first passing through the pulmonary circulation, accounting for the normal O_2 alveolar-arterial gradient $P(A\text{-}a)O_2$. The causes for this type of venous admixture include (1) the thebesian veins, which drain blood from the coronary circulation directly into the left atrium and, rarely, the left ventricle and (2) the bronchial vein, which provides the nutritive perfusion of the bronchial tree and pleura. Abnormal anatomic shunts include right-to-left atrial and ventricular septal defects and pulmonary arteriovenous malformations.

Hypoxemia that is the result of a physiologic or anatomic shunt cannot be corrected by having the patient breathe supplemental O_2. The hemoglobin in blood that perfuses alveoli with a $\dot{V}/\dot{Q}$ ratio of 1 will readily achieve 100% saturation; increasing the partial pressure of O_2 in these alveoli will minimally increase the O_2 content. Blood that perfuses alveoli with a $\dot{V}/\dot{Q}$ ratio of 0 will not be exposed to any O_2, no matter the fraction of inspired O_2 (Fio_2); therefore, no significant improvement in arterial oxygenation occurs (Figure 32-2).

As previously stated, the normal shunt fraction is less than 5%. Clinically significant shunts equal 10% to 20% of cardiac output, whereas potentially fatal shunts are usually greater than 30%. Seldom does a shunt result in an elevated $Paco_2$. Chemoreceptors sense elevations in $Paco_2$ and

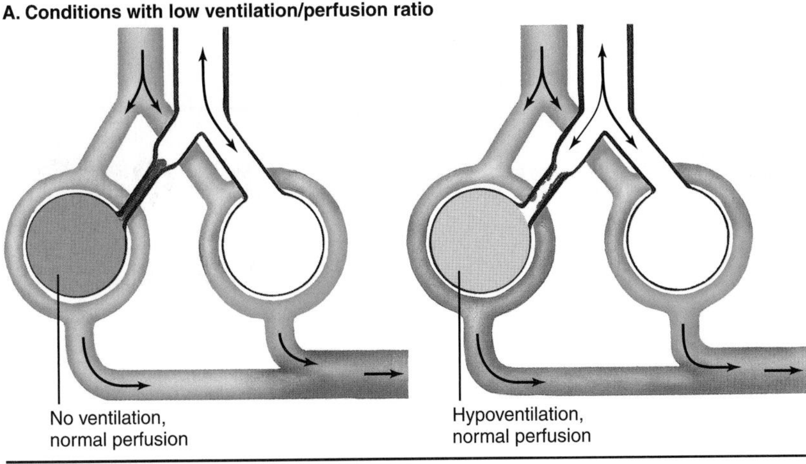

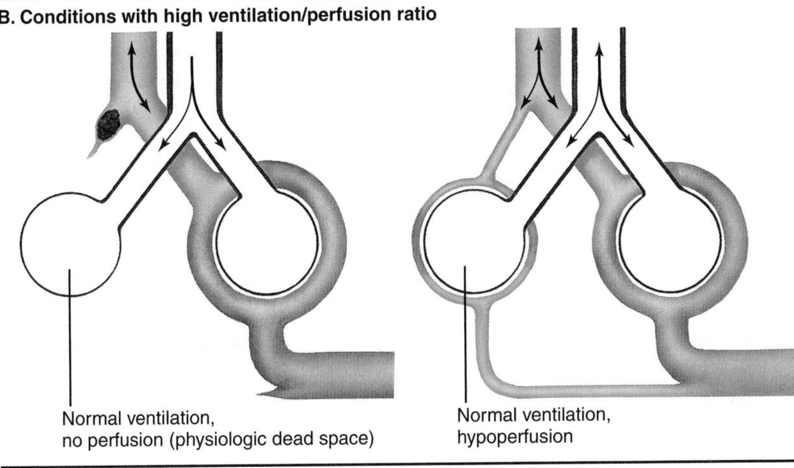

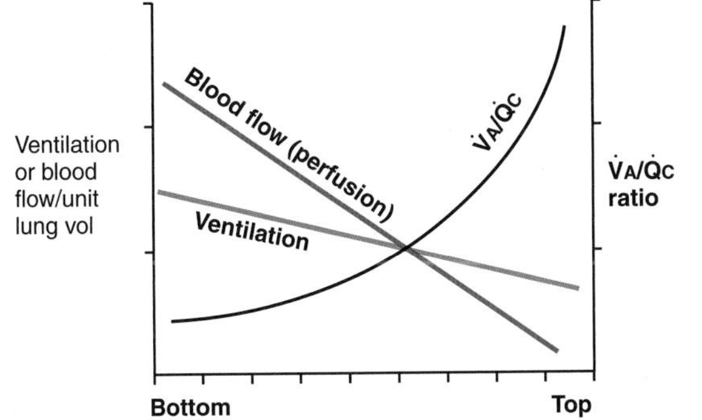

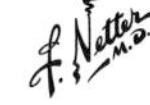

Figure 32-2 Ventilation-perfusion relationships. In the standing position, the effects of gravity result in gradients in both perfusion and ventilation of the lung from base to apex. Because the perfusion gradient is steeper than the ventilation gradient, the ratio of ventilation to perfusion ($\dot{V}A/\dot{Q}c$), is lowest at the bottom of the lung and greatest at the top of the lung (**B**). $\dot{V}A/\dot{Q}c$ is also affected by various other conditions affecting ventilation and perfusion (**A** and **B**). (Netter illustration from www.netterimages.com.)

increase ventilation. The $Paco_2$ of unshunted blood is reduced, and the overall $Paco_2$ is usually normal. If ventilatory drive related to a low Pao_2 produces significant hyperventilation, it is possible to actually have a $Paco_2$ that is less than normal.

Calculation of Shunt Fraction

The fraction of cardiac output that passes through the various shunts is expressed as the shunt fraction ($\dot{Q}s/\dot{Q}t$):

$$\dot{Q}s/\dot{Q}t = (Cco_2 - Cao_2)/(Cco_2 - C\bar{v}o_2)$$

where Cc equals the O_2 content of end-pulmonary capillary blood, Ca is the O_2 content of arterial blood, and $C\bar{v}$ represents the O_2 content of mixed venous blood. The O_2 content of arterial blood is calculated by:

$$Ca = 1.39\ (\text{hemoglobin concentration})\ (\%\ O_2\ \text{saturation}) + 0.003\ (Pao_2)$$

The O_2 contents of Cc and of $C\bar{v}$ are calculated by inserting the respective O_2 saturation and Pao_2 values into the equations.

When cardiac output and hemoglobin concentration are normal and the Pao_2 is greater than 175 mm Hg, the shunt fraction can be estimated by using the simplified formula:

$$\frac{P(A-a)O_2}{20}$$

Suggested Readings

Mark Evans A, Ward JP. Hypoxic pulmonary vasoconstriction—Invited article. *Adv Exp Med Biol*. 2009;648:351-360.

Spyer KM, Gourine AV. Chemosensory pathways in the brainstem controlling cardiorespiratory activity. *Philos Trans R Soc Lond B Biol Sci*. 2009;364:2603-2610.

Zoremba M, Dette F, Hunecke T, et al. The influence of perioperative oxygen concentration on postoperative lung function in moderately obese adults. *Eur J Anaesthesiol*. 2010;27:501-507.

CHAPTER 33

Cardiac Cycle: Control and Synchronicity

Brantley D. Gaitan, MD

The cardiac cycle describes the succession of atrial and ventricular events that make up a period of contraction (systole) followed by a period of relaxation (diastole) (i.e., a single heart beat). These periods are further subdivided into phases.

Systole comprises two phases: isovolumic contraction and ejection. On initiation of myocardial contraction, the ventricular pressure rises abruptly, closing the atrioventricular (AV) valves, and continues to increase for approximately 0.03 sec (isovolumic contraction). Once the ventricular pressure sufficiently exceeds the pressure in either the aorta or the pulmonary artery, the semilunar valves open, and ejection occurs.

At the end of systole, the second period, diastole, or relaxation of the ventricle—takes place during four phases: isovolumic relaxation, rapid inflow, diastasis, and atrial systole (the final three phases constitute ventricular filling) (Figures 33-1 and 33-2). During isovolumic relaxation, the ventricular pressure rapidly drops below that of the arterial pressure, and the semilunar valves snap shut. For approximately 0.06 sec, the ventricular pressure continues to decrease without any change in ventricular volume. Once the ventricular pressure drops below the atrial pressure, the AV valves open and blood rapidly fills the ventricles. This period of rapid blood inflow is augmented by a negative intracavitary pressure (diastolic suction) created by the rapid myocardial relaxation. Once relaxation is complete and elastic distention of the ventricle begins, the slowing of blood return, termed *diastasis,* immediately precedes atrial systole. Effective atrial systole contributes up to about 20% of ventricular filling and completes the period of diastole.

Control

The heart contains a specialized conduction system that comprises foci with automatic rhythmic electrical discharge (action potentials [APs]) that are

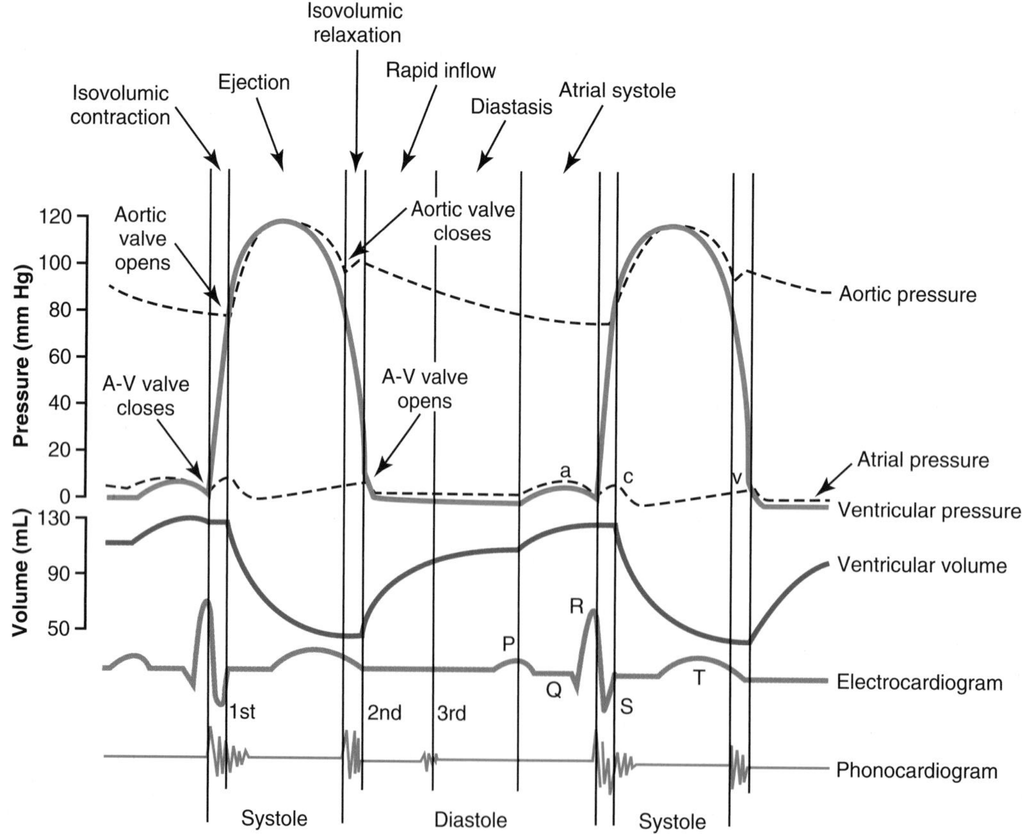

Figure 33-1 The simultaneous events of the cardiac cycle for left ventricular function, showing changes in left atrial pressure, left ventricular pressure, aortic pressure, ventricular volume, the electrocardiogram, and the phonocardiogram. (From Guyton AC, Hall JE. Textbook of Medical Physiology. 11th ed. Philadelphia: Elsevier Saunders; 2005.)

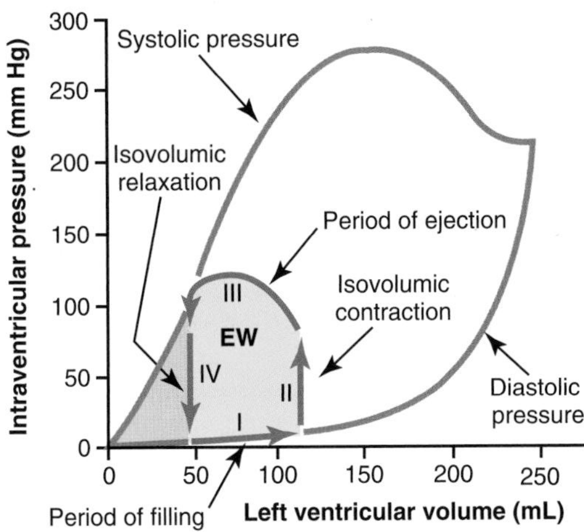

Figure 33-2 Relationship between left ventricular volume and intraventricular pressure during diastole and systole. The diastolic pressure curve is determined by filling the heart with blood and measuring the pressure immediately before ventricular contraction occurs. Until the volume of the left ventricle rises above ~ 150 mL the diastolic pressure changes minimally but above this volume the pressure increases rapidly because the myofibrils are stretched to their maximum.

During ventricular contraction the systolic pressure increases even at low ventricular volumes and reaches a maximum pressure at volumes of ~ 150 mL. At volumes >150 mL the systolic pressure may decrease as actin and myosin are so stretched that contraction is less than optimal.

The maximum systolic pressure for the left ventricle is between 250 and 300 mm Hg but varies widely between individuals. The heavy red lines show a volume-pressure curve during a normal cardiac cycle, with EW representing the net external work of the heart. (From Guyton AC, Hall JE. Textbook of Medical Physiology. 11th ed. Philadelphia: Elsevier Saunders; 2005.)

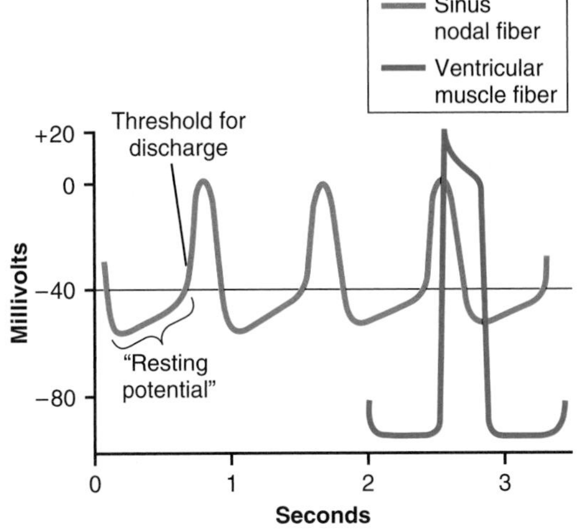

Figure 33-3 The action potential tracing of a sinus nodal fiber, compared with that of a ventricular muscle fiber. (From Guyton AC, Hall JE. Textbook of Medical Physiology. 11th ed. Philadelphia: Elsevier Saunders; 2005.)

conducted through both the atria and ventricles, controlling the cardiac cycle from beat to beat. Each normal cardiac cycle is initiated by spontaneous generation of an AP in the sinoatrial (SA) node (located in the posterior wall of the right atrium near the opening of the superior vena) that is conducted first through the atria, then to the ventricular system, resulting in well-coordinated myocardial contraction. Cardiac APs are the voltage changes that result from activation or inactivation of fast sodium channels, slow sodium-potassium channels, and potassium channels at different times that, together, create collective swings in voltage between a hyperpolarized and a depolarized state. APs higher up in the conduction system have a different morphology than do those in the ventricle, which explains why the control of the cardiac cycle resides in the more proximal or cephalad conducting system.

Rhythmicity of the cycle resides within the cells of the SA node because these cell membranes are inherently more "leaky" to Na^+ and Ca^{2+} ions than are cell membranes of the ventricular conduction system. The influx of Na^+ and Ca^{2+} creates a less negative resting membrane potential (−55 mV), a voltage at which many of the fast sodium channels have become inactivated. Therefore, depolarization is a result of the activation of the slow sodium-calcium channels, which results in a slower upslope of depolarization and a slower repolarization period in comparison with APs of ventricular muscle (Figure 33-3). The passive diffusion of Na^+ due to its high concentration in the extracellular fluid outside the nodal fibers continues to depolarize the membrane. Once the threshold of −40 mV is reached, the sodium-calcium channels are activated, and an AP is generated. The sodium-calcium channels are quickly inactivated, and potassium channels are opened and allow the positively charged K^+ ions to diffuse out of the cell until the resting membrane potential is hyperpolarized again at −55 mV. Finally, potassium channels close, with the inward-leaking Na^+ and Ca^{2+} ions counterbalancing the outward flux of K^+ ions. The process repeats itself, eliciting another cycle. The cells in the SA node control the heart rate because they depolarize more rapidly than does the rest of the conducting system (SA node rate, 70 to 80/min; AV node rate, 40 to 60/min; Purkinje fiber rate, 15 to 40/min).

The APs of ventricular myocytes have several key differences when compared with nodal APs. The intracellular potential is significantly more negative at −85 mV; depolarization occurs abruptly as a result of both fast sodium channels and slow sodium-calcium channels opening. Ventricular myocytes also exhibit a plateau phase of about 0.2 sec, which makes the AP last up to 15 times longer than in skeletal muscle. This plateau occurs because of the longer duration of activation of the slow sodium-calcium channels. The membrane of ventricular myocytes also becomes less permeable to K^+ ions than that of skeletal muscle cells so that, after activation, the efflux of K^+ is slowed and, thus, prevents early return of the AP voltage to its resting level. Once the slow sodium-calcium channels are inactivated at the end of the plateau, the permeability of the membrane to K^+ is simultaneously restored, and the AP is abruptly terminated with the return of the membrane potential to its baseline. Thus, the ventricular AP is much more rapid in onset and offset, has a plateau phase, and has a larger variation in membrane potential in comparison with nodal and conducting-system APs.

Physiologic Effects on Cardiac Cycle Control

Sympathetic nerves are distributed to all parts of the heart, especially the ventricular myocytes. These nerves (1) increase the rate of SA nodal discharge (chronotropy), (2) increase the rate of conduction plus excitability throughout the heart (dromotropy, synchronicity), and (3) increase the force of contraction of all myocytes (inotropy). (Maximal sympathetic outflow can triple the heart rate and double the strength of contraction.) Norepinephrine released at sympathetic nerve endings is believed to increase membrane permeability to Na^+ and Ca^{2+}, increasing the tendency of the membrane potential to drift upward to the threshold for excitation. Increased Ca^{2+} permeability causes increased inotropic effect.

Parasympathetic preganglionic fibers are distributed mainly to the SA and AV nodes and, to a much lesser extent, the atria and ventricles through the vagus nerve. Vagal stimulation releases acetylcholine from the axonal terminus of the preganglionic fibers, which (1) decreases the rate of SA node discharge and (2) decreases the excitability of AV junctional fibers, thus slowing the impulse transmission into the ventricles. Strong vagal stimulation can completely stop SA node discharge, leading to eventual ventricular escape beats from discharge of Purkinje fibers. Acetylcholine works by increasing the permeability of cells in the SA and AV nodes to K^+, thereby producing hyperpolarization (increased negativity of resting membrane potential, −70 to −75 mV); thus, conduction tissue is much less excitable and takes longer to spontaneously reach threshold.

The vasomotor center of the central nervous system (medullary-pontine area) contains neurons that affect chronotropic and inotropic responses from the heart. Vagal activity is reflex in origin and is aroused by impulses from carotid and aortic baroreceptors. The *nucleus ambiguus* contains vagal motor neurons that travel to the SA and AV nodes. Impulse activity depends mainly on baroreceptor input. Also, phasic input from the inspiratory center causes sinus arrhythmia (increased heart rate with inspiration, decreased heart rate with expiration).

Excess extracellular K^+ causes the heart to dilate and become flaccid and slows the heart rate. Larger quantities can cause conduction delays and AV blocks. The mechanism of this effect is that high extracellular K^+ concentration will decrease the resting membrane potential in myocytes (the membrane potential becomes less negative), which decreases the intensity of the AP and thereby decreases inotropy. Excess extracellular Ca^{2+}, on the other hand, can cause spastic contraction of the heart through the direct effect of Ca^{2+} in the contraction process. A deficiency of Ca^{2+} can cause flaccidity.

Body temperature has an effect on the control of the cardiac cycle as well. Heat increases the permeability of myocyte membranes to ions that control the heart rate; hyperthermia can double the heart rate, whereas hypothermia can slow the heart rate to a few beats per minute. The contractile function of the heart is initially augmented with hyperthermia, but this compensatory mechanism is soon exhausted, and the heart eventually becomes flaccid.

Synchronicity

The AP originating in the SA node spreads through the atrium at 0.3 m/sec; internodal pathways terminate in the AV node (1 m/sec). Delay occurs at the AV node, allowing time for the atria to empty before ventricular contraction begins. The impulse reaches the AV node 0.04 sec after its origin in the SA node. The prolonged refractory period of the AV node helps prevent arrhythmias, which can occur if a second cardiac impulse is transmitted into the ventricle too soon after the first is transmitted. Purkinje fibers lead from the AV node and divide into left and right bundle branches, spreading into the apex of the respective ventricles and then back toward the base of the heart. These large fibers have a conduction velocity of 1.5 to 4 m/sec (6 times that of myocytes and 150 times that of junctional fibers), which allows almost immediate transmission of cardiac impulses through the entire ventricular system. Thus, the cardiac impulse arrives at almost all portions of the ventricle simultaneously, exciting the first ventricular myocytes only 0.06 sec ahead of the last ventricular fibers. Effective pumping by both ventricles requires this synchronization of contraction.

The AP causes myocardial myocytes to contract by a mechanism known as *excitation-contraction coupling*. The AP passes into the myocytes along the transverse tubules, triggering release of Ca^{2+} into the cell from the sarcoplasmic reticulum as well as from the transverse tubules themselves. These Ca^{2+} ions promote the sliding of actin on myosin, which creates myofibril contraction. The transverse tubules can store a tremendous amount of Ca^{2+}; without this store, the sarcoplasmic reticulum of myocytes would not provide an adequate supply of Ca^{2+} ions for contraction to occur. Availability of extracellular Ca^{2+} directly impacts the availability of Ca^{2+} ions for release into the cellular sarcoplasm from the transverse tubules.

Suggested Readings

Guyton AC, Hall JE. *Textbook of Medical Physiology*. 11th ed. Philadelphia: WB Saunders; 2006:103-122.

Lake CL. Cardiovascular anatomy and physiology. In: Barash PG, Cullen BF, Stoelting RK, eds. *Clinical Anesthesia*. 5th ed. Philadelphia: Lippincott, Williams & Wilkins; 2006:856-885.

Opie LH. Mechanisms of cardiac contraction and relaxation. In: Braunwald E, ed. *Heart Disease: Textbook of Cardiovascular Medicine*. 8th ed. Philadelphia: WB Saunders; 2007:509.

CHAPTER 34

Physiologic Determinants of Cardiac Output

Amorn Vijitpavan, MD

Cardiac output (CO) is the quantity of blood that the heart pumps per minute. CO in a normal 70-kg individual with a heart rate (HR) of 70 to 80 beats/min is 5 to 6 L/min, but it decreases by approximately 25% when the individual is resting in the supine position and may increase approximately eightfold with exertion. The cardiac index (CI) normalizes a person's CO for body surface area (BSA):

$$CI\ (L \cdot min^{-1} \cdot m^{-2}) = CO/BSA$$

A normal CI varies between 2.5 and 3.5·L·min^{-1}·m^{-2}. The two major determinants of CO are stroke volume (SV) and HR:

$$CO\ (L/min) = SV \times HR$$

Heart Rate

The HR is determined primarily by the rate of spontaneous phase 4 depolarization of the sinoatrial (SA) node pacemaker cells, which are influenced by neural and humeral mechanisms. In children, HR is critically important for maintenance of CO, whereas in adults, both HR and SV contribute significantly to CO. In addition to an increase in CO from an increase in HR (as one would expect from the formula CO = HR × SV), an increase in HR increases contractility (positive inotropic effect); however, a HR exceeding 170 beats/min reduces CO because of decreased ventricular filling time.

Stroke Volume

The SV is the amount of blood ejected by the ventricle with each contraction. A normal SV is 70 to 80 mL. Determinants of SV include preload, afterload, and contractility.

Preload

Preload is directly proportional to end-diastolic myocardial fiber length, often represented as end-diastolic volume (EDV, with a normal value of ~120 mL). During normal cardiac muscle contraction, the sarcomere length is relatively short, but if EDV increases, the length of the sarcomere increases, and during subsequent contractions, more force is generated, the maximum rate of pressure development (dP/dt) increases, and SV increases proportionately (Figure 34-1).

Many factors affect preload, including primarily venous tone (which, in turn, is affected by total blood volume), intrathoracic pressure, body position, pulmonary vascular resistance, and atrial contraction. Impaired venous return (from, for example, peripheral vasodilation, hemorrhage, positive-pressure ventilation) decreases SV and CO. Although total blood volume is important to preload, the distribution of that blood volume between the extrathoracic and intrathoracic compartments is more important. The venous system has a very high capacity, and assuming no loss of volume from dehydration or hemorrhage, a large amount of blood can be shifted centrally from the periphery.

Ventricular volume can be measured using multiple techniques, including echocardiography, angiography, and scintigraphy, but, except for echocardiography, most are not helpful for clinically managing a patient. Transesophageal echocardiography is useful perioperatively to estimate EDV, but it has multiple limitations. Therefore, left ventricular end-diastolic pressure (LVEDP) is frequently used as a surrogate for EDV on the basis of a nonlinear, end-diastolic, pressure-volume relationship. More commonly, left atrial pressure, pulmonary artery occlusion pressure (PAOP), right atrial pressure (RAP), or central venous pressure (CVP) is used to estimate LVEDP and LVEDV.

The reliability of these cardiac pressures in estimating ventricular preload depends on ventricular compliance, the integrity of the cardiac valves, and intrathoracic pressure. Ventricular compliance (the distensibility of the chamber in response to changes in volume) is affected by coronary ischemia, ventricular hypertrophy, pericarditis, and cardiac tamponade, among others, all of which can result in a weak correlation between pressure and volume of the left ventricle. If compliance is decreased, then small increases in ventricular volume may be associated with large increases in ventricular pressure. PAOP and pulmonary artery pressure are most commonly used to estimate LV preload; CVP provides the poorest estimation of LV preload.

Afterload

Afterload is defined as the impedance to ejection, the force that resists muscle shortening during myocardial contraction. Systemic vascular resistance (SVR) accounts for about 95% of the resistance to ejection (the remainder is due to characteristics of the left ventricle and the LV outflow tract and aortic valve) and is often used clinically to estimate afterload.

$$SVR = 80 \times (MAP - RAP)/CO$$

where MAP is the mean arterial pressure and RAP is the right atrial pressure. Normal SVR is 900 to 1500 Dynes·sec^{-1}·cm^{-5}. Wood units are also used, most commonly in measuring pulmonary vascular resistance, and are calculated using the same equation but without multiplying ((MAP − RAP)/CO) by 80. Blood pressure is a poor estimation of afterload.

Afterload, as defined by ventricular wall stress, is represented by the Laplace law:

$$T = Pr/2h$$

where T is the tension in the LV wall, P is pressure, r is the radius, and h is wall thickness. From the Laplace law, it is apparent that ventricular volume, LV wall thickness, and systolic intraventricular pressure are primary determinants of afterload.

Intraventricular pressure has an important effect on afterload. A dilated thin-walled ventricle generates significantly greater wall stress than does a thicker-walled smaller ventricle. A failing ventricle will dilate and significantly increase afterload, which significantly reduces CO. Reducing afterload is an important goal in managing congestive heart failure.

Contractility

Contractility refers to the intrinsic ability of the myocardium to generate force at given end-diastolic fiber length and is closely related to the availability of intracellular calcium. Contractility is relatively easy to understand conceptually but difficult to define; measurements of cardiac performance include the dP/dt (Figure 34-2), isolated papillary muscle shortening, and the work generated by isolated or whole-heart preparations, but these definitions are not clinically useful.

No specific value represents normal contractility. Contractility may be assessed through echocardiography, angiography, and scintigraphy. A more clinically useful index of contractility is ejection fraction, the slope of the

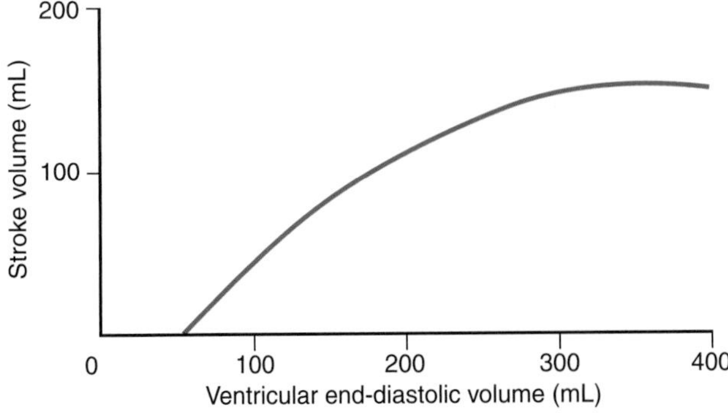

Figure 34-1 The Starling curve. As left ventricular end-diastolic volume (stretch of myofibrils) increases, myocardial contractility (stroke volume) increases.

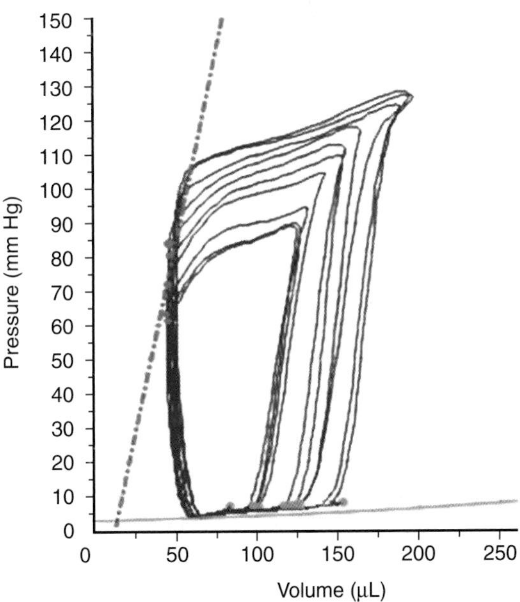

Figure 34-2 Several pressure-volume loops of the left ventricle. The slope of the red line connecting several of the loops at the point representing closure of the aortic valve correlates very well with left ventricular contractility and is independent of preload, afterload, and heart rate.

plot of SV against EDV. Although affected by changes in preload, afterload, and HR, ejection fraction is one of the most reliable and sensitive parameters of ventricular performance.

A change in contractility is considered to be a change in the contractile force of the heart in the presence of unchanged diastolic dimensions and pressure. Thus, it is a change in the myocardial force-velocity relation. Catecholamines, digitalis, and calcium ions increase contractility. The adrenergic nervous system exerts the most important influence on contractility. Hypoxia, acidosis, ischemia, and certain drugs (e.g., calcium channel blockers and β-adrenergic receptor blocking agents) decrease contractility.

Summary

The homeostasis of cardiac function and its instantaneous response to changing physiology are regulated by a delicate interplay among various determinants of CO. All of these factors work together to maintain sufficient CO to meet the metabolic needs of tissues. A persistent imbalance in any factor will lead to a structural adaptation of the myocardium. Although knowledge of CO is important, CO itself is not a sensitive indicator of LV performance because the circulation may temporarily adapt to maintain CO. Thus, CO should be considered in concert with other physiologic parameters to determine the correct course of therapy.

Suggested Readings

The determinants of cardiac output. In: Anderson RM. *The Gross Physiology of the Cardiovascular System*. Tucson: University of Arizona, Department of Biomedical Communications; 1980. http://cardiac-output.info/the-text/introduction.html. Accessed July 21, 2012.

Mohrman DE, Heller LJ. *Cardiovascular Physiology*. 7th ed. New York: McGraw-Hill Lange; 2010:48-66.

CHAPTER 35

Myocardial Oxygen Supply and Demand

David Layer, DO

The best way to achieve satisfactory perioperative cardiovascular outcome is to ensure that myocardial O_2 supply meets or exceeds myocardial O_2 demand.

O_2 SUPPLY

Coronary Blood Flow

Myocardial O_2 delivery depends on coronary blood flow (CBF) and arterial blood O_2 content (CaO_2) (Box 35-1). CBF is determined by the following equation (based on Ohm's law for calculating current flow in which current equals voltage divided by resistance):

$$Q \propto \Delta P/R$$

where Q is CBF; ΔP is the pressure across the coronary vascular bed, or coronary perfusion pressure (CPP); and R is total coronary resistance. CPP is usually defined as the aortic diastolic blood pressure (DBPAo) minus the left ventricular end-diastolic pressure (LVEDP). Thus, the foregoing equation may be rewritten as:

$$CBF \propto (DBP_{AO} - LVDEP)/R$$

Box 35-1 Determinants of O_2 Supply

- O_2 content
- Aortic root pressure
- Ventricular pressure
- Diastolic perfusion time (determined by heart rate)
- Local vascular resistance
- Autonomic innervation
- Autoregulation
- Coronary steal
- Exogenous and endogenous substances

Coronary Perfusion Pressure

CBF fluctuates with changes in aortic root blood pressure and changes in resistance to flow across the myocardium; the effect of coronary venous pressure is minimal. During the early part of systole (i.e., isovolumic contraction, before the aortic valve opens), the pressure at the coronary ostia is at end diastole and, by definition, is lower than the left ventricular systolic pressure. After the aortic valve opens, the pressure at the coronary ostia remains lower than peak systolic pressure because of the pressure gradient across the aortic valve creating a Venturi effect at the base of the aortic root. This pressure differential can be particularly pronounced in the presence of aortic stenosis.

High left ventricular pressures during systole further decrease flow to the left ventricle to less than 50% of the flow during diastole. The lower pressures in the right ventricle yield a more uniform CBF distribution during systole and diastole; however, disease states that elevate right ventricular pressures can produce a flow pattern similar to that of the left ventricle.

Because most CBF to the left ventricle occurs during diastole, the diastolic pressure, duration of diastole, and heart rate have been used to quantify O_2 supply using the diastolic perfusion index, calculated as the area beneath the diastolic pressure versus time curve multiplied by the heart rate. Factors that decrease aortic diastolic pressure, decrease the duration of diastole, or increase left ventricular diastolic pressure reduce CBF to the left ventricle (e.g., tachycardia, left ventricular failure [increased LVEDP], and aortic stenosis), which increases left ventricular pressures and decreases aortic root pressures.

Vascular Resistance

One of the most important extrinsic factors affecting coronary vascular resistance is extravascular compression of the intramyocardial portion of the coronary arteries. Extravascular coronary artery compression is greatest near the endocardium and lowest near the epicardium. Because intramyocardial pressure approaches ventricular pressure, the CPP is estimated by aortic pressure and ventricular pressure.

Vasoconstriction is the primary intrinsic factor contributing to coronary resistance; the autonomic nervous system and endogenous biochemicals account for the majority of vasoconstriction. Coronary autoregulation maintains CBF over a wide range of perfusion pressures (i.e., between approximately 50 and 150 mm Hg), primarily by metabolic coupling in vessels measuring less than 150 μm.

The critical metabolic control parameter appears to be hypoxia, which is mediated locally by adenosine. Specifically, decreased myocardial O_2 tension induces adenosine-mediated coronary vasodilation by modulating calcium flux into vascular smooth muscle. Parasympathetic stimulation induces direct coronary vasodilation. Sympathetically mediated coronary vasodilation results from increased myocardial O_2 consumption and local metabolite production (e.g., adenosine, nitric oxide, prostaglandins, endothelin).

Arterial Blood O_2 Content

The Cao_2 is determined primarily by the hemoglobin concentration (Hb) and O_2 saturation (Sao_2). Factors that affect the shape or position of the O_2 dissociation curve and availability of O_2 binding sites are also important.

$$Cao_2 = (Hb \times 1.39)(Sao_2) + (Pao_2)(0.003)$$

Other Factors

Atherosclerotic disease is the primary disease mechanism for increased coronary vascular resistance and inadequate O_2 delivery. In accordance with Poiseuille's law, reductions in flow are proportional to the length of the lesion and the fourth power of the radius of the lumen; seemingly small reductions in lumen size produce critical reductions in regional blood flow. Exogenous compounds that cause coronary vasodilation include calcium channel blockers, nitrates, and dipyridamole. Catecholamines have a dual effect. Stimulation of α-receptors leads to vasoconstriction, whereas β-receptor stimulation increases myocardial metabolism and causes vasodilation.

O_2 Demand

Models used to predict myocardial O_2 consumption require an estimate of basal myocardial O_2 consumption, ventricular wall tension, velocity of myofibril contraction, and energy consumed during contraction and relaxation (Box 35-2). Approximately 90% of myocardial O_2 consumption is for contractile activity, and less than 10% is necessary for the maintenance of cellular integrity and the electrical activity of the heart. In isolated muscle strips, O_2 consumption is proportional to the tension developed during a contraction. In the intact heart, pressure alone as a substitute for wall tension is a poor correlate of O_2 consumption. According to the Laplace law, ventricular tension is directly proportional to pressure (afterload) and chamber radius (preload) and is inversely proportional to wall thickness.

Box 35-2 Relationships That Determine Myocardial O_2 Consumption

Contractility (inotropy) = velocity of pressure development, dP/dt

$$\text{Wall tension} = \frac{(\text{pressure} \times \text{radius})}{(2 \times \text{wall thickness})}$$

Heart rate × stroke volume
Basal O_2 consumption
Work = area within ventricular pressure-volume loop (see Figure 34-2)

The systolic perfusion index, calculated by determining the area under the systolic pressure versus time curve and multiplying by the heart rate, is moderately correlated with O_2 demand. The velocity of tension development (inotropy or contractility) has also been shown to be an important determinant of O_2 consumption and can be estimated from the rate of change in pressure (dP/dt). The amount of work performed by the heart adds to its O_2 consumption and can be quantified by integrating the area under the pressure versus volume curve. In addition, the amount of work is a function of the frequency of contractions, or heart rate.

To accurately assess the effects of a given intervention or change in hemodynamics, myocardial O_2 consumption must take into account all of the aforementioned factors (see Box 35-2). In the clinical setting, crude estimates are often made on the basis of systolic pressure and heart rate, which, in and of themselves, are poor predictors of myocardial O_2 consumption.

Effects of Anesthetic Drugs

Determining the effects of a particular drug on the O_2 supply-demand ratio can be difficult because any particular drug can usually have multiple effects; it would be unusual for a drug to affect only one specific aspect of the supply-demand relationship (e.g., β-adrenergic receptor blocking agents are vasodilators but also increase myocardial O_2 consumption).

Suggested Readings

Ardehali A, Ports TA. Myocardial oxygen supply and demand. *Chest.* 1990;98: 699-705.

Odonkor PN, Grigore AM. Patients with ischemic heart disease. *Med Clin North Am.* 2013;97:1033-1050.

Tánczos K, Molnár Z. The oxygen supply-demand balance: A monitoring challenge. *Best Pract Res Clin Anaesthesiol.* 2013;27(2):201-207.

Weber KT, Janicki JS. The metabolic demand and oxygen supply of the heart: Physiologic and clinical considerations. *Am J Cardiol* 1979;44:722.

Zong P, Tune JD, Downey HF. Mechanisms of oxygen demand/supply balance in the right ventricle. *Exp Biol Med.* 2005;230:507-519.

CHAPTER 36

Tachyarrhythmias

Srikanth Hosur, MD, and Adebola Adesanya, MD, MPH

Tachyarrhythmias are classified as either narrow complex tachycardias (NCT) or wide complex tachycardias (WCT), based on the width of the QRS complexes. NCTs are further classified as atrioventricular (AV) node-passive or AV node-active tachycardias, based on whether the AV node is involved in the propagation and maintenance of the arrhythmia. AV node-passive tachycardias have a regular rhythm, as in atrial tachycardia or atrial flutter, or an irregular rhythm, as in multifocal atrial tachycardia, atrial flutter with varying conduction, or atrial fibrillation. (AV node reentry tachycardia [AVNRT]) or accessory pathway-dependent tachycardia. The accessory pathway conduction can be orthodromic (using the AV node as forward conduction) and, hence, have a narrow complex, or antidromic (using the accessory pathway as forward conduction and the AV node itself for retrograde conduction) and, hence, have a wide complex.

It is important to understand the mechanisms of these arrythmias because AV node-active tachycardias can usually be terminated by maneuvers that prolong AV node conduction, such as vagal maneuvers, or the administration of drugs, such as adenosine (Figure 36-1).

Narrow Complex Tachycardias

Treatment

NCTs can be treated medically or by cardioversion. The administration of adenosine and vagal maneuvers are helpful only in the termination of AV node-active tachycardias. Although all NCTs can be terminated using synchronized cardioversion, the use of cardioversion should be reserved for patients in whom the arrhythmia is accompanied by hemodynamic instability.

In patients with hemodynamically stable NCTs, diltiazem, 0.25 mg/kg, is preferred over β-adrenergic receptor blocking agents or verapamil because dilitiazem has less negative inotropy. Patients with a low ejection fraction are candidates for amiodarone administered intravenously as a

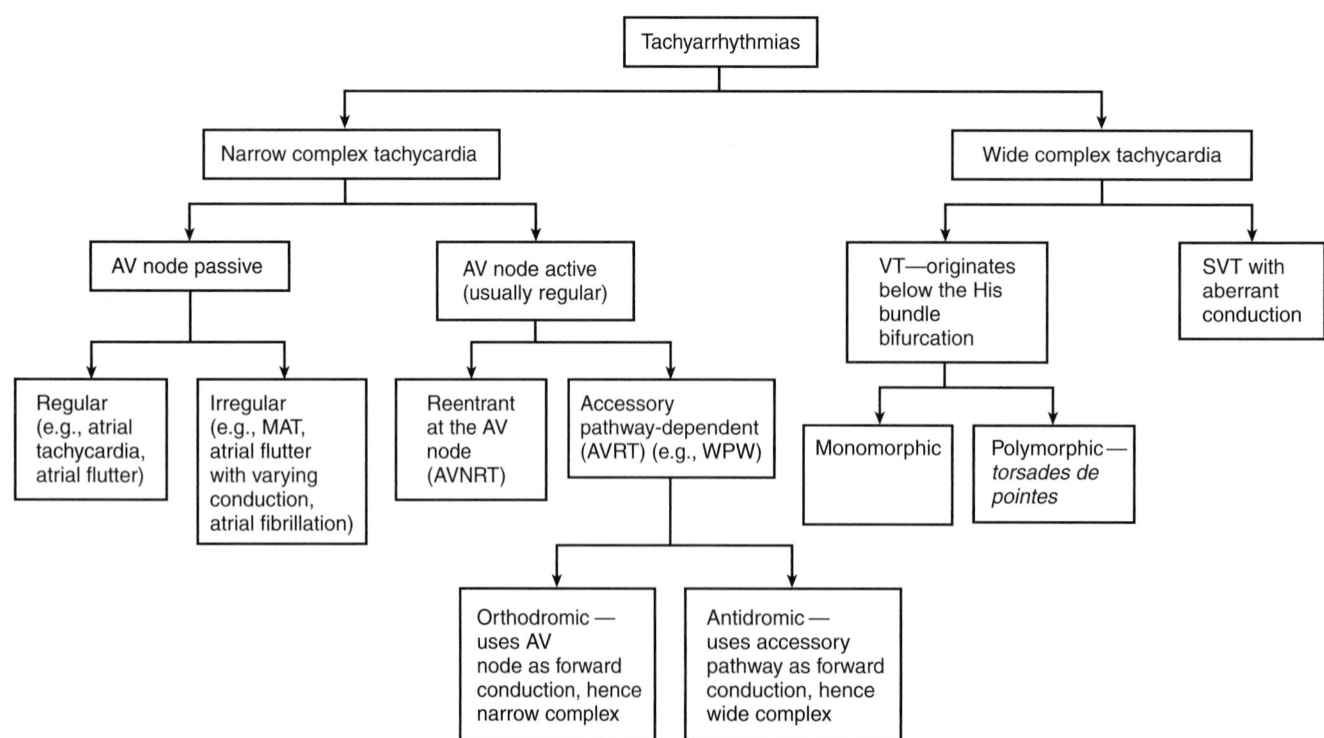

Figure 36-1 Classification of tachyarrhythmias into narrow complex and wide complex tachyarrhythmias and subtypes included within each category. AVNRT, Atrioventricular nodal reentrant tachycardia; AVRT, atrioventricular reentrant tachycardia; MAT, multifocal atrial tachycardia; SVT supraventricular tachycardia; VT, ventricular tachycardia; WPW, Wolff-Parkinson-White syndrome.

bolus of 150 mg that can be repeated. Procainamide is useful as a second-line agent in this situation.

Adenosine should be given in a central or antecubital vein at a dose of 6 to 12 mg. It is short acting, has a half-life of 12 to 18 sec, and can cause flushing, bronchospasm, and chest pain. Adenosine is antagonized by the administration of methylxanthines, such as aminophylline.

Wide Complex Tachycardias

WCTs are defined as arrhythmias with a QRS complex duration longer than 0.12 sec at a rate greater than 100 beats/min. WCTs are presumed to be ventricular tachycardias (VTs) until proved otherwise, although some supraventricular tachycardias (SVTs) can present as WCT (SVT with aberrancy). Differentiating between SVTs with a wide QRS complex and a VT is critical because the treatment is very different (Figures 36-2 to 36-11).

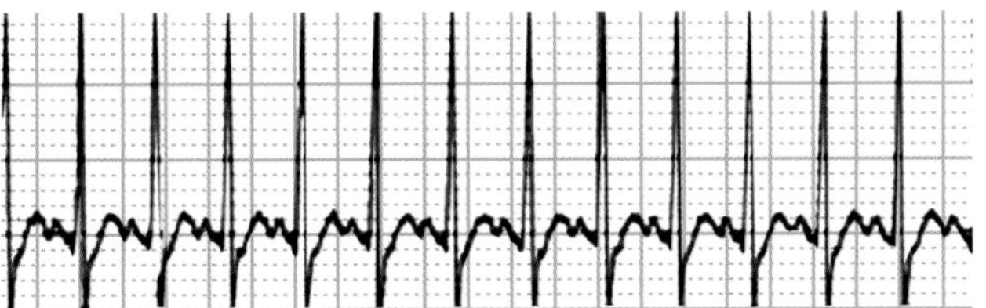

Figure 36-2 Atrial tachycardia originating from a single focus in the atrium. The electrocardiogram shows a regular rate of 150 to 250 beats/min. The P wave morphologic appearance is different from that seen in sinus tachycardia.

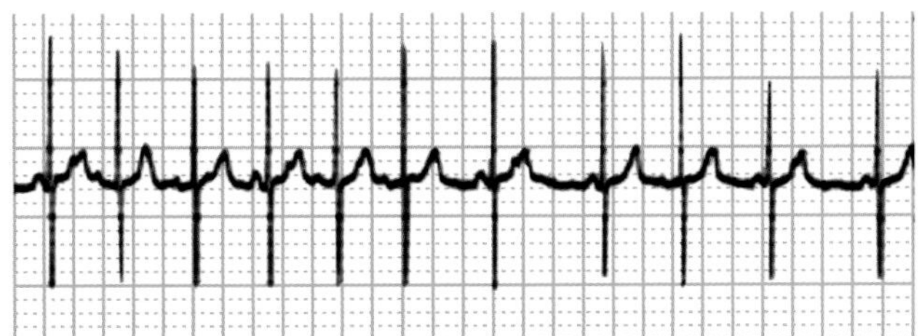

Figure 36-3 Multifocal atrial tachycardia (MAT) arising from multiple foci in the atria. MAT is seen in patients with pulmonary disease and excess ingestion of methylxanthine. The electrocardiogram shows an irregular rate with P waves of different morphologic appearances and varying PR intervals. MAT is not amenable to treatment with digoxin or adenosine.

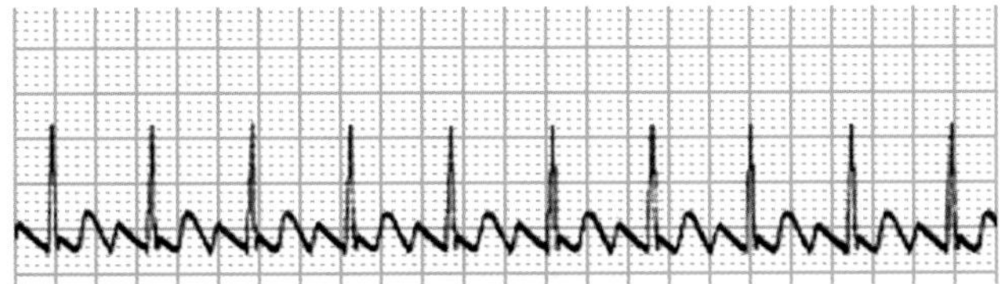

Figure 36-4 Atrial flutter originating in the reentry circuit in the atrium. The electrocardiogram shows sawtooth P flutter waves with variable conduction to the ventricles. The atrial rate is 250 to 300 beats/min.

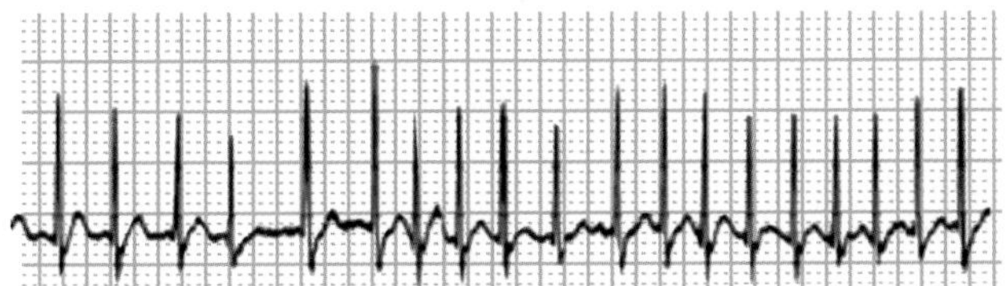

Figure 36-5 In atrial fibrillation, heterogeneous electrical remodeling causes multicircuit reentry in the atria, resulting in a lack of organized atrial activity and an irregular heart rhythm. Fibrillation waves can be seen in this example. P waves are absent.

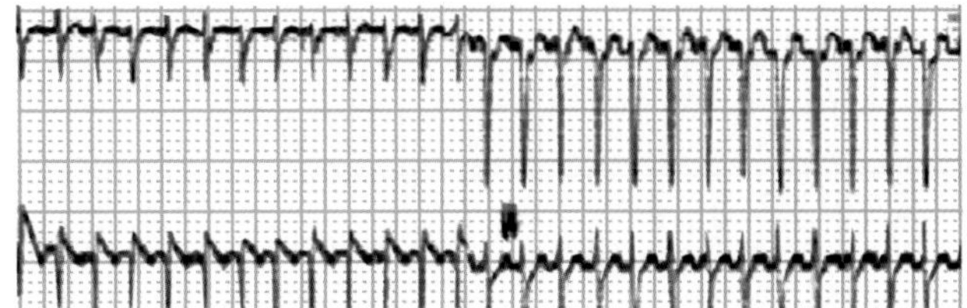

Figure 36-6 Atrioventricular (AV) node reentrant tachycardia (AVNRT) arises from an electrical loop involving the AV node and aberrant slower conducting tissue around the AV node. The ventricular rhythm is regular. In this example, the rate is 140 to 200 beats/min. P waves are absent or rarely seen after the QRS complex. AVNRT can be terminated using vagal maneuvers or adenosine.

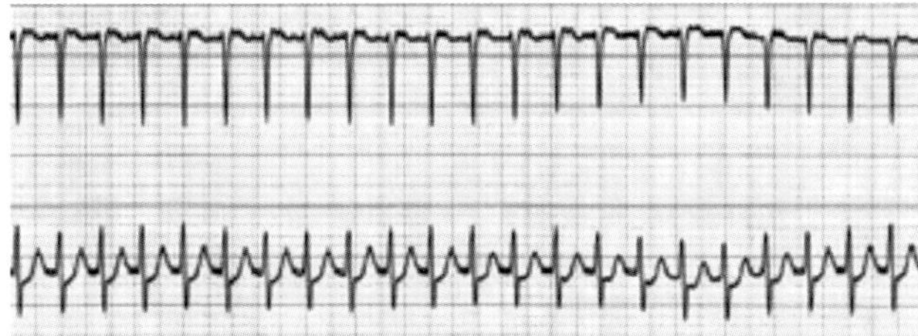

Figure 36-7 Atrioventricular (AV) reentrant tachycardia (AVRT), also known as reciprocating tachycardia. If conduction from the atria is through the AV node, this type of AVRT is orthodromic tachycardia (the most common variation, which has a narrow complex). If conduction is through the accessory pathway (AP), this is an antidromic tachycardia, which has a wide complex. The AP is between the atrial and ventricular myocardium and has a faster conduction but longer refractory period than does the AV node. An example is Wolff-Parkinson-White syndrome, in which the delta wave on the QRS complex is apparent when the heart rate is normal because of conduction through the AP (preexcitation).

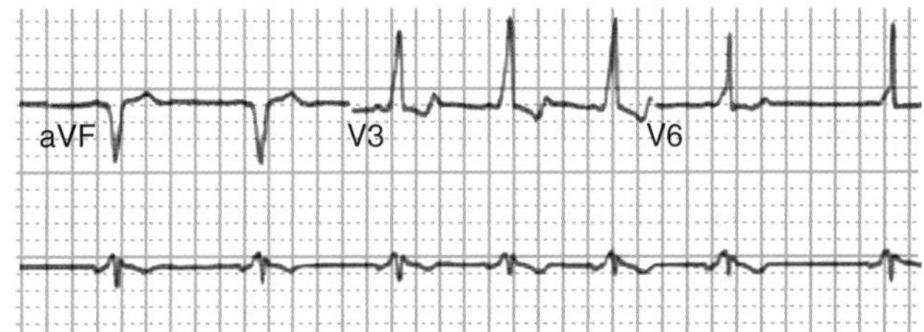

Figure 36-8 Wolff-Parkinson-White syndrome. In orthodromic conduction, the electrocardiogram shows narrow QRS complexes with rates of 150 to 200 beats/min and P waves not hidden but present on the ST segment/T wave. Treatment of hemodynamically stable patients with tachycardia is the same as for atrioventricular node reentrant tachycardia. In 1% to 15% of patients, adenosine can cause ventricular fibrillation; thus, resuscitation equipment should be kept readily available. The use of digoxin should be avoided in patients with Wolff-Parkinson-White syndrome because digoxin increases conduction through the accessory pathway and slows the atrioventricular node. In patients with antidromic wide complex tachycardia, the use of β-adrenergic receptor blocking agents and calcium channel blocking agents should be avoided.

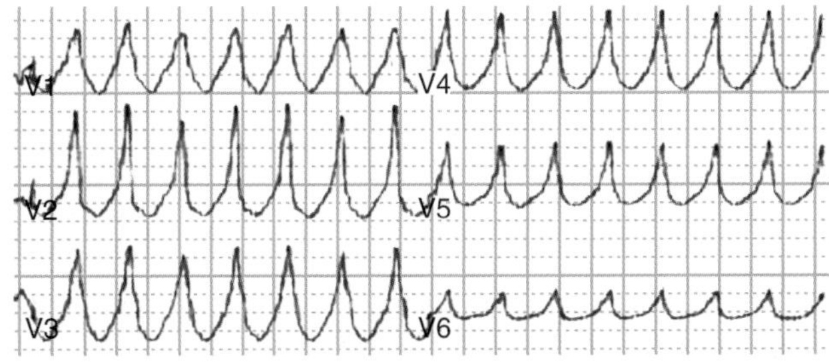

Figure 36-9 Ventricular tachycardia with positive concordance.

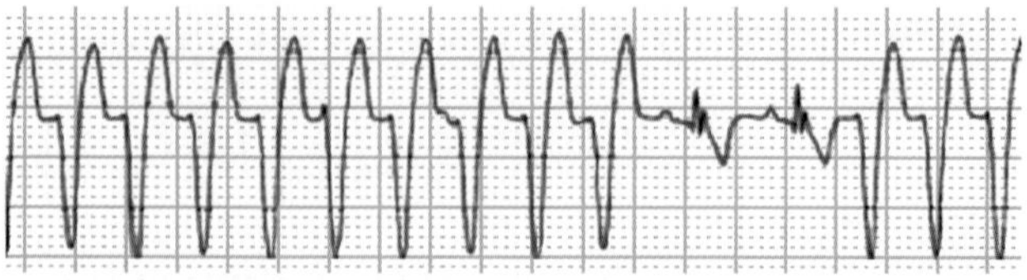

Figure 36-10 Ventricular tachycardia with fusion beats and atrioventricular dissociation.

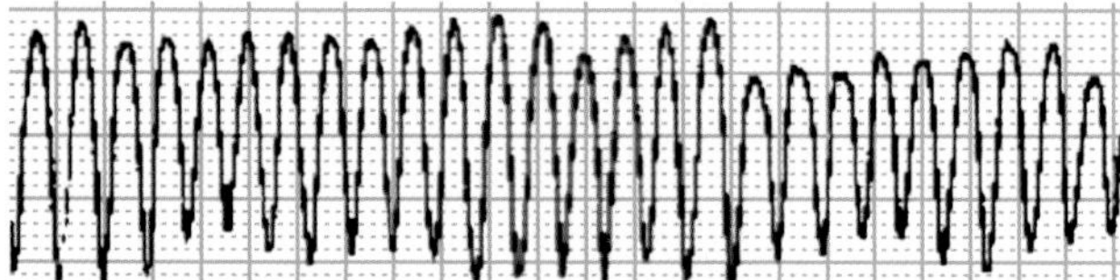

Figure 36-11 Polymorphic ventricular tachycardia.

Diagnosis

For the purpose of diagnosis, WCTs can be classified into four categories based on the following:

1. Origination above or below the bifurcation of the His bundle.
2. Presence of an SVT with aberrant ventricular conduction. SVT with aberrancy can be due to conduction slowing or bundle branch block. It can also be due to anterograde conduction over an accessory AV pathway (antidromic Wolff-Parkinson-White [WPW] syndrome).
3. Presence of a wide QRS waveform generated by ventricular pacing.
4. Presence of electrolyte abnormalities, such as hyperkalemia or hypokalemia, or the use of medications, such as tricyclic antidepressants and antihistamines (sodium channel blocking drugs).

WCTs associated with drug overdose usually have terminal alterations of the QRS complex with right-axis deviation (RV wave in lead aVR, and S waves in leads I and aVL). The diagnosis can be made by reviewing the patient's history and electrocardiogram. VT is more likely to occur in patients with coronary artery disease and signs of AV dissociation (cannon A waves). Hemodynamic stability does not rule out a diagnosis of VT.

A diagnosis of VT is likely when, on the 12-lead electrocardiogram, the QRS complex duration is longer than 160 ms, all of the QRS complexes in the precordial leads are positive or negative (positive or negative concordance), fusion beats or capture beats are seen, and AV dissociation is present. Polymorphic VT has beat-to-beat variations in morphologic appearance as a cyclic progressive change in cardiac axis. Polymorphic VT occurring in the setting of a prolonged QT interval is called torsades de pointes. VT that occurs with hyperkalemia is sinusoidal, is preceded by tall T waves, has short QT intervals, has prolonged PR intervals, and has flattened P waves. With tricyclic antidepressant toxicity, VT is characterized by a right-axis pattern with prominent S waves in leads I and aVL and an R wave in lead aVR.

Treatment

Regardless of the cause of WCT, electrical cardioversion with 100 to 200 J (monophasic) or 50 to 100 J (biphasic) is the treatment of choice in patients who are hemodynamically unstable.

The use of β-adrenergic receptor blocking agents, digitalis, and calcium channel blocking agents is recommended for patients with WCTs that are thought to be due to SVT with aberrancy but are contraindicated in patients with WPW syndrome. Procainamide and amiodarone are acceptable alternative choices because they are used to treat WCTs due to VT or SVT. Electrical cardioversion should be performed when the WCT does not respond to antiarrhythmic agents or if the patient is hemodynamically unstable. Torsades de pointes is treated with intravenously administered magnesium; the temporary use of transvenous overdrive pacing should be considered for patients with heart rates of 100 beats/min or greater and who do not respond to magnesium. Isoproterenol (2 μg/min in adults) can be infused with the same heart rate goal (≤100 beats/min) until pacing can be established.

Toxicity of sodium channel blocking agents, such as tricyclic antidepressants and antihistamines, should be treated with induction of alkalosis and diuresis. The administration of sodium bicarbonate infusions should be considered when the QRS intervals exceed 100 ms and the patient has persistent hypotension and arrhythmias. Hyperkalemia is treated with calcium, glucose-insulin infusions, β-agonists, and sodium bicarbonate.

Suggested Readings

Akhtar M. Electrophysiologic basis for wide QRS complex tachycardia. *Pacing Clin Electrophysiol.* 1983;6:81-98.

Drew BJ, Ackerman MJ, Funk M, et al. Prevention of torsades de pointes in hospital settings: a scientific statement from the American Heart Association and the American College of Cardiology Foundation. *Circulation.* 2010;121:1047.

Goldberger ZD, Rho RW, Page RL. Approach to the diagnosis and initial management of the stable adult patient with a wide complex tachycardia. *Am J Cardiol.* 2008;101:1456-1466.

Jacobson C. Narrow QRS complex tachycardias. *AACN Adv Crit Care.* 2007;18: 264-274.

Obel OA, Camm AJ. Supraventricular tachycardia ECG. Diagnosis and anatomy. *Eur Heart J.* 1997;18:C2-11.

Reising S, Kusumoto F, Goldschlager N. Life-threatening arrhythmias in the intensive care unit. *Intensive Care Med.* 2007;22:3-13.

CHAPTER 37

Bradyarrhythmias

Srikanth Hosur, MD, and Adebola Adesanya, MD, MPH

Bradycardia, typically defined as heart rate of less than 60 beats/min, may be physiologically normal in some individuals; however, heart rates less than 60 beats/min may be inadequate for others. Bradycardia becomes problematic when the heart rate results in a decrease in cardiac output that is inadequate for a specific clinical situation. Bradyarrhythmias can be due to sinus bradycardia, atrioventricular (AV) junctional rhythm, or heart block.

Regardless of the presentation, bradycardia should be treated immediately if hypotension or signs of hypoperfusion (e.g., acute altered mental status, seizures, syncope, ischemic chest pain, or congestive heart failure) are present. The goal of initial therapy is to administer a chronotropic drug, such as atropine or glycopyrrolate, that treats bradycardia of any cause. Patients with bradycardia that is unresponsive to atropine or glycopyrrolate are candidates for treatment with external or transvenous pacing if hypotension or hypoperfusion persists. Pacing devices provide controlled heart rate management without the risk of adverse effects associated with medications. Pharmacologic alternatives to atropine (second-line drug therapy) include dopamine, epinephrine, and isoproterenol, all of which can be titrated to the heart rate response. Isoproterenol, a pure β-sympathomimetic agent, increases myocardial oxygen demand and produces peripheral vasodilation, both of which are poorly tolerated in patients with acute myocardial ischemia. Glucagon can be used to treat patients with symptomatic bradycardia related to an overdose of β-receptor or calcium channel blocking agents (Table 37-1).

Patients with sinus bradycardia, AV junctional rhythm, or Mobitz I second-degree AV block (Figure 37-1) presenting with strong vagal tone and slow sinus node discharge or impaired AV node conduction will generally respond to treatment with atropine. Patients with complete heart block and an AV junctional escape rhythm will also respond to treatment with atropine. However, in patients with Mobitz II second-degree AV block (Figure 37-2) or new-onset wide QRS complex complete heart block (Figure 37-3), the heart block is usually infranodal, and increased vagal tone is not a significant cause of the bradycardia. These rhythms are less likely to respond to treatment with atropine; therefore, cardiac pacing is the treatment of choice.

Table 37-1 Intravenously Administered Pharmacologic Treatment of Bradycardia

Medication	Dose
Atropine*	0.5 mg q 3-5 min to a maximum total dose of 3 mg Doses of atropine sulfate of < 0.5 mg may paradoxically result in further slowing of the heart rate.
Dopamine	Initial: 5 $\mu g \cdot kg^{-1} \cdot min^{-1}$ Titrate to response
Epinephrine	Initial: 2-10 μg/min Titrate to response
Isoproterenol	Initial: 2 to 10 μg/min Titrate to response
Glucagon	Initial: 3 mg Infusion: 3 mg/h, if necessary

*Atropine administration should not delay implementation of external pacing for patients with poor perfusion.

Patients with Mobitz II second-degree AV block, even if asymptomatic, can progress without warning to complete heart block with a slow and unstable idioventricular rhythm; external pacing electrode pads or transvenous pacing electrodes should be placed prophylactically in this group of patients. Transcutaneous pacing is noninvasive but can be painful and may fail to produce effective mechanical capture. Transvenous (endocardial) pacing is accomplished by passing a pacing electrode into the right ventricle directly through a central vein catheter or through a pacing pulmonary artery catheter (if the catheter is already in place). The American Heart Association algorithm for bradycardia (Figure 37-4) provides a convenient framework for managing patients with bradycardia.

Intraoperative Bradycardia

Intraoperative bradycardia occurs commonly and can be hemodynamically significant, particularly in patients with preexisting heart disease. It is associated with hypotension (defined as a decrease in mean arterial pressure of >40% from baseline or a mean arterial pressure <60 mm Hg) in about 60% of cases. Factors associated with bradycardia under anesthesia include (1) age (bradycardia is more prevalent with increasing age above 50 years), (2) sex (male/female ratio of 60:40), (3) vagal stimulation (e.g., certain surgical procedures and laparoscopic inflation of the peritoneum), (4) opioid administration (fentanyl and remifentanil), (5) administration of high doses of inhalation anesthetic agents (particularly during inhalation induction), and (6) administration of high doses of propofol.

Other important factors to consider when symptomatic bradycardia occurs include hypoxemia and concomitant administration of neuromuscular blocking agents (NMBAs), β-adrenergic receptor blocking agents, calcium channel blocking agents, or digoxin. Because of its critical nature, hypoxemia should be excluded as the cause of bradycardia very early in the evaluation of a patient with symptomatic intraoperative bradycardia.

Opiates, such as fentanyl and morphine, have a direct action on the sinus node, in addition to having central nervous system effects that result in bradycardia. Inhaled anesthetic gases (i.e., isoflurane) directly depress sinus node activity by altering the slope of phase IV depolarization, an effect likely related to calcium flux across the cell membrane. Nondepolarizing NMBAs, such as vecuronium and rocuronium, lack the vagolytic effects that pancuronium has; succinylcholine, a depolarizing NMBA, causes bradycardia

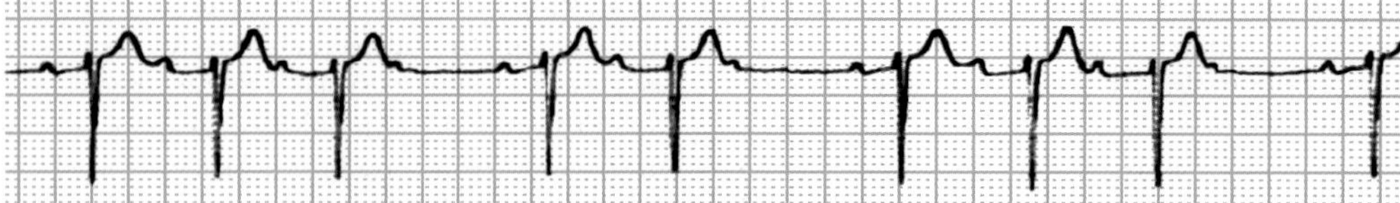

Figure 37-1 Second-degree atrioventricular block—Mobitz type I block.

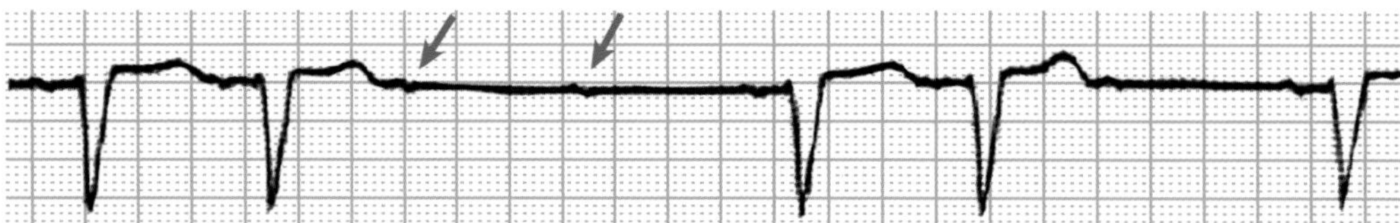

Figure 37-2 Second-degree atrioventricular block—Mobitz type II block.

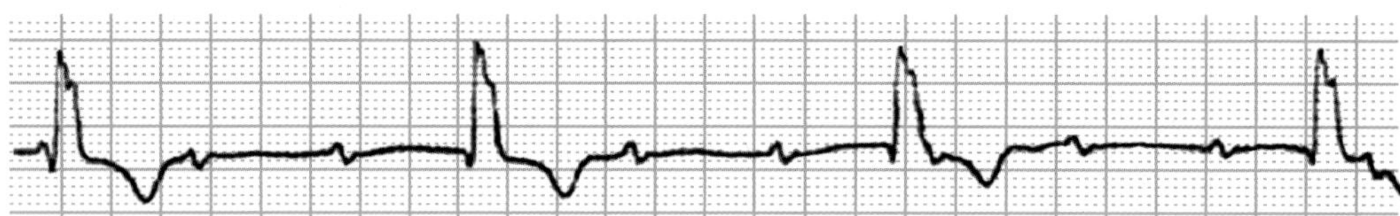

Figure 37-3 Complete (third-degree) atrioventricular block.

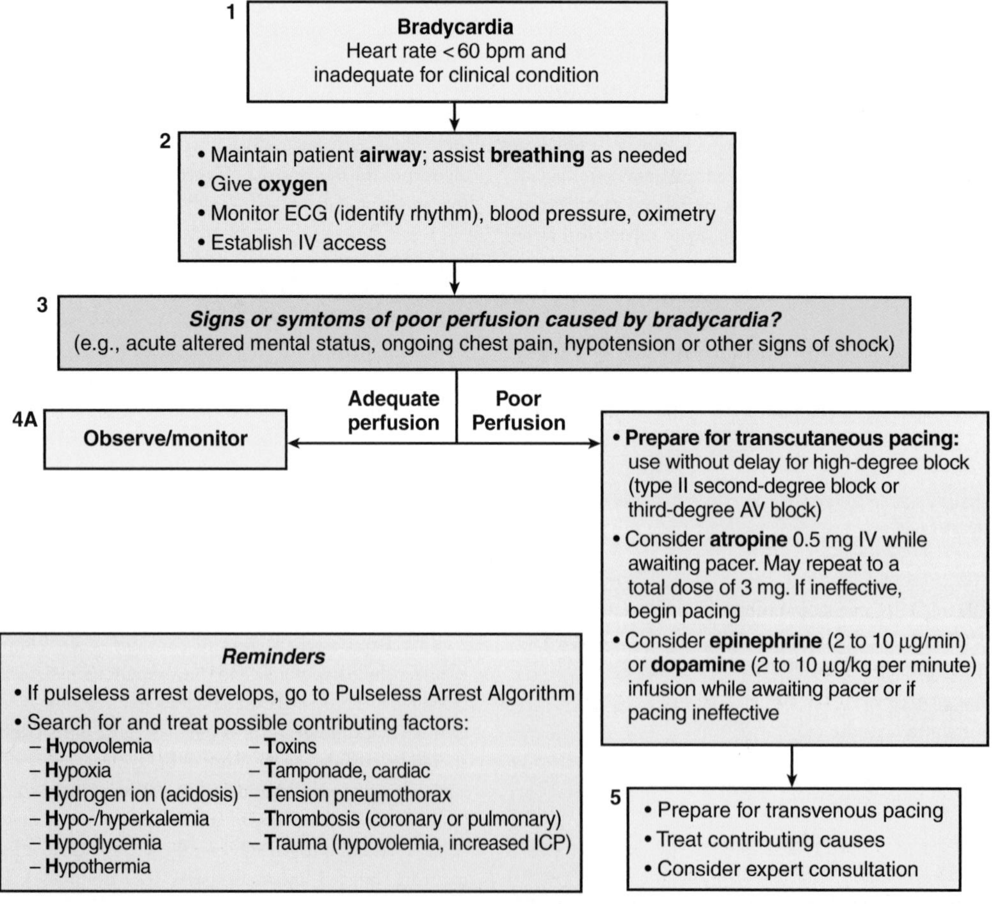

Figure 37-4 The American Heart Association algorithm for the treatment of bradycardia. Management of symptomatic bradycardia and tachycardia. bpm, Beats per minute; ECG, electrocardiogram; ICP, intracranial pressure; IV, intravenous. (From 2005 American Heart Association Guidelines for Cardiopulmonary Resuscitation and Emergency Cardiovascular Care. Part 7.3: Management of Symptomatic Bradycardia and Tachycardia. Circulation 2005;112:IV-67-77. Reprinted with permission of the American Heart Association.)

through mechanisms that include (1) release of choline molecules from the breakdown of succinylcholine, (2) direct stimulation of peripheral sensory receptors producing reflex bradycardia, and (3) direct stimulation of the sympathetic and parasympathetic nervous systems. Bradycardia may be observed after the first dose of succinylcholine is administered in children; in adults, however, bradycardia occurs more commonly after the second dose of succinylcholine, especially if it is given 5 minutes or more after the first dose is administered.

The incidence of bradycardia associated with the infusion of propofol has been reported to be between 5% (observations from case series) and 25% (data from randomized controlled trials). Children who undergo strabismus operations and who receive propofol seem to be particularly susceptible to the activation of the ocular cardiac reflex; bradycardia has been reported to occur in 6% to 16% of these patients, even if they are prophylactically treated with an anticholinergic drug.

Other causes of intraoperative bradycardia include vagal stimulation from manipulation of the oropharynx during laryngoscopy, intubation, or extubation. Surgical handling of extraocular muscles, bronchi, peritoneum, scrotum, and rectum can give rise to autonomic reflexes that include bronchospasm, bradycardia or tachycardia, hypotension or hypertension, and cardiac arrhythmias, especially in lightly anesthetized, hypoxic, or hypercapnic patients. The manifestations of vagal stimulation can be prevented or minimized by treatment with atropine, glycopyrrolate, topical anesthesia, intravenously administered local anesthetic agents, adrenergic blocking agents, deeper anesthesia, and vasoactive agents.

Hypothermia is known to cause bradycardia; however, the initial response to hypothermia is a transient increase in heart rate due to sympathetic stimulation. As temperature decreases below 34° C, the heart rate decreases proportionally. The resulting bradycardia is thought to result from the direct effect of hypothermia on the sinoatrial node. This bradycardia is not responsive to vagolytic maneuvers. Elevated intracranial pressure presenting alone—or as part of a triad of systemic hypertension, sinus bradycardia, and respiratory irregularities (Cushing syndrome)—is also a cause of bradycardia in the perioperative period.

Suggested Readings

Aghamohammadi H, Mehrabi S, Mohammad Ali Beigi F. Prevention of bradycardia by atropine sulfate during urological laparoscopic surgery: A randomized controlled trial. *Urol J*. 2009;6:92-95.

Brady WJ, Swart G, DeBehnke DJ, et al. The efficacy of atropine in the treatment of hemodynamically unstable bradycardia and atrioventricular block: Prehospital and emergency department considerations. *Resuscitation*. 1999; 41:47-55.

Chatzimichali A, Zoumprouli A, Metaxari M, et al. Heart rate variability may identify patients who will develop severe bradycardia during spinal anaesthesia. *Acta Anaesthesiol Scand*. 2011;55:234-241.

Love JN, Sachdeva DK, Bessman ES, et al. A potential role for glucagon in the treatment of drug-induced symptomatic bradycardia. *Chest*. 1998;114: 323-326.

Maruyama K, Nishikawa Y, Nakagawa H, et al. Can intravenous atropine prevent bradycardia and hypotension during induction of total intravenous anesthesia with propofol and remifentanil? *J Anesth*. 2010;24:293-296.

Tramer MR, Moore RA, McQuay HJ. Propofol and bradycardia: Causation, frequency and severity. *Br J Anaesth*. 1997;78:642-651.

Yorozu T, Iijima T, Matsumoto M, et al. Factors influencing intraoperative bradycardia in adult patients. *J Anesth*. 2007;21:136-141.

CHAPTER 38

Oculocardiac Reflex

Peter Radell, MD, PhD, and Sten G. E. Lindahl, MD, PhD, FRCA

The oculocardiac reflex (OCR) was first described by Aschner and Dagnini in 1908. Recently, with the understanding that stimulation of the trigeminal nerve in areas other than the ophthalmic branch (V_1) can occur, a more comprehensive term, trigeminocardiac reflex, has come into use.

Anatomy

The afferent limb of the fifth cranial nerve is trigeminal, and the efferent limb is vagal. Specifically, afferent impulses travel via short and long ciliary nerves to the ciliary ganglion. From there, afferent information is sent to the gasserian ganglion via the ophthalmic branch of the trigeminal nerve (V_1). Efferent impulses leave the brainstem by way of the vagus nerve (X) (Figure 38-1).

Triggering Stimuli

This reflex is triggered most commonly by traction on extraocular muscles (especially the medial rectus), direct pressure on the globe, ocular manipulation, and ocular pain. It may also be elicited by retrobulbar block, ocular trauma, and manipulation of tissue remaining in the orbital apex after enucleation. The reflex arc has even been described originating from other trigeminal afferent branches, for example, during sinus or nasal operations. The OCR seems to fatigue with repeated manipulation.

Manifestations

The most common manifestation of the OCR is sinus bradycardia. Other cardiac arrhythmias include ectopic beats, junctional rhythms, atrioventricular

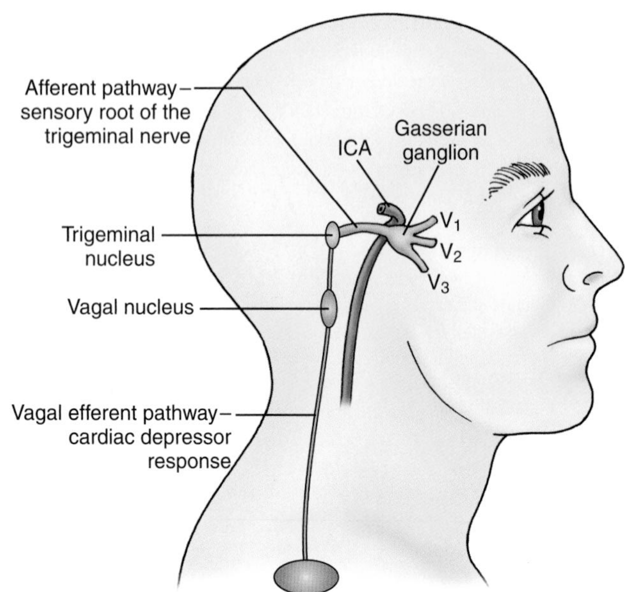

Figure 38-1 Trigeminocardiac reflex pathway. Divisions of the trigeminal nerve: V_1, ophthalmic; V_2, maxillary; V_3, mandibular. ICA, Internal carotid artery.

blockade, ventricular bigeminy, multifocal premature ventricular contractions, wandering pacemaker, ventricular tachycardia, and asystole.

Prevalence

The reported incidence of OCR during strabismus surgery is highly variable, ranging from 16% to 82%. The incidence is lower with the use of modern anesthetic agents, such as sevoflurane and desflurane, compared with older agents such as halothane. Children and young adults undergoing eye muscle operations under general anesthesia are the most susceptible to the development of OCR, but the incidence may also be increased in the elderly. Hypoxemia, hypercarbia, and acidosis increase the incidence and severity of the problem, and other risk factors include inadequate anesthetic depth and medication with β-adrenergic receptor blocking agents and potent opiates.

Intraoperative Management

The OCR may occur during local or general anesthesia. Peribulbar blocks may help prevent arrhythmias by blocking the afferent limb of the reflex arc. However, the injection of the anesthetic agent may itself stimulate the OCR. Hemodynamic effects are generally self-limited but, in combination with other illness, can be serious; for example, OCR in combination with undiagnosed Epstein-Barr virus myocarditis has led to malignant ventricular arrhythmias, cardiac arrest, and subsequent death.

If a cardiac arrhythmia appears, the initial course of action is to notify the surgeon that orbital stimulation should be halted. Next, the depth of anesthesia and adequacy of ventilation and oxygenation are optimized. Commonly, heart rate and rhythm will return to baseline within 20 seconds after these measures are initiated. However, if the initial cardiac arrhythmia is serious or if the reflex recurs, atropine should be intravenously administered in 0.02-mg/kg increments (smaller doses may have no effect or a paradoxical effect, worsening bradycardia) until resolution is achieved.

During pediatric strabismus operations, many advocate the intravenous administration of atropine (0.02 mg/kg) or glycopyrrolate (0.01 mg/kg) before the extraocular muscles are manipulated. The use of glycopyrrolate, as compared with atropine, may be associated with less tachycardia, but glycopyrrolate has a slower onset of action.

Postoperative Management

Onset time may be variable. For example, following retrobulbar block, the OCR may appear immediately or as late as 1.5 hours after an uncomplicated block. Retrobulbar hemorrhage can also result in delayed OCR because persistent bleeding gradually increases periocular pressure. Therefore, careful monitoring should continue for several hours after a suspected or known retrobulbar hemorrhage.

Suggested Readings

Choi SR, Park SW, Lee JH, et al. Effect of different anesthetic agents on oculocardiac reflex in pediatric strabismus surgery. *J Anesth.* 2009;23:489-493.

Hemmer LB, Afifi S, Koht A. Trigeminocardiac reflex in the postanesthesia care unit. *J Clin Anesth.* 2010;22:205-208.

Lübbers HT, Zweifel D, Grätz KW, Kruse A. Classification of potential risk factors for trigeminocardiac reflex in craniomaxillofacial surgery. *J Oral Maxillofac Surg.* 2010;68:1317-1321.

Oh AY, Yun MJ, Kim HJ, Kim HS. Comparison of desflurane with sevoflurane for the incidence of oculocardiac reflex in children undergoing strabismus surgery. *Br J Anaesth.* 2007;99:262-265.

Rodgers A, Cox RG. Anesthetic management for pediatric strabismus surgery: Continuing professional development. *Can J Anaesth.* 2010;57:602-617.

Yi C, Jee D. Influence of the anaesthetic depth on the inhibition of the oculocardiac reflex during sevoflurane anaesthesia for paediatric strabismus surgery. *Br J Anaesth.* 2008;101:234-238.

CHAPTER 39

The Autonomic Nervous System

James D. Hannon, MD

The autonomic nervous system (ANS) has also been called the visceral, the vegetative, or the involuntary nervous system. This self-controlling (autonomous) system comprises nerves, ganglia, and plexuses that innervate the heart, blood vessels, endocrine glands, visceral organs, and smooth muscle. It is widely distributed throughout the body and regulates functions that occur without conscious control. However, it does not function in a completely independent fashion; rather, it responds to somatic motor and sensory input.

The ANS is usually divided functionally into the sympathetic nervous system (SNS) and the parasympathetic nervous system (PNS). A third division, the enteric nervous system (ENS), has been added in light of the complexity of the innervation of the gastrointestinal tract and because the gastrointestinal tract is capable of functioning in isolation. Most visceral organs are innervated by both the SNS and the PNS, and the moment-to-moment level of activity of an individual organ represents the integration of the influences of the two systems. In addition, the actions of drugs that affect the myocardium, smooth muscle, and glandular tissue can be understood and classified according to their modifying or mimicking of the actions of neurotransmitters released by the ANS.

Anatomy

The Sympathetic Nervous System

Although the SNS is always active, an increase in its level of activity occurs in response to stresses that threaten normal homeostasis: intense physical activity, psychologic stress, blood loss, and disease processes. Activation of the SNS dilates the pupils, decreases blood flow to the gastrointestinal tract, increases cardiac output, and diverts blood flow to skeletal muscles (fight-or-flight response).

The physical arrangement of the main parts of the peripheral ANS, including the SNS, is illustrated in Figure 39-1. The SNS is widely distributed throughout the body. The cell bodies that give rise to the preganglionic fibers of the SNS lie in the intermediolateral columns of the thoracolumbar spinal cord from T1 to L2, and therefore, the SNS system is sometimes referred to as the thoracolumbar nervous system. The axons of these cells are carried in the anterior nerve roots and synapse with neurons lying in sympathetic ganglia found in three locations: paravertebral, prevertebral, and terminal. Preganglionic fibers may synapse with multiple postganglionic fibers at ganglia higher or lower than the level of their origin from the spinal cord, resulting in diffusion and amplification of the response. The 22 pairs of paravertebral ganglia lie on either side of the vertebral column and include the superior cervical, inferior cervical, and stellate ganglia. The unpaired prevertebral ganglia lie in the abdomen or pelvis near the ventral surface of the vertebral column (celiac, superior mesenteric, and inferior mesenteric). The terminal ganglia are found near the innervated organs (adrenal medulla). The cells of the medulla are embryologically and anatomically analogous to sympathetic ganglia.

The Parasympathetic Nervous System

The PNS is active during times of rest, causing the pupils to constrict, blood flow to the digestive tract to increase, and restorative processes that result in the conservation or accumulation of energy stores to predominate. The distribution of the PNS to effector organs is more limited than that of the SNS. Preganglionic fibers typically travel a greater distance than do those of the SNS, to the PNS ganglia proximal to innervated organs, and postganglionic cell bodies are located near or within innervated organs. In addition, the PNS has fewer postganglionic nerves for each preganglionic fiber and is able to produce discrete limited effects, in contrast with the diffuse mass effects characterizing SNS activation.

The preganglionic fibers of the PNS originate in the midbrain, the medulla (cranial), and the sacral part of the spinal cord. Therefore, it is also referred to as the craniosacral nervous system. Cranial parasympathetic fibers innervate the ciliary, sphenopalatine, sublingual, submaxillary, and otic ganglia. The vagus nerve (X) contains preganglionic fibers that do not synapse until they reach the many small ganglia lying in or on the organs of the thorax and abdomen. These include the heart, lungs, stomach, intestines, liver, gallbladder, pancreas, and ureters. Indeed, 75% of the activity within the PNS is mediated through the vagus nerve. Other cranial nerves (oculomotor [III], facial [VII], and glossopharyngeal [IX]) and the second, third, and fourth sacral nerves carry the rest of the PNS efferent function. Parasympathetic sacral outflow fibers form the pelvic nerves. These nerves synapse in ganglia near or within the bladder, rectum, and sexual organs.

The Enteric Nervous System

The ENS was originally considered to be a part of the PNS, and the nerves in its walls were thought to be postganglionic parasympathetic fibers. It is now known that the digestive tract contains about the same number of nerve fibers as the spinal cord and is capable of functioning independently of the SNS and PNS—although input from these systems is important for communication with the central nervous system.

Functional Effects

When the SNS is activated, the radial muscles of the iris contract, mydriasis occurs (α_1 receptor), and the ciliary muscles relax (β_2), enhancing distant vision. In the heart, there is increased inotropism (β_1), chronotropism (β_1), and dromotropism (increased conduction velocity; β_1). The SNS can vasodilate (β_1) or vasoconstrict (α_1) the coronary arteries. Similarly the SNS can cause vascular smooth muscles to contract (α_1) or relax (β_2). In the kidney, renin is secreted (β_1) and vasoconstriction occurs (α_1, α_2). Bronchial smooth muscles relax (β_2), allowing for decreased work of breathing and, therefore, an increased minute ventilation for the same amount of energy expenditure.

In the smooth muscle of the gastrointestinal system, both motility and tone are decreased (α_2), and sphincters contract (α_1). In the smooth muscle of the genitourinary system, the trigone and sphincter (α_1) contract, and the detrusor (β_2) relaxes. Glycogenolysis (α_1) takes place in the liver, and in adipose tissue, lipolysis (β_1, β_3) occurs. Other actions are outlined in Tables 39-1 and 39-2.

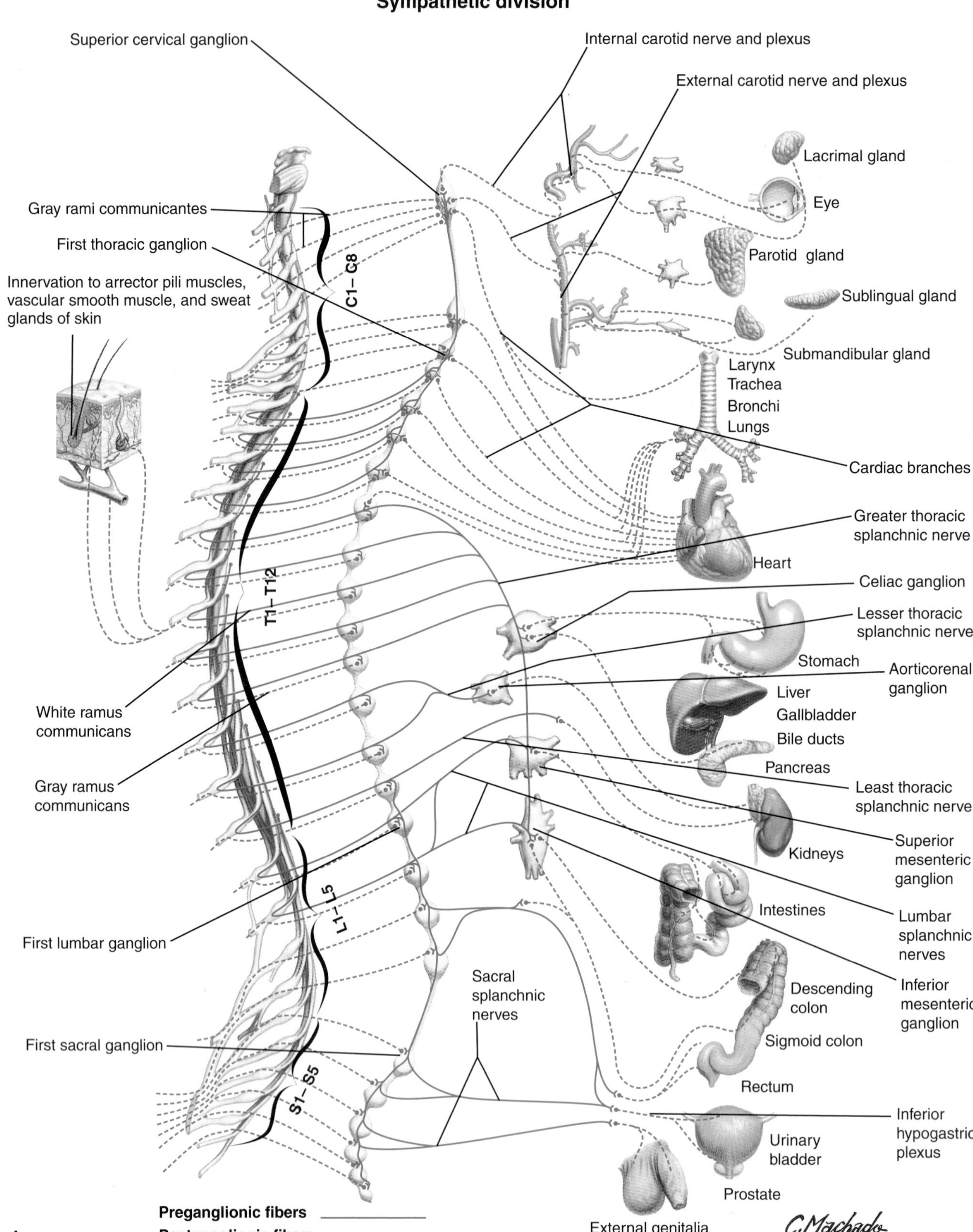

Figure 39-1 Schematic distribution of the, **A**, thoracolumbar (sympathetic) and, **B**, craniosacral (parasympathetic) nervous systems. (Netter illustrations from www.netterimages.com. © Elsevier Inc. All rights reserved.)

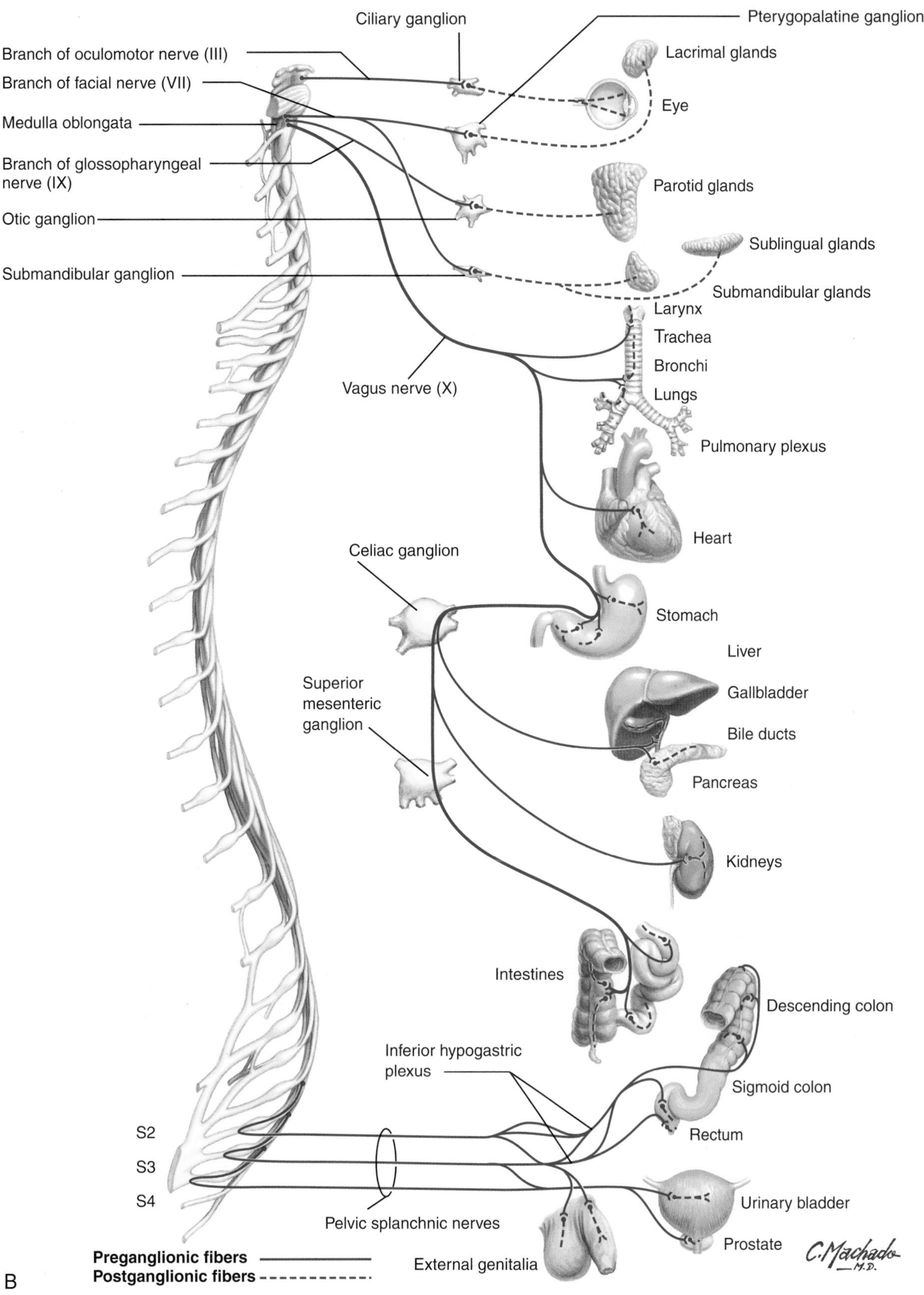
Parasympathetic division
Ciliary ganglion
Pterygopalatine ganglion
Branch of oculomotor nerve (III)
Lacrimal glands
Branch of facial nerve (VII)
Eye
Medulla oblongata
Branch of glossopharyngeal nerve (IX)
Parotid glands
Otic ganglion
Sublingual glands
Submandibular ganglion
Submandibular glands
Larynx
Trachea
Bronchi
Vagus nerve (X)
Lungs
Pulmonary plexus
Heart
Celiac ganglion
Stomach
Liver
Superior mesenteric ganglion
Gallbladder
Bile ducts
Pancreas
Kidneys
Intestines
Descending colon
Inferior hypogastric plexus
Sigmoid colon
S2
Rectum
S3
S4
Urinary bladder
Pelvic splanchnic nerves
Prostate
Preganglionic fibers
Postganglionic fibers
External genitalia
B
C. Machado M.D.

Figure 39-1, cont'd

Table 39-1 Other Effects of the Sympathetic Nervous System

Target	Action	Receptor
Endocrine pancreas	Inhibits production of insulin	α_2
	Inhibits release of glucagon	α_2
	Stimulates production of insulin	β_2
	Stimulates release of glucagon	β_2
Adrenergic nerve endings	Inhibits transmitter release	α_2
Salivary glands	Stimulates production of thick viscous secretions	α_1
Uterus		
Pregnant	Contracts	α_1
	Relaxes	β_2
Nonpregnant	Relaxes	β_2
Sex organs, male	Promotes ejaculation	α_1

Table 39-2 Actions of the Parasympathetic Nervous System

Target	Action
Eyes	Sphincter muscles of iris contract
	Miosis occurs
Heart	Chronotropism, dromotropism, and inotropism decrease
	Coronary arteries constrict
Vascular smooth muscle	Cerebral, pulmonary, skeletal muscle, and skin arterioles dilate
Bronchial smooth muscle	Contracts
Gastrointestinal smooth muscle	Motility and tone increase
	Sphincters relax
	Gallbladder contracts
Genitourinary smooth muscle	Detrusor contracts
	Trigone and sphincter relax
Endocrine pancreas	Insulin and glucagon secretions increase
Salivary glands	Produce profuse watery secretions
Sex organs, male	Penile erection

Suggested Readings

Barrett KE, Barman SM, Boitano S, Brooks H. The autonomic nervous system. In: Barrett KE, Barman SM, Boitano S, Brooks H, eds. *Ganong's Review of Medical Physiology*. 23rd ed. New York: McGraw-Hill; 2010;261-274.

Brunton LL, Lazo JS, Parker KL, eds. *Goodman and Gilman's: The Pharmacological Basis of Therapeutics*. 11th ed. New York: McGraw-Hill; 2006.

Glick DB. The autonomic nervous system. In: Miller RD, Eriksson LI, Fleisher LA, et al, eds. *Miller's Anesthesia*. 7th ed. Philadelphia: Elsevier; 2009;261-304.

Westfall TC, Westfall DP. Neurotransmission: The autonomic and somatic nervous systems. In: Brunton LL, Lazo JS, Parker KL, eds. *Goodman and Gilman's: The Pharmacological Basis of Therapeutics*. 11th ed. New York: McGraw-Hill; 2006:137-181.

CHAPTER 40

The Sympathetic Nervous System: Anatomy and Receptor Pharmacology

James D. Hannon, MD

Anatomy

The sympathetic nervous system (SNS) is widely distributed throughout the body. Although afferent pathways exist and are important in relaying visceral sensory information to the central nervous system, the most clearly defined portions of the SNS are the efferent preganglionic and postganglionic fibers and their associated paravertebral ganglia. The cell bodies that give rise to the preganglionic fibers of the SNS lie in the intermediolateral columns of the thoracolumbar spinal cord from T1 to L2 or L3 (hence, the SNS is sometimes referred to as the thoracolumbar nervous system).

The short myelinated preganglionic fibers leave the spinal cord in the anterior nerve roots, form white rami, and synapse in sympathetic ganglia lying in three locations outside the cerebrospinal axis. The gray rami arise from the ganglia and carry postganglionic fibers back to the spinal nerves for distribution to the sweat glands, pilomotor muscles, and blood vessels of the skin and skeletal muscle (Figure 40-1). The 22 sets of paravertebral ganglia are paired on either side of the vertebral column, connected to the spinal nerves by the white and gray rami communicans, and interconnected by nerve trunks to form the lateral chains. They include the upper and middle

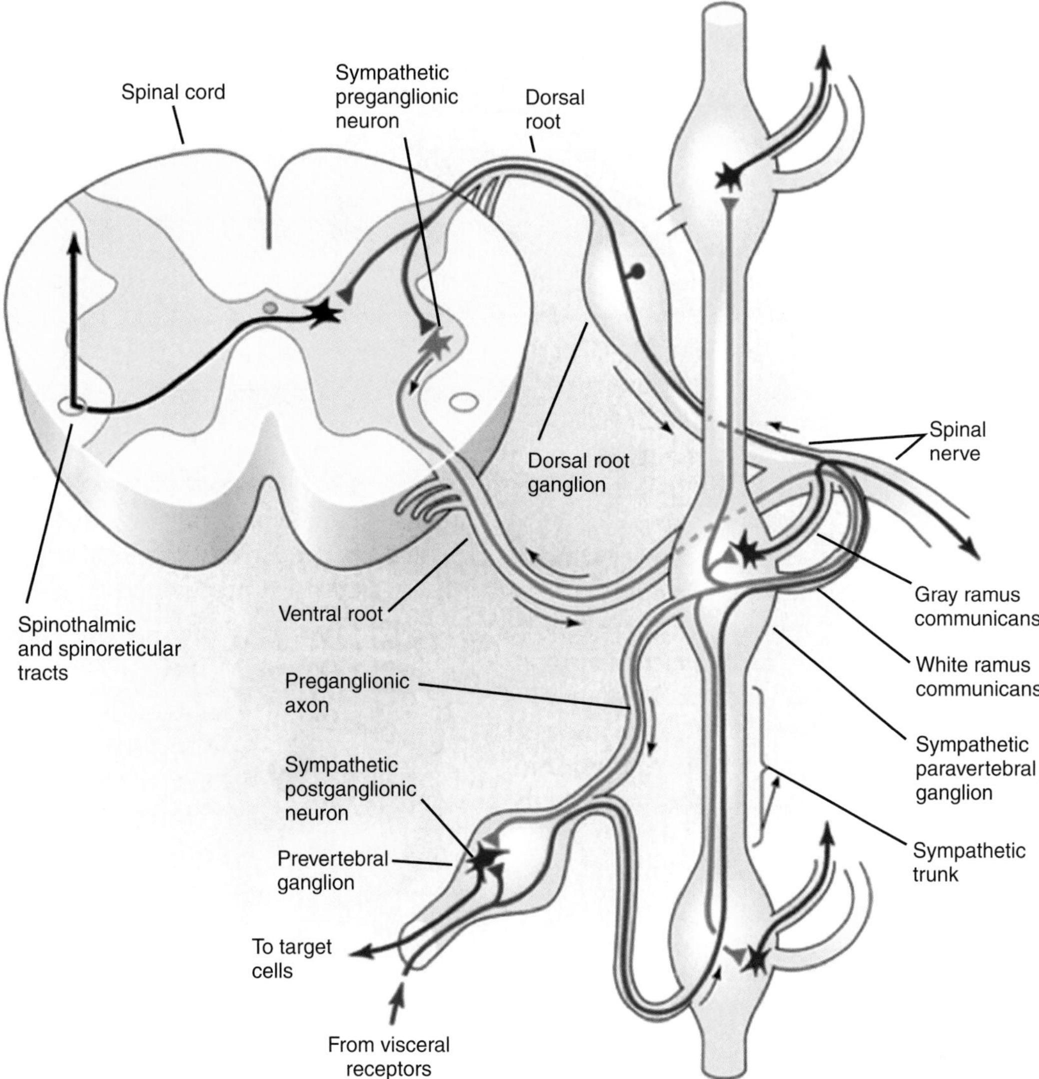

Figure 40-1 Anatomy of the preganglionic and postganglionic sympathetic nerve fibers and synapses. (Reprinted, with permission, from Boron WF, Boulpaep EL. Medical Physiology. New York: Elsevier; 2005.)

cervical ganglia, the stellate ganglia (fusion of inferior cervical and T1 ganglia), and the ganglia of the thoracic, abdominal, and pelvic sympathetic trunks. Unpaired prevertebral ganglia are found in the abdomen and pelvis near the ventral surface of the vertebral column. They are named according to the major branches of the aorta: for example, celiac, renal, and superior and inferior mesenteric ganglia. The terminal ganglia lie near the innervated organs (cervical ganglia in the neck, rectum, and bladder).

The cells of the adrenal medulla are analogous to sympathetic ganglia, except that the postganglionic cells have lost their axons and secrete norepinephrine, epinephrine, and dopamine directly into the bloodstream. Preganglionic fibers may pass through several paravertebral ganglia and synapse with multiple neurons in a ganglion, a characteristic that leads to a diffused output. Postganglionic fibers arising from the sympathetic ganglia may receive input from several preganglionic fibers and innervate visceral structures in the head, neck, thorax, and abdomen. They may pass to target organs through a nerve network along blood vessels or rejoin a mixed peripheral nerve.

Receptor Pharmacology

Neurotransmitters

Acetylcholine is the neurotransmitter of all preganglionic sympathetic fibers, including those that innervate the cells of the adrenal medulla. Norepinephrine is released by nearly all sympathetic postganglionic nerve endings; exceptions are the postganglionic cholinergic fibers that innervate sweat glands (sudomotor) and blood vessels in skeletal muscles (vasomotor). Increasing evidence indicates that neurons in the peripheral nervous system release two or more transmitters from individual nerve terminals when stimulated. Substances released with norepinephrine, such as adenosine triphosphate, may function as cotransmitters or neuromodulators of the response to norepinephrine.

Synthesis, Storage, Release, and Inactivation of Norepinephrine

The main site of norepinephrine synthesis is in the postganglionic nerve terminal. Tyrosine is transported actively into the axoplasm and converted to dihydroxyphenylalanine (rate-limiting step) and then to dopamine by cytoplasmic enzymes. Dopamine is transported into storage vesicles, where it is converted to norepinephrine (Figure 40-2). Exocytosis of norepinephrine is triggered by the increased intracellular calcium that accompanies an action potential. Active reuptake (uptake 1) of norepinephrine into the presynaptic terminal terminates the effect of norepinephrine at the effector site. This process accounts for nearly all of the released norepinephrine, which is then stored in vesicles for reuse. Monoamine oxidase is responsible for metabolism of the small amount of norepinephrine that enters the cytoplasm after neuronal reuptake without being taken up into vesicles. Monoamine oxidase

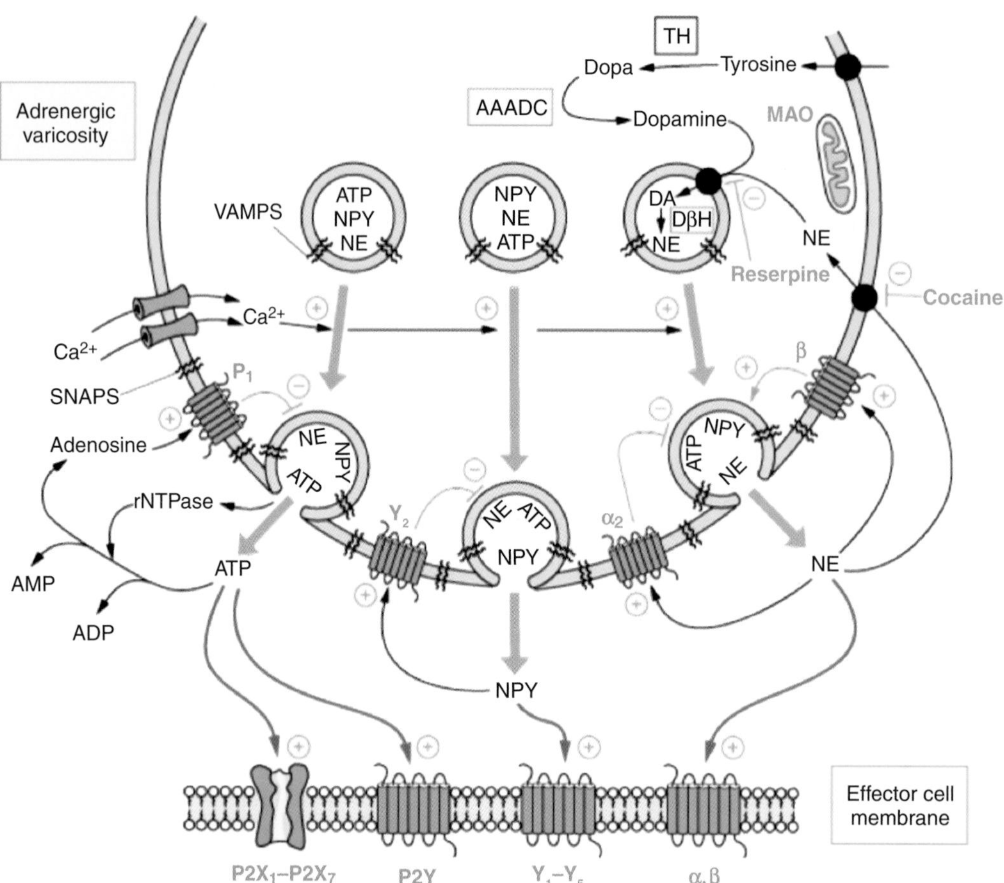

Figure 40-2 Diagram of the synthesis and disposition of norepinephrine and cotransmitters in adrenergic neurotransmission. AAADC, Aromatic L-amino acid decarboxylase; ADP, adenosine diphosphate; AMP, adenosine monophosphate; ATP, adenosine triphosphate; DA, dopamine; DβH, dopamine beta-hydroxylase; Dopa, dihydroxyphenylalanine; MAO, monoamine oxidase; NE, norepinephrine; NPY, neuropeptide Y; rNTPase, RNA nucleoside triphosphatase; SNAPS, synaptosomal; nerve associated proteins; TH, tyrosine hydroxylase; VAMPs, vesicle-associated membrane proteins. (Reprinted, with permission, from Westfall TC, Westfall DP. Adrenergic agonists and antagonists. In: Brunton LL, Lazo JS, Parker KL, eds. Goodman & Gilman's The Pharmacological Basis of Therapeutics. 11th ed. New York: McGraw-Hill; 2006.)

and catechol-O-methyltransferase are responsible for metabolism of norepinephrine that is not reabsorbed into neurons.

Receptor Subtypes

Acetylcholine activates nicotinic cholinergic receptors in the sympathetic ganglia and adrenal medulla. The primary sympathetic postganglionic neurotransmitter is norepinephrine. Epinephrine, the circulating hormone released by the adrenal medulla, and dopamine, the neurotransmitter of the less well characterized dopaminergic system, are the other naturally occurring catecholamines that interact with peripheral adrenergic receptors. The adrenergic receptors were initially classified as α and β according to their responsiveness to norepinephrine and epinephrine. Subsequent discovery of more selective agonists and antagonists allowed the α receptors to be subdivided into α_1 and α_2 and the β receptors into β_1, β_2, and β_3. Peripheral dopamine receptors have also been discovered; these are classified as DA_1 or DA_2. α_1-Receptors are found in the smooth muscle of blood vessels (contraction), the genitourinary system (contraction), and the intestine (relaxation) and in the liver (glycogenolysis, gluconeogenesis) and heart (increased contractile force, arrhythmias). α_2-Receptors are located in the pancreatic β cells (decreased insulin secretion), platelets (aggregation), nerve terminals (decreased norepinephrine release), and vascular smooth muscle (contraction). β_1-Receptors are found in the heart (increased force and rate of contraction and atrioventricular node conduction) and juxtaglomerular cells (increased renin secretion); β_2-receptors are in smooth muscles of the vascular, bronchial, gastrointestinal, and genitourinary systems (relaxation) and in skeletal muscle (glycogenolysis, uptake of K^+) and the liver (glycogenolysis, gluconeogenesis); and β_3-receptors, in adipose tissue (lipolysis).

Receptor Stimulation

The adrenergic receptors are coupled to regulatory proteins called G proteins that stimulate (β_1, β_2, β_3, DA_1) or inhibit (α_2, DA_2) adenylyl cyclase or stimulate (α_1) phospholipase C. Stimulation of adenylyl cyclase increases cyclic adenosine monophosphate, which results in protein phosphorylation. Stimulation of phospholipase C increases the production of inositol trisphosphate, which increases intracellular calcium, and diacylglycerol, which activates protein kinase C. Stimulation of presynaptic α_2-receptors and DA_2 receptors suppresses norepinephrine release from sympathetic nerve terminals, whereas stimulation of presynaptic β_2-receptors augments it.

Receptor Modulation

The responsiveness of catecholamine-sensitive cells can vary over time. Multiple mechanisms are responsible for regulating this responsiveness. *Homologous regulation* describes the case in which the responsiveness is altered by the adrenergic agonists themselves (decreased receptor density or affinity). *Heterologous regulation* is when the responsiveness is altered by other factors. The density of receptors can be increased (up-regulated) by chronic administration of β-receptor antagonists, by denervation, and by hyperthyroidism. Receptors may be down-regulated by continued β-adrenergic stimulation, hypothyroidism, and, possibly, corticosteroids.

Agonists

Sympathomimetic Amines

β-Phenylethylamine can be considered the parent compound. Compounds with hydroxyl groups at positions 3 and 4 of the benzene ring are called

Table 40-1 Adrenergic Agonists

Agent	Mode of Action						Dose
	α_1	α_2	β_1	β_2	DA_1	DA_2	
Natural							
Norepinephrine	++++	+++	++	+++			0.05-0.3 $\mu g \cdot kg^{-1} \cdot min^{-1}$
Epinephrine	+++	++	+++	+++	+		0.05-0.2 $\mu g \cdot kg^{-1} \cdot min^{-1}$
Dopamine							
Low dose					++++	++	1-5 $\mu g \cdot kg^{-1} \cdot min^{-1}$
Medium dose	+	?	++	+	++++		5-15 $\mu g \cdot kg^{-1} \cdot min^{-1}$
High dose	+++	?	++	+			> 15 $\mu g \cdot kg^{-1} \cdot min^{-1}$
Synthetic							
Metaproterenol			+	++++			MDI
Albuterol				++++			MDI
Terbutaline				++++			MDI
Isoproterenol	+		++++	++++			0.01-0.2 $\mu g \cdot kg^{-1} \cdot min^{-1}$
Dobutamine	+		+++	+			2.5-15 $\mu g \cdot kg^{-1} \cdot min^{-1}$
Mephentermine	++	?	+++	?			0.1-0.5 mg/kg
Ephedrine	++	?	++	+			0.2-1.0 mg/kg
Metaraminol	++++	?	++	?			10-102 μg/kg
Phenylephrine	++++		+				1-10 $\mu g \cdot kg^{-1} \cdot min^{-1}$
Methoxamine	++++						0.05-0.2 mg/kg
Dopexamine				++	+++	+	1-6 $\mu g \cdot kg^{-1} \cdot min^{-1}$
Fenoldopam					+++		0.1-0.8 $\mu g \cdot kg^{-1} \cdot min^{-1}$

++++, tremendous stimulation; +++, marked stimulation; ++, moderate stimulation; +, slight stimulation; ?, unknown.
DA, Dopamine; MDI, metered-dose inhaler.

Table 40-2 Antagonists of the Adrenergic Receptors

Receptor	Drug
$\alpha_1 = \alpha_2$ (nonselective)	Phenoxybenzamine (irreversible), phentolamine, tolazoline
α_1	Prazosin, terazosin, doxazosin, trimazosin
α_2	Yohimbine
$\beta_1 = \beta_2$ (nonselective)	Propranolol, timolol, nadolol, pindolol, sotalol, labetalol (weak α_1)
β_1	Metoprolol, atenolol, esmolol, acebutolol
β_2	Butoxamine
β_3	BRL 37344

catechols; catecholamines are catechols with an ethylamine side chain. Many directly acting sympathomimetic amines stimulate both α and β receptors (Table 40-1). The ratio of activities varies among agonists along a spectrum from predominantly α (phenylephrine) to predominantly β (isoproterenol). β-Receptor selectivity is enhanced by substitution of the amine group. Table 40-2 lists the antagonists of the adrenergic receptors, and Table 40-3 lists drugs that have a unique mechanism of action within the SNS.

Table 40-3 Drugs with Unique Mechanisms of Action Within the Adrenergic System

Drug	Action
Labetalol	α_1-Receptor selective and a more potent nonselective β-receptor blocker (5-10 times α_1 over β)
Carvedilol	α_1-Receptor selective and a more potent nonselective β-receptor blocker
Bretylium	Blocks NE release
Propafenone	β-Adrenergic receptor antagonist
Reserpine	Blocks vesicular uptake of NE
Guanethidine	Causes active release and then depletion of NE
Cocaine	Blocks neuronal reuptake of NE
TCA	Blocks neuronal reuptake of NE
Tyramine	Causes release of vesicular and nonvesicular stores of catecholamines

NE, Norepinephrine; TCA, tricyclic antidepressant.

Suggested Readings

Barrett KE, Barman SM, Boitano S, Brooks H. The autonomic nervous system. In: Barrett KE, Barman SM, Boitano S, Brooks H, eds. *Ganong's Review of Medical Physiology*. 23rd ed. New York: McGraw-Hill; 2010;261-272.

Glick DB. The autonomic nervous system. In: Miller RD, Eriksson LI, Fleisher LA, et al, eds. *Miller's Anesthesia*. 7th ed. New York: Elsevier; 2009;261-304.

Westfall TC, Westfall DP. Adrenergic agonists and antagonists. In: Brunton LL, Lazo JS, Parker KL, eds. *Goodman & Gilman's The Pharmacological Basis of Therapeutics*. 11th ed. New York: McGraw-Hill; 2006;277-334.

CHAPTER 41

The Parasympathetic Nervous System: Anatomy and Receptor Pharmacology

James D. Hannon, MD

Anatomy

The parasympathetic nervous system, often referred to as the craniosacral division of the autonomic nervous system, consists of preganglionic fibers—that originate in the midbrain, in the medulla oblongata, and in the sacral spinal cord—and their postganglionic connections. The preganglionic fibers are very long, whereas the postganglionic fibers are very short. The Edinger-Westphal nucleus (in the midbrain) gives rise to the preganglionic fibers of cranial nerve III, which travel to the ciliary ganglion in the orbit. Postganglionic fibers supply the ciliary muscle and the sphincter of the iris. The parasympathetic components of cranial nerves VII, IX, and X originate in the medulla. Preganglionic fibers in cranial nerve VII form the chorda tympani, which innervate the ganglia lying on the sublingual and submandibular salivary glands, and the greater superficial petrosal nerve, which innervates the sphenopalatine ganglion. Postganglionic fibers supply the sublingual, submandibular, and lacrimal glands. The parasympathetic component of cranial nerve IX innervates the otic ganglion, and postganglionic fibers supply the parotid gland. Cranial nerve X contains preganglionic fibers that do not synapse until they reach many small ganglia located directly on or in the viscera of the thorax and abdomen. It accounts for about 75% of the total parasympathetic activity and innervates the heart, tracheobronchial tree, liver, spleen, kidney, and the entire gut except the distal colon. Preganglionic vagal fibers synapse in the plexuses of Auerbach and Meissner in the intestinal wall. The preganglionic parasympathetic sacral outflow (S2, S3, S4) forms the pelvic nerves (nervi erigentes) that supply the distal colon, urinary bladder, and genitalia.

Receptor Pharmacology

Neurotransmitters

Acetylcholine (ACh) is the preganglionic and postganglionic neurotransmitter in the parasympathetic nervous system. Nerves that release ACh are said to be cholinergic. Increasing evidence indicates that neurons in the peripheral nervous system release two or more transmitters from individual nerve terminals when stimulated. Substances such as vasoactive intestinal peptide (VIP), released with ACh, may function as cotransmitters or neuromodulators.

Synthesis, Storage, Release, and Inactivation of Acetylcholine

Two enzymes, choline acetyltransferase (ChAT) and acetylcholinesterase (AChE), are involved in the synthesis and degradation of ACh. Two precursors are needed for synthesis: acetyl coenzyme A, formed in mitochondria from pyruvate, and choline, taken up from the extracellular space by active transport. ACh is formed by ChAT in the cytoplasm of the nerve terminal and sequestered in synaptic vesicles. ACh synthesis is capable of supporting a very high rate of synaptic release; uptake of choline is the rate-limiting step. Small amounts (quanta) of ACh are continuously released from the cholinergic nerve endings even without depolarization, resulting in miniature endplate potentials (MEPPs) in the postsynaptic membrane. MEPPs are below the threshold required to cause firing of the postsynaptic membrane. Depolarization of the nerve terminal by an action potential permits the influx of calcium ions, which facilitates the release of 100 or more quanta of ACh by exocytosis. ACh is not taken up by the cholinergic nerve endings. Instead, it is rapidly (almost immediately) hydrolyzed to choline by AChE, which is present in high concentrations at all cholinergic junctions (see Figure 19-1).

Receptor Subtypes

Cholinergic receptors are classified as nicotinic (N) or muscarinic (M), according to their response to nicotine and muscarine. N receptors can be subclassified as N_N and N_M types. N_M receptors are found at the neuromuscular junction in skeletal muscle; N_N receptors are found in autonomic ganglia (sympathetic and parasympathetic), the adrenal medulla, and the central nervous system (CNS). There are at least five different subtypes of M receptors, all found in the CNS. In the periphery, M_1 receptors are located in autonomic ganglia and various secretory glands. M_2 receptors are found mainly in the heart and also in smooth muscle. They slow spontaneous depolarization in the sinoatrial node, shorten the duration of the action potential in the atrium, and decrease conduction velocity in the atrioventricular node. They also may provide presynaptic regulation of ACh release from nerve endings in smooth muscle tissue and the CNS. M_3 receptors are located in smooth muscle, where they cause contraction, and in secretory glands, where they cause increased secretion. No agonists with a high degree of selectivity among receptor subtypes are currently available for clinical use.

Receptor Stimulation

N receptors are ligand-gated ion channels that respond rapidly when stimulated, causing increased permeability to Na^+ and Ca^{2+}, depolarization, and excitability. In contrast, M receptors belong to the class of G protein–coupled receptors, are slower to respond, and can cause either excitation or inhibition. Stimulation of M_1 and M_3 receptors activates intracellular phospholipase C, which, in turn, hydrolyzes phosphoinositides and mobilizes intracellular Ca^{2+}. Stimulation of M_3 receptors, which are located on endothelial cells within the lumen of blood vessels, causes the release of nitric oxide (NO), which diffuses to and relaxes adjacent smooth muscle cells. Activation of M_2 and M_4 receptors inhibits adenylyl cyclase and regulates ion channels through G proteins.

Receptor Modulation

If N receptor activation is prolonged, the effector response is abolished. ACh released from parasympathetic nerves inhibits release of norepinephrine from sympathetic nerve endings.

Cholinergic Agonist

ACh has a limited therapeutic value because of its widely distributed response, its lack of penetration into the CNS, and its rapid hydrolysis by AChE and plasma butyrylcholinesterase (also known as plasma cholinesterase and pseudocholinesterase). Nicotine is the prototypical ganglionic stimulant, but it is of limited clinical use because of its many side effects. Muscarinic agonists include synthetic analogs of ACh (e.g., methacholine, bethanechol, and carbachol) and natural alkaloids (e.g., pilocarpine, muscarine, and arecoline). Often, sustained cholinergic agonism is achieved with drugs that increase ACh by inhibiting AChE. Most of these drugs act on true cholinesterase (AChE) and butyrylcholinesterase, the exception being edrophonium. Neostigmine is used for antagonism of neuromuscular blockade; pyridostigmine is used to treat myasthenia gravis. Physostigmine, a tertiary amine that crosses the blood-brain barrier, is used to overcome atropine toxicity in the CNS through an indirect muscarinic effect. Organophosphate insecticides permanently block AChE, as do the chemical nerve agents (e.g., sarin).

Muscarinic Antagonists

All of the actions of ACh and cholinergic agonists at M receptors can be blocked by atropine and related drugs (belladonna alkaloids, e.g., scopolamine). In general, these antagonists cause little effect at N receptors. Tertiary amines, such as atropine and scopolamine, cross the blood-brain barrier (atropine less than scopolamine), whereas the quaternary amine glycopyrrolate does not. Ipratropium is a quaternary ammonium compound that, when inhaled, produces bronchodilation similar to that associated with the use of atropine but without inhibiting mucociliary clearance.

Nicotinic Antagonists

Nicotinic antagonists include neuromuscular blocking agents (e.g., curare, succinylcholine, pancuronium), which antagonize ACh at the neuromuscular junction but have variable potencies at the autonomic ganglia, and ganglionic blocking drugs (mecamylamine and trimethaphan), which were once used to control blood pressure in patients with dissecting aortic aneurysms because these drugs also inhibit sympathetic reflexes.

Suggested Readings

Barrett KE, Barman SM, Boitano S, Brooks H. The autonomic nervous system. In: Barrett KE, Barman SM, Boitano S, Brooks H, eds. *Ganong's Review of Medical Physiology*. 23rd ed. New York: McGraw-Hill; 2010, Chap. 17. http://www.accessmedicine.com. Accessed February 9, 2012.

Westfall TC, Westfall DP. Adrenergic agonists and antagonists. In: Brunton LL, Chabner BA, Knollmann BC, eds. *Goodman & Gilman's The Pharmacological Basis of Therapeutics*. 12th ed. New York: McGraw-Hill; 2011, Chap. 12. http://www.accessmedicine.com. Accessed February 9, 2012.

CHAPTER 42

Factors Affecting Cerebral Blood Flow

Kirstin M. Erickson, MD

Cerebral metabolic rate (CMR), autoregulation, CO_2 reactivity, and O_2 reactivity are the main factors affecting cerebral blood flow (CBF). The relationships among the latter three are depicted in Figure 42-1. Temperature and anesthetic medications also each influence CBF.

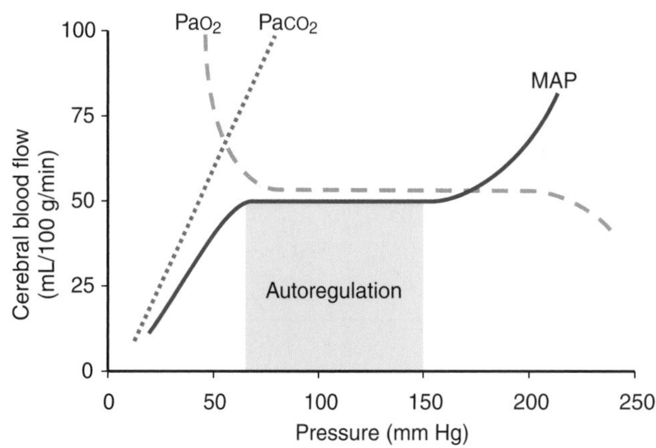

Figure 42-1 The relationship between cerebral blood flow (CBF) and mean arterial pressure (MAP) shows autoregulation of CBF across the range of MAP from 65 to 150 mm Hg. The relationship between $Paco_2$ and CBF is linear. The Pao_2 also influences CBF at extreme values.

The Cerebral Metabolic Rate

The brain consumes O_2 at a high rate. Although accounting for only about 2% of total body weight, the brain receives 12% to 15% of cardiac output. Normal CBF is approximately 50 mL·100 g^{-1}·min^{-1}. Normal CMR for O_2 ($CMRo_2$) is 3.0 to 3.5 mL·100 g^{-1}·min^{-1}. Increases in regional brain activity lead to local increases in CMR that, in turn, lead to proportional changes in CBF. This relationship is carefully maintained and is called flow-metabolism coupling.

Mechanisms involved are, as yet, undefined but appear to include local byproducts of metabolism (potassium, H^+, lactate, adenosine triphosphate), glutamate, and nitric oxide. Peptides (vasoactive peptide, substance P, and others) exert effects on the nerves that innervate cerebral vessels.

Neurogenic control of CBF occurs by sympathetic innervation and is independent of the influence of $Paco_2$.

The CMR decreases during sleep, increases with increasing mental activity, and may reach an extremely high level with epileptic activity. The CMR is globally reduced in coma and may be only locally impaired after brain injury.

Autoregulation

Autoregulation is defined as the maintenance of CBF over a range of mean arterial pressure (MAP) (see Figure 42-1). Cerebral vascular resistance (CVR) is adjusted to maintain constant CBF. Cerebral perfusion pressure equals MAP minus intracranial pressure (ICP). Because ICP (and therefore cerebral perfusion pressure) is not commonly available, MAP is used as a surrogate of cerebral perfusion pressure.

Autoregulation occurs when MAP is between 70 and 150 mm Hg in the normal brain (see Figure 42-1). This is a conservative estimate, given that considerable interindividual variation occurs. The lower limit of autoregulation (LLA) is the point at which the autoregulation curve deflects downward and CBF begins to decrease in proportion to MAP.

CVR varies directly with blood pressure to maintain flow, taking 1 to 2 min for flow to adjust after an abrupt change in blood pressure. In hypertensive patients, the autoregulatory curve is shifted to the right (Figure 42-2). A hypertensive patient may be at risk for developing brain ischemia at a MAP of 70 mm Hg, for example, because the LLA will be higher than in a nonhypertensive patient. Several weeks of blood pressure control may return the curve to normal. Following significant hypotension (lower than the LLA), autoregulation is impaired, and hyperemia may occur when MAP returns to the normal range. CO_2 reactivity remains intact, and inducing hypocapnia may attenuate hyperemia.

Autoregulatory vasodilation may be limited by background sympathetic vascular tone. Systemic vasodilators (nitroprusside, nitroglycerin, hydralazine, adenosine, and calcium channel blockers) may extend the lower limit of tolerable hypotension (shift the LLA to a lower pressure). Other than their effect on global cerebral perfusion pressure, β-adrenergic receptor blocking agents likely have no adverse effects on patients with intracranial pathology.

Autoregulation is impaired in areas of relative ischemia, surrounding mass lesions, after grand mal seizures, after head injury, and during episodes of hypercarbia or hypoxemia. Figure 42-3 shows how lost autoregulation may lead to dangerously low CBF. Regional or global ischemia may ensue.

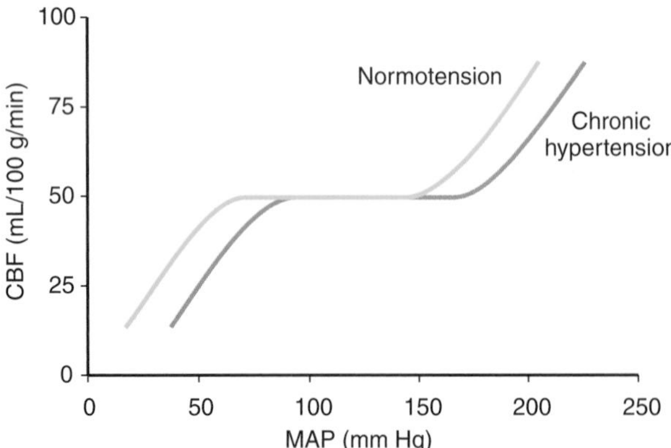

Figure 42-2 The relationship between cerebral perfusion pressure (CPP) and mean arterial pressure (MAP) shows autoregulation of CPP across a range of MAP. The curve is shifted to the right in patients with chronic hypertension. (From Erickson KM, Cole DJ. Arterial hypotension and hypertension. In: Brambrink A, Kirsch JR, eds. Neuroanesthesia and Critical Care Handbook. New York: Springer Publishing; 2010.)

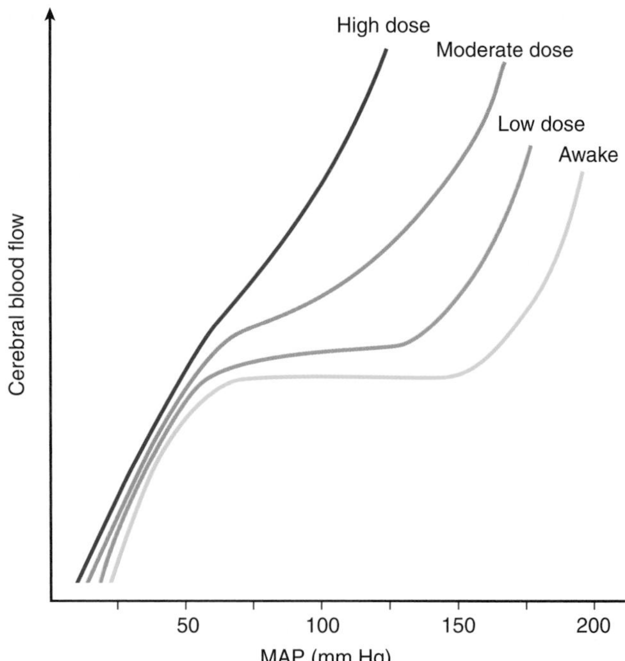

Figure 42-3 A representation of the effect of increasing the concentration of a inhalation anesthetic agent on autoregulation of cerebral blood flow. Dose-dependent cerebral vasodilation leads to attenuation of autoregulation, and both upper and lower thresholds are shifted to the left. MAP, Mean arterial pressure. (From Patel PM, Drummond J. Cerebral physiology and the effects of anesthetic drugs. In: Miller RD, ed. Miller's Anesthesia. 7th ed. Vol. 2. Philadelphia: Elsevier; 2009:309.)

CO_2 Reactivity

$Paco_2$ levels profoundly affect CBF by changing the H^+ concentration in the extracellular fluid surrounding smooth muscle in arteriolar cell walls. CBF varies directly with $Paco_2$ (see Figure 42-1). The effect is greatest in the normal physiologic range of $Paco_2$. CBF changes 1 to 2 $mL \cdot 100\ g^{-1} \cdot min^{-1}$ for each 1-mm Hg change in $Paco_2$. As $Paco_2$ increases from 30 to 60 mm Hg, for example, CBF doubles. Below a $Paco_2$ level of 25, the response is attenuated.

Mild hypocapnia ($Paco_2$ 30-34 mm Hg) in patients with large space-occupying lesions ("tight heads") undergoing craniotomy is used only selectively to facilitate surgical access. At a $Paco_2$ of 20 mm Hg, cerebral ischemia may occur because of a left shift in the oxyhemoglobin dissociation curve and decreases in CBF. With a $Paco_2$ below 20 mm Hg to 25 mm Hg, O_2 consumption decreases, and anaerobic metabolism ensues.

Changes in cerebral blood volume (CBV) due to $Paco_2$ occur in cerebral arterial vasculature. Hypercarbia has the greatest effect on vessels that are smaller than 100 μm in diameter.

The mechanism of CO_2 vasoactivity is thought to be secondary to changes in local H^+ in arteriolar walls on the brain side of the blood-brain barrier (BBB). Respiratory acidosis, not metabolic acidosis, leads to vasodilation because HCO_3^- does not initially cross the BBB but CO_2 does. The lowered pH of the periarteriolar cerebrospinal fluid causes vasodilation in 20 to 30 sec. The pH of the cerebrospinal fluid normalizes with active changes in HCO_3^- concentration, and CBF returns to normal in 6 to 8 h. CO_2 responsiveness in gray matter is greater than that in white matter owing to increased vascular density. Pathologic states, including trauma, tumor, or ischemia, decrease CO_2 responsiveness.

A "Robin Hood effect" may exist in which areas of focal ischemia (where CO_2 reactivity is likely lost) receive increased flow if normal vasculature is exposed to hypocapnia; however, this effect is unpredictable. Normocapnia should be maintained when regional ischemia is a risk. Following a period of hypocapnia, an abrupt return to normocapnia may cause acidosis in the cerebrospinal fluid and rebound in CBF and ICP. Cerebral ischemia is a risk if intracranial elastance is poor.

O_2 Reactivity

Pao_2 has little direct effect on CBF at values between 60 mm Hg and more than 300 mm Hg. A Pao_2 level below 60 mm Hg markedly increases CBF if blood pressure is maintained (see Figure 42-1). This effect is not well understood. A variety of chemoreceptors and local humeral effects may be involved. At Pao_2 levels above normal, up to 1 atm (760 mm Hg), only a very slight decrease in CBF has been measured.

Hypothermia

Hypothermia (between 28° C and 37° C) acutely reduces, but does not uncouple, $CMRo_2$ and CBF. CO_2 reactivity is also maintained during hypothermia. The effects of hypothermia on $CMRo_2$ are discussed in Chapter 131, Cerebral Protection.

Effects of Anesthetic Drugs

In general, anesthetic agents, except for ketamine and N_2O, depress CMR.

Intravenously Administered Anesthetic Agents

Intravenously administered anesthetic agents typically cause parallel declines in $CMRo_2$ and CBF, with preservation of $Paco_2$ responsiveness. Ketamine, however, increases both CBF and $CMRo_2$.

Propofol decreases $CMRo_2$ by approximately 50% and subsequently decreases CBF, CBV, and ICP. Autoregulation is preserved, even at propofol doses sufficient to produce burst suppression on the electroencephalogram.

Thiopental decreases $CMRo_2$ and CBF in a dose-dependent manner, up to 50% at induction of isoelectric electroencephalographic tracings. No further reduction in $CMRo_2$ results when additional thiopental is given after electroencephalographic suppression. This response suggests that thiopental and other depressant anesthetic agents reduce the component of cerebral metabolism associated with electrical brain activity, rather than with homeostasis. Autoregulation is preserved.

The effects of etomidate on $CMRo_2$ and CBF are similar to those of barbiturates. However, exacerbation of ischemic injury has been demonstrated, and on this basis, the use of etomidate is avoided. The effects of etomidate on autoregulation have not been studied. Etomidate is epileptogenic in patients with seizure disorders but not in patients without seizure disorders.

Benzodiazepines decrease $CMRo_2$ and CBF in a dose-dependent manner. Positron emission tomographic studies have shown selective decreases in brain regions associated with attention, arousal, and memory in patients treated with benzodiazepines.

Fentanyl modestly reduces $CMRo_2$ and CBF, although data on this topic are very limited. Sufentanil causes either a modest reduction in these parameters or no change. Alfentanil causes no change in $CMRo_2$ or CBF in dogs. Sedative doses of remifentanil can increase CBF slightly; large doses suppress CBF. High-dose fentanyl and sufentanil cause epileptiform activity, but smaller clinical doses are unlikely to precipitate seizures. Modest doses of alfentanil provoke seizures in patients with epilepsy. This property of alfentanil is occasionally used in the operating room to assist the surgeon in locating an epileptogenic focus for resection under general anesthesia.

Morphine depresses $CMRo_2$ and CBF by a small to moderate degree. Histamine release can cause cerebral vasodilation, and CBF and CBV will be dependent on MAP.

Dexmedetomidine reduces CBF and $CMRo_2$ in parallel. Reduction in MAP reduces the margin of safety in patients dependent on collateral perfusion pressure.

Mannitol causes a transient increase in CBV, which returns to normal after approximately 10 min.

Inhaled Anesthetic Agents

Inhaled anesthetic agents reduce $CMRo_2$ (see Chapter 67, Central Nervous System Effects of the Inhalation Agents). Decreases in $CMRo_2$ are dose dependent and nonlinear below 1 minimum alveolar concentration (MAC) of the agent; a precipitous drop is followed by a more gradual, linear decline as MAC is increased. Maximal reduction occurs with electroencephalographic suppression. Differences among the $CMRo_2$ effects of isoflurane, desflurane, and sevoflurane are minor.

Autoregulation is impaired by volatile anesthetic agents in a dose-dependent manner (see Figure 42-3). Sevoflurane impairs autoregulation less than does isoflurane or desflurane, which do so less than halothane. (This pattern follows the vasodilatory potency of each gas.)

Inhalation anesthetic agents are direct cerebral vasodilators. The correlation between CBF and CBV is not direct. With vasodilation induced by a inhalation agent, CBV increases, whereas CBF may be unchanged or reduced. Increased CBV may result in significant increases in ICP.

CO_2 responsiveness is preserved with the use of inhalation anesthetic agents. Hypocapnia attenuates the increased ICP caused by halothane when hypocapnia is instituted before the use of halothane, whereas the ICP effects of isoflurane and desflurane can be attenuated with simultaneous use of hypocapnia in patients with normal intracranial elastance. Hypocapnia may not effectively block a inhalation gas–induced increase in ICP in patients with intracranial tumors because impairments of normal brain physiology disable both $Paco_2$ responsiveness and autoregulation.

When administered alone, N_2O increases $CMRo_2$, CBF, and ICP. These effects are moderated or obliterated when N_2O is used in combination with intravenously administered drugs. The addition of N_2O to a inhalation anesthetic agent causes a moderate increase in CBF.

Suggested Readings

Drummond JC. The lower limit of autoregulation: Time to revise our thinking. *Anesthesiology*. 1997;86:1431-1433.

Fraga M, Maceiras P, Rodino S, et al. The effects of isoflurane and desflurane on intracranial pressure, cerebral perfusion pressure, and cerebral arteriovenous oxygen content differences in normocapnic patients with supratentorial brain tumors. *Anesthesiology*. 2003;98:1085-1090.

Kaisti K, Metsahonkala L, Teras M, et al. Effects of surgical levels of propofol and sevoflurane anesthesia on cerebral blood flow in healthy subjects studied with positron emission tomography. *Anesthesiology*. 2002;96:1358-1370.

Michenfelder JD. *Anesthesia and the Brain*. New York: Churchill Livingstone; 1988.

CHAPTER 43

Effects of Common Anesthetic Agents on Electroencephalograms

R. Doris Wang, MD

The electroencephalogram (EEG) is a depiction of the electrical activity occurring at the surface of the brain. This activity appears on the EEG recording as waveforms of varying frequency and amplitude measured in microvolts. Four categories of frequencies are the most clinically relevant (Table 43-1, Figure 43-1).

Intraoperative monitoring that employs raw EEG data is one of the traditional methods used to assess the adequacy of cerebral perfusion. Many electrical changes associated with increased doses of intravenously administered or inhalation anesthesia can mimic EEG changes associated with inadequate cerebral perfusion (i.e., brain ischemia).

Inhalation Anesthetic Agents

Inhalation anesthetic agents consistently increase slow-wave EEG activities. At doses lower than minimum alveolar concentration (MAC) levels, alpha rhythm disappears and the voltage of beta activity increases and becomes more widespread. As the end-tidal concentration of the inhalation agent increases, the EEG progressively increases in amplitude and decreases in frequency. During deep-inhalation anesthesia, burst suppression occurs. EEG changes vary somewhat depending on the specific anesthetic agent used, whether the agent is used alone or in combination with other anesthetic agents, whether hyperventilation is employed, and the patient's age. In addition, patients with increased baseline delta (slow-wave) activity resulting from underlying intracranial pathology can show relatively little or no change in the EEG with increasing anesthesia depth, but burst suppression may eventually become evident.

Table 43-1 Categories of the Most Clinically Relevant Electroencephalographic Frequencies

Wave Pattern	Frequency Range (Hz)	Level of Consciousness
Delta	0.5-4	Deep sleep
Theta	4-8	Drowsiness (also first stage of sleep)
Alpha	8-14	Relaxed but alert
Beta	14-30	Highly alert and focused

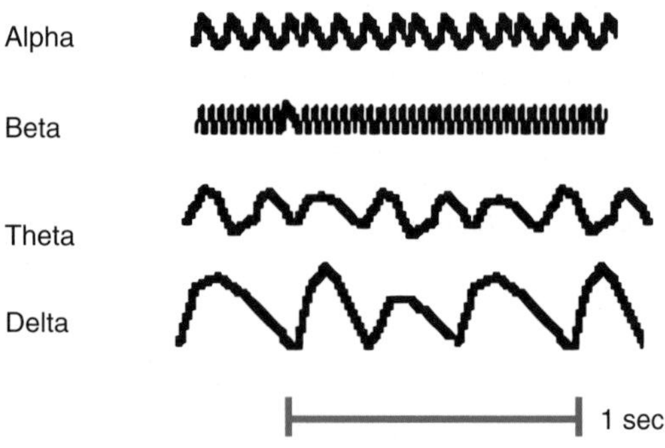

Figure 43-1 Examples of alpha, beta, theta, and delta electroencephalographic frequencies.

Halothane

Halothane produces 10-Hz to 20-Hz activity that persists until the patient loses consciousness. Theta and delta activity increase in a dose-dependent manner up to moderate doses of halothane (e.g., 1.5 MAC), at which point there is a modest decrease in theta rhythm. At 1 MAC of halothane (0.75%) and normocarbia, the dominant EEG frequencies are between 10 and 15 Hz. At 2 MAC, the predominant background rhythm is 7.5 Hz; at 2.5 MAC, it is 6 Hz. The use of halothane for EEG burst suppression is not practical because of the cardiovascular depression associated with the use of high-dose halothane (3-4 MAC).

Isoflurane

In patients receiving 0.5% isoflurane with 70% N_2O and O_2, 15-Hz to 20-Hz activity of low to moderate voltage is evident. With 2% isoflurane and O_2 or 1% isoflurane with 70% N_2O and O_2, the EEG exhibits 2-Hz to 6-Hz moderate-voltage to high-voltage activity with superimposed 10-Hz to 15-Hz activity. A burst-suppression pattern or total electrical silence usually occurs with isoflurane concentrations of greater than 2% in O_2 or 1.5% in 70% N_2O.

Sevoflurane

Epileptiform discharge during induction with inhaled sevoflurane—with or without hyperventilation—has been reported to occur in nonepileptic adults and children. Epileptiform discharge is seen in 50% to 100% of patients in whom anesthesia is maintained with 2 MAC of sevoflurane. The occurrence of epileptiform activity seems to be dose dependent, and the threshold is about 1.5 MAC. There appears to be no adverse clinical effect of this type of nonconvulsive epileptiform discharge.

Desflurane

Desflurane produces EEG changes comparable to those observed with equipotent doses of isoflurane. Burst suppression occurs at a MAC of at least 1.25. Substitution of N_2O for 0.42 MAC desflurane reduces the degree of EEG suppression relative to the equipotent administration of desflurane and O_2. Like isoflurane, desflurane does not generate epileptiform activity even at high inhaled concentrations or with the addition of hypocapnia and auditory stimulation.

Enflurane

Enflurane produces a loss of alpha activity and increased frontal beta activity at subanesthetic levels. Like sevoflurane, it can produce spike-and-wave activity at a MAC of greater than 1.5. Burst suppression is observed at greater than 1.5 MAC. Among all of the potent inhalation agents, enflurane is associated with the greatest probability of inducing spike activity (enflurane >> sevoflurane > isoflurane = desflurane).

N_2O

The initial change in EEG secondary to the use of N_2O is the progressive loss of alpha rhythm. As the patient loses consciousness, alpha waves disappear. Fast frontal oscillatory activity (>30 Hz) is observed with inspired N_2O concentrations greater than 50%. The fast activity is especially prominent in frontal regions. Theta waves increase in frequency and amplitude, particularly in the temporal region.

Barbiturates

In subanesthetic doses, barbiturates increase the frequency and amplitude of beta activity. Increased beta activity and theta/delta activities, with decreasing levels and frequency of alpha rhythm, are observed with increasing doses of barbiturates. Thiopental administration initially increases the amplitude of 18-Hz to 30-Hz activity. Loss of consciousness is associated with the appearance of 5-Hz to 12-Hz activity superimposed on faster activity, often occurring in spindle-shaped bursts. Burst-suppression patterns are also associated with high doses of barbiturates.

Etomidate

Fast frontal beta activity with transition to alpha activity is seen when etomidate is increased from a low to a moderate dose. As occurs with the use of propofol and thiopental, burst suppression is seen with administration of high-dose etomidate. However, side effects, such as adrenal suppression, and a higher incidence of postoperative nausea and vomiting on emergence, as compared with thiopental or propofol, preclude the routine use of etomidate to induce burst suppression.

Propofol

The EEG changes induced by increasing serum levels of propofol follow the pattern typical of the inhalation anesthetic agents and thiopental. Beta activity first increases and then slows to alpha and theta rhythms. Slow EEG activity increases with the appearance of delta activity. These EEG changes are more prominent in the frontocentral regions and tend not to interfere with the interpretation of routine EEGs or intraoperative electrocorticography during awake craniotomies. Propofol has both anticonvulsive and proconvulsive effects, depending on drug concentration. The rapid changes of propofol concentration in the brain at the beginning or end of anesthesia are thought to be crucial for the generation of seizures in susceptible patients.

Opioids

The use of opioids, such as fentanyl, sufentanil, or alfentanil, are usually not associated with beta activities but cause immediate EEG slowing with high-voltage, slow delta waves. Despite causing generalized EEG slowing, the use of an opioid anesthetic does not result in a burst-suppression pattern. In some patients, spindle-like activity with a frequency of 10 to 15 Hz appears predominately in the frontal leads. This sharp activity is not epileptiform in character and disappears after the opioid infusion is discontinued. Some patients show isolated sharp-wave activity after fentanyl induction. This phenomenon is more evident at high drug doses. For example, it is well established that opioid medications have the potential to induce epileptiform activity in both laboratory animals and humans. In patients undergoing nonlesional operations for the treatment of temporal lobe epilepsy, opioid-(particularly alfentanil and sufentanil) induced epileptiform activity facilitates intraoperative electrocorticography-guided localization of the epileptogenic zone. That is, opioids facilitate localization of the epileptogenic zone while minimizing resection of nonepileptogenic eloquent brain tissue.

Ketamine

Ketamine produces a dissociative state of anesthesia. Changes in EEG following ketamine administration bear a resemblance to arousal EEG (i.e., increases in beta activity), despite the sedative effects of ketamine. Administration of ketamine initially causes very fast (30-Hz to 40-Hz) activity in the frontal regions, followed by rhythmic theta activity and then periodic bursts of delta waves. In patients anesthetized with sevoflurane, paradoxical increases in data obtained from the bispectral index have been observed after administration of ketamine. However, the phenomenon is not observed when ketamine is given during stable propofol-remifentanil anesthesia. Burst suppression cannot be achieved with ketamine alone.

Benzodiazepines

Benzodiazepine derivatives potently enhance beta activity when administered at premedication doses. At high doses, benzodiazepines produce frontally dominant delta and theta activity. However, burst suppression cannot be achieved with benzodiazepines alone.

Dexmedetomidine

Dexmedetomidine induce a unique sleep-like state of sedation that can easily be reversed with verbal stimulation. EEG activity during dexmedetomidine sedation is similar to the activity of physiological stage 2 sleep with slight to moderate amount of slow-wave activity and abundant sleep-spindle activity. Dexmedetomidine does not appear to reduce seizure focus activity and may be a suitable adjunct during operations to treat seizures.

Suggested Readings

Faraoni D, Salengros J-C, Engelman E, et al. Ketamine has no effect on bispectral index during stable propofol-remifentanil anaesthesia. *Br J Anaesth.* 2009;102:336-339.

Hewitt PB, Chu DL, Polkey CE, Binnie CD. Effect of propofol on the electrocorticogram in epileptic patients undergoing cortical resection. *Br J Anaesth.* 1999;82:199-202.

Huupponen E, Maksimow A, Lapinlamp P, et al. Electronencephalogram spindle activity during dexmedetomidine sedation and physiological sleep. *Acta Anaesthesiol Scand.* 2008;52:289-294.

Isley MR, Edmonds HL, Stecker M. Guidelines for introperative neuromonitoring using raw (analogue or digital waveforms) and quantitative electroencephalography: A position statement by the American Society of Neurophysiological Monitoring. *J Clin Monit Comput.* 2009;23:369-390.

Julliac B, Guehl D, Chopin F, et al. Risk factors for the occurrence of electroencephalogram abnormalities during induction of anesthesia with sevoflurane in nonepileptic patients. *Anesthesiology.* 2007;106:243-251.

Lo SS, Sobol JB, Mallavaram N, et al. Anesthetic-specific electroencephalographic patterns during emergence from sevoflurane and isoflurane in infants and children. *Pediatr Anesth.* 2009;19:1157-1165.

Rampil IJ, Lockhart SH, Eger EI, et al. The electroencephalographic effects of desflurane in humans. *Anesthesiology.* 1991;74:434-439.

San-Juan D, Chiappa KH, Cole AJ. Propofol and the electroencephalogram. *Clin Neurophysiol.* 2010;121:998-1006.

Talke P, Stapelfeldt C, Garcia P. Dexmedetomidine does not reduce epileptiform discharges in adults with epilepsy. *J Neurosurg Anesthesiol.* 2007;19(3):195-199.

Vakkuri AP, Seitsonen ER, Jäntti VH, et al. A rapid increase in the inspired concentration of desflurane is not associated with epileptiform encephalogram. *Anesth Analg.* 2005;101:396-400.

Voss LJ, Ludbrook G, Grant C, et al. Cerebral cortical effects of desflurane in sheep: Comparison with isoflurane, sevoflurane and enflurane. *Acta Anesthesiol Scand.* 2006;50:313-319.

Wass CT, Grady RE, Fessler AJ, et al. The effects of remifentanil on epileptiform discharges during intraoperative electrocorticography in patients undergoing epilepsy surgery. *Epilepsia.* 2001;42:1340-1344.

CHAPTER 44

Physiology of Neuromuscular Transmission

Sorin J. Brull, MD, FCARCSI (Hon)

The Neuromuscular Junction

The neuromuscular junction is a synapse between the tightly apposed presynaptic motor neuron terminal and the postsynaptic muscle fiber; this is where a chemical process (release of acetylcholine [ACh] from the nerve ending) leads to an electrical event (muscle membrane depolarization) resulting in a mechanical effect (muscle contraction) (Figure 44-1). Large motor nerve axons branch as they course distally within skeletal muscle. Ultimately, the axons divide into 10 to 100 smaller terminal nerve fibers, lose their myelin sheath, and innervate a single muscle fiber. The combination of the terminal neural fibers that originate from 1 axon and the muscle fibers they innervate form a motor unit. The average number of muscle fibers innervated by a single motor neuron defines the innervation ratio, which, in humans, varies between 1:5 and 1:2000. For smaller muscles that are specialized in fine and precise movement (such as the hand and ocular muscles), the innervation ratio is low (1:5, or 5 muscle fibers per neuron), whereas large antigravity muscles have very high innervation ratios (1:2000). Transmission from nerve to muscle is mediated by ACh, which is synthesized in the nerve terminal and stored in specialized vesicles. Each nerve terminal contains approximately 500,000 vesicles (also called quanta, and each containing 6-10,000 ACh molecules) arranged in a specialized region of the membrane where the synaptic vesicles gather, the active zone. ACh is released by exocytosis into the junctional cleft after an appropriate nerve impulse reaches the nerve terminal and diffuses across the 50- to 70-nm cleft to bind the nicotinic cholinoceptors on the postjunctional muscle membrane and initiate muscle contraction.

Function of the Neuromuscular Junction

Acetylcholine Synthesis

ACh is synthesized from acetyl coenzyme A and choline under the catalytic influence of choline *O*-acetyltransferase (CAT) enzyme in the axoplasm (Figure 44-2). The ACh is transported into vesicles by a specific carrier-mediated system. Approximately 80% of the ACh present in the nerve terminal is located in the vesicles, with the remainder dissolved in the axoplasm.

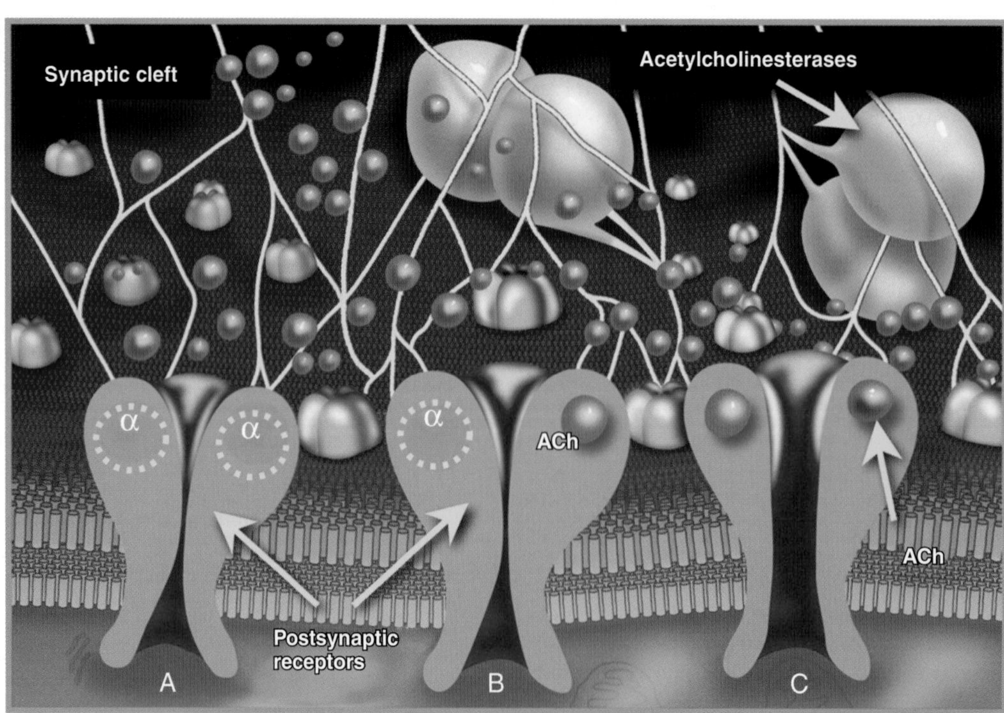

Figure 44-1 Normal neuromuscular junction. The synaptic cleft contains acetylcholinesterase enzyme that hydrolyzes acetylcholine (ACh). The receptors contain the ACh recognition site on the α subunits. Once both subunits are bound by ACh, the inactive (closed) receptors A and B undergo a conformational change and become active (open) by developing a central channel for cation exchange (receptor C).

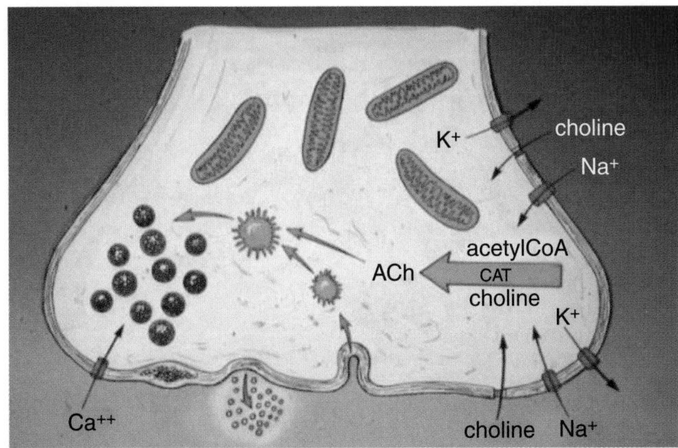

Figure 44-2 The nerve (presynaptic) terminal. Note the absence of a myelin sheath; acetylcholine (ACh) is synthesized from acetyl coenzyme A (acetyl CoA) and choline under the catalytic influence of choline *O*-acetyltransferase (CAT). Once formed, ACh is packaged into vesicles that are available for release into the cleft via exocytosis.

Nerve Terminal Depolarization

Depolarization of the nerve terminal follows the arrival of the nerve action potential and results from sodium influx through membrane sodium channels. The influx of sodium alters the membrane potential from −90 mV toward the membrane potential of sodium (+50 mV). However, at a membrane potential near 0 mV, potassium channels open and sodium channels begin to close, resulting in the membrane potential reaching +10 mV. During depolarization, calcium ions also enter the nerve terminal, where they are sequestered in the sarcoplasmic reticulum and mitochondria.

Acetylcholine Release

ACh is released spontaneously and tonically from the vesicles into the synaptic cleft, leading to small depolarizations (5 mV) at a frequency of 1 to 3 Hz, known as miniature end plate potentials. Each miniature end plate potential is thought to represent the effect of the contents of a single vesicle containing 6,000 to 10,000 ACh molecules, or 1 quantum. These miniature end plate potentials do not result in muscle contraction. However, a threshold action potential causes accelerated ACh release of 50 to 400 quanta by a voltage-gated calcium-dependent exocytosis process from the active zone into the synaptic cleft. The extent of calcium influx into the presynaptic neuron determines the number of ACh quanta released into the cleft and is a function of the duration of nerve depolarization. Only approximately 50% of the ACh released into the cleft reaches the postsynaptic receptors; the rest is either hydrolyzed by acetylcholinesterases (AChEs) contained within the cleft or diffuses out of the cleft. However, this amount of ACh is still 10 times greater than the minimum required to achieve postsynaptic ACh receptor threshold, such that sufficient postjunctional membrane depolarization occurs to produce a threshold end plate potential and activation of the excitation-contraction sequence that results in muscle contraction.

Transmitter Mobilization

The rate at which available ACh stores are replaced is termed *transmitter mobilization*. Evidence suggests that a positive feedback loop exists for ACh.

Postjunctional Events

Released ACh diffuses across the synaptic cleft and binds to a receptor on the postjunctional membrane (see later). This receptor forms a membrane ion channel. Two molecules of ACh must bind the receptor (one molecule to each of the two recognition sites—see later) before the receptor undergoes the conformational change necessary to open the receptor channel to ion flow. These channels are chemically sensitive but cannot discriminate between sodium and potassium ions. Once the channels are opened, ion flow makes the immediate area more positive. Each elementary current pulse is additive and summates to produce an end plate current. The end plate current depolarizes the end plate membrane to produce the end plate potential. Once the end plate potential reaches the critical threshold, a propagating action potential is triggered that is directed away from the end plate and results in the activation of muscle fiber contraction.

Junctional Cholinesterase

The neuromuscular junction contains two forms of acetylcholinesterase (AChE): a dissolved form in the nerve terminal axoplasm and a membrane-bound form anchored to the basement membrane of the junctional cleft. The enzyme acts to rapidly hydrolyze released ACh to choline and acetate. The kinetics of this enzyme in the neuromuscular junction is such that a single ACh molecule reacts with a single cholinoceptor before inactivation by the AChE.

Postsynaptic Receptors

The postsynaptic muscle membrane at the cleft contains multiple invaginations that markedly increase the membrane surface area. At the top of these folds are high concentrations (up to 10,000-20,000 receptors/μm^2) of nicotinic acetylcholine receptors (nAChRs). Outside the synaptic cleft area, the concentration of receptors is at least 1000 times lower. The nAChRs are pentameric proteins consisting of two α subunits (protomers), and one β, δ, and ϵ subunit each; the receptors are anchored to the postsynaptic muscle membrane by proteins such as agrin and rapsyn. In the adult mammal, the receptors are designated as $\alpha_2\,\beta$, δ and ϵ (Figure 44-3). Stereochemically, they are arranged in a counterclockwise order as α, ϵ, α, δ, β. The fetal nAChR is similar to that of the adult, except that the fetal nAChR has a γ protomer that is replaced in the adult by the ϵ protomer. The five subunits of the nAChR form a rosette surrounding a central transmembrane pore with a diameter of approximately 0.7 nm. Each α subunit possesses a recognition site for ACh at the $\alpha\epsilon$ and $\alpha\delta$ subunit interfaces. When ACh binds to the two α recognition sites, the receptor undergoes a conformational change and the central pore opens, allowing sodium flux that produces a brief (6.5-ms) current.

Presynaptic Receptors

A second type of nicotinic receptor is believed to exist on the nerve terminal. Similar to the postsynaptic receptors, these presynaptic receptors are also blocked by neuromuscular blocking agents (NMBAs) but are relatively selective for calcium fluxes. Their function is thought to help mobilize ACh during periods of high ACh demand, such as high-frequency (tetanic) stimulation. Blockade of these receptors is thought to account for the tetanic fade produced by partial nondepolarizing block.

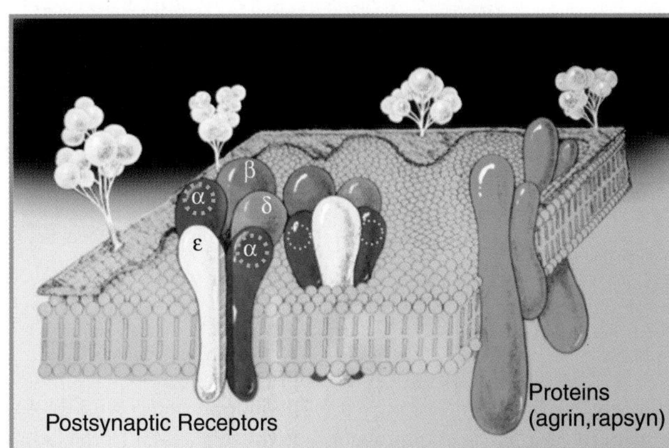

Figure 44-3 The postsynaptic receptors are pentameric proteins consisting of two α subunits and one β, δ, α, and ϵ subunit each. They are anchored to the postsynaptic membrane by agrin and rapsyn proteins. Anticholinesterases are tethered to the basement membrane.

Upregulation and Downregulation

Clinical hypersensitivity and hyposensitivity (resistance) to NMBAs are observed in a number of pathologic states. The concepts of upregulation and downregulation of receptor sites have been introduced to provide a cohesive theory of receptor-drug interaction that can explain a mechanism for abnormal effects of NMBAs in the clinical setting.

Upregulation

An increase in the number of nAChRs develops on the postjunctional membrane in conditions involving decreased stimulation of the neuromuscular junction over time (Box 44-1). Upregulation leads to hypersensitivity to the agonists ACh and succinylcholine (SCh) and decreased sensitivity to antagonists such as nondepolarizing NMBAs. Upregulation can lead to lethal potassium release from cells after SCh administration in patients with motor neuron lesions, burns, muscle atrophy from disuse, and severe trauma and infections, as well as in those who have received NMBAs over a prolonged period in the intensive care unit. The phenomenon can develop in 3 to 5 days when there is total loss of ACh activity at the end plate. Pretreatment with NMBAs does not predictably prevent SCh-induced hyperkalemia. In other conditions for which chronic anticonvulsant therapy is prescribed, such as cerebral palsy and epilepsy, resistance to NMBAs is seen without potassium release after SCh use.

Downregulation

Increased sensitivity to antagonists (e.g., NMBAs) and decreased sensitivity to agonists (e.g., SCh) develop in conditions of chronic agonist stimulation of receptors. These effects can occur with chronic reversible (e.g., neostigmine) or irreversible (e.g., organophosphates) cholinesterase inhibitor use. Most patients with myasthenia gravis have antibodies to ACh receptors that cause the neuromuscular junction to function as if it had fewer receptors. These patients are relatively resistant to SCh but extremely sensitive to NMBAs. Downregulation is also thought to occur in muscle groups that show a greater degree of paralysis after exercise conditioning.

Box 44-1 Conditions Associated with Acetylcholine Upregulation and Downregulation

Upregulation: ↑ agonist sensitivity, ↓ antagonist sensitivity

Upper and lower motor neuron lesions
Burns
Severe infection
Prolonged use of neuromuscular blocking agents
Muscle trauma
Cerebral palsy
Chronic use of anticonvulsant agents

Downregulation: ↓ agonist sensitivity, ↑ antagonist sensitivity

Myasthenia gravis
Organophosphate poisoning
Exercise conditioning

Acknowledgment

The author and editors would like to thank Jerald O. Van Beck, MD, for his work on this chapter in previous editions.

Suggested Readings

Bowman WC. Neuromuscular block. *Br J Pharmacol*. 2006;147:S277-S286.
Enoka RM. Morphological features and activation patterns of motor units. *J Clin Neurophysiol*. 1995;12:538-559.
Hirsch NP. Neuromuscular junction in health and disease. *Br J Anaesth*. 2007; 99:132-138.
Martyn JA, White DA, Gronert GA, et al. Up-and-down regulation of skeletal muscle acetylcholine receptors: Effects on neuromuscular blockers. *Anesthesiology*. 1992;76:822-843.
Zhai RG, Vardinon-Friedman H, Cases-Langhoff C, et al. Assembling the presynaptic active zone: A characterization of an active zone precursor vesicle. *Neuron*. 2001;29:131-143.

CHAPTER 45

Renal Physiology

Manoch Rattanasompattikul, MD, and Kamthorn Tantivitayatan, MD

Kidneys are essential organs for body homeostasis, especially in an organism in which cellular contents are not in continuous contact with the environment. In their vascular and tubular systems (Figure 45-1), the kidneys regulate water levels and electrolyte concentrations, excrete waste, and produce hormones. Within the smallest functional units of the kidney—the nephrons—glomerular filtration, tubular reabsorption, and tubular secretion take place (Figure 45-2).

Renal Blood Flow

Twenty percent of total cardiac output flows through both kidneys; of this amount, 80% goes to the cortex and 20% to the medulla. Renal blood flow (RBF) differs between sexes and in people of different ages. For example, men generally have higher RBF than do women: 1.21 ± 0.25 $mL{\cdot}min^{-1}{\cdot}1.73\ m^{-2}$ and 0.98 ± 184 $mL{\cdot}min^{-1}{\cdot}1.73\ m^2$, respectively. RBF declines after age 30; by the time individuals are approximately 90 years old, their RBF is about half the rate that it was when they were 20.

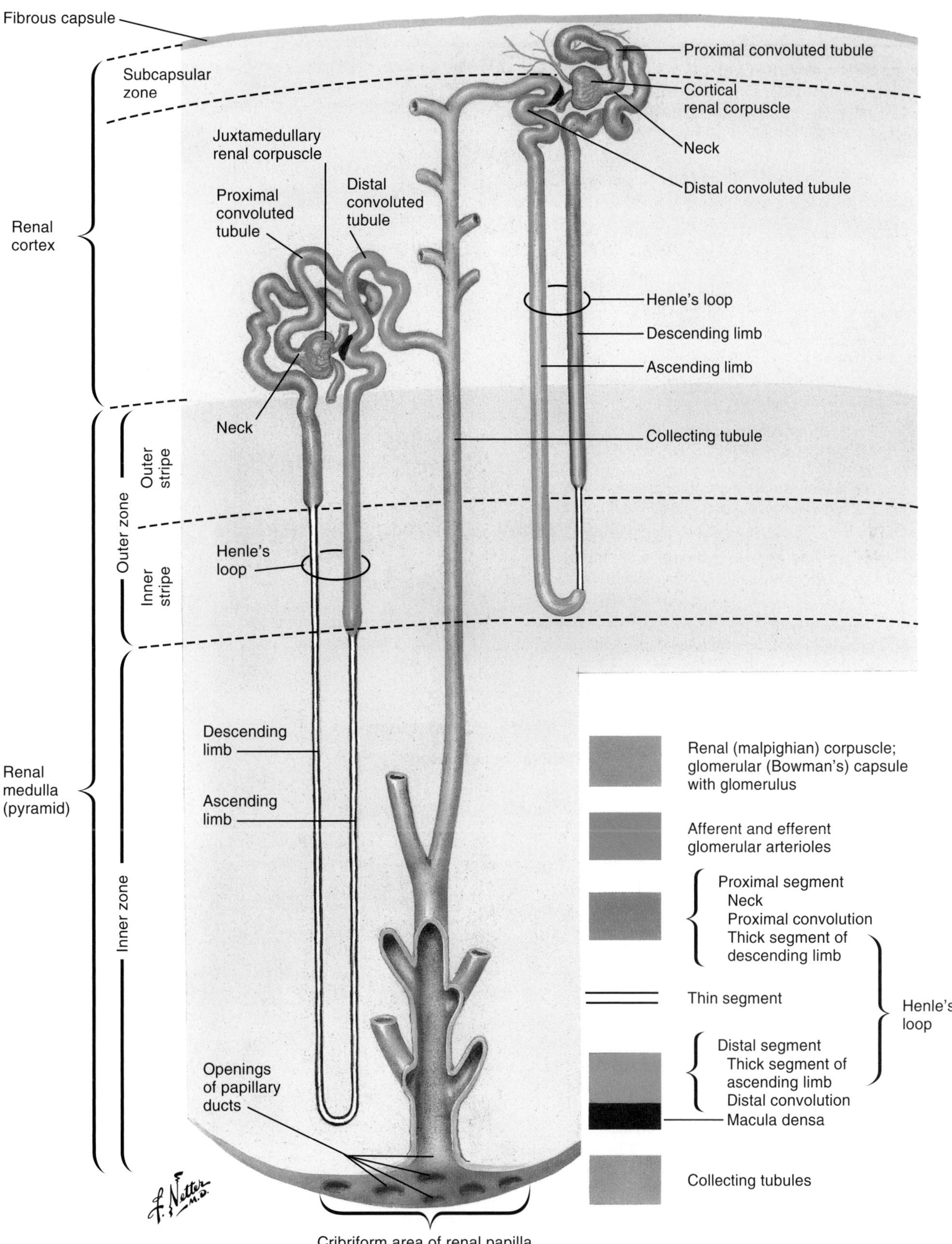

Figure 45-1 Schema of the nephron and collecting tubule. (Netter illustration from www.netterimages.com. © Elsevier Inc. All rights reserved.)

Glomerular Filtration and Peritubular Reabsorption

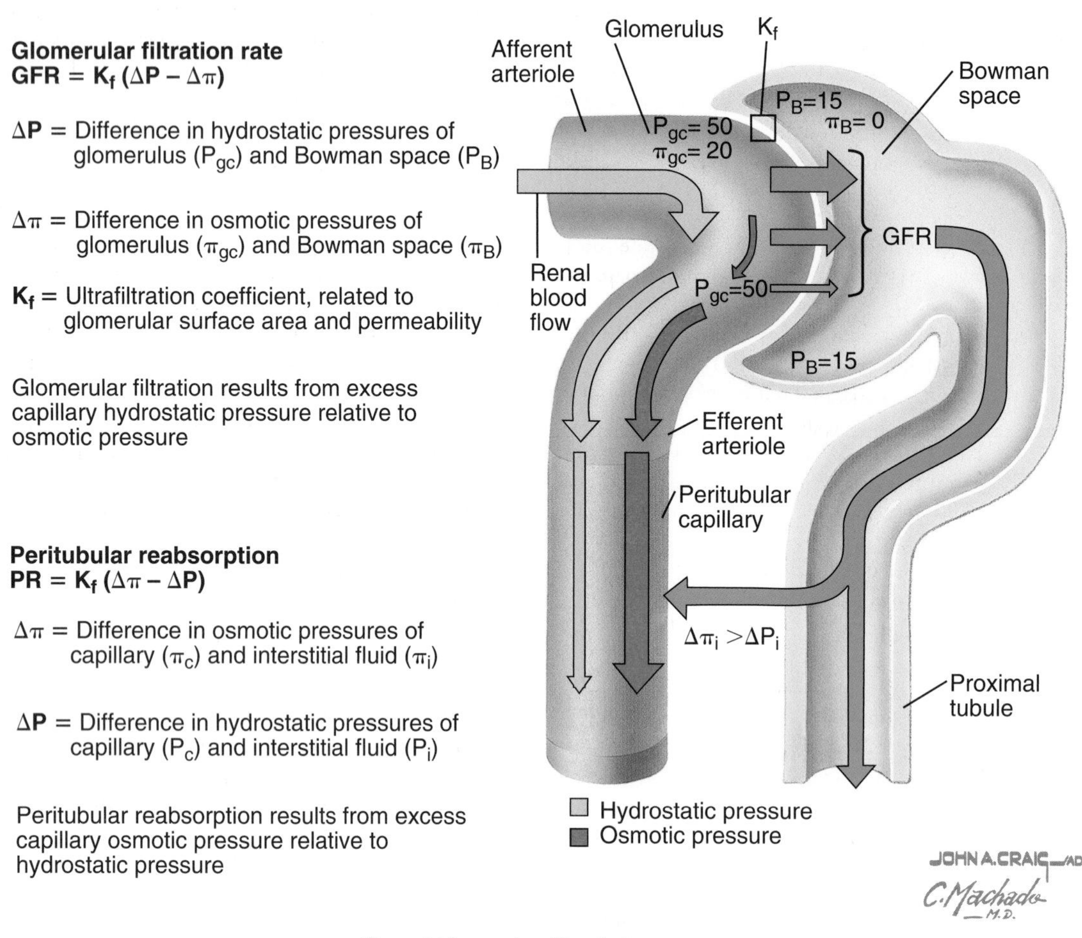

Renal Vascular Resistance

Arteriolar constriction

Increased afferent resistance

Decreased glomerular hydrostatic pressure

Afferent arteriole

GFR

Efferent arteriole

Decreased RBF

Decreased GFR, FF unchanged

Afferent arteriole

Increased glomerular hydrostatic pressure

GFR

Efferent arteriole

Increased efferent resistance

Decreased RBF

Increased GFR and FF

Filtration fraction FF = GFR/RPF

Figure 45-2 Glomerular filtration and peritubular reabsorption. (Netter illustration from www.netterimages.com. © Elsevier Inc. All rights reserved.)

Over a wide range of systemic blood pressure, RBF is maintained by autoregulation to keep a glomerular capillary pressure of approximately 60 to 70 mm Hg for a constant filtration rate and, thus, a proportionate salt loss. Myogenic receptors regulate afferent arteriolar tone by vasoconstriction to protect the glomerulus from too high blood pressure and vasodilation to allow greater blood flow to the glomerulus in times of hypotension. Tubuloglomerular feedback is another mechanism of autoregulation in which tubular fluid composition in the distal tubule (macula densa) affects the afferent arteriole (juxtaglomerular apparatus). Both autoregulatory mechanisms are impaired when mean arterial blood pressure drops below 70 mm Hg, resulting in hypoperfusion of the cortex and oliguria. Failure of renal autoregulation is associated with progressive hypertensive renal disease.

RBF is also regulated by renin-angiotensin-aldosterone system (RAAS), natriuretic peptides, and eicosanoids. During stress, RBF is shunted from cortical to medullary areas, which are under the influence of the sympathetic nervous system and many extrarenal (e.g., epinephrine, norepinephrine, vasopressin), perirenal (e.g., kinin, endothelin, adenosine), and intrarenal (e.g., nitric oxide, prostacyclin) biochemicals. During stress, these biochemicals and afferent nerve activity stimulate medullary mechanisms that increase O_2 consumption within the medulla, leading to the conservation of water and the production of concentrated urine. Functional magnetic resonance imaging studies have shown that furosemide increases O_2 consumption in these same areas and, depending on the adequacy of the O_2 supply, may create ischemic conditions.

Renal clearance of para-aminohippurate (PAH), which is almost completely removed from the blood in normal circumstances, can be used to estimate the renal plasma flow (RPF), which is the amount of plasma that flows through the kidney per minute and the primary determinant of glomerular filtration rate (GFR):

$$RPF_{PAH} = U_{PAH} \times V / P_{PAH}$$

where U_{PAH} and P_{PAH} are the urinary and plasma concentrations of PAH, respectively, and V is the volume of urine. Because the venous concentration of PAH is not 0, the calculated flow is referred to as an *effective RPF* and approximates 600 mL/min, an approximately 10% underestimation of the RPF.

RBF can then be derived from this calculated RPF using a known hematocrit value as follows:

$$RBF = RPF/(1 - Hct)$$

Glomerular Filtration Rate

The GFR, an index of renal function and an initial step in urine formation, involves hydrostatic and osmotic pressure gradients between the glomerular capillaries and the Bowman space (Figure 45-3). The hydrostatic pressure is higher than that of other vascular beds (~50 mm Hg), whereas that of the Bowman space is 10, yielding a net pressure of 40 mm Hg, which favors glomerular filtration. The ultrafiltrate has the same composition and osmolality as plasma but is protein free. The GFR of both kidneys, 120 mL/min, can increase if the glomerular capillary surface area, flow rate, or hydrostatic pressure increases. Polysaccharide inulin or endogenous creatinine concentration can be used to estimate the GFR because both substances are freely filtered in glomeruli and reabsorbed by nephrons but are not secreted or metabolized by renal tubules. Therefore, the filtration rate equals the excretion rate, and GFR equals the waste concentration in urine times the rate of urine output divided by the waste concentration in plasma: GFR = UV/P. The GFR is under the influence of many physiologic factors, such as RAAS, cardiac output, sympathetic innervation, hormone and vasoactive substances, and growth factors.

Tubular Reabsorption

Nutrients, electrolytes, urea, and water are reabsorbed in the renal tubules according to the body's needs (see Figure 45-3). Substances are passively or actively moved through tubular epithelia, interstitium, and peritubular capillary endothelia or are moved by facilitation, pinocytosis, or solvent drag ("bulk transport") via either transcellular or paracellular routes.

Primary active transport mechanisms—Na^+/K^+-ATPase, H^+-ATPase, H^+/K^+-ATPase, and Ca^{2+}-ATPase—require high energy; other secondary transport mechanisms use energy that is released from cotransport or countertransport of glucose, amino acids, and H^+. The proximal part of the renal tubule is the site of reabsorption of most water, whereas the loop of Henle and the proximal tubule are impermeable to water.

Tubular Secretion

In the renal tubule, selected byproducts of metabolism, such as some organic compounds bound to plasma proteins that are not filtered, are excreted. A few substances are secreted from peritubular capillaries into the tubular lumen in a process of active transport that is energy dependent. Tubular secretion of H^+ and NH_3, after formation and dissociation of NH_4^+ ions within the collecting ducts, is important in maintaining H^+ homeostasis, as is secretion of excess K^+ in distal tubules, a process that is controlled by aldosterone.

Conclusion

The kidney is the main organ of regulation of body fluid, nitrogen, and electrolyte balance. Its functions are subject to a number of regulatory influences from both intrinsic and extrinsic sources. The hydrostatic pressure in glomerular capillaries is dependent on blood pressure, resulting in a corresponding change in filtration and urine output with changes in blood pressure. Specialized regions of nephrons provide for three major processes in urine formation: glomerular filtration, tubular reabsorption, and tubular secretion. Specific characteristics of nephrons maintain the osmolarity of body fluids and blood while concentrating or diluting urine. Urine composition changes continuously to maintain fairly constant concentrations of a number of electrolytes, H^+, urea, and serum osmolarity. Renal clearance forms the basis for calculating RBF and GFR, providing assessments of renal function.

Suggested Readings

Cupples WA, Braam B. Assessment of renal autoregulation. *Am J Physiol Renal Physiol*. 2007;292:F1105-1123.

Hall JE, Guyton AC. *Guyton and Hall Textbook of Medical Physiology*. 12th ed. Philadelphia: Saunders/Elsevier; 2011.

Henke K, Eigsti J. Renal physiology: Review and practical application in the critically ill patient. *Dimens Crit Care Nurs*. 2003;22:125-132.

Stanton BA, Koeppen BM. The kidney. In: Berne RM, Levy MN, Koeppen BM, Stanton BA, eds. *Physiology*. 5th ed. St. Louis: Mosby; 2004:623-658.

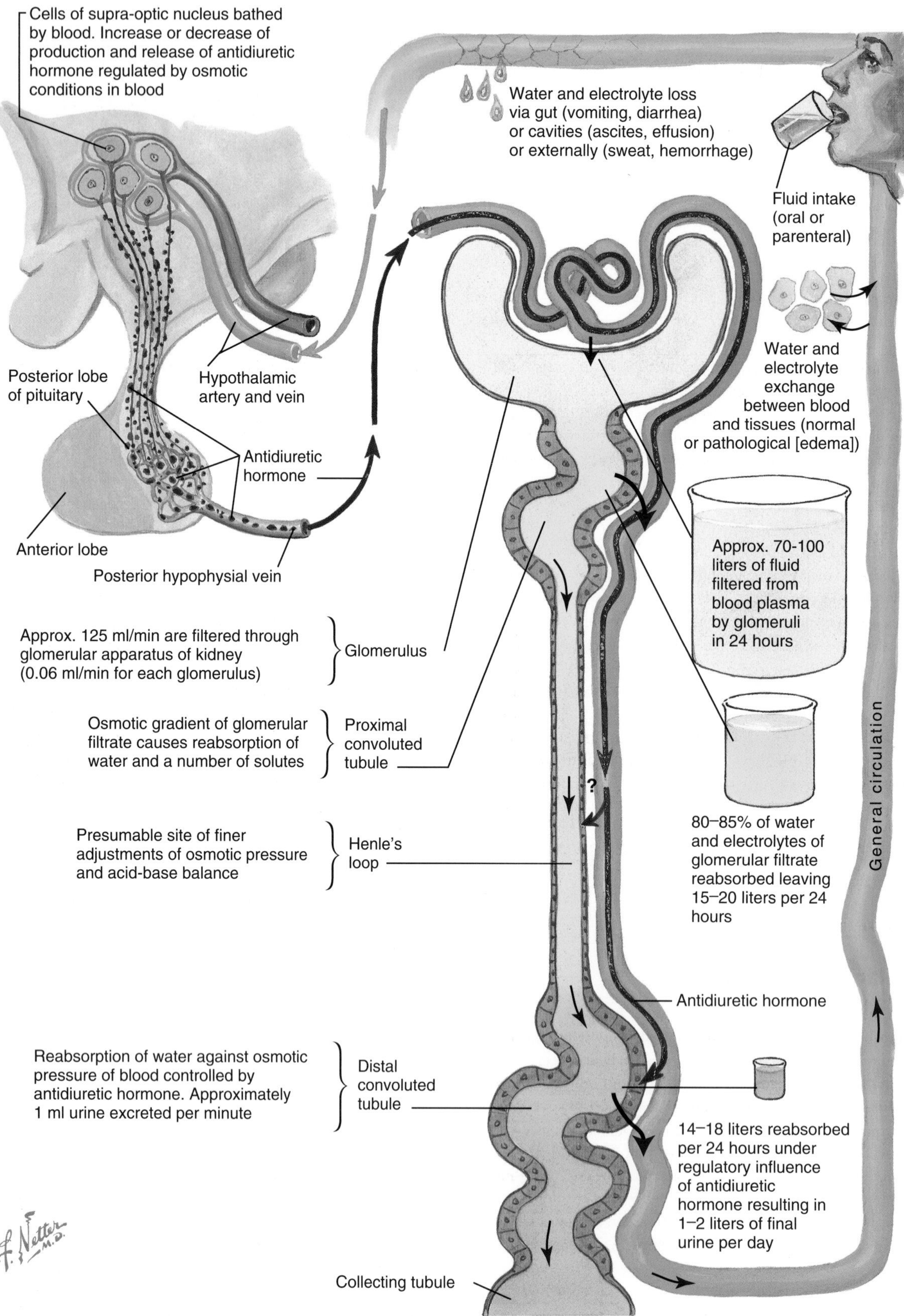
Regulation of Water Balance
Cells of supra-optic nucleus bathed by blood. Increase or decrease of production and release of antidiuretic hormone regulated by osmotic conditions in blood
Water and electrolyte loss via gut (vomiting, diarrhea) or cavities (ascites, effusion) or externally (sweat, hemorrhage)
Fluid intake (oral or parenteral)
Water and electrolyte exchange between blood and tissues (normal or pathological [edema])
Posterior lobe of pituitary
Hypothalamic artery and vein
Antidiuretic hormone
Anterior lobe
Posterior hypophysial vein
Approx. 70-100 liters of fluid filtered from blood plasma by glomeruli in 24 hours
Approx. 125 ml/min are filtered through glomerular apparatus of kidney (0.06 ml/min for each glomerulus)
Glomerulus
Osmotic gradient of glomerular filtrate causes reabsorption of water and a number of solutes
Proximal convoluted tubule
?
80–85% of water and electrolytes of glomerular filtrate reabsorbed leaving 15–20 liters per 24 hours
General circulation
Presumable site of finer adjustments of osmotic pressure and acid-base balance
Henle's loop
Antidiuretic hormone
Reabsorption of water against osmotic pressure of blood controlled by antidiuretic hormone. Approximately 1 ml urine excreted per minute
Distal convoluted tubule
14–18 liters reabsorbed per 24 hours under regulatory influence of antidiuretic hormone resulting in 1–2 liters of final urine per day
Collecting tubule
F. Netter M.D.

Figure 45-3 Regulation of water balance. (Netter illustration from www.netterimages.com. © Elsevier Inc. All rights reserved.)

CHAPTER 46

Renal Function Tests

C. Thomas Wass, MD

Glomerular function is characterized by glomerular filtration rate (GFR), whereas tubular functions include concentrating ability, water conservation, and electrolyte and pH homeostasis. For practical purposes, renal function tests can be stratified into clearance techniques that estimate GFR, tubular function tests, and assays that are largely used for clinical and laboratory investigation.

The Glomerular Filtration Rate

The GFR is the amount of plasma filtered through glomeruli per unit of time and is the single best index of functioning renal mass. Inulin is a sugar that is completely filtered by the glomerulus but is neither secreted nor reabsorbed by the tubule. Thus, the volume of intravenously administered inulin cleared from the plasma can be used to calculate the GFR. However, inulin clearance is seldom used clinically because the assay is cumbersome and time consuming to perform. Creatinine (Cr) is a metabolic end product of creatine phosphate in skeletal muscle that is cleared by the kidney in a manner similar to that of inulin. Creatinine clearance (CrCl), the most clinically useful measure of GFR, is estimated using the following formula:

$$\text{CrCl} = \frac{(140 - \text{age})(\text{body weight in kg})}{(\text{serum creatinine})(72)}$$

More precise measurement requires timed collections (over a period of 24 h) of urine and plasma samples and requires use of the following formula:

$$\text{CrCl} = \frac{(\text{UCr} \times \text{V})}{\text{PCr}}$$

where U is the urinary Cr concentration in mg/dL, V is the volume of urine in mL/min, and P is the plasma Cr concentration.

Normal GFR is 120 $\pm$ 25 mL/min in men and 95 $\pm$ 20 mL/min in women. Mild, moderate, and severe impairment have corresponding values of approximately 40 to 60 mL/min, 20 to 40 mL/min, and less than 20 mL/min, respectively. Serial GFR measurements are important in determining the severity of renal dysfunction, as well as in monitoring disease progression.

Tubular Function Tests

Fractional Excretion of Sodium

Measuring the urinary sodium concentration (U_{Na+}) is useful in assessing volume status. A U_{Na+} concentration of less than 20 mEq/L suggests intravascular volume depletion, whereas a U_{Na+} concentration of more than 40 mEq/L suggests a decreased ability of the renal tubules to reabsorb sodium (e.g., acute tubular necrosis). Fractional excretion of sodium (FE_{Na+}) reflects renal tubular sodium reabsorption. FE_{Na+} describes sodium clearance as a percentage of CrCl:

$$FE_{Na^+} = (\text{sodium clearance}/\text{CrCl})100\%$$

An FE_{Na+} less than 1% is seen in patients with a normal volume status or who are hypovolemic; an FE_{Na+} greater than 1% indicates tubular damage (e.g., acute tubular necrosis).

Urine-Concentrating and Urine-Diluting Ability

Urine-concentrating and urine-diluting abilities are assessed by measuring urine osmolality (normal is 300 mOsm/kg, but it can range from 50-1200 mOsm/kg) and can be evaluated as "appropriate" or "inappropriate" with respect to serum osmolality (or tonicity; normal range is approximately 278-298 mOsm/kg). Normally, as serum tonicity increases (e.g., dehydration or hypovolemia secondary to blood loss), release of antidiuretic hormone from the posterior pituitary causes water conservation and urine osmolality increases. The normal tubular response to hypovolemia is to generate a urine-to-plasma osmolality ratio of at least 1.5; a urine-to-plasma osmolality ratio of 1.0 implies loss of tubular function and supports the diagnosis of acute renal failure. The opposite occurs with dilution of the vascular space, with water diuresis causing urine osmolality to decrease.

Urinary Acidification Capacity

The kidneys excrete nonvolatile acids produced by protein catabolism, thereby preventing systemic acidosis. For patients consuming a typical American diet, the pH of a randomly obtained urine sample is usually less than 6.5. An acidification defect can be tested by orally administering ammonium chloride. If the urine pH is not less than 5.5 when serum pH is less than 7.35 and HCO_3^- is less than 20 mEq/L, a renal-tubule acidification defect is present.

Other Clinical and Laboratory Assays

Urinalysis

Urinalysis is a useful noninvasive diagnostic tool available to assess renal function. Testing includes visual inspection (Table 46-1); dipstick determination of pH (normal 4.5-8.0), blood, glucose, and protein; specific gravity (normal 1.003-1.030); and examination of urinary sediment. In patients with porphyria, urine is of normal color when fresh, but discolors over time when exposed to light (which is a pathognomonic observation). The pH is rarely diagnostic, but in conjunction with serum pH and bicarbonate values, it is useful in evaluating renal tubule acidification function. Dipstick determinations register glucose, but not other reducing sugars; elevations in urine glucose concentrations suggest a diagnosis of hyperglycemia or a tubule defect (e.g., Fanconi syndrome or isolated glycosuria). When the plasma glucose concentration is 180 mg/dL or less, all of the glucose filtered by

Table 46-1 Urine Colors

Color	Endogenous Cause	Exogenous Cause
Red	Hemoglobinuria, hematuria, myoglobinuria, porphyria	Beets, blackberries, chronic mercury or lead exposure, phenolphthalein, phenytoin, phenothiazines, propofol,* rhubarb, rifampin
Orange	Bilirubinuria, methemoglobinemia, uric acid crystalluria secondary to gastric bypass or chemotherapy	Carrots, carrot juice, coumadin, ethoxazene, large dose of vitamin C, phenazopyridine, rifampin
Brown/black	Bilirubinuria, cirrhosis, hematuria, hepatitis, methemoglobinemia, myoglobinuria, tyrosinemia	Aloe, cascara/senna laxatives, chloroquine, copper, fava beans, furazolidone, metronidazole, nitrofurantoin, primaquine, rhubarb, sorbitol, methocarbamol, phenacetin, phenol poisoning
Blue, blue-green, green	Biliverdin, familial hypercalcemia, indicanuria, urinary tract infection caused by *Pseudomonas* spp.	Asparagus, amitriptyline, chlorophyll breath mints, cimetidine, indomethacin, magnesium salicylates, metoclopramide, methylene blue, multivitamins, propofol, phenergan, phenol
White	Chyluria, phosphaturia, pyuria	
Purple	Urinary tract infection caused by *Providencia stuartii, Klebsiella pneumoniae, P. aeruginosa, Escherichia coli,* and enterococcus species; porphyria	Beets, iodine-containing compounds, methylene blue

*Pink color typically is found in people who are given propofol and those who abuse alcohol.

glomeruli is reabsorbed in the proximal tubules. Dipstick determination of glucose crudely indicates a blood glucose concentration of at least 230 mg/dL.

The presence of hemoglobin in the urine can be detected by a dipstick because peroxidase catalyzes the reaction of peroxide and chromogen to produce a colorimetric change. False-positive results may occur if the patient has myoglobin in the urine. Hemoglobin and myoglobin can be distinguished by dissolving 2.8 g of ammonium sulfate in 5 mL of urine, causing hemoglobin to precipitate. The two pigments can also be distinguished by spectrophotometry, electrophoresis, immunochemical methods, or looking for the presence or absence of red blood cells on microscopic examination. Protein testing is not sensitive for albumin on dipstick analysis.

Creatinine

An end product of skeletal muscle catabolism, Cr is excreted solely by the kidneys. Normal serum Cr ranges from 0.8 to 1.3 mg/dL for men and 0.6 to 1.1 for women (ranges vary due to sex-specific differences in muscle mass). Because Cr production is proportional to skeletal muscle mass, elderly patients who have decreased muscle mass, compared with younger patients, may have normal serum Cr concentrations despite substantial reductions in renal function.

Blood Urea Nitrogen

Blood urea nitrogen (BUN) is a byproduct of protein metabolism. Normal value ranges from 8 to 20 mg/dL. BUN values may increase independent of renal function as a result of dehydration, a high-protein diet, degradation of blood from a large hematoma or the gastrointestinal tract, or accelerated catabolism (e.g., a metabolic state observed in patients sustaining trauma, sepsis, or burns).

Both Cr and BUN values tend to be insensitive measures of changing renal function. That is, increases in their concentration typically do not occur until the GFR is reduced by as much as 75%. Accordingly, both are late indicators of impaired renal function. Dehydration is suspected in patients with a BUN/serum Cr ratio exceeding 20:1.

Suggested Readings

Cirillo M. Evaluation of glomerular filtration rate and of albuminuria/proteinuria. *J Nephrol.* 2010;23:125-132.

Giovanni FB. Urinalysis and microscopy. In: Davison AM, ed. *Oxford Textbook of Clinical Nephrology.* 3rd ed. New York: Oxford University Press; 2005:23-45.

Greenberg M. Verdoglobinuria. *Clin Toxicol.* 2008;46:485-486.

Lee J. Images in clinical medicine. Purple urine. *N Engl J Med.* 2007;357:e14.

Prigent A. Monitoring renal function and limitations of renal function tests. *Semin Nucl Med.* 2008;38:32-46.

CHAPTER 47

Acid-Base Status

Ian MacVeigh, MD

Recognizing, diagnosing, and treating acid-base disorders are absolutely essential skills for all anesthesia providers. Having a clear understanding of the terminology and physiology related to acid-base disorders and employing standard criteria for the assessment and diagnosis of these often-puzzling derangements results in quicker recognition and more effective treatment of acid-base disorders.

Terminology

Normal values of pH, defined as the negative logarithm of the hydrogen ion concentration $[H^+]$ (expressed in extracellular fluids in nanoequivalents per liter), range from 7.35 to 7.45. Changes in pH are inversely related to changes in $[H^+]$: a 20% increase in $[H^+]$ decreases the pH by 0.1; conversely, a 20% decrease in $[H^+]$ increases the pH by a 0.1 (Table 47-1).

The terms *acidemia* and *alkalemia* refer to the pH of blood. *Acidosis*, on the other hand, refers to the process that either adds acid or removes alkali from body fluids; conversely, *alkalosis* is the process that either adds alkali or removes acid from body fluids. *Compensation* refers to the body's homeostatic mechanisms that generate or eliminate $[H^+]$ to normalize pH in response to a pathologic acid-base disturbance. *Base excess*, an assessment of the metabolic component of an acid-base disturbance, quantifies the amount of acid that must be added to a blood sample to return the pH of the sample to 7.40 if the patient's $Paco_2$ were 40 mm Hg. A positive base excess value indicates that the patient has a metabolic alkalosis (acid would have to be added to the blood to reach a normal pH); a negative value indicates that the patient has a metabolic acidosis and alkali would have to be added to normalize the pH. Blood gas results are, by convention, reported as pH, $Paco_2$, Pao_2, HCO_3^-, and base excess; the latter two are calculated. The HCO_3^- is derived using the Henderson-Hasselbalch equation, which can be expressed as either of the following:

$$pH = pKa + \frac{PaCO_2}{HCO_3^-}$$

$$[H^+] = 24 \times \frac{PaCO_2}{HCO_3^-}$$

Tight control of the pH requires a fairly constant $Paco_2/HCO_3^-$ ratio, which allows one to check the validity of an arterial blood gas (ABG) sample (Table 47-2).

Table 47-1 pH for Given Hydrogen Ion Concentrations

pH	$[H^+]$ (nEq/L)
7.0	100
7.1	80
7.2	64
7.3	50
7.4	40
7.5	30
7.6	24
7.7	20

Types of Acid-Base Disorders

Acid-base disorders may be simple or mixed. Simple disorders include respiratory acid-base disorders, in which the primary change in pH is secondary to changes in $Paco_2$, and metabolic acid-base disorders, in which the primary change involves the $[H^+]$. Mixed disorders occur when more than one acid-base disorder coexists in the same patient. Remember that acid-base disorders are simply manifestations of underlying systemic disorders. Determining why the acid-base disorder is present requires the incorporation of information from the patient's history and the findings on physical examination.

Compensatory Responses

Every primary acid-base disorder should have an appropriate compensatory response. A primary respiratory (ventilatory) disorder induces a renal response—reabsorption of HCO_3^- in the proximal tubules is altered to compensate for the change in pH induced by the change in $Paco_2$. This process is slow, occurring over 24 to 36 h. A primary metabolic disorder, on the other hand, induces a much faster respiratory compensation, in which ventilation changes to

Table 47-2 Examples of the Use of Henderson-Hasselbalch Equation to Calculate H^+ Concentration with a Known HCO_3^- and $Paco_2$

$Paco_2$	HCO_3^-	$[H^+]$ (nEq/L) will be	Calculation $[H^+]$	pH
40	24	40	24 × 40/24 = 40	7.4
60	24	60	24 × 60/24 = 60	7.2
20	24	20	24 × 20/24 = 20	7.7
40	16	60	24 × 40/16 = 60	7.2
60	16	90	24 × 60/16 = 90	7.05
20	16	30	24 × 20/16 = 30	7.5

Table 47-3 Primary Change and Compensatory Response for the Primary Acid-Base Disorders

Primary Disorder	Primary Change	Compensatory Response*
Respiratory acidosis	↑ $Paco_2$	↑ HCO_3^-
Respiratory alkalosis	↓ $Paco_2$	↓ HCO_3^-
Metabolic acidosis	↓ HCO_3^-	↓ $Paco_2$
Metabolic alkalosis	↑ HCO_3^-	↑ $Paco_2$

*Homeostatic response in an attempt to maintain constant $Paco_2/HCO_3^-$ ratio.

increase or decrease $Paco_2$ (Table 47-3). The absence of compensation in a timely manner would probably indicate the presence of a secondary disturbance.

Metabolic Acidosis

Metabolic acidosis provokes stimulation of chemoreceptors, promoting an increase in ventilation. Winter's formula can be used to calculate the expected $Paco_2$ in patients with metabolic acidosis:

$$\text{Expected } Paco_2 = (1.5 \times [HCO_3^-]) + 8 \pm 2$$

If the measured $Paco_2$ is equal to the expected $Paco_2$, the patient has a compensated metabolic acidosis. If, on the other hand, the measured $Paco_2$ is greater than the expected $Paco_2$, compensation is inadequate, and the patient has a primary metabolic acidosis with superimposed respiratory acidosis. However, if the measured $Paco_2$ is lower than the expected $Paco_2$, the patient has a primary metabolic acidosis with superimposed respiratory alkalosis.

Metabolic Alkalosis

Metabolic alkalosis can be chloride responsive or resistant. Chloride-responsive states, which are associated with urinary chloride concentrations of less than 15 mEq/L, include vomiting, continuous nasogastric suctioning, and volume-contraction states—the latter being the most common in hospitalized postsurgical patients. Chloride-resistant disorders or conditions, associated with urinary chloride concentrations greater than 25 mEq/L, include hypercortisolism, hyperaldosteronism, sodium bicarbonate therapy, severe renal artery stenosis, hypokalemia, and the use of diuretics, in which case patients may have high urinary chloride concentrations, but the alkalosis nonetheless responds to the administration of chloride. The formula used to calculate the $Paco_2$ in patients with metabolic alkalosis is as follows:

$$\text{Expected } Paco_2 = (0.7 \times HCO_3^-) + 21 \pm 2$$

If the measured $Paco_2$ is equal to the expected $Paco_2$ the patient has a metabolic alkalosis. However, if the measured $Paco_2$ is greater than the expected $Paco_2$ the patient has a metabolic alkalosis with superimposed respiratory acidosis. Finally, if the measured $Paco_2$ is less than the expected $Paco_2$ the patient has a primary metabolic alkalosis with superimposed respiratory alkalosis.

Assessment of Acid-Base Disorders Secondary to Respiratory Mechanics

Although equations can be used to calculate the expected change in pH for changes in $Paco_2$, the easiest way to assess a patient for the influences of $Paco_2$ on pH is to remember that the pH changes inversely 0.08 for every 10-mm Hg change in $Paco_2$. For example, if the $Paco_2$ equals 50 mm Hg, the pH will be 7.32; if the $Paco_2$ is 30 mm Hg, the pH will be 7.48.

Acid-base disorders secondary to respiratory mechanics are the most common acid-base disorders seen in otherwise "healthy" patients anesthetized for surgical procedures.

If respiratory disorders are more longstanding (e.g., respiratory acidosis in a patient with chronic obstructive pulmonary disease or a ventilated patient in the intensive care unit retaining CO_2), then the kidneys will retain HCO_3^- to minimize the change in pH.

Acute respiratory acidosis prior to onset of renal compensation:

$$\text{Expected pH} = 7.40 - (0.008 \times Paco_2)$$
$$\Delta pH = 0.008 \times \Delta Paco_2$$

Acute respiratory alkalosis prior to onset of renal compensation:

$$\text{Expected pH} = 7.40 + [0.008 \times (40 - Paco_2)]$$
$$\Delta pH = 0.008 \times \Delta Paco_2$$

Chronic respiratory acidosis, renal compensation fully developed:

$$\text{Expected pH} = 7.40 - [0.003 \times (Paco_2 - 40)]$$
$$\Delta pH = 0.003 \times \Delta Paco_2$$

Chronic respiratory alkalosis, renal compensation fully developed:

$$\text{Expected pH} = 7.40 + [0.003 \times (40 - Paco_2)]$$
$$\Delta pH = 0.003 \times \Delta Paco_2$$

Respiratory Acidosis

Causes of respiratory acidosis include airway obstruction, central nervous system depression, the use of opioids, restrictive lung disease (kyphoscoliosis, fibrothorax), and neuromuscular diseases.

Respiratory Alkalosis

Causes of respiratory alkalosis include psychogenic hyperventilation, encephalitis, early pneumonia, early stages of bronchial asthma, pulmonary embolism, hepatic failure, early sepsis, and pregnancy. The lowest $Paco_2$ achieved by hyperventilation is approximately 16 mm Hg, and the pH is approximately 7.6 before renal compensatory changes occur.

Assessment of Acid-Base Disorders Secondary to Metabolic Disorders

Metabolic Acidosis

If, on an ABG analysis, the pH is less than 7.35 and the base excess is negative (a base deficit), then the patient has a metabolic acidosis, assuming that the $Paco_2$ is equal to 40 mm Hg. The first step is to calculate the anion gap (AG), which can be done by subtracting the sum of Cl^- and HCO_3^- from the Na^+ concentration. Normal values are 12 ± 4 mEq/L. This gap represents the unmeasured negatively charged ions (anions) that are balancing the electrical charge of the positively charged ions (cations) in human bodies.

Causes of an Increased Anion Gap

Causes of an increase in the AG (mnemonic, DARLINGS ARE IMP) include diabetic ketoacidosis (anions = acetoacetate, β-hydroxybutyrate), alcohol use, renal failure (anions = phosphate, sulfate), lactic acidosis, iron poisoning, no food (starvation), generalized seizures, sepsis, aspirin poisoning, rhabdomyolysis, ethylene glycol ingestion, the use of isoniazid (INH), and methanol or paraldehyde exposure.

Causes of a Decreased Anion Gap

Processes that decrease the unmeasured anions or increase the unmeasured cations will decrease the AG. Albumin is an anion and is responsible for approximately half of the normal AG of 12 mEq/L. If the albumin concentration is low, the AG will be lower than normal (i.e., <12 mEq/L), decreasing by approximately 2 to 3 units for every 1-g decrease in serum albumin concentration.

Conversely, immunoglobulins are cations, and if they increase (i.e., in paraproteinemias, such as multiple myeloma), the kidneys retain additional chloride to maintain electrical neutrality, and the AG decreases.

Causes of Non–Anion Gap Metabolic Acidosis

In metabolic acidosis without an AG, the loss of bicarbonate is compensated for by a rise in chloride. Primary causes of a metabolic acidosis without an AG include gastrointestinal losses (diarrhea, small bowel fistula, ileostomy, ureterosigmoidostomy, or an ileal conduit for an ureter), urinary losses (proximal and distal renal tubular acidosis, acetazolamide therapy, urinary obstruction, pancreatic fistula, or the correction phase of diabetic ketoacidosis), and infusion of isotonic saline.

ΔAnion Gap Strategy

The ΔAG strategy is used in patients with metabolic acidosis to detect the possibility of a superimposed metabolic disorder, either a metabolic alkalosis or a non-AG metabolic acidosis. The following three steps are required:

1. ΔAG = patient-calculated AG – normal AG (12 mEq/L)
2. Calculate the corrected HCO_3^- = measured HCO_3^- + ΔAG
3. Compare corrected HCO_3^- to a normal HCO_3^- = 24 mEq/L

If the corrected HCO_3^- is higher than the normal HCO_3^-, then the patient has a superimposed metabolic alkalosis; if the corrected HCO_3^- is lower than the normal HCO_3^-, then the patient has non-AG metabolic acidosis.

Suggested Readings

Constable PD. Hyperchloremic acidosis: The classic example of strong ion acidosis. *Anesth Analg*. 2003;96:919-922.

Gennari FJ, Adrogué HJ, Galla JH, Madias NE, eds. *Acid–Base Disorders and Their Treatment*. Boca Raton, FL: Taylor & Francis; 2005.

Poustie DA, Story S, Bellomo R. Quantitative physical chemistry analysis of acid-base disorders in critically ill patients. *Anaesthesia*. 2001;56:530-533.

Rastegar A. Use of the ΔAG/ΔHCO_3^- ratio in the diagnosis of mixed acid-base disorders. *J Am Soc Nephrol*. 2007;18:2429-2431.

CHAPTER 48

Electrolyte Abnormalities: Potassium, Sodium, Calcium, and Magnesium

Daniel R. Brown, MD, PhD, FCCM

Electrolytes are intimately involved in cellular electrophysiology as well as a myriad of cellular enzymatic processes. This chapter will focus on anesthetic implications of alterations in several important cations. The reader is encouraged to consult the suggested readings for additional details of associated pathophysiology and perioperative management.

Potassium

The total body potassium store in a 70-kg individual exceeds 3500 mEq, with less than 2% located in extracellular fluid. Potassium balance is primarily determined by oral intake and renal elimination. Extracellular potassium is dependent on multiple factors, including acid-base balance, activity of insulin, sodium-potassium ATP (adenosine triphosphate)-dependent exchange channels, and blood levels of insulin and catecholamines.

Hyperkalemia

The most significant clinical effect of hyperkalemia involves the electrical conduction system of the heart. These changes include gradual prolongation of the PR interval (with the eventual loss of the P wave), prolongation of the QRS complex, ST-segment elevation, and peaking of T waves, ultimately leading to ventricular arrhythmias (Figure 48-1). Cardiac conduction changes usually occur when plasma potassium concentration exceeds 6.5 mmol/L but may develop at lower levels in the setting of acute hyperkalemia. Options for acute management rely on membrane stabilization and intracellular shifting

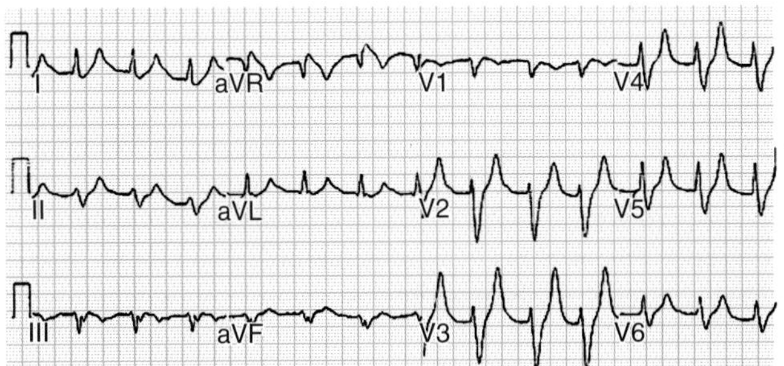

Figure 48-1 The marked widening of the QRS duration combined with tall peaked T waves is suggestive of advanced hyperkalemia. Note the absence of P waves, suggesting a junctional rhythm; however, in hyperkalemia, the atrial muscle may be paralyzed while the heart is still in sinus rhythm. (Courtesy of Frank G. Yanowitz, MD, Professor of Medicine, University of Utah School of Medicine, Medical Director, ECG Department, LDS Hospital, Salt Lake City, UT.)

of potassium and include administration of calcium chloride, sodium bicarbonate, and insulin or glucose.

Hypokalemia

For every 1 mmol/L decrease in plasma potassium concentration, the total body potassium store decreases by approximately 200 to 300 mmol. Characteristic electrocardiographic changes associated with hypokalemia include

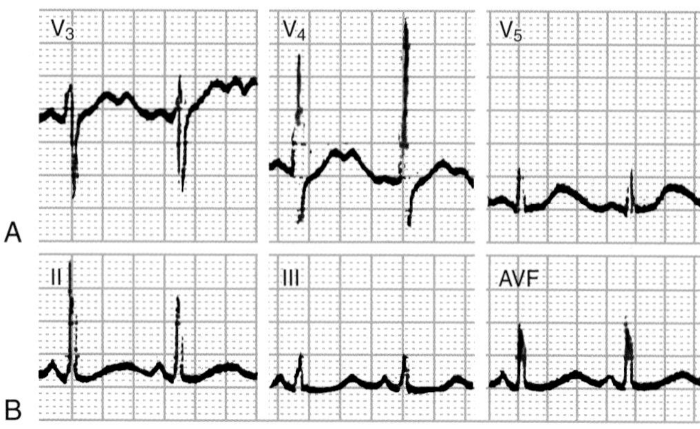

Figure 48-2 **A**, Note the prominent U wave in leads V_3 and V_4, giving the conjoined TU wave the appearance of a camel's hump. **B**, The "apparently" prolonged QT interval in leads S_2 and aVF is due to the fact that the T wave is actually a U wave with a flattened T wave merging into the following U wave. (Courtesy of Frank G. Yanowitz, MD, Professor of Medicine, University of Utah School of Medicine, Medical Director, ECG Department, LDS Hospital, Salt Lake City, UT.)

gradual QRS interval prolongation with the subsequent development of prominent U waves (Figure 48-2). Hypokalemia may also be associated with weakness and a greater effect of neuromuscular blocking agents. To treat hypokalemia, the clinician must take into account the patient's total body potassium levels and the chronicity of the hypokalemia. Chronic hypokalemia tends to be associated with a true decrease in total body potassium stores, whereas hypokalemia with normal body stores of potassium occurs more acutely. Treatment of hypokalemia involves oral or intravenous replacement of potassium. Intravenous potassium replacement should be gradual to avoid acute overcorrection and hyperkalemia. Respiratory and metabolic alkalosis should be avoided because alkalosis will worsen the degree of hypokalemia secondary to intracellular shifting.

Sodium

Serum sodium concentration is dependent on total body sodium levels as they relate to total body water. Therefore, the treatment of abnormal serum sodium concentrations must take into account both total body sodium stores and total body water. To a great extent, thirst and free water administration, sodium intake, and renal salt and water handling regulate water balance, although, in many clinical situations, the body's ability to regulate this relationship is impaired. When correcting sodium, changes in free water and sodium concentration are often difficult to predict; thus, frequent assessment of serum sodium concentration and volume status may be required.

Hypernatremia

Hypernatremia is defined as serum sodium concentration greater than 145 mmol/L and is often associated with a deficiency in total body water. Manifestations of hypernatremia include mental status changes, hyperreflexia, ataxia, and seizures. Free water deficit can be calculated as follows: free water deficit, in liters = (0.6 × weight, in kg) × ((serum sodium/140) – 1). Free water is administered to correct hypernatremia, although treatment of severe central diabetes insipidus may involve the use of subcutaneously or intravenously administered vasopressin. In the setting of hypervolemic hypernatremia, diuretics may be required to allow for both water and sodium elimination while free water is administered.

Hyponatremia

Hyponatremia is defined as a serum sodium concentration less than 135 mmol/L. Hyponatremia may present with mental status changes, lethargy, cramps, decreased deep tendon reflexes, and seizures. A serum sodium concentration of less than 120 mmol/L is a potentially life-threatening condition, with associated mortality rates reported to be as high as 50%. However, if the correction of hyponatremia occurs too rapidly, a demyelinating brainstem lesion—central pontine myelinolysis—may cause permanent neurologic damage. In severely symptomatic patients, the recommendation is to correct sodium at a rate of 1 to 2 $mmol \cdot L^{-1} \cdot h^{-1}$ until the serum sodium concentration reaches 125 to 130 mmol/L. In conditions of hypervolemic or euvolemic hyponatremia, hypertonic (2%–3%) saline may be used to treat symptomatic patients or in patients who would not tolerate additional intravascular volume. To avoid a hyperchloremic metabolic acidosis, it may be desirable to administer hypertonic saline formulated as 50% sodium chloride and 50% sodium acetate. When administering solutions with a saline concentration greater than 2%, clinicians should consider using central venous access. Management of hypervolemic hyponatremia may include administration of diuretics. Following administration of diuretics, the concentration of sodium in the urine may be as high as 70 to 80 mEq/L (one-half normal saline), thus resulting in loss of free water and thereby increasing serum sodium concentration.

Calcium

The total serum calcium concentration comprises three fractions: 50% protein-bound calcium, 5% to 10% anion-bound calcium, and 40% to 45% free, or ionized, calcium. Maintenance of a normal serum calcium concentration involves the parathyroid hormone and calcitonin, which regulate the release and uptake of calcium and phosphorus by the kidneys, bones, and intestines through negative-feedback regulation.

Hypercalcemia

Common causes of hypercalcemia include hyperparathyroidism and malignancies that increase mobilization of calcium from bone. Symptoms include nausea, polyuria, and dehydration. Electrocardiographic monitoring may demonstrate prolonged PR intervals, wide QRS complexes, and shortened QT intervals as hypercalcemia worsens. Avoidance of respiratory alkalosis may be beneficial because alkalosis lowers the plasma potassium concentration, potentially exacerbating cardiac conduction abnormalities. Management of hypercalcemia includes hydration and diuresis to promote renal elimination. In acute toxicity or renal failure, hemodialysis should be considered.

Hypocalcemia

Multiple factors contribute to the development of hypocalcemia. Acquired hypoparathyroidism following neck surgery is a common cause of hypocalcemia because of decreased parathyroid hormone levels. Respiratory or metabolic alkalosis induces hypocalcemia by increasing protein binding to calcium, thereby decreasing the amount of ionized calcium. Renal failure decreases the conversion of vitamin D into 1,25-dihydroxyvitamin D, thereby decreasing intestinal and bone absorption while increasing serum phosphate levels; the phosphate then combines with calcium and precipitates as $CaPO_4$. Massive blood transfusion may also result in hypocalcemia secondary to anticoagulants (the EDTA [ethylenediaminetetra-acetic acid] in transfused blood, which chelates calcium). Hypocalcemia is often asymptomatic, though severe hypocalcemia may be associated with prolonged QT interval, bradycardia, peripheral vasodilation, and decreased cardiac contractility, any of which can cause hypotension. Neurologic manifestations of hypocalcemia include perioral numbness, muscle cramps, tetany, hyperreflexia, and seizures. Several factors guide calcium-replacement therapy, including absolute serum calcium level, the rapidity of the drop in serum calcium concentration, and the underlying disease process. Calcium causes vasoconstriction, and extravascular infiltration may be associated with morbidity. In patients who have no symptoms, observation may be the most appropriate treatment. Calcium chloride contains three times the amount of calcium, compared with calcium gluconate.

Magnesium

Primary determinants of total body magnesium are intake and renal excretion. Determination of magnesium deficiency is difficult because magnesium is primarily an intracellular ion, and serum magnesium concentration may not reflect tissue levels. Nonetheless, therapy for magnesium disorders, almost exclusively hypomagnesemia, is often guided by serum magnesium concentration (normal 1.7-2.1 mg/dL).

Hypomagnesemia

Multiple factors may contribute to magnesium depletion, including decreased intake, impaired intestinal absorption, and increased gastrointestinal and renal losses. Hypomagnesemia is most often asymptomatic, but life-threatening neurologic and cardiac sequelae may develop. Hypomagnesemia may cause neuromuscular excitability, mental status changes, and seizures. Considerable evidence supports an association between hypomagnesemia and cardiac arrhythmias and potentiation of digoxin toxicity. Electrocardiographic changes include prolonged QT interval and atrial and ventricular ectopy. Magnesium has been advocated as a treatment for torsades de pointes and digoxin toxicity arrhythmias; indeed, evidence exists that a trial of $MgSO_4$ may be useful in the management of most arrhythmias. The cardiovascular effects of even rapid administration of intravenous $MgSO_4$ (4 g over 10 min) are minimal, with small decreases in blood pressure (<10%) being the most common effect. Replacement of potassium in the presence of hypomagnesemia is notoriously difficult, and it is often necessary to replace both ions simultaneously.

Hypermagnesemia

Hypermagnesemia most commonly develops in the setting of renal failure and occasionally with excessive magnesium intake (such as during magnesium therapy for preeclampsia). Manifestations of hypermagnesemia begin to occur when serum magnesium concentration exceeds 5 mg/dL and are primarily neurologic and cardiovascular. Hyporeflexia, sedation, and weakness are common. Electrocardiographic changes are variable but often include widened QRS complex and prolonged PR interval. Treatment includes enhancing renal excretion with loop diuretics and, in the setting of renal failure, dialysis. Calcium may be administered to temporarily antagonize the effects of hypermagnesemia.

Suggested Readings

Adrogué HJ, Madias NE. Hypernatremia. *N Engl J Med.* 2000;342:1493-1499.

Adrogué HJ, Madias NE. Hyponatremia. *N Engl J Med.* 2000;342:1581-1589.

Ghali JK. Mechanisms, risks, and new treatment options for hyponatremia. *Cardiology.* 2008;111:147-157.

Lindner G, Funk GC. Hypernatremia in critically ill patients. *J Crit Care.* 2013;28(2):216:e11-20.

Pokaharel M, Block CA. Dysnatremia in the ICU. *Curr Opin Critl Care.* 2011;17(6):581-593.

Tommasino C, Picozzi V. Volume and electrolyte management. *Best Pract Res Clin Anaesthesiol.* 2007;21:497-516.

Weiner M, Epstein FH. Signs and symptoms of electrolyte disorders. *Yale J Biol Med.* 1970;43:76-109.

Weisberg LS. Management of severe hyperkalemia. *Crit Care Med.* 2008;36:3246-3251.

CHAPTER 49

Hepatic Physiology and Preoperative Evaluation

Frank D. Crowl, MD

Patients with preexisting severe hepatic dysfunction are known to be at significant risk for experiencing perioperative death. Patients with mild to moderate hepatic dysfunction are at increased risk for death.

Some patients develop unexpected hepatic dysfunction (jaundice) in the postoperative period. The reported incidence of postoperative hepatic dysfunction, as demonstrated by abnormalities in liver function tests, is between 1 in 239 and 1 in 1091 anesthetics delivered. Interestingly, some of these patients had preexisting hepatic dysfunction that was not clinically apparent. One study found that 1 in 700 healthy asymptomatic ASA class I and II patients admitted for elective operations had unexplained abnormalities on preoperative liver function tests. After cancellation of their operations, one third of these patients developed clinical jaundice.

Metabolic Function

Glucose Homeostasis

The liver maintains glucose homeostasis through a combination of mechanisms: the conversion of fats and proteins to glucose by gluconeogenesis, glycogenesis (glucose → glycogen, 75 g stored in liver ~ 24-h supply), and the release of glucose from glycogen by glycogenolysis. Insulin stimulates glycogenesis and inhibits gluconeogenesis and the oxidation of fatty acids. Glucagon and epinephrine have the opposite effect by inhibiting glycogenesis and stimulating gluconeogenesis.

Fat Metabolism

Beta oxidation of fatty acids between meals provides a large proportion of body energy requirements and reduces the need for gluconeogenesis.

Protein Synthesis

All plasma proteins are produced in the liver, except gamma globulins, which are synthesized in the reticuloendothelial system, and antihemophiliac factor VIII, which is produced by vascular and glomerular endothelium and sinusoidal cells of the liver. Most drugs administered by anesthesia providers are metabolized by the liver, and many of the metabolites are excreted through the biliary system.

Hepatic Blood Flow

Total hepatic blood flow (HBF) is approximately 100 mL·100 g^{-1}·min^{-1}, 75% of which flows through the portal vein, which is rich in nutrients from the gut but is partially deoxygenated, and can therefore supply 50% to 55% of hepatic O_2 requirements. The hepatic artery supplies 25% of HBF and 45% to 50% of hepatic O_2 requirements.

Splanchnic vessels supplying the portal vein receive sympathetic innervation from T3 through T11. Hypoxemia, hypercarbia, and catecholamines produce hepatic artery and portal vein vasoconstriction and decrease HBF. β-Adrenergic blockade, positive end-expiratory pressure, positive-pressure ventilation (increased intrathoracic pressure increases hepatic vein pressure, which in turn decreases HBF), inhalation anesthetic agents, regional anesthesia with a sensory level above T5, and surgical stimulation (proximity of surgery to the liver determines the degree of HBF reduction) can all cause a reduction in HBF.

Preoperative Hepatic Assessment

Two indices are used to assess preoperative risk in patients with underlying advanced liver disease. The Child-Pugh score, the first scoring system used to stratify the severity of end-stage hepatic dysfunction, comprises five criteria: ascites, hepatic encephalopathy, INR (international normalized ratio), serum albumin, and bilirubin concentration. Patients are then stratified into three risk categories: A, minimal; B, moderate; C, severe.

The Model for End-stage Liver Disease (MELD) score, developed at the Mayo Clinic, uses only three laboratory values in its assessment of end-stage liver disease: INR, serum creatinine, and serum bilirubin concentration:

$$\text{MELD} = 3.78\,[\ln \text{bilirubin}] + 11.2\,[\ln \text{INR}] + 9.57\,[\ln \text{creatinine}] + 6.43$$

Patients with scores less than 10 are acceptable candidates for elective operations; in patients with scores of 10 to 20, operations are associated with increased risk; operations in patients with scores greater than 20 should be avoided unless other options have been exhausted. The MELD score is also used by the United Network for Organ Sharing (UNOS) to allocate cadaveric livers for transplantation.

Liver Function Tests

Preoperative assessment of liver function should not be performed routinely but, rather, should be based on the patient's history and findings on clinical examination that indicate that the patient has an increased risk for having or actually has hepatic disease.

Albumin

Serum albumin concentration is an indirect measure of the synthetic capacity of the liver and may have a predictive value for survival in hepatic disease. Because plasma half-life is 14 to 21 days, serum albumin concentrations change slowly with decreased synthesis. Albumin binds and transports neutral and acidic drugs, hormones, and bilirubin and helps maintain plasma oncotic pressure. Causes of decreased serum albumin concentration include liver disease, decreased synthesis (malnutrition), and increased losses (e.g., nephrotic syndrome, burns, ascites, and protein-losing enteropathies). Although malnutrition and hepatic dysfunction may decrease serum albumin concentration, the most common cause of decreased serum albumin concentration is severe illness. Decreased serum albumin may increase the free fraction of protein-bound drugs and decrease the amount of drug necessary to produce a desired effect. If the dose of a drug administered is not decreased in these circumstances, undesirable effects of the drug may be more frequent or pronounced. Total body albumin can be elevated in patients with cirrhosis who have a low serum albumin level but a large amount of albumin in ascitic fluid.

Prothrombin Time

The prothrombin time (PT) is the most important qualitative measure of the liver's ability to synthesize proteins. Factor VII half-life is 6 h; therefore, an abnormal PT value may indicate acute hepatic injury. The PT measures the entire extrinsic coagulation pathway. A PT that is prolonged by more than 4 sec is associated with a poor 6-month survival in patients with hepatic disease. Other causes of an increased PT include vitamin K deficiencies (e.g., malnutrition, cystic fibrosis), drug effects, decreased plasminogen levels, fibrinolysis, and disseminated intravascular coagulation.

Bilirubin

Unconjugated (indirect) bilirubin is water insoluble, minimally excreted by the kidneys, and a neurotoxin. In the liver, unconjugated bilirubin is rapidly conjugated (direct bilirubin) and secreted in bile. Because it is water soluble, conjugated bilirubin in plasma can be cleared and secreted by the kidneys. Serum levels of conjugated bilirubin do not begin to rise until the liver has lost at least half of its excretory capacity.

Unconjugated bilirubin is produced by the breakdown of heme (hemoglobin, myoglobin, and cytochrome enzymes) and is then bound to albumin for transport to the liver, where it is conjugated via glucuronyltransferase and subsequently excreted into biliary canaliculi. Overt jaundice, which occurs with total bilirubin levels above 3 mg/dL, may be accompanied by pruritus, encephalopathy, and renal insufficiency. Hemolysis causes an increase in unconjugated bilirubin, with a decrease in hemoglobin and an increase in reticulocyte count. Gilbert syndrome is a genetic defect in the conjugation pathway of bilirubin, resulting in an increase in unconjugated bilirubin without a decrease in hemoglobin and a decrease in free haptoglobin values (haptoglobin binds unconjugated bilirubin, limiting its neurotoxicity) or an increase in reticulocyte count. Intrinsic hepatic disease is reflected by an increase in conjugated bilirubin. Frequently, elevated bilirubin postoperatively can be attributed to hemolysis.

Transaminases

Transaminases are sensitive, but not specific, indicators of hepatic dysfunction. Transaminases are released in response to acute hepatic injury. The magnitude of rise in serum concentration does not always correlate with the severity of the disease. They are helpful in testing for regression or progression of hepatic disease. Higher levels are present in acute hepatic cell death (acute viral hepatitis A and B, overdose of acetaminophen, and shock). Mild elevations are seen in fatty liver disease (alcohol, diabetes, obesity), hepatitis C, hemochromatosis, Wilson disease, α_1-antitrypsin deficiency, autoimmune hepatitis, celiac sprue, Crohn disease, and ulcerative colitis. Transaminase levels may be normal or decreased in patients who undergo gastrointestinal bypass surgery and in patients with hemochromatosis, fatty liver of obesity, or end-stage hepatic disease. Skeletal muscle injury can produce marked increases in transaminase levels.

Alkaline Phosphatase

Alkaline phosphatase is present in bone, the gastrointestinal tract, pancreas, and placenta and is released from bile ducts when the ducts are obstructed (obstructive jaundice), which helps differentiate obstructive jaundice from jaundice due to parenchymal hepatic disease. An elevated alkaline phosphatase level can occur in the absence of hepatic disease (e.g., metastatic bone disease, hyperparathyroidism, rickets, osteomalacia, pregnancy, and pancreatic carcinoma). Biliary disease can be diagnosed by measuring serum levels of 5′-nucleotidase (released due to bile duct obstruction or impaired bile flow).

Table 49-1 Liver Function Tests and Differential Diagnosis

Hepatic Dysfunction	Bilirubin	Transaminase Enzymes	Alkaline Phosphatase	Causes
Prehepatic	Increased unconjugated fraction	Normal	Normal	Hemolysis Hematoma resorption Bilirubin overload from transfusion of red blood cells
Intrahepatic (hepatocellular)	Increased conjugated fraction	Markedly increased	Normal to slightly increased	Viral Drugs Sepsis Hypoxemia Cirrhosis
Posthepatic (cholestatic)	Increased conjugated fraction	Normal to slightly increased	Markedly increased	Stones Sepsis

Reprinted with permission from Marschall KE. Diseases of the liver and biliary tract. In: Hines RA, Marschall KE, eds. Stoelting's Anesthesia and Co-Existing Disease, 5th ed. Philadelphia: Churchill Livingstone; 2008:259-278.

Gamma-Glutamyltransferase

Gamma-glutamyltransferase (GGT) is principally found in the kidney, liver, and pancreas and is a very sensitive but not specific marker of liver and bile duct injury. Markedly elevated increases in GGT levels are indicative of a greater degree of liver damage. Disease of the bile ducts and liver, congestive heart failure, chronic alcohol use, and prescription and nonprescription drug use can increase GGT. For this reason, it is nonspecific and must be used with other tests and clinical findings to establish a specific diagnosis.

Summary

A liver biopsy remains the gold standard for the diagnosis, grading, and staging of liver disease. Liver function tests may be useful for the differential diagnosis of liver disease, as depicted in Table 49-1.

Suggested Readings

Hoteit MA, Ghazale AH, Bain AJ, et al. Model for end-stage liver disease score versus Child score in predicting the outcome of surgical procedures in patients with cirrhosis. *World J Gastroenterol*. 2008;14:1774-1780.

Marschall KE. Diseases of the liver and biliary tract. In: Hines RA, Marschall KE, eds. *Stoelting's Anesthesia and Co-Existing Disease*. 5th ed. Philadelphia: Churchill Livingstone; 2008:259-278.

Mushlin PS, Gelman S. Anesthesia and the liver. In: Barash PG, Cullen BF, Stoelting RK, eds. *Clinical Anesthesia*. 4th ed. Philadelphia: Lippincott Williams & Wilkins; 2001:1067-1101.

North PG, Wanamaker RC, Lee VD, et al. Model for end-stage liver disease (MELD) predicts nontransplant surgical mortality in patients with cirrhosis. *Ann Surg*. 2005;242:244-251.

Schemel WH. Unexpected hepatic dysfunction found by multiple laboratory screening. *Anesth Analg*. 1976;55:810-812.

CHAPTER 50

Mechanisms of Hepatic Drug Metabolism and Excretion

Wolf H. Stapelfeldt, MD

Drug clearance is defined as the theoretical volume of blood from which a drug is completely removed in a given time interval. Total drug clearance (CL_{total}) is the sum of clearances based on a variety of applicable elimination pathways (hepatic, renal, pulmonary, intestinal, plasma, other). A drug is considered to be hepatically eliminated if hepatic clearance ($CL_{hepatic}$) assumes a large proportion of the total body clearance ($CL_{hepatic} \approx CL_{total}$). This method is the case for most drugs metabolized in humans. Examples of a minority of drugs for which the metabolism is independent of hepatic function include esmolol (metabolized by esterases located in erythrocytes), remifentanil (metabolized by nonspecific esterases in muscle and intestines), and cisatracurium (metabolized by Hoffman elimination in plasma). However, most drugs depend, either directly or indirectly, on adequate hepatic function for metabolism and elimination.

Hepatic Clearance

$CL_{hepatic}$ is the volume of blood from which a drug is removed as it passes through the liver within a given time interval. Therefore, $CL_{hepatic}$ is limited by the volume of blood flowing through the liver within the same time interval ($\dot{Q}_{hepatic}$). Disease-induced or anesthetic-induced reductions in total hepatic blood flow are the principal causes for diminished hepatic clearance for a large number of drugs; the elimination of these drugs is termed *flow-limited.* Other factors affecting hepatic clearance include maximal hepatic metabolic activity, expressed as intrinsic clearance:

$$CL_{intrinsic} = V_m/k_m$$

where V_m = maximal metabolic rate (mg/min) and k_m (Michaelis constant) = drug concentration producing the half-maximal metabolic rate (mg/L). In this case drug elimination is termed *capacity-limited.* In this situation, unlike the flow-limited condition, drug elimination may change as a function of free-drug concentration that is available for hepatic metabolization and may, thus, be affected by the amount of protein binding and disease-induced changes in protein binding. Whether the hepatic elimination of a drug is flow-limited or capacity-limited depends on the ratio of the free plasma concentration of the drug to k_m (flow-limited if < 0.5) and that of the $CL_{intrinsic}$ to total hepatic blood flow ($\dot{Q}_{hepatic}$) of the drug, which determines the extraction ratio (ER) of the drug ($ER = CL_{hepatic}/\dot{Q}_{hepatic}$) according to the following formula (Figure 50-1):

$$ER = CL_{intrinsic}/(\dot{Q}_{hepatic} + CL_{intrinsic})$$

Depending on these ratios, different types of hepatic ERs have been described (Table 50-1).

High Extraction Ratio Elimination

$$CL_{intrinsic} >> \dot{Q}_{hepatic}\text{; therefore, } ER \approx 1\text{, and } CL_{hepatic} \approx \dot{Q}_{hepatic}$$

In drugs with a high ER elimination, $CL_{hepatic}$ is proportional to and principally limited by $\dot{Q}_{hepatic}$ (flow-limited). Drug elimination is diminished by conditions of decreased $\dot{Q}_{hepatic}$ (arterial hypotension; increased splanchnic vascular resistance, including hepatic cirrhosis; hepatic venous congestion). If drug administration rate is not adjusted for changes in hepatic clearance, resulting drug concentrations increase in a reciprocal fashion. Examples of highly extracted drugs include propofol, ketamine, fentanyl, sufentanil, morphine, meperidine, lidocaine, bupivacaine, metoprolol, propranolol, labetalol, verapamil, and naloxone.

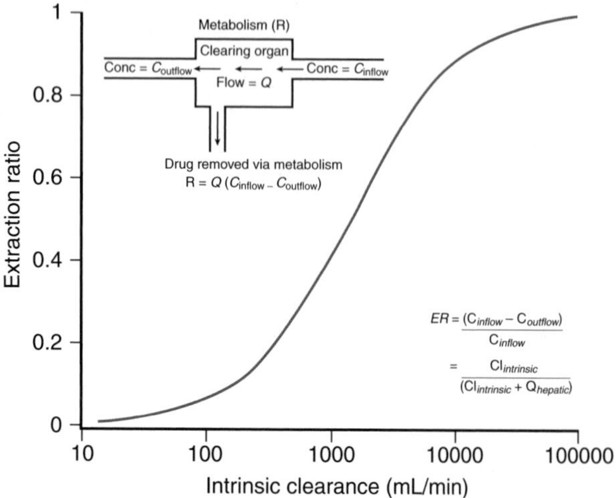

Figure 50-1 Relationship between intrinsic clearance ($CL_{intrinsic}$) and extraction ratio (ER), calculated for a liver blood flow of 1400 mL/min.

Table 50-1 Flow-Limited Versus Capacity-Limited Elimination of Drugs by the Liver

Type of Hepatic Elimination	Extraction Ratio (ER)	Rate of Hepatic Drug Metabolism
Flow-limited	*High*: At clinically relevant concentrations, most of the drug in the afferent hepatic blood is eliminated on first pass through the liver.	*Rapid*: Because drugs with a high ER are metabolized so rapidly, their hepatic clearances roughly equal their rates of transport to the liver (i.e., hepatic flow).
Capacity-limited	*Low*: Hepatic elimination of these drugs is determined by their plasma concentration.	*Slow*: When the capacity of the liver to eliminate a drug is less than the dosing rate, a steady state is unachievable; plasma levels of drug will continue to rise unless the dosing rate is decreased. Drug clearance has no real meaning in such settings.

Low Extraction Ratio Elimination

$$CL_{intrinsic} << \dot{Q}_{hepatic}\text{; therefore, } ER << 1$$

In this scenario, drug elimination is limited by the metabolic rate (capacity-limited) and is, thus, dependent upon hepatic enzyme activity and free-drug concentration (which may be affected by disease-induced changes in plasma transport protein concentrations for those drugs that are highly protein bound), whereas changes in $\dot{Q}_{hepatic}$ are of minimal significance. Hepatic enzyme activity may be affected (decreased or increased) by a variety of factors, including extremes of age, genetic factors (gene polymorphisms), environmental exposure (enzyme induction), and medication history (enzyme induction by phenobarbital, polycyclic hydrocarbons, rifampin, phenytoin, or chronic alcohol consumption; enzyme inhibition, by other substrates of the enzyme, or by drugs, such as cimetidine). Examples of poorly extracted drugs include thiopental, phenobarbital, hexobarbital, diazepam, lorazepam, phenytoin, valproic acid, ethanol, digitoxin, theophylline, acetaminophen, and warfarin.

Intermediate Extraction Ratio Elimination

Some drugs express an intermediate ER and variably depend on all three types of elimination ($\dot{Q}_{hepatic}$, hepatic enzyme activity, and free-drug concentration). Examples of these drugs are methohexital, midazolam, alfentanil, and vecuronium.

Hepatic Metabolic Reactions

Hepatic drug metabolism functions to remove drugs from the circulating plasma by enzymatically converting generally more or less lipophilic parent compounds to typically less pharmacologically active (mostly inactive), less toxic, and more water-soluble metabolites that are subject to biliary or renal excretion. Different types of reactions have been distinguished.

Phase 1 Reactions

Phase 1 reactions are oxidative, reductive, or hydrolytic reactions performed by more than 50 microsomal cytochrome P-450 enzymes (belonging to 17 distinct families, Figure 50-2) that are responsible for more than 90% of all hepatic drug biotransformation reactions. These processes act by inserting or unmasking polar OH, NH_2, or SH chemical groups through hydroxylation, *N*-dealkylation or *O*-dealkylation, deamination, desulfuration, *N*- or *S*-oxidation, epoxidation, or dehalogenation. The resulting more hydrophilic metabolites are passively returned to

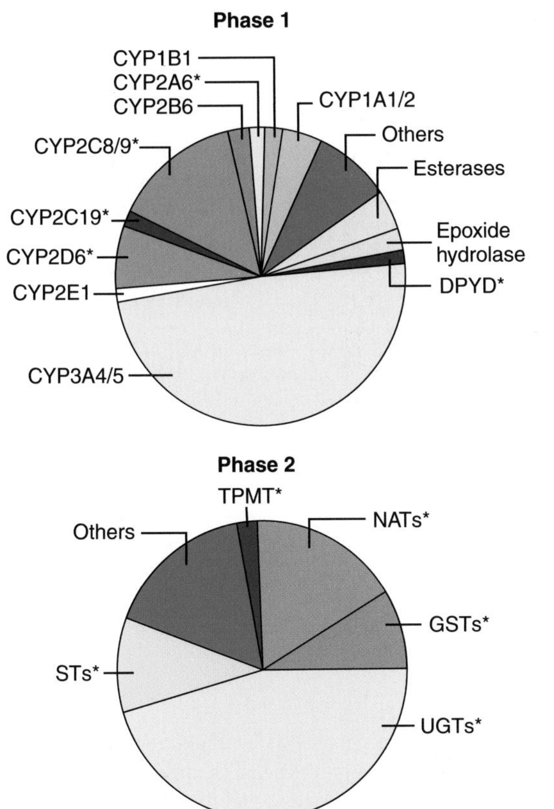

Figure 50-2 Proportion of drugs metabolized by major phase 1 or phase 2 enzymes. The relative size of each pie section indicates the estimated percentage of phase 1 (*top panel*) or phase 2 (*bottom panel*) metabolism that each enzyme contributes to the metabolism of drugs based on literature reports. *Indicates enzymes that have functional alleleic variants; in many cases, more than one enzyme is involved in a metabolism of a particular drug. CYP, Cytochrome P-450; DPYD, dihydropyridine dehydrogenase; GSTs, glutathione *S*-transferases; NATs, *N*-acetyltransferases; STs, sulfotransferases; TPMT, thiopurine methyltransferase; UGTs, uridine diphosphate glucuronosyltransferases. (Adapted from Wilkinson G. Pharmacokinetics: The dynamics of drug absorption, distribution, and elimination. In: Hardman JG, Limbird LE, Goodman GA, eds. Goodman and Gilman's The Pharmacological Basis of Therapeutics. 10th ed. New York: McGraw-Hill; 2001.)

blood, flow through the liver, and may serve as substrate for subsequent nonmicrosomal (phase 2) conjugation reactions. Phase 1 reactions are quite variable, exhibiting greater than fourfold differences in maximal metabolic rate, even among healthy people (due to genotype and drug or environmental exposure causing enzyme induction), and are further affected by nutrition status and hepatic disease, including a risk of oxidative stress related to the preferential centrilobular location of phase 1 reactions in zone 3, the area most vulnerable to the development of tissue hypoxia.

Phase 2 Reactions

Phase 2 reactions are conjugation reactions of drugs or metabolites with glucuronic acid, sulfate, or glycine in enzymatic processes that are catalyzed by uridine diphosphate (UDP) glucuronosyltransferases or several nonmicrosomal enzymes (glutathione *S*-transferase, *N*-acetyltransferase [NAT], or amino acid *N*-transferases). The resulting conjugates are typically less effective, less toxic, more hydrophilic, and more readily excreted via bile or urine. Some conjugates are the substrate for active extrusion via phase 3 reactions. Compared with phase 1 reactions, phase 2 reactions tend to be less variable (with the exception of NAT_2, which is responsible for isoniazid metabolism) and less affected by advanced stages of hepatocellular disease.

Phase 3 Reactions

Phase 3 reactions are energy-dependent transmembrane transport reactions utilizing various ATP (adenosine triphosphate)-binding transport proteins to actively extrude drug conjugates into bile. These reactions tend to be well preserved into advanced stages of hepatic disease as long as tissue oxygenation and hepatocellular energy production are maintained.

Extrahepatic Metabolic Reactions

Hepatic disease not only may affect drug metabolism within the confines of the liver parenchyma itself, but also may alter the pharmacokinetics of drugs that have a distribution or elimination that may depend on or be affected by hepatically synthesized proteins within the patient's plasma.

Butyrylcholinesterase (formerly called pseudocholinesterase) is responsible for the metabolism of drugs such as succinylcholine, mivacurium, and procaine local anesthetics. Enzyme activity is usually sufficient to terminate the action of these drugs in a clinically acceptable time frame until very advanced stages of chronic liver disease.

The concentration of pharmacologically active free (unbound) drug that is ultimately available for systemic distribution is related not only to the effect sites of the drug, but also to its sites of elimination (including in the liver) and may be affected by liver disease–induced changes in the plasma concentrations of transport proteins such as albumin or α_1-acid glycoprotein. To the extent that these proteins are decreased or increased, respectively, in advanced liver disease, as they often are, the apparent potency and elimination of highly protein-bound drugs with low hepatic extraction (such as thiopental bound to albumin) may be indirectly affected by concomitant changes in plasma protein binding.

Suggested Readings

Ibrahim AE, Feldman J, Karim A, Kharasch ED. Simultaneous assessment of drug interactions with low- and high-extraction opioids: Application to parecoxib effects on the pharmacokinetics and pharmacodynamics of fentanyl and alfentanil. *Anesthesiology*. 2003;98:853-861.

Sandner-Kiesling A, List WF. Anesthesia related physiologic and pharmacologic changes in the elderly. *Anaesthesiol Reanim*. 2003;28:60-68.

Sweeney BP, Bromilow J. Liver enzyme induction and inhibition: Implications for anaesthesia. *Anaesthesia*. 2006;61:159-177.

SECTION V Anatomy

CHAPTER 51

Anatomy of the Larynx

Douglas A. Dubbink, MD

Description

The larynx connects the inferior pharynx with the trachea and, in so doing, serves three functions (Box 51-1): to maintain a patent airway, to guard against aspiration of liquids or solids into the trachea, and to permit vocalization. It is about 5 cm in length and, in adults, lies at the level of C4 to C5. In cross-section at the level of the laryngeal prominence (Adam's apple), the larynx is triangular because of the shape of the thyroid cartilage. At the level of the cricoid cartilage, the larynx becomes more round. The larynx provides the area of greatest resistance to passage of air to the lungs.

Laryngeal Skeleton

The laryngeal skeleton has a total of nine cartilages (Table 51-1): three sets of paired cartilages (arytenoids, corniculates, cuneiforms) and three unpaired cartilages (thyroid, cricoid, and epiglottic) (Figure 51-1).

Joints, Ligaments, and Membranes of the Larynx

The joints of the larynx include the cricothyroid joint, which provides articulation between the lateral surfaces of the cricoid cartilage and the inferior horns of the thyroid cartilage, and the cricoarytenoid joint, which provides articulation between the bases of the arytenoid cartilage and the upper surface of the cricoid lamina. The thyrohyoid membrane is an extrinsic ligament that connects the thyroid cartilage to the hyoid bone. The larynx includes three sets of ligaments: the cricothyroid and cricotracheal, which connect the cricoid to the thyroid cartilage and first tracheal ring, respectively; the vocal ligament, which extends from the thyroid cartilage to the arytenoid cartilage; and the vestibular ligament, which extends from the thyroid cartilage to the arytenoid cartilage above the vocal fold.

Interior of the Larynx

The three divisions of the interior of the larynx include the vestibule, above the vestibular folds (false cords); the ventricle, between the vestibular folds above and the vocal folds (cords) below; and the infraglottic cavity, from the vocal folds to the tracheal cavity.

Box 51-1 Functions of the Larynx

Maintain a patent airway
Guard against aspiration of liquids or solids into the trachea
Permit vocalization

Table 51-1 Cartilages of the Larynx

Cartilage	Description and Location
Paired	
Arytenoid	Shaped like a three-sided pyramid that articulates with the upper border of the cricoid lamina
Corniculate	At apices of arytenoid cartilage in the posterior part of the aryepiglottic folds
Cuneiform	In the aryepiglottic folds, not always present
Unpaired	
Thyroid	Largest cartilage, comprising two laminae that are fused anteriorly to form the laryngeal prominence
Cricoid	Ring-shaped, with a posterior part (lamina) and anterior part (arch), located at the level of C6 in adults; the arytenoids articulate with the lateral parts of the superior border of the lamina
Epiglottic	Thin and leaflike, located behind the root of the tongue and in front of the inlet of the larynx; the mucous membrane covering the epiglottis is continued onto the base of the tongue, forming two depressions called the epiglottic valleculae

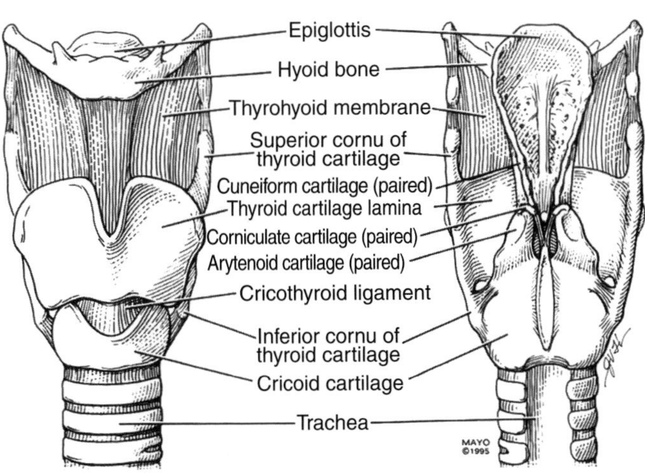

Figure 51-1 Anterior and posterior views of the larynx. (© Mayo Foundation for Medical Education and Research. All rights reserved.)

The vocal folds (vocal cords) consist of the vocal ligament, conus elasticus, vocalis muscle fibers, and a covering of mucous membrane. The rima glottidis is the opening between the vocal folds. The glottis comprises the vocal folds, the rima glottidis, and the narrow part of the larynx at the level of the vocal folds.

The vestibular folds are ligaments covered by folds of mucous membrane. They meet during swallowing to prevent aspiration. The rima vestibuli is the space between the false cords.

Innervation

Innervation to the larynx is supplied by the superior laryngeal nerve (Figure 51-2), a branch of the vagus nerve (X). This nerve has two terminal branches: the internal laryngeal nerve, which is purely sensory and has fibers from the mucosa of the tongue to the vocal folds (including the superior surface of these folds) and the external laryngeal nerve, which is purely motor and innervates the cricothyroid muscle. Another branch of cranial nerve X, the recurrent laryngeal nerve, provides branches to all of the muscles of the larynx, except the cricothyroid, and provides sensory innervation below the vocal cords. Its terminal branch, the inferior laryngeal nerve, has anterior and posterior branches.

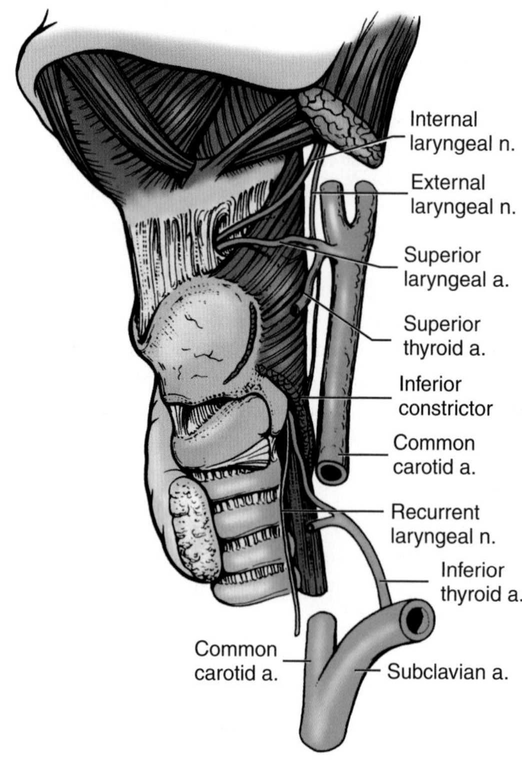

Figure 51-2 Vessels and nerves of the larynx. (From Silver CE. Surgery for Cancer of the Larynx and Related Structures. 2nd ed. Philadelphia: WB Saunders; 1996.)

Box 51-2 The Extrinsic Muscles of the Larynx
Depressors
Omohyoid Sternohyoid Sternothyroid
Elevators
Stylohyoid Digastrics Mylohyoid Geniohyoid Stylopharyngeus

Muscles

The extrinsic muscles comprise depressors and elevators (Box 51-2), which move the larynx as a whole. The intrinsic muscles, which are considered as functional groups, include the abductors and adductors. The abductors (the arytenoid muscle, aryepiglottic muscle, transverse arytenoid muscle, oblique arytenoid muscle, and thyroepiglottic muscle) open the inlet to the larynx and the adductor (lateral cricoarytenoid muscle) closes the vocal folds.

Blood Supply

The superior laryngeal artery is a branch of the superior thyroid artery off the external carotid artery. The inferior laryngeal artery is a branch of the inferior thyroid artery off the thyrocervical trunk off the subclavian artery.

Considerations with the Infant Larynx

The infant's larynx is more anterior than the adult's. The cricoid cartilage is at the level of C3 to C4 in the infant, compared with C4 to C5 in the adult. The infant's epiglottis is relatively longer, stiffer, and further away from the anterior pharyngeal wall, as compared with the adult epiglottis. The narrowest point is at the level of the cricoid cartilage. The tongue of an infant is relatively larger than the tongue of an adult.

Suggested Readings

Moore KL. *Clinically Oriented Anatomy*. 6th ed. Philadelphia: Lippincott, Williams & Wilkins; 2010.

Redden RJ. Anatomic considerations in anesthesia. In: Hagberg CA, ed. *Handbook of Difficult Airway Management*. Philadelphia: Churchill Livingstone; 2000: 1-13.

CHAPTER 52

Coronary Circulation and the Myocardial Conduction System

Harish Ramakrishna, MD, FASE

Coronary Circulation

The right and left main coronary arteries arise from ostia (small openings) located behind the right and left aortic valve cusps toward the more cephalad portion of the sinus of Valsalva (Figure 52-1). The third aortic cusp is named the posterior or noncoronary cusp. The left main coronary artery travels anteriorly and leftward from the left coronary sinus and, after a 2-mm to 10-mm course between the pulmonary trunk and the left atrium, divides into the left anterior descending (LAD) and left circumflex arteries. Occasionally, a diagonal branch is also present.

The LAD or left interventricular coronary artery is a direct continuation of the left main coronary artery, traveling anterior and caudad, descending in the anterior interventricular groove. This artery terminates in the inferior aspect of the cardiac apex. Branches of this artery include (1) the first diagonal, (2) the first septal perforator, (3) right ventricular branches (inconstant), (4) three to five additional septal perforators, and (5) two to six additional diagonal branches. The LAD provides blood to most of the ventricular septum (anterior two thirds); the anterior, lateral, and apical walls of the left ventricle; most of the right and left bundle branches; and the anterolateral papillary muscle (double blood supply—see later in the chapter) of the left ventricle. It can provide collateral vessels to the anterior right ventricle via the circle of Vieussens, to the ventricular septum via septal perforators, and to the posterior descending artery via the distal LAD artery or a diagonal branch.

The left circumflex artery (LCA) travels posteriorly around the heart in the left atrioventricular (AV) sulcus. In 85% to 90% of individuals, it terminates near the obtuse margin of the left ventricle; in the remaining 10% to 15%, it continues around to the crux of the heart to become the posterior descending artery. Branches include (1) a branch to the sinoatrial (SA) node in 40% to 50% of individuals, (2) a left atrial circumflex branch, (3) an anterolateral marginal branch, (4) a distal circumflex artery, (5) posterolateral marginal branches, and (6) the posterior descending artery, as noted. This artery provides blood to the left atrium, the posterior and lateral left ventricle, the anterolateral papillary muscle of the left ventricle, and the SA node, as noted earlier. If it continues as the posterior descending artery (in 10% to 15% of hearts), it also supplies blood to the AV node, the proximal bundle branches, the remainder of the inferoposterior left ventricle, the posterior interventricular septum, and the posteromedial papillary muscle of the left ventricle.

The right coronary artery (RCA) passes forward to emerge between the pulmonary trunk and the right atrium and then descends in the right AV sulcus. In most hearts, once it reaches the apex, the RCA continues traveling in the posterior AV sulcus around the posterior of the heart to terminate as a left ventricular branch or to anastomose with the LCA. Branches include (1) the conus artery, (2) the artery to the SA node (in 50% to 60% of hearts), (3) anterior right ventricular branches, (4) right atrial branches, (5) an acute marginal branch, (6) an artery to the AV node and proximal bundle branches, (7) the posterior descending artery (in 85% to 90% of hearts), and (8) terminal branches to the left atrium and left ventricle. The RCA supplies blood to the SA node (as noted earlier), the right ventricle, the crista supraventricularis, and the right atrium. If it provides the posterior descending artery, it also supplies blood to those areas discussed previously. The RCA provides collaterals to the LAD artery via the conus artery and septal perforators.

The coronary venous system consists of three primary systems: (1) the coronary sinus, (2) the anterior right ventricular veins, and (3) the thebesian veins (Figure 52-2). The coronary sinus is located in the posterior AV groove and receives blood from the great, middle, and small cardiac veins; the posterior veins of the left ventricle; and the left oblique atrial vein (oblique vein of Marshall). The coronary sinus drains blood primarily from the left ventricle and opens into the right atrium. The two to three anterior right ventricular veins originate in and drain blood from the right ventricular wall. These veins enter the right atrium directly or enter into a small collecting vein at the base of the right atrium. The thebesian veins are tiny venous outlets that drain directly into the cardiac chambers, primarily the right atrium and right ventricle.

Myocardial Conduction System

The conducting system of the heart is composed of specially differentiated cardiac muscle fibers that are responsible for initiating and maintaining normal cardiac rhythm as well as ensuring proper coordination between atrial and ventricular contraction. This system comprises the SA node, the AV node, the bundle of His, right and left branch bundles, and Purkinje fibers.

The SA node is a horseshoe-shaped structure located in the upper part of the sulcus terminalis of the right atrium (Figure 52-3). It extends through the atrial wall from epicardium to endocardium. SA nodal fibers have a higher intrinsic rate of depolarization than do any other cardiac muscle fibers and act as the pacemaker of the heart (see Chapter 33). Three internodal pathways facilitate conduction of impulses between the SA and AV nodes: the anterior (Bachmann bundle), middle, and posterior internodal tracts. The AV node lies in the medial floor of the right atrium at the base of the atrial septum above the orifice of the coronary sinus. The bundle of His begins at the anterior aspect of the AV node and penetrates through the central fibrous body. Here, the bundle of His divides into the left and right branch bundles. The division straddles the upper border of the muscular ventricular septum, and the bundles run superficially down

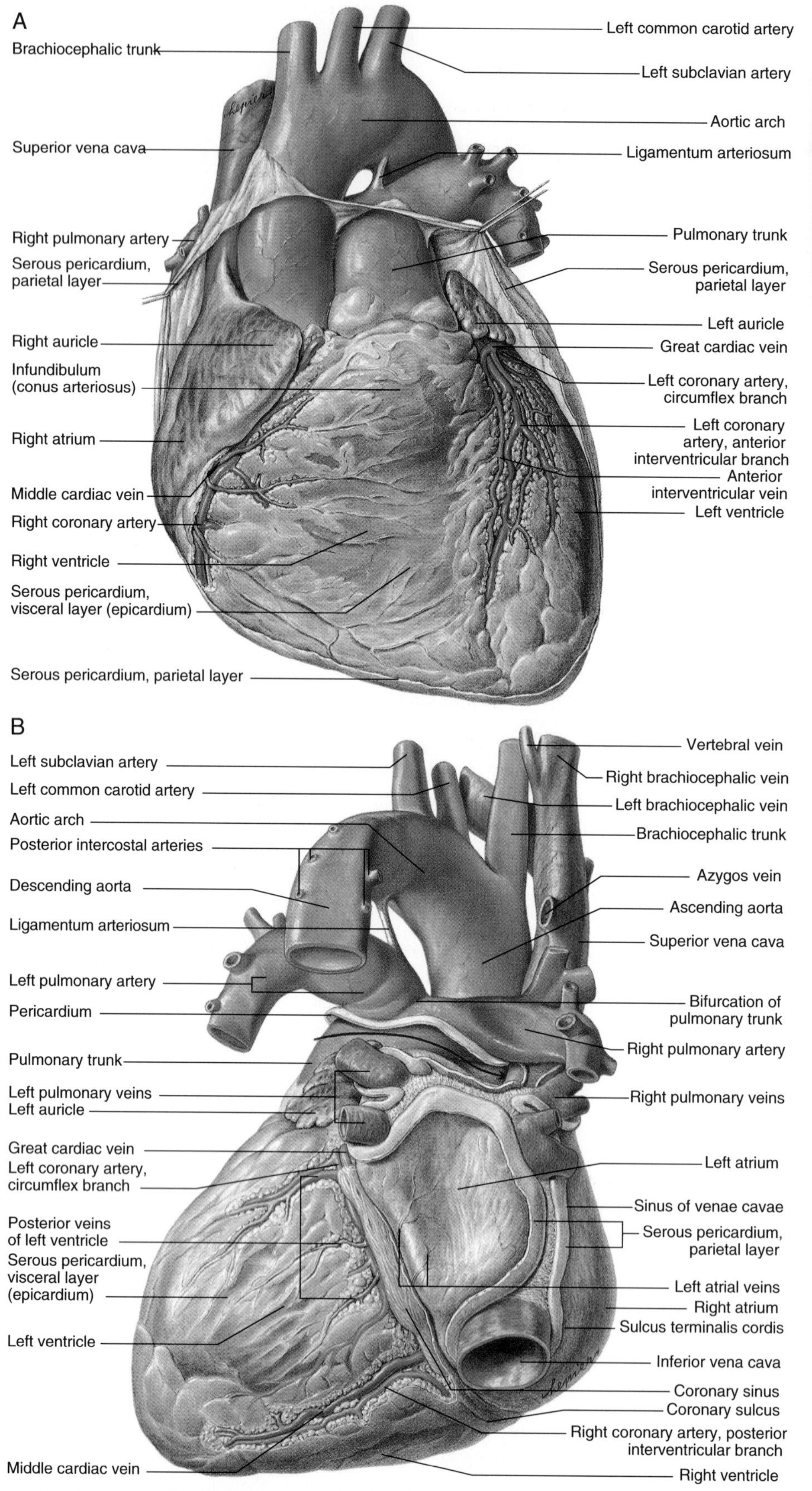

Figure 52-1 Coronary arterial distribution. **A,** Anterior view. The right and circumflex coronary arteries travel in the atrioventricular sulcus, adjacent to the tricuspid and mitral valves, respectively. The left anterior descending and posterior descending coronary arteries travel in the interventricular sulcus and demarcate the plane of the ventricular septum. **B,** Posteroinferior view showing right dominance. (From Standring S. The heart and great vessels. In: Gray's Anatomy. New York, Churchill Livingstone, 2008, Chap. 56.)

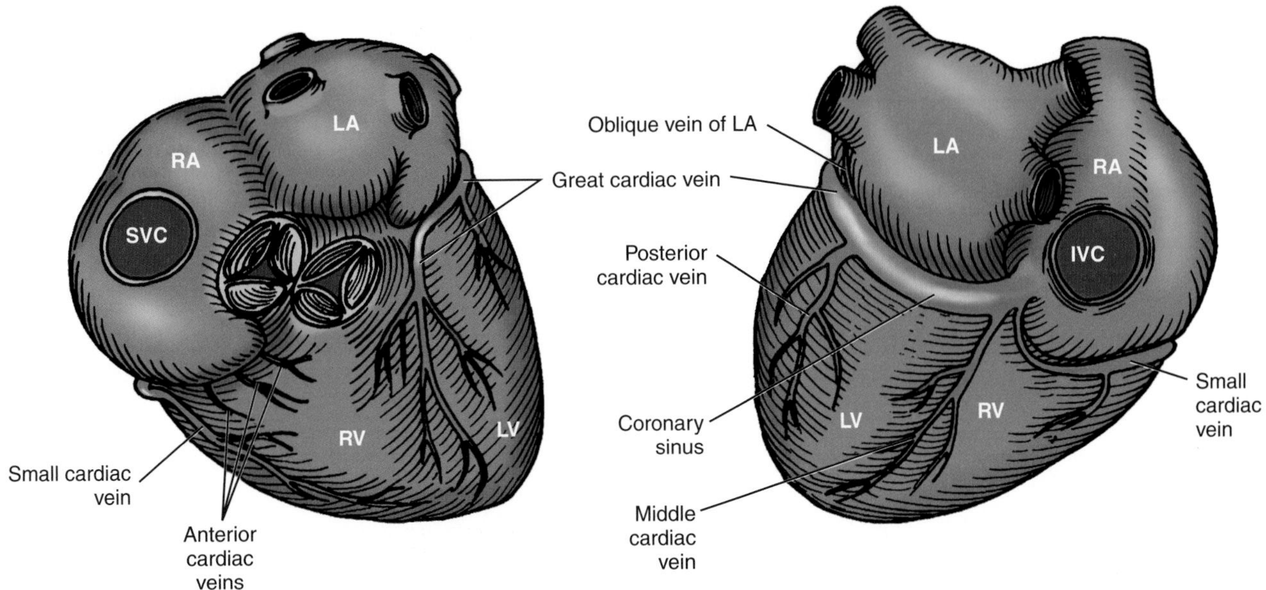

Figure 52-2 Coronary veins. The anterior cardiac veins empty into the right atrium, whereas the other major epicardial coronary veins drain into the coronary sinus. IVC, Inferior vena cava; LA, left atrium; LV, left ventricle; RA, right atrium; RV, right ventricle; SVC, superior vena cava. (Adapted from Williams PL, ed. The anatomical basis of medicine and surgery. In: Gray's Anatomy. 38th ed. New York, Churchill Livingstone, 1995.

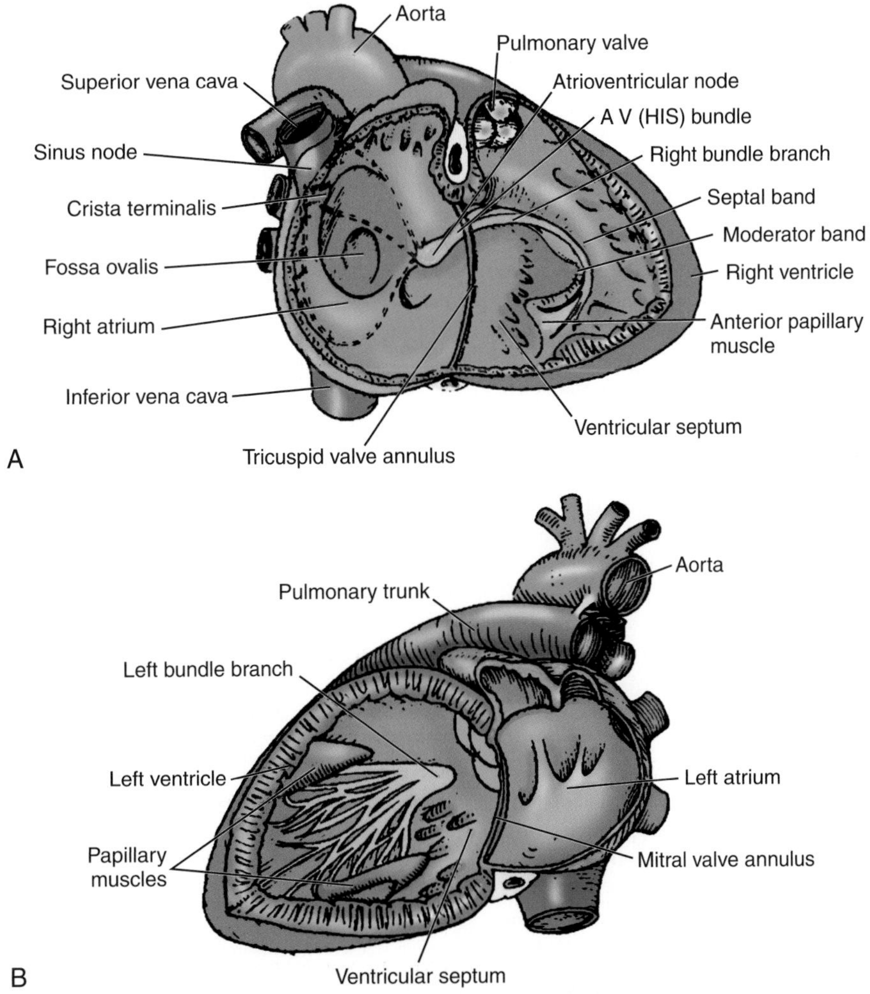

Figure 52-3 Cardiac conduction system. **A,** Right side of heart. The sinoatrial and atrioventricular (AV) nodes are both right atrial structures. **B,** Left side of heart. The left bundle branch forms a broad sheet that does not divide into distinct anterior and posterior fascicles. (Adapted from Williams PL, ed. The anatomical basis of medicine and surgery. In: Gray's Anatomy. 38th ed. New York, Churchill Livingstone, 1995.

either side of the septum. About midway to the apex, the left bundle divides into the anterior superior and posterior inferior fascicles. These fascicles continue to the base of the papillary muscles of the left ventricle, where they form plexuses of Purkinje fibers that distribute to all portions of the left ventricular myocardium. The right branch bundle continues to the anterior papillary muscle of the right ventricle, where it forms a plexus of Purkinje fibers that distribute to all portions of the right ventricular myocardium.

Suggested Readings

Murphy JG. Applied anatomy of the heart and great vessels. In: Murphy JG, Lloyd MA, eds. *Mayo Clinic Cardiology*. 3rd ed. Rochester, MN: Mayo Clinic Scientific Press; 2007, pp 27-54.

Standring S. The heart and great vessels. In: *Gray's Anatomy: The Anatomical Basis of Clinical Practice*. New York: Churchill Livingstone; 2008, Chap. 56.

Waller BF, Schlant RC. Anatomy of the heart. In: Alexander RW, Schlant RC, Fuster V, eds. *Hurst's The Heart*. 9th ed. New York: McGraw-Hill; 1998:19.

CHAPTER 53

Transesophageal Echocardiography: Anatomic Considerations

Kent H. Rehfeldt, MD, FASE, and Martin D. Abel, MD

Echocardiography typically uses ultrasound frequencies between 2 million and 10 million hertz (or 2-10 MHz), which is well above the audible range of humans (20-20,000 Hz). Sound waves are absorbed, reflected, and scattered to varying degrees by passage through human tissue. Reflected echoes are produced at boundaries between two inhomogeneous media (e.g., blood–soft tissue interface). More homogeneous tissues result in greater ultrasound scattering and less reflection.

Most transesophageal echocardiography (TEE) probes in use today have multiplane imaging capability. That is, the imaging plane of the transducer at the distal tip of the probe can be electronically rotated between 0 degrees (horizontal or transverse plane) and 180 degrees. The image obtained at 180 degrees represents a right-left mirror image of the view obtained at 0 degrees. Older probes and some pediatric probes are equipped with two transducers at their distal ends, one that generates transverse (or 0 degrees) imaging planes, with a second transducer producing longitudinal (or 90 degrees) imaging planes. The operator selects the desired imaging plane of these biplane probes by means of a button on the ultrasound machine itself.

Transesophageal Echocardiography Safety

Numerous complications have been attributed to TEE use, including vocal cord paresis, dysphagia or odynophagia, inadvertent manipulation of the tracheal tube, bronchospasm, arrhythmias, and vascular compression during flexion of the probe tip, particularly in infants. Minor trauma to the hypopharynx is not an uncommon finding following probe insertion. In one study, fiberoptic examination revealed hypopharyngeal hematoma or laceration in 24% of adult patients after typical blind insertion of the TEE probe, although no patients required treatment of these iatrogenic injuries. Probe insertion with direct visualization probably reduces the rate of hypopharyngeal injury. More serious complications, such as esophageal perforation, although fortunately rare, may occur more often than previously believed. In a recent study of more than 15,000 intraoperative TEE examinations, investigators reported 6 gastric or esophageal tears and 8 esophageal perforations, yielding an overall serious complication rate of about 1 in 1000 intraoperative examinations. Another study identified 7 esophageal perforations in more than 22,000 TEE examinations; 3 of those 7 patients died, giving an overall mortality rate of 0.014%.

Anatomic Correlations

Irrespective of the reason for the TEE study, a comprehensive examination is recommended for every patient, preferably before focusing on a specific question or application of TEE. It is beyond the scope of this brief description to detail all the anatomic views obtainable with TEE, and the reader is referred to other reviews of the subject.

Intraoperative Image Orientation

Transducer location and the near field (vertex) of the image sector are at the top of the display and far field at the bottom. At a multiplane angle of 0 degrees (horizontal or transverse plane), with the imaging plane directed anteriorly from the esophagus through the heart, the patient's right side appears in the left of the image display.

Basic Probe Movements

To generate desired images, manipulation of the TEE probe is required in addition to changing the multiplane or biplane angle (Figure 53-1). The basic probe movements include insertion or withdrawal of the probe within the esophagus or stomach. Anteflexion and retroflexion of the probe tip are controlled with the large wheel on the probe and result in cephalad or caudad angulation of the imaging plane, respectively. Left-side and right-side flexion can be achieved by manipulating the smaller wheel on the probe and

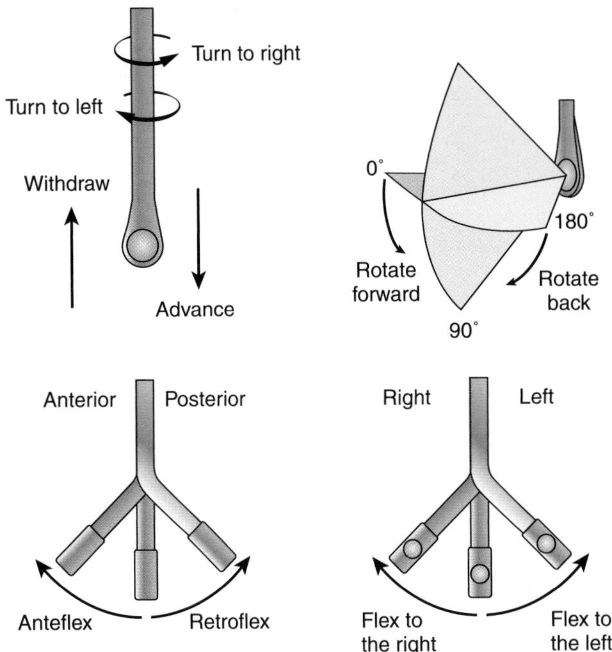

Figure 53-1 Basic probe movements, including anteflexion, retroflexion, side flexion, and withdrawal and advancement of the probe are demonstrated. (From Kahn RA, Shernan SK, Konstadt SN. Intraoperative echocardiography. In: Kaplan JA, ed. Kaplan's Cardiac Anesthesia. 5th ed. Philadelphia: Saunders Elsevier; 2006:451.)

cause deflection of the probe tip within a coronal plane. Rotation of the probe refers to clockwise or counterclockwise spinning of the probe shaft.

Standard Views

The American Society of Echocardiography and Society of Cardiovascular Anesthesiologists consensus task force defined the minimum recommended views that make up the standard intraoperative TEE examination. These standard views have been pictorially displayed, along with the associated icon depicting a typical multiplane angle at which the image may be generated, in Figure 53-2. It is important to remember that additional "off-axis" or nonstandard views may be required to adequately examine specific findings in any given patient. Furthermore, the multiplane angles suggested by the images should be considered a rough guide; the precise multiplane angle at which a given structure is best imaged varies among patients. A complete description of the probe maneuvers necessary to obtain these views is beyond the scope of this chapter. Readers are referred to the task force consensus statement.

When studying the images that make up the comprehensive multiplane intraoperative TEE examination, the use of several tips may prove helpful. First, in the majority of the midesophageal (ME) images, the structure closest to the probe (that is, the chamber at the apex of the image) is the left atrium. The only exception is when the probe is withdrawn above the left atrium and resides directly behind the great vessels. In this superior position, the probe is nearest the right pulmonary artery, which can be seen in long-axis (LAX) view, along with the pulmonary artery bifurcation in the ME

A ME four chamber
E TG two chamber
I ME AV LAX
M ME RV inflow-outflow
Q Desc aortic SAX
B ME two chamber
F TG basal SAX
J TG LAX
N TG RV inflow
R Desc aortic LAX
C ME LAX
G ME mitral commissural
K Deep TG LAX
O ME asc aortic SAX
S UE aortic arch LAX
D TG mid SAX
H ME AV SAX
L ME bicaval
P ME asc aortic LAX
T UE aortic arch SAX

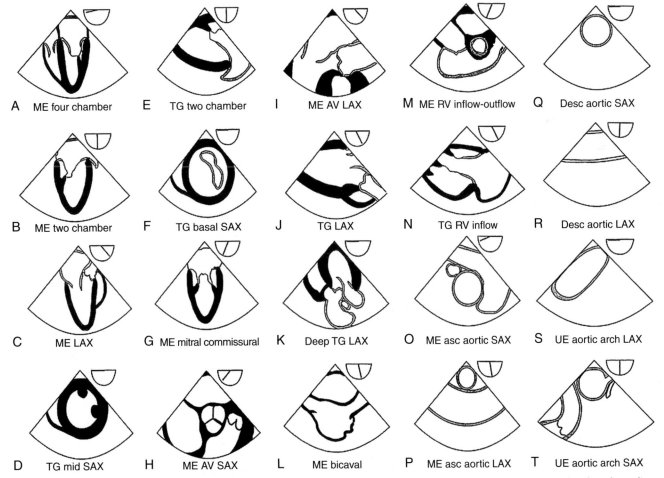

Figure 53-2 These 20 standard views make up the minimum comprehensive intraoperative TEE examination. asc, Ascending; AV, aortic valve; desc, descending; LAX, long axis; ME, midesophageal; RV, right ventricular; SAX, short axis; TG, transgastric; UE, upper esophageal. (Adapted from Kahn RA, Shernan SK, Konstadt SN. Intraoperative echocardiography. In: Kaplan JA, ed. Kaplan's Cardiac Anesthesia. 5th ed. Philadelphia: Saunders Elsevier; 2006:455-460.)

ascending aortic short-axis (SAX) view. Increasing the multiplane angle by approximately 90 degrees yields the ME ascending aortic LAX view, in which the right pulmonary artery is seen in SAX view. These two views demonstrate the orthogonal relationship between the ascending aorta and the right pulmonary artery. (The aortic and pulmonary valves also have a near-orthogonal relationship.) Second, the transgastric (TG) LAX views are most useful for placing a Doppler cursor in near-parallel alignment with the left ventricular outflow tract and aortic root. In this position, an aortic valve or left ventricular outflow tract velocity may be measured and used to calculate a pressure gradient across the aortic valve. Third, TG SAX views of the left ventricle, such as the TG midpapillary SAX views, are often selected when monitoring for ischemia, as myocardium perfused by the three major coronary arteries can be visualized in a single image. Ideally, regional wall motion abnormalities identified in the TG mid-SAX view are confirmed in other views, such as the ME four-chamber, two-chamber, or LAX planes.

Thoracic Aorta

Thorough intraoperative imaging of the thoracic aorta is important to detect conditions, such as severe atherosclerosis, that may modify the surgical approach (aortic cross-clamping) or to inform the decision to place mechanical support devices (intra-aortic balloon pump). A number of standard views image various aspects of the thoracic aorta. Both the ascending and descending aorta are generally imaged in both LAX and SAX views. The distal aortic arch and subclavian artery orifice are usually visualized as the probe is withdrawn slowly while keeping the aorta centered in the image. Occasionally, the left common carotid artery orifice may be seen. In contrast, however, the origin of the innominate artery and distal ascending aorta are rarely imaged owing to the interposition of the air-filled trachea between the esophagus and aorta, creating a "blind spot" for TEE.

Suggested Readings

Aviv JE, Di Tullio MR, Homma S, et al. Hypopharyngeal perforation near-miss during transesophageal echocardiography. *Laryngoscope*. 2004;114:821-826.

Michelena HI, Abel MD, Suri RM, et al. Intraoperative echocardiography in valvular heart disease: An evidence-based appraisal. *Mayo Clin Proc*. 2010; 85:646-655.

Piercy M, McNichol L, Dinh DT, et al. Major complications related to the use of transesophageal echocardiography in cardiac surgery. *J Cardiothor Vasc Anesth*. 2009;23:62-65.

Seward JB, Khandheria BK, Edwards WD, et al. Biplanar transesophageal echocardiography: Anatomic correlations, image orientation, and clinical applications. *Mayo Clin Proc*. 1990;65:1193-1213.

Seward JB, Khandheria BK, Freeman WK, et al. Multiplane transesophageal echocardiography: Image orientation, examination technique, anatomic correlations, and clinical applications. *Mayo Clin Proc*. 1993;68:523-551.

Seward JB, Khandheria BK, Oh JK, et al. Transesophageal echocardiography: Technique, anatomic correlations, implementation, and clinical applications. *Mayo Clin Proc*. 1988;63:649-680.

Shanewise JS, Cheung AT, Aronson S, et al. ASE/SCA guidelines for performing a comprehensive intraoperative multiplane transesophageal echocardiography examination: Recommendations of the American Society of Echocardiography council for intraoperative echocardiography and the Society of Cardiovascular Anesthesiologists task force for certification in perioperative transesophageal echocardiography. *Anesth Analg*. 1999;89:870-884.

CHAPTER 54

Transesophageal Echocardiography: Intraoperative Uses

Alina M. Grigore, MD, MHS, FASE

Transesophageal echocardiography (TEE) is an important tool for the management of cardiac and noncardiac patients throughout the perioperative period. Development of biplane, multiplane, and three-dimensional imaging and the addition of M-mode, color flow, spectral Doppler, and tissue Doppler have allowed the role of TEE to be expanded from a diagnostic tool to a monitoring device and a procedural adjunct.

Perioperative Indications and Contraindications

The American Society of Anesthesiologists (ASA) has developed evidence-based practice guidelines on the perioperative use of TEE (Box 54-1). Category I indications refer to severe life-threatening conditions in which the use of TEE is helpful in improving clinical outcome, whereas category II and III indications are supported by a weaker level of scientific evidence and expert opinion. TEE is a safe procedure, with a 0.01% to 0.03% mortality rate associated with its use and less than a 3% incidence of major complications (e.g., esophageal injury, vocal cord paralysis, arrhythmias, hemodynamic instability, seizure, and cardiac arrest).

Nonetheless, the risks associated with the use of TEE are related to the patient, the procedure, and the clinical settings and determine the appropriateness of performing TEE. Patients' coexisting medical conditions and anatomic issues (e.g., esophageal varices) define the risk for perioperative complications (Table 54-1). Certain surgical procedures could also increase the likelihood of complications. Clinical settings, defined by hospital variables, refer to the equipment and qualifications of medical personnel performing the intraoperative TEE. A careful assessment of these three

Box 54-1 Indications for the Perioperative Use of Transesophageal Echocardiography

Category I

Preoperative

For unstable patients with suspected thoracic aortic aneurysms, dissection, or disruption who need to be evaluated quickly
Assessment of aortic valve function in repair of aortic dissections with possible aortic valve involvement
Evaluation of pericardial window procedures
Assessment of repair of cardiac aneurysms
Evaluation of removal of cardiac tumors

Intraoperative

Evaluation of acute, persistent, and life-threatening hemodynamic disturbances in which ventricular function and its determinants are uncertain and have not responded to treatment
Valve repair
Congenital heart surgery for most lesions requiring cardiopulmonary bypass
Repair of hypertrophic obstructive cardiomyopathy
Endocarditis when preoperative testing was inadequate or extension of infection to perivalvular tissue is suspected

Intensive Care Unit

Unstable patients with unexplained hemodynamic disturbances, suspected valve disease, or thromboembolic problems*

Category II

Perioperative

In patients with increased risk of experiencing myocardial ischemia or infarction
In patients with increased risk of developing hemodynamic disturbances
Assessment of valve replacement

Preoperative

Assessment of patients with suspected acute thoracic aortic dissections, aneurysms, or disruption

Intraoperative

Detection of foreign bodies
Detection of air emboli during cardiotomy, heart transplant operations, and upright neurosurgical procedures
During intracardiac thrombectomy
During pulmonary embolectomy
For suspected cardiac trauma
During repair of thoracic aortic dissections without suspected aortic emboli
Evaluation of pericardectomy, pericardial effusions, or pericardial surgery
Evaluation of anastomotic sites during heart or lung transplantation

Monitoring

Placement and function of assist devices

Category III

Intraoperative

Evaluation of myocardial perfusion, coronary artery anatomy, or graft patency
During repair of cardiomyopathies other than hypertrophic obstructive cardiomyopathy
For uncomplicated endocarditis during noncardiac operations
Monitoring for emboli during orthopedic operations
Assessment of repair of thoracic aortic injuries
For uncomplicated pericarditis
Evaluation of pleuropulmonary disease
Monitoring of cardioplegia administration

Monitoring

Placement of intra-aortic balloon pumps, automatic implantable cardiac defibrillators, or pulmonary artery catheters

*If other tests or monitoring techniques have not confirmed the diagnosis or if patients are too unstable to undergo other tests.

Table 54-1 Intraoperative Transesophageal Echocardiography: Incidence of Complications

Complication	Incidence (%)
Lip injuries	13
Hoarseness	12
Esophageal perforation	0.01
Dental injury	0.03-0.1
Tracheal tube malposition	0.03-0.3
Odynophagia	1.8
Upper gastrointestinal complications	0.03

Box 54-2 Intraoperative Transesophageal Echocardiography: Contraindications

Esophageal pathology: stricture, diverticulum, varices, esophagitis, Mallory-Weiss tear
Gastric pathology: recent upper gastrointestinal hemorrhage, gastric ulcer, symptomatic hiatal hernia
Thoracic aortic aneurysm

variables and their interaction for a specific patient is mandatory to accurately determine the risk-benefit profile. For example, even though esophageal varices are known to increase the risk of bleeding associated with the use of TEE, in the setting of a patient with grade 1 to 2 esophageal varices who is hemodynamically unstable or undergoing a procedure that is associated with an increased risk of hemodynamic instability occurring, the benefit of TEE may outweigh the risk of bleeding. Moreover, the use of pediatric TEE probes and avoidance of manipulation at the gastroesophageal junction by using mainly midesophageal and upper esophageal imaging, minimizes the risk of bleeding in this particular patient population. According to the ASA's recently revised guidelines, absolute contraindications for the performance of TEE include esophageal stricture, tracheoesophageal fistula, recent esophageal surgery, and esophageal trauma (Box 54-2). Consensus has not been reached on the risks of the following conditions: Barrett esophagus, hiatal hernia, large descending thoracic aortic aneurysm, unilateral vocal cord paralysis, esophageal varices, postradiation therapy, previous bariatric surgery, Zenker diverticulum, colonic interposition, and dysphagia. Anticoagulation per se has not been shown to increase the risk of bleeding with the insertion and use of a TEE probe.

A change in the plan for a cardiac surgical procedure based on the findings on intraoperative TEE has been reported to vary from 3.4% to 27%. The ASA Task Force on Perioperative TEE recommends that TEE be used during all cardiac and thoracic surgical procedures.

Clinical Perioperative Applications

Assessment of Left Ventricular and Right Ventricular Function

Fractional area change and end-diastolic area (calculated as the end-diastolic area minus the end-systolic area divided by the end-diastolic area times 100; normal between 50% and 75%) are routinely used for the measurement of left ventricular (LV) and right ventricular (RV) function. Fractional area change is preload dependent and might not accurately estimate the ventricular intrinsic function. Stroke volume—calculated as the time velocity integral multiplied by the cross-sectional area of the valve through which the time velocity integral was measured (e.g., aortic valve)—can be used for the calculation of cardiac output (i.e., stroke volume times heart rate). Enlargement of the right ventricle—with change in shape from crescent to round, hypokinesis, or akinesis of the RV wall—can be used to qualify RV dysfunction.

Many people in the general population have diastolic dysfunction, and its prevalence increases with age. Traditional Doppler assessment in conjunction with tissue Doppler techniques allows for the assessment of diastolic dysfunction that is due to either impaired relaxation or decreased compliance.

Detection of Myocardial Ischemia

New-onset regional wall motion abnormalities, which can be detected with echocardiography, are among the earliest findings of myocardial ischemia and provide high sensitivity for the detection of myocardial ischemia. Unfortunately, regional wall motion abnormalities are assessed intermittently and are subject to interobserver variability but, when detected, allow earlier intervention to treat the ischemia.

Preload Assessment

TEE can provide accurate information related to LV end-diastolic pressure and can be used to guide fluid therapy. The ratio of transmitral early filling velocity to early mitral annular descent velocity—identified by tissue Doppler—can predict a range of LV end-diastolic pressures. Doppler tissue imaging of the mitral valve annulus is less dependent on the loading conditions and is more accurate in estimating LV end-diastolic pressure and pulmonary capillary occlusion pressure.

Cardiac Operations

TEE is useful for the assessment of valvular disease (insufficiency or stenosis) and can often provide diagnostic images for valvular vegetation and tumors and plays a significant role in assessing the adequacy of valve repair or replacement so that the surgeon or cardiologist can intervene during the same procedure to correct the problem. In the presence of hemodynamic instability associated with mitral valve repair, TEE is used to assess systolic anterior movement of the mitral valve, persistent LV outflow tract obstruction, and residual mitral regurgitation. Assessing the efficacy of routine measures (e.g., volume administration, increase in systemic vascular resistance), avoiding ventricular hypercontractility, and deciding whether surgical reintervention is necessary can also be guided by TEE.

Intraoperative TEE has a sensitivity of 83% to 90% for detecting congenital heart disease and can identify pathologic conditions not seen on transthoracic echocardiography in as many as 30% of cases. Intraoperative echocardiographic assessment of the repair of hypertrophic obstructive cardiomyopathy may lead to surgical reintervention for persistent gradients in up to 20% of cases.

Intraoperative TEE may also be used to detect LV aneurysms, locate cardiac tumors, detect constrictive pericarditis, evaluate the effectiveness of pericardectomy, and detect atrial or ventricular shunts.

The incidence of intracardiac thrombi detected by intraoperative TEE varies from 2% to 10%. Renal cell carcinoma often extends into the renal vein and cephalad into the inferior vena cava, extending all the way into the right atrium. Depending on how far cephalad the carcinoma extends into the inferior vena cava, intraoperative TEE can be used for management of the tumor resection. Air emboli, as small as 1 mm in diameter, can be detected by TEE with a high sensitivity.

Intraoperative TEE is also useful for placing and monitoring the function of intra-aortic balloon pumps; assessing the position, flow, and gradients of inflow and outflow cannulas of ventricular assist devices; placing coronary sinus catheters; and monitoring the distribution of cardioplegia. More recently, with the expansion and extension of noninvasive surgical procedures to the cardiac catheterization laboratory, TEE imaging is used to aid catheter-based closure of atrial septal defects, endovascular replacement of the aortic valves, and placement of automatic implantable cardiodefibrillators.

Thoracic Aortic Surgery

The use of intraoperative TEE for the emergent assessment of aortic dissection yields a high sensitivity (88%-100%) and specificity (77%-100%) and is more sensitive than transthoracic echocardiography. In the setting of suspected aortic trauma, TEE sensitivity and specificity are even higher, 100% and 94% to 100%, respectively. Echocardiographic imaging is also helpful for detecting and quantifying pleural fluid, which is potentially suggestive of ruptured aneurysm, and pericardial fluid for the diagnosis of pericardial effusion and pericardial tamponade. Assessment of regional wall motion abnormalities, particularly in the area around the right coronary artery, is also helpful to rule out acute dissection of coronary arteries (dissection more often affects the right coronary artery, as compared with the other coronary arteries). Intraoperative TEE also aids in the identification of the entry and exit sites of dissection and of the true and false lumina, assessment of aortic valve function, and determination of whether replacement of the aortic valve is necessary. With the institution of cardiopulmonary bypass, TEE imaging confirms adequate blood flow in the true lumen and decompression of the false lumen. Assessment of hemodynamic status, new onset of regional wall motion abnormalities at the time of aortic cross-clamping, LV loading conditions at the time of aortic declamping, and the adequacy of the aortic repair can also be achieved with intraoperative TEE.

When TEE is used for elective aortic operations, careful assessment of the aneurysm size and its position relative to the esophagus are mandatory prior to the insertion of the TEE probe. Rupture of a large aortic aneurysm could occur during manipulation of the TEE probe. In this particular case, the TEE probe should be inserted after the chest is open and cannulation for cardiopulmonary bypass is in place.

Endovascular aortic repair has recently gained significant popularity. TEE has value in identifying aortic disease, localizing the landing zone, and confirming the successful deployment of the graft. In addition, TEE and contrast-enhanced ultrasound studies are more sensitive in identifying leaks and thromboexclusion.

Atherosclerotic Disease of the Aorta

Atheromatous disease is present on intraoperative TEE in 9% of elderly patients and is associated with a change in therapy in 8% to 17% of cases. The clinical impact of these findings is still unclear. TEE examination of the aorta is not as accurate as is epiaortic scanning. It is highly recommended that TEE be used in conjunction with epiaortic scanning for the diagnosis and localization of plaques or ulcerations in patients in whom atherosclerotic disease of the aorta is likely.

Transplant Surgery

In cardiac transplantation, TEE is a sensitive tool for screening potential donor patients and for assessing ventricular and valvular function of the transplanted hearts, evaluating the integrity of the anastomosis, and estimating the pulmonary capillary occlusion pressure. In lung transplantation, TEE can be used to assess RV function, volume status, surgical anastomosis, and the patency of the pulmonary veins. Identification of pulmonary artery thrombi, patent foramen ovale, and atrial and septal defects is also achieved with intraoperative TEE examination.

Neurosurgery

TEE is used in neurosurgery, particularly for sitting craniotomies, due to its high sensitivity for detecting venous air embolism, its ability to detect paradoxical air embolism associated with patent foramen ovale, and its ability to help with placement of air aspiration catheters.

Use in the Emergency Department and Intensive Care Unit

TEE is a useful tool for the rapid assessment and diagnosis of hemodynamic instability following blunt or penetrating chest trauma. Myocardial contusion or rupture, atrial rupture, disruption or rupture of major aortic vessels, pericardial effusion or tamponade, mediastinal hematoma, tracheal or bronchial disruption, pleural effusion, and pneumothorax must all be considered and ruled out in the hemodynamically unstable patient. TEE, however, has limitations in patients with head trauma: cervical spine injuries and maxillofacial injuries can make probe placement difficult.

In the intensive care unit, TEE can be used for assessment of global myocardial function and regional wall motion abnormalities, determination of preload and afterload conditions, identification of valvular vegetation, assessment of valvular function and of the presence of systolic anterior movement, the differential diagnosis of shock (septic vs. cardiogenic), and the diagnosis of acute lung injury (to rule out cardiac dysfunction as the cause of the pulmonary edema). TEE is also useful to document correct placement of intra-aortic balloon pumps and percutaneous ventricular assist devices.

Suggested Readings

Desjardins G, Cahalan M. The impact of routine trans-esophageal echocardiography in cardiac surgery. *Best Pract Res Clin Anesthesiol.* 2009;23:263-271.

Kallmeyer IJ, Collard CD, Fox JA, et al. The safety of intraoperative transesophageal echocardiography: A case series of 7200 cardiac surgical patients. *Anesth Analg.* 2001;92:1126-1130.

Otto CM. *Textbook of Clinical Echocardiography.* 4th ed. Philadelphia: Elsevier Saunders; 2009.

Otto CM, Schwaegler RG. *Echocardiography Review Guide.* Philadelphia: Saunders Elsevier; 2008.

Perrino AC, Reeves ST. *Transesophageal Echocardiography.* 2nd ed. Philadelphia: Lippincott, Williams & Wilkins; 2003.

Practice guidelines for perioperative transesophageal echocardiography. An updated report by the American Society of Anesthesiologists and the Society of Cardiovascular Anesthesiologists Task Force on Transesophageal Echocardiography. *Anesthesiology.* 2010;112:1-11.

Spier BJ, Larue SJ, Teelin TC, et al. Review of complications in a series of patients with known gastro-esophageal varices undergoing transesophageal echocardiography. *J Am Soc Echocardiogr.* 2009;22:396-400.

Suriani RJ, Cutrone A. Intraoperative transesophageal echocardiography during liver transplantation. *J Cardiothorac Vasc Anesth.* 1996;10:699-707.

Swaminathan M, Lineberger CK, McCann RL, Mathew JP. The importance of intraoperative transesophageal echocardiography in endovascular repair of thoracic aortic aneurysms. *Anesth Analg.* 2003:97:1566-1572.

CHAPTER 55

Cerebral Circulation

Douglas A. Dubbink, MD

The brain receives its blood supply from the internal carotid arteries (80% of total cerebral flow) and the vertebrobasilar system (20% of total cerebral flow), which connect at the circle of Willis, a ring of vessels beneath the hypothalamus (Figure 55-1). The circle of Willis consists of the anterior communicating artery and the paired anterior cerebral, internal carotid, posterior communicating, and posterior cerebral arteries.

Anterior Circulation

The internal carotid artery enters the cranium through the carotid canal in the temporal bone, exits anteriorly, and then enters the posterior part of the foramen lacerum, eventually piercing the dural layers of the cavernous sinus. The carotid siphon refers to the S-shaped course of the artery within the sinus. The first branch is the ophthalmic artery, followed by the posterior communicating artery, and then the anterior choroidal artery. The internal carotid then terminates into the anterior and middle cerebral arteries.

Posterior Circulation

The vertebral arteries ascend through the transverse process of C6 to C1 before entering the skull through the foramen magnum. Branches of the vertebral arteries include the anterior spinal artery (single), posterior spinal arteries (paired), and the posterior inferior cerebellar artery. The vertebrobasilar system supplies the posterior cerebrum, midbrain, pons, medulla, and cerebellum.

Venous Drainage of the Head

Diploic veins are endothelium-lined canals draining the skull (Figure 55-2). The four main diploic veins on each side of the skull are named after the anatomic region being drained: frontal, anterior temporal, posterior temporal, and occipital. Emissary veins connect the venous sinuses and diploic veins to the veins on the surface of the skull.

Dural venous sinuses are located between the endosteal and meningeal layers of the dura mater. The sinuses receive blood from the brain, meninges, skull, and scalp.

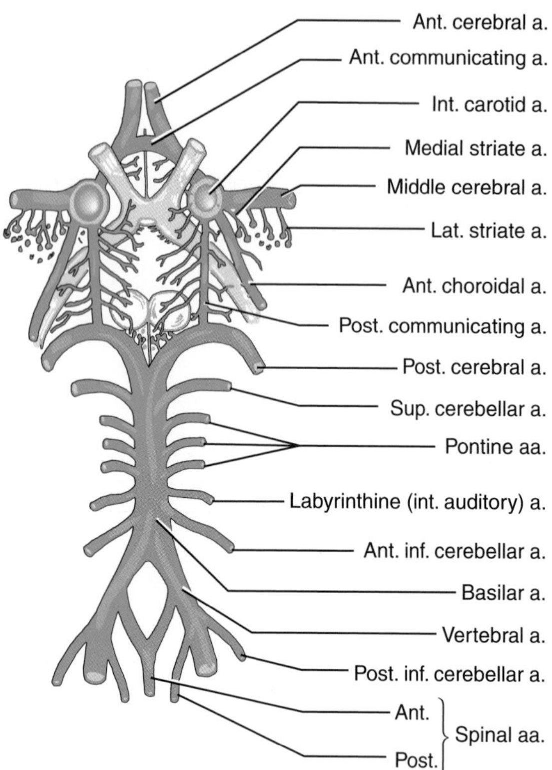

Figure 55-1 Diagram of the arterial supply to the brainstem and the constituents of the circle of Willis. (Reprinted, with permission, from Pansky B. Review of Gross Anatomy. 5th ed. New York: Macmillan; 1984.)

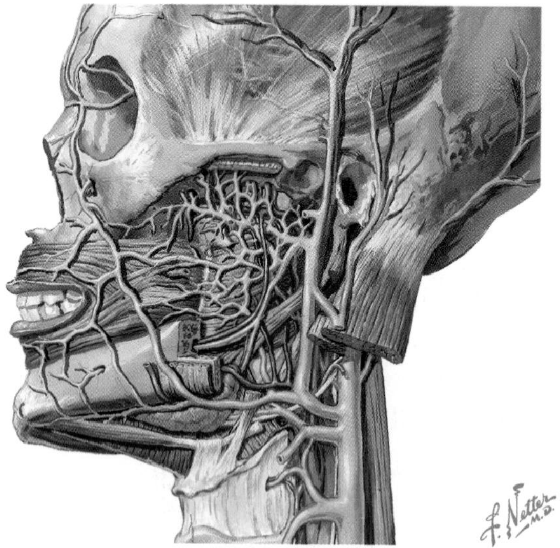

Figure 55-2 Venous drainage of the head. (Netter illustration from www.netterimages.com. © Elsevier Inc. All rights reserved.)

Clinical Considerations

Arterial anastomoses are quite numerous on the surface of the brain but are relatively rare within the brain parenchyma. Thus, occlusion or rupture of an intraparenchymal artery likely will cause more damage than a similar incident occurring on the surface of the brain.

Some 95% of all aneurysms can be found near the circle of Willis at one of five sites (see Figure 55-1 and Table 55-1). There are no valves in the dural venous sinuses or in the diploic, emissary, and meningeal veins; thus, infection from the scalp may spread to inside the intracranial vault.

Table 55-1 Common Sites of Aneurysms

Site of Aneurysm	Occurrence at This Site (%)
Anterior communicating artery	25
Middle cerebral artery	25
Internal carotid artery between posterior communicating and anterior choroidal arteries	22
Basilar bifurcation	7
Internal carotid bifurcation	4

Suggested Readings

Lassen NA. Control of cerebral circulation in health and disease. *Circ Res.* 1974;34:749-760.

McDonald DA, Potter JM. The distribution of blood in the brain. *J Physiol.* 1951; 114:356-371.

Vavilala MS, Lee LA, Lam AM. Cerebral blood flow and vascular physiology. *Anesthesiol Clin North Am.* 2002;20:247-264.

CHAPTER 56

Anatomy of the Posterior Fossa

Daniel J. Janik, MD

The posterior cranial fossa contains the brainstem (midbrain, pons, and medulla), cerebellum, and cranial nerves. Neurosurgical procedures in this area include resections of gliomas, meningiomas, acoustic neuromas, and arteriovenous malformations; microvascular decompressions; aneurysm repairs; and otologic operations.

Boundaries

The posterior fossa is bounded (1) in front by the dorsum sellae, the clivus, the posterior aspects of the sphenoid bone, and the basilar part of the occipital bone; (2) behind by the lower part of the occipital squama below the sulci for the transverse sinuses and internal occipital protuberance; (3) laterally by the petrous and mastoid parts of the temporal bones and lateral parts of the occipital bone; and (4) above and behind by the mastoid angles of the parietal bones. It contains all structures caudal to the tentorium cerebelli (Figure 56-1). The foramen magnum is in the floor of the posterior fossa.

Structures

In addition to the aforementioned cerebellum, midbrain, pons, and medulla oblongata, the fourth ventricle also lies within the posterior fossa (Figure 56-2). The nuclei of many cranial nerves and the cardiovascular and respiratory centers lie close to the anterior floor of the fourth ventricle.

Cranial nerves IV through XII either traverse or are contained within the posterior fossa (Figure 56-3).

Veins

The veins of the posterior fossa drain the cerebellum and brainstem and may be the source of bleeding, hematoma, or venous air embolism. As seen in Figure 56-4, the major venous structures include the great cerebral vein of Galen, petrosal vein, superior petrosal sinus, straight sinus, left and right transverse sinuses, lateral sinus, and occipital sinus.

Arteries

Arteries arising from the vertebrobasilar system (Figure 56-5) supply the pons, medulla, and cerebellum. Major arteries include the left and right vertebral arteries, basilar artery (formed from vertebrals), posterior inferior cerebellar artery, anterior inferior cerebellar artery, superior cerebellar artery, labyrinthine (internal auditory) artery, and posterior cerebral artery.

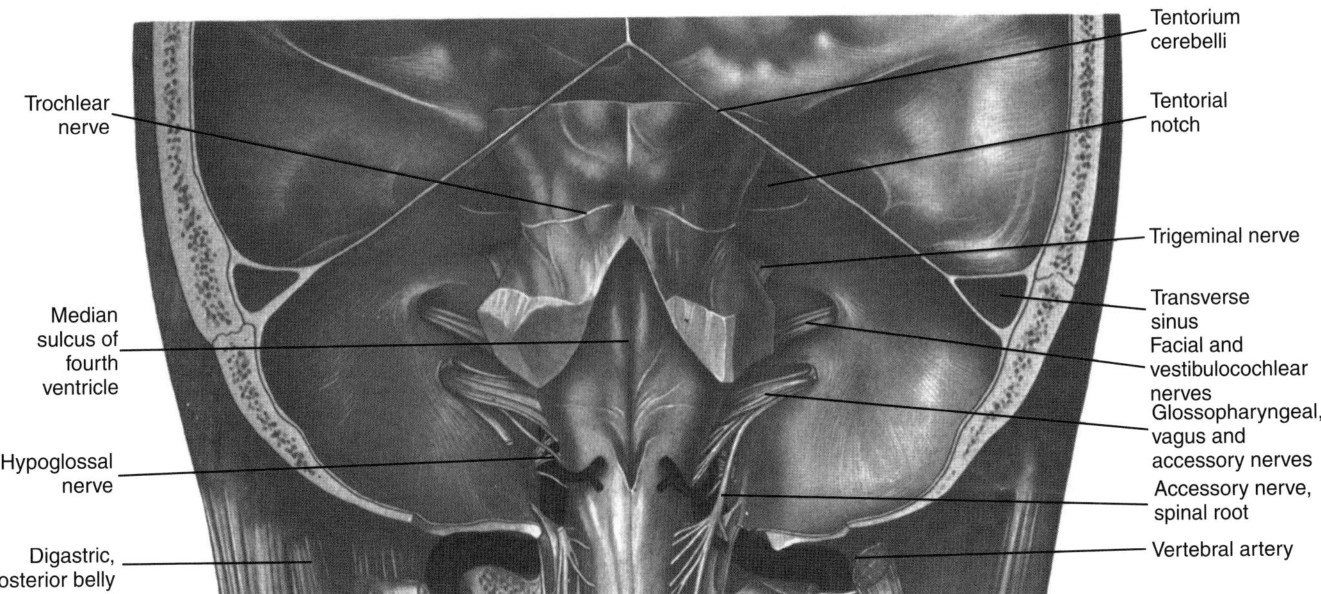

Figure 56-1 The posterior fossa, viewed from posterior in a coronal section with the cerebellar hemispheres removed.

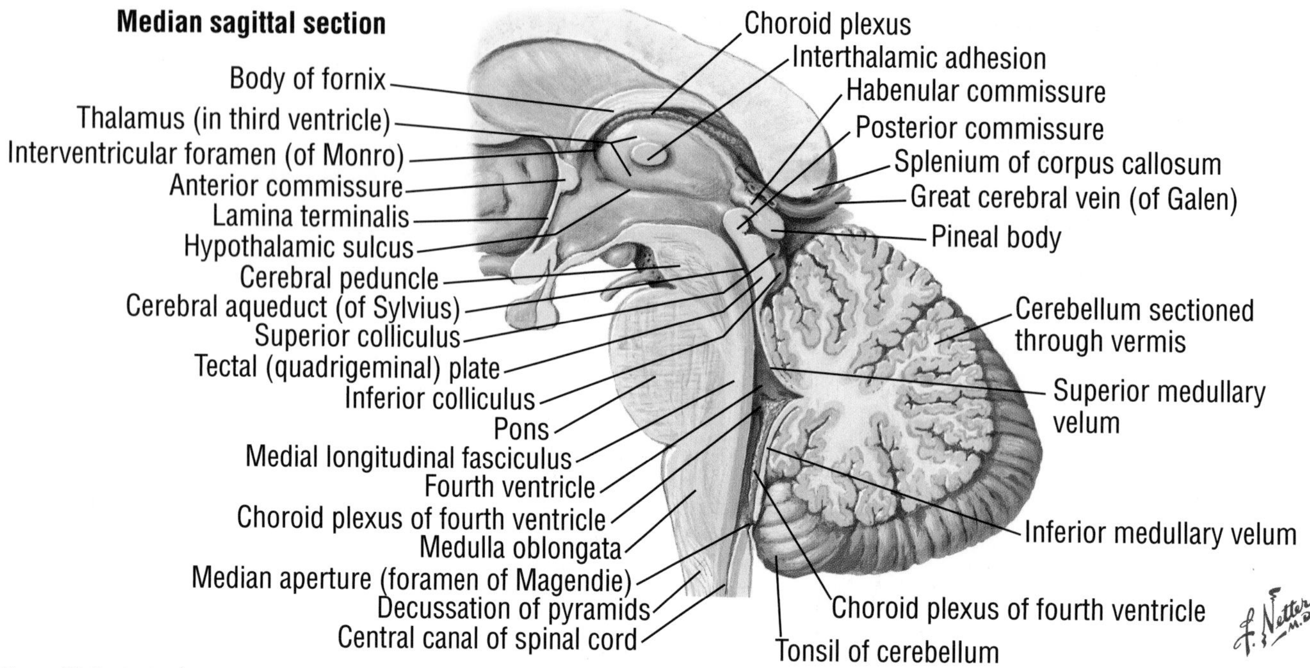

Figure 56-2 Sagittal section of the brainstem showing the fourth ventricle. (Netter illustration from www.netterimages.com. © Elsevier Inc. All rights reserved.)

Anterior view
Optic chiasm
Optic tract
Tuber cinereum
Cerebral crus
Lateral geniculate body
Posterior perforated substance
Pons
Middle cerebellar peduncle
Olive
Pyramid
Ventral roots of 1st spinal nerve (C1)
Decussation of pyramids
Olfactory tract
Anterior perforated substance
Infundibulum (pituitary stalk)
Mammillary bodies
Temporal lobe (*cut surface)*
Oculomotor nerve (III)
Trochlear nerve (IV)
Trigeminal nerve (V)
Abducent nerve (VI)
Facial nerve (VII) and intermediate nerve
Vestibulocochlear nerve (VIII)
Flocculus of cerebellum
Choroid plexus of 4th ventricle
Glossopharyngeal nerve (IX)
Vagus nerve (X)
Hypoglossal nerve (XII)
Accessory nerve (XI)

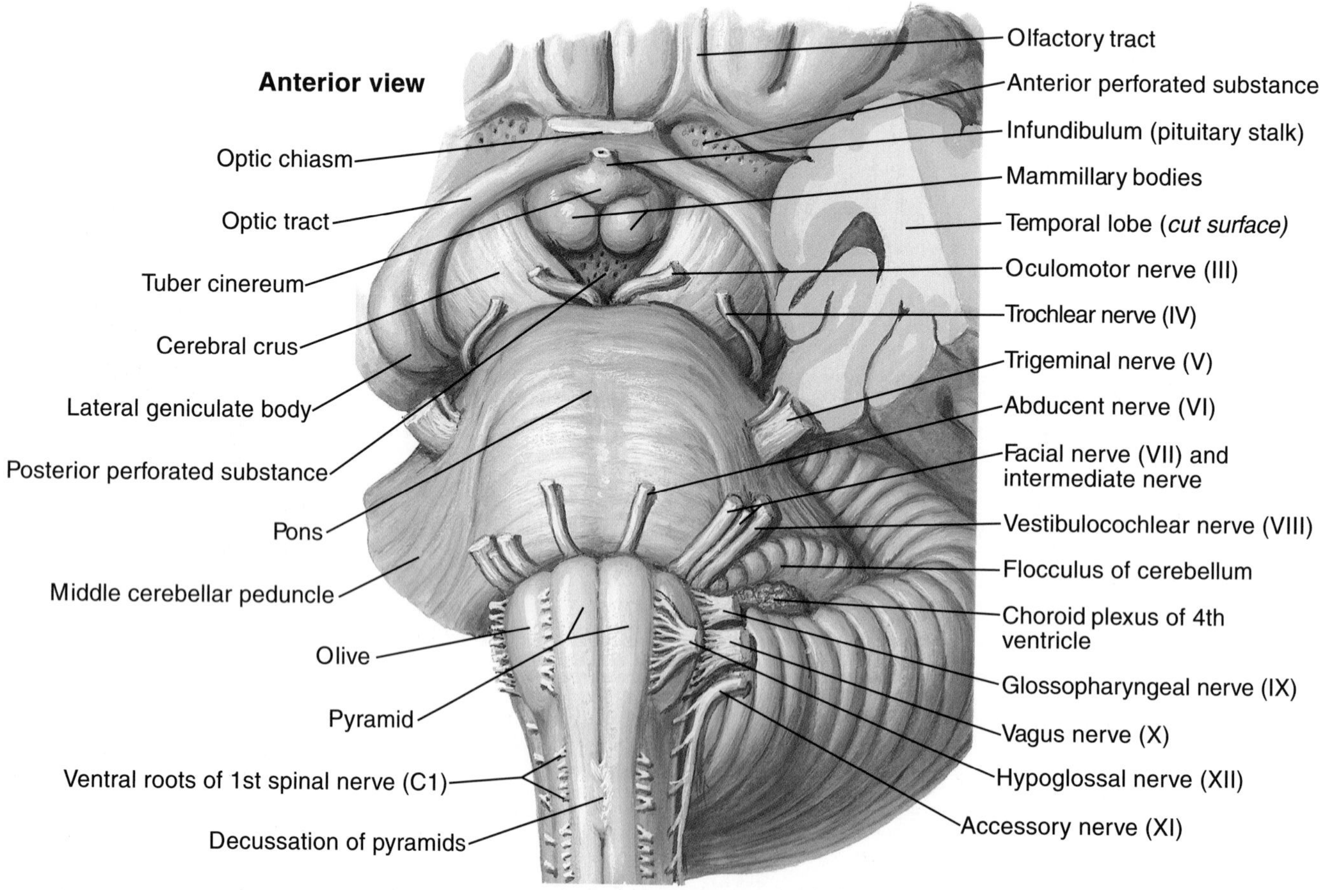

Figure 56-3 Anterior view of the brainstem showing the cranial nerves, which lie within and traverse the posterior fossa. (Netter illustration from www.netterimages.com. © Elsevier Inc. All rights reserved.)

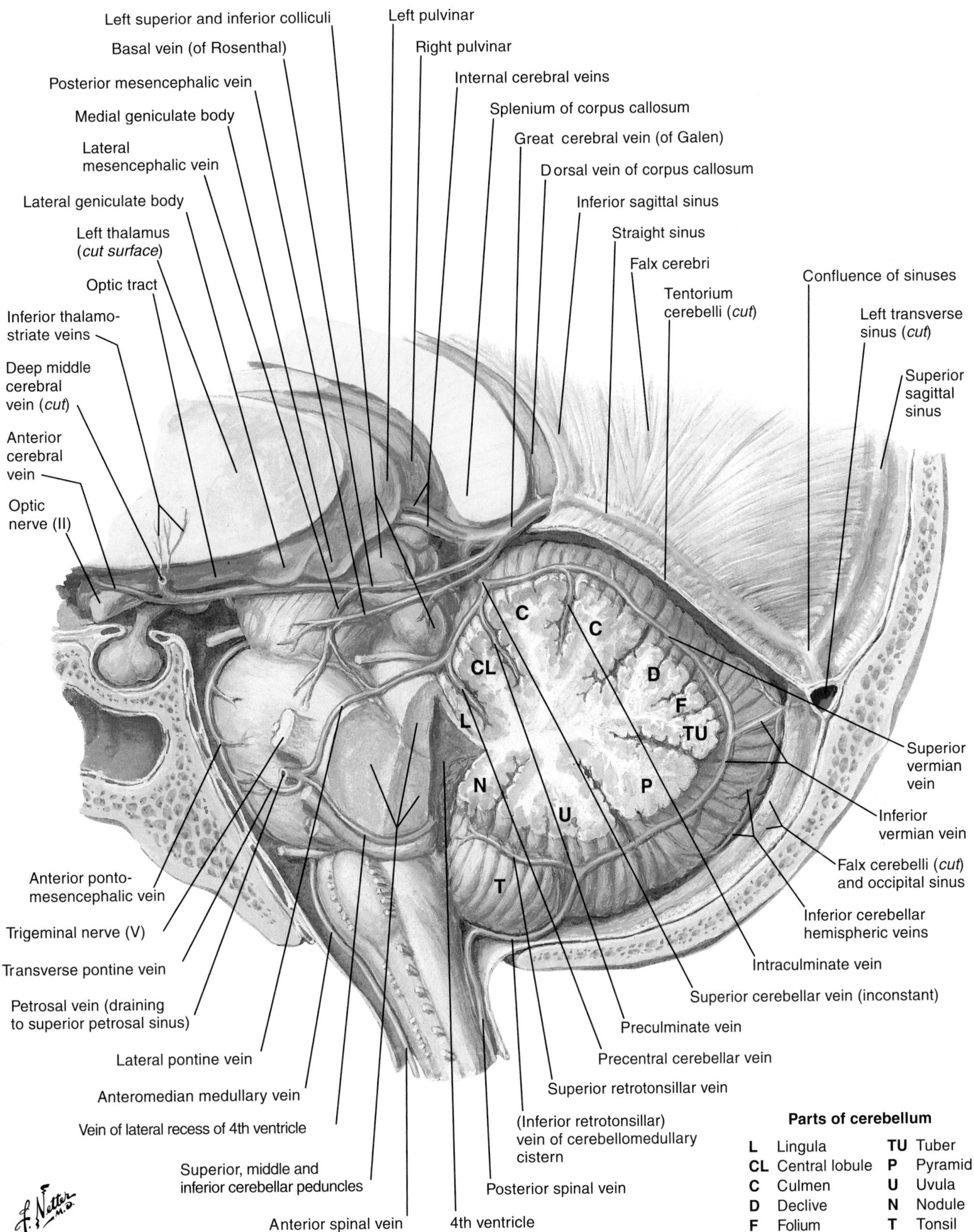
Left superior and inferior colliculi
Basal vein (of Rosenthal)
Posterior mesencephalic vein
Medial geniculate body
Lateral mesencephalic vein
Lateral geniculate body
Left thalamus (cut surface)
Optic tract
Inferior thalamo-striate veins
Deep middle cerebral vein (cut)
Anterior cerebral vein
Optic nerve (II)
Left pulvinar
Right pulvinar
Internal cerebral veins
Splenium of corpus callosum
Great cerebral vein (of Galen)
Dorsal vein of corpus callosum
Inferior sagittal sinus
Straight sinus
Falx cerebri
Tentorium cerebelli (cut)
Confluence of sinuses
Left transverse sinus (cut)
Superior sagittal sinus
C
C
CL
D
F
TU
L
N
P
U
T
Superior vermian vein
Inferior vermian vein
Falx cerebelli (cut) and occipital sinus
Inferior cerebellar hemispheric veins
Intraculminate vein
Superior cerebellar vein (inconstant)
Preculminate vein
Precentral cerebellar vein
Superior retrotonsillar vein
(Inferior retrotonsillar) vein of cerebellomedullary cistern
Posterior spinal vein
4th ventricle
Anterior spinal vein
Superior, middle and inferior cerebellar peduncles
Vein of lateral recess of 4th ventricle
Anteromedian medullary vein
Lateral pontine vein
Petrosal vein (draining to superior petrosal sinus)
Transverse pontine vein
Trigeminal nerve (V)
Anterior ponto-mesencephalic vein
Parts of cerebellum
L Lingula
CL Central lobule
C Culmen
D Declive
F Folium
TU Tuber
P Pyramid
U Uvula
N Nodule
T Tonsil
F. Netter M.D.

Figure 56-4 Venous drainage of the structures within the posterior fossa. (Netter illustration from www.netterimages.com.)

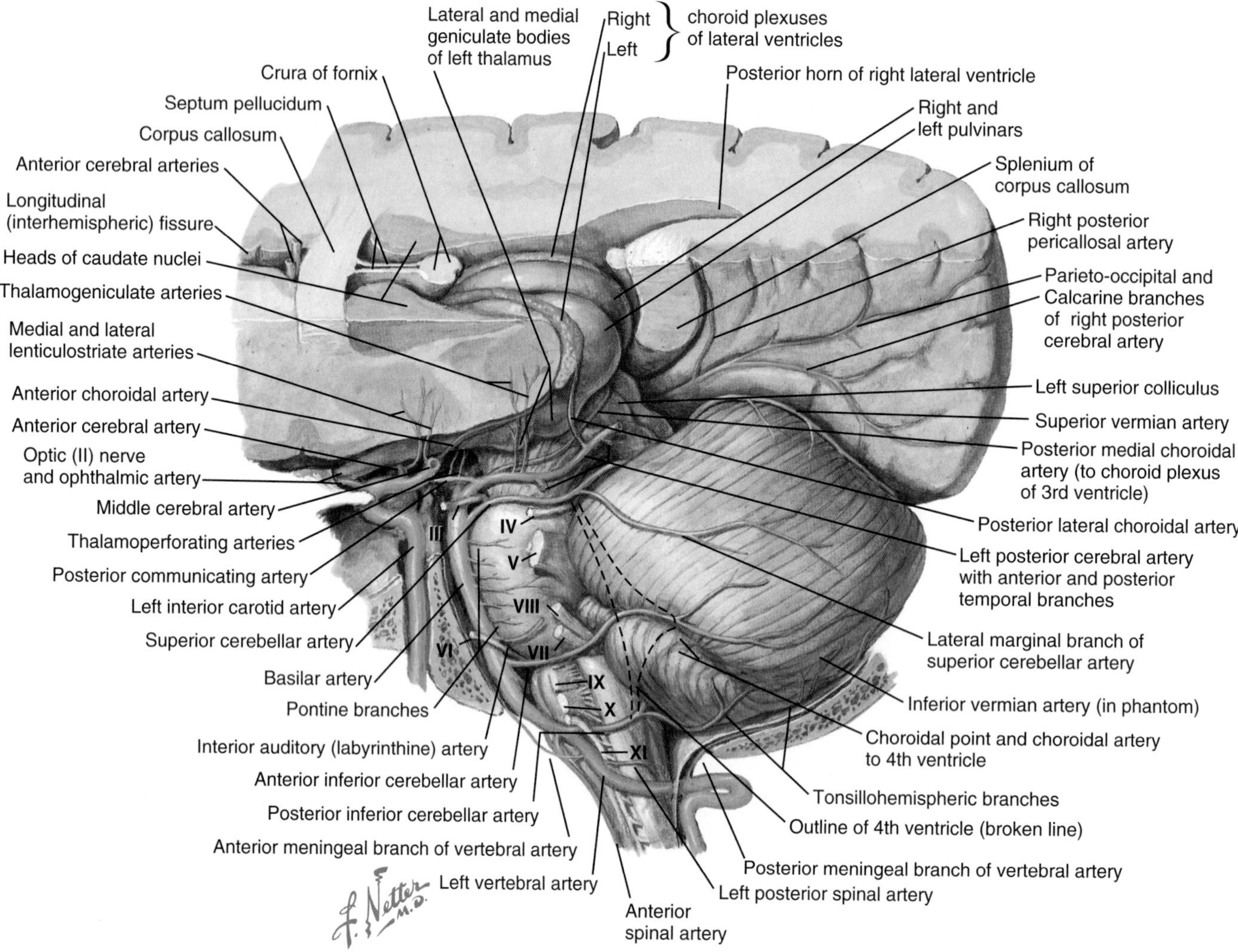

Figure 56-5 Arterial supply of the structures within the posterior fossa. (Netter illustration from www.netterimages.com.)

Suggested Readings

Artru AA, Cucchiara RF, Messick JM. Cardiorespiratory and cranial nerve sequelae of surgical procedures involving the posterior fossa. *Anesthesiology*. 1980; 52:83-86.

Netter F. *Atlas of Human Anatomy*. 3rd ed. Teterboro, NJ: Icon Learning Systems; 2003.

Snell RS. *Clinical Anatomy by Regions*. 8th ed. Philadelphia: Wolters Kluwer/ Lippincott, Williams & Wilkins; 2008:676-677.

Standring S. *Gray's Anatomy. The Anatomical Basis of Clinical Practice*. 40th ed. Philadelphia: Churchill Livingstone; 2008.

Winn HR. *Youman's Neurological Surgery*. 5th ed. Vol. 1. Philadelphia: WB Saunders; 1996:29-40.

CHAPTER 57

Spinal Cord Anatomy and Blood Supply

Adrian Gelb, MB ChB

Anatomy

The vertebral column encompasses the spinal cord and comprises 33 vertebrae—24 of which articulate (7 cervical, 12 thoracic, 5 lumbar) and 9 of which are fused (5 sacral and 4 coccygeal)—and 4 curvatures. Anteriorly, the cervical and lumbar curves are convex, whereas, in the thoracic and sacral areas, the vertebral column is concave (Figure 57-1). The stability and elasticity of the vertebral column is gained via several ligaments (Figure 57-2).

Ligaments

The supraspinous ligament is a band of longitudinal fibers interconnecting the tips of the spinous processes from the sacrum to C7. It is continuous with the interspinal ligament at all levels and with the ligamentum nuchae cephalad. The interspinous ligament is a thin membranous band that unites adjacent spinous processes and extends from the supraspinal ligament posteriorly to the ligamentum flavum anteriorly. The ligamentum flavum, the strongest of the ligaments, is the "yellow ligament" that runs from the base of the skull in front of and between the laminae all the way to the sacrum. The anterior and posterior longitudinal ligaments are the primary ligaments that provide vertebral column stability by binding the vertebral bodies.

Epidural Space

The epidural space surrounds the spinal meninges and contains fat, alveolar tissue, nerve roots, and extensive networks of arteries and venous plexuses. This space extends from the foramen magnum to the sacral hiatus and is widest in its posterior dimension. L2 is thought to be the widest part of the epidural space, measuring 5 to 6 mm at this level. The epidural space is bounded anteriorly by the posterior longitudinal ligament, laterally by the intervertebral foramina, and posteriorly by the ligamentum flavum.

Meninges

The spinal meninges are three individual membranes that surround the spinal cord: (1) The dura is the tough, fibroelastic, outermost membrane extending from the foramen magnum superiorly to the lower border of S2 inferiorly, where it is pierced by the filum terminales (i.e., the distal end of the pia mater). (2) The arachnoid is the middle membrane that is closely attached to the dura. This layer is very thin and avascular. (3) The pia is a highly vascular membrane that closely approximates the spinal cord. The space between the arachnoid and pia is the subarachnoid space. This space contains the spinal nerves and cerebrospinal fluid, as well as numerous delicate trabeculae that intertwine within this space. Lateral extensions of the pia mater, the denticulate ligaments, help support the spinal cord by binding to the dura.

The spinal cord begins at the level of the foramen magnum and ends below as the conus medullaris. At birth, the cord extends to L3, but it moves to its adult position at the lower border of L1 by age 1 year.

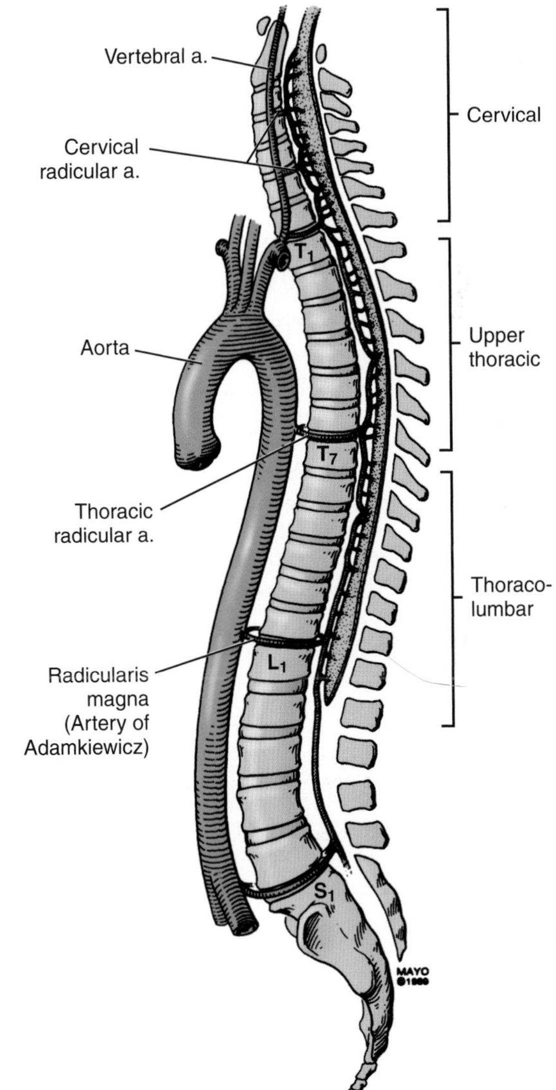

Figure 57-1 A lateral view of the vertebral column, illustrating its curvatures and the line and center of gravity of the body. Blood supply is via radicular arteries, which are variable in location but are shown here at T1, T7, L1, and S1. (Modified from Mahla ME, Horlocker TT. Vertebral column and spinal cord surgery. In: Cucchiara RF, Black S, Michenfelder JD, eds. Clinical Neuroanesthesia. 2nd ed. New York: Churchill Livingstone; 1998:403-448.)

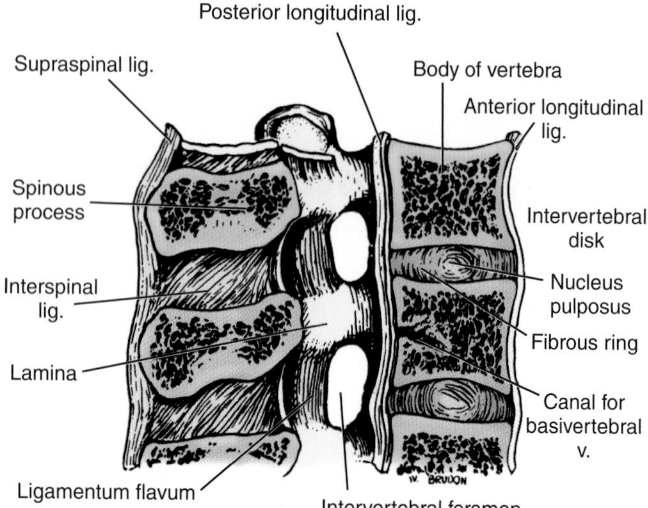

Figure 57-2 A median section of several vertebrae, illustrating the intervertebral disk and the ligaments of the column. (Modified from Woodburne RT. Essentials of Human Anatomy. 8th ed. Oxford, UK: Oxford University Press; 1988.)

Blood Supply

The spinal cord is supplied by one anterior spinal artery and two posterior spinal arteries. Throughout their length, these three spinal arteries receive contributions from radicular branches of intercostal arteries. The anterior spinal artery, which lies in the anterior median sulcus of the spinal cord, is formed at the level of the foramen magnum by the union of two radicular rami of the vertebral arteries (Figure 57-3, *A*). Although the anterior spinal artery is often considered to be a continuous structure, this is not the case; 8 to 12 medullary arteries join the anterior spinal artery through its course to the conus medullaris, and each forms an arborization pattern (Figure 57-3, *B*). Contributing to the anterior spinal artery system is a group of 8 to 12 radicular arteries (see Figure 57-1). In the cervical region, these arteries derive from the cervical branches of the vertebral and ascending cervical arteries. In the superior thoracic cord, contributions arise from the ascending and deep cervical arteries. The medullary arteries augmenting blood flow to the middle and lower thoracic cord are less prominent. The most caudal medullary artery is usually the largest, the arteria medullaris magna anterior (artery of Adamkiewicz). This artery has a variable origin along the spinal cord, arising between T5 and T8 in 15% of patients, between T9 and T12 in 60%, and between L1 and L5 in 25%.

The posterior spinal arteries arise from the vertebral or posterior inferior cerebellar arteries and descend as two branches, one anterior and the other posterior to the dorsal nerve root. These arteries are segmentally reinforced with radicular collaterals from the vertebral, cervical, and posterior intercostal arteries, and they provide better vascular continuity than does the anterior spinal arterial system.

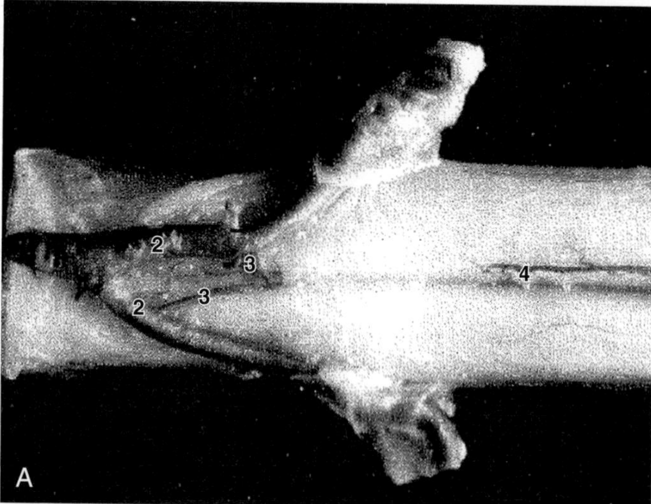

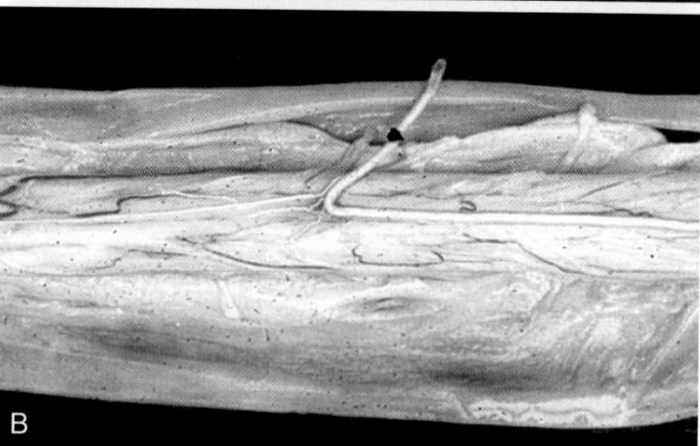

Figure 57-3 **A,** Formation of the anterior spinal artery (4) by rami (3) of the vertebral arteries (2). **B,** Arborization pattern formed by arteria medullaris magna anterior (medullary artery) as it joins the anterior spinal artery.

The peripheral border of the spinal cord receives its blood supply from ventral and dorsal penetrating vessels. Collateral circulation of the peripheral cord is adequate. However, within the spinal cord itself, there are no anastomoses, and the penetrating vessels are essentially end arterioles.

Suggested Readings

Mahla ME, Horlocker TT. Vertebral column and spinal cord surgery. In: Cucchiara RF, Black S, Michenfelder JD, eds. *Clinical Neuroanesthesia*. 2nd ed. New York: Churchill Livingstone; 1998:403-408.

Zhang T, Harstad L, Parisi JE, Murray MJ. The size of the anterior spinal artery in relation to the arteria medullaris magna anterior in humans. *Clin Anat.* 1995;8:347-351.

CHAPTER 58

Brachial Plexus Anatomy

David L. Brown, MD

Anesthesia providers should be familiar with the anatomy of the brachial plexus because they are frequently called upon to perform regional anesthetic techniques for the upper extremity. One challenge with visualizing this anatomy is that the traditional wiring diagram for the brachial plexus is often unnecessarily complex and intimidating (Figures 58-1 and 58-2).

Simplifying Brachial Plexus Anatomy

The brachial plexus is formed by the ventral rami of the fifth to eighth cervical nerves and the greater part of the ramus of the first thoracic nerve. Additionally, small contributions to the brachial plexus may come from the fourth cervical and the second thoracic nerves. The intimidating part of this anatomy is what happens from the point where these ventral rami emerge from between the middle and anterior scalene muscles until they end in the four terminal branches to the upper extremity: the musculocutaneous, median, ulnar, and radial nerves. Most of what happens to the roots on their way to becoming peripheral nerves is not clinically essential information for an anesthesia provider to understand, but having a familiarity with some broad concepts may help clinicians understand the brachial plexus anatomy more easily; that is the goal of this chapter.

After the roots pass between the scalene muscles, they reorganize into trunks—superior, middle, and inferior. The trunks continue toward the first rib. At the lateral edge of the first rib, these trunks undergo a primary anatomic division into ventral and dorsal divisions. This is also the point at which understanding of brachial plexus anatomy gives way to frustration and often unnecessary complexity. This anatomic division is significant because nerves destined to supply the originally ventral part of the upper extremity separate from those that supply the dorsal part. As these divisions enter the axilla, the divisions give way to cords. The posterior divisions of all three trunks unite to form the posterior cord, the anterior divisions of the superior and middle trunks form the lateral cord, and the medial cord is the anterior division of the inferior trunk. These cords are named according to their relationship to the second part of the axillary artery.

At the lateral border of the pectoralis minor muscle (which inserts onto the coracoid process), the three cords reorganize to give rise to the peripheral nerves of the upper extremity. Once again, in an effort to simplify, the branches of the lateral and medial cords are all "ventral" nerves to the upper extremity (see Figure 58-2). The posterior cord, in contrast, provides all "dorsal" innervation to the upper extremity. Thus, the radial nerve supplies all the dorsal musculature in the upper extremity below the shoulder. The musculocutaneous nerve supplies muscular innervation in the arm while providing cutaneous innervation to the forearm. In contrast, the median and ulnar nerves are nerves of passage in the arm, but in the forearm and hand, they provide the ventral musculature with motor innervation. These nerves can be further categorized; the median nerve innervates more heavily in the forearm, whereas the ulnar nerve innervates more heavily in the hand.

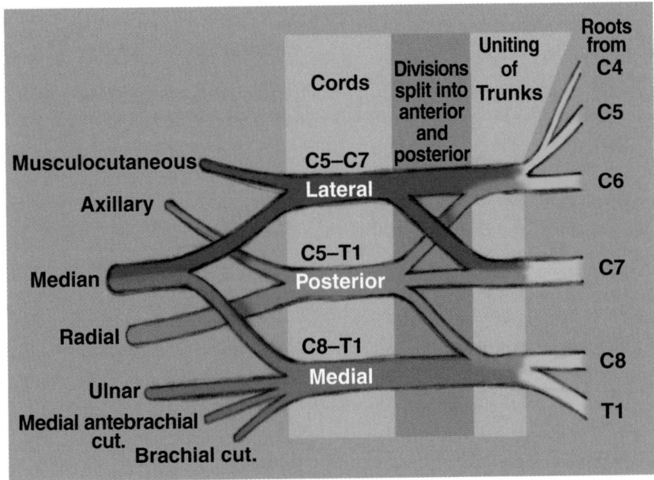

Figure 58-1 Brachial plexus anatomy displayed as a wiring diagram. Using terminology guides (from medial to lateral of roots—trunks—division—cords—peripheral nerves) simplifies communicating about the anatomy of the brachial plexus.

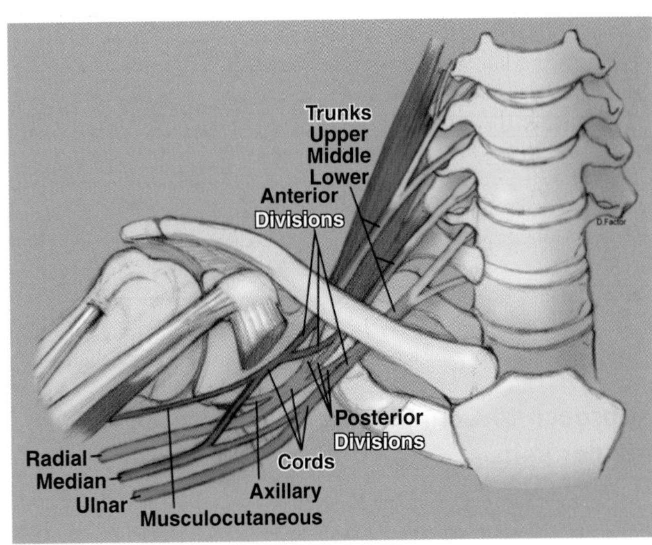

Figure 58-2 Anatomic relationships of the brachial plexus as it forms from medial to lateral.

Non-neural Brachial Plexus Anatomy

Although some of the brachial plexus neural anatomy of interest to anesthesia providers has been outlined, there are some additional anatomic details that need highlighting. As the cervical roots leave the transverse processes, on their way to the brachial plexus, they exit in the gutter of the transverse process immediately posterior to the vertebral artery. The vertebral arteries leave the brachiocephalic and subclavian arteries on the right and left, respectively, and travel cephalad to enter a bony canal in the transverse process typically at the level of C6 and above. One must be constantly aware of needle-tip location in relation to the vertebral artery during the performance of interscalene blocks. The vertebral artery lies anterior to the roots of the brachial plexus as the roots leave the cervical vertebrae.

Another structure of interest is the phrenic nerve. It is formed from branches of the third, fourth, and fifth cervical nerves and passes through the neck on its way to the thorax on the ventral surface of the anterior scalene muscle. The phrenic nerve is almost always blocked during an interscalene block and, less frequently, with supraclavicular techniques. Avoidance of phrenic blockade is important in only a small percentage of patients, although the location of the phrenic nerve should be kept in mind when performing blocks on patients with significantly decreased pulmonary function—that is, patients whose day-to-day activities are limited by their pulmonary impairment.

Suggested Readings

Brown DL. Upper extremity block anatomy: In: Brown DL. *Atlas of Regional Anesthesia*. 3rd ed. Philadelphia: Elsevier Saunders; 2006:25-36.

Kessler J, Schafhalter-Zoppoth I, Gray AT. An ultrasound study of the phrenic nerve in the posterior cervical triangle: Implications for the interscalene brachial plexus block. *Reg Anesth Pain Med*. 2008;33:545-550.

Neal JM. The upper extremity: Somatic blockade. In: Cousins MJ, Carr DB, Horlocker TT, Bridenbaugh PO, eds. *Cousins and Bridenbaugh's Neural Blockade in Clinical Anesthesia and Pain Medicine*. 4th ed. Philadelphia: Lippincott, Williams & Wilkins; 2009:316-342.

CHAPTER 59

Central Venous Cannulation

Michael J. Murray, MD, PhD

Central venous cannulas are frequently placed to measure central venous pressure; to administer fluid, blood products, parenteral nutrition, and vasoactive drugs; and to provide access for insertion of pulmonary artery catheters and transvenous cardiac pacing electrodes. Anesthesia providers most often cannulate the internal jugular vein (IJV), subclavian vein, or femoral vein, although the latter is not commonly used because cannulating the femoral vein increases the risk of infection. This chapter discusses placement of a cannula in the IJV.

Because the IJV is readily accessible, cannulating the IJV is easier than cannulating other sites (and is therefore associated with a lower rate of complications), resulting in the IJV being most anesthesia providers' preferred site for obtaining central venous access. Although either side may be used, the favored approach is from the right because the angle of entry into the right IJV is close to 180 degrees (resulting in a slightly higher success rate and, therefore, a slightly lower complication rate), whereas, on the left, the angle is closer to 90 degrees. In addition, the performance of this technique on the right is easier for right-handed operators.

Approach to Cannulation of the Internal Jugular Vein

An important landmark in cannulating the IJV is the triangle formed by the sternal and clavicular heads of the sternocleidomastoid muscle and the clavicle. With the patient's head turned 20 to 30 degrees to the side opposite the site of insertion, the apex of the triangle is identified by palpating the juncture of the two heads of the muscle. (Turning the head further than 30 degrees tends to compress the IJV and pulls it posteriorly and medially so that it lies behind the internal carotid artery.) The IJV lies just medial to the lateral head of the sternocleidomastoid muscle at a depth of 1 to 3 cm.

The traditional approach to cannulating the IJV was to place the patient in the Trendelenburg position, sterilize the skin with a povidone-iodine topical antiseptic, and drape the patient after drawing a line along the medial aspect of the lateral sternocleidomastoid and a line along the lateral aspect of the medial sternocleidomastoid. Where the two lines intersected was the point typically chosen to infiltrate a small amount of local anesthetic and the site for insertion of a "finder" needle that was attached to a 3-mL to 5-mL syringe. While applying negative pressure, the syringe with needle attached was advanced at a 45-degree angle to the skin toward the ipsilateral breast. If deoxygenated blood was not aspirated after penetrating to a depth of 3 to 5 cm, the needle was withdrawn and moved 1 to 2 mm medially or laterally and another attempt was made. More cephalad or caudal insertion sites were typically avoided because the carotid artery lies anterior to the IJV high in the neck and the cupola of the lung lies low in the neck. With this technique, many clinicians palpated the carotid artery before performing a venipuncture to verify the position of the artery in relationship to the IJV.

The Seldinger approach was developed 6 decades ago, with a modified version used most often today to obtain central venous access. With the traditional Seldinger technique, an 18G thin-wall needle is inserted into the IJV, a guidewire is passed, the needle is removed, a dilator is threaded over the guidewire, the dilator is removed, a cannula (or introducer) is inserted over the guidewire, the guidewire is removed, the cannula or introducer is sutured in place, and a dressing is applied. The modified version is identical except that, rather than using a bare thin-wall needle to initially access the IJV, a thinner needle with an overlying catheter is inserted, and once venous blood is aspirated, the catheter is advanced into the IJV and the needle is withdrawn. The advantage of using the modified Seldinger technique is that many consider it easier to use manometry or waveform analysis to confirm entry into the vein with a catheter than with an 18G thin-wall needle in place. Once venous pressure is confirmed, the remainder of the procedure is as described here—a guidewire is inserted through the catheter, the catheter removed, a dilator advanced over the guidewire, and so on.

Placement and maintenance of central venous cannulas is associated with a number of complications, most specifically, bloodstream infections, carotid artery puncture and cannulation, and pneumothorax.

Reducing the Morbidity and Mortality Rates Associated with Central Venous Cannulation

Several clinical practice guidelines have recently been developed to decrease the morbidity (and mortality) associated with the placement of central venous cannulas. To decrease the incidence of central line–associated bloodstream infections, the Centers for Disease Control and Prevention published *Guidelines for the Prevention of Intravascular Catheter-Related Infections* in 2011. These guidelines recommend that inserters of central lines use surgical handwashing, maximal sterile barriers during insertion (hat and mask, sterile gloves and gown, and sterile drape—large enough to entirely cover the patient), and 2% chlorhexidine with isopropyl alcohol to sterilize the skin and that inserters allow the antiseptic to dry before inserting the catheter.

In 2012, the American Society of Anesthesiologists Task Force on Central Venous Access likewise released a report with several recommendations to decrease complications and to improve the success rate of central venous cannulation. Although the literature was ambivalent about the best site for accessing central venous circulation, the task force did indeed recommend the IJV as the optimum site for cannulation and agreed that, when clinically appropriate and feasible, central venous access should be attempted while the patient was in the Trendelenburg position. The task force made no recommendation regarding the Seldinger technique (using a wire through a thin-wall needle) versus a modified Seldinger technique (using a catheter over the needle and wire through the catheter). Instead, the task force recommended that the choice of technique be based on the clinical situation and the skill of the anesthesia provider.

The most significant change in these guidelines was the recommendation that static ultrasonography be used for identifying the IJV prior to skin puncture and that real-time ultrasonography be used for needle, wire, and catheter placement into the IJV. Documentation of intravenous placement of the needle prior to insertion of the large-bore catheter could also be by (1) manometry, (2) pressure waveform analysis, (3) venous blood gas, (4) fluoroscopy, (5) continuous electrocardiography, (6) transesophageal echocardiography, or (7) chest radiography.

Many anesthesiologists and anesthesia departments have incorporated the recommendations from the Centers for Disease Control and Prevention and the American Society of Anesthesiologists into protocols for the placement of central venous cannulas. There is little debate about the use of the Centers for Disease Control and Prevention guidelines in decreasing the risk of infection, but there is some concern about the use of ultrasonography for identifying the IJV and placing central venous cannulas during emergency situations in which an ultrasound machine may not be immediately available, or when time is so critical that the experienced clinician considers that the time required for the use of ultrasonography is not justified. Evidence from the United Kingdom indicates that, since the use of ultrasound for central venous access became widespread in 2004, the chance of success in emergency situations has decreased when using the traditional anatomic approach. This has been found to be especially true for individuals who have trained after 2004, individuals who simply do not have the experience that their predecessors had with the anatomic approach.

This conundrum is ironic because, over the last several years, the health care system has been emulating the airline industry, emphasizing training on simulators, crew resource management, and situational awareness to improve patient outcomes. Perhaps clinicians can learn from a report released by the Federal Aviation Administration in 2010 following an analysis of more than 700 incidents. The report concluded that too great a reliance on technology and not enough emphasis on fundamental skills was a hazard in the emergency incidents that were reviewed. In a similar light, clinicians could justifiably conclude that they must use their judgment to identify patients in whom they can safely use the anatomic approach for cannulation of the IJV so that they can maintain the skills and experience necessary to perform competently in emergency situations.

Suggested Readings

O'Grady NP, Alexander M, Burns LA, et al. *Guidelines for the prevention of intravascular catheter-related infections, 2011*. Atlanta, GA: Centers for Disease Control and Prevention. http://www.cdc.gov/hicpac/pdf/guidelines/bsi-guidelines-2011.pdf. Accessed January 12, 2013.

Rupp SM, Apfelbaum JL, Blitt C, et al. Practice guidelines for central venous access: A report by the American Society of Anesthesiologists Task Force on Central Venous Access. *Anesthesiology*. 2012;116:539-573.

SECTION VI Pharmacology

CHAPTER 60

Molecular and Cellular Mechanisms of Anesthesia

Carlos B. Mantilla, MD, PhD, and Gilbert Y. Wong, MD

Despite considerable advances in the field of anesthesia, our understanding of the underlying mechanisms of general anesthesia is still incomplete. A general anesthetic state is obtained with a combination of hypnosis, amnesia, analgesia, and lack of motor response to painful stimuli. Different anesthetic drugs display varying potencies in attaining these behavioral end points, but all of them result in loss of consciousness.

Potent anesthetic agents include small molecules (e.g., nitrous oxide), alcohols, halogenated ethers, and complex compounds (e.g., barbiturates, etomidate, alkyl phenol, and propofol). The diversity in chemical structure of these agents suggests multiple modes of action. Anesthetic agents share certain characteristics, including hydrophobicity (i.e., low water solubility, expressed as a lipid-to-water partition coefficient) and lack of specific antagonists capable of reversing anesthetic effects. Thus, anesthetic agents have, until recently, generally been considered to act nonspecifically on lipid membranes in the central nervous system (CNS). However, recent findings indicate that most anesthetic agents have specific effects on membrane proteins, which depend on hydrophobic, electrostatic, and size properties, all of which contribute to complex mechanisms of action.

A unitary hypothesis of anesthesia proposed the existence of a common mechanism for the action of all anesthetics. Based on the strong correlation between lipid solubility and anesthetic potency, it was thought that anesthetics act nonselectively on neuronal membranes (the Meyer-Overton rule; Figure 60-1). According to this theory, hydrophobic anesthetic agents concentrate in lipid membranes, which contain proteins required for electrical conduction. Once in the lipid membrane, anesthetic agents would change the order and fluidity of the neuronal lipid bilayer, interact with membrane proteins, or alter the protein-lipid interface. At the cellular level, any of these effects may alter neuronal function. Although this hypothesis is attractive, our current understanding of the molecular and cellular basis of consciousness, perception, memory, and sleep suggests diverse anesthetic effects and thus does not support this hypothesis.

Lipid-Based Hypotheses

Based on the Meyer-Overton rule (Figure 60-1, *A*), the lipid-solubility hypothesis suggests that anesthesia is produced when sufficient numbers of molecules disrupt neuronal lipid membranes. However, several findings are inconsistent with the lipid-solubility hypothesis. First, some hydrophobic molecules, chemically similar to anesthetic agents, are either much less potent than predicted or have no anesthetic properties. Second, application of increased pressure to membranes does not alter the lipid solubility of anesthetic agents, whereas this increased pressure does antagonize the anesthetic state (a phenomenon termed the *pressure-reversal effect*). Third, n-alcohols exhibit increasing anesthetic potency and hydrophobicity as the carbon chain is elongated, but an additional carbon molecule past 12 or 13 is associated with complete loss of anesthetic action (the *cutoff effect*).

Modifications of the lipid-solubility hypothesis attempt to account for these phenomena by including lipid-perturbation effects. The critical-volume hypothesis suggests that anesthesia occurs when anesthetic agents cause lipid-membrane expansion, thereby disrupting membrane-protein function. At clinically relevant concentrations of anesthetic agents, the membrane expands approximately 0.4%, similar to the effect of a 1°C increase in temperature, which is not associated with anesthesia. In addition, although this hypothesis would explain the pressure-reversal effect, it still fails to explain the anesthetic cutoff effect. The lipid-fluidity hypothesis arises from the disordering effect that anesthetic agents exert on membranes, which could interfere with the function of membrane proteins. Anesthetic potency correlates with the disordering effect on cholesterol membranes. The cutoff parallels the altered membrane-disordering ability of alcohols, and increased pressure reverses anesthetic-induced changes in membrane fluidity. Nevertheless, the assumption that changes in the lipid membrane alter protein function lacks experimental support.

Protein-Based Hypotheses

Recent evidence suggests that anesthetic effects result from their actions on proteins. First, general anesthetic potency correlates well with inhibition of several specific proteins (Figure 60-1, *B*). Anesthetic binding to hydrophobic pockets in proteins explains both the correlation of potency with hydrophobicity and the anesthetic cutoff effect. In addition, multiple anesthetic drugs—including barbiturates, ketamine, and isoflurane—display stereoselective effects (e.g., the S-isomer is more potent than the R-isomer) consistent with protein binding. Finally, the steep dose-response curve for inhalation anesthetic agents suggests receptor occupancy (i.e., 1 MAC [minimum alveolar concentration] is effective in 50% of subjects, whereas 1.3 MAC is effective in 95% of subjects).

Most evidence indicates that anesthetic drugs act specifically at ion channels (Figure 60-2). For example, multiple anesthetic drugs (e.g., barbiturates and inhalation anesthetic agents) potentiate γ-aminobutyric acid (GABA) activity. Propofol and etomidate also act by potentiating $GABA_A$ receptors, and mutations in the $GABA_A$ receptor are now known to modulate anesthetic effects in vitro and in animal models. Several anesthetic agents prolong inhibitory chloride currents at GABA receptors and shift the GABA dose-response curve leftward, enhancing receptor sensitivity to GABA.

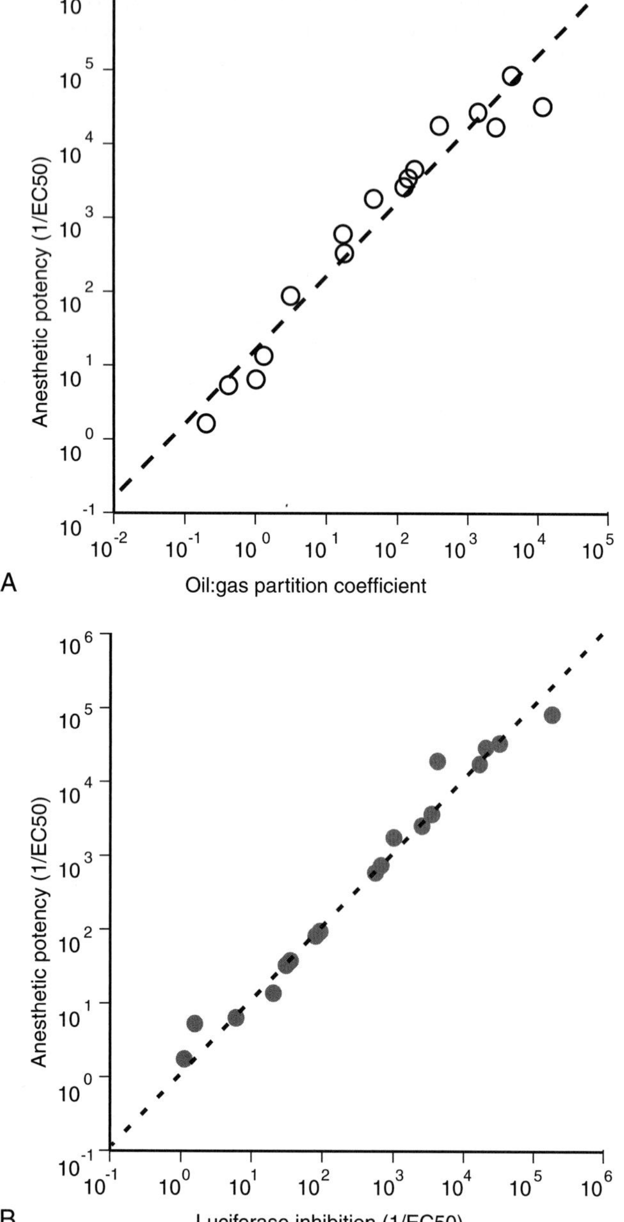

Figure 60-1 Anesthetic drugs exhibit a strong correlation between their potency (i.e., reciprocal of their minimum alveolar concentration, [MAC]) and their hydrophobicity (**A**). This relationship supports the lipid-solubility hypothesis of anesthetic action (Meyer-Overton rule). In addition, there is a strong correlation between the potency of different anesthetic drugs and their inhibition of the firefly enzyme luciferase (**B**), supporting a protein-based hypothesis of anesthetic action. (Adapted from Campagna JA, Miller KW, Forman SA. Mechanisms of actions of inhaled anesthetics. N Engl J Med. 2003;348:2110-2124 and Franks NP. Molecular targets underlying general anaesthesia. Br J Pharmacol. 2006;147(Suppl 1):S72-81.)

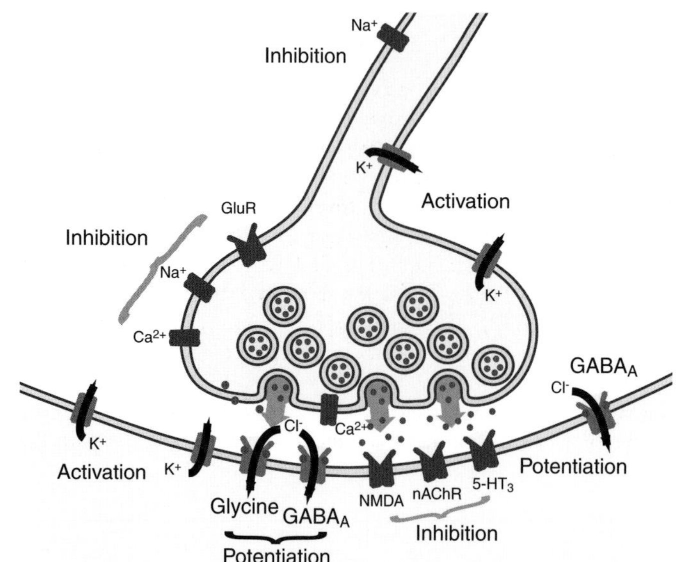

Figure 60-2 Potential sites of anesthetic action include presynaptic and postsynaptic targets (shown in large filled circles). Presynaptic inhibition of Ca^{2+} entry in the axon terminal following the action potential and direct inhibition of neurotransmitter vesicle release can lead to decreased availability of neurotransmitter in the synaptic cleft and reduced impulse transmission. Postsynaptic effects are mediated by modulation of ion channels, including ligand-gated ion channel receptors. Potentiation of $GABA_A$ (γ-aminobutyric acid) and glycine receptors enhances inhibitory neurotransmission. Activation of presynaptic or postsynaptic two-pore K^+ channels causes cell hyperpolarization and reduces cellular excitability. Inhibition of glutamate (via ionotropic glutamate receptors [GluR], including NMDA [*N*-methyl-D-aspartate] receptors), serotonin (via 5-HT_3 receptors), or acetylcholine (via neuronal nicotinic receptors—nAChR) impairs excitatory neurotransmission. Anesthetic effects on ion channels likely result from specific interactions at hydrophobic pockets within transmembrane proteins, leading to altered protein function, rather than from the direct effects on the lipid membrane or lipid-protein interface.

All inhalation anesthetic agents potentiate glycine receptors, the second most important inhibitory neurotransmitter after GABA. In addition, two-pore domain K^+ channels, which modulate baseline neuronal excitability, are activated by inhalation anesthetic agents.

Nitrous oxide, xenon, and ketamine act by antagonism of the excitatory N-methyl-D-aspartate (NMDA) subtype of glutamate receptors. Despite the effects of general anesthetic agents on Ca^{2+}, Na^+, and K^+ channels at high concentrations, neuronal voltage-gated channels are largely insensitive to the effects of anesthetic agents. However, direct effects on voltage-gated Ca^{2+} and K^+ channels may underlie anesthetic effects in the heart, including the negative inotropic and chronotropic effects and proarrhythmogenic properties. Ischemic preconditioning correlates with anesthetic effects on ATP (adenosine triphosphate)-sensitive K^+ channels.

Cellular Effects

Modulation of ion channels present in the membranes of excitable cells, including neurons, determines the effect of an anesthetic agent. Anesthetic effects on ion channels likely result from direct effects on hydrophobic pockets within transmembrane proteins rather than effects at the lipid membrane or lipid-protein interface.

Synaptic transmission is sensitive to the effects of anesthetic agents. Inhalation anesthetic agents potentiate inhibitory neurotransmission acting on GABA or glycine receptors and inhibit excitatory transmission acting on NMDA receptors. Synaptic transmission may be affected at both presynaptic and postsynaptic sites (see Figure 60-2). Presynaptically, anesthetic agents decrease neurotransmitter release to a small degree, probably by decreasing Ca^{2+} entry into cells. Postsynaptically, anesthetic agents potentiate inhibitory currents, block excitatory neurotransmission, or both. Anesthetic agents may also act at extrajunctional GABA receptors and K^+ channels that modulate neuronal function, causing cell hyperpolarization and, thus, reduced neuronal excitability. However, axonal conduction is not altered by clinically relevant concentrations of anesthetic agents.

Central Nervous System Effects

Consistent with their effects at the molecular and cellular level, anesthetic drugs have been shown to exert inhibitory and excitatory effects on various CNS structures. These varying effects depend on whether synaptic transmission is blocked or enhanced at inhibitory or excitatory nuclei in the CNS. Indeed, increasing evidence from studies using clinically relevant concentrations of anesthetic agents suggests a selective mechanism of anesthetic action on a limited number of CNS targets. In general, anesthetic agents inhibit the brainstem reticular formation, resulting in loss of consciousness. Inhibitory effects at the spinal cord mediate the anesthetic-induced lack of movement in response to surgical stimuli and pain. At low concentrations, anesthetic agents also have excitatory supraspinal effects, resulting in euphoria, excitation, and hyperreflexia. The interaction between inhibitory and excitatory effects on various CNS structures determines the behavioral and physiologic changes observed during anesthesia. In summary, although anesthetic agents may act at a molecular and cellular level on different ion channels, anesthetic agents may result in similar effects on neuronal pathways, e.g., interrupting thalamocortical connectivity and, thus, eliminating transmission of sensory stimuli to the cortex.

Suggested Readings

Campagna JA, Miller KW, Forman SA. Mechanisms of actions of inhaled anesthetics. *N Engl J Med*. 2003;348:2110-2124.

Franks NP. General anaesthesia: From molecular targets to neuronal pathways of sleep and arousal. *Nat Rev Neurosci*. 2008;9:370-386.

Franks NP. Molecular targets underlying general anaesthesia. *Br J Pharmacol*. 2006;147(Suppl 1):S72-81.

Mihic SJ, Ye Q, Wick MJ, et al. Sites of alcohol and volatile anaesthetic action on $GABA_A$ and glycine receptors. *Nature*. 1997;389:385-388.

CHAPTER 61

Factors Affecting Anesthetic Gas Uptake

David P. Shapiro, MD

Uptake

The solubility of the inhalation anesthetic agent, the patient's cardiac output, and the partial pressure difference of the gas between the alveoli and pulmonary vein are the three major factors affecting uptake and distribution. Their relationship is expressed by the formula:

$$\text{Uptake} = \lambda \cdot Q \cdot \frac{P_A - P_{\bar{v}}}{P_B}$$

where λ is solubility, Q is the cardiac output, $P_A - P_{\bar{v}}$ is the alveolar-venous partial pressure difference, and P_B is the barometric pressure.

Solubility

The solubility of an anesthetic agent is defined by its blood-gas partition coefficient. It describes the relative affinity of an inhaled anesthetic agent for the blood. For example, isoflurane has a blood-gas partition coefficient of 1.4. This means that, at equilibrium, the isoflurane concentration in the blood would be 1.4 times the concentration in the gas (alveolar) phase. By definition, the partial pressures of the agent in blood and gas are identical at equilibrium, but the blood would contain more isoflurane. The blood-gas partition coefficients of commonly used inhalation anesthetic agents are listed in Table 61-1.

The higher the blood-gas partition coefficient, the greater the amount of anesthetic agent dissolved in blood at equilibrium, and onset of anesthesia is delayed because it is *not* the total amount of drug in the blood, but the partial pressure of inhalation agent in the blood and, therefore, in the brain that induces anesthesia. For agents with a high coefficient, it takes a relatively long time to "fill the tank" before the partial pressure begins to rise high enough to induce anesthesia. Gases with a high coefficient, because the gas diffuses so quickly into blood, have a relatively low alveolar/inspired gas ratio (F_A/F_I) (Figure 61-1), which also delays onset. Uptake of the more soluble inhalation agents can be increased by anesthetic overpressuring, that is, delivering a concentration of inspired gas two to four times the MAC (minimum alveolar concentration).

Table 61-1 Partition Coefficients at 37°C

Anesthetic Agent	Blood-Gas Partition Coefficient
Desflurane	0.45
Nitrous oxide	0.47
Sevoflurane	0.65
Isoflurane	1.4
Enflurane	1.8
Halothane	2.5
Diethyl ether	12.0
Methoxyflurane	15.0

Modified from Eger EI II. Effect of inspired anesthetic concentration on the rate of rise of alveolar concentration. Anesthesiology. 1963;24:153-157.

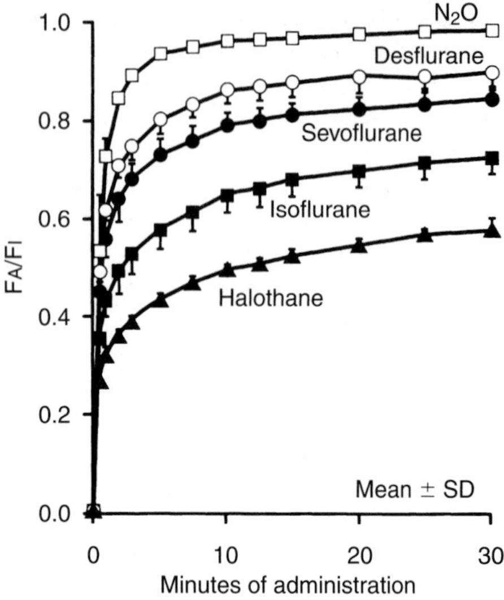

Figure 61-1 The pharmacokinetics of modern inhalation anesthetic agents defined as the ratio of end-tidal anesthetic concentration (FA) to inspired anesthetic concentration (FI) (mean ± SD). The rate of rise of FA/FI over time for most agents correlates inversely with the relative solubility of the anesthetic agents. (From Yasuda N, Lockhart SH, Eger EI, et al. Comparison of kinetics of sevoflurane and isoflurane in humans. Anesth Analg. 1991;72:316-324.)

Cardiac Output

As cardiac output increases, more blood travels through the lungs, thereby removing more anesthetic from the gas phase and resulting in a lower FA and a slower rate of FA increase. Changes in cardiac output have the most pronounced effect on the uptake of more soluble anesthetic gases. The alveolar-venous anesthetic gradient results from tissue uptake. As this gradient approaches 0 and tissues are fully saturated, uptake of anesthetic by the blood ceases, and the FA/FI ratio more rapidly approaches unity.

With decreased cardiac output, less blood flows through the lungs. Less anesthetic agent is taken up by the blood, and alveolar concentration increases more rapidly. Again, highly soluble agents are most affected. With a less soluble anesthetic, the rate of FA/FI increase is rapid regardless of the cardiac output and, thus, is little affected by a decrease in cardiac output. With highly soluble agents, a potentially dangerous positive feedback exists in that anesthetic-induced cardiac depression decreases uptake, increases alveolar concentration, and further depresses cardiac output.

The anesthetic agent in the blood is initially distributed to the vessel-rich tissues (Table 61-2). Soon after blood returns to the lungs, depending on its blood-gas partition coefficient, it has the same partial pressure that it had on leaving the lungs. As the gradient for the uptake of anesthetic approaches 0, less agent is taken up, and alveolar concentration rises (PI ~ PA ~ PBLOOD). Because children have greater perfusion of the vessel-rich group than do adults, FA/FI rises more rapidly in children, so anesthesia is achieved more rapidly in these patients.

Table 61-2 Tissue Group Characteristics

Characteristic	Group			
	Vessel-Rich	Muscle	Fat	Vessel-Poor
Percentage of body mass	10	50	20	20
Perfusion as percentage of cardiac output	75	19	6	0

From Eger EI II. Effect of inspired anesthetic concentration on the rate of rise of alveolar concentration. Anesthesiology. 1963;24:153-157.

An increased functional residual capacity results in slower uptake of the inhalation agent simply because there is a greater volume of lung that must be filled. This volume dilutes the concentration of inhalation agent, therefore slowing induction. Conversely, uptake is more rapid for patients with disease conditions that reduce functional residual capacity.

A ventilation-perfusion mismatch tends to increase the alveolar anesthetic partial pressure and decrease the arterial anesthetic partial pressure. With the less soluble anesthetic agents, the arterial partial pressure of the agent decreases markedly because of mixing with blood from areas with inadequate ventilation. With more highly soluble anesthetic agents, blood from the relatively hyperventilated alveoli contains more anesthetic agent, which compensates for blood emerging from underventilated alveoli, resulting in less effect on the arterial partial pressure.

A left-to-right cardiac shunt in the presence of normal tissue perfusion does not affect anesthetic uptake. With a right-to-left shunt, a fraction of blood does not pass through the lungs and cannot take up anesthetic. This type of shunt results in a slower rate of increase in arterial concentration of anesthetic agent and slower induction of anesthesia, with the least soluble agents affected most.

Ventilation

The PA of an anesthetic agent influences the partial pressure in the brain. The FI of the anesthetic gases and alveolar ventilation are the two factors influencing the rate at which the alveolar concentration of the anesthetic agent increases. Increasing the FI of an inhalation agent or increasing alveolar ventilation facilitates the rate of increase of the anesthetic gas in the alveoli. The rate of FA increase is also influenced by the concentration effect and the second-gas effect.

Concentration effect describes how increasing the FI of a gas produces a more rapid rise in alveolar concentration of that gas. This phenomenon is the sum of two components. The first is confusingly termed the *concentrating effect;* the second is an effective increase in alveolar ventilation.

As the inhalation agent is taken up by the blood, the total lung volume is decreased by the amount of gas taken up by the blood, concentrating (hence, the concentrating effect) the agent remaining within the lung. The magnitude of this effect is influenced by the initial concentration of gas within the lung—the higher the concentration, the greater the effect. For example, when the lung is filled with 1% N_2O, if one half is taken up, then the remaining concentration is 0.5% (0.5 part in 99.5 parts). If the same lung is filled with 80% N_2O and one half is taken up, then the remaining concentration is 67%, not 40% (40 parts in a total of 60).

The effective increase in alveolar ventilation occurs as uptake of N_2O into the blood causes a decrease in volume within the lung, causing additional gas to be drawn in via the trachea to replace N_2O lost by uptake. This decreases the FI/FA concentration difference because inspired gas (as in the second example earlier) contains 80% N_2O, thus further raising the alveolar concentration of N_2O from 67% to 72%.

Second-Gas Effect

The phenomenon known as the *second-gas effect* results from large volumes of a first gas (usually N_2O) being taken up from alveoli, as described in the concentrating effect, increasing the rate of increase in alveolar concentration of the second gas given concomitantly. Factors responsible for the concentration effect also govern the second-gas effect. The effective increase in alveolar ventilation should increase the alveolar concentration of all concomitantly inspired gases regardless of their

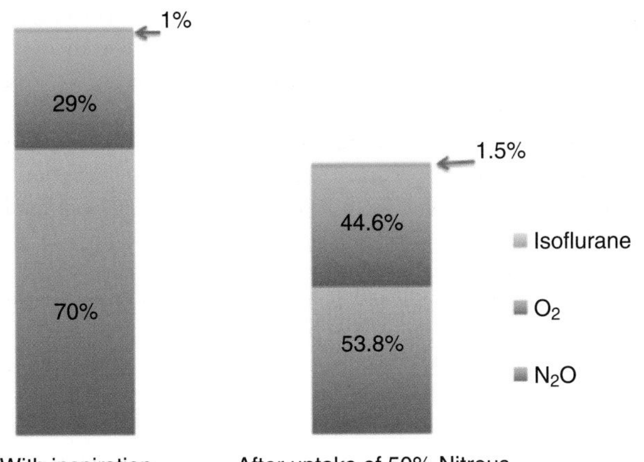

Figure 61-2 A lung is filled with 80% N_2O and 1% of a second gas. Uptake of 50% of the N_2O increases the concentration of the second gas to 1.5%. Restoration of the lung gas volume by addition of more of the original 80% to 1% mixture changes the second-gas concentration to 1.4%. (Reprinted, with permission, from Eger EI II. Effect of inspired anesthetic concentration on the rate of rise of alveolar concentration. Anesthesiology. 1963;24:153-157.)

inspired concentration. Moreover, uptake of the first gas reduces the total gas volume, thereby increasing the concentration of the second gas (Figure 61-2).

The fractional uptake of the second gas determines the relative importance of increased ventilation versus the concentrating effect. Increased ventilation plays the greater role in raising the second-gas concentration when the fraction of the second gas removed by uptake into the blood is large (i.e., with more soluble second gases). The concentrating effect plays the greater role when uptake into the blood is small (i.e., with less soluble agents).

Both the concentration and second-gas effects speed inhalation inductions (i.e., increase the rate of FA/FI increase). Uptake of large volumes of anesthetic agent, usually N_2O, concentrates the remaining gases regardless of whether they are N_2O (concentration effect) or a second gas concomitantly administered (second-gas effect). Uptake of large volumes also increases the effective alveolar ventilation. The concentrating action plus the increase in alveolar ventilation tend to increase the concentration of both N_2O and a second gas.

During hyperventilation, more anesthetic agent is delivered to the lungs, increasing the rate of FA/FI increase. This change is more pronounced with more soluble anesthetic agents because a large portion of highly soluble anesthetic agent delivered to the lungs is taken up by the blood. During hypoventilation, the rate of increase in the alveolar concentration is slowed because of decreased delivery of anesthetic gas to the lungs.

Although acknowledging the usefulness of the original description of the concentration and second-gas effects for teaching purposes, Korman and Mapleson suggested that these explanations are too simplistic and do not consider alternative volume effects of gas uptake. A study by Carette and colleagues in 2007 suggests that the second-gas effect may persist well past the phase of uptake of large volumes of N_2O. It should also be pointed out that a 1999 study by Sun and associates reported that N_2O did not affect the alveolar or blood concentrations of a second gas (enflurane) under controlled constant-volume ventilation (leading the authors to conclude that the second-gas effect is not a valid concept), whereas another study by Taheri and Eger in the same year using N_2O and desflurane effectively demonstrated the predicted effects of the concentration and second-gas effects.

Suggested Readings

Carette R, Hendrickx JFA, Lemmens HJ, DeWolf AM. Large volume N_2O uptake alone does not explain the second gas effect of N_2O on sevoflurane during constant inspired ventilation. *Acta Anaesthesiol Belg*. 2007;58:146.

Eger EI II. *Anesthetic Uptake and Action*. Baltimore: Williams & Wilkins; 1974.

Eger EI II. Effect of inspired anesthetic concentration on the rate of rise of alveolar concentration. *Anesthesiology*. 1963;24:153-157.

Eger EI II. Uptake and distribution. In: Miller RD, ed. *Anesthesia*. 5th ed. Philadelphia: Churchill Livingstone; 2000:74-95.

Korman B, Mapleson WW. Concentration and second gas effects: Can the accepted explanation be improved? *Br J Anaesth*. 1997;78:618-625.

Mapleson WW, Korman B. Concentration and second-gas effects in the water analogue. *Br J Anaesth*. 1998;81:837-843.

Stoelting RK, Eger EI II. An additional explanation for the second gas effect: A concentrating effect. *Anesthesiology*. 1969;30:273-277.

Sun X, Su F, Shi YQ, Lee C. The "second gas effect" is not a valid concept. *Anesth Analg*. 1999;88:188-192.

Taheri S, Eger EI II. A demonstration of the concentration and second gas effect in humans anesthetized with nitrous oxide and desflurane. *Anesth Analg*. 1999;89:774-780.

Yasuda N, Lockhart SH, Eger EI, et al. Comparison of kinetics of sevoflurane and isoflurane in humans. *Anesth Analg*. 1991;72:316-324.

CHAPTER 62

Minimum Alveolar Concentration

Anna E. Bartunek, MD

Dosing for most drugs is based on mass of drug per kilogram of patient body weight. However, for inhalation anesthetic agents, the mass of drug and patient weight have little to do with the intensity of the drug effect. Therefore, a method for quantifying the amount of inhalation agent necessary for anesthesia has been devised. Minimum alveolar concentration (MAC) is the alveolar concentration of an inhalation anesthetic agent at 1 atm and at steady-state concentration necessary to suppress a gross purposeful movement in 50% of patients in response to a skin incision.

MAC has been determined in different age groups, under different conditions, and for all inhalation anesthetic agents (Table 62-1), allowing for comparison of the potency of the different agents. MAC is inversely related to anesthetic potency and, therefore, with its lipid solubility (Meyer-Overton theory). MAC is analogous to the pharmacologic effective dose (ED_{50}) of drugs.

Important Concepts Related to Minimum Alveolar Concentration

Alveolar Concentration

The MAC value of an inhalation anesthetic agent is expressed as a percentage of its alveolar concentration that, at steady state, should approximate the end-tidal concentration, which is measured continuously throughout anesthesia. Alveolar partial pressure of an anesthetic agent is its fractional pressure in the alveolus. The sum of the partial pressures of all components of the alveolar gas mixture equals the total ambient pressure, which is 1 atm or 760 mm Hg at sea level.

Steady State

At equilibrium, the end-tidal concentration approximates the alveolar concentration, which, in turn, approximates the anesthetic concentration at the anesthetic site of action in the central nervous system. Equilibrium is present when end-tidal, alveolar, blood, and brain anesthetic partial pressures are equal. Based on the high cerebral blood flow and low blood solubility of modern anesthetic agents, equilibration is approached after end-tidal concentration has been kept constant for 10 to 15 min. For example, if at sea level and at equilibrium end-tidal N_2O concentration is 60%, then its partial pressure in the alveolus, blood, and brain equals 0.6 atm or 456 mm Hg.

Ambient Pressure

MAC values are conventionally given as a percentage of alveolar anesthetic concentration at 1 atm. They either have been determined at sea level or, ideally, have been corrected to sea level when determined at higher altitudes. One has to bear in mind that anesthetic potency and uptake are directly related to the partial pressure of the anesthetic agent (see Table 62-1). At higher altitude, as compared with at sea level, the same concentration of an inhalation anesthetic agent will exert a lower partial pressure within the alveolus and, consequently, a reduced anesthetic effect. Modern variable bypass vaporizers compensate for this effect because, although the dials are marked in "percent," partial pressure is what is actually determined. At an altitude at which the pressure is one half of sea level, a variable bypass vaporizer set to 1% would deliver 2%, though the actual partial pressure of anesthetic agent delivered would be the same. For example, at sea level, with a barometric pressure of 760 mm Hg, the partial pressure of the agent would be 7.6 mm Hg; at an altitude with a barometric pressure of 380 mm Hg, a variable bypass vaporizer set at 1% would actually deliver 2% of the agent (2% of 380 = 7.6 mm Hg partial vapor pressure).

Stimulus

Skin incision is the standard stimulus used to define MAC in humans. As the intensity of the stimulus decreases, so too does the MAC necessary to block a defined response: intubation > skin incision > tetanic stimulation > laryngoscopy > trapezius squeeze > vocal command.

Response

A positive response, in the classic determination of anesthetic potency, is gross purposeful muscular movement of the head or extremities. Other responses can be eye opening to command or sympathetic adrenergic reaction (increase in blood pressure and heart rate) to noxious stimuli (see later in this chapter).

Determination of Minimum Alveolar Concentration

MAC can be determined in humans by anesthetizing them with the inhalation anesthetic agent alone in O_2 and allowing 15 min for equilibration at a preselected target end-tidal concentration. A single skin incision is made, and the patient is observed for the presence or absence of purposeful movement. A group of patients must be tested in this fashion over a range of anesthetic

Table 62-1 Minimum Alveolar Concentration (MAC) and MAC_{awake} of Inhalation Anesthetics at Ambient Pressure of 760 mm Hg

	Isoflurane	Desflurane	Sevoflurane	N_2O	Xenon
MAC in O_2 (vol%)	1.3	6.0	2.1	105	71
MAC in 70% N_2O and 30% O_2 (vol%)	0.6	2.5	0.7	—	—
MAC Awake (vol%)	0.4	2.4	0.6	71	33
MAC in O_2 (mm Hg)	9.7	45.6	15.6	798	540

concentrations that allows and prevents patient movement. The percentage of patients in groups of four or more that show a positive response to surgical stimulation is plotted against the average alveolar concentration for that group. Drawing a best-fit line through these points results in the concentration at which half of the subjects move with skin incision and thus MAC is determined. Another approach is to plot the individual end-tidal anesthetic concentrations against the probability of no response by nonlinear regression analysis. This results in a typical dose-response curve, whereas the concentration that corresponds to the 0.5 probability of no response estimates the MAC value.

Dose-Response Relationship

The dose-response curve allows for an extrapolation to that anesthetic concentration at which 95% of the patients do not respond to the applied noxious stimulus with movement. Although the ED_{95} seems to be the more clinically relevant value, it is seldom used to describe the anesthetic potency. The dose-response curves for inhalation anesthetic agents are steep; 1 MAC prevents skeletal muscle movement on incision in 50% of patients, whereas 1.3 MAC prevents movement in 99% of patients (ED_{99}). The dose-response curves for different inhalation anesthetic agents are parallel, implying that they share a common mechanism or site of action. This observation is supported by the fact that MAC values are additive. If 0.7 MAC N_2O is administered with 0.7 MAC isoflurane, the resulting effect is 1.4 MAC.

Factors Affecting Minimum Alveolar Concentration

Numerous physiologic and pharmacologic factors, disease states, and conditions can change the anesthetic sensitivity and, therefore, raise or lower MAC (Table 62-2). Not all the underlying mechanisms are yet clear (decrease of MAC in pregnancy or increase in redheads). Nevertheless, anesthetic requirements seem to correlate with cerebral metabolic rate, whereas factors decreasing cerebral metabolic rate (temperature, age, severe hypoxia, hypotension, various drugs) decrease MAC.

MAC is age dependent (Figure 62-1). The MAC value is highest in infants 3 to 6 months of age. For patients older than 1 year, MAC decreases by approximately 6% to 7% with each increasing decade of life.

MAC decreases linearly with decreasing temperature; a 1° C decrease in body temperature reduces anesthetic requirement by approximately 4% to 5%. Factors that do not change MAC include duration of anesthesia, arterial blood pressure greater than 50 mm Hg, sex, and patient size.

Anesthetic Requirement to Blunt Responses to Various Stimuli

The classic MAC value gives a measure of the anesthetic requirement to suppress movement to skin incision. MAC variants have been determined in an effort to define the optimal concentrations of inhalation anesthetic agents to allow for various clinically essential stimuli, such as laryngoscopy, intubation, laryngeal mask insertion, laryngeal mask removal, and extubation. The MAC variants are often depicted as multiples or fractions of the classic MAC value.

MAC_{awake} is the concentration of an inhaled anesthetic agent at which half of patients will open their eyes to command. It is an index of the hypnotic potency of an inhaled anesthetic agent. The knowledge of MAC_{awake} is helpful to prevent intraoperative awareness. The MAC_{awake} is approximately one third of MAC for isoflurane, desflurane, and sevoflurane but is higher for N_2O and xenon (see Table 62-1). Differences in the ratio of MAC to MAC_{awake} among different anesthetic agents probably reflect different mechanisms of action. The decrease of MAC_{awake} with age is parallel to that of MAC itself. Drugs that suppress central nervous system activity (e.g., fentanyl and clonidine) reduce the MAC_{awake}.

The MAC necessary to blunt the adrenergic or cardiovascular response in 50% of individuals who have a skin incision is known as the MAC_{BAR}.

Table 62-2 Impact of Pharmacologic Agents and Physiologic Factors on Minimum Alveolar Concentration (MAC)

Decreased MAC ↓	MAC ↑
Medications	
Opioids	Inhibition of catecholamine reuptake (amphetamines, ephedrine)
Benzodiazepines	
Barbiturates	
Propofol	
Ketamine	
α_2-Agonists	
Intravenously administered local anesthetic agents	
Alcohol	
Acute ethanol ingestion	Chronic ethanol abuse
Physiologic Conditions	
Increasing age for patients >1 year of age	In the first months of life for infants <6 months of age
Pregnancy	
Pathophysiologic Conditions	
Hypothermia	Hyperthermia
Severe hypotension	Hyperthyroidism
Severe hypoxemia	Increased extracellular Na^+ in central nervous system
Severe anemia	
Acute metabolic acidosis	
Sepsis	
Genetic Factors	
None established*†	Genotype related to red hair

*Gender does not change MAC except in elderly Japanese population in whom MAC might be slightly lower in women.
†No good data comparing MAC in different ethnic groups exist.

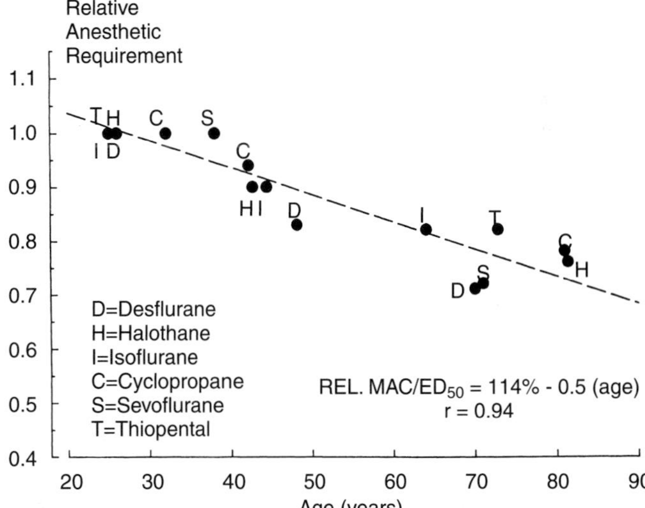

Figure 62-1 Anesthetic requirements decrease with advancing age. Dose is expressed as minimum alveolar concentration (MAC) for inhalation anesthetic agents and as the relative median effective dose (ED_{50}) for intravenously administered agents. (From Muravchick S. Anesthesia for the elderly. In: Miller RD, ed. Anesthesia. 5th ed. Philadelphia: Churchill Livingstone; 2000:2140-2156.)

However, different harmful stimuli result in different degrees of hemodynamic responses, with intubation being more noxious than skin incision. The prevention of sympathetic stimulation and hemodynamic responses (heart rate and blood pressure increase) during surgery is especially important in patients with coronary heart disease. The MAC_{BAR} typically is considerably greater than the classic MAC value. This creates a conundrum for the clinician; administering a MAC_{BAR} to produce acceptable hemodynamic response during periods of intense surgical stimulation results in unacceptably low blood pressure during times when there is minimal stimulation. Opioids, even in small doses, and N_2O markedly decrease the MAC_{BAR}. This effect is the reason why N_2O and opioids are frequently coadministered with halogenated anesthetics as part of a "balanced" anesthetic.

The anesthetic concentrations that allow laryngoscopy (LS), intubation (IT), and laryngeal mask insertion (LMI) in 50% of individuals are defined as MAC_{LS}, MAC_{IT}, and MAC_{LMI}. The MAC_{IT} values are about 30% greater than the classic MAC values. The MAC_{IT} and MAC_{LMI} for sevoflurane have been extensively studied because inhaled sevoflurane is frequently used to induce anesthesia in children.

Clinical Relevance

By definition, 1 MAC of an inhaled anesthetic agent alone is insufficient to provide adequate anesthesia because half of patients will respond with movement after skin incision. Nevertheless, the MAC value became the principal measure to compare the potencies of different inhalation agents. Consequently, the applied dose of an inhaled anesthetic agent often is stated in multiples or fractions of MAC. Several gas analyzers convert end-tidal concentrations of inhalation agents to MAC values; the monitor either adjusts for age and body temperature or assumes a default state of 40 years of age and a normal body temperature.

Owing to the many identified and unidentified factors affecting MAC (see Table 62-2), individual anesthetic requirements vary widely. It is therefore important to remember that MAC is an average value for a selected population rather than an absolute value for each individual.

Suggested Readings

Eger EI II. Age, minimum alveolar anesthetic concentration, and minimum alveolar anesthetic concentration-awake. *Anesth Analg*. 2001;93:947-953.

Eisenkraft JB. Anesthesia delivery system. In: Longnecker DE, Brown DL, Newman MF, eds. *Anesthesiology*. New York: McGraw-Hill; 2008:767-820.

Forman SA, Mashour GA. Pharmacology of inhalational anesthetics. In: Longnecker DE, Brown DL, Newman MF, eds. *Anesthesiology*. New York: McGraw-Hill; 2008:739-766.

Quasha AL, Eger EI, Tinker JH. Determination and applications of MAC. *Anesthesiology*. 1980;53:315-334.

Zbinden AM, Petersen-Felix S, Thomson DA, et al. Anesthetic depth defined using multiple noxious stimuli during isoflurane/oxygen anesthesia. II. Hemodynamic responses. *Anesthesiology*. 1994;80:261-267.

CHAPTER 63

Effect of Intracardiac Shunts on Inhalation Induction

David J. Cook, MD, and Eduardo S. Rodrigues, MD

Intracardiac shunts may alter the rate of induction of inhaled anesthetic agents. This alteration depends on the direction and size of the shunt and on the solubility of the anesthetic agent used.

Induction of anesthesia is a function of the equilibration of three factors: the rate of anesthetic inflow into the lungs and equilibration with alveolar gas (as determined by tidal volume, respiratory rate, inspired fraction of anesthetic agent, and functional residual capacity), the rate of transfer of the anesthetic agent from lungs to arterial blood, and the rate of transfer of the anesthetic agent from blood to brain:

$$P_A \leftrightarrow Pa \leftrightarrow Pb$$

where P_A equals the alveolar partial pressure of the inhaled anesthetic agent; Pa, the arterial partial pressure of the inhaled anesthetic agent; and Pb, the brain partial pressure of the inhaled anesthetic agent. $P\bar{v}$ equals the mixed venous partial pressure of the inhaled anesthetic agent.

Cardiac shunts primarily alter the effect of the uptake of the anesthetic agent by pulmonary arterial blood. The determinants of anesthetic uptake from alveoli are the blood-gas partition coefficient of the anesthetic agent, the cardiac output (CO), and the alveolar to mixed venous partial pressure difference of the anesthetic agent ($P_A - P\bar{v}$).

The blood-gas partition coefficient is the distribution ratio of the anesthetic agent between blood and alveolar gas at equilibrium (relative solubility). For a highly soluble agent, it usually takes several passes of the blood volume through the lung before enough of the agent is absorbed that the blood is saturated to the point that the necessary Pa of the agent to achieve anesthesia is reached. A highly soluble agent, then, has a much slower induction time, compared with an agent that is not soluble (see following discussion). Assuming no change in ventilation or inspired fraction of anesthetic agent and normal tissue perfusion, the rate of induction is determined primarily by anesthetic solubility and the effective pulmonary blood flow.

Right-to-Left Shunt

With a right-to-left shunt, a portion of the CO bypasses the lung, slowing induction because less anesthetic agent can be transferred from the alveoli to systemic blood per unit of time. The rate of induction for an insoluble agent

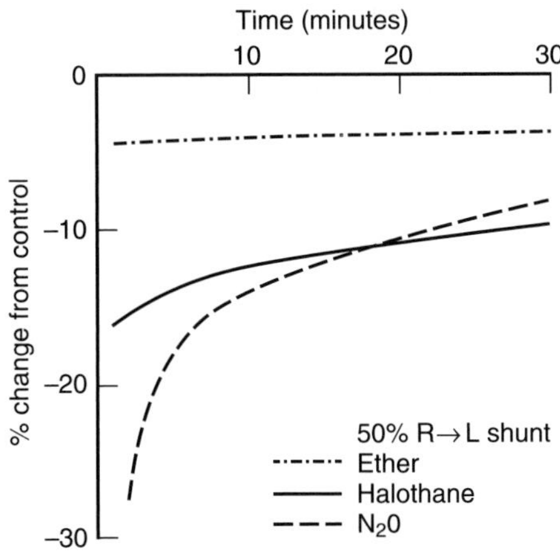

Figure 63-1 Decrease in arterial-to-inspired concentration ratio caused by a 50% right-to-left shunt from control for three anesthetic agents of different solubility (ether, halothane, and N_2O). (From Tanner G. Effect of left-to-right, mixed left-to-right, and right-to-left shunts on inhalation induction in children: A computer model. Anesth Analg. 1985;64:101-107.)

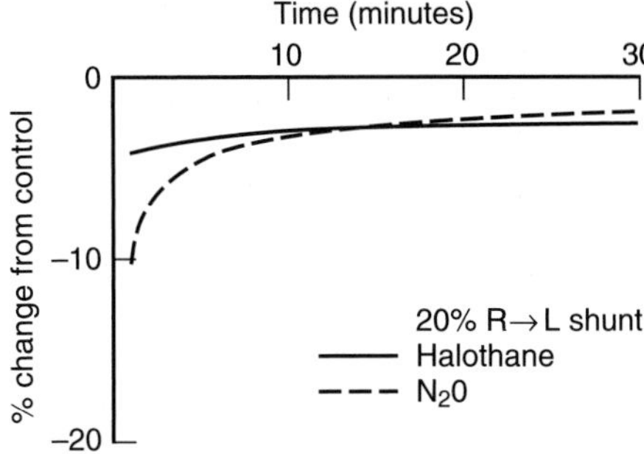

Figure 63-2 Decrease in arterial-to-inspired concentration ratio from control for two anesthetic agents (halothane and N_2O) caused by a 20% right-to-left shunt. (From Tanner G. Effect of left-to-right, mixed left-to-right, and right-to-left shunts on inhalation induction in children: A computer model. Anesth Analg. 1985;64:101-107.)

is proportional to the degree of shunting (i.e., the greater the shunt, the slower induction). The impact of the shunt is less pronounced for a soluble anesthetic agent. Using ether as an example, with a blood-gas partition coefficient of 12, 1 L of blood would have to absorb 12 times more ether than 1 L of gas. If ventilation were 5 L/min with 10% ether, then 500 mL of ether would be delivered to the alveoli per minute. At equilibrium, the entire blood volume would have to absorb 6 L of ether before equilibrium was reached. In this scenario, ventilation slows induction because only 0.5 L of ether is delivered to the alveoli; it would take 12 min for 6 L to be delivered to the alveoli. If there were a 50% right-to-left shunt and pulmonary blood flow was only 2.5 L (half of the "normal" 5 L/min), pulmonary blood flow would still take up the 0.5 L of ether.

However, for a poorly soluble anesthetic agent (e.g., N_2O, with a blood-gas partition coefficient of 0.47), if ventilation is 5 L/min with 50% N_2O, then 2.5 L of N_2O is delivered to the alveoli per minute. The entire blood volume would have to absorb approximately 1.25 L of N_2O before equilibrium was reached. If the patient had a 50% shunt, the 2.5 L of blood flowing through the lungs would absorb 1.25 L of N_2O but would then mix with the 2.5 L of blood that bypassed the lung, resulting in a concentration of only 0.625 L of N_2O. Induction time would take at least twice as long.

These examples demonstrate that, with highly soluble agents, such as ether, uptake is limited primarily by ventilation. With poorly soluble agents, such as N_2O, uptake is limited primarily by blood flow. Subsequently, the impact of shunting is greater with agents of lower solubility (Figures 63-1 and 63-2).

Left-to-Right Shunt

With a left-to-right shunt, no significant change occurs in the speed of induction, assuming that systemic blood flow is normal. If tissue perfusion is decreased because of the left-to-right shunt, then induction will initially be slowed because less anesthetic agent will be delivered to the brain per unit of time. CO usually increases to compensate for the shunting, and local control of vasculature maintains cerebral perfusion and minimizes the effect of the shunt (Figure 63-3).

Mixed Shunt (Right-to-Left and Left-to-Right)

A left-to-right shunt attenuates the slowed anesthetic induction that may occur with right-to-left shunting because of an increase in effective pulmonary blood flow.

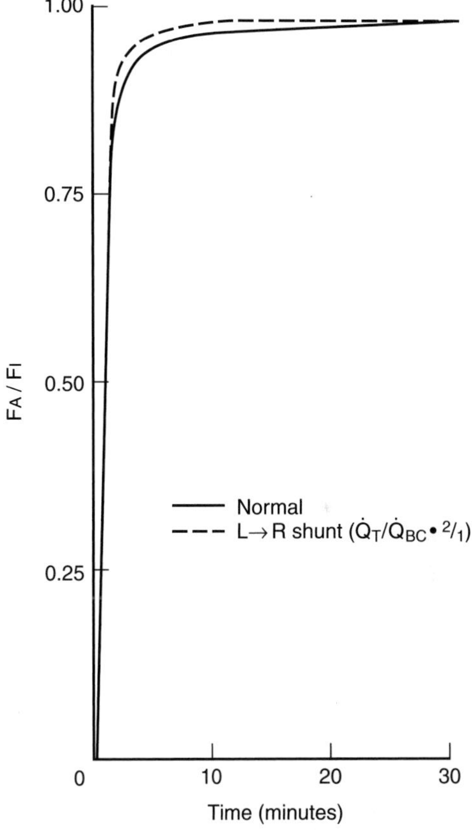

Figure 63-3 Arterial-to-inspired concentration (FA/FI) ratio for N_2O modeled with and without a 50% left-to-right shunt and normal tissue perfusion. For the normal simulation, $\dot{Q}_{BC}$ = 3.0 L/min, $\dot{Q}_T$ = 3.16 L/min, $\dot{Q}_{LR}$ = 0.16 L/min, and $\dot{Q}_S$ = 0.16 L/min. For the left-to-right shunt simulation, $\dot{Q}_{BC}$ = 3.0 L/min, $\dot{Q}_T$ = 6.0 L/min, $\dot{Q}_{LR}$ = 3.0 L/min, and $\dot{Q}_S$ = 0.3 L/min. $\dot{Q}_{BC}$, Blood flow perfusing body compartments; $\dot{Q}_{LR}$, left-to-right shunt; $\dot{Q}_S$, right-to-left shunt; $\dot{Q}_T$, total cardiac output. (From Tanner G. Effect of left-to-right, mixed left-to-right, and right-to-left shunts on inhalation induction in children: A computer model. Anesth Analg. 1985;64:101-107.)

Suggested Readings

Eger EI II. *Anesthetic Uptake and Action*. Baltimore: Williams & Wilkins; 1974.

Tanner G. Effect of left-to-right, mixed left-to-right, and right-to-left shunts on inhalation induction in children: A computer model. *Anesth Analg*. 1985; 64:101-107.

CHAPTER 64

Inhalation Anesthetic Agents

Bradley Anderson, MD, and Michael J. Murray, MD, PhD

The inhaled anesthetic agents form a cornerstone for modern anesthetic delivery. Their roots run deep into medical history as they have helped pave the way toward modern-day surgical procedures. Today, four main inhaled anesthetic agents are in use in the United States: N_2O, isoflurane, sevoflurane, and desflurane. Each possesses differing characteristics in their relative pharmacokinetic and pharmacodynamic profiles, making them uniquely suitable for use in different situations.

Originally used in nineteenth-century dentistry, N_2O, a colorless gas at room temperature, is commonly referred to as *laughing gas*. Although N_2O is not often used today, when it is used, it is in combination with other inhalation anesthetic agents rather than as a sole agent.

Desflurane, sevoflurane, and isoflurane are all fluorinated inhalation anesthetic agents. Compared with ether, inhalation anesthetic agents that have been halogenated with fluorine have reduced flammability as well as greater molecular stability. The use of desflurane and sevoflurane is gradually replacing that of older inhalation anesthetic agents because desflurane and sevoflurane result in the fastest and second-fastest respectively, induction and emergence times (because of their low blood solubility).

Pharmacokinetics

The pharmacokinetics of a drug refers to its absorption, distribution, excretion, and metabolism inside the body. For inhaled anesthetic agents, absorption is accomplished through the alveoli in the lungs. As these drugs are inhaled, they are exposed to the rich vascular supply of the lungs (i.e. the pulmonary capillary beds), where they are absorbed and distributed systemically. The partial pressure of the inhalation anesthetic agent in the central nervous system (PCNS) is proportional to the arterial partial pressure (Pa), which, in turn, is proportional to the alveolar pressure (PA) at equilibrium. Therefore, at equilibrium, the PCNS is directly proportional to the PA.

Uptake

The uptake of an anesthetic agent from the lung into the bloodstream is dependent on three main factors (excluding the concentration and second-gas effects) (Box 64-1). The first is the alveolar–mixed venous partial pressure difference $P(A - \bar{v})$. The next is the solubility of the anesthetic agent in the blood, defined as the blood-gas partition coefficient (λ), and the last is cardiac output (CO). Using these factors, a simple calculation can be used to help determine the uptake of any given inhaled anesthetic agent. From this equation, it is apparent that, if any of the three factors is increased, the result will be a larger uptake of the anesthetic agent:

$$\text{Uptake} = P(A - \bar{v}) \times \lambda \times CO$$

Box 64-1 Factors Affecting the Uptake of an Anesthetic Agent into the Bloodstream

- Alveolar–venous partial pressure difference
- Solubility of the anesthetic agent in the blood
- Cardiac output

Excretion

Excretion of inhalation anesthetic agents relies on both alveolar ventilation and urinary and gastrointestinal elimination of byproducts of metabolism. During emergence, as ventilation increases, so too does the amount of anesthetic agent removed from the body. Metabolism of the inhaled anesthetic agents varies and, as such, has variable effects on the rate of decrease of the PA. For highly metabolized anesthetic agents, alveolar ventilation plays less of a role in the elimination of the inhaled anesthetic agents, but it is still the primary means of excretion.

Distribution

Tissues inside the body vary greatly in their relative blood flow distributions. Tissues that receive the greatest perfusion are labeled the vessel-rich group and include the brain, heart, liver, and kidneys. Although the vessel-rich group makes up about 10% of the total body mass, these organs receive an overwhelming majority of the CO. The muscle group and fat group come in second and third place, respectively, in their blood flow distributions. These tissues receive smaller fractions of the CO even though they make up a much larger proportion of body mass.

Minimum Alveolar Concentration

Minimum alveolar concentration (MAC), the concentration of an inhalation anesthetic agent that will prevent movement in response to a surgical stimulus in 50% of patients, is expressed as a percentage of the partial pressure of the anesthetic drug in relation to the barometric pressure. More simply stated, if the MAC of isoflurane is 1.14 at sea level, the partial pressure of isoflurane at steady state must be 0.0114 × 760 mm Hg, which is 8.66 mm Hg. For N_2O with a MAC of 104, the partial pressure would be 790.4 mm Hg—a partial pressure that could only be obtained under hyperbaric conditions. Using this terminology, inhalation anesthetic agents can be compared using multiples of MAC (e.g., 0.5, 1.0, 1.2) to express their relevant effects at a given concentration. It is far easier to compare inhalation anesthetic agents in terms of their MAC than their partial pressures, which can vary greatly, depending on the agent, the altitude, and other factors.

Just as a MAC can be determined for the absence of a response to surgical stimulus, the MAC can also be determined for additional depths of anesthesia. For example, the MACs needed to prevent verbal as well as autonomic responses have been identified. Conveniently, the standard deviation of the MAC is approximately 10%; therefore, 1.2 MAC is roughly

Table 64-1 Pharmacologic Characteristics of Inhalation Anesthetic Agents

	Agent			
Characteristic	**N_2O**	**Desflurane**	**Sevoflurane**	**Isoflurane**
Molecular weight	44.02	168.04	200.05	184.5
MAC	104	6.0	2.05	1.14
Partition coefficient				
Blood-gas	0.47	0.42	0.63	1.4
Brain-blood	1.1	1.3	1.7	1.6
Muscle-blood	1.2	2.0	3.1	2.9
Fat-blood	2.3	27	48	45

MAC, minimum alveolar concentration.

the concentration required to prevent response to a surgical stimulus in 97% of patients.

When fluorinated hydrocarbon agents are used in combination with N_2O, their MACs are additive. For example, if a patient inhales 0.75 MAC of N_2O, then only 0.25 MAC of a second inhalation anesthetic (e.g., isoflurane) is required to achieve a combined MAC of 1.0.

Blood-Gas Partition Coefficient

The λ describes the relative solubility of an anesthetic agent in blood, compared with its solubility in a gas (Table 64-1). Simply put, it is the concentration of anesthetic agent in the blood divided by the concentration in gas when the two phases are in equilibrium with one another. Soluble anesthetic agents, or ones that have a high λ, have higher concentrations in the blood phase than in the gas phase. Therefore, for a soluble anesthetic agent to exert a partial pressure in the blood phase equal to that of the gas phase, a relatively large number of molecules must be absorbed into the blood, translating into a slower rate of rise of the PA.

Just as the λ describes the solubility of anesthetic agents in blood compared with solubility in gas, the tissue-blood coefficient is used to describe the solubility of anesthetic agents in tissue, compared with their solubility in blood. Tissues with high tissue-blood coefficients (e.g., fat) require more molecules of anesthetic agent to be dissolved into them for equilibrium with the blood to be reached.

Concentration Effect and Second-Gas Effect

When anesthetic agents are combined, two phenomena—known as the *concentration effect* and *second-gas effect*—occur. When N_2O is delivered in combination with other gases, the higher the inspired N_2O concentration is, the faster the alveolar concentrations of N_2O and the other gases will approach their respective inspired concentrations (PI concentration effect) (Figure 64-1). For example, patients receiving a PI of 80% N_2O will experience a more rapid increase in their PA/PI ratio, as compared with patients receiving 60% N_2O. As pulmonary capillary blood removes N_2O from the alveoli, the gases in the anatomic dead space (e.g., bronchi) will be entrained into the alveoli, which results in an even faster rise in the alveolar concentration of the agent (second-gas effect).

Shunts

Right-to-left intracardiac shunts slow the rate of rise of the anesthetic PA during induction. This delay is due to the dilution of pulmonary blood entering the left side of the heart with venous blood that has not been exposed to the inhalation anesthetic agent within the lungs. Right-to-left intracardiac shunts therefore slow an inhalation induction.

Left-to-right intracardiac shunts deliver pulmonary blood containing inhalation anesthetic agents back to the pulmonary circulation for a second pass. As a result, a smaller amount of inhalation anesthetic agent diffuses from the alveoli to capillary blood. From a clinical standpoint, the induction rate is unchanged if there is only a left-to-right shunt. However, when combined right-to-left and left-to-right intracardiac shunts are present, depending on the anatomic location and size of the shunts, left-to-right shunts can affect induction times. The normally delayed induction experienced with a right-to-left shunt can be offset by a left-to-right shunt because unsaturated blood from the right side going into the left side has the opportunity to pass back to the right side, perfuse alveoli, and take up anesthetic drug.

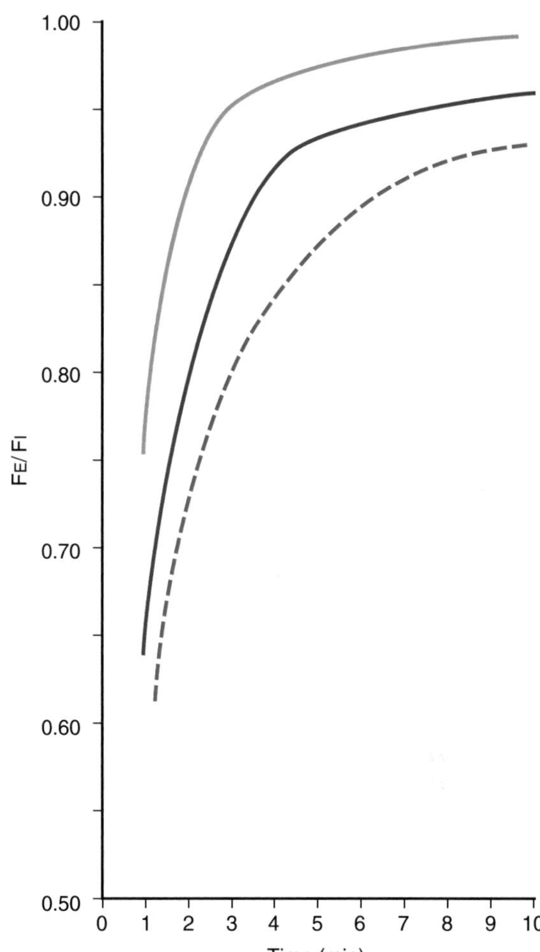

Figure 64-1 The concentration effect. By raising the concentration of inhaled N_2O, the rate of rise of the end-tidal (FE) concentration in relation to the inspired (FI) concentration is increased. The dashed, blue, and green lines correspond with 10%, 50%, and 85% concentrations, respectively. (From Eger EI. Effect of inspired anesthetic concentration on the rate of rise of alveolar concentration. Anesthesiology. 1963;24:153-157.)

Alveolar—Mixed Venous Partial Pressure Difference

The relationship between the PA compared with the partial pressure of gases in the mixed venous blood returning to the lungs ($P\bar{v}$) is known as the alveolar–mixed venous partial pressure difference: $P(A - \bar{v})$. During induction, the $P(A - \bar{v})$ is at its highest. Blood has not yet been exposed to anesthetic agents, and the high PA created by the inhaled gases leads to a large $P(A - \bar{v})$. Over time, more anesthetic agent in the alveoli equilibrates with pulmonary capillary blood until, eventually, blood returning to the lungs carries back some of the anesthetic agent, resulting in a smaller $P(A - \bar{v})$. As various tissues in the body become more saturated, the $P\bar{v}$ increases even further, and the amount of anesthetic agent taken up at the alveolar-capillary interface progressively declines because of the decrease in the P(A − v̄). This decrease in anesthetic uptake necessitates a decrease in the amount of anesthetic agent administered to the patient over time.

The Effect of CO on Uptake and Emergence

CO plays a major role in the uptake and induction time of inhaled anesthetic agents: uptake of the inhaled anesthetic agent is directly proportional to the CO. With a greater CO, more blood is delivered into the pulmonary capillary beds per unit of time; more blood absorbs more anesthetic agent, slowing the rate of rise of the agent and its pressure within the alveoli (Pa). Similarly, in patients with a high CO, even though more anesthetic agent is absorbed, it is dissolved in a larger volume of blood, leading to a lower Pa (and thus a lower PCNS) of the inhaled agent. In patients with a low CO, the opposite occurs: blood spends more time in the pulmonary circulation, allowing for the anesthetic agent to equilibrate with the smaller volume of blood, and the anesthetic agent in the alveoli achieves steady state more quickly. Because the PA of the drug reaches equilibrium more quickly, so too does the Pa of the blood, and as this blood is delivered to the tissues, it translates into a more rapid rise in the PCNS.

Suggested Readings

Eger EI, Saidman LJ. Illustrations of inhalation anesthetic uptake, including intertissue diffusion to and from fat. *Anesth Analg*. 2005;100:1020-1033.
Eger EI, Stoelting RK. An additional explanation for the second gas effect: A concentrating effect. *Anesthesiology*. 1969;30:273-277.
Giorgio T. Inhalation anesthetics: A review. *Minerva Anesth*. 2010;75:215-228.

CHAPTER 65

Nitrous Oxide

Renee E. Caswell, MD

Nitrous oxide (N_2O), a colorless, inorganic, odorless gas is not flammable but will support combustion as actively as does O_2. It is relatively insoluble, with a blood-gas partition coefficient of 0.47 and is the least potent inhalation anesthetic agent used in practice, with a minimum alveolar concentration of 104%. N_2O is most often used in concentrations of 50% to 70% as an adjuvant to more potent inhaled anesthetic agents or in addition to intravenously administered anesthetic agents. N_2O does not produce skeletal muscle relaxation but does have analgesic effects. It has been used in clinical anesthetic practice for more than 150 years. Despite this long record of use, controversy and concern continue to exist regarding the effect of N_2O on cellular function via inactivation of vitamin B_{12}, expansion or increased pressure of air-filled spaces, effects on embryonic development, and effect on postoperative nausea and vomiting.

Systemic Effects

Respiratory System

N_2O decreases tidal volume and increases respiratory rate in spontaneously breathing patients and reduces the ventilatory response to CO_2 and hypoxia.

Central Nervous System

Although not a potent anesthetic, N_2O has good analgesic properties. Maximum analgesic effects are noted at a concentration of 35%; when N_2O is administered at a concentration of 75%, half of patients are unaware of their surroundings. Concentrations exceeding 60% can increase cerebral blood flow and potentially increase intracranial pressure.

Cardiovascular System

Compared with other inhalation agents, N_2O has only minimal cardiovascular effects. The slight direct myocardial depression is usually offset by sympathetic stimulation, so that little effect is observed. Adjuvant opioids can block the sympathomimetic effects of N_2O, and mild circulatory depression can be seen when opioids are used with N_2O. However, despite this scientific rationale, most cardiovascular anesthesiologists avoid the use of N_2O in patients with pulmonary hypertension because of concern about the sympathetic stimulation that may lead to an increase in pulmonary vascular resistance.

Metabolism

N_2O is primarily excreted unchanged through the lungs, with a small amount diffusing through the skin and metabolized in the bowel.

Postoperative Nausea and Vomiting

N_2O may increase the incidence of postoperative nausea and vomiting. In the ENIGMA trial (Evaluation of Nitrous Oxide in the Gas Mixture for Anaesthesia: A Randomised Controlled Trial), the incidence of severe nausea and vomiting within 24 h of surgery was reduced from 23% in the N_2O group to 10% in the N_2O-free group. This result is consistent with findings from other trials.

Toxicity

N_2O inactivates methionine synthase by oxidizing the cobalt in vitamin B_{12}. Methionine synthase is a ubiquitous cytosolic enzyme that plays a crucial role in the synthesis of DNA, RNA, myelin, catecholamines, and other products. Decreased methionine synthase activity can result in both genetic and protein aberrations. Liver biopsies have demonstrated a 50% reduction in methionine synthase activity at 45 to 90 min in patients administered 70% N_2O.

Hematologic and Immune Toxicity

Inhibition of methionine synthase may lead to megaloblastic anemia. N_2O exposure for 2 to 6 h in seriously ill patients can cause megaloblastic bone marrow changes. The elderly are particularly vulnerable to developing this complication because up to 20% of the elderly are deficient in cobalamin. N_2O has also been implicated in impairment of immune function by decreasing neutrophilic chemotaxis and mucociliary transport. The multicenter ENIGMA trial demonstrated postoperative benefits with high concentrations of O_2 (80%), compared with 70% N_2O. Differences included the rates of wound infection, fever, pneumonia, and atelectasis. It is not known whether these differences relate to the high concentrations of inspired O_2, the avoidance of N_2O, or a combination of both.

Occupational Exposure

Retrospective epidemiologic studies have shown an increased incidence of spontaneous abortion in women working in operating rooms. Most of these occupational exposure studies predated the modern use of scavenging and operating room ventilation. Occupational exposure limits for N_2O of 25 to 50 ppm have been established. Occupational exposure limits are expressed as an 8-hour time-weighted average. No cause-and-effect relationship has been proven to support a fetotoxic or genotoxic effect of N_2O exposure in humans.

Neurologic Toxicity

Neurologic injury has been seen in patients with cobalamin deficiency, although the injury may not be apparent for several weeks. In addition, patients with unsuspected vitamin B_{12} deficiency have been diagnosed with myeloneuropathy 2 to 6 weeks after they have received N_2O anesthesia. N_2O abusers can present with altered mental status, paresthesia, ataxia, and weakness and spasticity of the legs. There are no experimental data to suggest that postoperative cognitive dysfunction is attributable to the use of N_2O, although exposure to anesthesia remains a possible risk factor.

Myocardial Effects

The use of N_2O has been associated with increased perioperative myocardial risks. These risks have been attributed to increased homocysteine levels. Further studies are needed to clarify the impact of N_2O on perioperative cardiac outcomes.

N_2O and Closed Air Spaces

N_2O can diffuse into closed air spaces with significant clinical consequences. Although relatively insoluble compared with other anesthetic agents, N_2O is 30 times more soluble than N_2. The blood-gas coefficient of N_2O is 0.47, whereas that of N_2 is 0.015. N_2O diffuses quickly, whereas N_2 diffuses more slowly. As a result, at any given partial pressure, far more N_2O can be carried to or removed from a closed gas space. The air space will expand, increasing volume in distensible spaces, increasing pressure in nondistensible spaces, or causing a combination of both effects.

Compliant Spaces Increase Volume

The maximum change in volume that can result is related to the concentration of N_2O in the alveoli (Figure 65-1):

$$\text{Change in volume (\%)} = \text{FA}N_2O/1 - \text{FA}N_2O$$

$$50\%\ N_2O: \frac{0.5}{1-0.5} = 100\% \uparrow \text{ in volume}$$

$$80\%\ N_2O: \frac{0.8}{1-0.8} = 400\% \uparrow \text{ in volume}$$

Alveolar nitrous oxide concentration = 50%

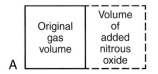

A

Original gas volume

Volume of added nitrous oxide

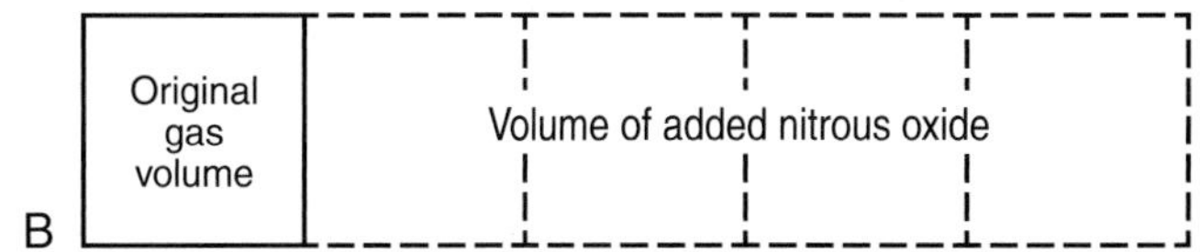

Figure 65-1 Volume changes in a closed space when alveolar N_2O is 50% **(A)** or 80% **(B)**. (From Eger EI II, Saidman LJ. Hazards of nitrous oxide anesthesia in bowel obstruction and pneumothorax. Anesthesiology. 1965;26:61-66.)

Noncompliant Spaces Increase Pressure

The maximum change in pressure is arithmetically related to the partial pressure of N_2O in the alveoli:

50% N_2O increases pressure 0.5 atm
75% N_2O increases pressure 0.75 atm

These principles hold true for any anesthetic gas used, but they are clinically relevant for N_2O because of its low solubility and the high concentrations used (i.e., isoflurane would not have a significant effect on closed air spaces because it is used at only 1% to 2% concentration).

Examples

Bowel Gas and Bowel Obstruction

The bowel usually contains small volumes of gas, so the increase in volume is of no consequence. For example, 100 mL of bowel gas resulting from swallowing and bacteria could increase two to three times without causing clinical problems. On the other hand, the stomach and intestine can contain up to 5 to 10 L of air, and 1 to 2 L of air is not uncommon. Doubling or tripling this volume can crowd the operative field, limit movement of the diaphragm, compromise respiration, make abdominal closure difficult, and increase abdominal pressure during laparoscopy with CO_2 inflation. Even with obstruction, changes in volume occur slowly. Operations lasting less than 1 h will cause only insignificant changes in volume.

Pneumothorax and Communicating Blebs

Because of the high blood flow in the lungs, the effect of N_2O on a pneumothorax occurs rapidly. N_2O (75%) can double the size of a pneumothorax in 10 min, and triple it in 30 min.

Venous Air Emboli

The lethal dose for a volume of air embolism is reduced significantly in the presence of N_2O. If N_2O is being used intraoperatively, it should be discontinued immediately when the presence of a venous air embolism is suspected.

Balloon-Tipped Catheters

It has been observed that, when the anesthesia provider is attempting to float a pulmonary artery catheter in a patient anesthetized with N_2O, a greater volume of air can be withdrawn from the balloon than was injected. The volume change in the catheter tip is maximal at 5 to 10 min, depending on the N_2O mixture. This increased volume can cause a problem if an occluded balloon is expanded. It is advisable to deflate the balloon and reinflate it every few minutes if N_2O is being used and to always deflate the balloon after the occlusion pressure has been determined.

Tracheal Tube Cuffs

N_2O can also diffuse into tracheal tube cuffs, causing increases in volume and pressure. Overexpansion of tracheal tube cuffs secondary to N_2O diffusion may cause airway obstruction and glottic or subglottic trauma. Volume increase depends on the concentration of N_2O and the length of time during which the patient is exposed to N_2O. Three hours of pure N_2O (100%) can increase cuff volume by approximately 300%.

Middle Ear

N_2O enters the middle ear cavity, elevating middle ear pressure. Normally, any increase in middle ear pressure is vented via the eustachian tube into the nasopharynx. Narrowing of the eustachian tube by acute inflammation, scar tissue, or surgery in the vicinity of the eustachian tube impairs this venting. Increases in pressure can lead to changes in the outcome of previous middle ear operations and displacement of the tympanic membrane graft during tympanoplasty operations.

Intraocular Pressure

Sulfur hexafluoride and perfluoropropane are sometimes injected into the vitreous cavity at varying concentrations in the surgical management of retinal disease, including retinal detachments and macular holes. N_2O is 117 times more soluble than sulfur hexafluoride. Pressure has been shown to increase by 14 to 30 mm Hg if N_2O is used. This increased pressure can compromise retinal blood flow and cause retinal ischemia or infarction. Reabsorption of N_2O from the ocular cavity may cause underfilling of the therapeutic gas mixtures and, thus, potentially compromise the success of the operation.

Dural Closure

Despite these concerns about N_2O in closed spaces, it is not necessary to discontinue N_2O before closing the dura during craniotomy to avoid expanding intracranial air and increasing intracranial pressure.

Suggested Readings

Fernández-Guisasola J, Gómez-Arnau JI, Cabrera Y, del Valle SG. Association between nitrous oxide and the incidence of postoperative nausea and vomiting in adults: A systematic review and meta-analysis. *Anaesthesia*. 2010;65:379-387.

Irwin MG, Trinh T, Yao CL. Occupational exposure to anaesthetic gases: A role for TIVA. *Expert Opin Drug Saf*. 2009;8:473-483.

Myles PS, Leslie K, Chan MT, et al. Avoidance of nitrous oxide for patients undergoing major surgery: A randomized controlled trial. *Anesthesiology*. 2007;107:221-231.

Sanders R, Weimann J, Maze M. Biologic effects of nitrous oxide: A mechanistic and toxicologic review. *Anesthesiology*. 2008;109:707-722.

CHAPTER 66

Cardiovascular Effects of the Inhalation Agents

Timothy S.J. Shine, MD, and Neil G. Feinglass, MD, FCCP, FASE

There is no one perfect anesthetic agent, though inhalation agents come closest to providing the components of a complete anesthetic (i.e., analgesia, amnesia, hypnosis, and muscle relaxation) as a single agent. All of the inhalation agents depress the cardiovascular system in a dose-dependent fashion (Figure 66-1) through one or more mechanisms, the overall effect of which is a decrease in mean arterial pressure.

Systemic Vascular Resistance

The decrease in blood pressure that occurs with the use of halothane is due to a reduction in myocardial contractility, heart rate, and systemic vascular resistance (SVR). Isoflurane, sevoflurane, and desflurane decrease blood pressure primarily by decreasing SVR. Isoflurane and desflurane are potent vasodilators (Figure 66-2), with halothane causing a more modest reduction in SVR at equipotent doses. Isoflurane causes up to a 50% reduction in SVR at 1.9 minimum alveolar concentration.

Heart Rate

Isoflurane, sevoflurane, and desflurane may increase heart rate (Figure 66-3). Halothane may cause no change or a decrease in heart rate because it impairs baroreceptor function. Isoflurane is less depressant to the baroreflex, and, with a decrease in SVR, a compensatory increase occurs in heart rate even though isoflurane also depresses sympathetic nervous system activity; however, halothane has less effect on the parasympathetic system than on the sympathetic nervous system. Isoflurane anesthesia appears, clinically, to have less effect on cardiac chronicity in patients younger than 40 years of age, as compared with older patients.

Myocardial Contractility

As mentioned previously, halothane directly depresses myocardial contractility and stroke volume by altering concentrations of intracellular calcium (Ca^{2+}) at several subcellular targets, whereas the inhalation agents currently used in the United States have fewer or no effects on myocardial contractility (isoflurane = desflurane = sevoflurane) (Table 66-1). Isoflurane can decrease stroke volume, but if a compensating increase in heart rate occurs, cardiac output is maintained. Unfortunately, many patients receive potent opioids that often decrease cardiac chronotropy, and, as noted above, older patients, even in the absence of opioids, most commonly do not have a compensating increase in heart rate. Because cardiac output is preserved with the use of isoflurane, desflurane, and sevoflurane, perfusion of the myocardium and brain are relatively preserved during anesthesia with these agents.

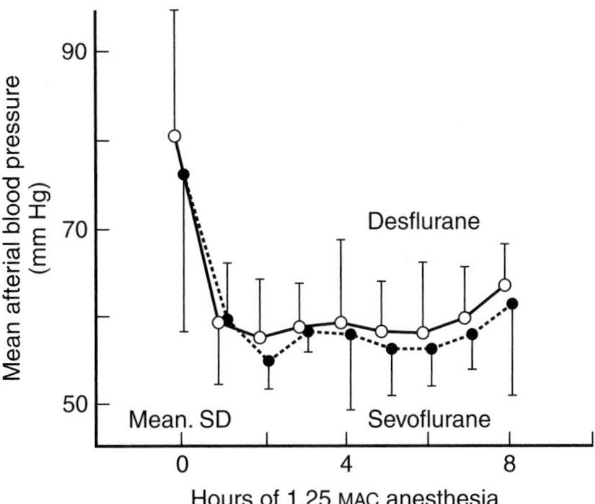

Figure 66-1 Mean arterial pressure decreases significantly within one hour of the onset of anesthesia with equivalent MAC doses of either sevoflurane or desflurane, without any difference between the two compounds. (Eger EI, et al. Recovery and kinetic characteristics of desflurane and sevoflurane in volunteers after 8-h exposure, including kinetics of degradation products. Anesth. 1997; 87:517-526.)

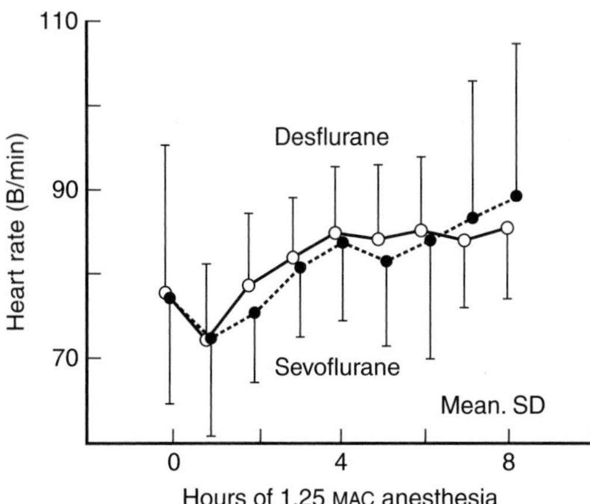

Figure 66-3 Heart rate increases significantly within one hour of the onset of anesthesia with equivalent MAC doses of either sevoflurane or desflurane, without any difference between the two compounds. (Eger EI, et al. Recovery and kinetic characteristics of desflurane and sevoflurane in volunteers after 8-h exposure, including kinetics of degradation products. Anesth. 1997;87: 517-526.)

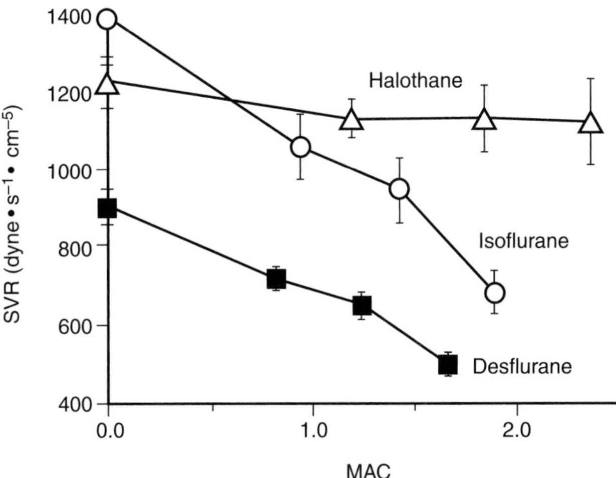

Figure 66-2 Comparison of the effects of desflurane (■) with those of isoflurane (O) and halothane (Δ) on systemic vascular resistance (SVR) in healthy young men. *MAC,* Minimum alveolar concentration. (From Weiskopf RB, Cahalan MK, Eger EI II, et al. Cardiovascular actions of desflurane in normocarbic volunteers. Anesth Analg. 1991;73:143-156.)

Table 66-1 Cardiovascular Effects of Inhalation Anesthetic Agents

Agent	Contractility	PVR	SBP
Halothane	↓	—	↓
Enflurane	↓	↓	↓↓
Isoflurane, desflurane, sevoflurane	—	↓	↓

PVR, Peripheral vascular resistance; *SBP,* systolic blood pressure.

Sensitivity to Epinephrine

All of the inhalation agents sensitize the myocardium to the effects of epinephrine, with halothane having the greatest effect, as compared with isoflurane and desflurane. Children are less likely to exhibit this effect than are adults. Drugs that block the reuptake of norepinephrine, such as cocaine and ketamine, also increase the arrhythmogenicity of the inhalation agents. One half the dose of epinephrine required to produce three or more premature ventricular contractions is considered safe (e.g., 1 μg/kg of epinephrine during halothane anesthesia and 3 μg/kg during isoflurane anesthesia are unlikely to cause arrhythmias) (Figure 66-4).

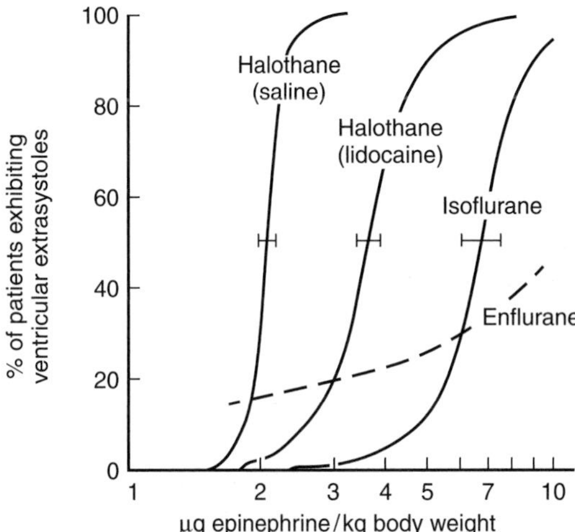

Figure 66-4 Results of a subcutaneous dose of epinephrine showing the percentage of patients with at least three ventricular extrasystoles. (From Johnston RR, Eger EI II, Wilson C. A comparative interaction of epinephrine with enflurane, isoflurane, and halothane in man. Anesth Analg. 1976;55:709-712.)

Coronary Vasodilation

Halothane and isoflurane have been shown to have some coronary vasodilating properties. In isolated vessels, halothane relaxes coronary arteries more than isoflurane does. As in myocytes, the mechanism of coronary artery relaxation is through an effect on intracellular Ca^{2+} regulation at several locations. At one time, controversy existed as to whether isoflurane might "steal" coronary blood flow away from areas of myocardial ischemia, but researchers have now shown that coronary steal with isoflurane does not occur. Several studies have shown that isoflurane and halothane do not change collateral-dependent or ischemic-zone myocardial blood flow when diastolic arterial pressure is kept constant.

Anesthetic Effect on Diastolic Dysfunction

In vivo diastolic relaxation is impaired by the use of inhalation anesthetic agents. The primary effect is from dose-dependent isovolumetric relaxation (the greatest time for myocardial blood flow to myocardium). The measured early filling (E wave by Doppler) is decreased in rate and extent by the inhalation anesthetic agents without appreciable change in intrinsic myocardial stiffness or elasticity. Clinically, however, the inhalation anesthetic agents seem to improve overall filling dynamics in patients with heart failure. This effect may be due to the combination of reduced preload and afterload, which, in essence, shifts left ventricular performance to a more favorable position on the pressure-volume (Starling) curve.

Right Ventricular Function

The crescent-shaped right ventricle operates under different parameters than does the left ventricle. Data suggest that inhalation anesthetic agents may have two different effects on right ventricular performance: (1) they adversely affect cardiac autonomic nervous system activity, and (2) they may impair coordination of right ventricular contractility.

Suggested Readings

Bollen BA, Tinker JH, Hermsmeyer K. Halothane relaxes previously constricted isolated porcine coronary artery segments more than isoflurane. *Anesthesiology*. 1987;66:748-752.

Eger EI II. Isoflurane (Forane). *A Compendium and Reference*. 2nd ed. Madison, WI: Anaquest; 1988.

Johnston RR, Eger EI II, Wilson C. A comparative interaction of epinephrine with enflurane, isoflurane, and halothane in man. *Anesth Analg*. 1976;55:709-712.

Pagel PS, Grossman W, Haering JM, Warltier DC. Left ventricular diastolic function in the normal and diseased heart: Perspectives for the anesthesiologist. *Anesthesiology*. 1993;79:836-854.

Sill JC, Bove AA, Nugent M, et al. Effects of isoflurane on coronary arteries and coronary arterioles in the intact dog. *Anesthesiology*. 1987;66:273.

Weiskopf RB, Cahalan MK, Eger EI II, et al. Cardiovascular actions of desflurane in normocarbic volunteers. *Anesth Analg*. 1991;73:143-156.

CHAPTER 67

Central Nervous System Effects of the Inhalation Agents

Michael J. Murray, MD, PhD

Inhalation anesthetic agents induce anesthesia by depressing brain function via a dose-dependent reversible mechanism that is associated with alterations in cerebral metabolic rate (CMR), in cerebral blood flow (CBF), of the electroencephalogram (EEG), and of evoked potentials. The alterations in CMR and CBF can be attenuated to some extent, but not completely, and therefore can adversely affect outcome in patients with neurologic diseases and in patients undergoing neurosurgical procedures.

Flow-metabolism coupling is defined as a matching of O_2 and glucose delivery to metabolic demand; CBF increases or decreases in concordance with changes in CMR. A misconception about the inhalation anesthetic agents is that, because they increase CBF and decrease CMR, they "uncouple" flow and metabolism. In fact, although increasing concentrations of inhalation anesthetic agents result in a higher CBF for a given CMR, a coupled relationship between these variables persists (Figure 67-1).

This relationship between CMR and CBF is apparent only if adequate blood pressure is maintained; if blood pressure is allowed to decrease, the increase in CBF will be attenuated or abolished because inhalation anesthesia agents inhibit autoregulation in a dose-dependent fashion (Figure 67-2). However, inhalation anesthetic agents do not inhibit CO_2 reactivity and, if anything, may actually exaggerate the response. Thus, in the normal brain, the cerebral vasodilation that occurs in response to an inhalation anesthetic agent can be blunted, abolished, or reversed by decreasing CO_2 levels; however, these responses may not apply in the presence of abnormal intracranial anatomy or physiology.

Because the inhalation agents cause an increase in CBF (and in cerebral blood volume [CBV]), the use of these anesthetics in patients at risk for developing or who have increased intracranial pressure (ICP) is a concern. However, numerous studies have confirmed that hypocapnia

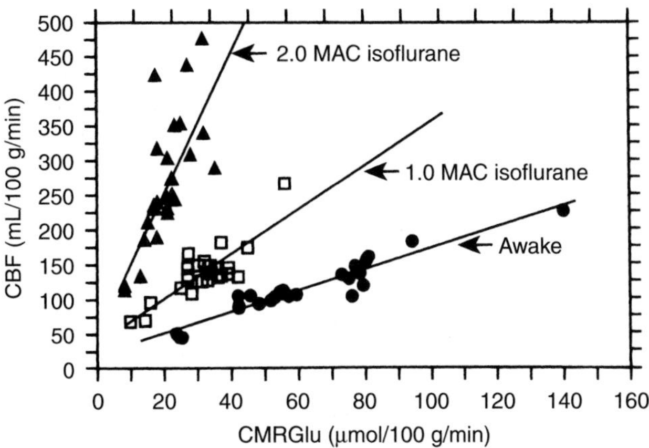

Figure 67-1 Regression plots of regional cerebral metabolic rate for glucose (CMRGlu) versus regional cerebral blood flow (CBF) in the rat. As the concentration of isoflurane is increased, the slope of the regression line increases (i.e., a higher CBF for a given CMRGlu value). This indicates that isoflurane is a cerebrovasodilator in the rat brain but that it does not uncouple flow and metabolism, even at 2 MAC (minimum alveolar concentration). (From Todd MM, Warner DS, Maktabi MA. Neuroanesthesia: A critical review. In: Longnecker DE, Tinker JH, Morgan GE Jr, eds. Principles and Practice of Anesthesiology. 2nd ed. Vol. 2. St. Louis: Mosby; 1998:1607-1658. Data from Maekawa T, Tommasino C, Shapiro HM, et al. Local cerebral blood flow and glucose utilization during isoflurane anesthesia in the rat. Anesthesiology. 1986;65:144-151.)

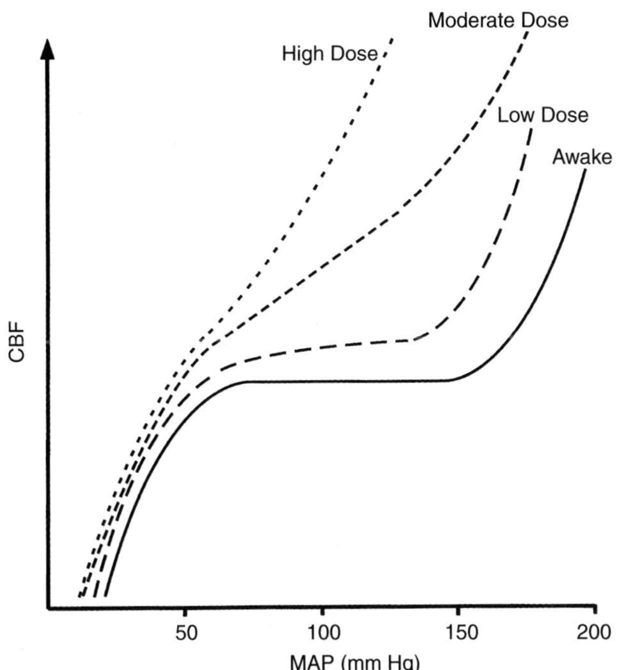

Figure 67-2 Schematic representation of the effect of a progressively increased dose of a typical inhalation anesthetic agent on cerebral blood flow (CBF) autoregulation. Both upper and lower thresholds are shifted to the left. MAP, Mean arterial pressure. (From Drummond JC, Patel PM. Cerebral physiology and the effects of anesthetic techniques. In: Miller RD, ed. Anesthesia. 5th ed. New York: Churchill Livingstone; 2000:695-734.)

attenuates or blocks the increase in ICP that otherwise would occur in at-risk patients.

Anesthesia-induced EEG changes follow a common pattern. When anesthesia is induced with an inhalation agent, the frequency and amplitude of the EEG waveforms increase, and the measurements throughout the cortex are more uniform, such that waveforms measured on the EEG appear to synchronize. At about 1 minimum alveolar concentration (MAC), the EEG slows progressively; depending on the anesthetic agent, burst suppression, an isoelectric pattern, or seizures may evolve as the anesthetic concentration increases.

Michenfelder defined critical regional CBF as "that flow below which the majority of subjects develop ipsilateral EEG changes indicative of ischemia within 3 min following carotid occlusion." Table 67-1 lists the critical CBF rates of various inhalation anesthetic agents.

Table 67-1 Critical Regional Cerebral Blood Flow for Anesthetic Agents in Patients Receiving an Inhalation Anesthetic Agent with N_2O

Agent	Cerebral Blood Flow Rate
Isoflurane	$10\ mL \cdot 100\ g^{-1} \cdot min^{-1}$
Desflurane	$\leq 10\ mL \cdot 100\ g^{-1} \cdot min^{-1}$
Sevoflurane	$11.5\ mL \cdot 100\ g^{-1} \cdot min^{-1}$

The inhalation agents also affect evoked potentials, but only minimally so at concentrations below 1 MAC. All anesthetic agents tend to increase latencies and decrease amplitudes of evoked potentials at concentrations greater than 1 MAC. Evoked potentials of cortical origin are particularly sensitive to the effects of inhalation anesthetic agents; brainstem auditory evoked potentials are the most resistant. Although more sensitive to the effects of inhalation anesthetic agents, somatosensory evoked potentials can be adequately monitored at less than 1 MAC of the inhalation anesthetic agent.

Nitrous Oxide

Cerebral Metabolic Rate and Cerebral Blood Flow

Although N_2O is perceived to be physiologically and pharmacologically inert, it is a cerebral vasodilator that can significantly increase ICP in patients with increased intracranial elastance. The effect of N_2O on ICP is blocked or blunted by opioids, barbiturates, and hypocapnia. Most data suggest that N_2O increases CMR.

Electroencephalogram

Most subjects lose consciousness at N_2O concentrations of approximately 50%, when alpha activity is replaced by fast-wave activity on the EEG. As the concentration of N_2O approaches 75%, slow-wave activity (4 to 8 Hz) appears on the EEG, with some background fast-wave activity still present. If the partial pressure of N_2O continues to increase (as is possible in a hyperbaric environment), fast-wave activity is abolished, with progressive slowing demonstrated on the EEG.

Evoked Potentials

An N_2O concentration below 1 atm has a minimal effect on evoked potentials. Its primary effect is to decrease the amplitude of the evoked response; it has little or no effect on latency.

Pneumocephalus

Pneumocephalus can occur during posterior fossa or cervical spine operations performed with the patient in the sitting position. When the dura is open, gravity can cause the cerebrospinal fluid (CSF) to continuously drain; the CSF is subsequently replaced by air (an effect known as the inverted pop-bottle phenomenon), resulting in a progressive accumulation of air in the ventricles, over the cortical surfaces, or both. If used as part of the anesthetic, N_2O will equilibrate with any air-filled space in the body. Because the blood solubility of N_2O is 30 times greater than that of nitrogen, a significant, albeit transient, net increase of gas molecules will occur in the air-filled space, and hence, the volume or pressure will increase once the dura is closed. Thus, the use of N_2O may cause tension pneumocephalus of sufficient significance to produce major cerebral compromise, manifested by seizures, altered consciousness, or specific neurologic deficits.

If a tension pneumocephalus is suspected, the use of N_2O should be discontinued. Patients receiving a second anesthetic within the first 3 weeks after undergoing supratentorial craniotomy are at risk for developing complications if N_2O is used because a number of these patients will still have significant intracranial air collection.

Isoflurane

Cerebral Metabolic Rate and Cerebral Blood Flow

Of the inhalation agents, isoflurane is the least potent cerebral vasodilator. CO_2 reactivity and autoregulation are maintained with the use of isoflurane. As do all of the inhalation agents, isoflurane depresses CMR; CMR decreases by 50% at 2.0 MAC of isoflurane, the point at which the EEG becomes isoelectric. Doubling the isoflurane concentration to 4.0 MAC has been shown to cause no further decrease in CMR. There is no evidence of toxicity associated with the use of deep levels of isoflurane anesthesia.

Intracranial Pressure

The potential of isoflurane to increase ICP can be blocked by simultaneous induction of hypocapnia, although it is not necessary to induce hypocapnia before administering isoflurane. Isoflurane has no effect on CSF production, and it decreases the resistance to CSF reabsorption.

Electroencephalogram

See the previous discussion of CMR and CBF.

Evoked Potentials

Evoked potentials can be measured at isoflurane concentrations below 1 MAC.

Desflurane

Cerebral Metabolic Rate and Cerebral Blood Flow

The cerebral metabolic and vascular effects of desflurane are similar to those of isoflurane. Desflurane is a cerebral arteriolar dilator and produces a dose-dependent decrease in cerebrovascular resistance and CMR. Similar to isoflurane, it may be used to induce controlled hypotension, but its use is more often associated with a compensatory tachycardia than is the use of isoflurane.

Intracranial Pressure

As is true for all inhalation anesthetic agents, desflurane may increase ICP in certain patients, but because CO_2 reactivity is maintained with desflurane, the increase can be attenuated or blocked by inducing hypocapnia. However, one study in humans showed a sustained elevation in lumbar CSF pressure after administration of 1 MAC desflurane despite previous establishment of hypocapnia. Desflurane has been shown to produce an increase in CSF formation without any significant effect on CSF reabsorption in dogs.

Electroencephalogram

Desflurane produces a dose-related depression of EEG activity. In swine, prominent burst suppression has been observed at MAC levels above 1.24. Although EEG tolerance to the cerebral effects of desflurane has been observed in dogs, it has not been seen in humans.

Sevoflurane

Cerebral Metabolic Rate and Cerebral Blood Flow

The effects of sevoflurane on CMR and CBF resemble those of isoflurane. In most animal models in which it has been studied, sevoflurane produces little change in global CBF independent of CO_2 levels. Cerebral autoregulation and cerebrovascular responsiveness to changes in CO_2 are preserved in patients with cerebrovascular disease up to a concentration slightly below 1 MAC.

Intracranial Pressure

Institution of hypocapnia prior to administration of sevoflurane blocks the potential of the agent to increase ICP at concentrations up to 1.5 MAC in dogs.

Electroencephalogram

Slowing on the EEG begins at concentrations of 1.2% sevoflurane, and burst suppression in seen at approximately 2 MAC. Therefore, other agents should be used for maintenance of anesthesia if EEG will be monitored intraoperatively.

Suggested Readings

Grady RE, Weglinski MR, Sharbrough FW, Perkins WJ. Correlation of regional cerebral blood flow with electroencephalographic changes during sevoflurane-nitrous oxide anesthesia for carotid endarterectomy. *Anesthesiology*. 1998;88:892-897.

Michenfelder JD. *Anesthesia and the Brain*. New York: Churchill Livingstone; 1988.

Reasoner DK, Todd MM, Scamman FL, Warner DS. The incidence of pneumocephalus after supratentorial craniotomy: Observations on the disappearance of intracranial air. *Anesthesiology*. 1994;80:1008-1012.

CHAPTER 68

Renal Effects of the Inhalation Agents

Richard L. Applegate II, MD

Inhalation anesthetic agents can alter renal function through physiologic effects or through toxic effects of the agents or their breakdown products. Physiologic effects of inhalation anesthetics are typically transient. The risk for renal toxicity with modern inhalation agents is low.

Physiologic Effects

Autoregulation of renal blood flow appears to be maintained during administration of modern inhalation anesthetic agents, though the use of these agents associated with changes in cardiovascular function that may include decreases in cardiac output and arterial pressure. If prolonged, these decreases may adversely affect renal function. However, perioperative renal dysfunction is most commonly caused by intravascular volume depletion and anemia, leading to hypoperfusion of the kidney, with intracellular hypoxia. The impact of surgical stress may add to renal ischemia, as the kidney has few β_2-adrenergic receptors; therefore, catecholamine stimulation leads to unopposed renal vasoconstriction. Additionally, positive-pressure ventilation during anesthesia is associated with reversible decreases in renal perfusion pressure, creatinine clearance, and sodium excretion, as is abdominal insufflation during laparoscopic procedures.

Toxicity

Metabolic Products

The halogenated anesthetic agents undergo varying degrees of metabolic degradation. The metabolic pathways differ depending on the agent, with the production of a number of intermediate metabolites and the release of fluoride (F^-). Inhaled anesthetic gases may also undergo chemical degradation in CO_2 absorbers to produce a number of compounds, including fluoromethyl-2, 2-difluoro-1-(trifluoromethyl) vinyl ether (FDVE), known as compound A, from sevoflurane. CO may also be produced from the breakdown of desflurane and, to a lesser degree, from other halogenated anesthetic agents currently in use. These products of metabolism and degradation may contribute to postoperative renal dysfunction.

When methoxyflurane was clinically available and used, its metabolism led to release of F^-; a F^- concentration above 50 μmol/L was identified as a risk factor for anesthesia-related renal dysfunction and raised concern about the renal safety of all halogenated anesthetic agents that release F^- as a product of metabolism. Elevated F^- concentrations after prolonged exposure to enflurane (which is also no longer available in the United States) may be associated with transient renal dysfunction, but following exposure to other halogenated agents (isoflurane and sevoflurane), these levels are not associated with clinical renal damage in humans. Investigation into long administration ($>$10 h) of inhaled anesthetic agents at a fresh-gas flow of 1 L/min or less has shown no association with significant renal dysfunction, although transient elevation of sensitive markers of renal damage may occur.

Published evidence indicates that the renal damage associated with methoxyflurane administration is caused by O-demethylation to produce F^- and DCAA (dichloroacetic acid), which is nephrotoxic, especially in the presence of F^-. It is also possible that intrarenal metabolism is responsible for renal dysfunction following methoxyflurane administration. Other currently available halogenated anesthetic agents (isoflurane, sevoflurane, desflurane) are not metabolized in renal cells, nor are they metabolized to DCAA, and their use is not associated with clinically significant renal dysfunction.

Breakdown Products

Sevoflurane can degrade in some CO_2 absorbers to produce compound A (FDVE) and other products. This degradation is more likely to occur at low fresh-gas flow rates. Compound A is nephrotoxic in rats. The amount of compound A that is generated varies with the type of absorbent, with newer absorbent materials producing little to no compound A, compared with absorbents, such as soda lime, that have larger amounts of strong bases (KOH, NaOH). Current U.S. Food and Drug Administration labeling suggests limiting sevoflurane exposure to 2 minimum alveolar concentration hours at fresh-gas flow rates of 1 to 2 L/min and discourages the administration at fresh-gas flow rates under 1 L/min because this will minimize exposure to compound A. However, numerous reports of longer administration have been published showing no difference in renal function or sensitive markers of renal damage following the administration of sevoflurane, when compared with other inhaled anesthetic agents.

Suggested Readings

Keijzer C, Perez RSGM, De Lange JJ. Compound A and carbon monoxide production from sevoflurane and seven different types of carbon dioxide absorbent in a patient model. *Acta Anaesthesiol Scand*. 2007;51:31-37.

Kharasch ED. Adverse drug reactions with halogenated anesthetics. *Nature*. 2008;84:158-162.

Kharasch ED, Schroeder JL, Liggitt HD, et al. New insights into the mechanism of methoxyflurane nephrotoxicity and implications for anesthetic development. Part 1: Identification of the nephrotoxic metabolic pathway. *Anesthesiology*. 2006;105:726-736.

Kharasch ED, Schroeder JL, Liggitt HD, et al. New insights into the mechanism of methoxyflurane nephrotoxicity and implications for anesthetic development. Part 2: Identification of the nephrotoxic metabolites. *Anesthesiology*. 2006;105:737-745.

Sear JW. Kidney dysfunction in the postoperative period. *Br J Anaesth*. 2005; 95:20-32.

Wagener G, Brentjens TE. Renal disease: The anesthesiologist's perspective. *Anesthesiol Clin*. 2006;24:523-547.

CHAPTER 69

Hepatic Effects of the Inhalation Agents

Wolf H. Stapelfeldt, MD

Inhaled anesthetic agents have a propensity to affect hepatic function both directly and indirectly. Direct effects on hepatic parenchyma include interactions of anesthetic agents with hepatic enzymes and the generation of metabolic products with toxic or allergenic properties. Indirect effects include decreased hepatic blood flow and, consequently, altered hepatic drug clearance and O_2 delivery to hepatocytes. An understanding of the latter requires a review of the anatomy and physiology of the hepatic blood supply.

Hepatic Blood Supply

The normal liver contains approximately 10% to 15% of the total blood volume and receives approximately 25% of the normal total cardiac output (1 mL/min of blood flow per gram of liver). Only one third of the afferent blood supply is arterial via the hepatic artery and its branches—the remaining two-thirds come from the portal vein and its branches. However, each of these two afferent blood supply systems provides approximately 50% of the O_2 consumed by the liver. This dual blood supply is highly regulated via several mechanisms.

Pressure-flow autoregulation is a myogenic response of the hepatic artery that actively adjusts vascular smooth muscle tone to varying passive wall stretch to maintain blood flow in the presence of changing hepatic perfusion pressure. This mechanism appears to be in effect predominantly in the postprandial state, less so in the fasted state.

Metabolic control mediates arterial vasoconstriction in response to hypocarbia or alkalemia (which is the reason why excessive hyperventilation should be avoided if hepatic perfusion is of concern) as well as vasodilatation in response to hypercarbia, acidemia, or hypoxemia—direct responses that may be offset by the indirect effect of reflex increases in sympathetic vasoconstrictor tone. Therefore, near normocarbia and a physiologic pH are generally considered optimal with regard to maintaining hepatic arterial blood flow.

Hepatic arterial buffer responses provide for reciprocal (active) changes in hepatic arterial blood flow in response to (passive) changes in portal venous blood flow, with the goal of maintaining total hepatic blood flow. This physiologic mechanism is believed to be mediated by varying adenosine washout, is selectively inhibited by halothane (but not, however, by isoflurane, sevoflurane, or desflurane [see following discussion]), and is abolished by splanchnic hypoperfusion or the presence of endotoxemia.

Parasympathetic autonomic activity is mediated through the vagus nerve, whereas sympathetic autonomic control is exerted by splanchnic vasoconstrictor nerve (T3-T11) activity; the effects on the autonomic nervous system are mediated by hepatic arterial and hepatic venous α_1-, α_2-, and β_2-adrenergic receptors, as well as portal venous α_1- and α_2-adrenergic receptors. β-Adrenergic antagonists are being used clinically to treat portal hypertension attributable to increased mesenteric blood flow caused by excessive β_2-adrenergic receptor activity.

Humoral control includes a profound arterial vasodilatory response to glucagon, hepatic arterial and portal venous constrictive properties of angiotensin II, and decreased mesenteric blood flow produced by somatostatin, as well as a differential response to vasopressin, which simultaneously causes splanchnic arterial vasoconstriction and portal venous dilatation, making vasopressin an effective adjuvant in the treatment of portal hypertension.

Inhaled Anesthetic-Induced Changes in Hepatic Blood Flow

Inhaled anesthetic agents produce concentration-dependent decreases in portal venous blood flow, which passively reflect their effect on arterial blood pressure, causing decreased mesenteric blood flow. To the extent that cardiac output is maintained and hepatic arterial blood flow is increased (via an intact hepatic arterial buffer response), total hepatic blood flow is maintained in the presence of isoflurane, sevoflurane, and desflurane, but previously used anesthetics (enflurane or halothane) produced hepatic arterial vasoconstriction and obliteration of the hepatic arterial buffer response (Figure 69-1, *A*). The resulting anesthetic-induced net changes in hepatic arterial O_2 delivery (Figure 69-1, *B*) mirrored the respective anesthetic changes in total hepatic blood flow.

Hepatic Metabolism of Inhaled Anesthetic Agents

Although most of the total amount of modern inhaled anesthetic agent taken up by blood and tissues in the course of clinical anesthesia is ultimately eliminated unchanged through exhalation via the lungs, a fraction taken up by hepatic parenchyma is subject to metabolism by members of the hemoprotein cytochrome P-450 enzyme superfamily. The fractional contribution of hepatic metabolism to elimination depends on the concentration of agent in contact with hepatic enzymes as a result of equilibration with blood flowing through the liver, reflecting the blood solubility of the agent (isoflurane 0.2%; desflurane 0.01%). An exception is sevoflurane, which, despite comparatively low blood solubility, undergoes 3% to 5% metabolism. All halogenated agents principally undergo oxidative metabolism selectively catalyzed by CPY2E1, releasing fluoride anions in the process. However, only enflurane and sevoflurane cause noticeable and potentially clinically significant (>50 μM) increases in plasma fluoride concentration; this increase typically occurs after prolonged anesthesia (several minimum alveolar concentration hours) or with prior induction of the CPY2E1 enzyme (isoniazid treatment, chronic alcohol consumption, or obesity). Such increases in plasma fluoride concentration can temporarily impair renal tubular concentrating ability (temporary nephrogenic diabetes insipidus) without causing any other lasting renal compromise. Only in rare instances have the newer inhaled halogenated anesthetic agents been demonstrated to cause hepatic toxicity analogous to that documented for halothane. This toxicity is believed to be due to the lesser fractional metabolism of the less soluble agents, as well as the fact that, unlike the other agents, halothane undergoes both oxidative (catalyzed by CPY2E1 and, to a lesser extent, CPY2A6) and reductive (Figure 69-2) metabolism (within a hypoxic environment, catalyzed by CPY2A6 and CPY3A4, the most ubiquitous cytochrome P-450 enzyme). In contrast with the newer anesthetic agents, halothane produces fluoride anions as a result of reductive metabolism; oxidative metabolism releases only bromide anions (which may contribute to prolonged sedation following halothane anesthesia). Reductive metabolism of halothane can produce highly reactive radicals that are thought to account for hepatic toxicity that is observed under hypoxic conditions. This hepatic toxicity is not to be confused with halothane hepatitis, a distinct condition that is encountered in approximately 1 in 10,000 adults or 1 in 200,000 children anesthetized with halothane. Based on factors such as a previous exposure and the presence of eosinophilia, as well as demonstration of antibodies against trifluoroacetic acid

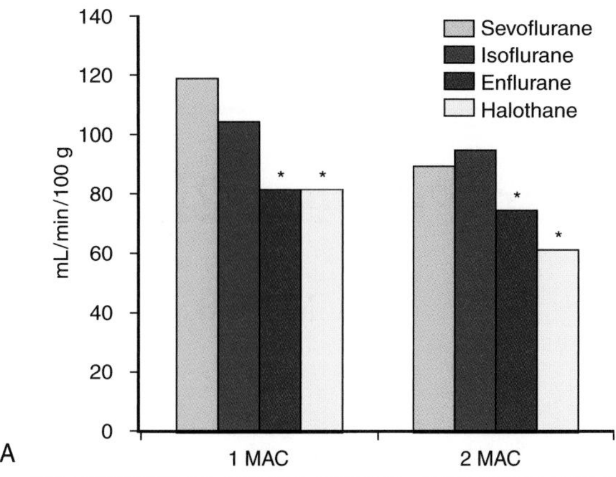

Impact of halothane, enflurane, isoflurane, and sevoflurane at 1.0 and 2.0 minimum alveolar concentration (MAC) on total hepatic blood flow (THBF) in dogs. THBF decreased with increasing anesthetic concentrations of each volatile agent. Sevoflurane and isoflurane were similar in their modest effect of THBF, whereas halothane caused a dramatic decrease in THBG, especially at 2-MAC exposure.

*Differs from sevoflurane and isoflurane at comparable values ($P < 0.05$).

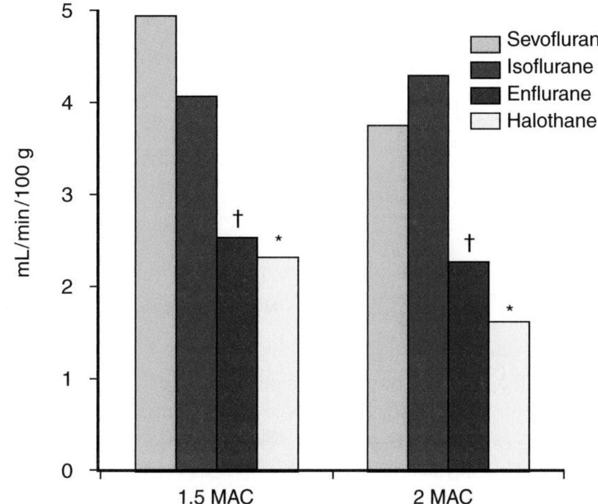

Impact of halothane, enflurane, isoflurane, and sevoflurane at 1.5 and 2.5 minimum alveolar concentration (MAC) on hepatic arterial oxygen delivery in chronically instrumented dogs. Halothane produced the greatest reduction in hepatic arterial oxygen delivery, whereas sevoflurane and isoflurane has insignificant effects on oxygen delivery at an MAC level.

*Differs from isoflurane and sevoflurane at comparable MAC values ($P < 0.05$).

†Differs from sevoflurane at comparable MAC values ($P < 0.05$).

Figure 69-1 Effect of inhaled anesthetics on hepatic arterial blood flow and O_2 delivery.

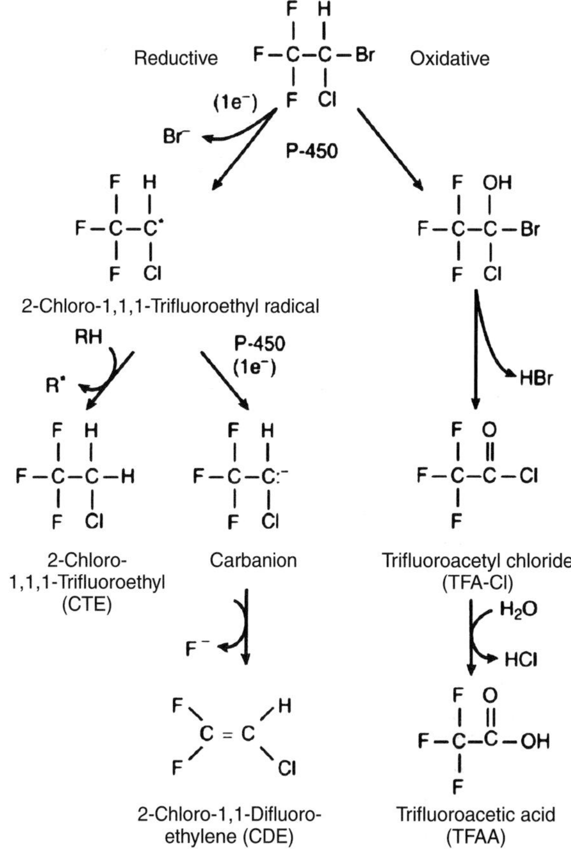

Figure 69-2 Major byproducts of oxidative and reductive halothane metabolism.

acylated haptens, it is believed to be an allergic response to oxidative (trifluoroacetic acid) metabolites.

Extrahepatic Degradation of Inhaled Anesthetic Agents

In addition to enzymatic metabolism in the liver, inhaled anesthetic agents are also subject to spontaneous degradation in the presence of CO_2 absorbents (sodalime and previously Baralyme), producing potentially toxic degradation products as well as a risk of ignition due to significant heat produced by these exothermic chemical reactions. Concerns depend on the particular agent.

Sevoflurane uniquely causes the formation of compound A, a vinyl ether with nephrotoxic properties. The threshold for renal injury appears to be approximately 150 ppm-hours of exposure, which is a potential concern only after prolonged sevoflurane anesthesia, causing glucosuria and enzymuria without any demonstrable effects on blood urea nitrogen or creatinine levels. To limit the concentration of compound A to which patients are exposed, fresh gas flows of not less than 2 L/min are recommended during sevoflurane anesthesia.

All inhaled halogenated anesthetic agents, in particular desflurane, enflurane, and isoflurane (in this order of propensity), can produce carbon monoxide as a result of a chemical interaction with strong bases. Besides the choice of anesthetic agent (the risk being negligible with sevoflurane or halothane), other determining factors include the anesthetic concentration as well as the type (risk greater with Baralyme, which, for these reasons, has been taken off the market), temperature, and most importantly, the degree of dryness (water content) of the CO_2 absorbent. The risk of significant carbon monoxide production is minimized by keeping fresh-gas flows low (to prevent desiccation of the absorbent) or, if necessary, by replacing or rehydrating desiccated absorbent.

Both of these risks are completely eliminated by using one of the newer, calcium hydroxide–based absorbents (such as Amsorb or DrägerSorb Free), which are devoid of strong bases and, thus, are chemically inert with regard to the abovementioned reactions with inhaled anesthetic agents.

Suggested Readings

Bedirli N, Ofluoglu E, Kerem M, et al. Hepatic energy metabolism and the differential protective effects of sevoflurane and isoflurane anesthesia in a rat hepatic ischemia-reperfusion injury model. *Anesth Analg.* 2008;106(3):830-837.

Dykes MH. Postoperative hepatic dysfunction in perspective. 1970. *Int Anesthesiol Clin.* 1998;36(4):155-162.

Eger EI II, Gong D, Koblin DD, et al. Dose-related biochemical markers of renal injury after sevoflurane versus desflurane anesthesia in volunteers. *Anesth Analg.* 1997;85(5):1154-1163.

Fee JP, Thompson GH. Comparative tolerability profiles of the inhaled anaesthetics. *Drug Saf.* 1997;16:157-170.

Gatecel C. Losser MR. Payen D. The postoperative effects of halothane versus isoflurane on hepatic artery and portal vein blood flow in humans. *Anesth Analg.* 2003;96(3):740-745.

Kang JG, Ko JS, Kim GS, et al. The relationship between inhalational anesthetic requirements and the severity of liver disease in liver transplant recipients according to three phases of liver transplantation. *Transplantat Procs.* 2010;42(3):854-857.

Picker O, Beck C, Pannen B. Liver protection in the perioperative setting. *Best Pract Res Clin Anaesthesiol.* 2008;22(1):209-224.

CHAPTER 70

Effects of pK_a, pH, and Protein Binding

Mary B. Weber, MD

pK_a and pH

Most drugs are either weak acids or bases and, therefore, exist in both the ionized and nonionized forms at physiologic pH. The extent of ionization depends on the pH of the solution and the dissociation constant (pK_a) of the drug. The pK_a is defined as the pH at which a compound exists as 50% ionized and 50% nonionized. When the pK_a of the drug is close to the pH of the surrounding milieu, smaller changes in pH produce greater changes in the degree of ionization. Basic drugs tend to be highly ionized at a low pH, whereas acidic drugs are highly ionized at a high pH. The Henderson-Hasselbalch equation allows the calculation of the ratio of the nonionized to ionized drug, depending upon the pH,

$$\mathrm{p}K_a - \mathrm{pH} = \log \frac{[\text{protonated form}]}{[\text{unprotonated form}]}$$

which, for a weak acid, would be the ratio of the nonionized, or nondissociated, acid to the ionized, or dissociated, compound.

The nonionized form of a drug molecule is more lipid soluble and can traverse the lipid component of cell membranes. Therefore, a nonionized drug is more readily absorbed from the gastrointestinal tract and reabsorbed from renal tubules.

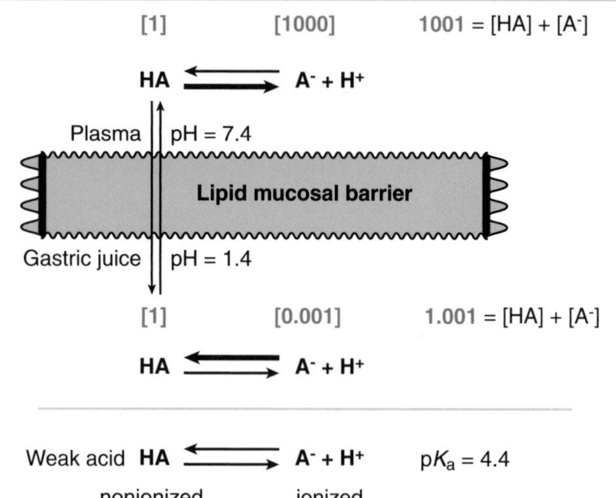

Figure 70-1 The influence of pH on the distribution of a weak acid between plasma and gastric juice separated by a lipid barrier. (From Brunton LL, Lazo JS, Parker KL, eds. Goodman and Gilman's The Pharmacological Basis of Therapeutics. 11th ed. New York, McGraw-Hill, © 2006. All rights reserved. Available at: http://www.accessmedicine.com.)

Ion Trapping

When a pH gradient exists across a membrane, the concentration of total drug may be quite different on each side (Figure 70-1). The nonionized fraction traverses the membrane freely and equilibrates, but the ionized form, which does not easily cross the membrane, is trapped on the side with a pH that favors ionization. For a weak acid, the drug will accumulate on the more basic side of the membrane; for a weak base, the drug will accumulate on the acidic side of the membrane. This mechanism is known as ion trapping. For example, the nonionized fraction of a local anesthetic agent (a weak base) crosses the placenta, where it is changed to the ionized fraction in the relatively acidic fetus. The ionized fraction cannot leave the placenta; nonionized drug continues to enter the fetal circulation, where it is ionized and maintains a gradient across the placenta.

Protein Binding

Drugs exist in the blood in two forms, either dissolved in plasma or bound to proteins. The two main plasma proteins that bind with drugs are albumin, which is the major carrier for acidic drugs, and α_1-acid glycoprotein (AAG), the major carrier for basic drugs.

Protein binding affects drug distribution and action because, generally, only the free portion traverses cell membranes and reaches its site of action. By limiting drug excursion into the tissues, extensive protein binding results in a small calculated volume of distribution. Protein binding also influences clearance of drug because it is the unbound fraction of drug that is available for metabolism and clearance by the liver and kidney. The percentage of bound drug depends on the concentration of protein, the concentration of drug, and the number and affinity of binding sites on the protein molecule for the drug.

These reactions occur quite rapidly, with half-lives of a few milliseconds, because the complex is maintained by a weak ionic bond. As the concentration of unbound drug decreases through whatever process, bound drug immediately dissociates from its protein-binding site to restore equilibrium.

As mentioned, albumin is the primary protein in the body binding acidic drugs (e.g., thiopental and midazolam), whereas AAG binds many basic drugs, including many opioids, propranolol, verapamil, quinidine, and local anesthetic agents. Certain drugs (e.g., fentanyl and sufentanil) can bind to both proteins. The degree of protein binding is higher with drugs having higher lipid solubility. Acid-base disturbances also affect drug binding.

Changes in protein binding have a much greater effect on drugs that are highly protein bound. For example, a decrease in binding from 98% to 94% will triple the fraction of free drug, whereas a decrease in binding from 68% to 64% results in a much smaller percentage increase of free drug.

Factors Affecting Drug Binding

Age and Sex

As people age, their plasma concentration of albumin decreases, whereas that of AAG increases. These small changes are not clinically important. Sex-related differences are nonexistent.

Renal Disease

Albumin levels may be decreased with renal disease. In addition, it is thought that renal failure alters the albumin molecule, thereby reducing binding with organic acids. On the other hand, binding of basic drugs with AAG is variable, depending on the type of renal disease.

Maternal and Neonatal Effects

Albumin levels are decreased in pregnant women, whereas AAG levels are unchanged. In neonates, levels of both albumin and AAG are decreased.

Hepatic Disease

Plasma albumin levels are frequently decreased in patients with liver disease, and qualitative changes in the albumin molecule decrease the affinity for drugs. Therefore, free fractions of drugs that are typically bound to albumin are increased. Free fractions of basic drugs that are normally bound to AAG are unaffected.

Miscellaneous

Because AAG is an acute-phase reactant, its plasma concentration is increased in patients experiencing the physiologic stress of surgery, trauma, myocardial infarction, neoplastic disease, or inflammatory disease, resulting in decreased free fractions of drugs that bind to AAG. In contrast, albumin levels decrease in patients with neoplastic disease, in critically ill patients, and in those who have undergone operations or have experienced trauma.

Suggested Readings

Buxton ILO. Pharmacokinetics and pharmacodynamics. In: Brunton L, Lazo J, Parker K, eds. *Goodman and Gilman's The Pharmacological Basis of Therapeutics*. 11th ed. New York: McGraw-Hill; 2006:1-40.

Fuguet E, Ràfols C, Bosch E, Rosés M. A fast method for pKa determination by capillary electrophoresis. *Chem Biodivers*. 2009;6:1822-1827.

CHAPTER 71

Thiopental

C. Thomas Wass, MD

Thiopental is no longer available in the United States because the governments of countries in which it is manufactured refuse to allow it to be exported to countries in which it is used for lethal injection. However, anesthesia providers should be familiar with the use of thiopental because, (1) from a historical perspective, for decades it was the most widely used intravenous drug to induce anesthesia and (2) thiopental is a core medicine on the World Health Organization's Essential Drugs List. Thiopental is still widely used outside the United States, and anesthesia providers who travel to practice outside the United States for whatever reason must remain familiar with its pharmacokinetics and pharmacodynamics.

Barbituric acid (2,4,6,-trioxyhexahydropyrimidine) (Figure 71-1) was first synthesized by Adolph von Bäyer (founder of what was to become the Bayer chemical company) in 1864. Although this molecule is the structural framework from which barbiturates are derived, it is devoid of anesthetic properties. Structural modification at the number 2 and 5 carbon atoms results in barbiturate drugs that have sedative-hypnotic properties. For example, addition of a benzene ring at the C5 position results in phenobarbital, a drug first used for its sedative properties in the early 1900s and still one of the most widely used drugs in the world to treat seizure disorders. With the lack of thiopental in the United States, intensive care physicians are using phenobarbital to induce barbiturate coma in patients with raised intracranial pressure unresponsive to other therapies. Replacement of the oxygen atom with a sulfur atom at the C2 position and adding a large aliphatic carbon group to the C5 atom transforms barbituric acid into thiopental. Clinically, sodium thiopental was first administered in 1934 by Ralph Waters at the University of Wisconsin, Madison, and by John Lundy at the Mayo Clinic in Rochester, MN.

Commercially available thiopental [5-ethyl-5-(1-methyl-butyl)-2-thiobarbituric acid] is a racemic mixture of stereoisomers [the S(−) isomer

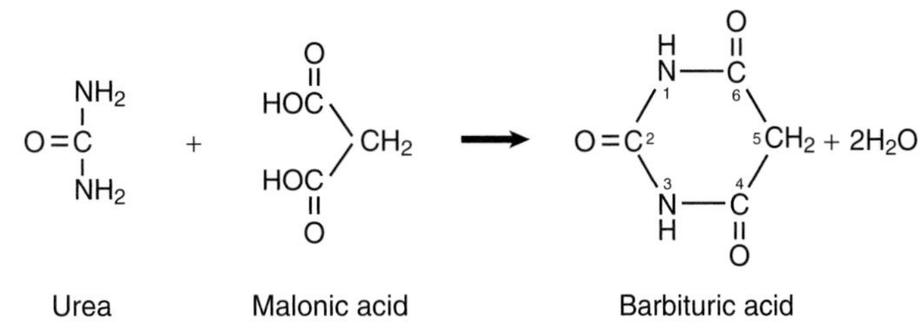

Urea + Malonic acid → Barbituric acid + $2H_2O$

Figure 71-1 Barbiturates are hypnotically active drugs that are derivatives of barbituric acid (2,4,6-trioxyhexahydropyrimidine), a hypnotically inactive pyrimidine nucleus that is formed by the condensation of malonic acid and urea.

is twice as potent as the R(+) counterpart] that is water soluble and highly alkaline (pK_a of 7.6 and pH of 10.5). Decreased pH (e.g., mixing with opioids, catecholamines, or neuromuscular blocking agents) may result in precipitation. Reconstitution with Ringer's lactate solution is not recommended. Refrigerated thiopental is stable for approximately 1 week following reconstitution with sterile water. Both isomers exert their biologic activity by enhancing and mimicking the action of γ-aminobutyric acid (GABA) at $GABA_A$ receptors.

Pharmacokinetics

Distribution of intravenously administered drugs throughout body tissues is determined by tissue blood flow, blood-tissue concentration gradient, lipid solubility, extent of protein binding, and degree of ionization. Thiopental is very lipid soluble and, thus, readily crosses the blood-brain barrier. Other pharmacokinetic properties of thiopental are listed in Table 71-1. Decreased protein binding (e.g., in patients with uremia or cirrhosis) increases the free fraction of drug available to interact with GABA receptors in the brain.

Because the brain is a highly perfused (i.e., belongs to the vessel-rich organ group) relatively low-volume organ, cerebral thiopental concentrations equilibrate rapidly with the central blood pool (Figure 71-2), resulting in depressed electroencephalographic activity—and induction of anesthesia—within 20 to 40 sec.

After achieving maximal concentration within the central nervous system, thiopental follows its concentration gradient into the central blood pool and is subsequently redistributed to a relatively large skeletal muscle reservoir. As a result, electroencephalographic activity returns toward baseline—and patients emerge from anesthesia—within 5 to 8 min. That is, redistribution is the primary mechanism responsible for prompt awakening following an induction dose of thiopental. But when thiopental is administered in multiple doses or as a continuous infusion, skeletal muscle becomes progressively saturated and eventually equilibrates with the central blood pool, thereby preventing further uptake by this large tissue reservoir. At that point, further decreases in blood thiopental concentrations occur more slowly and become dependent on uptake by less well perfused organs (e.g., adipose) as well as hepatic metabolism.

Thiobarbiturate metabolism occurs primarily in hepatic endoplasmic reticulum; however, a small fraction of drug may undergo extrahepatic (e.g., kidney) biotransformation. Biologic reactions responsible for the production of inactive water-soluble metabolites include oxidation of substituents on the C5 atom, desulfurization on the C2 atom, and hydrolytic opening of the barbituric acid ring. Of additional interest, hepatic clearance is characterized as a low hepatic extraction ratio, and thus, thiopental metabolism is more dependent on hepatic enzyme (e.g., P-450 oxidase) activity than on hepatic blood flow.

Finally, thiopental is eliminated from the body by renal excretion (99% as inactive metabolites, 1% unchanged as active metabolite). The degree of protein binding substantially affects renal glomerular filtration and tubular reabsorption. For example, competitive displacement of thiopental from plasma proteins (primarily albumin) by aspirin, phenylbutazone, or uremic toxins results in enhanced drug effect because of increased free-drug fraction and greater renal tubular reabsorption.

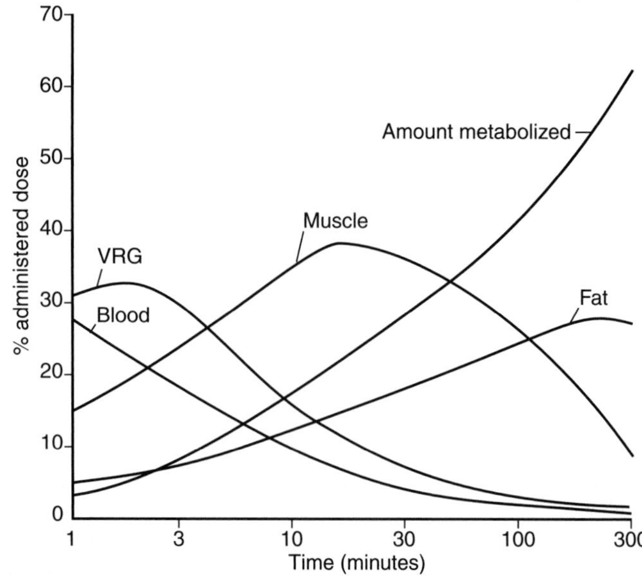

Figure 71-2 Distribution, redistribution, and metabolism of thiopental following intravenous bolus. VRG, Vessel-rich group. (Modified from Stoelting RK, Hillier SC. Barbiturates. In: Stoelting RK, ed. Handbook of Pharmacology and Physiology in Anesthetic Practice. 4th ed. Philadelphia: Lippincott Williams & Wilkins; 2005:119-131.)

Table 71-1 Induction Dose, Half-Life, and Metabolism/Route of Elimination for Commonly Used Intravenous Anesthetic Agents

Drug	Induction Dose	Elimination Half-Life (h)	Metabolism/ Elimination
Etomidate	0.1-0.3 mg/kg	2.9-5.3	Hepatic Renal
Fentanyl	10-20 μg/mg	0.25	Hepatic Renal
Ketamine	1-2 mg/kg	2.5-2.8	Hepatic Renal
Midazolam	1-2 mg/kg	1.7-2.6	Hepatic Renal
Morphine	1 mg/kg	2-4	Hepatic Renal
Propofol	1-3 mg/kg	4-7	Hepatic Renal
Thiopental	3-5 mg/kg	7-17	Hepatic Renal

Side Effects and Adverse Effects

Transient hypotension following an intravenously administered bolus of thiopental is primarily due to peripheral vasodilation resulting from decreased sympathetic tone. Cardiac output is minimally affected. Decreased activity in the medullary and pontine ventilatory centers produce dose-dependent respiratory depression. Barbiturates can stimulate δ-aminolevulinic acid synthetase, which can precipitate a crisis in patients with acute intermittent porphyria.

Inadvertent intra-arterial injection of thiopental causes intense vasoconstriction and pain along the arterial distribution. Tissue damage occurs as a result of (1) reactive vasoconstriction, (2) occlusive thiopental crystal formation, and (3) inflammatory mediated arteritis. Treatment consists of immediate dilution (with 0.9% saline solution) and vasomotor relaxation (e.g., lidocaine, papaverine, or phenoxybenzamine) injected into the offending catheter. Sympathectomy (e.g., brachial plexus or stellate ganglion block) may also alleviate vasoconstriction.

Suggested Readings

Stoelting RK, Hillier SC. Barbiturates. In: Stoelting RK, ed. *Handbook of Pharmacology and Physiology in Anesthetic Practice*. 4th ed. Philadelphia: Lippincott Williams & Wilkins; 2005:119-131.

CHAPTER 72
Propofol

Michael J. Murray, MD, PhD

Propofol (2,6,-diisopropylphenol), an intravenously administered anesthetic agent, belongs to the family of sterically hindered phenols (Figure 72-1). Because propofol is water insoluble, it must be formulated in a 1% lipid emulsion, which is similar to that used in parenteral nutrition: it contains 10% soybean oil, 2.25% glycerol, and purified 1.2% egg phosphatide. The emulsion has not been reported to cause histamine release. Although patients who are allergic to egg whites have received propofol and have not experienced allergic reactions, propofol should probably not be administered to patients who have had an anaphylactic reaction to eggs.

Because thiopental is no longer available in the United States, propofol has become the most commonly used intravenously administered anesthetic induction agent; its advantages are a rapid onset and offset, a rapid redistribution such that little drug accumulates even with continuous infusions, and a very low rate of postoperative nausea and vomiting associated with its use. The antiemetic effects and clear emergence are most pronounced when anesthesia is maintained with an intravenously administered infusion of propofol. The antiemetic effects are so pronounced that 10 to 20 mg of propofol are occasionally administered in the postanesthetic care unit as rescue therapy for patients with postoperative nausea and vomiting.

Compared with the other intravenously administered anesthetic agents, propofol causes the most injection site pain and the most hypotension. The prevalence of pain on injection ranges from 10% to 50%, although the incidence of thrombophlebitis is low. Pain on injection can be attenuated by the intravenous use of local anesthetic agents and slow administration of the propofol into a large vein with rapidly running intravenous fluids.

Propofol infusion syndrome has been described in pediatric patients and in younger neurosurgical patients in the intensive care unit in whom propofol was infused at very high rates (>150 to 200 $\mu g \cdot kg^{-1} \cdot min^{-1}$) for hours to days; these patients developed profound metabolic acidosis, progressive bradyarrhythmias, cardiac arrest unresponsive to therapy, and death. The cause is unknown, though several mechanisms have been proposed.

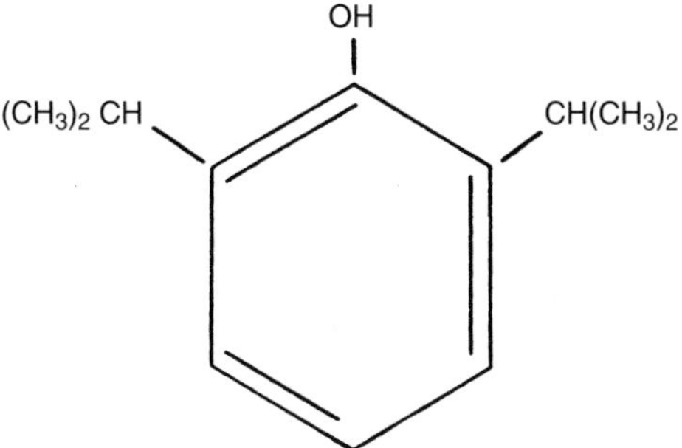

Figure 72-1 Chemical structure of propofol (2,6,-diisopropylphenol).

Effects on Major Organ Systems

Central Nervous System

The exact mechanism of action of propofol has yet to be fully elucidated; however, stimulation of γ-aminobutyric acid (GABA) receptors is likely responsible for the anesthetic properties of this drug. Propofol, injected intravenously as a bolus dose of 2 mg/kg, induces unconsciousness in less than 1 min, a rate that is similar to that of thiopental, etomidate, and methohexital. Induction is smooth, with excitatory effects seen less often than with methohexital, although more often than with thiopental. An induction bolus of propofol will produce anesthesia lasting approximately 4 min, a duration comparable with that of thiopental. Propofol produces electroencephalographic changes characteristic of general anesthesia. This decrease in cerebral function is accompanied by decreased cerebral metabolism, cerebral blood flow, and intracranial pressure.

Cardiovascular System

Propofol causes a dose-dependent decrease in blood pressure secondary to, primarily, decreased systemic vascular resistance, though myocardial contractility decreases at higher doses, resulting in a fall in cardiac output.

Respiratory System

Propofol produces a dose-dependent depression of central respiratory drive that ultimately results in apnea. As with the other anesthetic drugs, the ventilatory response to CO_2 is decreased.

Other Organ Systems

Propofol has little to no effect on liver function, renal function, coagulation, and steroidogenesis. Administration of propofol increases the depth, but not the duration, of neuromuscular blockade.

Pharmacokinetics and Pharmacodynamics

The concentration of propofol decreases rapidly following an intravenously administered bolus dose because of redistribution of drug (i.e., $t_{1/2\alpha}$ = 2 to 8 min). The elimination half-life ($t_{1/2\beta}$ = approximately 1 h) is markedly shorter than that of thiopental ($t_{1/2\beta}$ = approximately 11 h). Both two-compartment and three-compartment models have been proposed. The volume of distribution is large but becomes significantly smaller as the age of the patient increases. Thus, dosages should be reduced in elderly patients.

Propofol is excreted as glucuronide and sulfate conjugates, primarily in the urine. Prolonged infusions can result in green urine (which is of no clinical significance) because of the presence of a phenolic or quinol metabolite. Because clearance of propofol exceeds hepatic blood flow, extrahepatic mechanisms have been proposed.

Blood concentrations of 2.5 to 6 $\mu g/mL$ are required for patients undergoing major operations; concentrations of 1.5 to 4.5 $\mu g/mL$ are adequate for minor operations. Movement on skin incision is prevented in 50% of premedicated patients (on 66% N_2O) by blood levels of 2.5 μg/mL of propofol.

Doses

The dose for induction of anesthesia is 1.5 to 2.5 mg/kg, which should be reduced in patients who are elderly, are hypovolemic, or have poor cardiac reserve. Anesthesia can also be induced with 20 to 40 mg of propofol given every 10 sec until onset of unconsciousness. Anesthesia can be maintained with frequent, intermittent, 0.5-mg/kg boluses of propofol, titrated to clinical effect, or with a propofol infusion of 100 to 200 $\mu g \cdot kg^{-1} \cdot min^{-1}$. A recommended starting dose for conscious sedation is 50 $\mu g \cdot kg^{-1} \cdot min^{-1}$.

Suggested Reading

Schuttler J, Ihmsen H. Population pharmacokinetics of propofol: A multicenter study. *Anesthesiology*. 2000;92:727-738.

CHAPTER 73

Etomidate

Heidi A. Hadley, MD

Etomidate (R-(+)-phenylethyl-1H-imidazole-5 carboxylate sulfate) (Figure 73-1), an intravenously administered anesthetic drug, was initially described in 1964 and was approved for clinical use 10 years later. Its benefits include rapid onset, rapid offset, minimal cardiovascular effects, and cerebral protection. Water soluble at an acidic pH and lipid soluble at physiologic pH, it is available in the United States as a 0.2% solution with 35% propylene glycol. In this preparation, it has a pH of 6.9 and a p*K* of 4.2, making it a weak base. The *d* isomer is responsible for its anesthetic effects: hypnosis and sedation, notably without analgesia. By binding to $GABA_A$ (γ-aminobutyric acid type A) receptors—predominately at the β_2 and β_3 subunits (Table 73-1)—etomidate causes neuronal hyperpolarization and subsequent depression of the reticular activating system through the inhibition of neural signals. Additionally, etomidate increases the affinity of GABA receptors for the GABA molecule.

Table 73-1 $GABA_A$ Subunit Binding Sites of Propofol and Etomidate

Subunit binding site	Drug
α	Propofol
β_1	Propofol
β_2	Propofol, etomidate
β_3	Propofol, etomidate
γ_2	Propofol

$GABA_A$, γ-Aminobutyric acid type A.

Pharmacokinetics

Distribution

Following an intravenous administration of a bolus, 99% of etomidate exists in the nonionized form in plasma, 75% of which is protein bound, primarily to albumin. The high lipid solubility results in a fast onset of action (within 1 min of intravenous injection) and a large volume of distribution (2.5-4.5 L/kg). Redistribution is responsible for rapid offset due to an initial decrease in plasma concentration. Renal or hepatic disease, resulting in low plasma protein levels, causes an increased duration of effect and a doubling of the half-life of etomidate.

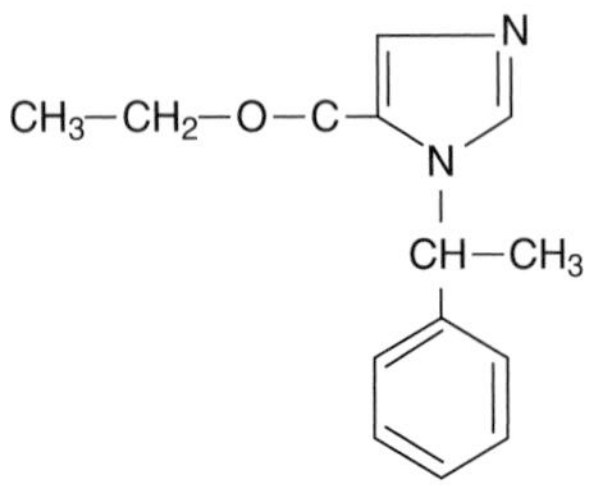

CH3—CH2—O—C N N CH—CH3

Figure 73-1 Chemical structure of etomidate.

Metabolism

Etomidate is metabolized via ester hydrolysis (both plasma and hepatic), converting the ethyl side chain into a carboxylic acid ester, rendering it water soluble and inactive. The metabolism of etomidate is five times faster than that of thiopental metabolism.

Elimination

The majority of inactive metabolite is renally excreted, with an elimination half-life of 2.9 to 5.3 h and a clearance rate of 18 to 35 $mL \cdot kg^{-1} \cdot min^{-1}$.

Pharmacodynamics

Dosing

The induction dose of etomidate is 0.3 mg/kg (range: 0.2-0.6 mg/kg), with loss of consciousness occurring in the patient within 2 min following an intravenously administered bolus of etomidate. A linear relationship exists between dose and duration of action. Decreased doses are used if patients are premedicated with opioids or benzodiazepines. Elderly patients require a reduction in the dose of etomidate ($\leq$0.2 mg/kg) owing to their smaller volume of distribution and decreased clearance rates. Maintenance of anesthesia with etomidate can be achieved via initial infusion rates of 100 $\mu g \cdot kg^{-1} \cdot min^{-1}$, which may be later reduced to 10 to 20 $\mu g \cdot kg^{-1} \cdot min^{-1}$, after 10 minutes, with the goal of maintaining plasma levels between 300 and 500 ng/dL.

Effects on Major Organ Systems

Central Nervous System

Etomidate provides cerebral protection by decreasing cerebral metabolic rate, with a proportional decrease in cerebral blood flow, thus maintaining an appropriate O_2 supply/demand ratio. Because mean arterial pressure is unaffected, a stable cerebral perfusion pressure is preserved. Intracerebral pressure is initially decreased with the use of etomidate; however, it will later return to baseline, unless high infusion rates are utilized.

Electroencephalographic changes that occur with the use of etomidate are similar to those seen with barbiturates except that etomidate does not induce beta waves, as do barbiturates. Epileptiform activity on the electroencephalogram or a grand mal seizure can be induced; the use of etomidate is therefore avoided in patients with a history of seizures. It can be used to intentionally trigger an epileptiform focus on the electroencephalogram to aid with localization during surgical interventions for seizures. Conversely, etomidate, at induction doses, can also be used to treat status epilepticus, but it is not a first-line drug.

Cardiovascular System

Etomidate is best known for its mild cardiovascular depressant effects, as compared with other induction agents, and is therefore often used in patients with hemodynamic instability, decreased ejection fraction, coronary artery disease, or valvular heart disease who require a stable cardiac output and mean arterial pressure (Table 73-2). Although peripheral vascular resistance is decreased with the use of etomidate, blood pressure is minimally affected; etomidate does not affect cardiac output or myocardial contractility. Coronary blood flow will be decreased, as will the myocardial O_2 requirement, preserving the O_2 supply/demand ratio.

Respiratory System

Etomidate causes only minimal respiratory depression. It will decrease tidal volume, but a compensatory increase in respiratory rate is typically observed, both of which will be affected for only 3 to 5 minues. Apnea is typically only observed when etomidate is administered at high doses and combined with opioids.

Adverse Drug Effects

Endocrine Effects

Corticoadrenal suppression is the most significant adverse effect that occurs with the use of etomidate and is the primary factor limiting its use for continuous infusion. Etomidate inhibits the function of 11β-hydroxylase (converts 11-deoxycortisol into cortisol), resulting in a reversible dose-dependent inhibition of cortisol and aldosterone synthesis (Figure 73-2). The time to maximal suppression is 4 h after intravenous injection, and suppression typically resolves within 24 h. Corticoadrenal suppression was initially observed in patients in the intensive care unit; however, the inhibition of 11β-hydroxylase is also present at induction bolus doses. Etomidate is a desirable intubation agent in patients who are septic because of life-threatening cardiovascular compromise, but these are patients who would least tolerate any suppression of cortisol production.

Risks and benefits must be weighed on an individual patient basis, placing emphasis on acute maintenance of adequate blood pressure. Use of exogenous corticosteroids is debatable; however, long-term infusions or multiple boluses of etomidate should not be administered because of the proven increased risk of death. Two new etomidate derivatives that are in development (methoxycarbonyl-etomidate and carboetomidate) maintain the cardiovascular benefits of etomidate while avoiding the undesirable corticoadrenal suppression.

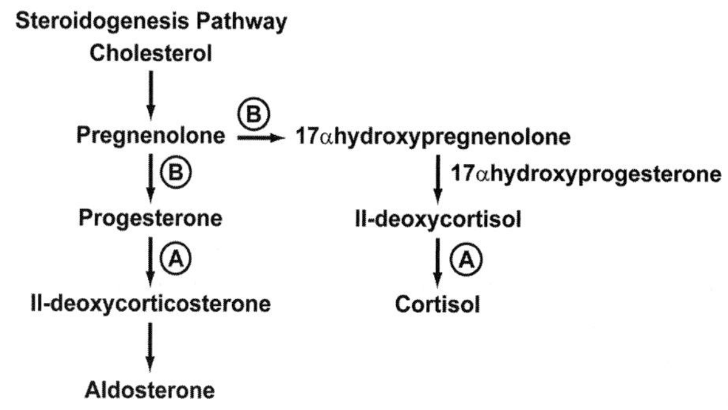

Figure 73-2 The major steps in the production of cortisol and aldosterone in the adrenal glands that are inhibited by etomidate.

Table 73-2 Benefits and Adverse Drug Effects of Major Intravenously Administered Induction Agents

Agent	Cardio depressant	Decreased ICP	Respiratory Depression	Continuous Infusion	Analgesia	Thrombo-phlebitis	Adrenocortico suppression	Porphyria	Broncho-relaxation	Myoclonus
Propofol	Yes	Yes	Yes	Yes	No	Yes	No	No	No	No*
Thiopental	Yes	Yes	Yes	No†	No	No	No	Yes	No	No
Midazolam	Yes	No	No	Yes	No	Yes	No	No	No	No
Etomidate	No‡	Yes	No§	No	No	Yes	Yes	Yes	No	Yes
Ketamine	No‡	No¶	No	Yes	Yes	No	No	No	Yes	No*

*Rare reports of myoclonus.
†Used only to maintain barbiturate coma.
‡Will cause cardiodepression only at high doses.
§Synergistic with opioids.
¶Increases intracranial pressure (ICP).

Additional Effects

The central nervous system effects of etomidate result in an imbalance of the inhibitory and stimulatory signals between the thalamus and the cortex. The resulting stimulation can produce myoclonus in 30% to 60% of patients. The risk of myoclonus can be decreased with concomitant opioid or midazolam use.

Etomidate causes pain with intravenous injection, which can be prevented by administering intravenous lidocaine or opioids prior to injection or use of a central vein. Lipid emulsions are available in Europe as an alternative to the propylene glycol solution and are reported to decrease injection site pain. Thrombophlebitis, which can occur 24 to 48 h after the use of etomidate, appears in up to 25% of patients.

The central nervous system effects of etomidate have been associated with increased rates of postoperative nausea and vomiting; however, the results of a study that compared an etomidate-lipid infusion and propofol in patients with a history of postoperative nausea and vomiting showed no differences between the two drugs.

Etomidate should not be used in patients with a history of porphyria because, similar to thiopental, it can induce a porphyria attack. Cases of etomidate-induced hypersensitivity are rare (1/50,000-1/450,000) and are associated with anaphylactoid reactions. Additionally, etomidate can cause postoperative hiccups and a sense of restlessness.

Suggested Readings

Evers AS, Maze M. Intravenous anesthetics. In: Evers AS, Maze M, eds. *Anesthetic Pharmacology—Physiologic Principles and Clinical Practice*. Philadelphia: Churchill Livingstone; 2003:395-416.

Jackson WL. Should we use etomidate as an induction agent for endotracheal intubation in patients with septic shock? A critical appraisal. *Chest*. 2005; 127;1031-1038.

Malerba G, Romano-Girard F, Cravoisy A, et al. Risk factors of relative adrenocortical deficiency in intensive care patients needing mechanical ventilation. *Intensive Care Med*. 2005;31:388-392.

Sneyd JR, Rigsby-Jones AE. New drugs and technologies, intravenous anesthesia is on the move (again). *Br J Anesth*. 2010;105:246-254.

Stoelting RK. Non-barbituate induction drugs. In: Stoelting RK, ed. *Pharmacology and Physiology in Anesthetic Practice*. 3rd ed. Philadelphia: Lippincott-Raven; 1999:145-148.

CHAPTER 74

Ketamine

Gilbert A. Blaise, MD

The ketamine molecule (2-(*o*-chlorophenyl)-2-methylamino-cyclohexamine) is chemically related to phencyclidine and contains a chiral center (C2 carbon of the cyclohexanone ring) with two optical isomers. The S-isomer is four times more potent, is associated with a faster recovery, and has a low incidence of psychomimetic effects, compared with the R-isomer. However, in North America, ketamine is sold primarily as a racemic mixture (Figure 74-1). It also contains benzethonium chloride as a preservative compound.

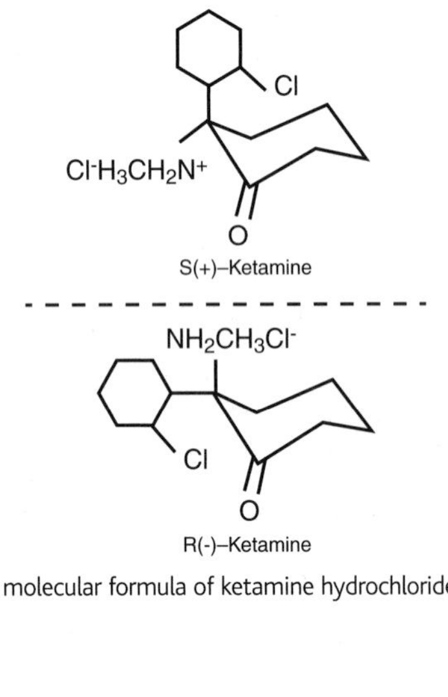

Figure 74-1 The molecular formula of ketamine hydrochloride, $C_{13}H_{16}ClNO{\cdot}HCl$.

Designed to become the ideal anesthetic at a time when other anesthetic agents were particularly toxic and not easy to use, ketamine was introduced as a complete anesthetic agent in 1960. Its popularity was established in the mid-1970s during the Vietnam War, where it was deemed to be an "exceptional battlefield anesthetic."

Administered intravenously or intramuscularly, it can evoke profound analgesia, loss of consciousness, amnesia, and immobility. The anesthesia produced by ketamine is termed *dissociative* because patients appear to be dissociated from their environment rather than simply nonreactive. Under ketamine anesthesia, the thalamus is no longer synchronized with the limbic system. Ketamine has a very high therapeutic index compared with other anesthetic medications. Ketamine is also a recreational drug of abuse (best known under the names vitamin K and special K).

Mechanisms of Action

Ketamine is not a particularly selective drug, with multiple sites of action, including those in the central and peripheral nervous systems. The properties of ketamine are primarily mediated by noncompetitive antagonism at N-methyl-D-aspartate (NMDA) receptors, but the drug also has local anesthetic properties. The NMDA receptors consist of five subunits surrounding a central ion channel that is permeable to Ca^{2+}, Na^{+}, and K^{+} (Figure 74-2). Binding sites for Mg^{2+} and ketamine have been found inside this channel.

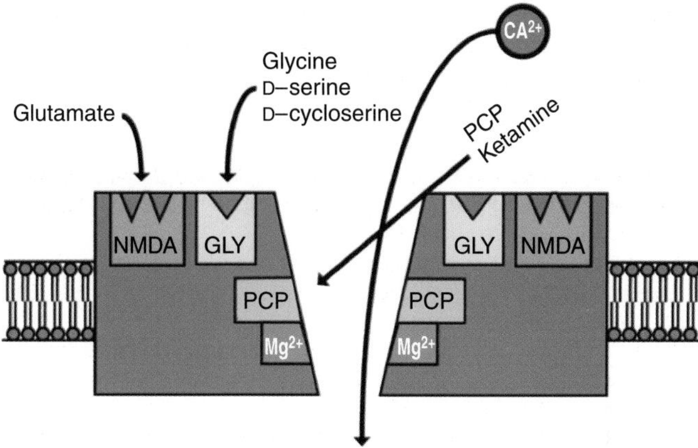

Figure 74-2 The properties of ketamine are primarily mediated by noncompetitive antagonism at NMDA receptors, which consist of five subunits surrounding a central ion channel that is permeable to Ca^{2+}, Na^{+}, and K^{+}. GLY, Glycine; NMDA, *N*-methyl-D-aspartic acid; PCP, phencyclidine.

Glutamate is the most prominent excitatory amino acid in the body, and NMDA receptor activation is a major mechanism of the effect of glutamate on the central nervous system, on the peripheral nervous system, and in many other organs and tissues (e.g., lungs, inflammatory cells). NMDA receptors have been implicated in the mechanism of anesthesia, pain transmission, morphine tolerance, memory and cognitive function, long-term potentiation, long-term depression, neuronal toxicity, and chronic neurologic diseases (e.g., Alzheimer disease and major depression) as well as inflammatory responses.

At clinical concentrations, ketamine can also bind to phencyclidine receptors. Ketamine has even been reported to interact with μ, δ, and κ opioid receptors. Ketamine inhibits reuptake of the monoamines epinephrine, dopamine, and serotonin. It is an agonist of purinergic neurotransmission and interacts with adenosine receptors.

Ketamine anesthesia is reversed by anticholinesterases, an antagonistic outcome that is likely to elevate acetylcholine concentrations. There is evidence that ketamine interacts with muscarinic and nicotinic receptors, based on the fact that it produces anticholinergic symptoms (postanesthetic delirium, bronchodilation, and sympathomimetic effects). Ketamine interaction with voltage-sensitive Ca^{2+} channels has been studied extensively, and the local anesthetic effect of ketamine has been explained by its interaction with Na^{+} channels.

Systemic Effects

Cardiovascular System

The cardiovascular response to ketamine mimics sympathetic nervous system stimulation, causing increased blood pressure, cardiac output, and myocardial O_2 consumption. Heart rate changes depend on baroreflex activity. This initial action of ketamine on the cardiovascular system is due to amine reuptake inhibition.

Respiratory System

Ketamine alone does not induce respiratory depression, so airway patency is well maintained during ketamine anesthesia; however, if ketamine is combined with respiratory-depressing agents, such as benzodiazepines or opioids, respiratory depression and upper airway obstruction can occur. Because of its anticholinergic and adrenergic effects, ketamine induces bronchodilation and has been administered with success as a sedative to treat patients with asthma.

Central Nervous System

Ketamine, a cerebral vasodilator, causes an increase in cerebral blood flow and intracranial pressure in patients with space-occupying intracranial lesions. Intracranial pressure elevation is minimal if ventilation is controlled.

Emergence delirium is reported to occur in 5% to 30% of patients who are administered ketamine as an anesthetic agent; the incidence of delirium is increased in patients over the age of 16 years if the dosage exceeds 2 mg/kg, if the drug is administered rapidly, or if patients have preexisting personality problems. Emergence reactions usually occur early during emergence from anesthesia and may persist for a few hours but can be prolonged to more than 24 h in some patients. These reactions are characterized by visual, auditory, proprioceptive, and confusional illusions, often with associated feelings of excitement, fear, or euphoria (schizophrenia-like reactions).

Clinical Use

Ketamine is the only effective NMDA blocker that is available as a medication that can be administered by several routes: intravenously, intramuscularly, subcutaneously, intranasally, sublingually, orally, rectally, cutaneously (patches, ointment on wounds), intrathecally, and epidurally. Ketamine is being studied in perioperative pain management, chronic pain management, inflammatory-response mediation, and the treatment of depression. Because NMDA antagonists have an additive or synergistic action with opioids by reducing hyperalgesia induced by opioids, decreasing tolerance elicited by continuous morphine administration, or reversing opioid-mediated tolerance, ketamine is being used increasingly to provide perioperative analgesia. Ketamine may have a preemptive effect and, if added to another form of multimodal analgesia, could diminish secondary hyperalgesia and the prevalence of chronic pain after abdominal operations. Combining ketamine with opioids improves postoperative analgesia and reduces side effects.

Ketamine has been used as an intravenously administered analgesic or locally applied ointment with some success in the treatment of severe complex regional pain syndrome. Fibromyalgia and chronic fatigue syndrome could be due to pathologic NMDA receptor activation, and if so, ketamine may have a role in treating patients with these disorders. Blocking NMDA receptors is effective therapeutically in severe depression that is unresponsive to standard treatments.

Ketamine, a modulator of inflammatory responses, has been shown to be neuroprotective in several animal models of neurologic ischemia-reperfusion injury.

Several animal studies have shown that ketamine causes apoptosis in developing brains and produces long-term cognitive impairment. Phencyclidine compounds can model irreversible schizophrenic disease in rodents. Delirium can create long-term cognitive deficits in susceptible patients. However, at a low dose, ketamine can prevent postoperative delirium.

Because of the occurrence of emergence reactions, the use of ketamine as an anesthetic agent has declined. This decline has been facilitated by the availability of new anesthetic agents, better monitoring, and the improved knowledge and skills of anesthesiologists. As an anesthetic, ketamine remains useful as an agent well suited for short and very painful procedures performed outside the operating room (e.g., in austere environments, emergency departments, diagnostic clinics) where monitoring and support are limited. Ketamine is still used for induction of anesthesia in hemodynamically unstable patients.

Several questions remain unanswered regarding ketamine; the many effects associated with its use require balancing the beneficial actions of this pharmacologic agent with its potential adverse effects.

Suggested Readings

Hudetz JA, Patterson KM, Iqbal Z, et al. Ketamine attenuates delirium after cardiac surgery with cardiopulmonary bypass. *J Cardiothorac Vasc Anesth*. 2009; 23:651-657.

Lois F, De Kock M. Something new about ketamine for pediatric anesthesia? *Curr Opin Anaesthesiol*. 2008;21:340-344.

Wu GJ, Chen TL, Ueng YF, Chen RM. Ketamine inhibits tumor necrosis factor-α and interleukin-6 gene expressions in lipopolysaccharide-stimulated macrophages through suppression of toll-like receptor 4-mediated c-Jun N-terminal kinase phosphorylation and activator protein-1 activation. *Toxicol Appl Pharmacol*. 2008;228:105-113.

CHAPTER 75

Opioid Pharmacology

Halena M. Gazelka, MD, and Richard H. Rho, MD

According to Goodman and Gilman's, "the term *opioid* refers broadly to all compounds related to opium, a natural product derived from the poppy. Opiates are drugs derived from opium and include the natural products morphine, codeine, and thebaine and many synthetic derivatives. Endogenous opioid peptide endorphins are the naturally occurring ligands for opioid receptors. Opiates exert their effects by mimicking these peptides. The term *narcotic* is derived from the Greek word for *stupor*; it originally referred to any drug that induced sleep, but it now is associated with opioids."

Opiates may be classified into three major groups based on pharmacodynamic activity: pure opioid agonists, pure antagonists (e.g., naloxone), and mixed agonists/antagonists (e.g., butorphanol, nalbuphine). All of the opiates share common structural characteristics, and small changes in molecular shape of these compounds can convert an agonist to an antagonist.

The clinical effects of a particular opiate depend on which specific opioid-receptor type or types (μ_1, μ_2, κ, δ, and σ) that it binds. The primary mechanism of action of opiates is via μ-receptor agonism. These opioid-receptor subtypes have been characterized according to their differences in affinity, anatomic location, and functional responses, as shown in Table 75-1.

The analgesic effects from systemic administration of opioids may result from receptor activity at several different nervous system sites, including the sensory neuron of the peripheral nervous system; the dorsal horn (layer 4 and 5 of the substantia gelatinosa) of the spinal cord, which inhibits the transmission of nociceptive information; the brainstem medulla, which potentiates descending inhibitory pathways that modulate ascending pain signals; and the cortex of the brain, which decreases the perception and emotional response to pain. Opioid-receptor activation inhibits the presynaptic release and postsynaptic response to excitatory neurotransmitters (glutamate, acetylcholine, and substance P).

Opioids can be administered by many routes—oral, parenteral, intramuscular, transcutaneous, subcutaneous, transmucosal, epidural, and intrathecal—making them adaptable for use in most clinical situations. The distribution half-lives of all opioids are fairly short, approximately 5 to 20 min. The highly lipid-soluble opiates, such as fentanyl and sufentanil, have a rapid onset and short duration of action.

The liver is responsible for the biotransformation of most opioids; many, including morphine and meperidine, have metabolites—morphine-6-glucoronide and normeperidine, respectively—that are as equally active as the parent compound. These metabolites must be eliminated by the kidneys, and adjustment of doses of these medications is imperative for patients with renal failure. The metabolites of fentanyl, sufentanil, and alfentanil are inactive, however.

Table 75-1 Opioid Receptor Subtypes, Clinical Effects, and Example Agonists

Receptor	Clinical Effects	Example Agonist(s)
μ_1	Supraspinal analgesia Bradycardia Sedation Pruritus Nausea and vomiting	Morphine Meperidine
μ_2	Respiratory depression Euphoria Physical dependence Pruritus Constipation	Morphine Meperidine
κ	Spinal analgesia Respiratory depression Sedation Miosis	Fentanyl Morphine Nalbuphine
δ	Spinal analgesia Respiratory depression	Oxycodone β-Endorphin Leu-enkephalin

Effects

Central Nervous System Effects

High doses of opioids may cause deep sedation or hypnosis; however, opioids do not reliably produce amnesia. Opioids reduce the minimum alveolar concentration of Inhalation anesthetic agents required during balanced general anesthesia.

Seizures can result from the neuroexcitatory effects of normeperidine, a metabolite of meperidine. Normeperidine-induced seizures are more likely to occur in patients who have received chronic meperidine therapy, have received large doses of meperidine over a short period, or have impaired renal function with decreased ability to eliminate this metabolite.

Opioids can reduce cerebral metabolic O_2 requirements, cerebral blood flow, and intracranial pressure if alveolar ventilation is unchanged. Opioids cause miosis by stimulating the Edinger-Westphal nucleus of the oculomotor nerve. In patients in whom ventilation is not controlled, opioid-induced respiratory depression can produce hypoxemia, resulting in pupillary dilation and an increase in intracranial pressure due to hypercarbia.

Opioids stimulate the chemoreceptor trigger zone located in the area postrema of the brain stem, which can result in nausea and vomiting.

Respiratory Effects

Opioid administration decreases minute ventilation by decreasing the respiratory rate (as opposed to decreasing the tidal volume). These medications

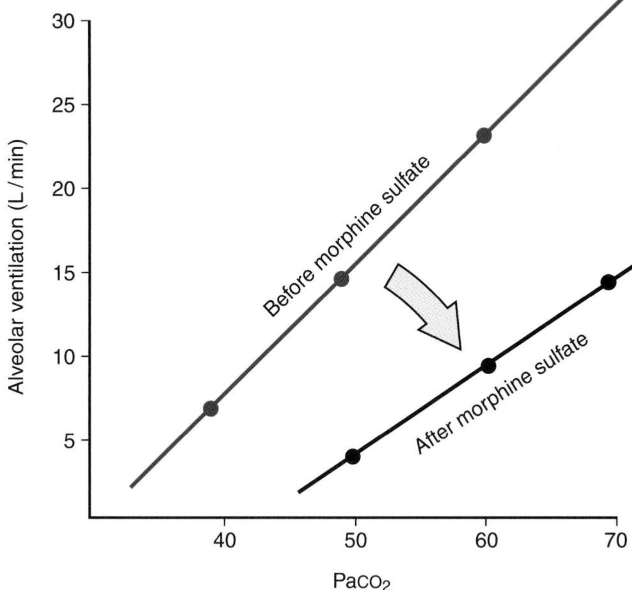

Figure 75-1 Opiates depress ventilation. This graph illustrates the shifting of the CO_2 response curve down and to the right. (Modified from Nonvolatile anesthetic agents. In: Morgan GE, Mikhail MS, Murray MJ: Clinical Anesthesiology. 4th ed. New York: Lange Medical Books/McGraw-Hill Medical Publishing Division; 2005:195. Available at: http://www.accessmedicine.com.)

have a direct effect on the respiratory centers in the medulla, producing a dose-dependent depression of the ventilatory response to CO_2. A decreased slope and rightward shift is noted on the CO_2 response curve when opioids are administered (Figure 75-1). The apnea threshold, defined as the highest $Paco_2$ without ventilatory effort, is increased with the use of opioids. They also blunt the increase in ventilation in response to hypoxemia. Further, morphine and meperidine can cause histamine-induced bronchospasm.

Musculoskeletal Effects

Opioids can produce generalized skeletal muscle rigidity, a phenomenon associated with the more-potent opiates, e.g., fentanyl, sufentanil, and carfentanil. Loss of chest-wall compliance and contraction of laryngeal and pharyngeal muscles can be severe, resulting in ventilatory difficulty even with positive-pressure ventilation. The mechanism of opioid-induced muscle rigidity is believed to be mediated by the μ receptors at the supraspinal level by increasing dopamine synthesis and by inhibiting γ-aminobutyric acid activity. This muscle rigidity can be prevented by decreasing the rate of opioid administration or by concomitantly administering a neuromuscular blocking agent and controlling ventilation.

Postoperative shivering can be attenuated with meperidine, which may act through a κ-receptor mechanism. Only 12.5 to 25 mg of meperidine, administered intravenously as a slow push, is usually needed to produce this effect in an adult.

Cardiovascular Effects

At clinically relevant doses, opioids do not cause significant myocardial depression; however, opioids can cause a dose-dependent bradycardia resulting in decreased cardiac output. One exception is meperidine, which may cause tachycardia because of its structural similarities to atropine. Meperidine may also cause a decrease in myocardial contractility because it has negative inotropic effects. Most opioids exert their cardiovascular effects both by sympatholysis via vasomotor centers in the medulla and by increased parasympathetic tone via vagal pathways. Prolongation of the QT interval has been noted with both meperidine and methadone administration.

Gastrointestinal Effects

Opioids increase nonperistaltic smooth muscle tone in the small and large bowel via vagal and peripheral mechanisms; however, this ineffective nonpropulsive activity leads to an overall increase in bowel transit time and can result in ileus.

Hormone Effects

Opioids may decrease the stress response to pain and surgery by acting on the hypothalamus. The inhibition of gonadotropin-releasing hormone and corticotropin-releasing factor results in decreased release of endogenous cortisol.

Histamine Release

Although true allergic responses to opioids are rare, opioids may cause a non–IgE-mediated release of histamine from mast cells, decreasing systemic vascular resistance, with resultant decreases in blood pressure and tachycardia. This response is most evident with meperidine and morphine.

It is worth noting that, due to its many associated toxicities (many of them noted previously), meperidine has fallen out of favor for use as a pain reliever. However, meperidine is still widely utilized in the management of postoperative shivering.

Opioid-Induced Hyperalgesia

Increasing evidence suggests that opioids, which are intended to treat pain, may actually make patients more sensitive to pain and may worsen preexisting pain states. Initially, opioids provide clear analgesic effects but then can become associated with states of hyperalgesia (increased sensitivity to noxious stimuli). Opioid-induced hyperalgesia was first noted in patients chronically consuming these medications, but it has now been recognized in patients receiving opioids for durations as short as the length of a surgical procedure. An example is remifentanil, an ultra–short-acting opiate used as an infusion during surgical procedures. Hyperalgesia has been noted after 60- to 90-min infusions with this opioid agonist. The mechanism is thought to be secondary to increased nociceptive signal processing at the level of the spinal cord. Coadministration of ketamine abolishes the hyperalgesia induced by remifentanyl, implying an underlying NMDA-receptor (*N*-methyl-D-aspartate) mechanism.

Dependence and Tolerance

Dependence and tolerance are two significant problems with long-term administration of opioids. Dependence refers to the presence of withdrawal symptoms if a drug is withheld and can be either physical or psychological. Psychological dependence refers to craving for a drug and is synonymous with addiction. Tolerance is the need to increase the dose of an opioid over time to maintain the desired analgesic effect, reflecting the desensitization of the antinociceptive pathways to opiates and the upregulation of opioid-binding receptors.

Suggested Readings

Angst MS, Clark JD. Opioid-induced hyperalgesia: A qualitative systematic review. *Anesthesiology*. 2006;104:570-587.

Brunton L, Blumenthal D, Buxton I, Parker K. *Goodman and Gilman's Manual of Pharmacology and Therapeutics*. New York: McGraw-Hill; 2008:349.

Joly V, Richebe P, Guignard B, et al. Remifentanil-induced postoperative hyperalgesia and its prevention with small-dose ketamine. *Anesthesiology*. 2005; 103:147-155.

Kalso E. Opioids in chronic non-cancer pain: Systematic review of efficacy and safety. *Pain*. 2004;112:372-380.

Trescot AM, Helm S, Hansen H, et al. Opioids in the management of chronic non-cancer pain: An update of American Society of the Interventional Pain Physicians' (ASIPP) guidelines. *Pain Physician*. 2008;11(2 Suppl):S5-62.

CHAPTER 76

Cardiovascular Effects of Opioids

Kent H. Rehfeldt, MD, FASE

Anesthesiologists frequently administer opioids preoperatively, intraoperatively, and postoperatively, most often to provide analgesia or as part of a balanced anesthetic. A predominantly opioid-based anesthetic may be selected for hemodynamically unstable patients because, compared with other classes of anesthetic drugs, opioids usually cause fewer unwanted changes in the hemodynamic profile. Nonetheless, opioids, especially in large doses, can alter hemodynamics. Changes in heart rate, cardiac conduction, blood pressure, and myocardial contractility are possible. Whether these effects are beneficial or detrimental depends on the clinical setting.

Heart Rate

The administration of opioids (with the exception of meperidine) usually results in decreased heart rate. The tendency of meperidine to increase heart rate has been attributed to its atropine-like structure or to the effect of its principal metabolite, normeperidine. The reduction in heart rate that typically accompanies the use of opioids other than meperidine is seen in conjunction with reduced sympathetic tone and may be desirable in some patients, such as those at risk for developing coronary ischemia. When compared with the use of fentanyl and sufentanil, the use of alfentanil less reliably prevents increases in heart rate and blood pressure in response to surgical stimulation during cardiac operations. Additionally, opioids directly stimulate μ receptors in medullary vagal nuclei, an effect that can be attenuated by bilateral vagotomy. Some investigators have also noted decreases in heart rate with the use of remifentanil, even in the absence of enhanced parasympathetic tone, suggesting a direct effect on cardiac conduction tissue. Severe bradycardia and even asystole have been reported following the administration of opioids, such as remifentanil; fortunately these serious reactions are rare and may be more likely to occur when remifentanil is given as a bolus or when administered to patients who are also receiving β-adrenergic receptor or calcium channel blocking agents. Similarly, profound bradycardia may be more likely to occur when opioids are given during vagotonic procedures. For example, fentanyl, sufentanil, and alfentanil significantly augment the oculocardiac reflex, contributing to intraoperative bradycardia during some eye operations. Pretreatment with drugs such as pancuronium or atropine diminishes the likelihood of occurrence of opioid-induced decreases in heart rate.

Blood Pressure

Besides causing bradycardia, opioid administration can also lower blood pressure. Decreased sympathetic tone probably accounts for most of the blood pressure reduction. The tone of both venous capacitance vessels and arteriolar resistance vessels may decrease. Hypotensive effects are most prominent in patients with increased sympathetic tone, such as those with congestive heart failure or hypovolemia. Blood pressure changes are less common in isovolemic supine patients. However, orthostatic hypotension may be seen in patients with autonomic nervous system impairment (e.g., autonomic neuropathy in patients with diabetes). Besides reducing sympathetic tone, a direct opioid effect on vascular smooth muscle has also been observed when sufentanil and remifentanil have been administered in experimental settings. These direct effects on vascular smooth muscle appear to be independent of a neurogenic or systemic mechanism and may contribute to the hypotension sometimes encountered when sufentanil and remifentanil are used clinically. Interestingly, pretreatment with glycopyrrolate may attenuate the decrease in blood pressure that can accompany remifentanil administration.

In addition to reducing sympathetic tone and direct vascular effects, morphine and meperidine also activate mast cells and trigger histamine and tryptase release, which can contribute to vasodilatation and hypotension. The use of fentanyl, sufentanil, alfentanil, and remifentanil does not promote histamine release.

Hypertension is occasionally observed in patients receiving opioid medications intraoperatively. Most frequently seen in patients with preserved left ventricular function, hypertensive responses probably result from either too low of an opioid dose or inadequate administration of other types of anesthetic agents.

Myocardial Contractility

The inotropic effects of opioids are probably not clinically important in most settings when typical doses are used. However, some investigators have noted dose-dependent increases in myocardial contractility with the use of agents such as fentanyl and sufentanil, possibly related to direct myocardial adrenergic stimulation. The use of alfentanil may increase myocardial contractility by augmenting the sensitivity to calcium. On the other hand, meperidine may have detectable negative inotropic effects. Variable effects on myocardial contractility have been reported in response to morphine use.

Opioids and Myocardial Ischemia

Opioids are often selected for patients who currently have or have a history of ischemic heart disease. In fact, morphine is included in advanced cardiac care algorithms for the treatment of patients presenting with acute myocardial ischemia. The benefits of morphine in these patients include a reduction in sympathetic tone, lowering of the heart rate, and vasodilatation, resulting in reduced preload without altering the responsiveness of large coronary arterioles to vasoactive agents. Overall, a more favorable myocardial oxygen supply/demand ratio is maintained. Similarly, opioid-based anesthetic agents promote a more favorable myocardial oxygen supply/demand ratio when compared with inhalation-based anesthesia. Opioid use is not associated with coronary steal. Although it is not well established clinically, the use of opioids may confer an ischemic preconditioning benefit similar to that seen with the use of inhalation anesthetic agents.

Electrophysiologic Effects

Anesthesiologists are frequently asked to provide care for patients undergoing catheter-based electrophysiology investigations and procedures. Thus, an understanding of the impact of commonly used sedative and anesthetic drugs on electrophysiology parameters is essential. As noted, opioids typically reduce sympathetic outflow and enhance parasympathetic tone by direct stimulation of vagal nuclei. The enhanced vagal tone that follows fentanyl administration may manifest during electrophysiology procedures as prolonged sinus node recovery time, which is a measure of sinus node automaticity. Remifentanil also prolongs sinus node recovery time, increases sinoatrial conduction time, and prolongs the ventricular effective refractory period. Ideally, the use and possible effects of opioids on measured electrophysiology parameters should be discussed with the interventional cardiologist prior to beginning the procedure.

Opioids and the Long QT Syndrome

The impact of perioperatively administered drugs on the QT interval and the possible promotion of torsades de pointes in patients with congenital long QT syndrome have recently been reviewed. A few reports link the use of sufentanil and high-dose methadone to QT prolongation or torsades de pointes. On the other hand, remifentanil seems to have no effect on the QT interval, at least, as has been shown in a large animal model. Although conflicting evidence exists, fentanyl and morphine may be the preferred opioids for use in patients with congenital long QT syndrome.

Suggested Readings

Arnold RW, Jensen PA, Kovtoun TA, et al. The profound augmentation of the oculocardiac reflex by fast acting opioids. *Binocul Vis Strabismus Q*. 2004;19:215-222.

Blunk JA, Schmelz M, Zeck S, et al. Opioid-inducted mast cell activation and vascular responses is not mediated by μ-opioid receptors: An in-vivo microdialysis study in human skin. *Anesth Analg*. 2004;8:364-370.

Ebert TJ, Ficke DJ, Arain SR, et al. Vasodilation from sufentanil in humans. *Anesth Analg*. 2005;101:1677-1680.

Fujii K, Iranami H, Nakamura Y, et al. Fentanyl added to propofol anesthesia elongates sinus node recovery time in pediatric patients with paroxysmal supraventricular tachycardia. *Anesth Analg*. 2009;109:456-460.

Graham MD, Hopkins PM, Harrison SM. The effects of alfentanil on cytosolic Ca^{2+} and contraction in rat ventricular myocytes. *Anesth Analg*. 2004;98:1013-1016.

Kies SM, Pabelick CM, Hurley HA, et al. Anesthesia for patients with congenital long QT syndrome. *Anesthesiology*. 2005;102:204-210.

Noseir RK, Ficke DJ, Kundu A, et al. Sympathetic and vascular consequences from remifentanil in humans. *Anesth Analg*. 2003;96:1645-1650.

Robbins GR, Wynands JE, Whalley DG, et al. Pharmacokinetics of alfentanil and clinical responses during cardiac surgery. *Can J Anaesth*. 1990;37:52-57.

Zaballos M, Jimeno C, Almendral J, et al. Cardiac electrophysiological effects of remifentanil: Study in a closed-chest porcine model. *Br J Anaesth*. 2009;103:191-198.

CHAPTER 77

Opioid Side Effects: Muscle Rigidity and Biliary Colic

Richard L. Applegate II, MD

Neuromuscular Effects of Opioids

Muscle rigidity can occur following administration of opioidergic agents. The rigidity can be in the muscles of the trunk or extremities and may involve muscles of the upper airway. Skeletal muscle rigidity can present as dyskinesia, hoarseness, or difficulty breathing.

When opioid-induced muscle rigidity occurs during induction of anesthesia, rigidity can prevent adequate mask ventilation. The ventilation difficulty can cause hypercarbia, hypoxia, or both. Severe rigidity can be associated with insufflation of gas into the stomach if excessive pressures are used in an attempt to ventilate the lung.

Intubated patients in the intensive care unit who have received intravenously administered opioids may develop muscle rigidity that impairs positive-pressure ventilation. Several reports in neonates suggest that opioid-induced rigidity may hinder airway management. Endoscopic studies demonstrate that the primary cause of this difficulty in ventilation is obstruction at the level of the vocal cords.

Mechanism

The mechanism of opioid-induced rigidity in adults is not completely understood. Results from studies of rat models suggest that activation of central μ_1 receptors trigger this effect, whereas δ and κ receptors—sites where μ_1 receptors are plentiful—may antagonize the effect. Central nervous system sites that may be involved in this rigidity include the basal ganglia, locus coeruleus, and the periaqueductal gray matter.

Risk Factors

A number of risk factors are proposed, including extremes of age (neonates and octogenarians), the presence of neurologic disorders such as Parkinson disease, and critical illness.

Incidence

The reported incidence of difficulty with mask ventilation on induction of anesthesia following the administration of opioids varies widely, from 0% to 100% of subjects. Early studies reported the incidence to be as high as more than 80%, with many later reports showing the incidence to be between 20% and 40%. This range appears to reflect differences in dosage, administration rates, and pretreatment with nondepolarizing neuromuscular blocking agents or benzodiazepines and differences among the various opioids. Interestingly, the incidence of rigidity following opioid administration appears to be decreasing over time. A recent comparison study reported an incidence of rigidity of only 4 of 1229 remifentanil recipients and 0 of 1209 fentanyl recipients. This is much lower than had been reported earlier, which may reflect the impact of practice improvement and education on the risk presented by rapid administration of opioids at the time of anesthesia induction.

Opioids That May Cause Rigidity

It appears that any μ-agonist opioid can induce this condition, with reports of muscle rigidity occurring after administration of fentanyl, sufentanil, alfentanil, remifentanil, and morphine. The more potent the opioid, the greater the likelihood of rigidity occurring at an equipotent dose; however, despite this widely held belief, a meta-analysis demonstrated no significant differences in the incidence of rigidity among these drugs. Doses of fentanyl as low as 1 μg/kg have been reported to cause ventilatory difficulty, but the incidence appears to be greater with more rapid administration of higher doses. Bolus administration of potent opioids such as remifentanil may present an increased risk for developing this complication, and muscle rigidity is perhaps more pronounced in the postoperative period.

Treatment

The treatment of opioid-induced muscle rigidity includes administration of nondepolarizing neuromuscular blocking agents, anesthesia induction agents (propofol, thiopental), and benzodiazepines (midazolam, diazepam). Prevention measures include pretreatment with nondepolarizing neuromuscular blocking agents or benzodiazepines and slow administration of the potent opioids.

Biliary Effects of Opioids

The common biliary duct terminates at the sphincter of Oddi in the wall of the duodenum. Contraction of the sphincter can be triggered by a wide range of agents, including cholecystokinin, opioids, vagus nerve transmission, and a range of endogenous transmitters that may be released by local gastrointestinal stimulation following a meal. Importantly, administration of μ-receptor agonists can lead to increases in sphincter of Oddi contraction, with increases in common bile duct pressure and delayed emptying of the gallbladder or bile duct. If this occurs intraoperatively during cholangiography, a mistaken diagnosis of biliary stone or stricture could be made. This assumption, in turn, may lead to unnecessary surgical exploration of the common bile duct. However, the clinical significance of intraoperative opioid-induced increases in sphincter of Oddi contraction and bile duct pressure is not clear.

Opioids That May Cause Biliary Spasm

All opioids have the potential to cause an increase in motor tone in the sphincter of Oddi, with a resultant increase in common bile duct pressure. The relative potency for this effect among various agents has been compared in a number of studies, with varying findings. Traditionally, morphine has been found to be a more potent stimulant for this contraction, as compared with meperidine. Remifentanil appears to delay gallbladder emptying, with a short duration of effect after the infusion is stopped. Agonist-antagonist agents have lesser effects on gallbladder emptying and bile duct pressures, whereas naloxone will reverse the biliary effects of μ-receptor agonists.

Treatment

A variety of agents can be given to reverse opioid-induced biliary spasm. Although naloxone will completely reverse the biliary effects, the abrupt antagonism of analgesia may be undesirable. Anticholinergic agents, calcium channel blockers, nitroglycerin, isosorbide, and glucagon are reported to be effective in lowering bile duct pressure in the presence of morphine-induced biliary spasm.

Suggested Readings

Bennett JA, Abrams JT, Van Riper DF, Horrow JC. Difficult or impossible ventilation after sufentanil-induced anesthesia is caused primarily by vocal cord closure. *Anesthesiology*. 1997;87:1070-1074.

Bosch A, Pena LR. The sphincter of Oddi. *Dig Dis Sci*. 2007;52:1211-1218.

Gallantine EL, Meert TF. Antinociceptive and adverse effects of mu and kappa opioid receptor agonists: A comparison of morphine and U50488-H. *Basic Clin Pharmacol Toxicol*. 2008;103:419-427.

Komatsu R, Turan AM, Orhan-Sungur M, et al. Remifentanil for general anaesthesia: A systematic review. *Anaesthesia*. 2007;62:1266-1280.

Marsh DF, Hodkinson B. Remifentanil in paediatric anaesthetic practice. *Anaesthesia*. 2009;64:301-308.

Nakada J, Nishira M, Hosoda R, et al. Priming with rocuronium or vecuronium prevents remfentanil-mediated muscle rigidity and difficult ventilation. *J Anesth*. 2009;23:323-328.

Wu S, Zhang Z, Jin J, et al. Effects of narcotic analgesic drugs on human Oddi's sphincter motility. *World J Gastroenterol*. 2004;10:2901-2904.

CHAPTER 78

Nondepolarizing Neuromuscular Blocking Agents

Mark T. Keegan, MB, MRCPI, MSc

The introduction of nondepolarizing neuromuscular blocking agents (NMBAs) into clinical practice marked a significant advance in anesthesia and surgery. The past 20 years have seen a significant evolution in nondepolarizing NMBAs, with the appearance of new drugs, free from many of the undesirable side effects of their predecessors. Some of these new agents have threatened the position of succinylcholine as the drug of choice for rapid-onset, short-acting muscle relaxation.

Mechanism of Action

By competing with acetylcholine (ACh) for binding to nicotinic receptor α subunits, nondepolarizing NMBAs cause receptor inhibition, thus resulting in skeletal muscle relaxation. The nondepolarizing NMBAs may also be capable of directly blocking the ion channel, stopping the flux of Na^+ through the ion pore. Some nondepolarizing NMBAs block Na^+ channels on prejunctional nicotinic ACh receptors, interfering with mobilization of ACh from sites of synthesis. Calcium-dependent release of ACh is not affected.

Characteristics of Neuromuscular Nondepolarizing Blockade

Muscle relaxation caused by nondepolarizing NMBAs is characterized clinically by a train of four T4:T1 ratio less than 1 (with <0.7 representing adequate surgical relaxation), tetanic "fade," post-tetanic potentiation, absence of fasciculations, potentiation by other nondepolarizing NMBAs, and antagonism of the block by acetylcholinesterase inhibitors. Blockade by nondepolarizing NMBAs occurs more rapidly in laryngeal adductors, diaphragm, and masseter than in the adductor pollicis. The ED_{95} is the dose needed to produce 95% suppression of a single-twitch response evoked by a peripheral nerve stimulator in the presence of NO_2-barbiturate-opioid anesthesia and is used as a measure of potency. Administration of one to three times the ED_{95} allows tracheal intubation. The speed of onset of blockade is inversely proportional to the potency of the NMBA.

Alterations in Sensitivity

Enhanced NMBA effects occur with administration of inhalation anesthetics, local anesthetics, diuretics, antiarrhythmics, aminoglycosides, magnesium, and lithium. Hypothermia, acidosis, and hypokalemia also increase the potency of nondepolarizing NMBAs. Patients with myasthenia gravis are very sensitive to the effects of nondepolarizing NMBAs. In contrast, patients with burn injuries are resistant to the effects owing to proliferation of nicotinic receptors (upregulation). Administration of 10% of the intubating dose of an NMBA 2 to 4 min before the full intubating dose is given is known as priming. Priming may accelerate the onset of muscle relaxation to approximately 60 sec.

Chemical Structure and Pharmacokinetics

Currently used nondepolarizing NMBAs are benzylisoquinolinium and aminosteroid compounds, both of which have one or more positively charged quaternary ammonium groups (Tables 78-1 and 78-2). (ACh has a single quaternary ammonium.) The presence of a quaternary ammonium group on nondepolarizing NMBAs means that they are highly ionized water-soluble compounds at physiologic pH. Lipid solubility is limited, so nondepolarizing NMBAs do not easily cross lipid-membrane barriers such as the blood-brain barrier. After a single dose, the volume of distribution is similar to the extracellular fluid volume; the volume of distribution, plasma clearance, and elimination may be affected by patient age or the presence of renal or hepatic dysfunction. Although many nondepolarizing NMBAs rely on hepatic or renal clearance, or both, some are eliminated in an unusual fashion (see following discussion).

Nonrelaxant Side Effects

Nonrelaxant side effects of nondepolarizing NMBAs include histamine release and cardiovascular and autonomic effects. Such side effects are detailed in Chapter 79.

Commonly Used Nondepolarizing Neuromuscular Blocking Agents

Vecuronium

Vecuronium is a monoquaternary aminosteroid NMBA. At an ED_{95} of 0.05 mg/kg, its onset of action is 3 to 5 min and its duration of action is 20 to 35 min. The drug is supplied in powder form because it is unstable in solution. Vecuronium is metabolized by the liver and cleared by the kidney.

Table 78-1 Nondepolarizing Neuromuscular Blocking Agents by Duration of Action

Structural Class	Short-Acting Agent	Intermediate-Acting Agent	Long-Acting Agent
Benzylisoquinolinium	Mivacurium*	Atracurium Cisatracurium	*d*-Tubocurarine* Metocurine* Doxacurium*
Aminosteroid	Rapacuronium*	Vecuronium Rocuronium	Pancuronium
Asymmetrical mixed-onium chlorofumarate	Gantacurium*		

*Not available in the United States.

Table 78-2 Characteristics of Commonly Used Neuromuscular Blocking Agents

Agent	Intubating Dose (mg/kg)	Infusion Rate ($\mu g \cdot kg^{-1} \cdot min^{-1}$)	Onset (sec)*	Duration of Action	Vagolysis	Histamine Release	Elimination	Comments
Succinylcholine	1.5	NA	30-90	Very short	Variable	Slight	Butyrylcholinesterase	Depolarizing muscle relaxant
Mivacurium	0.15	3-12	90-150	Short	No	Yes	Butyrylcholinesterase	No longer available in U.S.
Rapacuronium	1.5	NA	45-90	Short	Yes	Yes	Kidney, ester hydrolysis	No longer available
Rocuronium	0.9-1.2	9-12	60-90	Intermediate	Yes	No	Liver, kidney	
Cisatracurium	0.15-0.2	1-3	90-120	Intermediate	No	No	Hofmann degradation	
Atracurium	0.5	3-12	90-150	Intermediate	No	Yes	Hofmann degradation, ester hydrolysis	
Vecuronium	0.08-0.12	1-2	90-150	Intermediate	No	No	Liver, kidney	
Pancuronium	0.08-0.12	NA	Slow	Long	Yes	No	Kidney, liver	
Gantacurium	0.4-0.6	NA	90-120	Very short	No	Yes	Cysteine adduction, ester hydrolysis	Still investigational

*Time to intubation.
NA, not applicable.

Biliary excretion also plays a role in its elimination. Repeated dosing of vecuronium causes a cumulative effect that is less than that of pancuronium but greater than that of atracurium. Vecuronium has minimal, if any, cardiovascular effects.

Atracurium

Atracurium is an intermediate-acting NMBA, which is a mixture of 10 stereoisomers. At an ED_{95} dose of 0.2 mg/kg, its onset and duration of action are 3 to 5 min and 20 to 35 min, respectively. Atracurium is metabolized and eliminated independent of the liver and kidney. It undergoes spontaneous nonenzymatic in vivo degradation (Hofmann elimination) at normal body pH and temperature. The drug also undergoes hydrolysis by nonspecific plasma esterases, unrelated to butyrylcholinesterase. One third of administered atracurium is degraded by Hofmann elimination and two thirds by ester hydrolysis. Both pathways produce laudanosine, which, although not active as an NMBA, may cause central nervous system excitation at high doses in animals. At doses of atracurium used clinically in humans, laudanosine does not appear to have significant effects. Repeated supplemental doses of atracurium do not produce a significant cumulative drug effect because of the rapid clearance of the drug from plasma. Accordingly, there is consistency of time to recovery of neuromuscular function. Atracurium causes a dose-dependent histamine release, which is significant at doses greater than 0.5 mg/kg. The use of atracurium should be avoided in patients with asthma.

Cisatracurium

One of the 10 stereoisomers of atracurium, the 1R-cis, 1R′-cis form, makes up approximately 15% of the atracurium mixture. The purified preparation, known as cisatracurium, is an NMBA that is four times more potent than the parent compound. Cisatracurium does not cause histamine release; hence, it has minimal cardiovascular effects. Metabolism is by the Hofmann degradation, but nonspecific esterases have no role in its elimination.

Pancuronium

Pancuronium, a bisquaternary aminosteroid, is the most commonly administered long-acting NMBA. It has an ED_{95} of 0.07 mg/kg, with an onset of action of 3 to 5 min and duration of action of 60 to 90 min. The drug is mainly excreted unchanged in the urine, although there is a small component of hepatic metabolism. Renal failure may increase its duration of action. Pancuronium causes a vagolytic effect, leading to a modest increase in heart rate, blood pressure, and cardiac output. For this reason, it may be a good choice in patients undergoing cardiac operations, especially when a high-dose opioid technique is being used.

The Search for a Replacement for Succinylcholine

Although the *depolarizing* NMBA succinylcholine is widely used, its significant side effects have led to the search for an NMBA with an equivalent rapid onset and short duration of action.

Rocuronium

Rocuronium is a monoquaternary aminosteroid with a structure similar to that of vecuronium. When administered at three times ED_{95}, rocuronium has an onset of action similar to that of succinylcholine, although the laryngeal muscles are relatively more resistant to the effects of rocuronium. Doses used for rapid tracheal intubation (0.9 to 1.2 mg/kg) typically cause neuromuscular blockade that may last for an hour or more. Sugammadex, a modified γ-cyclodextrin, is not a muscle relaxant but, instead, is the first selective relaxant binding agent. It is capable of reversing any depth of neuromuscular blockade induced by rocuronium and, to a lesser extent, vecuronium. The drug does not yet have U.S. Food and Drug Administration approval for general use, but it has the potential to change rocuronium from an intermediate-acting NMBA to a short-acting NMBA.

Rapacuronium and Mivacurium

Rapacuronium, a monoquaternary synthetic steroid NMBA that has a rapid onset of action, was introduced as a replacement for succinylcholine. However, its tendency to cause life-threatening bronchospasm led to its withdrawal from clinical use. Mivacurium also has a rapid onset of action and is hydrolyzed by plasma cholinesterase at 80% of the rate of succinylcholine metabolism. Histamine-induced bronchospasm was also problematic with mivacurium, and it is no longer available in the United States, though it is still used elsewhere.

Gantacurium

Gantacurium, an NMBA currently under investigation, represents a new class of nondepolarizing NMBAs known as the asymmetrical mixed-onium chlorofumarates. It is degraded by two nonenzymatic chemical reactions, cysteine adduction and ester hydrolysis. Gantacurium has a pharmacodynamic profile similar to that of succinylcholine. Gantacurium has undergone phase 1 and 2 trials but has not been approved by the Food and Drug Administration at present.

Suggested Readings

Abrishami A, Ho J, Wong J, et al. Sugammadex, a selective reversal medication for preventing postoperative residual neuromuscular blockade. *Cochrane Database Syst Rev*. 2009:CD007362.

Claudius C, Garvey LH, Viby-Mogensen J. The undesirable effects of neuromuscular blocking drugs. *Anaesthesia*. 2009;64(Suppl 1):10-21.

Martyn JA, Fagerlund MJ, Eriksson LI. Basic principles of neuromuscular transmission. *Anaesthesia*. 2009;64(Suppl 1):1-9.

Naguib M, Brull SJ. Update on neuromuscular pharmacology. *Curr Opin Anaesthesiol*. 2009;22:483-490.

Perry JJ, Lee JS, Sillberg VA, Wells GA. Rocuronium versus succinylcholine for rapid sequence induction intubation. *Cochrane Database Syst Rev*. 2008: CD002788.

Stoelting RK, Hillier SC. *Pharmacology and Physiology in Anesthetic Practice*. 4th ed. Philadelphia: Lippincott, Williams & Wilkins; 2006:208-250.

CHAPTER 79

Nonrelaxant Side Effects of Nondepolarizing Neuromuscular Blocking Agents

Mark T. Keegan, MD

In addition to their action on the neuromuscular junction, nondepolarizing neuromuscular blocking agents (NMBAs) produce a variety of nonrelaxant effects. Many of these "side effects" may be unwanted and potentially harmful; nondepolarizing NMBAs are commonly implicated in medication-related adverse perioperative events. Some nonrelaxant effects may be used to the advantage of the patient and the practitioner.

Interference with Autonomic Function

Nondepolarizing NMBAs may interact with nicotinic and muscarinic cholinergic receptors in the sympathetic and parasympathetic nervous systems. The length of the carbon chain separating the two positively charged ammonium groups influences the specificity of a nondepolarizing NMBA for nicotinic receptors at autonomic ganglia (versus nicotinic receptors at the neuromuscular junction). The so-called "autonomic margin" reflects the difference between the dose of a nondepolarizing NMBA that causes neuromuscular blockade and the dose that leads to circulatory effects. For example, blockade of autonomic ganglia leading to hypotension occurs with the use of *d*-tubocurarine, an older nondepolarizing NMBA, at doses slightly higher than those required for blockade of the neuromuscular junction. However, the ED_{95} doses for neuromuscular blockade with the use of cisatracurium, vecuronium, and rocuronium are significantly lower than the doses that cause autonomic effects, so these drugs are said to have a wide autonomic margin.

The effects of nondepolarizing NMBAs on the parasympathetic muscarinic receptors in the heart may be clinically significant. Pancuronium, for example, produces a vagolytic action on nodal cells mediated through muscarinic receptors. This action occurs at doses used clinically for neuromuscular blockade, leading to an increase in heart rate.

The sympathetic nervous system contains at least three sets of muscarinic receptors. Blockade of these receptors on dopaminergic interneurons decreases modulation of ganglionic traffic (disinhibition), and blockade of adrenergic neurons results in removal of a negative feedback system for catecholamine release. Muscarinic blockade at sympathetic adrenergic neurons leading to inhibition of norepinephrine uptake represents the mechanism behind the exaggerated response sometimes seen with pancuronium during light anesthesia. The drug may cause norepinephrine release independent of muscarinic blockade. Thus, pancuronium may cause tachycardia and a predisposition to arrhythmias because of vagal block with shift toward adrenergic tone, indirect sympathomimetic activation, and atrioventricular nodal blockade (greater than sinoatrial nodal blockade).

Histamine Release

The benzylisoquinolinium compounds cause nonimmunologic release of histamine, and possibly other mediators, from mast cells. Histamine release is a function of dose and rate of administration. The physiologic effects of histamine include positive chronotropy (H_2 receptors), positive inotropy (H_2 receptors), positive dromotropy (H_1 receptors), coronary artery effects (H_1 receptors, vasoconstriction; H_2 receptors, vasodilation), and peripheral vasodilation. Erythema of the face, neck, and torso may occur. Bronchospasm is rare, but may be severe, and has been a limiting factor in the use of some nondepolarizing NMBAs. Rapid administration of atracurium in doses greater than 0.4 mg/kg and mivacurium at doses greater than 0.15 mg/kg has been associated with histamine-related hypotension. In general, however, histamine release causes minimal effects in healthy patients. If clinical manifestations occur, they are usually of short duration (lasting 1 to 5 min), and the response undergoes rapid tachyphylaxis, so subsequent doses of nondepolarizing NMBAs cause little, if any, effect. Vecuronium, at doses of 0.1 to 0.2 mg/kg, may rarely cause severe bronchospasm, probably because of competitive inhibition of histamine-*N*-methyltransferase, thus inhibiting the

Table 79-1 Approximate Autonomic Margins of Safety of Nondepolarizing Neuromuscular Blocking Agents*

Drug	Vagus†	Sympathetic Ganglia†	Histamine Release‡
Benzylisoquinolinium Compounds			
Mivacurium	>50	>100	3.0
Atracurium	16	40	2.5
Cisatracurium	>50	>50	None
d-Tubocurarine§	0.6	2	0.6
Aminosteroid Compounds			
Vecuronium	20	>250	None
Rocuronium	3-5	>10	None
Pancuronium	3	>250	None

*Number of multiples of the ED_{95} for neuromuscular blockade required to produce the autonomic side effect (ED_{50}).
†In the cat.
‡In human subjects.
§No longer available.
ED, Effective dose.
Reproduced, with permission, from Naguib M, Lien CA. Pharmacology of muscle relaxants and their antagonists. In: Miller RD, Eriksson LI, Fleisher LA, et al, eds. Miller's Anesthesia. 7th ed. Philadelphia, Churchill Livingstone, 2009, Table 29.10.

Table 79-2 Clinical Autonomic Effects of Nondepolarizing Neuromuscular Blocking Agents

Drug	Autonomic Ganglia	Cardiac Muscarinic Receptors	Histamine Release
Benzylisoquinolinium Compounds			
Mivacurium	None	None	Slight
Atracurium	None	None	Slight
Cisatracurium	None	None	None
d-Tubocurarine*	Blocks	None	Moderate
Aminosteroidal Compounds			
Vecuronium	None	None	None
Rocuronium	None	Blocks weakly	None
Pancuronium	None	Blocks moderately	None

*No longer available.
Reproduced, with permission, from Naguib M, Lien CA. Pharmacology of muscle relaxants and their antagonists. In: Miller RD, Eriksson LI, Fleisher LA, et al, eds. Miller's Anesthesia. 7th ed. Philadelphia: Churchill Livingstone; 2009: Table 29.11.

degradation of histamine. Table 79-1 shows the approximate autonomic margins of safety of nondepolarizing NMBAs, and Table 79-2 illustrates the clinical autonomic effects of nondepolarizing NMBAs and the effects on histamine.

Respiratory Effects

In addition to the effects of histamine on the respiratory system described here, nondepolarizing NMBAs may directly affect autonomic receptors in the lungs. At least three types of muscarinic receptors are found in the airways, as shown in Figure 79-1. Nondepolarizing NMBAs have different antagonistic activities at both the M_2 and M_3 receptors. Blockade of M_2 receptors on airway smooth muscle causes an increased release of acetylcholine, which will act on M_3 receptors and cause bronchoconstriction. Blockade of M_3 receptors causes bronchodilation by inhibiting vagally mediated bronchoconstriction. Rapacuronium, a nondepolarizing NMBA, blocks M_2 receptors to a much greater extent than it

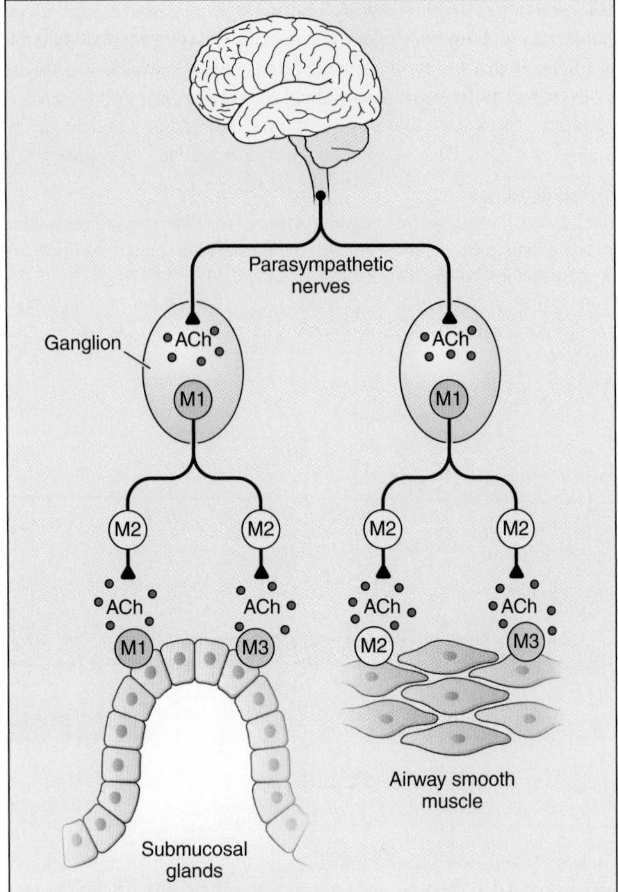

Figure 79-1 The muscarinic M_3 receptors are located postsynaptically on airway smooth muscle. Acetylcholine (ACh) stimulates M_3 receptors to cause contraction. M_2 muscarinic receptors are located presynaptically at the postganglionic parasympathetic nerve endings, and they function in a negative feedback mechanism to limit the release of ACh. (From Naguib M, Lien CA. Pharmacology of muscle relaxants and their antagonists. In: Miller RD, Eriksson LI, Fleisher LA, et al, eds. Miller's Anesthesia. 7th ed. Philadelphia; Churchill Livingstone; 2009: Fig. 29.21.)

blocks M_3 receptors. This causes an unacceptably high incidence of bronchospasm and led to the withdrawal of rapacuronium from the market.

Allergic Reactions

Although the development of anaphylaxis during anesthesia is very unusual, NMBAs are frequently implicated in such reactions. NMBAs were the most common causative agents in a large study of anesthesia-related anaphylaxis in France published in 2003. The quaternary ammonium ions found in nondepolarizing NMBAs may cross-react with food, cosmetics, industrial materials, and disinfectants. If a patient has reacted to one nondepolarizing NMBA, there is a significant risk of cross-reactivity to other NMBAs. The reactions are mediated through IgE.

Other Nonrelaxant Side Effects of Nondepolarizing Neuromuscular Blocking Agents

Teratogenicity and Carcinogenicity

NMBAs are highly ionized, but they and their metabolites are able to cross the placenta in small amounts. Nonetheless, at clinically relevant doses, human teratogenic effects—if they exist—are unproved. There are no data in the literature concerning carcinogenic effects of NMBAs.

Critical Illness Polymyoneuropathy

Medium-term and long-term administration of infusions of nondepolarizing NMBAs—especially those that are steroid based—in critically ill patients can lead to profound weakness, requiring prolonged periods of rehabilitation. Such weakness can occur in patients with multiorgan failure even in the absence of NMBA use, but weakness is more likely to occur when continuous infusions of nondepolarizing NMBAs are used.

Toxic Metabolites

Laudanosine, a metabolite of atracurium, causes central nervous system stimulation and possibly seizures, in high concentrations. Typically administered doses of atracurium and cis-atracurium, however, do not cause such problems.

Drug Interactions

Pancuronium inhibits butyrylcholinesterase and leads to an extremely prolonged action of mivacurium.

Suggested Readings

Kampe S, Krombach JW, Diefenbach C. Muscle relaxants. *Best Pract Res Clin Anaesthesiol*. 2003;17:137-146.

Mertes PM, Laxenaire MC, Alla F. Anaphylactic and anaphylactoid reactions occurring during anesthesia in 1999-2000. *Anesthesiology*. 2003;99:536-545.

Stoelting RK, Hillier SC. Neuromuscular blocking drugs. In: Stoelting RK, Hillier SC, eds. *Pharmacology and Physiology in Anesthetic Practice*. 4th ed. Philadelphia: Lippincott, Williams & Wilkins; 2006:208-250.

CHAPTER 80
Succinylcholine Side Effects

Aaron J. Mancuso, MD

Succinylcholine, a depolarizing neuromuscular blocking agent (NMBA) acts at the postjunctional neuromuscular membrane to produce rapid skeletal muscle relaxation. Although use of this drug is widespread, there are some limitations to its use. Several side effects have been associated with succinylcholine administration, including massive hyperkalemia, malignant hyperthermia, anaphylaxis, cardiac arrhythmia, prolonged apnea, phase II blockade, and postoperative myalgia, as well as increases in intraocular, intragastric, and intracranial pressures.

Massive Hyperkalemia

Depolarizing neuromuscular blocking NMBAs produce sustained opening of the nicotinic cholinergic receptor channel. Under normal conditions, postjunctional membrane depolarization results in leakage of potassium ions from the interior of cells sufficient to produce an average increase of 0.5 to 1.0 mEq/L in serum potassium concentration (Figure 80-1). However, when succinylcholine depolarizes muscle that has been traumatized (e.g., crush injury, thermal trauma) or denervated (e.g., upper motor neuron lesion), enough potassium may extrude from cells to produce systemic hyperkalemia and cardiac arrest. This susceptibility to hyperkalemia is thought to be caused by proliferation of junctional and extrajunctional cholinergic receptors. Receptor upregulation provides more postjunctional sites with which succinylcholine interacts, causing increased release of potassium. Patients with upper motor neuron lesions resulting from stroke, brain or spinal cord tumors, other intracerebral or spinal cord mass lesions, closed head injury, or encephalitis are at increased risk for developing succinylcholine-induced hyperkalemia. Other disease processes implicated in predisposing patients to developing succinylcholine-induced hyperkalemia include unhealed third-degree burns, severe intra-abdominal infections, severe metabolic acidosis with hypovolemia, crush injuries, and prolonged nondepolarizing muscle blockade or immobility. Because the precise point at which succinylcholine induces hyperkalemia after burns and other trauma cannot be known with certainty, it is advisable to not administer succinylcholine to such patients beyond the first 24 h after injury. Pretreatment with a defasciculating dose of neuromuscular blocking drug does *not* seem to influence the magnitude of potassium release evoked by succinylcholine.

Rhabdomyolysis

Patients with Duchenne muscular dystrophy may develop rhabdomyolysis, hyperkalemia, and cardiac arrest after receiving succinylcholine. This scenario has led to death in a number of children with undiagnosed Duchenne muscular dystrophy. In males younger than 5 years, the use of succinylcholine should be reserved for situations in which the drug is clearly indicated, such as emergency pediatric intubations and laryngospasm. Additionally, case reports of masseter muscle rigidity have also been associated with the subsequent development of rhabdomyolysis.

Malignant Hyperthermia

Succinylcholine is a known triggering agent for malignant hyperthermia (MH) and should be avoided in the anesthetic management of all patients known to be susceptible to or who have a strong family history of MH. Diseases and enzyme deficiencies associated with the development of MH include Noonan syndrome, osteogenesis imperfect, arthrogryposis, King-Denborough syndrome, carnitine palmitolytransferase II deficiency, and myophosphorylase deficiency (McArdle disease). In general, when administering anesthesia to patients with rare enzymopathies, it is best to first discuss the disease with known specialists, review the literature, or access online information regarding the potential for developing MH with the use of succinylcholine, even if there is no known association between the enzyme deficiency and MH. The gold standard test for MH susceptibility involves open muscle biopsy with contracture testing with caffeine-halothane contracture testing (used in North America) or in vitro contracture testing (used in Europe). New genetic tests for susceptibility for MH do exist, and a number of genetic mutations have been identified. Sequence variations in

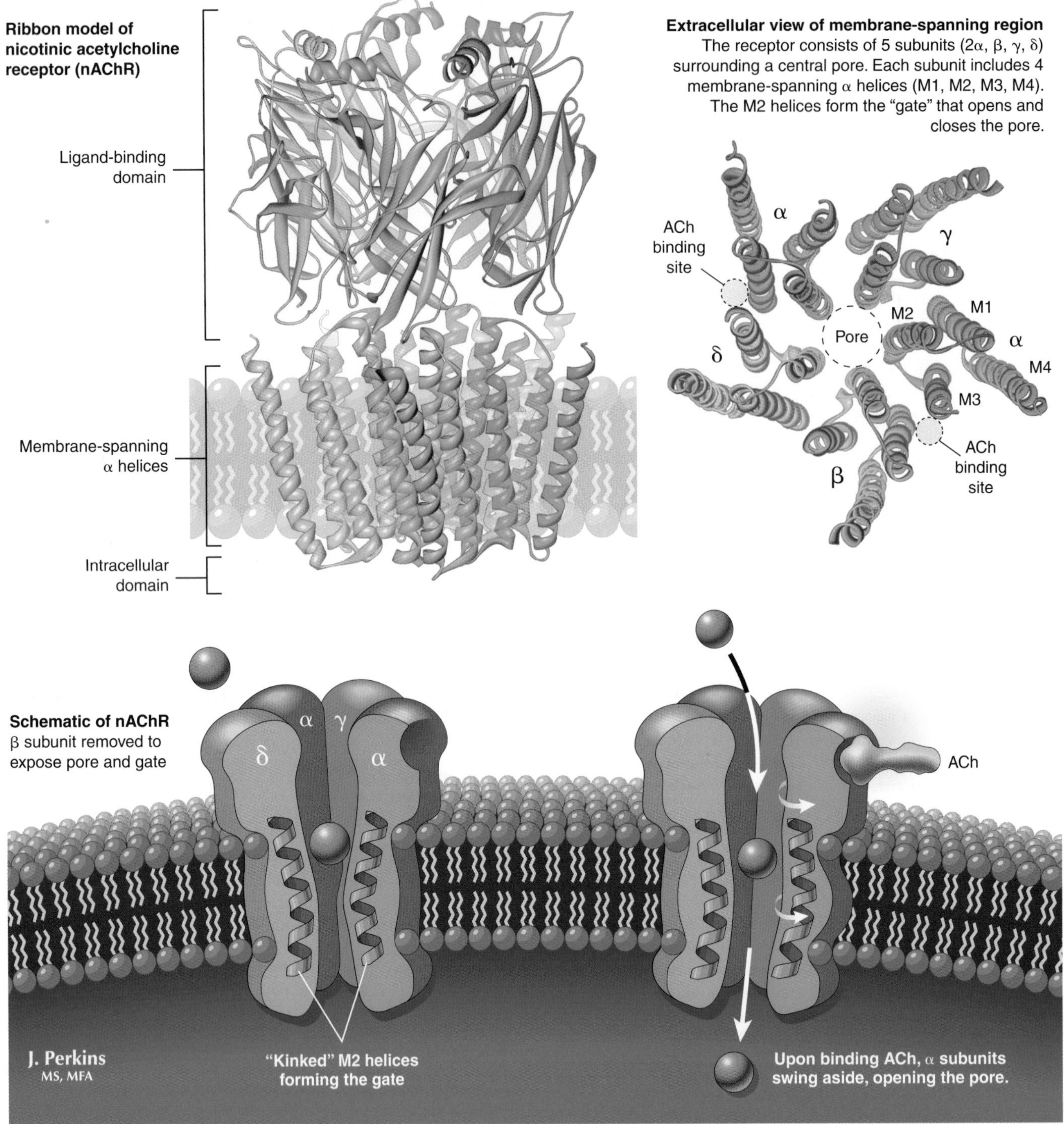

Figure 80-1 Nicotinic acetylcholine receptor. (Netter illustration from www.netterimages.com. © Elsevier Inc. All rights reserved.)

the ryanodine receptor gene (*RYR1*) in skeletal muscle have been described as the primary locus of MH susceptibility. (See Chapter 245 for more information on MH.)

Anaphylactic Reactions

Numerous case reports describe severe, and sometimes fatal, reactions to succinylcholine. Mortality rates have been reported between 3.5% and 4.7% even with prompt recognition and treatment of anaphylactic reactions. Several studies have demonstrated the reliability of skin testing, leukocyte histamine-release assay, and detection of IgE antibodies to succinylcholine in aiding in the diagnosis of allergic reactions to succinylcholine, even when these tests are performed several years after the initial anaphylactic reaction.

Cardiac Arrhythmias

Succinylcholine is capable of producing diverse cardiac arrhythmias. Not only does it directly stimulate muscarinic receptors of the sinus node, but it also stimulates muscarinic and nicotinic receptors in both sympathetic and parasympathetic ganglia. Therefore, children, who are sympathotonic, will be prone to developing bradycardia after receiving a single dose of succinylcholine, whereas adults, who are relatively vagotonic, will likely experience increased heart rate.

In addition, it has been demonstrated that successive boluses of succinylcholine, given 2 to 10 min apart, can result in sinus bradycardia, junctional rhythms, and even sinus arrest. This relationship of the second dose suggests a possible role of the succinylcholine metabolites succinylmonocholine and choline in enhancing the slowing of heart rate. Administration of a nondepolarizing drug approximately 3 min before the first dose of succinylcholine greatly reduces the incidence of bradycardia.

Succinylcholine-Associated Apnea

Some patients who receive a conventional dose of succinylcholine experience a prolonged neuromuscular block due to the presence of atypical plasma cholinesterase. More than 30 different variants of plasma cholinesterase have been described, though not all of them are associated with prolonged apnea after administration of succinylcholine. Homozygotes of this atypical enzyme (approximately 1 in every 3200 patients) can have a greatly prolonged duration of succinylcholine-induced neuromuscular blockade, whereas heterozygotes (approximately 1 in every 480 patients) will experience only a modest prolongation. Dibucaine, an amide-linked local anesthetic agent, inhibits 80% of the activity of normal plasma cholinesterase, compared with only a 20% inhibition of the homozygote atypical enzyme. A dibucaine number of 80 (i.e., percentage of inhibition) thus confirms the presence of normal plasma cholinesterase. However, the dibucaine number does not reflect the *quantity* of pseudocholinesterase present but, rather, the *quality* of the enzyme and its ability to hydrolyze succinylcholine.

Phase II Blockade

Infusion of large doses of succinylcholine over a prolonged period of time may result in a phase II blockade ("desensitizing succinylcholine neuromuscular blockade"). Clinically similar to the neuromuscular block produced by nondepolarizing NMBAs, phase II blockade may produce unexpected weakness on emergence from anesthesia. On a cellular level, the muscle cell membrane repolarizes gradually, but neuromuscular transmission remains blocked. The response of a phase II blockade to reversal is unpredictable.

Postoperative Myalgia

Skeletal muscle myalgia of the neck, back, and abdomen can occur after succinylcholine administration. These myalgias may be secondary to fasciculation-induced muscle-spindle stretching, or they may result from prejunctional repetitive firing of motor nerves. Myoglobinuria may also occur. A meta-analysis looking at postoperative myalgia and fasiculations with succinylcholine use revealed that higher doses, compared with lower doses, of succinylcholine may in fact decrease the risk of myalgia. Small doses of a nondepolarizing NMBA which acts presynaptically to suppress these repetitive discharges, will attenuate muscle fasciculations. Debate still persists, however, as to whether preventing fasciculations necessarily correlates with a reduction in succinylcholine-induced muscle aches.

Intraocular Pressure Increase

Succinylcholine causes a modest transient increase in intraocular pressure that persists for 5 to 10 min after administration. The proposed mechanisms include choroidal vascular dilatation or a decrease in drainage secondary to elevated central venous pressures. Although patients with treated glaucoma are at minimal risk, administration of succinylcholine to patients with recent ocular incisions or with penetrating eye injuries may result in vitreous expulsion and visual loss. Many case reports have been published and studies have been conducted to identify a pretreatment agent to obviate this adverse effect; results have been mixed with the use of nondepolarizing NMBAs, opioids, propanolol, lidocaine, and others.

Intragastric Pressure Increase

Succinylcholine can cause, on average, a 40-cm H_2O increase in intragastric pressures, presumably due to abdominal muscle contraction. Studies have shown that pretreatment with a nondepolarizing neuromuscular blocking agent decreases this rise in pressure. It has been shown that lower esophageal sphincter pressure also increases following the administration of succinylcholine, resulting in maintained gastroesophageal barrier pressures. Whether the administration of succinylcholine during induction causes increased susceptibility to esophageal reflux and possible pulmonary aspiration (secondary to increased intragastric pressures) remains debatable.

Intracranial Pressure Increases

The results of several studies have suggested that succinylcholine may increase intracranial pressure, whereas others have been unable to demonstrate this phenomenon. This ambiguity has spawned a variety of clinical recommendations and considerable debate. The mechanism responsible for this phenomenon has yet to be fully elucidated, but proposed mechanisms include decreased venous effluent from the brain due to fasciculation-induced increases in intrathoracic pressure, neck muscle contraction with resultant jugular venous compression, and succinylcholine-induced increases in afferent muscle spindle activity that cause increased cerebral blood flow, cerebral blood volume, and intracranial pressure. However, succinylcholine should not be deleted from the therapeutic armamentarium for emergency airway management based solely on concerns about increased intracranial pressure.

Acknowledgment

The author and editors would like to thank Thomas J. Christopherson, MD, for his work on this chapter in previous editions.

Suggested Readings

Benca J, Hogan K. Malignant hyperthermia, coexisting disorders, and enzymopathies: Risks and management options. *Anesth Analg*. 2009;109:1049-1053.

Didier A, Benzanti M, Senft M, et al. Allergy to suxamethonium: Persisting abnormalities in skin tests, specific IgE antibodies, and leukocyte histamine release. *Clin Allergy*. 1987;17:385-392.

El-Orbany M, Connolly LA. Rapid sequence induction and intubation: Current controversy. *Anesth Analg*. 2010;110:1318-1325.

Li Wan Po A, Girard T. Succinylcholine: Still beautiful and mysterious after all these years. *J Clin Pharm Ther*. 2005;30:497-501.

Martyn J, Durieux ME. Succinylcholine: New insights into mechanisms of action of an old drug. *Anesthesiology*. 2006;104:633-634.

Martyn JA, Richtsfeld M. Succinylcholine-induced hyperkalemia in acquired pathologic states: Etiologic factors and molecular mechanisms. *Anesthesiology*. 2006;104:158-169.

Perry JJ, Lee JS, Sillberg VA, Wells GA. Rocuronium versus succinylcholine for rapid sequence induction intubation. *Cochrane Database Syst Rev*. 2008(2):CD002788.

Robinson R, Carpenter D, Shaw MA, et al. Mutations in RYR1 in malignant hyperthermia and central core disease. *Hum Mutat*. 2006;27:977-989.

Schreiber JU, Lysakowski C, Fuchs-Buder T, Tramèr MR. Prevention of succinylcholine-induced fasciculation and myalgia: A meta-analysis of randomized trials. *Anesthesiology*. 2005;103:877-884.

CHAPTER 81

Prolongation of Succinylcholine Effect

Mark T. Keegan, MB, MRCPI, MSc

Pharmacology

At the motor nerve ending, the nerve action potential normally causes calcium channels to open, leading to the release of acetylcholine (ACh) from storage vesicles. ACh diffuses across the junctional cleft to react with receptor proteins in the end plate to initiate muscle contraction. Molecules of ACh released from the end plate are quickly (in less than 1 ms) metabolized by acetylcholinesterase molecules that are attached to the end plate outside the cell via stalks of collagen.

Succinylcholine consists of two molecules of ACh linked by methyl groups (Figure 81-1). Succinylcholine attaches to the nicotinic cholinergic receptor and mimics the action of ACh, thus producing depolarization of the postjunctional membrane. Compared with ACh, the hydrolysis of succinylcholine is slow, resulting in a sustained depolarization. Yet, compared with other neuromuscular blocking agents, the duration of action of succinylcholine is brief (3 to 5 min), owing to hydrolysis by butyrylcholinesterase (BChE), also known as plasma cholinesterase or pseudocholinesterase. This rapid breakdown of succinylcholine, to succinylmonocholine and choline, allows only a fraction (approximately 5%-10%) of the administered dose of the drug to reach the neuromuscular junction. The initial metabolite, succinylmonocholine, is 1/20 to 1/90 as potent as the parent compound. Succinylmonocholine is subsequently hydrolyzed to succinate and choline. There is little or no BChE at the neuromuscular junction, so the action of succinylcholine is terminated by diffusion from the end plate to extracellular fluid. Thus, by controlling the rate at which succinylcholine is hydrolyzed before it reaches, and after it leaves, the neuromuscular junction, BChE influences the onset and duration of action of the drug.

BChE is a serine hydrolyase capable of hydrolyzing esters, including ACh, succinylcholine, mivacurium, trimethaphan, and ester-type local anesthetics. BChE is found in plasma, liver, pancreas, heart, and brain. It is distinct from acetylcholinesterase, which is found in nerve endings and in red blood cells. BChE is an α_2-receptor globulin, weighing 320 kD, that exists in aggregate form, usually as a tetramer. The four subunits are identical, each having an active catalytic site. The enzyme is coded by exons located on chromosome 3q36 and is synthesized by the liver. The serum half-life is 8 to 16 h. The concentration of BChE in plasma is about 5 mg/L. The physiologic role of BChE is obscure, but it may be involved in lipid metabolism, choline homeostasis, or slow nerve conduction. Low levels or even complete absence of BChE are compatible with normal health and development.

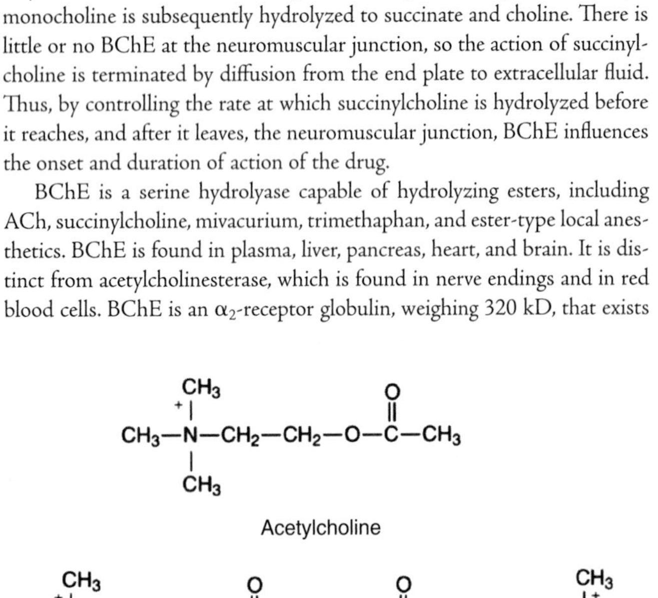

$$CH_3-\overset{+}{N}(CH_3)_2-CH_2-CH_2-O-\overset{O}{\overset{\|}{C}}-CH_3$$

Acetylcholine

$$CH_3-\overset{+}{N}(CH_3)_2-CH_2-CH_2-O-\overset{O}{\overset{\|}{C}}-CH_2-CH_2-\overset{O}{\overset{\|}{C}}-O-CH_2-CH_2-\overset{+}{N}(CH_3)_2-CH_3$$

Succinylcholine

Figure 81-1 Chemical structures of acetylcholine and succinylcholine.

Succinylcholine Apnea

Clinical interest in BChE abnormalities and pharmacology stemmed from observations that certain patients given succinylcholine develop prolonged apnea. The enzyme present in the plasma of affected individuals differs from normal BChE. Mutations of the gene coding for BChE give rise to a variety of biochemical phenotypes. Most of the variant alleles are the result of single-nucleotide polymorphisms, which have been elucidated by DNA techniques. Clinically significant BChE abnormalities are uncommon, with succinylcholine-induced prolonged apnea occurring in 1 in 2500 patients. Viby-Mogensen studied patients with prolonged apnea after succinylcholine administration and found that 66% had an inherited BChE abnormality. Succinylcholine apnea from the various abnormal BChE phenotypes is usually of shorter duration than the surgical procedure.

Skeletal muscle paralysis of excessive duration caused by succinylcholine requires maintenance of mechanical ventilatory support and continuation of anesthesia or sedation, typically in the postanesthesia care unit or the intensive care unit, until neuromuscular function returns. Some have advocated transfusion of fresh frozen plasma to replace BChE, but the risks of transfusion are far higher than those associated with a few hours of mechanical ventilation. Neostigmine inhibits the degradation of succinylcholine by BChE, and administration is not appropriate in these circumstances.

Measurement of Butyrylcholinesterase Activity

The activity of BChE refers to the number of succinylcholine molecules hydrolyzed per unit of time, expressed in international units. The BChE proteins produced by genetic variations may differ in enzyme amount (quantitative difference) or in enzyme performance (qualitative difference) when compared with normal BChE. Changes in either quantity or quality of the enzyme will cause alterations in BChE activity. The presence of succinylcholine interferes with both quantitative and qualitative assays; therefore, it is preferable to postpone testing until the day after an episode of prolonged neuromuscular blockade associated with the use of succinylcholine to ensure accurate results. Figure 81-2 illustrates the correlation between the duration of succinylcholine action and BChE activity. There is a wide normal range of BChE activity; prolonged muscle relaxation after administration of succinylcholine is clinically significant only with extreme depression of BChE activity.

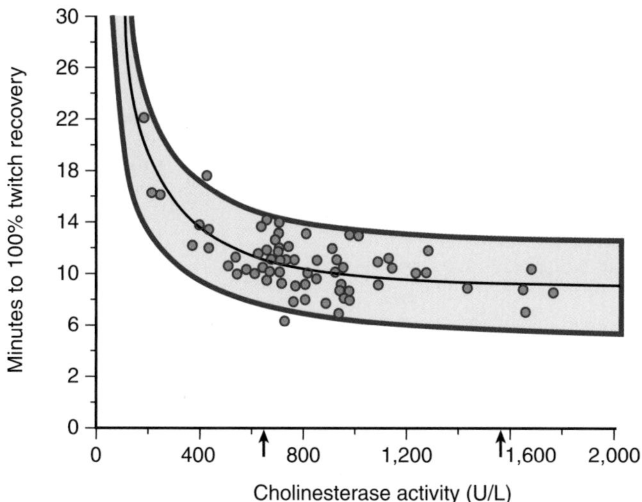

Figure 81-2 Correlation between the duration of succinylcholine neuromuscular blockade and butyrylcholinesterase activity. The normal range of activity lies between the arrows. (Modified from Viby-Mogensen J. Correlation of succinylcholine duration of action with plasma cholinesterase activity in subjects with the genotypically normal enzyme. Anesthesiology. 1980;53:517-520.)

Quantitative Analysis

The two major methods of quantitative analysis use either benzoylcholine or a thiocholine ester as the substrate for a colorimetric analysis. Quantitative BChE activity from a patient's serum is compared with that in pooled control serum to determine units of activity.

Qualitative Analysis

Qualitative tests of BChE activity involve assessment of enzyme function in the presence of a variety of inhibitors, including dibucaine, fluoride, and a number of others. Qualitative testing allows identification of a number of BChE variants.

Atypical variants were originally described by Kalow, who identified individuals whose BChE could not metabolize succinylcholine but were only partially inhibited by dibucaine, a local anesthetic. Whereas a normal individual's hydrolysis of benzoylcholine was inhibited 70% to 80% by dibucaine, affected individuals showed only 20% to 30% inhibition of hydrolysis (Table 81-1). The dibucaine number is defined as the percentage inhibition of BChE in the presence of 40 μmol/L of dibucaine:

$$\text{Dibucaine number} = \frac{\text{Total activity} - \text{Activity in presence of inhibitor}}{\text{Total activity}} \times 100$$

Table 81-1 Dibucaine Number and Duration of Succinylcholine or Mivacurium Neuromuscular Blockade

Butyrylcholinesterase Type	Prevalence	Dibucaine No.	Response to Succinylcholine or Mivacurium
Homozygous, typical	Normal	70-80	Normal
Heterozygous, atypical	1/480	50-60	Lengthened by 50-100%
Homozygous, atypical	1/3200	23-30	Prolonged to 4-8 h

Adapted, with permission, from Naguib M, Lien CA. Pharmacology of muscle relaxants and their antagonists. In: Miller RD, Eriksson LI, Fleisher LA, et al, eds. Miller's Anesthesia. 7th ed. Philadelphia: Churchill Livingstone; 2009: Table 29.1.

Table 81-2 Human Butyrylcholinesterase Variants

Common Name	Phenotypic Description	Amino Acid Alteration	DNA Alteration
Usual	Normal	None	None
Atypical	Dibucaine-resistant	70 Asp → Gly	nt 209 (GAT → GGT)
Silent-1	Silent, no activity	117 Gly → frameshift	nt 351 (GGT → GGAG)
Silent-2	Silent, no activity	6 Ile → frameshift	nt 16 (ATT → TT)
Silent-3	Silent, no activity	500 Tyr → stop	nt 1500 (TAT → TAA)
Fluoride-1	Fluoride-resistant	243 Thr → Met	nt 728 (ACG → ATG)
Fluoride-2	Fluoride-resistant	390 Gly → Val	nt 1169 (GGT → GTT)
K variant	K polymorphism	539 Ala → Thr	nt 1615 (GCA → ACA)
H variant	H polymorphism	142 Val → Met	nt 424 (GTG → ATG)
J variant	J polymorphism	497 Glu → Val 539 Ala → Thr	nt 1490 (GAA → GTA) nt 1615 (GCA → ACA)

nt, Nucleotide.

Reprinted, with permission, from Bartels CF, Jensen FS, Lockridge O, et al. DNA mutation associated with the human butyrylcholinesterase K-variant and its linkage to the atypical variant mutation and other polymorphic sites. Am J Hum Genet. 1992;50:1086-1103.

Total Activity

The dibucaine number correlates with the duration of action of succinylcholine in a reciprocal fashion (i.e., low dibucaine number implies reduced activity of BChE and a prolonged duration of action of succinylcholine).

Fluoride-resistant (F) variants have been found, the enzyme of which is resistant to inhibition by sodium fluoride. People with one of several extremely rare silent (S) variant genes produce little or no BChE. Individuals with K (Kalow) variants inherit genes producing low levels of normal BChE; similar J and H variants also have been discovered. High-activity (C5) variant families have been identified with cholinesterase activity three times normal. Human BChE variants are shown in Table 81-2.

Other Causes of Butyrylcholinesterase Abnormalities

A variety of physiologic conditions and drugs can lead to BChE abnormalities (Box 81-1).

Physiologic Variances in Butyrylcholinesterase Activity

From birth to age 6 months, the activity of BChE is 50% of that in nonpregnant adults. Activity reaches 70% of adult activity by age 6 years and normal adult levels at puberty. Pregnancy is associated with a 25% to 30% decrease in BChE activity from week 10 to postpartum week 6. This reduction has no clinical significance.

Acquired Butyrylcholinesterase Defects

Decreased BChE activity can be seen in a number of disease states and with administration of various drugs. Hepatitis, cirrhosis, malnutrition, cancer, and hypothyroidism are associated with decreased BChE activity in plasma. The alteration in BChE activity may be useful as a marker of hepatic synthetic

Box 81-1 Causes of Changes in Butyrylcholinesterase Activity

Inherited

Genetic variants that lead to decreased or increased activity

Physiologic

Decreases in last trimester of pregnancy
Reduced activity in the newborn

Acquired Decreases

Liver diseases
Cancer
Debilitating diseases
Collagen diseases
Uremia
Malnutrition
Hypothyroidism

Acquired Increases

Obesity
Alcoholism
Hyperthyroidism
Nephropathy
Psoriasis
Electroconvulsive therapy

Drug-Related

Neostigmine
Pyridostigmine
Chlorpromazine
Echothiophate iodide
Cyclophosphamide
Monoamine oxidase inhibitors
Pancuronium
Oral contraceptives
Organophosphates
Hexafluorenium
Bambuterol
Esmolol

Other Causes of Decreased Activity

Plasmapheresis
Extracorporeal circulation
Tetanus
Radiation therapy
Burns

Adapted, with permission, from Whittaker M. Plasma cholinesterase variants and the anaesthetist. Anaesthesia. 1980;35:174-197.

function. Certain drugs, including acetylcholinesterase inhibitors, pancuronium, procaine, hexafluorenium, and organophosphate insecticides inhibit BChE, whereas other drugs, including chemotherapeutic agents, can cause decreased BChE synthesis. BChE measurements can be used as a marker of occupational exposure to insecticides. Decreasing BChE activity to 25% of the control level, as seen in severe liver disease, prolongs succinylcholine duration of action from 3.0 ± 0.15 min to 8.6 ± 0.7 min, an increase that is usually undetectable in the clinical setting. Other diseases, such as thyrotoxicosis and nephrotic syndrome, are associated with increased BChE activity that is probably of no clinical significance.

Phase I Versus Phase II Block

A phase II neuromuscular blockade can cause prolongation of the action of succinylcholine; it is a risk of using repeated doses or an infusion of the drug. Phase II blockade may occur when the dose (usually >6 mg/kg) or duration (>30 min continuous infusion) of succinylcholine use is excessive. The exact mechanism for the transition from phase I to phase II blockade is not known but is thought to occur when the postjunctional membrane has become repolarized but still does not respond normally to ACh. The onset of phase II block coincides with tachyphylaxis, as more succinylcholine is required for the same effect. Phase II blockade can be avoided if succinylcholine administration is stopped when train-of-four fade becomes evident. Reversal of a phase II blockade is controversial; it should not be attempted until spontaneous recovery of the twitch has occurred. Administration of neostigmine or edrophonium when spontaneous recovery of the twitch response has been observed for 20 to 30 min and has reached a plateau has been suggested to promote return of the train of four to normal. Characteristics of phase I, transition, and phase II neuromuscular blockade during succinylcholine infusion are shown in Table 81-3.

Table 81-3 Clinical Characteristics of Phase I, Transition, and Phase II Neuromuscular Blockade during Succinylcholine Infusion

Characteristic	Phase I	Transition	Phase II
Tetanic stimulation	No fade	Slight fade	Fade
Posttetanic facilitation	None	Slight	Moderate
Train-of-four			
Fade	None	Moderate	Marked
Ratio	>0.7	0.4-0.7	<0.4
Edrophonium	Augments	Has little effect	Antagonizes
Recovery	Rapid	Rapid to slow	Increasingly prolonged
Dose requirements (mg/kg)*	2-3	4-5	>6
Tachyphylaxis	No	Yes	Yes

*Cumulative dose of succinylcholine given by intravenous infusion with patient under N_2O anesthesia supplemented with intravenously administered agents. The dose required to cause a phase II block is lower in the presence of potent inhalation anesthetic agents.
Modified, with permission, from Lee C, Katz RL. Neuromuscular pharmacology. A clinical update and commentary. Br J Anaesth 1980;52:173-188.

Suggested Readings

El-Orbany MI, Joseph NJ, Salem MR, Klowden AJ. The neuromuscular effects and tracheal intubation conditions after small doses of succinylcholine. *Anesth Analg*. 2004;98:1680-1685.

Goodall R. Cholinesterase: Phenotyping and genotyping. *Ann Clin Biochem*. 2004; 41:98-110.

Stoelting RK, Hillier SC. Neuromuscular blocking drugs. In: Stoelting RK, Hillier SC, eds. *Pharmacology and Physiology in Anesthetic Practice*. 4th ed. Philadelphia: Lippincott, Williams & Wilkins; 2006:208-250.

Ramsey FM, Lebowitz PW, Saverese JJ, Ali HH. Clinical characteristics of long-term succinylcholine neuromuscular blockade during balanced anesthesia. *Anesth Analg*. 1980;59:110-116.

Viby-Mogensen J. Correlation of succinylcholine duration of action with plasma cholinesterase activity in subjects with the genotypically normal enzyme. *Anesthesiology*. 1980;53:517-520.

CHAPTER 82

Anticholinesterases and the Reversal of Neuromuscular Blocking Agents

Claudia C. Crawford, MD

Classification

Acetylcholinesterase (AChE) inhibitors (neostigmine, pyridostigmine, physostigmine, and edrophonium) are reversible inhibitors and are commonly administered to accelerate the reversal of nondepolarizing neuromuscular blockade of nicotinic receptors in the neuromuscular junction. AChE the enzyme that metabolizes acetylcholine (ACh) into choline and acetic acid, is one of the most efficient enzymes known; a single molecule has the capacity to hydrolyze an estimated 300,000 molecules of ACh per minute. When the enzyme is inhibited, the concentration of ACh in the neuromuscular junctional cleft is increased, allowing ACh to compete for ACh receptor sites from which neuromuscular blocking agents (NMBAs) have dissociated (Figure 82-1).

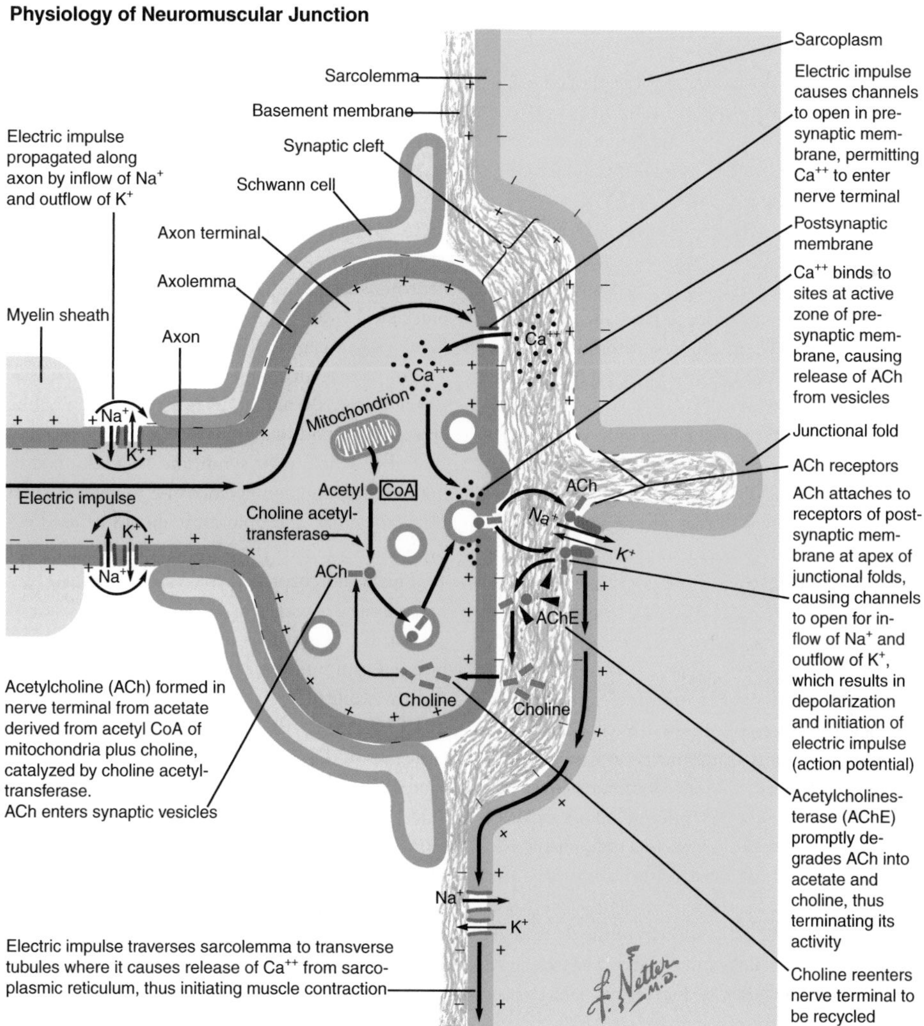

Figure 82-1 The physiology of the neuromuscular junction. (Netter illustration from www.netterimages.com.)

Structure

The active center of the AChE molecule consists of a negatively charged subsite that attracts the quaternary group of choline through both coulombic and hydrophobic forces, and an esteratic subsite, where nucleophilic attack occurs.

Unlike physostigmine, neostigmine, pyridostigmine, and edrophonium are quaternary ammonium ions that do not cross the blood-brain barrier. Neostigmine and pyridostigmine bind to the AChE molecule through formation of a carbamyl-ester complex at the esteratic site of the enzyme. Edrophonium has neither a carbamate nor an ester group but, instead, binds to the AChE molecule by virtue of its electrostatic attachment to the anionic site of the molecule and is further strengthened by hydrogen bonding at the esteratic site. This blockade is of brief duration; it is the duration of the drug in the body, rather than the duration of molecular action, that is important for edrophonium's duration of action. Individual edrophonium molecules leave the enzyme rapidly but are immediately replaced by another molecule as long as the drug is present in the body.

Pharmacokinetics and Pharmacodynamics

Edrophonium, neostigmine, and pyridostigmine do not differ in terms of pharmacokinetics. This similarity means that the difference in their potencies is most likely explained on a pharmacodynamic basis.

Because all three drugs are quaternary ammonium ions, they are poorly lipid soluble and do not effectively penetrate lipid cell–membrane barriers, such as the gastrointestinal tract or blood-brain barrier. In contrast, lipid-soluble drugs with AChE activity, such as physostigmine (a tertiary amine) and organophosphates and chemical nerve agents, are readily absorbed from the gastrointestinal tract and other mucous membranes and have predictable central nervous system effects. Neostigmine, pyridostigmine, and edrophonium have very large volumes of distribution because of extensive tissue storage in organs such as the liver and kidneys.

The reported shorter onset of action of edrophonium may reflect a presynaptic (i.e., ACh release) rather than a postsynaptic (i.e., AChE inhibition) action. Neostigmine has been shown to be more rapid and effective than edrophonium in reversing profound neuromuscular blockade, especially when the NMBA being reversed is pancuronium or vecuronium. These differences are decreased if a larger (1.0 mg/kg) dose of edrophonium is administered.

Renal excretion accounts for about 50% of the elimination of neostigmine and about 75% of the elimination of pyridostigmine and edrophonium. All three agents have similar elimination half-lives. The prolongation of their elimination half-lives by renal failure is similar to that affecting clearance of the NMBAs; thus "recurarization" is rarely a problem in patients with renal disease.

Pharmacologic Effects

Although the nicotinic effects produced by the increased amounts of available ACh are desirable for reversing neuromuscular blockade, the muscarinic effects of the ACh on the gastrointestinal, pulmonary, and cardiovascular systems can be problematic. The predominant effect on the heart is bradycardia from slowed conduction velocity of the cardiac impulse through the atrioventricular node. Hypotension may result, reflecting decreases in peripheral vascular resistance. AChE drugs enhance secretion of gastric fluid and motility of the entire gastrointestinal tract, probably caused by accumulated ACh at the ganglion cells of the Auerbach plexus and on smooth muscle cells. Bronchial, lacrimal, salivary, gastric, and sweat gland secretion are also increased. These muscarinic effects are blocked by administration of anticholinergic drugs such as atropine or glycopyrrolate.

Clinical Uses

Routine use of AChE antagonists is somewhat controversial. The drugs have side effects, as do the anticholinergic medications used with them. The degree of motor blockade by NMBAs is not always accurately assessed; even when the train-of-four response on a peripheral nerve stimulator appears normal, up to 70% of the postjunctional receptors may be occupied by nondepolarizing NMBAs. Because of the latter observation, however, reversal of NMBAs, when they are used, has become the standard of care unless one can demonstrate spontaneous return of the T4:T1 ratio of at least 0.9.

Recommendations for the Use of Acetylcholinesterase Antagonists

Anesthesia providers typically maintain neuromuscular blockade at 70% to 90% twitch depression throughout surgical procedures for which neuromuscular block is indicated. Profound blockade is rarely necessary for surgical procedures and will render antagonists ineffective. At the end of the surgical procedure, AChE reversal agents should be used only after the return of 10% of a control twitch or of T1 that is perceptible using tactile perception of a muscular twitch using a train-of-four monitor.

Neostigmine is the AChE drug most frequently used. If only T1 is present, the maximum dose of neostigmine should be used, 70 μg/kg up to a recommended maximum of 5 mg; if T2 is present, 50 μg/kg should be used; if T3 is present, use 30 μg/kg. (Commonly recommended doses are 30-70 mg/70 kg for edrophonium and 10-20 mg/70 kg for pyridostigmine.)

Clinical assessment should be performed in addition to the use of peripheral nerve stimulators to assess the adequacy of reversal. The maximum inspiratory pressure and sustained head lift of at least 5 sec are recommended clinical guides. A maximum inspiratory pressure of at least −25 cm H_2O is sufficient for adequate ventilation. A maximum inspiratory pressure of −45 cm H_2O approximately correlates with a normal CO_2 response curve and sustained head lift.

Factors that may delay or inhibit antagonism of blockade include hypothermia, respiratory acidosis, presence of certain antibiotics (e.g., aminoglycosides), hypokalemia, and hypocalcemia. The time required to antagonize neuromuscular blockade depends on at least four factors: (1) the degree of blockade, (2) the pharmacokinetics and pharmacodynamics of the NMBA, (3) the specific antagonist used, and (4) the dose of the antagonist.

Another AChE with application for anesthesiologists is physostigmine (Antilirium). Because it is a tertiary amine, not a quaternary amine, it crosses the blood-brain barrier and, therefore, can be useful for treatment of central anticholinergic syndrome. In addition, it has shown utility in treating sedation and somnolence due to general anesthetics, benzodiazepines, phenothiazines, and opioids. It should be used with caution because it can precipitate a seizure if administered intravenously too rapidly.

Finally, no chapter on reversal of NMBAs would be complete without mentioning a new class of selective neuromuscular blocker-binding agents that are capable of rapid reversal of both shallow and profound aminosteroid-induced neuromuscular blockade. Rather than increasing the amount of free ACh available to bind receptor sites, this class of drug forms a tight bond with the NMBA itself, neutralizing it both at the binding site and in peripheral tissues, eliminating the side effect profile of the AChE-anticholinergic reversal model—and minimizing the risk of recurarization. One such drug, sugammadex, is used outside the United States; as of late 2013, the Food and Drug Administration has not approved its use in the United States because of concerns about hypersensitivity and allergic reactions.

Suggested Readings

Naguib M, Brull SJ. Update on neuromuscular pharmacology. *Curr Opin Anesthesiol.* 2009;22:1-8.

Stoelting RK. Anticholinesterase drugs and cholinergic agonists. In: Stoelting RK, Hillier SC, eds. *Pharmacology and Physiology in Anesthetic Practice.* 4th ed. Philadelphia: Lippincott, Williams & Wilkins; 2006:251-265.

CHAPTER 83
Anticholinesterase and Anticholinergic Poisoning

Michael J. Murray, MD, PhD

Anesthesia providers are likely to assist in caring for patients with anticholinesterase poisoning either because of their knowledge of cholinergic pharmacology and physiology or because of their expertise in managing the airway and ventilators.

Cholinergic Physiology

The neurotransmitter acetylcholine (ACh) is found at preganglionic and postganglionic fibers in the parasympathetic system, in the preganglionic fibers in the sympathetic nervous system, and in the neuromuscular junction (nicotinic sites). Acetylcholinesterase (AChE), which is found in the synaptic cleft of the aforementioned sites, rapidly (<1 ms) hydrolyzes ACh, thereby terminating its action.

Butyrylcholinesterase, also called plasma cholinesterase or pseudocholinesterase, is synthesized by the liver, is released into the circulation ($t_{1/2} \sim 23$ h), and hydrolyzes biochemicals similar to ACh and, in particular, succinylcholine, mivacurium, and ester local anesthetic agents.

Anticholinesterase Poisoning

Anticholinesterase drugs inhibit AChE, thereby increasing the concentration of ACh at cholinergic sites; the excess ACh results in prolonged stimulation of muscarinic and nicotinic receptors. Anesthesia providers use carbamates, anticholinesterase drugs such as neostigmine, to reverse the effects of neuromuscular blocking agents at the end of a procedure. The muscarinic side effects of neostigmine are mitigated by simultaneously infusing an anticholinergic agent, such as atropine or glycopyrrolate, with the neostigmine.

Pesticides (with the exception of sevin, a carbamate) and the chemical nerve agents are organophosphate compounds, irreversible inhibitors of AChE; once released, ACh remains at its site of action, resulting in prolonged stimulation of muscarinic and nicotinic receptors. Muscarinic signs and symptoms include salivation, lacrimation, urination, diaphoresis, gastrointestinal upset, and emesis (i.e., the mnemonic SLUDGE; or DUMBELS—diarrhea, urination, meiosis, bronchorrhea/bronchoconstriction, emesis, lacrimation, salivation). Bradycardia (or tachycardia) and hypotension are signs of severe poisoning, as are confusion and shock. Nicotinic effects occur at the neuromuscular junction; skeletal muscle initially fasciculates and then becomes weak or paralyzed because the myofibril cell membrane is unable to repolarize (Box 83-1). Severe reactions, termed *cholinergic crisis*, may lead to ventilatory failure and death within minutes to hours following exposure.

Box 83-1 Signs and Symptoms of Anticholinesterase Poisoning Based on Type of Cholinergic Receptor Stimulated

Muscarinic

Pinpoint pupils/blurred vision
Hypersecretion—rhinorrhea, salivation, bronchorrhea
Bradycardia
Nausea, vomiting, diarrhea/incontinence

Nicotinic

Muscle twitching followed by weakness/paralysis
Tachycardia/hypertension
Central nervous system effects
Irritability/ataxia/seizures

Organophosphates

The most common clinical scenario of anticholinesterase toxicity is insecticide poisoning in agriculture workers. When used as commercial insecticides, organophosphate compounds are usually applied as aerosols or dusts, whereas when used in chemical warfare (e.g., nerve agents, such as tabun and sarin), they are dispersed in liquid form, though some of the agent will vaporize. They are rapidly absorbed through the skin and mucous membranes or, if inhaled, through alveolar membranes. Organophosphates are also used for medical purposes; for example, echothiophate is used to treat glaucoma.

Therapy

When treating organophosphate poisoning, the first line of therapy is termination of exposure (e.g., relocating the patient and removing contaminated clothing). If the patient has come in contact with the organophosphate, as opposed to inhaling the vapor of the anti-AChE, the patient should undergo a "wet" decontamination, being washed with copious amounts of water and 0.5% hypochlorite (active agent in household bleach). The severity of the poisoning can be classified as mild, moderate, or severe based on the symptoms and signs of exposure (Table 83-1).

Pharmacologic intervention to reverse muscarinic symptoms for patients with moderate to severe poisoning includes 2 to 4 mg of intravenously administered atropine, a competitive muscarinic antagonist (repeated as needed). No nicotinic antagonists exist; therefore, the AChE needs to be reactivated to treat nicotinic manifestations of poisoning. Pralidoxime chloride (2-PAM CL), the only oxime commercially available in the United States, reactivates AChE by removing the organophosphoryl moiety but

Table 83-1 Signs and Symptoms of Anticholinesterase Poisoning Based on Severity

Mild	Moderate	Severe
Headache Meiosis Rhinorrhea Salivation	Same as for mild, PLUS: Rhinorrhea is severe Dyspnea Muscle fasciculations	Same as for moderate, PLUS: Severe respiratory difficulty Urinary incontinence Weakness, paralysis Convulsions

must be administered as soon as possible after exposure because, with time, the bond between the organophosphate and the AChE "ages," permanently inhibiting the AChE. Nicotinic muscle weakness is reversed within a few minutes following intravenous administration of 50 mg/kg (1-5 g) of 2-PAM CL over 5 min.

Prophylaxis in anticipation of "nerve gas" exposure is usually achieved using pyridostigmine. The theory that pyridostigmine will occupy a percentage of receptors on AChE, preventing them from binding with organophosphates, has been demonstrated in experimental animals. However, data in humans are limited to our experience during the Gulf War. Many Gulf War veterans reported experiencing pyridostigmine-induced side effects (e.g., gastrointestinal upset); however, symptoms were generally mild, and combat and daily function were rarely compromised.

Anticholinergic Poisoning

Inhibition of cholinergic function most often occurs because of ingestion of plants (Box 83-2) or foods that contain high concentrations of atropine or related compounds. Central anticholinergic effects are biphasic, beginning with central nervous system excitation followed by depression. Signs include fragmentary speech patterns, visual hallucinations, atypical behavior, ataxia, and fever. Peripheral anticholinergic effects include decreased saliva, sweat (further contributing to fever), and tearing. Other peripheral symptoms include loss of accommodation, blurred vision, mydriasis, tachycardia, and decreased gastrointestinal motility and urinary bladder tone. A mnemonic summarizes many central and peripheral effects of anticholinergic poisoning (Box 83-3).

Clinical Considerations

Common causes of anticholinergic poisoning are eating the seeds or flowers of one of the plants listed in Box 83-2 or drinking a tea made from one or more of these plants. One historical treatment for asthma was to inhale the smoke from burning jimsonweed. The active ingredient in that folk remedy was ipratropium, a well-known antimuscarinic bronchodilator.

Box 83-2 Plants That May Cause Anticholinergic Poisoning

Atropa belladonna (deadly nightshade)
Datura stramonium (jimsonweed)
Hyoscyamus niger (henbane)
Mandragora officinarum (mandrake)

Box 83-3 Mnemonic for Remembering the Signs and Symptoms of Anticholinergic Poisoning

"Hot as a hare"	Fever
"Blind as a bat"	Loss of accommodation and blurred vision
"Red as a beet"	Flushed appearance
"Dry as a bone"	No saliva, sweat, or tears
"Mad as a hatter"	Central nervous system excitation, hallucinations, ataxia

Therapy

Treatment of anticholinergic poisoning begins with induced vomiting or gastric lavage plus activated charcoal. Physostigmine, the first-line drug therapy, is chosen because of its ability to reverse both central (it has a tertiary amine group that readily crosses the blood-brain barrier) and peripheral effects. Possible consequences of physostigmine administration include hypotension, asystole, and bronchospasm.

Suggested Readings

Centers for Disease Control and Prevention (CDC). Acute illnesses associated with insecticides used to control bed bugs—seven states, 2003-2010. *MMWR Morb Mortal Wkly Rep*. 2011;60:1269-1274.

Chen Y. Organophosphate-induced brain damage: Mechanisms, neuropsychiatric and neurological consequences, and potential therapeutic strategies. *Neurotoxicology*. 2012;33:391-400.

Collombet JM. Nerve agent intoxication: Recent neuropathophysiological findings and subsequent impact on medical management prospects. *Toxicol Appl Pharmacol*. 2011(15);255:229-241.

Mercey G, Verdelet T, Renou J, et al. Reactivators of acetylcholinesterase inhibited by organophosphorus nerve agents. *Acc Chem Res*. 2012;45:756-766.

Sanaei-Zadeh H. Atropine dosage in patients with severe organophosphate pesticide poisoning. *Am J Emerg Med*. 2012;30:628.

Sawyer TW, Mikler J, Tenn C, et al. Non-cholinergic intervention of sarin nerve agent poisoning. *Toxicology*. 2012;294:85-93.

Weissman BA, Raveh L. Multifunctional drugs as novel antidotes for organophosphates poisoning. *Toxicology*. 2011;290:149-155.

CHAPTER 84

The Pharmacology of Atropine, Scopolamine, and Glycopyrrolate

Niki M. Dietz, MD

Atropine

Atropine is a naturally occurring tertiary amine capable of inhibiting the activation of muscarinic receptors that are found primarily on autonomic effector cells innervated by postganglionic parasympathetic nerves but also present in ganglia and on some cells. At usual doses of the drug, the principal effect of atropine is competitive antagonism of cholinergic stimuli at muscarinic receptors, with little or no effect at nicotinic receptors.

Atropine is derived from flowering plants in the family Solanaceae (e.g., deadly nightshade [*Atropa belladonna*, named for Atropos, the Fate of Greek mythology who cuts the thread of life], mandrake [*Mandragora officinarum*], or jimsonweed [*Datura stramonium*]). Venetian women dropped the juice of deadly nightshade into their eyes to produce mydriasis, which was thought to enhance beauty (hence, the name belladonna, which, translated from Italian, is *beautiful woman*). Though atropine is used today to treat pesticide poisoning, Solanaceae plants have been used since 200 AD as a biologic weapon to poison, among other substances, wells and wine.

Pharmacokinetics

Absorption

Atropine is well absorbed from the gastrointestinal tract (i.e., from the upper small intestine). It is also well absorbed following intramuscular administration or from the tracheobroncheal tree following inhalation.

Distribution

Atropine undergoes rapid distribution throughout the body, and 50% is plasma protein bound. Atropine crosses the blood-brain barrier and the placenta.

Elimination

The plasma half-life of atropine is 2 to 3 h; it is metabolized in the liver, with 30% to 50% of the drug excreted unchanged in the urine.

Pharmacologic Properties

Gastrointestinal System

Atropine reduces the volumes of saliva and gastric secretions. The motility of the entire gastrointestinal tract, from esophagus to colon, is decreased, prolonging transit time. Atropine causes lower esophageal sphincter relaxation through an antimuscarinic mechanism.

Cardiovascular System

The effect of atropine on the heart is dose dependent. An intravenously administered dose of 0.4 to 0.6 mg causes a transient decrease in heart rate of about 8 beats/min, which was once thought to be due to central vagal stimulation but is now known to be mediated through an unknown mechanism. Larger doses of atropine cause progressively increasing tachycardia by blocking vagal effects on M_2 receptors on the sinoatrial node; by the same mechanism, atropine can reverse sinus bradycardia secondary to extracardiac causes but has little or no effect on sinus bradycardia caused by intrinsic disease of the sinoatrial node. Atropine at high doses (>3 mg) may cause cutaneous vasodilation.

Respiratory System

Atropine reduces the volume of secretions from the nose, mouth, pharynx, and bronchi. Along with many other anticholinergic drugs (e.g., ipratropium), it relaxes smooth muscles of bronchi and bronchioles, with resultant decreases in airway resistance.

Central Nervous System

Atropine is one of the few anticholinergic agents that crosses the blood-brain barrier, stimulating the medulla and higher cerebral centers. Higher doses are associated with restlessness, irritability, disorientation, and delirium. Even higher doses produce hallucinations and coma. This constellation of symptoms and signs, called central anticholinergic syndrome, can be treated with physostigmine.

Genitourinary System

Atropine decreases the tone and amplitude of ureter and bladder contractions, one of the reasons that belladonna and opium suppositories are administered to patients who have bladder spasms in response to a urinary catheter. The relaxation effect is more pronounced in neurogenic bladders. Bladder capacity is increased and incontinence is relieved as uninhibited contractions are reduced. The renal pelves, calyces, and ureters are dilated.

Ophthalmic Response

Atropine blocks responses of the sphincter muscle of the iris and the accommodative muscle of the ciliary body of the lens to cholinergic stimulation, resulting in mydriasis (pupil dilation) and cycloplegia (paralysis of lens accommodation). It usually has little effect on intraocular pressure except in patients with angle-closure glaucoma, in whom intraocular pressure may increase.

Scopolamine

Scopolamine, another belladonna alkaloid, sometimes referred to as hyoscine, has stronger antisalivary actions and much more potent central nervous system effects than does atropine (Table 84-1). It is a strong amnesic that usually also produces sedation. Restlessness and delirium are not unusual and can

Table 84-1 Duration of Action and Effects of Atropine, Scopolamine, and Glycopyrrolate

	Duration		Effect			
Drug	**IV**	**IM**	**CNS**	**GI Tone**	**Antisialagogue**	**HR**
Atropine	5-30 min	2-4 h	Stimulation	−−	+	+++*
Scopolamine	0.5-1 h	4-6 h	Sedation†	−	+++	0/+*
Glycopyrrolate	2-4 h	6-8 h	None	−−−	++++	+

CNS, Central nervous system; GI, gastrointestinal; HR, heart rate; IM, intramuscular; IV, intravenous.
*May decelerate initially.
†CNS effects often manifest as sedation before stimulation.
Adapted, with permission, from Lawson NW, Meyer J. Autonomic nervous system physiology and pharmacology. In: Barash PG, Cullen BF, Stoelting RF, eds. Clinical Anesthesia. 3rd ed. Philadelphia; Lippincott Williams & Wilkins: 1997:243-327.

make patients difficult to manage. Elderly patients who take scopolamine are at risk for incurring injury from falls when unsupervised. Scopolamine produces less cardiac acceleration than does atropine, and both drugs can produce paradoxical bradycardia when used in low doses, possibly through a weak peripheral cholinergic agonist effect.

Scopolamine in a transdermal patch has become popular as a treatment for motion sickness. The proposed mechanism for motion sickness is a disturbance in the balance between the cholinergic and adrenergic systems in the central nervous system. Because the vomiting center is activated by stimulation of cholinergic receptors in the vestibular nuclei and reticular formation neurons by impulses transmitted in response to vestibular stimulation, drugs that inhibit the cholinergic system have been proved to be effective in preventing motion sickness and are occasionally used to prevent or treat postoperative nausea and vomiting.

Glycopyrrolate

Glycopyrrolate is a synthetic antimuscarinic with a quaternary ammonium with anticholinergic properties similar to those of atropine (see Table 84-1); however, unlike atropine, glycopyrrolate is completely ionized at physiologic pH.

Pharmacokinetics

Absorption

With intravenous injection, the typical onset of action of glycopyrrolate occurs within 1 min; with intramuscular administration, it is approximately 15 to 30 min, with peak effects occurring within approximately 30 to 45 min. Compared with atropine and scopolamine, glycopyrrolate is a more potent antisialogogue (effects persisting for up to 7 h) and has a longer duration of action (vagal-blocking effects persist for 2-3 h).

Distribution

The in vivo metabolism of glycopyrrolate in humans has not been studied.

Elimination

After intravenous administration, the mean half-life of glycopyrrolate is 45 to 60 min, and after intramuscular administration, it is 30 to 75 min.

Pharmacologic Properties

Gastrointestinal System

Glycopyrrolate completely inhibits gastrointestinal motility but does not change gastric pH or the volume of gastric secretions.

Cardiovascular System

Glycopyrrolate has minimal effects on heart rate.

Central Nervous System

The structure of glycopyrrolate prevents it from crossing lipid barriers; therefore, unlike atropine and scopolamine, glycopyrrolate does not cross the blood-brain barrier, and the resultant effects on the central nervous system are limited.

Suggested Readings

Renner UD, Oertel R, Kirch W. Pharmacokinetics and pharmacodynamics in clinical use of scopolamine. *Ther Drug Monit.* 2005;27:655-665.
Simpson KH, Smith RJ, Davies LF. Comparison of the effects of atropine and glycopyrrolate on cognitive function following general anaesthesia. *Br J Anaesth.* 1987;59:966-969.
Stoelting RK, Hiller SC. *Pharmacology and Physiology in Anesthetic Practice.* 4th ed. Philadelphia: Lippincott, Williams & Wilkins; 2005.
Takizawa E, Takizawa D, Al-Jahdari WS, et al. Influence of atropine on the dose requirements of propofol in humans. *Drug Metab Pharmacokinet.* 2006;21: 384-388.

CHAPTER 85
Benzodiazepines

Eric G. Cornidez, MD

Benzodiazepines promote the binding of the major inhibitory neurotransmitter γ-aminobutyric acid (GABA) to $GABA_A$ receptors. The benzodiazepinergic enhancement of the inhibitory effect of GABA on neuronal excitability is the result of increased neuronal membrane permeability to chloride ions, leading to hyperpolarization and a less excitable state. Most of the effects of benzodiazepines (sedation, anxiolysis, muscle relaxation, anterograde amnesia, and anticonvulsant activity) are consequences of the impact of these drugs on the central nervous system. Benzodiazepines are used to treat insomnia, alcohol withdrawal, and seizures and, most importantly from the anesthesia provider's perspective, are frequently used to provide sedation and amnesia in the perioperative setting. Major side effects can include lightheadedness, motor incoordination, confusion, and impairment of motor and mental functions. Benzodiazepines have recently been associated with the development of delirium in the intensive care unit (Table 85-1).

Midazolam

Midazolam is a short-acting water-soluble benzodiazepine with sedative, anxiolytic, amnesic, and anticonvulsant properties. It may be given orally, intravenously, intramuscularly, or intranasally. Because of its rapid and reliable onset of action and short half-life and because it can be administered orally, midazolam is frequently used in the pediatric and adult perioperative setting to provide preoperative anxiolysis, conscious sedation during surgery, and induction or supplementation of general anesthesia.

Pharmacology

Midazolam causes virtually no local irritation after injection and can be mixed with other drugs commonly used as premedication agents. Its onset of action is among the fastest in its group (intravenous [IV], 1-5 min; intramuscular [IM], 15 min; oral [PO], 15 min). Similar to diazepam, it is highly bound to plasma proteins (95% protein binding). Rapid redistribution from the brain to other tissues and rapid metabolism by the liver account for the short duration of action.

Metabolism

Midazolam is hydroxylated and conjugated in the liver to two active derivatives that are renally excreted, and, therefore, patients in renal failure have prolonged pharmacodynamic effects. The elimination half-life of midazolam is 1 to 4 h and is prolonged with cirrhosis, congestive heart failure, obesity, and advanced age; similarly, as mentioned, the half-life of the metabolites is prolonged in patients with renal failure.

Effects on Organ Systems

Cardiovascular System

An intravenously administered 0.2-mg/kg dose of midazolam produces an increase in heart rate and decrease in blood pressure similar to that of an induction dose of thiopental (3-4 mg/kg). Hypotension is more common in pediatric patients or patients with hemodynamic instability and is more prominent when the patient also has received opioids because of synergism between the opioids and benzodiazepines.

Respiratory System

Ventilation is depressed by 0.015 mg/kg of midazolam, especially in patients with chronic obstructive pulmonary disease. Transient apnea may occur, especially when large doses of midazolam are given in conjunction with opioids.

Central Nervous System

The administration of midazolam results in dose-related decreases in cerebral blood flow and cerebral O_2 consumption. As do most benzodiazepines, midazolam may impair physical, mental, or both physical and mental abilities. Patients should be advised not to participate in activities that require mental alertness and rapid physical response time (e.g., driving) for at least 24 h after receiving midazolam.

Placenta

Midazolam crosses the placenta and enters the fetal circulation. Its effects on the fetus are not known; however, studies have demonstrated a teratogenic risk when midazolam is administered to pregnant patients early in pregnancy.

Diazepam

Diazepam is a water-insoluble benzodiazepine used to treat acute alcohol withdrawal and seizures; to provide preoperative anxiolysis, intravenous sedation, and skeletal muscle relaxation; and for maintenance of general anesthesia. The safety and efficacy of diazepam in children younger than 2 years of age has not been studied.

Pharmacology

Because of its insolubility in water, diazepam is dissolved in propylene glycol and sodium benzoate; the solution may cause pain when injected using an IV or IM route. Diazepam is taken up rapidly into the brain because of its high lipid solubility and then redistributed extensively to other tissues. Its oral form has absorption of 85% to 100%, making it more reliable than IM administration. Diazepam is highly protein bound; therefore, diseases associated with hypoalbuminemia may increase its effects.

Metabolism

Diazepam is metabolized by hepatic microsomal enzymes, producing two main metabolites, desmethyldiazepam and oxazepam. Desmethyldiazepam is slightly less potent than diazepam and is metabolized more slowly, contributing to sustained effects. Elimination half-life ranges from 21 to 37 h in healthy persons, increases progressively with age, and increases markedly

Table 85-1 Commonly Used Benzodiazepines

Drug	Route(s)	Common Use(s)	Comments	Half-life
Midazolam	Oral, IV, IM	Anesthetic premedication	Rapid onset	2.5
Temazepam	Oral	Insomnia	Short-term therapy	8.8
Alprazolam	Oral	Anxiety	Withdrawal symptoms may be especially severe	11.2-16.3
Lorazepam	Oral, IV, IM	Anxiety; anesthetic premedication, alcohol withdrawal	Metabolized solely by conjugation	14
Clonazepam	Oral	Seizure disorders; adjunctive treatment in acute mania and certain movement disorders	Tolerance	20-50
Diazepam	Oral, IV, IM, rectal	Anxiety, status epilepticus, skeletal muscle relaxation; anesthetic premedication	Decreases metabolism of cytochrome P-450–dependent drugs.	30-60

IM, Intramuscular; *IV*, intravenous.

in the presence of cirrhosis. The elimination half-life of nordazepam is 48 to 96 h.

Effects on Organ Systems

Cardiovascular System

Diazepam given in IV doses of 0.3 to 0.5 mg/kg results in mild reductions in blood pressure, peripheral vascular resistance, and cardiac output. Occasionally, hypotension will occur after even small doses of diazepam.

Respiratory System

Diazepam causes a decreased slope of the ventilatory response to CO_2, but the CO_2 response curve is not shifted to the right, as it is after opioid administration. Occasionally, small doses of diazepam may result in apnea.

Skeletal Muscle

Diazepam reduces skeletal muscle tone through its action on spinal internuncial neurons.

Anticonvulsant Activity

Diazepam (0.1 mg/kg) abolishes seizure activity in status epilepticus and alcohol withdrawal, although the effect is short-lived. It also increases the threshold for local anesthetic-induced seizure activity.

Placenta

Diazepam crosses the placenta easily. An increased risk of congenital malformations has been associated with the use of diazepam during pregnancy.

Lorazepam

Lorazepam is a relatively long-acting benzodiazepine that is a more potent amnesic than is diazepam or midazolam. The cardiovascular, ventilatory, and neuromuscular blocking effects of lorazepam resemble those of diazepam and midazolam. Its elimination half-life is 10 to 20 h. Lorazepam is used clinically for preoperative sedation and anterograde amnesia but is seldom used for induction of anesthesia or IV sedation because of its slow onset.

Pharmacology

The onset of action depends on the route of administration: IV, 5 min; IM, 20 to 30 min; PO, 30 to 60 min.

Metabolism

Lorazepam is metabolized by hepatic microsomal enzymes to inactive compounds, which are then eliminated in urine. The elimination half-life ranges from 10.5 h in older children or adults, to approximately 16 h in the elderly, to 40 h in neonates. Because its metabolites are inactive, the use of lorazepam is recommended over midazolam for patients in the intensive care unit who require anxiolysis for longer than 24 h.

Other Benzodiazepines

The benzodiazepines oxazepam (Serax), clonazepam (Klonopin), flurazepam (Dalmane), temazepam (Restoril), triazolam (Halcion), and quazepam (Doral) are used most commonly to treat insomnia or anxiety. Though these drugs are not typically used in the perioperative setting, patients may present for anesthesia who may be taking these medications; therefore, clinicians will need to consider the actions of these drugs when formulating an anesthetic plan.

Benzodiazepine Antagonist

Flumazenil

Flumazenil is a specific antagonist of the central nervous system effects of benzodiazepine because it binds to specific sites on the $GABA_A$ receptor, where it competitively inhibits the binding of the neurotransmitter, GABA, to this receptor. Flumazenil is eliminated almost entirely by hepatic metabolism to inactive products, and its clinical effects usually last 30 to 60 min. Therefore, flumazenil may need to be readministered after 30 min should sedation reappear. Small incremental doses are preferable to a single bolus: 1 mg of flumazenil given over 1 to 3 min should abolish most effects of therapeutic doses of benzodiazepines. Patients suspected of having a benzodiazepine overdose should respond to a cumulative dose of 1 to 5 mg of flumazenil administered over 2 to 10 min. Should the sedated patient not respond to 5 mg of flumazenil, a cause of sedation other than benzodiazepines should be investigated. Some clinicians have successfully used flumazenil to reverse some of the sequelae of hepatic encephalopathy.

Tolerance, Dependence, and Withdrawal

Tolerance to the anxiolytic effect of benzodiazepines is controversial. Even though most patients who chronically use benzodiazepines report experiencing decreased drowsiness over a few days, they do not convincingly demonstrate a tolerance to the impairment of some measures of psychomotor performance (e.g., visual tracking). On the other hand, tolerance has been demonstrated to the anticonvulsant, neuromuscular blocking, and ataxic effects of benzodiazepines. Dependence on benzodiazepines has been shown to occur. Abrupt discontinuation of benzodiazepines after prolonged administration of high doses may result in symptoms of withdrawal (one third of patients in the intensive care unit who receive benzodiazepines for 7 days or longer have been reported to exhibit signs of withdrawal) such as dysphoria, irritability, sweating, tremors, unpleasant dreams, and temporary intensification of insomnia or anxiety.

Suggested Readings

Aston A. Guidelines for the rational use of benzodiazepines: When and what to use. *Drugs*. 1995;48:25-40.

Charney DS, Mihic SJ, Harris RA. Hypnotics and sedatives. In: Brunton L, Chabner B, Knollman B, eds. *Goodman & Gilman's The Pharmacological Basis of Therapeutics*. 12th ed. New York: McGraw-Hill Education, Inc. 2011:457-480.

Riva J, Lejbusiewicz G, Papa M, et al. Oral premedication with midazolam in paediatric anaesthesia. Effects on sedation and gastric contents. *Paediatr Anaesth*. 1997;7:191.

CHAPTER 86

Dexmedetomidine

Gavin D. Divertie, MD

Dexmedetomidine—an intravenously administered α_2-agonist with sedative, analgesic, sympatholytic, and anxiolytic properties—is relatively unique in its ability to preserve respiratory drive and airway reflexes. Dexmedetomidine has been approved by the U.S. Food and Drug Administration for use in two situations: (1) as a short-term (<24 h) infusion in intubated and mechanically ventilated adults in the intensive care unit and (2) in nonintubated adults before or during operations or other procedures requiring sedation. Many off-label uses have also been reported (Box 86-1).

A water-soluble imidazole compound, dexmedetomidine is the pharmacologically active dextroisomer (*S*-enantiomer) of medetomidine (Figure 86-1). This highly selective α_2-agonist has an eight times greater affinity for the α_2-receptor than does clonidine and has α_2:α_1 activity of 1620:1. Presynaptic α_2-adrenoceptor activation, primarily in the spinal cord, inhibits release of norepinephrine, terminating the propagation of pain signals. Postsynaptic α_2-adrenoceptor activation in the central nervous system, primarily the locus coeruleus, both inhibits sympathetic activity and modulates vigilance (Figure 86-2). Combined, these effects produce analgesia, sedation, and anxiolysis and, similar to clonidine, may decrease blood pressure and heart rate.

Pharmacokinetics

Dosage and Administration

Packaged in a glass vial containing 200 μg/2 mL (100 μg/mL) of drug, dexmedetomidine is diluted in 0.9% NaCl prior to administration, with the final concentration being 4 μg/mL. For sedation in the intensive care unit, 0.5 to 1.0 μg/kg is given as a bolus over at least 10 min, followed by a maintenance infusion of 0.2 to 0.7 $\mu g \cdot kg^{-1} \cdot h^{-1}$ for up to 24 h. Omitting the loading dose minimizes the hemodynamic changes associated with the use of dexmedetomidine and has become common practice in treating critically ill patients. An infusion rate of 0.2 to 1.4 $\mu g \cdot kg^{-1} \cdot h^{-1}$ for up to 5 days has been reported to have been used without the development of tolerance, rebound hypertension, tachycardia, or other adverse sequelae.

Box 86-1 Off-Label Uses of Dexmedetomidine

As an adjunct
- To local, regional, and general anesthesia
- In labor analgesia and cesarean delivery

To facilitate awake fiberoptic intubation in patients with difficult airways
In combination with propofol, to provide anesthesia for infants undergoing microlaryngeal surgery
To alleviate preoperative anxiety and emergence delirium in children*
To blunt the cardiovascular effects of cocaine intoxication
To treat drug and alcohol withdrawal syndromes

*Administered intranasally (2 μg/kg).

For procedural sedation, an intravenous bolus of 0.5 to 1.0 μg/kg administered over at least 10 min is followed by a maintenance infusion initiated at 0.6 $\mu g \cdot kg^{-1} \cdot h^{-1}$ and titrated to effect between 0.2 and 1.0 $\mu g \cdot kg^{-1} \cdot h^{-1}$. Infusion rates of up to 10 $\mu g \cdot kg^{-1} \cdot h^{-1}$ have been reported to have been used in the operating room.

Compatibility of coadministration of dexmedetomidine with blood, serum, or albumin has not been established; coadministration with amphotericin B or diazepam has been shown to be incompatible. Atipamezole completely antagonizes the effects of dexmedetomidine but is not available for human use.

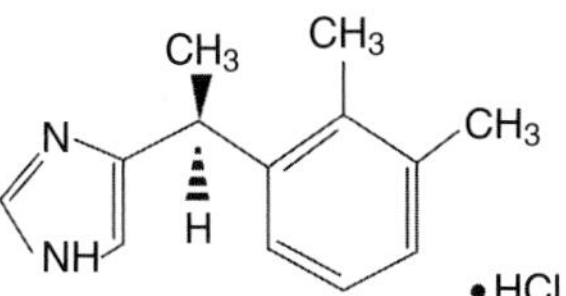

Figure 86-1 Chemical structure of dexmedetomidine.

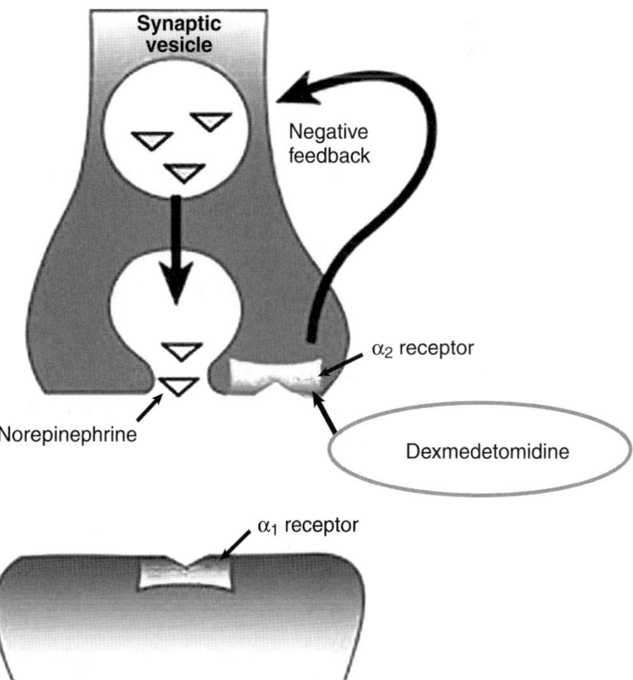

Figure 86-2 Proposed mechanism of action of dexmedetomidine at the synaptic cleft in the central nervous system.

Onset of Action

Dexmedetomidine produces sedation within 5 min of intravenous administration and reaches its maximum effect within 15 min. The vasoconstrictive effect of dexmedetomidine occurs even sooner, with the transient increase in blood pressure beginning at 1 min and peaking within 3 min of intravenous administration.

Duration of Action

Dexmedetomidine redistributes rapidly, with a $t_{1/2\alpha}$ of 6 min and steady-state volume of distribution of 118 L. Duration of action is 4 h, with an elimination half-life ($t_{1/2\beta}$) of approximately 2 h.

Metabolism

Dexmedetomidine undergoes almost complete biotransformation in the liver via direct glucuronidation and cytochrome P-450 metabolism, with very little excretion of unchanged drug. Therefore, decreasing the dose in patients with hepatic failure may be warranted. The pharmacokinetics of the active dexmedetomidine molecule does not change in patients with renal failure; however, because 95% of dexmedetomidine metabolites are excreted in the urine, accumulation of metabolites may occur. The intrinsic activity of these metabolites is unknown.

Systemic Effects

Cardiovascular System

Dexmedetomidine does not have any direct cardiac effects. A biphasic cardiovascular response to a 1-µg/kg bolus of dexmedetomidine has been described. A transient increase in blood pressure, with a decrease in baroreceptor-mediated reflex in heart rate, occurs initially; is explained by peripheral α_2-adrenoceptor vasoconstriction and can be attenuated by infusing the bolus over 10 min or more. The initial response lasts for 5 to 10 min and is followed by a decrease in blood pressure and a stabilization of heart rate. The final result is that both the blood pressure and heart rate fall 10% to 20% below baseline values. These effects are caused by inhibition of central sympathetic outflow and activation of the presynaptic α_2-adrenoceptor, leading to decreased release of norepinephrine and epinephrine. Hypotension, bradycardia, and varying degrees of heart block may occur; the use of dexmedetomidine should therefore be avoided in patients with hypovolemia, hypotension, bradycardia, fixed stroke volume, or advanced heart block. Treatment with fluid, atropine, pacing, or temporary discontinuation of the drug is usually successful.

Central Nervous System

Patients who have received therapeutic doses of dexmedetomidine appear to be asleep but are easily aroused and have preserved psychomotor function. Interestingly, dexmedetomidine produces less amnesia than do GABA-receptor agonists, such as the benzodiazepines. Several other central nervous system effects have also been reported. Dexmedetomidine lowers intracranial pressure, cerebral blood flow, and cerebral metabolic O_2 consumption, with preservation of cerebral blood flow/cerebral metabolic O_2 consumption coupling. Dexmedetomidine also lowers the seizure threshold but not to a clinically significant degree. The use of dexmedetomidine attenuates cerebrovascular reactivity to isoflurane, sevoflurane, and CO_2, but not to hypoxia, and may be neuroprotective under ischemic conditions.

Respiratory System

During dexmedetomidine infusion, airway reflexes are preserved. Depression of respiratory drive is minimal and not clinically significant. However, coadministration of dexmedetomidine with other sedatives, anesthetic agents, hypnotics, or opioids may have synergistic effects.

Miscellaneous Effects

Activation of peripheral α_2-adrenoceptors results in decreased salivation, inhibition of renin release, increased glomerular filtration rate, a mild diuretic effect, decreased intraocular pressure, and decreased insulin release from pancreatic islets, resulting in more frequent episodes of hyperglycemia in critically ill patients. Activation of central α_2-adrenoceptors inhibits thermoregulatory responses and lowers the shivering threshold. Adjunctive use of dexmedetomidine during general anesthesia reduces postoperative shivering rates by 70%. Similar to the action of other α_2-adrenoceptor agonists, dexmedetomidine prolongs neural blockade, including brachial plexus block. Our understanding of the mechanism behind this prolongation is incomplete. Dexmedetomidine has no effect on the duration of action of neuromuscular blocking agents, adrenal steroidogenesis (compared with the suppression of steroidogenesis observed with the use of etomidate), or neutrophil function (compared with the neutrophil-inhibiting effects of GABA agonists). Dexmedetomidine crosses the placenta, but drug concentrations in the newborn are low and devoid of clinical effects.

Adverse Effects

Overall, the most common treatment-emergent adverse effects that occur in patients in the intensive care unit who receive dexmedetomidine infusion for sedation include hypotension, hypertension, nausea, bradycardia, fever, vomiting, hypoxia, tachycardia, and anemia.

Suggested Readings

Candiotti KA, Bergese SD, Bokesch PM, et al. Monitored anesthesia care with dexmedetomidine: A prospective, randomized, double-blind, multicenter trial. *Anesth Analg.* 2010;110:47-56.

Coursin DB, Coursin DB, Maccioli GA. Dexmedetomidine. *Curr Opin Crit Care.* 2001;7:221-226.

Riker RR, Shehabi Y, Bokesch PM, et al. Dexmedetomidine vs midazolam for sedation of critically ill patients: A randomized trial. *JAMA.* 2009;301:489-499.

CHAPTER 87

Inotropes

Steven T. Morozowich, DO, FASE

Inotropy (contractility) refers to the force and velocity of cardiac muscle contraction and the term *inotrope* generally refers to a drug that produces positive inotropy (increased contractility). Inotropes differ from vasopressors (see Chapter 88), which primarily produce vasoconstriction and a subsequent rise in systemic vascular resistance (SVR) and mean arterial pressure (MAP). However, some inotropes have vasopressor properties as well, and the predominant effect is usually dose dependent. Inotropes and vasopressors are collectively referred to as *vasoactive agents*. Vasoactive agents have been in use since the 1940s, but few controlled clinical trials have compared these drugs or documented improved patient outcomes with their use; therefore, their use is guided largely by expert opinion. In the setting of circulatory shock characterized by low cardiac output (CO; e.g., cardiogenic, as opposed to distributive shock), the main clinical benefit of increasing contractility with inotropes is to increase stroke volume (SV), thereby increasing CO that, in turn, increases blood flow and delivery of oxygen ($\dot{D}O_2$) to vital organs until definitive therapy can be initiated. These agents are, by definition, used as supportive therapy by anesthesia providers, with the assumption that clinical recovery will be facilitated by their temporary use.

Physiology

Circulatory shock is defined as inadequate $\dot{D}O_2$ to the tissues. Low CO characterizes most causes of circulatory shock. CO is the product of SV and heart rate (HR) and, along with arterial O_2 content (CaO_2), is a major determinant of MAP and $\dot{D}O_2$:

$$CO = SV \times HR$$
$$MAP = CO \times SVR$$
$$\dot{D}O_2 = CaO_2 \times CO \text{ (in dL/min)}$$

Thus, optimizing SV will improve CO, MAP, and $\dot{D}O_2$ if HR, SVR, and CaO_2 remain constant. One must remember that SV and overall myocardial performance are determined by five other factors, in addition to inotropy, that require consideration: (1) HR and rhythm (atrioventricular synchrony), (2) myocardial blood flow, (3) preload, (4) afterload, and (5) diastolic function.

Clinical Implications

The resuscitation goals intended to preserve $\dot{D}O_2$ in all types of circulatory shock are (1) primary resuscitation, which involves rapidly reestablishing normal organ perfusion pressure with a MAP of at least 65 mm Hg; and (2) secondary resuscitation, which involves rapidly reestablishing adequate $\dot{D}O_2$.

A MAP of greater than 65 mm Hg must be achieved in primary resuscitation to maintain cerebral and coronary perfusion. Because CO is a determinant of both MAP and $\dot{D}O_2$, further resuscitation focused on augmenting CO is preferred. Secondary resuscitation involves first ensuring adequate volume status (correcting hypovolemia, ideally with blood if hemoglobin levels are $<$8-9 g/dL) and then, if CO remains inadequate, administering vasoactive agents while monitoring resuscitation end points.

All inotropes increase CO by increasing the force of contraction of cardiac muscle, but the other determinants of myocardial performance are variably affected. For example, some inotropes directly increase HR and some indirectly decrease HR (reflex), whereas others have no effect on HR. Some inotropes increase arterial tone (SVR) and venous tone (venoconstriction), whereas others decrease vascular tone through vasodilation, and some improve diastolic function. Any given agent, therefore, may have multiple effects, many of which are dose dependent. The anesthesia provider must have a thorough understanding of the etiologic and pathophysiologic factors of cardiogenic shock in an individual patient and of the pharmacokinetics and pharmacodynamics of the vasoactive agents. In the future, one will also have to take into account an individual's pharmacogenetic makeup, but lacking that information in current practice mandates that the clinician have clearly defined goals of therapy in mind when selecting an agent and then carefully monitor an individual patient's response to any given agent. Assessment of this response is probably as important as the selection of a specific agent.

In cardiogenic shock, the failing ventricle is very sensitive to afterload, so inotropes that produce systemic vasodilation (*inodilators*) should be considered as first-line agents as long as systemic hypotension does not occur. Although supraphysiologic goals for CO have not been shown to improve outcome and may cause harm, if maximal doses of a first-line agent are inadequate to meet the previously defined goals, then an alternative drug should be considered or a second-line drug should be added to the first—in the latter situation, consideration should be given to using agents with different mechanisms of action to maximize the potential to achieve goals. When assessing the effectiveness of any given agent, the anesthesia provider must monitor for side effects of these drugs with equal diligence, titrating the drug to the minimally effective dose.

Classification

Inotropes are broadly classified here by their clinical effects as (1) inodilators, agents that produce inotropy and vasodilation or (2) inoconstrictors, agents that produce inotropy and vasoconstriction. Further classification of these drugs is illustrated in Figure 87-1. The commonly used drugs stimulate adrenergic receptors in the myocardium (Table 87-1) to produce their effects. The standard dosing of inotropes, their receptor binding (or mechanism of action), and adverse effects are listed in Table 87-2.

Specific Drugs

Inodilators

Isoproterenol

Isoproterenol has potent β_1-receptor and β_2-receptor activity with virtually no α-receptor activity, resulting in inotropy, chronotropy, and systemic and pulmonary vasodilation. Despite the inotropy of isoproterenol, the venodilation associated with its use decreases venous return (preload), resulting in a

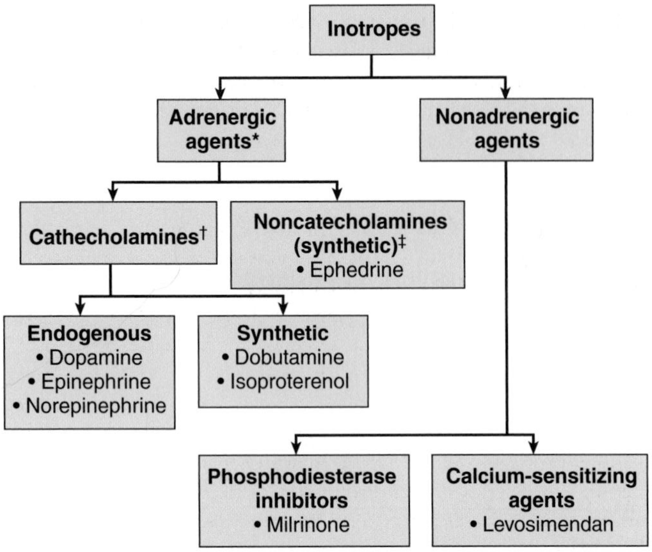

Inotropes
Adrenergic agents*
Nonadrenergic agents
Cathecholamines†
Noncatecholamines (synthetic)‡
• Ephedrine
Endogenous
• Dopamine
• Epinephrine
• Norepinephrine
Synthetic
• Dobutamine
• Isoproterenol
Phosphodiesterase inhibitors
• Milrinone
Calcium-sensitizing agents
• Levosimendan

Figure 87-1 Inotrope classification. *Adrenergic agents mimic sympathetic nervous system stimulation and are also termed *sympathomimetics*. †Catecholamines structurally contain a catechol group and are rapidly metabolized by catechol-*O*-methyltransferase (COMT) and monoamine oxidase, corresponding to their short duration of action (1-2 min), making them ideal agents for titration. ‡Noncatecholamines have longer durations of action (approximately 5-15 min) because they are not metabolized by COMT.

Table 87-1 Adrenergic Receptors with Cardiovascular Effects

Adrenergic Receptor	Location	Cardiovascular Effect(s)
β_1	Myocardium	Inotropy (increased contractility) Chronotropy (increased heart rate) Dromotropy (increased conduction)
β_2	Systemic arterioles Pulmonary arterioles Veins	Vasodilation
α_1	Systemic arterioles (receptor density*): Skin (high) Skeletal muscle (high) Abdominal viscera/ splanchnic (moderate) Kidney (moderate) Myocardium (minimal) Brain (minimal) Pulmonary arterioles Veins	Vasoconstriction

*Vasoconstriction of vascular beds with moderate and high α^1 receptor density allows the redistribution of blood flow to vital organs with minimal receptor density (brain and myocardium) and is the basis for adrenergic vasopressor use (e.g., epinephrine) in cardiopulmonary resuscitation.

Table 87-2 Standard Dosing of Inotropes, Their Receptor Binding (or Mechanism of Action), and Adverse Effects

Drug	IV Infusion Dose*	Receptor Activity or Mechanism of Action: α_1	β_1	β_2	Dopamine	Adverse Effect(s)
Isoproterenol	>0.15 μg·kg⁻¹·min⁻¹	0	++	++	0	Arrhythmias, myocardial ischemia, hypotension
Milrinone	Loading dose of 20-50 μg/kg, then 0.25-0.75 μg·kg⁻¹·min⁻¹	Phosphodiesterase inhibitor				Hypotension
Levosimendan	Loading dose of 12-24 μg/kg, then 0.05-0.2 μg·kg⁻¹·min⁻¹	Calcium sensitizer				Hypotension
Dobutamine	2-20 μg·kg⁻¹·min⁻¹	−	++	+	0	Arrhythmias, tachycardia, myocardial ischemia, hypotension
Dopamine	1-5 μg·kg⁻¹·min⁻¹	−	−	−	++	Arrhythmias, myocardial ischemia, hypertension, tissue ischemia
	5-10 μg·kg⁻¹·min⁻¹	+	++	+	++	
	10-20 μg·kg⁻¹·min⁻¹	++	++	+	++	
Epinephrine	0.01-0.03 μg·kg⁻¹·min⁻¹	−	++	+	0	Arrhythmias, myocardial ischemia, hypertension, hyperglycemia, hypermetabolism/lactic acidosis
	0.03-0.1 μg·kg⁻¹·min⁻¹	+	++	+	0	
	>0.1 μg·kg⁻¹·min⁻¹	++	++	+	0	
Norepinephrine	Start 0.01 μg·kg⁻¹·min⁻¹ (max. 30 μg/min)	++	++	−	0	Arrhythmias, hypertension, tissue ischemia

*Doses are guidelines, and the actual administered dose should be determined by patient response: ++, potent; +, moderate; −, minimal; 0, none.

minimal increase in CO and a drop in MAP. Because of this, the use of isoproterenol is limited to situations in which hypotension and shock result from bradycardia or heart block. Because a transplanted heart is denervated, isoproterenol is commonly used following cardiac transplantation to maintain an elevated HR and CO.

Milrinone

Milrinone, by inhibiting phosphodiesterase, augments intracellular concentrations of cyclic adenosine monophosphate (cAMP) in myocytes and vascular smooth muscle cells, resulting in increased myocardial contractility and smooth muscle relaxation in the pulmonary and systemic circulation. Thus, milrinone improves right ventricular function in the setting of pulmonary hypertension, more so than do the adrenergic inodilators. In addition, milrinone uniquely improves diastolic relaxation (lusitropy). Because milrinone is a nonadrenergic agent, decreased myocardial β-adrenergic activity—whether secondary to the use of β-adrenergic receptor blocking agents or chronic heart failure—does not diminish its effectiveness and does not produce the adverse events associated with β-receptor stimulation.

The vasodilatory properties of milrinone limit its use in hypotensive patients, and its 30-min to 60-min half-life is significantly longer than that of the adrenergic inodilators.

Levosimendan

Levosimendan is a nonadrenergic calcium-sensitizing agent that produces inotropy by calcium sensitization of myocardial contractile proteins, without increasing intracellular calcium, and produces vasodilation within the systemic and pulmonary circulation by activation of adenosine triphosphate–sensitive potassium channels. Levosimendan produces similar clinical effects to milrinone, but is also limited by hypotension and a long duration of action (80 h due to active metabolites). Levosimendan is not currently approved for use in the United States.

Dobutamine

Dobutamine primarily stimulates β_1-receptors and β_2-receptors, resulting in increased chronotropy, inotropy, and systemic and pulmonary vasodilation, and ultimately increasing HR and CO and decreasing SVR with or without a small reduction in MAP. Dobutamine is frequently used to treat low CO following cardiac surgery and is considered a first-line agent in early cardiogenic shock without evidence of organ hypoperfusion; if organ hypoperfusion is present, an inoconstrictor (e.g., dopamine) should be used to restore organ perfusion pressure.

Inoconstrictors

Epinephrine

Epinephrine, in low doses, increases CO because β_1 inotropic and chronotropic effects predominate, whereas the minimal α_1 vasoconstriction is offset by β_2 vasodilation, resulting in increased CO with decreased SVR and variable effects on the MAP. At higher doses, α_1 vasoconstrictive effects predominate, producing increased SVR, MAP, and CO. Thus, in the acutely failing ventricle (e.g., low CO syndrome after cardiac surgery), epinephrine maintains coronary perfusion pressure and CO. Epinephrine is recommended for cardiopulmonary resuscitation to restore coronary perfusion pressure, and as a second-line agent in septic or refractory circulatory shock. It is the drug of choice in anaphylaxis because of its efficacy in maintaining MAP, partly due to its superior recruitment of splanchnic reserve (about 800 mL), compared with other vasoactive agents, which helps to restore venous return and CO. Consequently, the degree of splanchnic vasoconstriction appears to be greater than with equipotent doses of norepinephrine or dopamine in patients with severe shock, thus limiting its liberal use.

Norepinephrine

Norepinephrine has potent α_1, modest β_1, and minimal β_2 activity, resulting in intense vasoconstriction and a reliable increase in SVR and MAP but a less pronounced increase in HR and CO. The increase in SVR is not well tolerated by a left ventricle with minimal reserve; therefore, caution must be used in the setting of the failing left ventricle. Reflex bradycardia usually occurs in response to the increased MAP, such that its modest β_1 chronotropic effect is mitigated and the HR remains relatively unchanged. Based on recent recommendations, norepinephrine is most commonly used to treat septic shock and may be the drug of choice in hyperdynamic (normal or increased CO) septic shock because of its ability to increase SVR and MAP, thus correcting the physiologic deficit in organ perfusion pressure, compared with other drugs that increase MAP by increasing CO (e.g., dobutamine). Norepinephrine has been recommended for use in cardiogenic shock with severe hypotension (systolic blood pressure <70 mm Hg) to improve coronary and organ perfusion pressure.

Dopamine

Dopamine is the immediate metabolic precursor to norepinephrine and is characterized by dose-dependent effects that are due to both direct receptor stimulation and indirect effects because of its conversion to norepinephrine. Doses of less than 5 $\mu g \cdot kg^{-1} \cdot min^{-1}$ stimulate dopamine receptors and have minimal cardiovascular effects. At doses between 5 and 10 $\mu g \cdot kg^{-1} \cdot min^{-1}$, dopamine begins to bind to β_1-receptors, promotes norepinephrine release, and inhibits norepinephrine reuptake in presynaptic sympathetic nerve terminals, resulting in increased inotropy and chronotropy and a mild increase in SVR via α_1-adrenergic receptor stimulation. At doses of 10 to 20 $\mu g \cdot kg^{-1} \cdot min^{-1}$, α_1-receptor–mediated vasoconstriction dominates. Dopamine is used less frequently than are other inotropes owing to its indirect effects because significant variations in plasma concentrations in patients receiving the same dose have been found and because studies have demonstrated a higher mortality rate with its use. However, despite this, dopamine is recommended as a first-line agent in patients with early cardiogenic shock who have a systolic blood pressure of 70 to 100 mm Hg and signs or symptoms of end-organ compromise, instead of dobutamine, because the α_1 activity of dopamine will correct the deficit in organ perfusion pressure, whereas the β_2-mediated vasodilation of dobutamine would further impair organ perfusion pressure.

Ephedrine

Ephedrine acts primarily on α-receptors and β-receptors but is less potent than epinephrine. Ephedrine also releases endogenous norepinephrine from sympathetic neurons and inhibits norepinephrine reuptake, accounting for additional indirect α-receptor and β-receptor effects. The combined effects of ephedrine result in an increased HR, CO, and MAP. Ephedrine is a noncatecholamine; because of its longer duration of action, its dependence on endogenous norepinephrine for its indirect effects, and its potential to therefore deplete norepinephrine, it is not ideal for use as an infusion and is therefore rarely used except in the setting of transient anesthetic-related hypotension.

Suggested Readings

Dellinger RP, Levy MM, Rhodes A, et al. Surviving Sepsis Campaign: International guidelines for management of severe sepsis and septic shock, 2012. *Intensive Care Med.* 2013;39:165-228.

Overgaard CB, Dzavik V. Inotropes and vasopressors: Review of physiology and clinical use in cardiovascular disease. *Circulation.* 2008;118:1047-1056.

Pinsky MR. Goals of resuscitation from circulatory shock. *Contrib Nephrol.* 2004;144:94-104.

Pinsky MR. Hemodynamic evaluation and monitoring in the ICU. *Chest.* 2007; 132:2020-2029.

Pinsky MR, Vincent JL. Let us use the pulmonary artery catheter correctly and only when we need it. *Crit Care Med.* 2005;33:1119-1122.

Rivers E, Nguyen B, Havstad S, et al. Early goal-directed therapy in the treatment of severe sepsis and septic shock. *N Engl J Med.* 2001;345:1368-1377.

CHAPTER 88

Vasopressors

Steven T. Morozowich, DO, FASE

Vasopressors are drugs that produce vasoconstriction and a subsequent increase in systemic vascular resistance (SVR) and mean arterial pressure (MAP). Vasopressors differ from inotropes (see Chapter 87), which primarily produce increased cardiac contractility (inotropy). However, some vasopressors have inotropic properties as well; the predominant effect is usually dose dependent. Vasopressors and inotropes, collectively referred to as vasoactive agents, have been in use since the 1940s, but few controlled trials have assessed their efficacy in improving patient outcomes; their use is largely guided by expert opinion. Vasopressors are used in cardiopulmonary resuscitation, in the treatment of circulatory shock, and in any clinical situation in which the goal is to increase the MAP to restore organ perfusion pressure. In cardiopulmonary resuscitation, vasopressors are used to constrict the peripheral vasculature, preferentially increasing coronary perfusion pressure in an attempt to restore myocardial blood flow, oxygen delivery ($\dot{D}O_2$), and the return of spontaneous circulation. In circulatory shock characterized by refractory hypotension, vasopressors are used in a supportive context until definitive therapy can be initiated, with the assumption that clinical recovery will be facilitated by temporarily restoring and maintaining normal organ perfusion pressure. In certain clinical situations (e.g., vasospasm following rupture of a cerebral aneurysm or during cardiopulmonary bypass) vasopressors may be infused continuously to increase MAP to a predetermined level.

Physiology

Circulatory shock is typically defined as the presence of profound hypotension such that $\dot{D}O_2$ is inadequate to meet demand. Depending on the underlying cause, the sympathetic nervous system compensation intended to restore normal organ perfusion pressure is manifested in different ways (Table 88-1). In distributive (i.e., septic) shock, the underlying pathophysiology prevents the compensatory increase in SVR seen in most types of circulatory shock, resulting in refractory hypotension despite a normal or elevated cardiac output (CO) and $\dot{D}O_2$. Although the $\dot{D}O_2$ is normal, a MAP below the autoregulatory range (e.g., MAP <65 mm Hg) results in impaired organ blood flow. This occurs because the absolute organ perfusion pressure (or driving pressure) is too low and the normal autoregulatory decrease in organ vascular resistance is insufficient to restore normal organ blood flow. This relationship is expressed by relating Ohm's law to fluid flow:

$$\text{Organ blood flow} = \frac{\text{Organ perfusion pressure}}{\text{Organ vascular resistance}}$$

Organ perfusion pressure is the difference between organ arterial and venous pressure. Because normal organ venous pressure is typically negligible, the organ perfusion pressure is usually equal to the organ arterial pressure, which is the MAP, thus demonstrating the direct relationship between organ blood flow and MAP:

$$\text{Organ blood flow} = \frac{\text{MAP}}{\text{Organ vascular resistance}}$$

Clinical Implications

The resuscitation goals intended to preserve $\dot{D}O_2$ to the organs in all types of circulatory shock are (1) primary resuscitation, which involves rapidly reestablishing normal organ perfusion pressure with a MAP of at least 65 mm Hg; and (2) secondary resuscitation, which involves rapidly reestablishing adequate $\dot{D}O_2$.

A MAP of greater than 65 mm Hg must be maintained to perfuse the cerebral and coronary vasculature. Because CO is a determinant of both MAP and $\dot{D}O_2$, further resuscitation focused on augmenting CO is preferred. However, MAP is the product of CO and SVR; therefore, transiently increasing the SVR with vasopressors to achieve a MAP of greater than 65 mm Hg is acceptable while secondary resuscitation is ongoing. Secondary resuscitation involves ensuring adequate hemoglobin levels and intravascular volume status and then administering other vasoactive agents to achieve the resuscitation end points. The selection of a vasoactive agent is based on correcting the underlying physiologic deficits; the agent ultimately chosen probably does not matter as long as these goals are achieved. In this regard, the indication for vasopressor therapy is classically demonstrated in the example of distributive shock, in which vasopressors correct the underlying deficit in SVR, thus restoring organ perfusion pressure. The importance of organ perfusion pressure has recently been emphasized; vasopressors are now being recommended as secondary agents when the indication is less obvious—circulatory shock characterized by low CO and persistent hypotension that is refractory to conventional treatment. Historically, vasopressors were used with extreme caution in this setting to avoid the complications associated with excessive vasoconstriction (increasing SVR and organ vascular resistance beyond normal physiologic values) such that CO, $\dot{D}O_2$, and organ blood flow were impaired, possibly worsening outcome. However, excessive vasoconstriction primarily occurs when vasopressors are given in the setting of inadequate volume resuscitation, with or without preexisting low CO. Considering this, patients receiving vasopressors require careful monitoring and frequent reevaluation so that these agents can be titrated to the minimum effective dose.

Classification

Vasopressor agents are broadly classified here by their clinical effect as either pure vasoconstrictors or inoconstrictors (vasoconstrictors with inotropic properties). Further classification of these agents is illustrated in Figure 88-1, and their standard dosing, receptor binding, and adverse effects are listed in Table 88-2. Although some adrenergic agents stimulate many receptors, producing various cardiovascular effects, their vasopressor actions are mediated via α_1-receptors, resulting in arterial and venous vascular smooth muscle contraction and an increase in SVR, pulmonary vascular resistance, and venous return. The only nonadrenergic agent currently in use is vasopressin, which exerts its vasopressor effects through V_1-receptor stimulation, resulting in vascular smooth muscle contraction.

Table 88-1 Types of Circulatory Shock and Associated Clinical Picture

Type of Shock	MAP	CO	$\dot{D}O_2$	CVP	MPAP	PAOP	SVR	Common Clinical Examples	Treatment*
Hypovolemic	↓→	↓	↓	↓	↓	↓	↑	Hemorrhage Capillary leak	Volume resuscitation
Obstructive	↓	↓	↓	↑	↑	↑→	↑→	Pulmonary embolus Tension pneumothorax	Inotropes†
Cardiogenic	↓→	↓	↓	↑	↑	↑	↑	Myocardial infarction Arrhythmia	Inotropes†
Distributive	↓	↑	↑	↓	↓	↓	↓	SIRS‡ Anaphylaxis	Vasopressors†

*Treatment of the underlying cause of circulatory shock is the primary objective, and pharmacologic therapy with vasopressors, inotropes, or both is used as a temporizing measure to maintain organ perfusion pressure (MAP >65 mm Hg) and CO while the underlying process is corrected.
†Adequate intravascular volume is required, especially with distributive shock, before use of a vasoconstrictor.
‡Includes sepsis and trauma.
CO, Cardiac output; CVP, central venous pressure; $\dot{D}O_2$, delivery of O_2; MAP, mean arterial pressure; MPAP, mean pulmonary artery pressure; PAOP, pulmonary artery occlusion pressure; SIRS, systemic inflammatory response syndrome; SVR, systemic vascular resistance; ↑, increased; ↓, decreased; →, no change.

Table 88-2 Standard Dosing of Vasopressors, Their Receptor Binding (or Mechanism of Action), and Adverse Effects

		Receptor Activity or Mechanism of Action				
Drug	**IV Infusion Dose***	α_1	β_1	β_2	**Dopamine**	**Adverse Effects**
Vasopressin	0.01-0.04 unit/min	V_1 receptor agonist				Hypertension, excessive vasoconstriction
Phenylephrine	0.15-0.75 $\mu g \cdot kg^{-1} \cdot min^{-1}$	++	0	0	0	Bradycardia, hypertension, excessive vasoconstriction
Norepinephrine	Start 0.01 $\mu g \cdot kg^{-1} \cdot min^{-1}$ and titrate to effect (max. 30 μg/min)	++	++	−	0	Arrhythmias, hypertension, tissue ischemia
Epinephrine	0.01-0.03 $\mu g \cdot kg^{-1} \cdot min^{-1}$ 0.03-0.1 $\mu g \cdot kg^{-1} \cdot min^{-1}$ >0.1 $\mu g \cdot kg^{-1} \cdot min^{-1}$	− + ++	++ ++ ++	+ + +	0 0 0	Arrhythmias, myocardial ischemia, hypertension, hyperglycemia, hypermetabolism/lactic acidosis
Dopamine	1-5 $\mu g \cdot kg^{-1} \cdot min^{-1}$ 5-10 $\mu g \cdot kg^{-1} \cdot min^{-1}$ 10-20 $\mu g \cdot kg^{-1} \cdot min^{-1}$	− + ++	− ++ ++	− + +	++ ++ ++	Arrhythmias, myocardial ischemia, hypertension, tissue ischemia

*Doses are guidelines, and the actual administered dose should be determined by patient response: ++, potent; +, moderate; −, minimal; 0, none.
IV, intravenous.

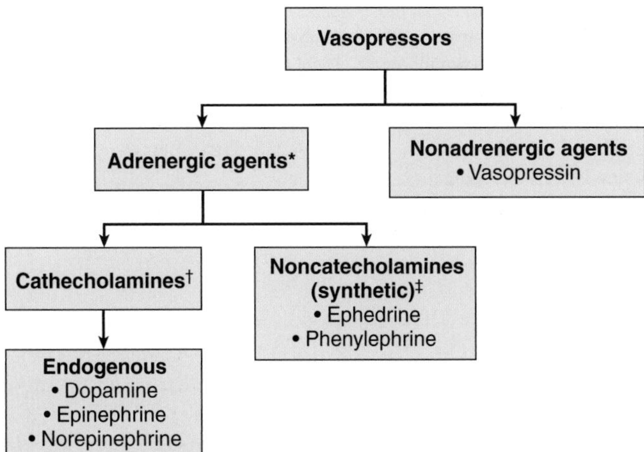

Figure 88-1 Vasopressor classification. *Adrenergic agents mimic sympathetic nervous system stimulation and are also termed *sympathomimetics*. †Catecholamines structurally contain a catechol group and are rapidly metabolized by catechol-O-methyltransferase (COMT) and monoamine oxidase, corresponding to their short duration of action (1-2 min), making them ideal agents for titration. ‡Noncatecholamines have longer durations of action (approximately 5-15 min), because they are not metabolized by COMT.

Specific Agents

Pure Vasoconstrictors

Vasopressin

Vasopressin (antidiuretic hormone) levels are increased in response to early shock to maintain organ perfusion, but levels fall dramatically as shock progresses. Unlike the adrenergic agents, vasopressin does not stimulate adrenergic receptors, its use is not associated with the adverse effects associated with the use of adrenergic agents, and its vasopressor effects are relatively preserved during hypoxemic and acidemic conditions, making it useful in refractory circulatory shock and cardiopulmonary resuscitation, specifically asystole. The use of vasopressin is primarily indicated in distributive shock, usually as a secondary agent, but its ability to increase MAP and not adversely impact CO has recently been demonstrated in refractory cardiogenic shock, underscoring the physiologic importance of maintaining organ (myocardial) perfusion pressure. Its 30-min to 60-min duration of action is much longer than that of adrenergic agents, making titration more difficult.

Phenylephrine

Phenylephrine stimulates only α-receptors, resulting in arterial and venous vasoconstriction, clinically producing an increase in SVR, MAP, venous return, and baroreceptor-mediated reflex bradycardia. The increase in SVR (afterload) and reflex bradycardia may decrease CO, so phenylephrine should only be used transiently, in general, and with caution in patients with preexisting cardiac dysfunction (low CO). Perioperatively, phenylephrine is used to correct hypotension, improve venous return, and decrease heart rate in patients with various cardiac conditions (e.g., aortic stenosis and hypertrophic cardiomyopathy). The reflex bradycardia associated with the use of phenylephrine may prove useful in the treatment of hypotension caused by tachyarrhythmias or when tachyarrhythmias occur in response to other vasoactive agents used in the treatment of circulatory shock.

Inoconstrictors

Norepinephrine

Norepinephrine has potent α_1, modest β_1, and minimal β_2 activity. Thus, norepinephrine produces powerful vasoconstriction and a reliable increase in SVR and MAP but a less pronounced increase in HR and CO, compared with epinephrine. Therefore, caution must be used in the setting of the failing ventricle. Reflex bradycardia usually occurs in response to increased MAP, such that the modest β_1 chronotropic effect is mitigated and the heart rate remains relatively unchanged. Based on recent recommendations, norepinephrine is most commonly used to treat septic shock and may be the drug of choice in hyperdynamic (normal CO) septic shock because of its ability to increase SVR and MAP, thus correcting the physiologic deficit in organ perfusion pressure, compared with other agents (e.g., dopamine) that, instead, increase MAP by increasing CO. In addition, its use has been recommended in cardiogenic shock with severe hypotension (systolic blood pressure < 70 mm Hg) to improve coronary and organ perfusion pressure.

Epinephrine

Epinephrine, in low doses, increases CO because β_1 inotropic and chronotropic effects predominate, whereas the minimal α_1 vasoconstriction is offset by β_2 vasodilation, resulting in increased CO with decreased SVR and variable effects on the MAP. At higher doses, α_1 vasoconstrictive effects predominate, producing increased SVR, MAP, and CO. Thus, in the acutely failing ventricle (e.g., low CO syndrome after cardiac surgery), epinephrine maintains coronary perfusion pressure and CO. Epinephrine is used in cardiopulmonary resuscitation as a second-line agent in septic or refractory circulatory shock, and is the drug of choice in anaphylaxis because of its efficacy in maintaining MAP (partly due to its superior recruitment of splanchnic reserve, compared with other vasoactive agents), which helps to restore venous return and CO. Consequently, the degree of splanchnic vasoconstriction associated with the use of epinephrine appears to be greater than with equipotent doses of norepinephrine or dopamine in patients with severe shock, thus limiting its liberal use.

Dopamine

Dopamine is the immediate precursor to norepinephrine and is characterized by dose-dependent effects that are due to both direct receptor stimulation and indirect effects due to norepinephrine conversion and release. Doses of less than 5 $\mu g \cdot kg^{-1} \cdot min^{-1}$ stimulate dopamine receptors and have minimal cardiovascular effects. At moderate doses, between 5 and 10 $\mu g \cdot kg^{-1} \cdot min^{-1}$, dopamine weakly binds to β_1-adrenergic receptors, promotes norepinephrine release, and inhibits norepinephrine reuptake in presynaptic sympathetic nerve terminals, resulting in increased inotropy and chronotropy and a mild increase in SVR via stimulation of α_1-adrenergic receptors. At higher doses, 10 to 20 $\mu g \cdot kg^{-1} \cdot min^{-1}$, α_1-receptor-mediated vasoconstriction dominates. Dopamine is used less frequently than are other agents due to its indirect effects, because significant variations in plasma concentrations in patients receiving the same dose have been found, and because of controversial studies demonstrating higher mortality rate with its use. However, despite this, dopamine has recently been recommended as a first-line treatment of septic shock, particularly in patients with hypodynamic (low CO) septic shock because it increases CO and MAP with minimal increases in the SVR.

Ephedrine

Like epinephrine, ephedrine acts primarily on α-receptors and β-receptors but with less potency. Ephedrine also releases endogenous norepinephrine from sympathetic neurons and inhibits norepinephrine reuptake, accounting for additional indirect α-receptor and β-receptor effects. The combined effects of ephedrine result in an increased heart rate, CO, and MAP. Ephedrine is a noncatecholamine and because of its longer duration of action, its dependence on endogenous norepinephrine for its indirect effects, and its potential to therefore deplete norepinephrine, it is not ideal for infusion and is therefore rarely used except in the setting of transient anesthesia-related hypotension.

Suggested Readings

Dellinger RP, Levy MM, Rhodes A, et al. Surviving Sepsis Campaign: International guidelines for management of severe sepsis and septic shock, 2012. *Intensive Care Med.* 2013;39:165-228.

Overgaard CB, Dzavik V. Inotropes and vasopressors: Review of physiology and clinical use in cardiovascular disease. *Circulation.* 2008;118:1047-1056.

Pinsky MR. Goals of resuscitation from circulatory shock. *Contrib Nephrol.* 2004;144:94-104.

Pinsky MR. Hemodynamic evaluation and monitoring in the ICU. *Chest.* 2007; 132:2020-2029.

Pinsky MR, Vincent JL. Let us use the pulmonary artery catheter correctly and only when we need it. *Crit Care Med.* 2005;33:1119-1122.

Rivers E, Nguyen B, Havstad S, et al. Early goal-directed therapy in the treatment of severe sepsis and septic shock. *N Engl J Med.* 2001;345:1368-1377.

CHAPTER 89

Sodium Nitroprusside

Scott A. Gammel, MD

Sodium nitroprusside (SNP), one of the most effective arteriolar vasodilators, is composed of a ferrous ion, five cyanide groups, and a nitrosyl group (Figure 89-1). The latter moiety is responsible for its vasodilator action, whereas cyanide is responsible for most of its toxicity.

Mechanism of Action

When given intravenously, SNP reacts with oxyhemoglobin in erythrocytes. Nitric oxide (NO) and cyanide are released, and methemoglobin is formed. NO rapidly diffuses out of the erythrocyte into the plasma and across vascular smooth muscle cell (VSMC) membranes. Within the VSMCs, NO reacts with the heme moiety in soluble guanylate cyclase, leading to a greater than 100-fold increase in the conversion of guanosine triphosphate to the secondary messenger cyclic guanosine monophosphate [cGMP]) (Figure 89-2). cGMP induces smooth muscle relaxation by multiple mechanisms: (1) inhibition of calcium entry into VSMCs, (2) activation of K^+ channels (VSMC membrane hyperpolarization), and (3) stimulation of a cGMP-dependent protein kinase, which, in turn, activates myosin light chain phosphatase, the enzyme that dephosphorylates myosin light chains, and leads to VSMC relaxation.

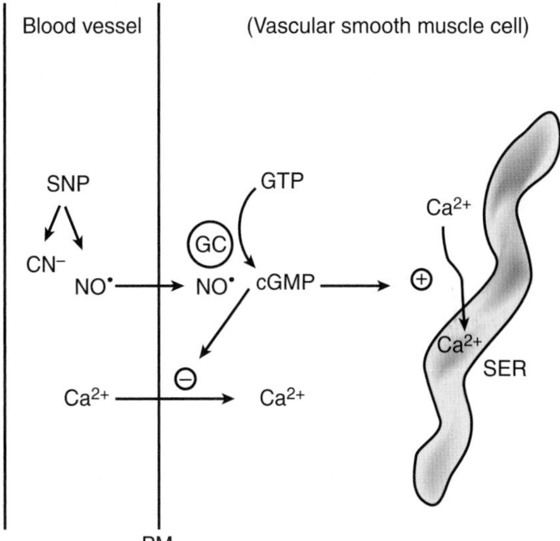

Figure 89-2 Mechanism of action of sodium nitroprusside. A decrease in intracellular free calcium concentration leads to relaxation. Ca^{2+}, Calcium ion; cGMP, cyclic guanosine monophosphate; CN^-, cyanide ion; GC, guanylate cyclase; GTP, guanosine triphosphate; $NO^{\bullet}$, nitric oxide radical; PM, plasma membrane; SER, smooth endoplasmic reticulum; SNP, sodium nitroprusside. (Adapted from Friederich JA, Butterworth JF IV. Sodium nitroprusside. Twenty years and counting. Anesth Analg. 1995;81:152-162.)

Pharmacokinetics

Taken orally, SNP is not absorbed to any extent, so this drug must be administered intravenously. Once infused, SNP is rapidly distributed with a volume of distribution equal to the volume of the extravascular space. As described previously, SNP is cleared through its reaction in erythrocytes; the circulatory $t_{1/2}$ is approximately 2 min. The NO that is formed has a $t_{1/2}$ of a few seconds. The cyanide that is released binds with hydrogen ions

$$CN^- + H^+ \Leftrightarrow HCN$$

to form hydrogen cyanide (HCN, prussic acid), but 99% of it binds to the iron in methemoglobin (hemoglobin with the iron in the ferric state [Fe^{3+}] as opposed to the ferrous state [Fe^{2+}]) of erythrocytes. Normal levels of methemoglobin are 1% or less and can only bind a small amount of the cyanide released during the metabolism of SNP. Unbound HCN is detoxified in the liver by the enzyme rhodanese using a sulfur donor to produce thiocyanate with a volume of distribution of approximately 0.25 L/kg and a serum $t_{1/2}$ of about 3 days; elimination is mainly renal (Figure 89-3). Thiocyanate toxicity does not represent a therapeutic problem; its formation is a zero-order kinetic process. The limiting factor is a sulfur donor, principally thiosulfate (thiosulfate reacts with the thiol group on the amino acid cysteine to form a disulfide that, in turn, reacts with cyanide to produce thiocyanate), which is usually present in small quantities—enough to detoxify SNP if infused at no greater than 2 $\mu g \cdot kg^{-1} \cdot min^{-1}$. Thiosulfate can be infused to decrease the toxicity of SNP infusions greater than 2 $\mu g \cdot kg^{-1} \cdot min^{-1}$ (Table 89-1); however, if the concentration of HCN exceeds the concentration of thiosulfate, the excess HCN remains in plasma and is recirculated to cells in which the cyanide poisons the electron transfer processes within mitochondria—where oxidation-inhibited metabolic acidosis rapidly develops.

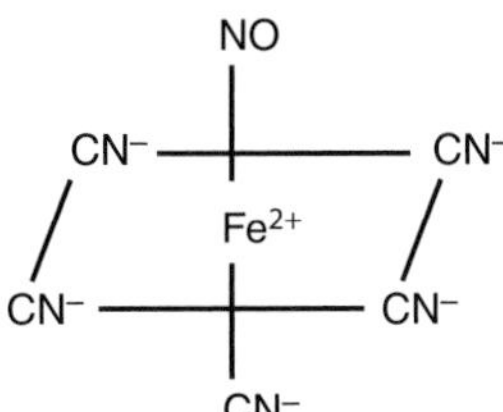

Figure 89-1 Chemical structure of sodium nitroprusside.

The essential features of SNP metabolism are as follows: (1) one molecule of SNP combines with methemoglobin to produce one molecule of cyanmethemoglobin, four CN^- ions, and one molecule of NO; (2) rhodanese combines cyanide with a disulfide to produce thiocyanate; (3) thiocyanate is eliminated in the urine; and (4) CN^- that is not otherwise metabolized binds to cytochromes inhibiting cellular respiration.

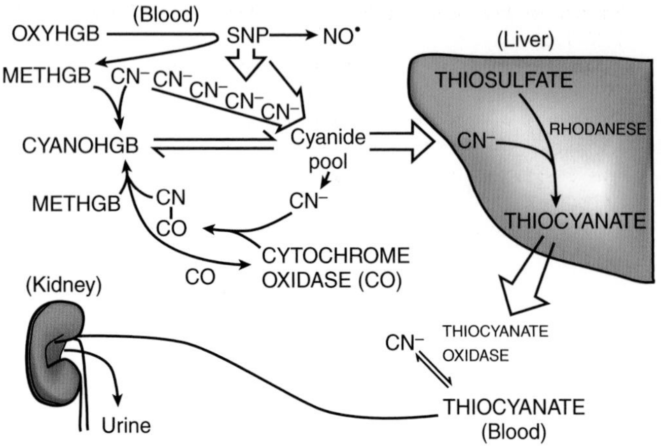

Figure 89-3 Primary pathways of sodium nitroprusside (SNP) metabolism. CN^-, Cyanide ion; CYANOHGB, cyanmethemoglobin; METHGB, methemoglobin; $NO^•$, nitric oxide radical; OXYHGB, oxyhemoglobin. (Adapted from Friederich JA, Butterworth JF IV. Sodium nitroprusside. Twenty years and counting. Anesth Analg. 1995;81:152-162.)

Table 89-1 Signs, Symptoms, and Treatment of Toxicity Due to Byproducts of Sodium Nitroprusside Metabolism

Byproduct	Signs and Symptoms	Treatment
Cyanide*	Tachyphylaxis, metabolic acidosis Increased Svo_2, mental status changes	Stop infusion, administer 100% O_2 Correct metabolic acidosis with $NaHCO_3$
	Seizures, coma	Administer Sodium thiosulfate, 150 mg/kg IV over 15 min Sodium nitrate, 5 mg/kg, slow IV 3% sodium nitrite, 5 mg/kg by slow IV Hydroxocobalamin α, 25 mg/h, up to 100 mg max
Thiocyanate†	Fatigue, nausea, vomiting, tinnitus, miosis, hyperreflexia, confusion, psychosis, seizures, coma, hypothyroidism	Dialysis can facilitate clearance
Methemoglobinemia‡	Evidence of impaired oxygenation, despite adequate cardiac output and arterial Pao_2	Methylene blue, 1-2 mg/kg IV over 5 min, up to 7-8 mg/kg

*May cause reddish discoloration of the skin and mucous membranes.
†Rare. One hundred times less toxic than cyanide.
‡Rare. Pulse oximetry readings tend toward 86% to 88%.

Pharmacodynamics

Cardiovascular Effects

By relaxing smooth muscles in arterioles, SNP decreases systemic vascular resistance and blood pressure; by relaxing smooth muscle in venules, SNP decreases right atrial pressure. Because the predominant effects are on the arterial side, the decrease in systemic blood pressure can result in a reflex tachycardia due to increased sympathetic efferent activity, which will also increase myocardial contractility. The increased heart rate, the increased contractility, and the decreased systemic vascular resistance (decreased afterload) can all increase cardiac output. The increase in myocardial O_2 consumption and the decrease in diastolic blood pressure can lead to myocardial ischemia and infarction, so SNP should be used with some caution in patients with coronary artery disease (Box 89-1).

Box 89-1 Dosage and Administration of Sodium Nitroprusside

Preparation*

50 mg in 250 mL of D_5W (200 μg/mL)

Intravenous Infusion

Initial: 0.3-0.5 $\mu g \cdot kg^{-1} \cdot min^{-1}$ up to 10 $\mu g \cdot kg^{-1} \cdot min^{-1}$†
Bolus: 1-2 μg/kg

Example for a 75-kg Adult

For a 0.5 $\mu g \cdot kg^{-1} \cdot min^{-1}$ infusion:
The infusion would be 37.5 μg/min or 11.25 mL/h
For a 2 $\mu g \cdot kg^{-1} \cdot min^{-1}$ infusion:
The infusion would be 150 μg/min or 45 mL/h

*Protect from light to reduce degradation to hydrogen cyanide.
†Maximum infusion rate should not be administered for longer than 10 min.
D_5W, 5% dextrose in water.

Pulmonary Effects

The use of SNP is known to attenuate hypoxic pulmonary vasoconstriction. The resulting increase in shunt fraction is likely to be greater in patients with normal lungs versus those with chronic obstructive pulmonary disease, in whom the shunt fraction is already increased.

Central Nervous System Effects

SNP has no known direct effects on the central or autonomic nervous systems. SNP does, however, dilate capacitance vessels regardless of anesthetic background and dilates resistance vessels when autoregulation has been blunted (e.g., by inhalation anesthetic agents) so that cerebral blood flow and cerebral blood volume increase, thereby increasing intracranial pressure, particularly if there is a preexisting decreased intracranial compliance. Intracranial pressure increases maximally with moderate reduction (<30%) in mean arterial pressure, which can have a significant impact on cerebral perfusion pressure. Cyanide ions in cerebrospinal fluid cross the blood-brain barrier, causing cyanide encephalopathy and toxic edema or even brain damage, particularly in patients with impaired autoregulation and reduced cerebral blood flow and poor collateral circulation.

Coagulation Effects

SNP decreases the number and aggregation of platelets 1 to 6 h after infusion in patients with congestive heart failure. Platelet count and function return to preinfusion values in 24 h. Controlled hypotension using SNP reduces epinephrine-induced (and spontaneous) aggregation of platelets. During general anesthesia, systemic SNP significantly reduces blood flow to free musculocutaneous flaps, but local infusion into the flap significantly increases flow.

Toxicity

The toxicity of the cyanide ions in SNP has already been discussed. As with most hepatic reactions, the conversion of cyanide ion to thiocyanate is slowed by hypothermia; metabolism also requires adequate levels of vitamin B_{12} (thought to be deficient in Leber optic atrophy and tobacco amblyopia).

Children or young adults have a greater risk of developing toxicity because they have pronounced baroreceptor reflexes, necessitating larger doses of SNP. β-Adrenergic receptor blocking agents, angiotensin-converting enzyme inhibitors, and inhalation anesthetic agents blunt receptor reflexes and reduce the amount of SNP needed. Infusions of SNP should be discontinued if tachyphylaxis, metabolic acidosis, or increased mixed venous O_2 saturation develops.

Suggested Readings

Aronson S, Dyke CM, Stierer KA, et al. The ECLIPSE trials: Comparative studies of clevidipine to nitroglycerin, sodium nitroprusside, and nicardipine for acute hypertension treatment in cardiac surgery patients. *Anesth Analg*. 2008;107: 1110-1121.

Haas CE, LeBlanc JM. Acute postoperative hypertension: A review of therapeutic options. *Am J Health Syst Pharm*. 2004;61:1661-1675.

Sass N, Itamoto CH, Silva MP, et al. Does sodium nitroprusside kill babies? A systematic review. *Sao Paulo Med J*. 2007;125:108-111.

Thomas JE, Rosenwasser RH, Armonda RA, et al. Safety of intrathecal sodium nitroprusside for the treatment and prevention of refractory cerebral vasospasm and ischemia in humans. *Stroke*. 1999;30:1409-1416.

CHAPTER 90 Nitroglycerin

Suneerat Kongsayreepong, MD

Mechanism of Action for Vasodilation

Nitroglycerin (glycerol trinitrate) is metabolized to NO in the vascular smooth-muscle wall and acts to stimulate cyclic guanosine monophosphate (cGMP) production. Increased cGMP leads to the reduction of cytosolic Ca^{2+}, dephosphorylation of the myosin light chain, and smooth muscle relaxation and vasodilation. Because sulfhydryl groups are needed to produce the NO, vascular tolerance can occur when an excessive number of sulfhydryl groups are metabolized by prolonged exposure to nitroglycerin. Nitroglycerin is reported to have greater effects as a venodilator because of greater uptake in veins, as compared with arteries.

Metabolism

Metabolism of nitroglycerin occurs in the liver by hepatic glutathione organic nitrate reductase; inactivated metabolites are excreted by the kidney. Nitroglycerin, with a half-life of 1.9 to 2.6 min, also appears to be taken up by and metabolized in the endothelium of vessel walls.

Cardiovascular Effects

Because of the aforementioned greater uptake of nitroglycerin by the venous endothelium, nitroglycerin acts primarily on venous capacitance vessels, causing peripheral and splanchnic pooling of blood, decreased preload, decreased cardiac ventricular wall tension, and decreased heart size. With increased concentrations of nitroglycerin, relaxation of arterial vessels occurs, first affecting conductance vessels and then the smaller resistance vessels.

The effect of nitroglycerin on cardiac performance depends on the patient's underlying cardiac status. In patients with a normal or low ventricular filling pressure, cardiac output may decrease because of inadequate preload. In those with congestive heart failure (CHF), cardiac output increases as a result of decreased preload, reduced systolic wall tension, and, at higher doses of nitroglycerin, a decrease in afterload. For similar reasons, nitroglycerin, at high doses, also improves cardiac output in patients with mitral regurgitation. In patients with coronary artery disease, nitroglycerin causes decreased wall tension and decreased myocardial O_2 demand, which, in turn, results in increased myocardial contractility and cardiac output.

Myocardial blood flow is affected indirectly via hemodynamic changes and directly by coronary arterial dilation. Coronary perfusion increases more from the lowering of left ventricular end-diastolic pressure than from improved flow during diastole. A decrease in left ventricular end-diastolic pressure also reduces extrinsic tissue compression of coronary vessels in the subendocardium. Nitroglycerin is a potent epicardial coronary vasodilator in both normal and diseased vessels. Therapeutic doses of nitroglycerin dilate large coronary arteries but not coronary arterioles, improving collateral and subendocardial blood flow to ischemic areas. Nitroglycerin produces less coronary steal than do agents that produce intense vasodilation of the small coronary resistance vessels. High doses of nitroglycerin (9-32 $\mu g \cdot kg^{-1} \cdot min^{-1}$) cause direct coronary arteriolar vasodilation, overriding any coronary autoregulation. Part of the action of nitroglycerin on coronary vasodilation may involve its effects on stimulating the production and release of prostacyclin.

Nitroglycerin causes vasodilation of pulmonary arteries and veins, resulting in a decrease in right atrial, pulmonary artery, and pulmonary artery occlusion pressure. Nitroglycerin may reduce the pulmonary artery hypertension associated with various disease states and congenital heart disease. Nitroglycerin also dilates renal arteries, cerebral arteries, and cutaneous vessels. Blood flow to the kidney and brain may decrease if adequate systemic blood pressure is not maintained.

Therapeutic Uses

The cause of the antianginal effects of nitroglycerin is multifactorial. The use of nitroglycerin reduces the preload and systolic wall tension, resulting in decreased myocardial O_2 demand, and dilates the coronary arteries, resulting in increased O_2 delivery. The benefit of nitroglycerin in patients who have a partial occlusion of the coronary arteries likely occurs through a decrease in myocardial O_2 consumption; for those patients with total occlusion, the benefit occurs via redistribution of coronary artery blood flow. Nitroglycerin also relaxes vessels that are in spasm. The use of nitroglycerin was once considered to be contraindicated in patients with acute myocardial infarction because of the hypotension and tachycardia associated with its use; however, studies now show that the use of nitroglycerin increases collateral blood flow to ischemic regions and decreases infarction size. Maximum benefit is probably attained when CHF coexists. As long as hypotension is avoided, patients with acute myocardial infarction without CHF also benefit. Nitroglycerin works if it is instituted within 10 h of the ischemic event, at a starting dose of 0.5 $\mu g \cdot kg^{-1} \cdot min^{-1}$.

Perioperative indications for the use of nitroglycerin include myocardial ischemia, CHF, systemic and pulmonary hypertension, and coronary artery spasm. Preoperative oral or transcutaneous nitrates are continued until the time of the operation. Transcutaneous administration is probably not effective intraoperatively because absorption is not reliable. Intranasally administered nitroglycerin has been used to treat the pressor response to tracheal intubation and the hypertensive response that occurs after suprarenal aortic cross-clamping of abdominal aortic aneurysms. Inhaled nitroglycerin (2.5 μ/kg) has been used selectively to target pulmonary vasculature in the treatment of pulmonary hypertension—with a significant decrease in systolic, diastolic, and mean pulmonary artery pressure related to the decrease in pulmonary vascular resistance—without significant effects on systemic hemodynamics in adults and children undergoing cardiac operations.

Intraoperative indications for the intravenous administration of nitroglycerin include hypertension greater than 20% of preoperative levels in patients with coronary artery disease, left ventricular end-diastolic pressure greater than 18 to 20 mm Hg, ST-segment changes greater than 1 mm, and acute right or left ventricular dysfunction. Intraoperative doses of less than 1.0 $\mu g \cdot kg^{-1} \cdot min^{-1}$ are not considered to be effective.

In open surgical repair of an aortic aneurysm, intravenous administration of nitroglycerin maintains preaortic cross-clamp perfusion pressure and peripheral blood flow. Intravenously administered nitroglycerin also helps to control blood pressure during deployment of aortic endovascular stent grafts. Controlled hypotension to decrease blood loss during surgery can be achieved with intravenously administered nitroglycerin, either alone or combined with a drug to combat the reflex tachycardia.

The infusion of a single, intravenous, 100-μg bolus of nitroglycerin has been suggested for acute tocolysis when fetal bradycardia occurs following uterine hypertonicity after administration of combined spinal-epidural analgesia. Intravenously administered nitroglycerin can provide uterine relaxation during fetal surgery without affecting placental blood flow.

The prophylactic use of nitroglycerin has been evaluated in patients with coronary disease who have undergone a variety of operations. Although the use of nitroglycerin reduces the incidence of wall-motion abnormalities, as detected by transesophageal echocardiography, several studies have shown that the prophylactic use of nitroglycerin is ineffective in reducing the rate of ischemia, as evidenced by electrocardiography.

Polyethylene tubing is recommended for administration of nitroglycerin because polyvinylchloride tubing absorbs nitroglycerin.

Adverse Effects

A number of adverse effects are associated with the use of nitroglycerin. Nitrate tolerance may occur with a depletion of sulfhydryl groups, neurohumoral activation, volume expansion, downregulation of nitrate receptors, or any combination thereof. This tolerance may occur with all forms of nitrate administration that maintain continuous blood levels of the drug. If tolerance develops after prolonged exposure, physiologic responsiveness may be achieved with higher doses of nitroglycerin. Intermittent dosing with a nitrate-free interval each day or night can maintain a patient's responsiveness to nitroglycerin. Cross-tolerance can occur, with a possible decreased effect in patients who previously received isosorbide dinitrate.

Discontinuation of the drug after prolonged exposure may result in a rebound phenomenon, possibly resulting in coronary vasospasm and myocardial ischemia or infarction. Metabolism of nitroglycerin by liver nitrate reductase produces a nitrite that oxidizes the ferrous iron of hemoglobin to the ferric form of methemoglobin. Nitroglycerin doses of 5 $mg \cdot kg^{-1} \cdot day^{-1}$ or higher should be avoided to prevent significant methemoglobinemia.

Nitroglycerin has been reported to interfere with platelet aggregation and to reduce the ability of platelets to adhere to damaged intima at doses as low as 1.19 $\mu g \cdot kg^{-1} \cdot min^{-1}$. Inhibition returns to baseline values within 15 min of discontinuation of the infusion.

Contraindications

The use of nitroglycerin is contraindicated in patients who have used sildenafil, vardenafil, or tadalafil within the previous 24 to 48 h. Because these drugs inhibit phosphodiesterase, which degrades cGMP, nitroglycerin-mediated vasodilatation is markedly enhanced and prolonged, resulting in cases of profound hypotension, myocardial infarction, and death. Relative contraindications to the use of nitroglycerin include increased intracranial pressure, hypovolemia, and angina associated with aortic stenosis, idiopathic hypertrophic subaortic stenosis, and tachyarrhythmias.

Suggested Readings

Bernard EO, Schmid ER, Lachat ML, Germann RC. Nitroglycerin to control blood pressure during endovascular stent-grafting of descending thoracic aortic aneurysms. *J Vasc Surg*. 2000;31:790-793.

Calvey TN, Williams NE, eds. *Principle and Practice of Pharmacology for Anaesthetists*. 5th ed. Malden, MA: Wiley-Blackwell; 2008:287-306.

Degoute CS. Controlled hypotension: A guide to drug choice. *Drugs*. 2007;67:1053-1076.

Van de Velde M, Vercauteren M, Vandermeersch E. Fetal heart rate abnormalities after regional analgesia for labor pain: The effect of intrathecal opioids. *Reg Anesth Pain Med*. 2001;26:257-262

Goyal P, Kiran U, Chauhan S, et al. Efficacy of nitroglycerin inhalation in reducing pulmonary arterial hypertension in children with congenital heart disease. *Br J Anaesth*. 2006;97:208-214.

Michel T. Treatment of myocardial ischemia. In: Brunton LL, ed. *Goodman & Gilman's The Pharmacological Basis of Therapeutics*. 11th ed. New York: McGraw-Hill; 2006:823-844.

Opie LH, Gersh BJ, eds. *Drugs for the Heart*. 6th ed. Philadelphia: WB Saunders; 2005:33-49.

Royster RL, Butterworth J, Groban L, et al. Cardiovascular pharmacology. In: Kaplan JA, Reich DL, Lake CL, Konstadt SN, eds. *Kaplan's Cardiac Anesthesia*. 5th ed. Philadelphia: WB Saunders; 2006:213-280.

Singh R, Choudhury M, Saxena A, et al. Inhaled nitroglycerin versus inhaled milrinone in children with congenital heart disease suffering from pulmonary artery hypertension. *J Cardiothorac Vasc Anesth*. 2010;24:797-891.

Yoshikawa F, Kohase H, Umino M, Fukayama H. Blood loss and endocrine responses in hypotensive anaesthesia with sodium nitroprusside and nitroglycerin for mandibular osteotomy. *Int J Oral Maxillofac Surg*. 2009;38:1159-1164.

Yurtseven N, Karaca P, Kaplan M, et al. Effect of nitroglycerin inhalation on patients with pulmonary hypertension undergoing mitral valve replacement surgery. *Anesthesiology*. 2003;99:855-858.

CHAPTER 91

β-Adrenergic Receptor Blocking Agents

Ian MacVeigh, MD

β-Adrenergic receptor antagonists are a heterogeneous group of drugs widely used in managing hypertension and cardiac disease. Key to understanding their physiologic effects is knowledge of the molecular mechanism of action of the β-adrenergic receptor.

β-Receptors are divided into β_1-receptors, found primarily in the heart, and β_2-receptors, found in the smooth muscle of the vasculature and bronchi.

The β_1-adrenergic receptor located on the cardiac sarcolemma is coupled to adenyl cyclase via a G protein. When activated, adenyl cyclase converts adenosine triphosphate (ATP) to cyclic adenosine monophosphate (cAMP), a secondary intracellular messenger, that stimulates protein kinase A to phosphorylate membrane calcium channels, leading to an increase in cytoplasmic Ca^{2+}. The consequences of β_1-adrenergic stimulation are positive inotropy, chronotropy, dromotropy, and lusitropic relaxant effect (the latter by increasing the reuptake of cytosolic calcium into the sarcoplasmic reticulum). Because the secondary messenger cAMP is metabolized by phosphodiesterase, phosphodiesterase inhibitors augment β_1 activity, which is manifested by sympathomimetic effects. Because of inhibition of G protein (e.g., vagal [muscarinic] stimulation), the coupling with adenyl cyclase is interrupted, resulting in attenuation of the effects described previously—the similar effects observed with inhibition of the β-receptor itself (Figure 91-1).

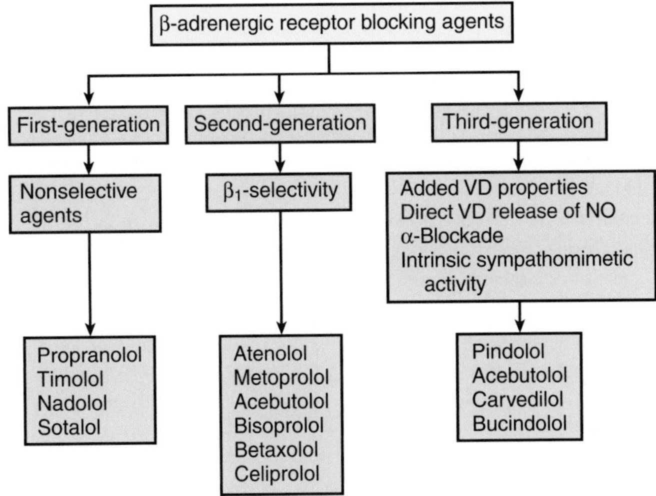

Figure 91-1 β-Adrenergic receptor blocking agents differ with regard to their β_1-selectivity, lipid solubility, and intrinsic sympathomimetic activity. NO, Nitric oxide; VD, vasodilatory.

Indications for β-Adrenergic Receptor Blockade

Because β-adrenergic receptor blocking agents have negative inotropy and chronotropy—decreasing myocardial oxygen demand and improving myocardial perfusion—they are used in the treatment of a number of conditions. β-Adrenergic receptor blocking agents reduce the exercise-induced increase in contractility and blood pressure; therefore, they are used to treat all classes of angina except variant or Prinzmetal angina. When β adrenergic receptor blocking agents are administered correctly, patients will ideally have heart rates between 50 and 60 beats/min at rest and no more than 100 beats/min with exercise.

For similar reasons, β-adrenergic receptor blocking agents are very effective in reducing the frequency and number of ischemic episodes in patients with myocardial ischemia or acute coronary syndromes. By decreasing inotropy and chronotropy, heart rate, contractility, afterload, and myocardial wall stress are all decreased, which optimizes myocardial O_2 supply/demand. Current recommendations for patients with acute coronary syndromes are for β-adrenergic receptor blocking agents to be started early, along with statins, antiplatelet drugs, and angiotensin-converting enzyme inhibitors. This quadruple therapy has been associated with a 90% reduction in mortality rates at 6 months following the diagnosis of acute coronary syndrome. In patients who have had an acute myocardial infarction, β-adrenergic receptor blocking agents are specifically indicated to treat ongoing pain, tachycardia, hypertension, or ventricular rhythm instability. The initiation of β-adrenergic receptor blocking agents early after infarction and continued long-term has been associated with a reduction in mortality rate by as much as 25%.

β-Adrenergic receptor blocking agents lower blood pressure by decreasing cardiac output and peripheral vascular resistance and are specifically indicated to treat hypertension in patients with congestive heart failure, with coronary artery disease, and after myocardial infarction. Patients with congestive heart failure, even if they are not hypertensive, can benefit from β-blockade; the administration of carvedilol and of metoprolol have been reported to improve cardiac ejection fraction, reverse abnormal patterns of gene expression toward normal, and decrease mortality rate.

Because of their negative dromotropy, inhibitory effects in the sinus and atrioventricular nodes, and other antiarrhythmic properties (Table 91-1), β-adrenergic receptor blocking agents are recommended to acutely and chronically treat a number of tachyarrhythmias. They are indicated to treat supraventricular tachycardias, to control the rate in patients with atrial fibrillation, and to treat ventricular tachyarrhythmias (specifically metoprolol and sotalol [class III antiarrhythmic]). β-Adrenergic receptor blocking agents also counteract the arrhythmogenic effects of excess catecholamine stimulation, as seen, for example, in patients after myocardial infarction.

β-Adrenergic receptor blocking agents are recommended to treat hypertrophic obstructive cardiomyopathy to decrease systolic anterior motion of

Table 91-1 Characteristics of Commonly Used β-Adrenergic Receptor Blocking Agents

Drug	Bioavailability (%)	Protein Binding (%)	Elimination Half-life (h)	Major Elimination Pathway	Other Properties
Atenolol	50	15	6-9	Renal	β_1-Selective
Carvedilol	30	95	7-10	Hepatic	Antioxidant
Labetalol	30	50	3-6	Hepatic	α-Blocker/γ-blocker ratio: 1/4
Metoprolol	50	10	3-6	Hepatic	β_1-Selective
Esmolol*	100	55	0.15	Blood esterases	β_1-Selective
Sotalol	100	0	10-15	Renal	Class III antiarrhythmic
Bisoprolol	80	30	9-12	Renal	β_1-Selective
Nadolol	30	30	14-24	Renal	Water-soluble
Propranolol	35	90	3-5	Hepatic	—

*Available only as intravenously administered agent.

the anterior mitral valve leaflet. In patients with mitral stenosis, by decreasing the heart rate both at rest and during exercise, β-blockade prolongs diastolic filling time and, therefore, improves cardiac output. In patients with mitral valve prolapse, β-adrenergic receptor blocking agents are recommended to treat any associated arrhythmias. β-Blockade is indicated in patients with dissecting aortic aneurysms to decrease pulse pressure and sheer stress on the aortic wall.

The cyanotic spells associated with the tetralogy of Fallot are decreased in frequency and severity by the administration of β-adrenergic receptor blocking agents. In patients with congenital long QT syndrome, β-blockade restores the imbalance between the left and right stellate ganglia.

In patients with thyrotoxicosis, β-adrenergic receptor blocking agents control the associated tachycardia, palpitations, and anxiety. The use of β-adrenergic receptor blocking agents is strongly recommended to treat hypertension and tachycardia in patients with thyroid storm, if left ventricular function is normal.

Patients coming to the operating room may be on β-adrenergic receptor blocking agents for other reasons, such as to treat anxiety, essential tremor, neurocardiogenic syncope, and open-angle glaucoma and for prophylaxis of migraine headaches.

Of particular importance for anesthesia providers, β-adrenergic receptor blocking agents should be used in patients at high risk for experiencing a coronary event and who are undergoing noncardiac and vascular operations, but this recommendation is not without risk if the patient has not been on β-adrenergic receptor blocking agents before the operation. The POISE study demonstrated that extended-release metoprolol decreased the rate of myocardial events but was associated with an increased risk of stroke and a higher mortality rate at 30 days. However, patients who are on β-adrenergic receptor blocking agents preoperatively but have not taken their usual daily dose should receive a β-adrenergic receptor blocking agent preoperatively.

Pharmacology of β-Adrenergic Receptor Blocking Agents

Multiple β-adrenergic receptor blocking agents are available, differing in β_1 cardioselectivity, lipid solubility, and whether or not they have intrinsic sympathomimetic activity (see Table 91-1).

Intrinsic Sympathomimetic Activity

β-Adrenergic receptor blocking agents with intrinsic sympathomimetic activity cause mild peripheral vasodilation without reducing cardiac output. β-Adrenergic receptor blocking agents without intrinsic sympathomimetic activity lower blood pressure by decreasing cardiac output and inhibiting renin release and central sympathetic outflow.

Lipid Solubility

Lipid-soluble drugs, such as propranolol, carvedilol, and penbutolol, are metabolized by the liver, have a short duration of action, and are capable of entering the brain. Metoprolol, pindolol, and timolol have intermediate lipid solubility. Atenolol, esmolol, sotalol, nadolol, and betaxolol are the least lipid soluble and, therefore, have the least central nervous system penetration and activity and the longest duration of action because they are renally excreted.

β_1 Cardioselectivity

The cardioselectivity of the β-adrenergic receptor blocking agents can be found in standard textbooks, but because none of the β-adrenergic receptor blocking agents are 100% β_1 selective, the American College of Chest Physicians has recommended that β-adrenergic receptor blocking agents not be first-line agents in patients with reactive airways disease and that, when these drugs are used in such patients, the risks of precipitating an asthmatic attack must be weighed against the benefits of the drug.

Side Effects

Because of their mechanism of action, β-adrenergic receptor blocking agents are associated with a number of symptoms and signs that are not truly side effects but, rather, sequelae of their mechanism of action. These sequelae include bradycardia, hypotension, and central nervous system effects, which include sedation, fatigue, (combination of peripheral and central effects), sleep disturbances, depression, and hallucinations. In men, β-adrenergic receptor blocking agents increase the incidence of impotence. As mentioned, the use of even the most cardioselective β-adrenergic receptor blocking agents is associated with bronchospasm in patients with a history of asthma. They may mask hypoglycemic symptoms in patients with diabetes and increase triglyceride and reduce high-density lipoprotein levels.

Abrupt discontinuation of β-adrenergic receptor blocking agents is associated with rebound hypertension and tachycardia, which can result in myocardial ischemia or infarction. With respect to specific side effects, labetalol has been associated with an increase in concentration of liver enzymes, an increased concentration of antinuclear and antimitochondrial antibodies, pruritus of the scalp, and positive tests for pheochromocytoma because it interferes with assays of metanephrine and catecholamines. Contraindications to the use of β-adrenergic receptor blocking agents are listed in Box 91-1.

Anesthesia providers should use β-adrenergic receptor blocking agents sparingly and with caution in patients taking digitalis, calcium channel blockers, or disopyramide. Levels of β-adrenergic receptor blocking agents metabolized by the liver (propranolol, metoprolol, carvedilol, labetalol) are increased by cimetidine, which decreases hepatic blood flow. In patients who have taken an accidental or intentional overdose of β-adrenergic receptor blocking agents, the side effects can be mitigated by glucagon, 100 mg/kg, administered intravenously over 1 min, then 1 to 5 mg/h; isoproterenol, up to 0.1 $g \cdot kg^{-1} \cdot min^{-1}$; or dobutamine, 15 $\mu g \cdot kg^{-1} \cdot min^{-1}$.

Box 91-1 Contraindications to the Use of β-Adrenergic Receptor Blocking Agents

Absolute

Severe bradycardia
Sinus node dysfunction or high-grade atrioventricular block
Overt ventricular systolic failure
Severe asthma or active bronchospasm
Severe peripheral vascular disease with rest ischemia
Severe depression

Relative

Systolic blood pressure ≤ 100 mm Hg
Raynaud phenomenon
Insulin-dependent diabetes mellitus
Mild asthma or severe chronic obstructive pulmonary disease
Hyperlipidemia
Pregnancy, may decrease placental blood flow
Liver disease*

*Avoid agents with high hepatic clearance (e.g., propranolol, carvedilol, timolol, metoprolol).

Suggested Readings

Fleisher LA, Beckman JA, Brown KA, et al. ACC/AHA 2006 guideline update on perioperative cardiovascular evaluation for noncardiac surgery: Focused update on perioperative beta-blocker therapy—A report of the American College of Cardiology/American Heart Association Task Force on Practice Guidelines (Writing Committee to Update the 2002 Guidelines on Perioperative Cardiovascular Evaluation for Noncardiac Surgery). *Anesth Analg*. 2007;104:15-26.

Lindenauer PK, Pekow P, Wang K, et al. Perioperative beta-blocker therapy and mortality after major noncardiac surgery. *N Engl J Med*. 2005;353:349-361.

London MJ. Con: Beta-blockers are indicated for all adults at increased risk undergoing noncardiac surgery. *Anesth Analg*. 2007;104:11-14.

POISE Study Group. Effects of extended-release metoprolol succinate in patients undergoing non-cardiac surgery (POISE trial): A randomised controlled trial. *Lancet*. 2008;371:1839-1847.

Urban MK, Markowitz SM, Gordon MA, et al. Postoperative prophylactic administration of β-adrenergic blockers in patients at risk for myocardial ischemia. *Anesth Analg*. 2000;90:1257-1261.

Wiesbauer F, Schlager O, Domanovits H, et al. Perioperative β-blockers for preventing surgery-related mortality and morbidity: A systematic review and meta-analysis. *Anesth Analg*. 2007;104:27-41.

CHAPTER 92

Calcium Channel Blockers

Ian MacVeigh, MD

Calcium channel blockers (CCBs), also known as calcium entry blockers or calcium channel antagonists, are a heterogeneous group of drugs that selectively inhibit the influx of extracellular calcium through L-type voltage-gated calcium channels (VGCCs). This type of calcium channel plays an important role in signal transduction on excitable cells such as myocytes and neurons. For cells to use adenosine triphosphate as an energy source, the concentration of intracellular Ca^{2+} must be quite low, otherwise the Ca^{2+} would precipitate with phosphorus. When an action potential on the cell surface opens VGCCs, the flux of Ca^{2+} that passes into the cytoplasm is relatively large compared with the tiny amount of intracellular Ca^{2+}; the electrical signal that depolarized the cell membrane is thereby converted to an ion-coded signal. The Ca^{2+} functions as a secondary messenger—its divalent charge is sufficient to produce conformational change in a number of cytoplasmic proteins, such as actin-myosin, for example. VGCCs close rapidly by a voltage-dependent mechanism, and the intracellular Ca^{2+} quickly dissipates, allowing for precise intracellular signaling. VGCCs require either a low voltage (T-type) or high voltage to open. High-voltage calcium channels are identified as N-type (present on neurons) or L-type (so named because when investigators studying VGCCs replaced Ca^{2+} with Ba^{2+} in organ baths, there was a large unitary conductance to Ba^{2+}).

Mechanism of Action

The currently available CCBs effectively inhibit the opening of L-type VGCCs, and, when inward flux of calcium is inhibited, contraction of smooth muscle cells in peripheral arterial blood vessels decreases, arteries vasodilate, systemic vascular resistance (SVR) decreases, and blood pressure falls. CCBs have no effect on venous blood vessels but are particularly effective in dilating larger more noncompliant arteries, one of the most common causes of systolic hypertension in elderly patients.

Inotropy also decreases because the amount of calcium available for each myocardial contraction is less. The combination of decreased SVR (afterload) and decreased inotropy optimizes myocardial O_2 demand-supply, decreasing the incidence and severity of angina pectoris.

In addition, CCBs decrease electrical activity in the conducting system within the heart by inhibiting VGCCs during phase 0 of the slow-response sinoatrial and atrioventricular nodal cells and during phase 2 of the action potential of the fast-response Purkinje fibers, producing a negative chronotropic effect (i.e., decreased heart rate) and dromotropic effect (i.e., decreased conduction). The combination of effects is one of the reasons that CCBs are commonly used to treat atrial fibrillation and atrial flutter in patients for whom heart rate control is a primary goal.

Classes of Drugs

The two main types of CCBs are the dihydropyridine (DHP) and the nondihydropyridine (N-DHP) compounds. The DHPs have a similar chemical structure and have similar pharmacologic effects, different from those that result from administration of the N-DHPs, partly explained by the fact that the two classes of drugs bind to different sites on the L-type VGCCs. There is some rationale, therefore, for using certain drugs (e.g., a DHP and an N-DHP [diltiazem]) in combination.

The DHPs have more vascular selectivity than do the N-DHPs, and because they have little chronotropic effect, a β-adrenergic receptor blocking agent is sometimes used to counteract the reflex tachycardia that can be seen when certain DHPs are administered. As a class, DHPs are not used to treat angina, with the exception of amlodipine, nicardipine, and nifedipine, which are approved to treat stable angina as well as angina caused by vasospasm in the coronary arteries.

The N-DHPs have chronotropic and dromotropic effects for the reasons described above. As a consequence, the N-DHPs increase the potential for heart block and should be used judiciously, if at all, in patients with cardiomyopathies. The N-DHP drugs have either a phenylalkylamine or a benzothiazepine chemical structure. Verapamil, the best-known phenylalkylamine, is relatively selective for the heart and, for the reasons mentioned earlier, reduces myocardial O_2 demand and reverses coronary artery spasm; therefore, this drug is used to treat angina. Diltiazem, the best-known benzothiazepine, has cardiac effects that are somewhat similar to those of verapamil but are not as pronounced. Diltiazem has some effects on the peripheral vasculature, similar to those of the DHPs, reducing SVR but without producing the same degree of reflex tachycardia as is seen with the use of the DHPs.

General Indications

Except for nimodipine, which is only approved to prevent or treat vasospasm associated with subarachnoid hemorrhage, all of the CCBs are approved to treat hypertension either by themselves or in combination with other drugs. CCBs have also been used (off label) to treat some of the sequelae of Raynaud syndrome, migraine and cluster headaches, high-altitude pulmonary edema, and hypertension associated with the use of nonsteroidal anti-inflammatory agents, cyclosporine, and other drugs. Some (see following discussion) have been approved to treat angina and others to treat atrial arrhythmias.

Dihydropyridines

With the exception of sublingual nifedipine, these drugs have a long duration of action. Nifedipine, nicardipine, and felodipine have some negative inotropy, whereas amlodipine and lacidipine have no, or very little, cardiac-depressant activity.

Nifedipine

The use of sublingual capsules of nifedipine has been associated with myocardial ischemia and death when given to patients with coronary artery disease. Because sublingual nifedipine may cause a rapid peripheral vasodilation that decreases blood pressure and myocardial O_2 supply, along with a reflex tachycardia that results in an increased myocardial O_2 demand, the U.S. Food and Drug Administration requires the labeling to include a warning against the use of sublingual nifedipine to treat hypertension. All other formulations of nifedipine are approved for the treatment of hypertension, effort angina, and vasospastic angina. These formulations have approximately 60% bioavailability, are 95% protein bound, have high first-pass hepatic metabolism by CYP-450 enzymes, and have a half-life of 2 to 5 h. Its metabolites are excreted by the kidneys and in feces. Because nifedipine is such a potent vasodilator, its use is contraindicated in patients with aortic stenosis, hypertrophic obstructive cardiomyopathy, and severe left ventricular dysfunction; the vasodilation results in its primary side effects: headaches and ankle edema.

Nicardipine

Nicardipine is commonly administered intravenously to treat hypertension in patients in the operating room and intensive care unit. It is injected as a bolus of 0.625 to 2.5 mg followed by a continuous infusion of 0.5 to 5 mg/h. The advantages of nicardipine are its lack of effect on heart rate and preload and the fact that its use is not associated with rebound hypertension upon discontinuation.

Amlodipine

Amlodipine has a slow onset of 1 to 2 h and a long duration of action, with an elimination half-life of 35 to 48 h. Its major clinical uses are for the treatment of hypertension and effort angina.

Nimodipine

Nimodipine is the only CCB approved for preventing and for treating cerebral vasospasm after subarachnoid hemorrhage or after cerebral aneurysm clipping. This drug is usually administered as a 30-mg to 40-mg oral dose every 4 h.

Nondihydropyridines

Verapamil

Verapamil, a phenylalkylamine, is indicated to treat essential hypertension, effort-induced angina, vasospastic angina, and atrial arrhythmias, usually at an oral dose of 180 to 480 mg/day or as an intravenous bolus of 2.5 to 10 mg. When verapamil is administered orally, its bioavailability is only 10% to 20%, and it has a protein binding of approximately 90%. Similar to the other CCBs, it has high first-pass hepatic metabolism by P-450 CYP3A4, an active metabolite (norverapamil), and an elimination half-life of 3 to 7 h. Metabolites are excreted by the kidneys (75%) or in the gastrointestinal tract (25%). Because of its mechanism of action, the use of verapamil is contraindicated in patients with sick sinus syndrome, preexisting atrioventricular nodal disease, severe left ventricular myocardial depression, or digoxin toxicity. Patients with Wolff-Parkinson-White syndrome with concomitant atrial fibrillation are at risk of developing antegrade conduction through the bypass tract, manifested usually within a few minutes of administration as a wide-complex ventricular tachycardia that can rapidly deteriorate into ventricular fibrillation. Patients receiving β-adrenergic receptor blocking agents should not receive verapamil because these patients have a high risk of developing severe bradycardia. The side effects of verapamil include headache, facial flushing, dizziness, and constipation. Verapamil also interacts with several drugs, increasing blood levels of digoxin, atorvastatin, simvastatin, lovastatin, ketoconazole, cyclosporine, carbamazepine, and theophylline.

Verapamil toxicity can be treated with calcium administered intravenously either as the chloride salt or as calcium gluconate. Glucagon and levosimendan have also been successfully used to treat toxicity, as have isoproterenol and atropine. For patients with acute heart block that is unresponsive to pharmacologic therapy, temporary pacing should be considered. Because CCBs can block the effect of insulin, insulin supplementation may be required.

Diltiazem

Diltiazem, a benzothiazepine, is often administered intravenously as a bolus dose of 0.25 mg/kg followed by a continuous infusion of 5 to 15 mg/min to treat acute supraventricular tachycardias and to decrease the ventricular response rate in atrial fibrillation or flutter. It is approximately 85% protein bound, metabolized in the liver to an active metabolite, desacetyl diltiazem; metabolites are 35% excreted in urine, with the remainder excreted in the gastrointestinal tract. Diltiazem has a low incidence of side effects, but the same care should be taken when this drug is administered to patients taking β-adrenergic receptor blocking agents, and it should be used with caution, if at all, in patients with cardiomyopathy or atrioventricular nodal disease.

Toxicity

Most of the toxicity associated with CCBs is mild and can be treated by discontinuing the drug. As mentioned earlier, severe toxicity can be treated with intravenous calcium, inotropes, isoproterenol, glucagon, or other drugs. Similar to the toxicity seen when verapamil is used in combination with a β-adrenergic receptor blocking agent, the side effects seen with the CCBs are agent specific. However, because these are all potent vasodilators, headache, lightheadedness or dizziness, flushing, and peripheral edema can be seen in 10% to 20% of patients. One of the adverse side effects of verapamil is constipation, reported in 25% of patients taking the drug. Interestingly, however, peripheral edema is less common with verapamil than it is with the other compounds. As mentioned previously, patients using a short-acting nifedipine are at increased risk of experiencing myocardial infarction and dying; therefore, this drug should not be used in patients with known coronary artery disease. In 1995, a report suggested that the use of even long-acting CCBs is associated with an increased risk of myocardial infarction; however, more recent studies have failed to confirm these findings. Other studies associating the use of CCBs with gastrointestinal bleeding and malignancy in the elderly have likewise been flawed. CCBs can be safely used for most patients with hypertension, angina, Raynaud syndrome, hypertension and asthma, or hypertension in patients that is not controlled with other medications.

Anesthetic Considerations in Patients Taking Calcium Channel Blockers

Inhalation anesthetic agents decrease the availability of intracellular calcium, which, in turn, increases the negative inotropic, chronotropic, and dromotropic effects of CCBs. The inhibition of calcium influx into myocytes potentiates the effects of all neuromuscular blocking agents. There are reports of patients who were on verapamil preoperatively who developed cardiovascular collapse when they were given dantrolene intraoperatively for presumed malignant hyperthermia. CCBs have also been reported to impair hypoxic pulmonary vasoconstriction and, because of their vasodilating properties, to increase intracranial pressure.

Suggested Readings

Abernethy DR, Schwartz JB. Calcium antagonist drugs. *N Engl J Med.* 1999;341:1447-1455.

Duminda N, Wijeysundera W, Beattie S. Calcium channel blockers for reducing cardiac morbidity after noncardiac surgery: A meta-analysis. *Anesth Analg.* 2003;97:634-641.

Elliott WJ, Venkata C, Ram S. Calcium channel blockers. *J Clin Hypertens.* 2011;13:687-689.

Tsien RW, Barrett CF. A brief history of calcium channel discovery. In: *Madame Curie Bioscience Database*. Austin: Landes Bioscience; 2000. *British Journal of Pharmacology.* 2006;147(1):S56-S62.

Varpula T, Rapola J, Sallisalmi M, Kurola J. Treatment of serious calcium channel blocker overdose with levosimendan, a calcium sensitizer. *Anesth Analg.* 2009;108:790-792.

CHAPTER 93

Renin-Angiotensin-Aldosterone Inhibition

Ian MacVeigh, MD

The renin-angiotensin-aldosterone system (RAAS) is important for homeostasis because it helps regulate intravascular volume and systemic vascular resistance (SVR), thereby affecting cardiac function because of its effects on preload (intravascular volume) and afterload (SVR). The kidneys retain sodium and water when the RAAS is activated, which increases preload, and arteriolar blood vessels constrict, thereby increasing SVR; if cardiac output (CO) is unchanged by the increased afterload, blood pressure (BP) will increase (BP = CO × SVR). Early in the development of heart failure, these compensatory mechanisms are beneficial (see Chapter 142), but over time, left ventricular remodeling occurs; therefore, the risks of unopposed RAAS activation outweigh its benefits. Several drug classes have been developed to modify the RAAS, including angiotensin-converting enzyme (ACE) inhibitors, angiotensin receptor blockers (ARBs), inhibitors of aldosterone (e.g., spironolactone), and direct renin inhibitors (e.g., aliskiren).

Physiology

Renin, a protease, is released by juxtaglomerular cells adjacent to the afferent arterioles of renal glomeruli in response to hypotension and β_1-adrenergic receptor activation. The macula densa of distal tubules, which lie in close proximity to the juxtaglomerular cells, also release renin (e.g., in response to decreased levels of sodium in the renal tubules).

Renin released into the blood metabolizes angiotensinogen, an α_2 globulin of hepatic origin, to the decapeptide angiotensin I. The vascular endothelium of many organs, but particularly within the lung, contains an enzyme, ACE, that cleaves two amino acids from angiotensin I to form the octapeptide angiotensin II. Angiotensin II can bind to two receptor subtypes that have different internal signaling pathways: angiotensin 1 (AT_1) receptors are responsible for most of the effects of angiotensin II seen in adults, and angiotensin 2 (AT_2) receptors are thought to be responsible for most of its antigrowth effects seen in the fetus. The binding of angiotensin II to AT_1 receptors on smooth muscle cells within peripheral arteriolar resistance vessels stimulates the muscles to contract, resulting in vasoconstriction, and thereby increasing SVR and arterial blood pressure. Angiotensin II also stimulates the adrenal cortex to release aldosterone, which, in turn, promotes the retention of sodium and free water within the distal tubules of the kidneys and the excretion of potassium. In patients with hypertensive heart disease, the release of aldosterone may accelerate hypertrophy, fibrosis, and diastolic dysfunction. Angiotensin II has additional endocrine effects (e.g., stimulation of the posterior pituitary to release vasopressin, a potent vasoconstrictor and antidiuretic hormone). In addition, angiotensin II potentiates central and peripheral sympathetic noradrenergic activity; in the periphery, the postganglionic sympathetic release of norepinephrine by nerve cells is enhanced, and the reuptake of norepinephrine is inhibited, thereby producing additional peripheral vasoconstriction. Through mechanisms independent of those mentioned, angiotensin II also stimulates cardiac hypertrophy and vascular hypertrophy (Figure 93-1).

Since the first ACE inhibitor, captopril, was marketed in 1982, a diverse number of medications that affect the RAAS have been developed and marketed for an equally diverse number of indications. Most commonly, patients receive one or more ACE inhibitors that modulate the RAAS for the treatment of hypertension and heart failure and, in diabetics, to decrease the incidence of diabetic nephropathy. However, because ACE inhibitors have been reported to be effective in preventing migraine headaches, for treating hyperuricemia, and in patients with hypertension to decrease their likelihood of developing Alzheimer disease, patients who present for an anesthetic may be taking drugs that alter the RAAS for a multitude of sometimes interrelated problems. Anesthesia providers should understand the pharmacokinetics and pharmacodynamics of these drugs because, even though only one parenteral ACE inhibitor is available (i.e., enalapril), if patients who are taking drugs that modulate the RAAS develop perioperative complications, the clinician may have to parenterally administer a substitute medication that has similar effects.

Angiotensin-Converting Enzyme Inhibitors

ACE inhibitors are considered peripheral vasodilator drugs that work by inhibiting the production of angiotensin II. In patients with normal left ventricular function, ACE inhibitors decrease SVR with minimal effect on heart rate, cardiac output, and pulmonary artery occlusion pressure. In patients with decreased left ventricular function, ACE inhibitors decrease preload, afterload, and systolic wall stress.

These drugs were originally used as second-line agents to treat hypertension but are now considered to be first-line agents if the patient also has heart failure, has had a myocardial infarction, has a high risk of developing coronary artery disease, has diabetes, has kidney disease, or has had a stroke. The Heart Outcomes Prevention Evaluation (HOPE) Study, which was not limited to the study of hypertensive patients, demonstrated that the ACE inhibitor ramipril decreased the number of cardiovascular events (e.g., death, myocardial infarction, stroke) in patients with prior cardiac events or with diabetes. The European Trial on Reduction of Cardiac Events with Perindopril in Stable Coronary Artery Disease (EUROPA) study in which perindopril, another ACE inhibitor, was administered to patients with stable coronary disease but no evidence of heart failure, found fewer subsequent cardiovascular events. Over time, the indications for the use of ACE inhibitors has increased, and they are currently recommended for the treatment of heart failure of any stage, for use during the early phase of acute myocardial infarction, and for postinfarction left ventricular dysfunction (to limit adverse remodeling). In addition to their effects in patients with myocardial and vascular disease, ACE inhibitors decrease the risk of nephropathy in diabetic patients and in patients with proteinuric renal disease.

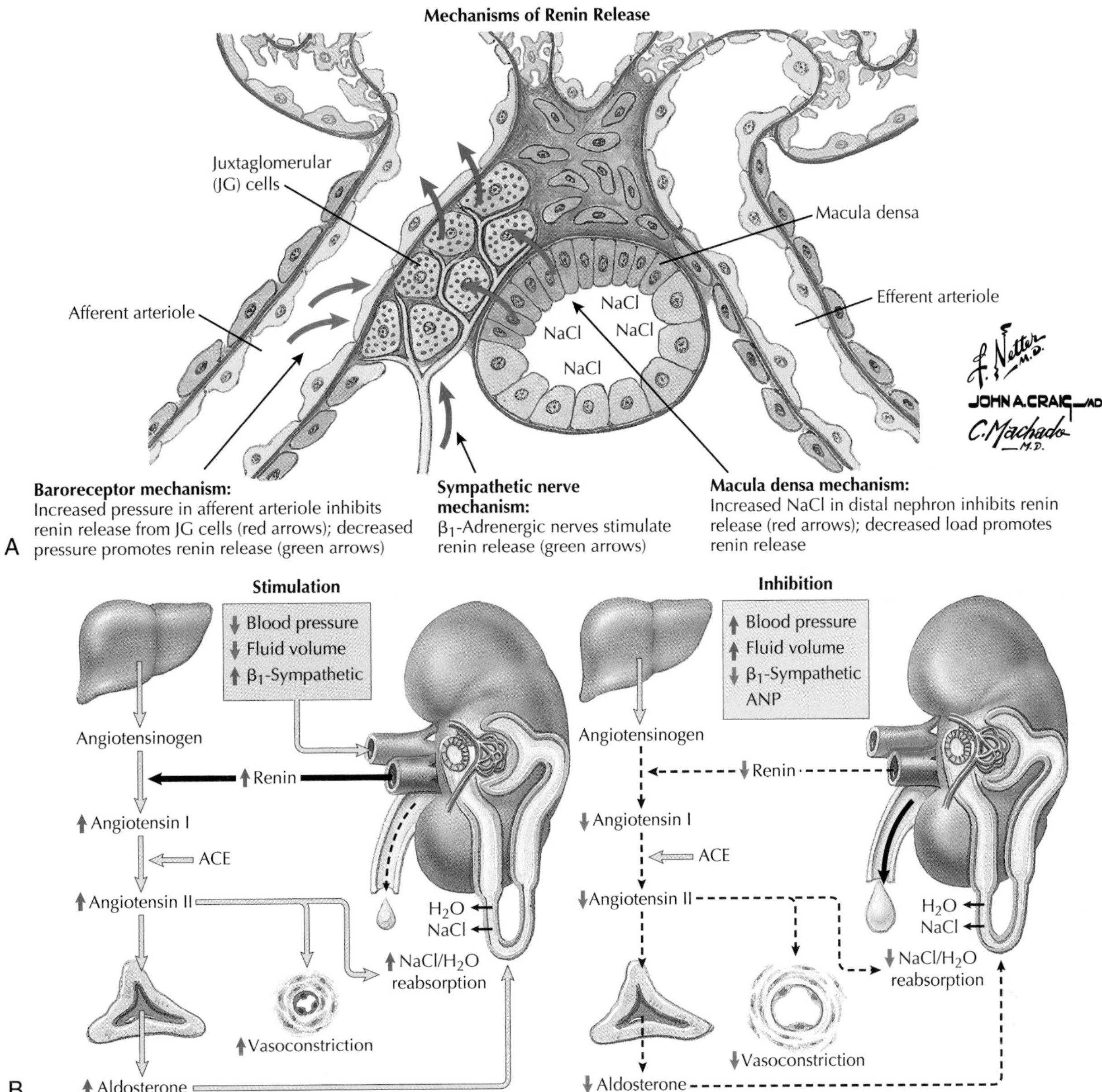

Figure 93-1 Mechanism of renin secretion and factors regulating the renin-angiotensin-aldosterone system. The cascade of events initiated to promote sodium and water reabsorption is illustrated in **A**. Renin is secreted from the juxtaglomerular cells in response to reduced sodium concentration and flow in the distal tubule (**B**). (Netter illustration from www.netterimages.com.)

Classification of Angiotensin-Converting Enzyme Inhibitors

ACE inhibitors differ in potency, bioavailability, half-life, and route of elimination (Table 93-1).

Class I: Directly Active Agents

Captopril, the original ACE inhibitor, has the shortest half-life of any of the available drugs and is the only agent that contains a sulfhydryl group in its chemical structure (which may confer additional properties because it is the only ACE inhibitor that is also a free radical scavenger). The presence of the sulfhydryl group may also result in some of its specific side effects: skin rash, loss of taste, neutropenia, and proteinuria.

Class II Drugs

The drugs in this class (the majority of ACE inhibitors: enalapril, ramipril, perindopril, benazepril, cilazapril, delapril, fosinopril, quinapril, trandolapril) are all prodrugs that are converted to active drugs by hepatic metabolism.

Class III Drugs

Lisinopril, the only drug in this class, is not a prodrug, is water soluble, and does not undergo hepatic metabolism but is excreted unchanged by the kidneys.

Side Effects

A number of side effects are associated with these drugs—some are associated with increased bradykinin levels because ACE inhibitors also increase its formation, and others are due to the decrease in angiotensin II levels. The most commonly reported side effect is a nonproductive cough, with an incidence of 5% to 10%. More worrisome is angioedema, with an incidence 0.3% to 0.6%, and neutropenia—mostly seen in patients on high-dose captopril in association with renal failure and collagen vascular diseases—both of which can be life threatening. As might be expected based on their mechanism of action, the ACE inhibitors are associated with orthostatic hypotension (especially so in patients with hyponatremia), hyperkalemia (more commonly seen with concomitant use of potassium-sparing diuretics or in the presence of renal failure), and reversible renal failure (which can be precipitated by situations that

Table 93-1 Pharmacokinetics of Angiotensin-Converting Enzyme Inhibitors

Drug	Usual Dose (mg)	Duration of Action (h)	Absorption (%)	Prodrug	Peak Concentration (Active Component) (h)	Route of Elimination	Plasma Half-life (h)	Dose Reduction in Renal Disease
Captopril (G)	12.5-50 bid/tid	6-12	60-75	No	1	Kidney	2	Yes
Benazepril	10-20 qd	24	37	Yes	1-2	Kidney/liver	10-11	Yes
Enalapril	5-10 qd/bid	12-24	55-75	Yes	3-4	Kidney	11	Yes
Lisinopril	20-40 qd	24	25	Yes	6-8	Kidney	12	Yes
Moexipril	7.5-15 qd/bid	24	>20	Yes	1-2	Kidney	2-9	Yes
Quinapril	20-40 qd	24	60	Yes	2	Kidney	25	Yes
Ramipril	2.5-20 qd/bid	24	50-60	Yes	2-4	Kidney/liver	13-7	Yes
Trandolapril	2-4 qd	24	70	Yes	4-10	Kidney/liver	16-24	Yes
Fosinopril	20-40 qd/bid	24	36	Yes	3	Kidney/liver	12	No

bid, Twice a day; PO, by mouth (*per os*); tid, three times daily; qd, every day.

decrease renal blood flow: hypotension, hypovolemia, severe congestive heart failure, severe hyponatremia, and unilateral renal artery stenosis). The use of ACE inhibitors is contraindicated in patients with bilateral renal artery stenosis, hyperkalemia, and serum creatinine levels of 2.5 mg/dL or greater. They are also contraindicated in pregnant patients because they are teratogenic in the first and second trimesters of pregnancy, and their use in the third trimester is associated with an ACE inhibitor fetal nephropathy.

Angiotensin Receptor Blockers

ARBs, also known as angiotensin II receptor antagonists, AT_1-receptor antagonists, or sartans, directly block the AT_1 receptor and have the theoretical advantage of blocking the effects of angiotensin II formed by non-ACE pathways. ARBs have no effect on bradykinin metabolism, and, therefore, their use is associated with a significantly reduced incidence of cough and angioedema, as compared with ACE inhibitors. Originally used to treat hypertension in patients intolerant of ACE inhibitors, they are now being used to treat patients with heart failure (data supporting candesartan) and migraine (candesartan) and hypertensive patients with type II diabetes (irbesartan and losartan), in whom these drugs may delay the progression of diabetic nephropathy (Table 93-2). Because they have the same hemodynamic effects as the ACE inhibitors but have fewer side effects, ARBs will increasingly be used to treat the same conditions as the ACE inhibitors. The most common side effect with ARBs is dizziness.

Aldosterone Antagonists

Spironolactone, which had fallen out of use, is increasingly coming back into use; therefore, it is likely that an anesthesia provider will see patients for whom they are providing care who have been taking this medication. Spironolactone, which interferes with the aldosterone-dependent sodium-potassium exchange site in the distal convoluted renal tubule, is administered as a diuretic in patients with hypertension because it increases the amounts of sodium and water to be excreted, while potassium is retained.

Direct Renin Inhibitors

In 2007 aliskiren, a direct renin inhibitor that is available as an oral drug, was approved by regulatory bodies in Europe and the United States for treatment of hypertension. By attaching to the S3bp binding site of renin, it prevents the conversion of angiotensinogen to angiotensin I thereby also lowering the plasma concentrations of angiotensin II and angiotensin. Because this drug is only available in an oral form, it is unlikely to be used by anesthesia providers in the perioperative period. However, patients who have been taking this drug may present for anesthesia, and clinicians should be aware that the use of aliskiren has been associated with an increased incidence of nonfatal stroke, renal complications, hyperkalemia, and hypotension in patients with diabetes and renal impairment.

Anesthetic Considerations for Patients on Renin-Angiotensin-Aldosterone System Inhibitors

Nonsteroidal anti-inflammatory drugs (NSAIDs) may decrease the antihypertensive action of ACE inhibitors, an effect that is more common in the presence of low renin levels. Therefore, patients on an NSAID and an ACE inhibitor or ARB might not have the same response as someone who is not taking an NSAID. However, whether or not a patient is also taking an

Table 93-2 Pharmacokinetics of Angiotensin Receptor Blocking Agents

Drug	Usual Dose (mg)	Half-life (h)	Bioavailability (%)	Active Metabolite	Route of Elimination
Losartan	25-50 PO bid	2	33	Yes	Kidney/liver
Candesartan	8-16 PO bid	4	42	Yes	Kidney/liver
Irbesartan	75-300 qd	11-15	70	No	Kidney/liver
Valsartan	40-80 PO bid	6	25	No	Kidney/liver
Telmisartan	40-80 PO qd	24	43	No	Liver >> kidney
Eprosartan	400-800 qd	5-7	15	No	Liver > kidney
Olmesartan	20-40 qd	13	26	Yes	Kidney/liver

bid, Twice a day; PO, by mouth (*per os*); qd, every day.

NSAID, hypotension is more likely to occur during induction and maintenance of anesthesia in patients treated with ACE inhibitors or ARBs simply because these patients, as compared with patients not taking these drugs, are more likely to have decreased intravascular volumes because of the mechanism of action of the medications. Even so, hypotension is more likely to occur in sodium-depleted patients, in those undergoing regional anesthesia (particularly neuraxial anesthesia), in patients taking other diuretics in addition to spironolactone, in those undergoing major operations with large fluid shifts, and during cardiopulmonary bypass. The hypotensive episodes can be refractory to indirect-acting sympathomimetic agents and may require aggressive fluid administration, norepinephrine, vasopressin, or terlipressin. The decision to administer an ACE inhibitor or ARB on the morning of a patient's operation remains controversial and should be individualized. Most centers withhold these medications 24 h prior to anesthesia. However, if patients have taken their usual dose of an ACE inhibitor or ARB the day of surgery, they are more likely to become hypotensive following induction of anethesia. Therefore, some authorities recommend administering an intravenous bolus of 250 mL to 1 L of crystalloid solution prior to the induction of anesthesia to decrease the incidence and severity of hypotension.

Suggested Readings

Allikmets K. Aliskiren – an orally active renin inhibitor. Review of pharmacology, pharmacodynamics, kinetics, and clinical potential in the treatment of hypertension. *Vasc Health Risk Manag.* 2007;3(6):809-815.

Bertrand M, Godet G, Meersschaert K, et al. Should the angiotensin II antagonists be discontinued before surgery? *Anesth Analg.* 2001;92:26-30.

Bullo M, Tschumi S, Bucher BS, et al. Pregnancy outcome following exposure to angiotensin-converting enzyme inhibitors or angiotensin receptor antagonists: A systematic review. *Hypertension.* 2012;60:444-450.

Francis GS. ACE inhibition in cardiovascular disease. *N Engl J Med.* 2000;342: 201-202.

Solomon SD, Skali H, Anavekar NS, et al. Changes in ventricular size and function in patients treated with valsartan, captopril, or both after myocardial infarction. *Circulation.* 2005;111:3411-3419.

van Vark LC, Bertrand M, Akkerhuis KM, et al. Angiotensin-converting enzyme inhibitors reduce mortality in hypertension: A meta-analysis of randomized clinical trials of renin-angiotensin-aldosterone system inhibitors involving 158, 998 patients. *Eur Heart J.* 2012;33:2088-2097.

White HD. Should all patients with coronary disease receive angiotensin converting enzyme inhibitors? *Lancet.* 2003;362:755-757.

CHAPTER 94

Bronchodilators

Suneerat Kongsayreepong, MD

Three major classes of bronchodilators are used to treat bronchoconstriction: β-adrenergic receptor agonists, methylxanthines, and anticholinergic agents. The β-adrenergic receptor agonists are further divided into catecholamines, resorcinols, and saligenins.

β-Adrenergic Receptor Agonists

Selective β_2-receptor agonists relax bronchioles and uterine smooth muscle without affecting the heart via β_1-receptor stimulation. These drugs activate adenyl cyclase, which converts adenosine triphosphate (ATP) to cyclic adenosine 3′-5′-monophosphate (cAMP), which in turn causes relaxation of smooth muscle, resulting in bronchodilation. Nonselective β-receptor agonists used for bronchodilation include epinephrine, isoproterenol, and isoetharine. Selective β_2-receptor agonists include albuterol, terbutaline, metaproterenol, and others (Table 94-1). Side effects associated with the use of nonselective medications include increased heart rate, contractility, and myocardial O_2 consumption. Selective β_2-receptor agonists may also produce some cardiac effects, especially if administered subcutaneously or intravenously. Hypokalemia and hyperglycemia may also occur. Chronic use can be associated with tachyphylaxis.

Therapeutic aerosols may be administered, preferably, by a metered-dose inhaler (MDI) or as a wet aerosol from a nebulizer containing the medication. Only particles with a diameter of 1 to 5 μm are efficiently deposited in the lower respiratory tract, which is one of the primary reasons that 13% of the output from MDIs, compared with only 1% to 5% of the output from nebulizers, reaches the lower respiratory tract. Propellants used in MDIs are blends of liquefied gas chlorofluorocarbons (CFCs) that can damage the earth's ozone layer; in addition, some patients are sensitive to these propellants, resulting in bronchospasm. Because of these concerns, some MDIs use hydrofluoroalkanes (HFAs) as the propellant. The HFA formulations of albuterol and ipratropium bromide have been shown to be equivalent to their respective CFC formulations. However, the delivered dose of HFA-formulated beclomethasone dipropionate is five times greater than the dose delivered with the original CFC formulation.

A breath-activated nebulizer, a new type of jet nebulizer, has a low dead-space volume and nebulizes only on inspiration. With this type of nebulizer, waste during exhalation should be completely eliminated. The delivered dose can be more than three times greater than the dose delivered with continuous nebulization.

The use of continuous bronchodilator therapy is sometimes necessary for the treatment of severe bronchospasm, such as for status asthmaticus. In such situations, a low dose of a bronchodilator (e.g., albuterol, 10-15 mg/h) should be used, and the patient should be continuously monitored for side effects (e.g., tachycardia, arrhythmias, hypokalemia) and worsening of symptoms.

Dry-powder inhalers (DPIs) deliver drugs in powder form to the lung. When using this type of inhaler, patients must generate sufficient inspiratory flow rate (≥50 L/min). Generating this level of inspiratory flow rate may be difficult for patients to achieve if they are in acute respiratory distress, especially during severe asthmatic attack.

Table 94-1 Bronchodilators

Drug	Trade Name(s)	Delivery Mode/Route	Mechanism of Action
β-Adrenergic Receptor Agonists			
Isoproterenol 0.05%	Isuprel	Nebulizer	Prototypical β-adrenergic receptor agonists, significant β_1 side effects
Albuterol 0.5%	Ventolin Proventil	Oral, DPI MDI/nebulizer	β_2-Adrenergic receptor agonists, increase in cAMP
Isoetharine hydrochloride, 1%	Bronkosol	MDI/nebulizer	β_2-Adrenergic receptor agonists, increase in cAMP
Metaproterenol sulfate 5%	Alupent Metaprel	MDI/nebulizer/ oral	β_2-Adrenergic receptor agonists, increase in cAMP
Terbutaline 0.1%		Oral/SQ/ Nebulizer/IV	β_2-Adrenergic receptor agonists
Methylxanthines			
Aminophylline	Somophyllin	Oral/IV	Inhibition of cAMP breakdown by phosphodiesterase
Theophylline	Respbid, Slo-Bid, Theo-24 Theolair	Oral/IV	Adenosine antagonism
Anticholinergics			
Atropine sulfate 2% or 5%	Abboject	SQ, IM, IV, Nebulizer	Cholinergic blocker, decreased cGMP
Ipratropium bromide 0.02%	Atrovent	MDI/nebulizer	Cholinergic blocker, decreased cGMP

cAMP, Cyclic adenosine monophosphate; *cGMP,* cyclic guanosine monophosphate; IM, intramuscular; *IV,* intravenous; *MDI,* metered-dose inhaler; SQ, subcutaneous.
Adapted, with permission, from Peruzzi WT, Shapiro BA. Respiratory care. In: Murray MJ, Cousin DB, Pearl RG, Prough DS, eds. Critical Care Medicine: Perioperative Management. 2nd ed. Philadelphia: Lippincott-Raven; 2002:428-446.

Catecholamines

Catecholamines are potent and effective bronchodilators that have a rapid onset of action, reach their peak effect quickly, and have a short duration of action (0.5-3 h). These drugs are useful when rapid onset is needed.

Epinephrine has both α-adrenergic and β-adrenergic properties. A dose of 0.3 to 0.5 mg given subcutaneously is commonly used to treat acute bronchospasm. The effects are rapid, peaking in 5 to 25 min, and improvements in pulmonary function are seen for up to 4 h. Side effects include increased heart rate, cardiac output, and systolic blood pressure and decreased diastolic blood pressure and systemic vascular resistance.

Of the sympathomimetics, isoproterenol is the most potent β-adrenergic receptor agonist. It is effective when administered intravenously or inhaled. However, it has essentially been replaced by selective β_2-adrenergic receptor agonists.

Resorcinols

Resorcinols are β-adrenergic receptor agonists with a rapid onset and longer duration of action. These are well absorbed from the gastrointestinal tract and can be given orally.

Metaproterenol, a selective β_2-adrenergic resorcinol, is available as a solution for aerosol delivery, as a tablet, as a syrup, and for use in an MDI. Onset is 5 to 15 min, with a peak effect at 30 to 60 min and a duration of 3 to 4 h. As a resorcinol, metaproterenol has hydroxyl groups at the 3 and 5 positions of the phenyl ring (as opposed to catecholamines, which have them at the 3 and 4 positions). It is, therefore, resistant to metabolism by catechol-O-methyltransferase (COMT) and has a longer duration of action than most catecholamines. It has enough structural similarities to isoproterenol that metaproterenol has substantial cardiac side effects.

Terbutaline, a selective β_2-adrenergic receptor agonist, has an onset of action in 5 to 15 min, a peak of action over 30 to 60 min, and a duration of action lasting 4 to 6 h. A dose of 0.25 mg administered subcutaneously is an alternative treatment for acute severe bronchospasm when the cardiac effects of epinephrine must be avoided. However, when given subcutaneously, terbutaline will have some β_1-adrenergic effects and may cause ventricular arrhythmias in patients who have been anesthetized with halothane.

Saligenins

Saligenins are the most recently developed β-adrenergic receptor agonists and have the most β_2-receptor specificity. Drugs in this group have a rapid onset of action and a duration of action of about 4 to 6 h.

Albuterol, a selective β_2-adrenergic receptor agonist, has very few side effects; cardiac effects are unlikely when the dose of albuterol is less than 400 μg. Its onset of action is 15 min, with a peak effect in 30 to 60 min and a duration of 4 to 6 h. Albuterol is available as a syrup, oral tablet, extended-release tablet, nebulizer solution, MDI, and DPI.

Salmeterol is a very lipophilic, selective β_2-adrenergic receptor agonist that must diffuse through the phospholipid membrane before reaching the receptor site. Its onset of action is very slow; therefore, this drug cannot be used as a rescue medication. Salmeterol has a very long duration of action.

Formoterol is a selective β_2-adrenergic receptor agonist with a rapid onset of action (within 2-3 min) and a long duration of action (12 h). However, this medication cannot be used as a rescue drug because of potential toxicity.

Methylxanthines

Theophylline is a poorly soluble methylxanthine found in high concentrations in tea leaves. Methylxanthines inhibit the breakdown of cAMP by phosphodiesterase. Aminophylline is the water-soluble salt of theophylline that can be administered orally (3-6 mg/kg) or intravenously (loading dose of 5 mg/kg, followed by 0.5-1.0 $mg \cdot kg^{-1} \cdot h^{-1}$). Therapeutic plasma concentrations of theophylline are between 5 and 15 μg/mL, although levels as low as 5 μg/mL have been shown to be clinically effective.

Aminophylline works in vitro by inhibiting phosphodiesterase and, thereby, cAMP breakdown. The in vivo mechanism of aminophylline is less clear. Antiinflammatory actions on neutrophils, sympathetic stimulation, and adenosine antagonism are possible mechanisms. The narrow therapeutic range of aminophylline and the potential for arrhythmias developing in patients with the use of this drug have made its use in the perioperative setting controversial. Theophylline is principally metabolized by the liver, and 10% is excreted unchanged in urine. Smokers metabolize the drug faster than do nonsmokers. Heart failure, liver disease, and severe respiratory obstruction all slow the metabolism of theophylline and increase the likelihood of toxicity. Metabolism is slowed by cimetidine and β-adrenergic receptor antagonists.

Theophylline improves pulmonary function and resolves obstruction, in a dose-dependent manner, in patients with reactive airway disease. The drug decreases pulmonary vascular resistance and increases cardiac output. The cardiac-stimulating effects of theophylline are still seen in the presence of β blockade because xanthines are not receptor dependent. Theophylline and caffeine have been shown to decrease the number and duration of apneic episodes in preterm infants.

Side effects with the use of theophylline are often seen when plasma levels exceed 20 μg/mL. The most frequent side effects are nausea and vomiting. Seizures may result from toxic levels and are likely to occur when plasma concentrations exceed 40 μg/mL. Tachycardia and other arrhythmias may also occur with high plasma levels. Theophylline facilitates neuromuscular transmission; thus, patients receiving theophylline may require higher than normal doses of nondepolarizing neuromuscular blocking agents.

Anticholinergic Agents

Cholinergic mechanisms play a major role in mediating reflex bronchoconstriction, and anticholinergic drugs may be used to reduce these responses. These medications have been found to be somewhat more effective than β-adrenergic receptor agonists in some patients with chronic bronchitis and emphysema. In the management of asthma, anticholinergic agents are generally less effective than are β-adrenergic receptor agonists, but in acute asthma, a combination of the two types of agents may produce a greater response. Atropine sulfate, a parasympatholytic that can relax airway smooth muscle, can also be given by nebulizer. Because atropine reduces mucociliary clearance and causes other central nervous system and cardiovascular side effects, even at low doses, this medication is not commonly used as a bronchodilator.

Ipratropium bromide, a quaternary amine delivered by nebulizer or MDI, has little systemic absorption. Its bronchodilator effects begin within minutes, with a peak effect in 1 to 2 h. Ipratropium has little or no effect on mucociliary clearance from the lung and little or no effect on heart rate, blood pressure, and gastrointestinal tract. Ipratropium is also available in combination with albuterol.

Antiinflammatory Agents

Antiinflammatory agents, such as cromolyn sodium, which stabilize mast cell membranes and thereby intervene in the inflammatory process, are frequently used to treat bronchospastic diseases. Corticosteroids block both the initial immune response and the subsequent inflammatory process. Corticosteroids do not have direct effects on bronchial smooth muscle relaxation but do facilitate the effects of β_2-adrenergic receptor agonists. Even though the cellular and biochemical effects are immediate, the full clinical effects take longer; the increase in β-adrenergic receptor agonist response occurs within 2 h and β-adrenergic receptor agonist density increases within 4 h. Systemically administered steroids, such as hydrocortisone or methylprednisolone, may be required in patients with poor responses to β_2-adrenergic receptor agonists over 1 to 2 h. Inhaled corticosteroids, such as beclomethasone, flunisolide, and triamcinolone, which are available as MDIs, DPIs, and nebulizer solutions, are then used to minimize systemic side effects. Symptoms usually improve in the 1 to 2 weeks, with maximal response most often occurring in 4 to 8 weeks

Adjunctive Medication

Although the exact mechanism by which $MgSO_4$ relaxes airway smooth muscle is not completely understood, it is thought that is does so through blockade of voltage-dependent calcium channels and thereby inhibiting Ca^{2+} influx. Intravenously administered $MgSO_4$ (2 g) is a safe and effective adjunct for the treatment of acute asthma and bronchospasm in both adults and children. Nebulized $MgSO_4$ has been used, but this treatment is controversial and warrants further studies.

Inhalation anesthetic agents, such as isoflurane, in subanesthetic doses have been used to relieve bronchospasm after extubation and in patients with status asthmaticus. They have also occasionally been used long term (i.e., 2-3 days) in the intensive care unit in patients with status asthmaticus.

Suggested Readings

Blitz M, Blitz S, Hughes R, et al. Aerosolized magnesium sulfate for acute asthma: A systematic review. *Chest.* 2005;128:337-344.

Chung KF, Caramori G, Adcock IM. Inhaled corticosteroids as combination therapy with β-adrenergic agonists in airways disease: Present and future. *Eur J Clin Pharmacol.* 2009;65:853-871.

Colbert BJ, Kennedy BJ. *Integrated Cardiopulmonary Pharmacology.* 2nd ed. Upper Saddle River, NJ: Prentice Hall; 2008.

Fink J. Aerosol drug therapy. In: Wilkin RL, Stroller JK, Kacmarek RM, eds. *Egan's Fundamentals of Respiratory Care.* 9th ed. St Louis: Mosby; 2009:801-842.

Mohammed S, Goodacre S. Intravenous and nebulized magnesium sulphate for acute asthma: Systematic review and meta-analysis. *Emerg Med J.* 2007; 24:823-830.

Woods BD, Sladen RN. Perioperative considerations for the patient with asthma and bronchospasm. *Br J Anaesth.* 2009;103(Suppl 1):i57-65.

CHAPTER 95

Sodium Bicarbonate

Anna E. Bartunek, MD, and Wolfgang Schramm, MD

Sodium bicarbonate ($NaHCO_3$) is an inorganic salt that readily dissociates into Na^+ and HCO_3^- to bind acids and strong bases; when reacting with acids, the sodium salt of the acid, H_2O, and CO_2 are the byproducts. $NaHCO_3$ has been used for centuries in foods, animal feeds, and industrial processes. In vertebrate animals, the HCO_3^- ion is the principal buffer in extracellular and interstitial fluid. Because of its ability to neutralize acid, $NaHCO_3$ has been frequently ingested by mouth as an antacid and administered intravenously to treat metabolic acidosis. Because of its effect on blood pH, $NaHCO_3$ is used to treat a variety of drug overdoses (chlorpropamide, phenobarbital, cocaine, and class Ia and Ic antiarrhythmic agents), to treat metabolic acidosis induced by ingestion of methanol (and to enhance formate elimination by the kidneys) and ethylene glycol poisoning, and to alkalinize urine (e.g., in patients with rhabdomyolysis).

Although anesthesia providers commonly use $NaHCO_3$ to treat metabolic acidosis, the indications for doing so are not universally accepted.

Acid-Base Balance

The precise functions of enzymes and proteins within cells are dependent on pH; therefore, a number of mechanisms exist to maintain hydrogen ion concentration ($[H^+]$) within a very narrow range in the face of CO_2, H^+, and OH^- production during normal metabolism and despite physiologic and pathologic challenges. Intracellular and extracellular chemical buffering, transcellular diffusion or transport of electrically charged ions, and excretion or retention of acid or alkali by the kidneys and of CO_2 by the lungs maintain acid-base homeostasis. The most important buffer in the extracellular space is $NaHCO_3$, also referred to as the carbonic acid/bicarbonate buffer.

The Carbonic Acid/Bicarbonate Buffering System

Because CO_2 is not sufficiently soluble in blood, a number of mechanisms have had to evolve over time to facilitate the transport of CO_2 from the periphery to the lungs (Chapter 22). The most efficient of these mechanisms combines CO_2 with H_2O to form carbonic acid, which in turn dissociates into hydrogen ions and bicarbonate ions.

The reactions are reversible and subject to the law of mass action:

$$H_2O + CO_2 \leftrightarrow H_2CO_3 \leftrightarrow H^+ + HCO_3^-$$

In peripheral tissues—where CO_2 is continuously produced—the reaction proceeds from the left to the right, whereas in the lung the reaction proceeds in the opposite direction. The H^+ created by the reaction must be buffered in order to preserve physiologic pH.

The Carbonic Acid/Bicarbonate Buffer

A buffer is typically a weak acid in equilibrium with its conjugate base that minimizes changes in the pH of a solution when an acid or a base is added; bicarbonate in the previous reaction is the conjugate base of carbonic acid. The Henderson-Hasselbalch equation describes the effects of changes in carbonic acid and bicarbonate on pH. Because the blood concentration of H_2CO_3 is so low, it can be replaced by $\alpha \times Pco_2$, wherein α is the solubility coefficient for CO_2 in plasma:

$$pH = pK + \log\frac{HCO_3^-}{\alpha \times Pco_2}$$

In human plasma, pK is 6.1, $\alpha = 0.03\ mmol \cdot L^{-1} \cdot mm \cdot Hg^{-1}$ and pH is 7.4 at a body temperature of 37°C. This yields:

$$7.4 = 6.1 + \log\frac{HCO_3^-}{0.03 \times Pco_2}$$

The amount of hydrogen any chemical can buffer is highest when its pH equals pK. Yet, in human plasma, the pK of 6.1 of the carbonic acid $[CO_2]$/bicarbonate buffer is not within the optimal buffer range. Therefore, the buffering capacity is dependent on the HCO_3^-/Pco_2 ratio, which is kept in a narrow range by means of neuroventilatory Pco_2 control. To preserve a pH of 7.4, the ratio of bicarbonate to partial pressure of CO_2 must be maintained at 20:1 because the log of 20 is 1.3 (1.30103). Indeed, this is the case because the normal HCO_3^- concentration is 24 mEq/dL and the normal $Paco_2$ is 40 mm Hg. Substituting in the preceding equation yields

$$\begin{aligned} pH &= 6.1 + \log \text{ of } [24/(0.03 \times 40)] \\ &= 6.1 + \log \text{ of } [24/1.2] \\ &= 6.1 + \log \text{ of } 20 \\ &= 6.1 + 1.3 \\ &= 7.4 \end{aligned}$$

Box 95-1 Causes of Metabolic Acidosis

- Inadequate O_2 delivery to tissues → lactic acidosis
  - Hypovolemia
    - Hemorrhage
    - Hypohemoglobinemia
    - Exsiccosis
    - Inadequate volume substitution
    - Sepsis
  - Inadequate cardiac output
    - Deterioration of preexisting cardiac disease
    - Cardiac failure during or after cardiac surgery
  - Hypoxia due to ventilatory failure
  - Aortic cross-clamping
  - Malignant hyperthermia
  - During liver transplantation (reduced cardiac output and disrupted lactate metabolism)
- Renal insufficiency
  - Mild to moderate renal insufficiency, e.g., renal tubular acidosis (impaired H^+ secretion and/or HCO_3^- reabsorption)
  - Severe renal insufficiency: accumulation of endogenous acids such as sulfate, fomate, phosphate
- Infusion of large amounts of crystalloid → "dilutional acidosis"
- Hyperchloremia
  - Excessive administration of any chloride-rich solution
    - 0.9% saline
    - Hetastarch formulated in saline
  - Renal dysfunction
  - Hyperventilation
- Acetazolamide medication → bicarbonate excretion increased
- Ketoacidosis
- Diarrhea
- Various intoxications
  - Methanol
  - Salicylates

Metabolic Acidosis

Several causes of metabolic acidosis (Box 95-1) may occur simultaneously in patients with critical illness. Acidemia may impair cardiac contractile function, constrict pulmonary arteries, and reduce adrenergic receptor responsiveness to catecholamines; therefore, many clinicians often restore the HCO_3^-/Pco_2 ratio to 20 by administering bicarbonate. Treatment of the underlying problem is then undertaken to ultimately restore and maintain a pH of 7.4.

Formulation

$NaHCO_3$ is available for injection as an 8.4% solution. It is a highly hypertonic sodium solution in which Na^+ is 1 mEq/mL and HCO_3^- is 1 mEq/mL.

Therapeutic Uses of Sodium Bicarbonate

$NaHCO_3$ is administered intravenously to patients to treat a variety of conditions, including, but not limited to, lactic acidosis, metabolic acidosis during cardiopulmonary resuscitation, circulatory failure in infants and children, neonatal acidosis from apnea and circulatory collapse, hemodynamic instability during aortic surgery, postreperfusion syndrome during liver transplantation, acidosis associated with malignant hyperthermia, as a buffer during cardiopulmonary bypass, diabetic ketoacidosis, and others.

Lactate Acidosis

Lactate acidosis caused by anaerobic glycolysis due to inadequate O_2 delivery (see Box 95-1) is probably the most common cause of metabolic acidosis faced by the anesthesia provider. If the pH is below 7.2 to 7.25 or is decreasing to those levels despite all measures to restore O_2 delivery (e.g., normalization of blood volume and composition, restoration of adequate ventilation, or pharmacologic or mechanical support of cardiac function), many clinicians will administer $NaHCO_3$.

The following rules must be carefully observed when $NaHCO_3$ is used: (1) it is more important to treat the underlying problem than to correct pH; (2) only severe acidosis should be corrected (i.e., base excess less than −14 (3) pH should not be reversed to normal but to about 7.25 to 7.3 (overcorrection should be avoided); (4) adequate ventilation to remove the generated CO_2 is crucial; (5) $NaHCO_3$ must be administered slowly or in several small doses; and (6) treatment with $NaHCO_3$ must be guided by repeated blood gas measurements.

Dose Recommendations

One formula to calculate an $NaHCO_3$ dose to treat a metabolic acidosis established by the base excess (BE) is determined from an arterial blood gas measurement and body weight (BW):

$$NaHCO_3\ (mEq) = 0.3 \cdot BW\ (kg) \cdot BE\ (mEq/L)$$

Initially only half of the calculated dose should be administered; administration of the second half of the calculated dose should be guided by a repeat blood gas analysis or the initial dose should be 1 mEq/kg $NaHCO_3$ and may be followed by 0.5 mEq/kg if justified by a repeat arterial blood gas analysis. In severe circulatory failure, arterial blood gas analysis may not reflect the severity of the tissue and venous acidosis.

Metabolic Acidosis During Cardiopulmonary Resuscitation

In the past, $NaHCO_3$ has been used to reverse acidosis during cardiopulmonary resuscitation. Because there is no evidence to show that its administration improves outcome, the most current Advanced Cardiac Life Support Guidelines do not recommend routine administration of $NaHCO_3$ during cardiopulmonary resuscitation or after restoration of spontaneous circulation. The guidelines do acknowledge that administration of $NaHCO_3$ may be considered during resuscitation if the patient has associated hyperkalemia, preexisting metabolic acidosis, or tricyclic antidepressant overdose (see following discussion).

Circulatory Failure in Infants and Children

As in adults, metabolic acidosis usually improves when oxygenation of tissues is restored by appropriate resuscitation. Administration of $NaHCO_3$ may be considered in patients with prolonged shock or cardiac arrest, provided adequate ventilation is ensured.

Neonatal Acidosis from Apnea and Circulatory Collapse

Reversal of acidosis by the use of $NaHCO_3$ in the apneic newborn has been common practice for many years, although evidence of its beneficial effect on outcome has not been shown. The administration of $NaHCO_3$ increases the risk of intracranial hemorrhage in the newborn, probably due to increased plasma osmolarity and decreased neuronal and glial pH.

If metabolic acidosis (pH $<$7.10) does not improve despite intubation and ventilation, the use of $NaHCO_3$ might be considered. Hyperosmolar 8.4% $NaHCO_3$ should be diluted 1:1 with sterile water. $NaHCO_3$, at a dose of 2 mEq/kg, can be administered initially but should not be injected more quickly than 1 mEq/min and only in the presence of adequate ventilation.

Hemodynamic Instability During Aortic Operations

During open repair of aortic dissections or resection of aortic aneurysms that require cross-clamping of the aorta, the ischemia below the level of the cross-clamp often leads to lactic acidosis and release of toxic cytokines. Following cross-clamp removal and reperfusion of caudal tissue and organs, these substances enter the bloodstream, return to the central circulation, and precipitate moderate to severe hypotension and, occasionally, circulatory collapse. Because there is no time to measure arterial blood pH, some clinicians will administer 50 to 100 mEq of $NaHCO_3$ prophylactically to try to attenuate, if not prevent, the vascular instability associated with cross-clamp removal.

Postreperfusion Syndrome During Liver Transplantation

Lactic acidosis develops during the anhepatic phase of liver transplantation because of reduced cardiac output and lack of lactate clearance. During the reperfusion of the transplanted liver, $NaHCO_3$ is often administered to treat metabolic acidosis and hyperkalemia to attenuate the severity of postreperfusion syndrome.

Acidosis Associated with Malignant Hyperthermia

The symptoms of malignant hyperthermia include metabolic acidosis and hyperkalemia, both of which respond to treatment with $NaHCO_3$.

As a Buffer During Cardiopulmonary Bypass

$NaHCO_3$ is used in the priming fluid for cardiopulmonary bypass. During extracorporeal circulation, base deficits below −5 should be corrected with $NaHCO_3$ while the underlying cause of the acidosis is addressed.

Diabetic Ketoacidosis

Acidosis improves when treated adequately with volume replacement, electrolyte replacement, and administration of insulin. $NaHCO_3$ might be required if arterial blood pH remains below 7.1 despite standard treatment. One must bear in mind the same considerations as when one treats a patient with lactate acidosis.

Other Uses of Sodium Bicarbonate

Hyperkalemia

Because alkalosis shifts K^+ from the plasma into cells, $NaHCO_3$ is a primary agent for acute treatment of hyperkalemia.

Alkalinization of the Urine

Administration of $NaHCO_3$ intravenously increases the pH of urine and is therefore used in a variety of circumstances (e.g., to increase renal clearance of toxic substances or overdoses of drugs and to prevent precipitation of certain biochemicals in the renal tubules).

When used to increase the pH of urine, the administration of $NaHCO_3$ should be guided by repeated measurements of urinary and plasma pH. Serum K^+ and Na^+ must also be measured continually and replaced if necessary. Hypokalemia is of particular concern, not only because of its effect on the heart, but also because the kidneys will compensate for the hypokalemia by absorbing K^+ accompanied by the elimination of H^+, which in turn decreases urinary pH.

$NaHCO_3$ is administered and urinary output is maintained at higher-than-normal levels by administering increased amounts of intravascular fluid. Indications for such therapy include rhabdomyolysis, hemolytic transfusion reaction, and to enhance renal excretion of certain drugs.

Rhabdomyolysis

The administration of $NaHCO_3$, acetazolamide, or both is recommended by some to treat rhabdomyolysis when creatine kinase levels are above 20,000 to 30,000 U/L. The goal is to maintain urinary pH above 6.5, which decreases the chances of myoglobin precipitating in the renal tubules leading to acute tubular necrosis. There are few clinical data that show that the administration of $NaHCO_3$ results in better outcomes than what can be achieved with intravenous administration of fluid only.

Hemolytic Transfusion Reaction

Increasing urinary pH to 8 by administering $NaHCO_3$, in addition to large-volume crystalloid infusion, minimizes hemoglobinuric renal damage after a transfusion reaction.

Renal Drug Elimination

A high urinary pH enhances renal elimination of certain acidic drugs, such as salicylates, chlorpropamide, and phenobarbital and prevents precipitation of methotrexate in the renal tubules.

Methanol Toxicity

Ingested methanol is converted to formaldehyde by alcohol dehydrogenase, which, in turn, is metabolized to formic acid by aldehyde dehydrogenase. Formic acid impairs cellular respiration through its inhibition of mitochondrial cytochrome c oxidase, resulting in a profound metabolic acidosis. Treatment is with other compounds (ethanol or fomepizole) that compete with methanol for binding to alcohol dehydrogenase, allowing the methanol to be excreted by the kidneys. Depending on the degree of toxicity, $NaHCO_3$ is administered to correct the metabolic acidosis.

Contrast-Induced Nephropathy

Angiography in patients with preexisting renal insufficiency necessitates the implementation of preemptive measures to reduce the likelihood of contrast-induced nephropathy. Isotonic concentrations of $NaHCO_3$ to alkalinize the urine, infused over several hours, have been shown to exert a protective effect.

Sodium Channel Blocker Toxicity

Increasing blood pH and sodium concentration, both of which can be achieved by the administration of $NaHCO_3$, reverse, in part, the sodium channel blockade–induced membrane-depressant effects (manifested by QRS prolongation on the electrocardiogram) of several drugs. The administration of $NaHCO_3$ is therefore recommended in cases of overdosage with tricyclic antidepressants, class Ia and Ic antiarrhythmic drugs, propranolol, propoxyphene, and diphenhydramine.

Local Anesthetics Agents

Raising the pH of local anesthetic solutions results in a higher concentration of local anesthetic in its uncharged form. The addition of $NaHCO_3$ to a local anesthetic agent used for regional anesthesia increases its rate of diffusion across the cell membrane, reducing the time of onset of neural blockade and producing a more complete block. The addition of $NaHCO_3$ to a local anesthetic solution also reduces the pain of injection, most likely because it decreases the acidity of the solution.

Toxicity

Treatment with $NaHCO_3$ is not without side effects, which include but are not limited to cellular dysfunction, central nervous system acidosis and impaired adrenergic activity, metabolic alkylosis, hypernatremia and hyperosmolarity, and milk alkali syndrome.

Cellular Dysfunction

In plasma, bicarbonate combines with hydrogen ions to form bicarbonic acid, which quickly dissociates to CO_2 and H_2O. CO_2 crosses cell membranes readily, whereas the entry of HCO_3^- into cells is much slower. Potentially, a high concentration of intracellular CO_2 can worsen the preexisting acidosis, further impairing cellular function, especially in the brain and heart.

Central Nervous System Acidosis and Impaired Adrenergic Activity

During cardiac arrest, CO_2 increases in venous blood; administration of $NaHCO_3$ with distribution during chest compressions without restoration of normal cardiac function may worsen the central venous acidosis and may impair the action of endogenous and exogenous catecholamines.

Metabolic Alkalosis

Administration of too much bicarbonate overcorrects metabolic acidosis resulting in a metabolic alkalosis that reduces the unloading of O_2 from hemoglobin by shifting the O_2-hemoglobin dissociation curve to the left. The physiologic response of a decrease in minute ventilation (raising the P_{CO_2} to lower pH to the physiologic range) is not well tolerated in some patients with pulmonary disease.

Hypernatremia and Hyperosmolarity

The high sodium content in $NaHCO_3$ solution may result in plasma hyperosmolarity and hypernatremia, which can worsen congestive heart failure when intravascular volume increases to maintain iso-osmolality of the blood. Chronic administration of $NaHCO_3$ can worsen hypertension because of the associated hypernatremia.

Milk-Alkali Syndrome

If patients have hypercalcemia from whatever cause—metastatic bone disease, hyperparathyroidism, ingestion of calcium (high-calcium or dairy-rich diet, calcium supplements, or calcium-containing antacids such as calcium carbonate)—raising blood pH above a certain level can result in the milk-alkali syndrome in which calcium binds to phosphate, resulting in metastatic calcification, renal calculi, and renal failure.

Suggested Readings

American Heart Association. Advanced Life Support. *Circulation*. 2005;112(Suppl I): III-25-III-54. http://circ.ahajournals.org/cgi/content/full/112/22_suppl/III-25. Accessed July 27, 2012.

Aschner JL, Poland RL. Sodium bicarbonate: Basically useless therapy. *Pediatrics*. 2008;122:831-835.

Merten GJ, Burgess WP, Gray LV, et al. Prevention of contrast-induced nephropathy with sodium bicarbonate: A randomized controlled trial. *JAMA*. 2004; 291:2328-2334.

Nicolaou DD, Kelen GD. Acid-base disorders. In: Tintinalli JE, Kelen GD, Stapczynski JS, et al, eds. *Tintinalli's Emergency Medicine*. 7th ed. New York: McGraw-Hill; 2004:128-139.

CHAPTER 96

Monoamine Oxidase Inhibitors

Lisa A. Seip, MD

Monoamine oxidase inhibitors (MAOIs) bind (through an irreversible covalent bond) and inactivate monoamine oxidase (MAO). MAO is primarily found on mitochondrial membranes and is responsible for the metabolism of endogenous and exogenous biogenic amines in the presynaptic nerve terminal, liver, and intestinal mucosa. Two forms of this enzyme exist, MAO-A and MAO-B. MAO-A is responsible for the degradation of norepinephrine, epinephrine, and serotonin. MAO-B degrades phenylethylamine. Dopamine and tyramine are substrates of both MAO-A and MAO-B. By blocking the metabolism of these biogenic amines, MAOIs increase the intraneuronal levels of amine neurotransmitters. MAOIs are not often used in current practice because safer options are available, but they are still used in some patients with depression, Parkinson disease, and panic attacks whose symptoms do not respond or who become refractory to other therapies. Anesthesia providers should be aware of the side effects and potential life-threatening interactions that may occur when patients undergoing an anesthetic have been taking an MAOI.

MAOIs are classified as either hydrazide or nonhydrazide derivatives. Additionally, they are either selective or nonselective inhibitors of MAO. The MAOIs available for use in the United States include phenelzine, tranylcypromine, isocarboxazid, selegiline, and rasagiline (Table 96-1). Phenelzine, tranylcypromine, and isocarboxazid inhibit the activity of both MAO-A and MAO-B. Selegiline and rasagiline block MAO-B and are used for the treatment of Parkinson disease. Although selegiline and rasagiline are selective inhibitors of MAO-B, they lose their selectivity in a dose-dependent fashion. The lowest strength (6-mg) selegiline patch is efficacious in the treatment of depression without the need for dietary modification. This mode of drug delivery allows selegiline to bypass first-pass hepatic metabolism and be delivered to the brain in a concentration that inhibits both MAO-A and MAO-B.

Adverse Effects

Orthostatic Hypotension

Orthostatic hypotension is the most common adverse effect associated with the use of MAOIs (Box 96-1). Octopamine, a false neurotransmitter, is formed by the β-hydroxylation of tyramine in the sympathetic nerve terminal and is stored within the presynaptic storage vesicle, displacing norepinephrine. Neural impulses that normally would stimulate the release of norepinephrine from these storage vesicles now release less norepinephrine along with some octopamine, which has very little α- and β-receptor activity. When an individual taking MAOIs assumes an upright position, the presence of this false neurotransmitter manifests itself by causing less vasoconstriction than normally would occur, resulting in hypotension.

Hepatic Enzymes

The MAOIs inhibit hepatic microsomal enzymes. The use of hydrazide derivatives has been linked to cases of hepatocellular injury and even fulminant hepatic failure. The mechanism is idiosyncratic.

Food and Drug Interactions

Tyramine Reaction

Patients should avoid consuming foods that contain tyramine (aged cheese, liver, fava beans, avocados, and Chianti wine) while they are taking MAOIs and for 2 weeks after discontinuation of MAOIs. Ingested tyramine is normally metabolized prior to entering the systemic circulation by MAO in the intestinal mucosa and liver. If a patient on an MAOI ingests a tyramine-rich food, the tyramine that is absorbed in the intestine escapes intestinal and hepatic metabolism. The delivery of large amounts of tyramine, a monoamine with indirect-acting sympathomimetic activity to the nerve terminal, results in the release of a supranormal amount of norepinephrine into the synaptic cleft. Profound hypertension may develop and, in some patients, may cause a myocardial infarction or cerebrovascular accident.

Indirect-Acting and Direct-Acting Sympathomimetics

The increased stores of catecholamines in a patient taking an MAOI sensitize the patient to the effects of not only tyramine, but also other indirect-acting sympathomimetics, including ephedrine, cocaine, and ephedra, which may also cause a severe hypertensive reaction. Patients on MAOIs will also have an exaggerated response to the direct-acting sympathomimetics because of receptor hypersensitivity, but to a much lesser extent. Direct-acting sympathomimetic drugs can be used in patients on MAOIs, usually at a lower dose and titrated to effect.

Opioids

MAOIs, when combined with opioids, can precipitate excitatory or depressive reactions. Fentanyl, sufentanil, and alfentanil have been reported to interact with MAOIs to produce such reactions, but these reactions are much more likely to occur with meperidine. Meperidine blocks neuronal reuptake of serotonin and, when administered to a patient on an MAOI, can result in agitation, muscle rigidity, headache, fever, convulsions, and coma from excess serotonergic activity. The situation is further complicated because MAOIs inhibit hepatic microsomal enzyme activity, hepatic metabolism of meperidine is slowed, and plasma concentrations of meperidine rise, resulting in an increased incidence of hypotension, respiratory depression, and coma.

Anesthetic Management

Because of the covalent bond that the MAOI forms with the enzyme, the inhibition of MAO persists even after the MAOIs are no longer detectable in plasma. The resumption of MAO activity depends upon de novo synthesis of the enzyme, a process that takes approximately 8 to 12 days to restore 50% of pretreatment activity. Therefore, if an MAOI is going to be stopped prior to surgery, it should be discontinued for at least 2 weeks prior to a surgical procedure to allow for resumption of normal enzyme activity.

Table 96-1 Monoamine Oxidase Inhibitors Most Commonly Used in the United States

Drug	Hydrazide vs. Nonhydrazide	Selectivity*	Clinical Use
Phenelzine	Hydrazide	A and B	Antidepressant
Tranylcypromine	Nonhydrazide	A and B	Antidepressant
Isocarboxazid	Hydrazide	A and B	Antidepressant
Selegiline—oral	Nonhydrazide	B	Antiparkinsonian
Selegiline—patch	Nonhydrazide	A and B	Antidepressant
Rasagiline	Nonhydrazide	B	Antiparkinsonian

*The two forms of the monoamine oxidase enzyme are designated A and B.

Box 96-1 Adverse Effects Associated with the Use of Monoamine Oxidase Inhibitors

Anorgasmia	Orthostatic hypotension
Hepatitis	Paresthesias
Insomnia	Sedation
Impotence	Weight gain

However, it is debatable whether MAOIs should be discontinued prior to elective operations. If the patient's clinical condition will deteriorate upon halting therapy, the MAOI should probably be continued. If the MAOI must be continued or the operation is an emergency, the anesthetic should be tailored to avoid adverse drug interactions.

Regional anesthesia and general anesthesia are acceptable anesthetic modalities in these patients. One benefit of a regional technique is the decreased postoperative opioid requirement. If a regional technique is utilized, the local anesthetic solution should not contain epinephrine.

Intraoperative fluctuations in blood pressure are common in patients taking MAOIs. Orthostatic hypotension is common for the reasons described previously. A direct-acting sympathomimetic may be used to maintain mean arterial pressure in hypotensive patients. The dose should be titrated to effect in small increments because patients can have an exaggerated response to treatment. Indirect-acting sympathomimetics may induce a severe hypertensive response, and their use should be avoided. Ketamine and pancuronium are not used because they enhance sympathetic activity.

MAOIs also decrease plasma cholinesterase activity. If succinylcholine is chosen for neuromuscular blockade, its duration of action may be prolonged. The use of opioids should be limited and, when used, the patient should be closely monitored for adverse effects. If an opioid is required, morphine is the preferred agent because its use has not been associated with the serotonergic syndrome in patients taking MAOIs.

Caution must be exercised when administering medications that are metabolized by the liver because MAOIs inhibit hepatic microsomal enzymes. Prolonged or exaggerated depressant effects may be seen with the use of drugs such as benzodiazepines or barbiturates in combination with an MAOI. Rarely, patients taking MAOIs develop liver failure.

Suggested Readings

Mendelsohn, JM. Monoamine oxidase inhibitors. In: Ford MD, Delaney KA, Ling JL, et al, eds. *Clinical Toxicology*. Philadelphia: WB Saunders; 2001:546-554.

Stoetling RK, Hillier SC. Drugs used for psychopharmacologic therapy. In: Stoetling RK, Hillier SC. *Pharmacology and Physiology in Anesthetic Practice*. 4th ed. Philadelphia: Lippincott, Williams & Wilkins; 2006:406-407.

Tobe EH. Transdermal selegiline: New opportunity for managing depression. In: Brunton LL, Lazo JS, Parker KL, eds. *Goodman and Gilman's The Pharmacologic Basis of Therapeutics*. 11th ed. New York: McGraw-Hill; 2006:242.

CHAPTER 97

Nonsteroidal Antiinflammatory Drugs

Jack L. Wilson, MD

Nonsteroidal antiinflammatory drugs (NSAIDs) are valuable medications for the treatment of pain in the perioperative period. They can be utilized as sole agents or in a multimodal analgesic regimen. Although these medications have potent antiinflammatory and analgesic properties, their use is not without risk.

Mechanism of Action

The antiinflammatory effects of NSAIDs are largely secondary to the reversible competitive inhibition of prostaglandin G/H synthase enzymes (cyclooxygenases). This inhibition prevents the formation of inflammatory mediators such as prostaglandins and thromboxanes. Some NSAIDs also inhibit lipoxygenase, preventing production of leukotrienes (Figure 97-1).

Two clinically relevant forms of cyclooxygenase are described. The first, cyclooxygenase-1 (COX-1), is found in all tissues, including gastric mucosa, where the byproducts of its metabolism of arachidonic acid are thought to play a protective role. Inhibition of this enzyme almost exclusively results in the unwanted gastrointestinal effects of NSAIDs. Inhibition of the second, cyclooxygenase-2 (COX-2), is largely responsible for the antipyretic,

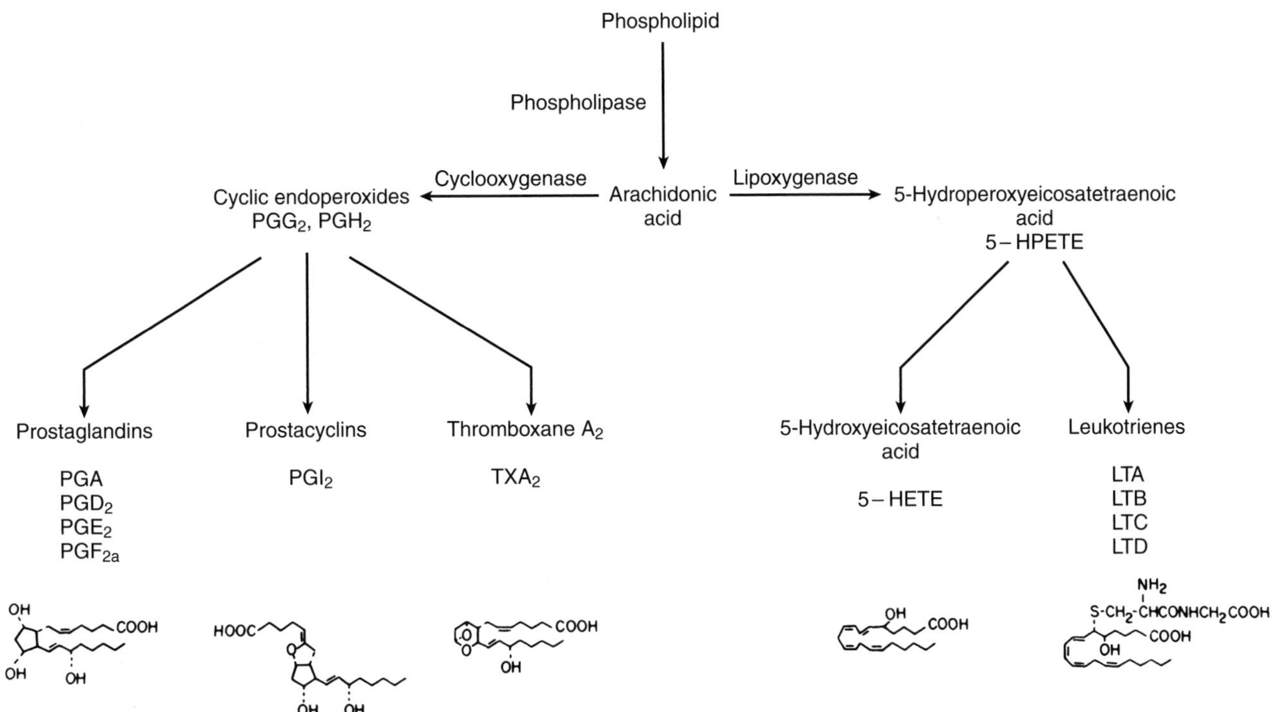

Figure 97-1 Arachidonic acid metabolism. Five major groups of metabolites are formed: prostaglandins (PGs), prostacyclins, thromboxanes, 5-hydroxyeicosatetraenoic acid, and leukotrienes (LTs). (From Katz N, Ferrante FM. Nociception. In: Ferrante FM, VadeBoncouer TR, eds. Postoperative Pain Management. New York: Churchill Livingston; 1993:17-67.)

Table 97-1 Toxicities of NSAID Subtypes

NSAID Subtype	GI Toxicity	Platelet Function	Renal Function	Cardiac Protection	Hypertension
Aspirin	Possible in susceptible patients	Irreversible platelet inhibition (7-10 days)	No effect	Positive cardioprotective effect at low doses	No effect
Nonselective	Possible in susceptible patients	Reversible platelet inhibition (hours)	Possible renal failure in susceptible patients	No reliable effect	Possible exacerbation
COX-2 selective inhibitors	Limited potential	No effect	Possible renal failure in susceptible patients	Increased risk of stroke or MI in susceptible patients	Possible exacerbation

COX, Cyclooxygenase; GI, gastrointestinal; MI, myocardial infarction; NSAID, nonsteroidal antiinflammatory drug.

antiinflammatory, and analgesic properties of traditional NSAIDs (Table 97-1). Traditional NSAIDs, such as ibuprofen and naproxen, block both forms of the COX enzyme. In an effort to reduce adverse gastric events, COX-2 inhibitor-specific drugs were introduced in the late 1990s.

Traditionally, it was believed that NSAIDs exerted an antiinflammatory effect in the periphery, preventing production of localized inflammatory mediators. It is now understood that NSAIDS may have a central analgesic mechanism as well. Following spinal NMDA (*N*-methyl-D-aspartate) receptor activation, accumulation of arachidonic acid metabolites (compounds known collectively as eicosanoids, e.g., prostaglandins, thromboxanes, and leukotrienes) occurs. NSAIDs injected intrathecally in rats have resulted in decreased pain behaviors following intraperitoneal injection of an irritant. There may be a role for intrathecal use in humans, particularly for conditions related to central sensitization, a concept that remains in the investigational stage (see Chapter 210).

Indications

Acute and chronic pain conditions may both respond to NSAIDs, and these medications have a strong role in the outpatient pain clinic and outpatient surgery facilities. The latter is a particularly good match for NSAID use, given the lack of unwanted side effects such as sedation, pruritus, respiratory depression, nausea, and reduced gut motility with the use of NSAIDs. Chronic use of NSAIDs necessitates repeated patient follow-up and observation for toxicity.

A large variety of NSAIDs are available for clinical use. The majority of these medications are administered orally, but other forms of delivery are available, including intravenous and transdermal routes. Given individual pharmacogenomic variability, lack of clinical response to one class of NSAIDs may be met with success when substitution of another is made.

Toxicity

NSAIDs are some of the most widely prescribed medications, and millions of people use nonprescription forms of these drugs; however, the toxicities of NSAIDs are potentially life threatening. The most clinically relevant toxicities relate to the gastrointestinal, renal, hematologic, cardiovascular, and hepatic systems. A review of NSAID subtype effects on these systems is presented in Table 97-2.

Gastrointestinal System

Dyspepsia is commonly related to NSAID use. Silent ulceration, gastrointestinal bleeding, and perforation are also associated with NSAID use.

Table 97-2 Nonselective NSAIDs Available in the United States by Prescription

Generic Name	Brand Name(s)
Diclofenac	Cataflam, Voltaren, Arthrotec (combination with misoprostol)
Diflunisal	Dolobid
Etodolac	Lodine, Lodine XL
Fenoprofen	Nalfon, Nalfon 200
Flurbiprofen	Ansaid
Ibuprofen*	Motrin, Motrin IB, Motrin Migraine Pain, Advil, Advil Migraine Liqui-gels, Ibu-Tab 200, Medipren, Cap-Profen, Tab-Profen, Profen, Ibuprohm, Children's Elixsure, Vicoprofen (combination with hydrocodone), Combunox (combination with oxycodone)
Indomethacin	Indocin, Indocin SR, Indo-Lemmon, Indomethegan
Ketoprofen*	Oruvail, Orudis, Actron
Ketorolac	Toradol
Mefenamic acid	Ponstel
Meloxicam	Mobic
Nabumetone	Relafen
Naproxen*	Aleve, Naprosyn, Anaprox, Anaprox DS, EC-Naproxyn, Naprelan, Naprapac (copackaged with lansoprazole)
Oxaprozin	Daypro
Piroxicam	Feldene
Salsalate	Disalcid
Sulindac	Clinoril
Tolmetin	Tolectin, Tolectin DS, Tolectin 600

*This prescription medication is also available in over-the-counter formulations.
NSAID, Nonsteroidal antiinflammatory drug.

Careful monitoring for these complications is required. The risk of gastrointestinal toxicity increases linearly with patient age. Other risk factors include a history of peptic ulcer disease, corticosteroid use, excessive alcohol use, and concurrent use of anticoagulant medications, bisphosphonates, or other NSAIDs. Dyspepsia resulting from NSAIDs can generally be treated empirically with an H_2-receptor antagonist or a proton-pump inhibitor. If the use of NSAIDs is strongly indicated and effective but the patient has risk factors for gastrointestinal toxicity, misoprostol or a proton-pump inhibitor can be used concurrently. Alternatively, the patient can be treated with a COX-2 selective antagonist. Although the lack of inhibition of COX-1 receptors will preserve prostaglandin-mediated gastrointestinal mucosal protection, COX-2 selective agents may still block COX-1 at clinically recommended doses, thus retaining gastrointestinal toxicity potential.

Renal System

Reduced renal blood flow resulting in medullary ischemia may occur when patients with prostaglandin-regulated renal blood flow receive NSAIDs. This group may include patients with heart failure, renal insufficiency, cirrhosis, and true volume-depletion states. In these cases, the patients are more dependent on the prostaglandin vasodilation effects on renal vasculature. Allergic nephritis and tubulointerstitial nephritis may also result from NSAID use. Hemodynamically mediated acute renal failure, as well as allergic nephritis and nephrotic syndrome, can be induced by any of the NSAIDs, including COX-2 selective drugs.

Hepatic System

Although elevations in serum liver enzymes are not uncommon in patients treated with NSAIDs, liver failure is quite rare. If aminotransferase levels rise significantly or the patient has a significant drop in serum albumin levels or increases in the prothrombin time, NSAID-induced hepatic toxicity should be suspected, and the medications should be withheld. Patients with systemic lupus erythematosus are at increased risk for developing NSAID-induced liver toxicity.

Hematologic System

Aspirin irreversibly impairs platelet function for the life of the platelet (7 to 10 days). Other NSAIDs reversibly inhibit platelets for their duration of action (a matter of hours). The mechanism of this decreased platelet function relates to COX-1–mediated inhibition of thromboxane A_2 synthesis, a prostaglandin involved in platelet aggregation and adhesion. COX-2 selective inhibitors have little or no effect on platelet function. NSAID use appears to present no significant risk to the patient undergoing epidural or spinal anesthesia. When NSAIDs are used concurrently with other antiplatelet medications, bleeding complications may be more likely to occur, although data on this combination are lacking.

Cardiovascular System

Although low-dose aspirin (75-325 mg/day) provides a degree of cardioprotection via inhibition of platelet aggregation, the traditional NSAIDs possess no reliable cardioprotective properties. The use of selective COX-2 inhibitors is associated with an increased risk of stroke and heart attack in susceptible patients, including those with rheumatoid arthritis and conditions that place them at risk for developing thrombosis. The mechanism of this thrombosis is inhibition of PGI_2, without effect on thromboxane A_2. The use of NSAIDs (including COX-2 selective agents) can result in hypertension and attenuation of the effects of antihypertensive medications, with the exception of calcium channel blockers.

Respiratory System

NSAIDs can precipitate a potentially life-threatening exacerbation of reactive airway disease with severe respiratory compromise in patients with aspirin-induced asthma. These patients typically have a history of perennial vasomotor rhinitis and are found to have nasal polyps on examination.

Pregnancy/Lactation

Although no evidence of teratogenicity exists relating to NSAID use during pregnancy, chronic use may lead to oligohydramnios and constriction of the fetal ductus arteriosus. The use of NSAIDs during the third trimester of pregnancies must be weighed against these risks. There are no reported harmful effects on neonates who are breastfeeding from women taking NSAIDs.

Bone Healing

Reports from animal and in vitro studies have linked impaired bone healing and tendon-to-bone healing with the concurrent use of traditional NSAIDs. Studies of COX-2 selective antagonists have revealed mixed results. Further clinical study is required to understand this complex interaction and the clinical implication in surgical cases involving fracture healing, tendon attachments, and bone fusions.

Suggested Readings

Barden J, Derry S, McQuay HJ, Moore RA. Single dose oral ketoprofen and dexketoprofen for acute postoperative pain in adults. *Cochrane Database Syst Rev.* 2009;(4):CD007355.

Bulley S, Derry S, Moore RA, McQuay HJ. Single dose oral rofecoxib for acute postoperative pain in adults. *Cochrane Database Syst Rev.* 2009;7;(4):CD004604.

Clarke R, Derry S, Moore RA. Single dose oral etoricoxib for acute postoperative pain in adults. *Cochrane Database Syst Rev.* 2012;4:CD004309.

Derry C, Derry S, Moore RA, McQuay HJ. Single dose oral ibuprofen for acute postoperative pain in adults. *Cochrane Database Syst Rev.* 2009;(3):CD001548.

Derry C, Derry S, Moore RA, McQuay HJ. Single dose oral naproxen and naproxen sodium for acute postoperative pain in adults. *Cochrane Database Syst Rev.* 2009;(1):CD004234.

Derry CJ, Derry S, Moore RA. Single dose oral ibuprofen plus paracetamol (acetaminophen) for acute postoperative pain. *Cochrane Database Syst Rev.* 2013;6:CD010210.

Derry P, Derry S, Moore RA, McQuay HJ. Single dose oral diclofenac for acute postoperative pain in adults. *Cochrane Database Syst Rev.* 2009;(2):CD004768.

Derry S, Best J, Moore RA. Single dose oral dexibuprofen [S(1)-ibuprofen] for acute postoperative pain in adults. *Cochrane Database Syst Rev.* 2013;10:CD007550.

Derry S, Derry CJ, Moore RA. Single dose oral ibuprofen plus oxycodone for acute postoperative pain in adults. *Cochrane Database Syst Rev.* 2013;6:CD010289.

Derry S, Karlin SM, Moore RA. Single dose oral ibuprofen plus codeine for acute postoperative pain in adults. *Cochrane Database Syst Rev.* 2013;3:CD010107.

Derry S, Moore RA. Single dose oral celecoxib for acute postoperative pain in adults. *Cochrane Database Syst Rev.* 2012;3:CD004233.

Derry S, Moore RA. Single dose oral celecoxib for acute postoperative pain in adults. *Cochrane Database Syst Rev.* 2013;10:CD004233.

Derry S, Moore RA. Single dose oral aspirin for acute postoperative pain in adults. *Cochrane Database Syst Rev.* 2012;4:CD002067.

Derry S, Moore RA, McQuay HJ. Single dose oral codeine, as a single agent, for acute postoperative pain in adults. *Cochrane Database Syst Rev.* 2010;(4):CD008099.

Edwards J, Meseguer F, Faura C, Moore RA, McQuay HJ, Derry S. Single dose dipyrone for acute postoperative pain. *Cochrane Database Syst Rev.* 2010;(9):CD003227.

Hall PE, Derry S, Moore RA, McQuay HJ. Single dose oral lornoxicam for acute postoperative pain in adults. *Cochrane Database Syst Rev.* 2009;(4):CD007441.

Kakkar M, Derry S, Moore RA, McQuay HJ. Single dose oral nefopam for acute postoperative pain in adults. *Cochrane Database Syst Rev.* 2009;(3):CD007442.

Lloyd R, Derry S, Moore RA, McQuay HJ. Intravenous or intramuscular parecoxib for acute postoperative pain in adults. *Cochrane Database Syst Rev.* 2009;(2):CD004771.

Moll R, Derry S, Moore RA, McQuay HJ. Single dose oral mefenamic acid for acute postoperative pain in adults. *Cochrane Database Syst Rev.* 2011;(3):CD007553.

Moore OA, McIntyre M, Moore RA, Derry S, McQuay HJ. Single dose oral tenoxicam for acute postoperative pain in adults. *Cochrane Database Syst Rev.* 2009;(3):CD007591.

Moore RA, Derry S, McQuay HJ. Single dose oral aceclofenac for postoperative pain in adults. *Cochrane Database Syst Rev.* 2009;(3):CD007588.

Moore RA, Derry S, McQuay HJ. Single dose oral acemetacin for acute postoperative pain in adults. *Cochrane Database Syst Rev.* 2009;(3):CD007589.

Moore RA, Derry S, McQuay HJ. Single dose oral dexibuprofen [S(1)-ibuprofen] for acute postoperative pain in adults. *Cochrane Database Syst Rev.* 2009;(3):CD007550.

Moore RA, Derry S, McQuay HJ. Single dose oral fenbufen for acute postoperative pain in adults. *Cochrane Database Syst Rev.* 2009;(4):CD007547.

Moore RA, Derry S, McQuay HJ. Single dose oral meloxicam for acute postoperative pain in adults. *Cochrane Database Syst Rev.* 2009;(4):CD007552.

Moore RA, Derry S, McQuay HJ. Single dose oral sulindac for acute postoperative pain in adults. *Cochrane Database Syst Rev.* 2009;(4):CD007540.

Moore RA, Derry S, McQuay HJ, Wiffen PJ. Single dose oral analgesics for acute postoperative pain in adults. *Cochrane Database Syst Rev.* 2011;(9):CD008659.

Moore RA, Derry S, Moore M, McQuay HJ. Single dose oral nabumetone for acute postoperative pain in adults. *Cochrane Database Syst Rev.* 2009;(4):CD007548.

Moore RA, Derry S, Moore M, McQuay HJ. Single dose oral tiaprofenic acid for acute postoperative pain in adults. *Cochrane Database Syst Rev.* 2009;(4):CD007542.

Roy YM, Derry S, Moore RA. Single dose oral lumiracoxib for postoperative pain in adults. *Cochrane Database Syst Rev.* 2010;(7):CD006865.

Tirunagari SK, Derry S, Moore RA, McQuay HJ. Single dose oral etodolac for acute postoperative pain in adults. *Cochrane Database Syst Rev.* 2009;(3):CD007357.

Toms L, Derry S, Moore RA, McQuay HJ. Single dose oral paracetamol (acetaminophen) with codeine for postoperative pain in adults. *Cochrane Database Syst Rev.* 2009;(1):CD001547.

Toms L, McQuay HJ, Derry S, Moore RA. Single dose oral paracetamol (acetaminophen) for postoperative pain in adults. *Cochrane Database Syst Rev.* 2008;(4):CD004602.

Traa MX, Derry S, Moore RA. Single dose oral fenoprofen for acute postoperative pain in adults. *Cochrane Database Syst Rev.* 2011;(2):CD007556.

Tzortzopoulou A, McNicol ED, Cepeda MS, Francia MB, Farhat T, Schumann R. Single dose intravenous propacetamol or intravenous paracetamol for postoperative pain. *Cochrane Database Syst Rev.* 2011;(10):CD007126.

Wasey JO, Derry S, Moore RA, McQuay HJ. Single dose oral diflunisal for acute postoperative pain in adults. *Cochrane Database Syst Rev.* 2010;(4):CD007440.

CHAPTER 98

Antiemetic Agents

Robert J. Trainer, DO, MBA

Nausea and vomiting represent an extremely distressing and financially costly problem, the risk of which has increased as the fields of anesthesia, surgery, and cancer chemotherapy have advanced. Many drugs are now available to treat and provide prophylaxis against the myriad of situations that give rise to nausea and vomiting (Figures 98-1 and 98-2).

From studies in the 1950s, a model of the emetic reflex emerged (which has been subsequently validated), consisting of a chemoreceptor trigger zone (CTZ) in the area postrema and a vomiting center in the brainstem. Nausea and vomiting result from chemical or neural stimulation of the vomiting center. Chemical activation is mediated via the CTZ, which is sensitive to the presence of toxins and poisons in the bloodstream (see Figure 98-1). Neural activation occurs as a result of information coming directly from the frontal lobes of the brain, the digestive tract, and the balancing mechanism of the inner ear.

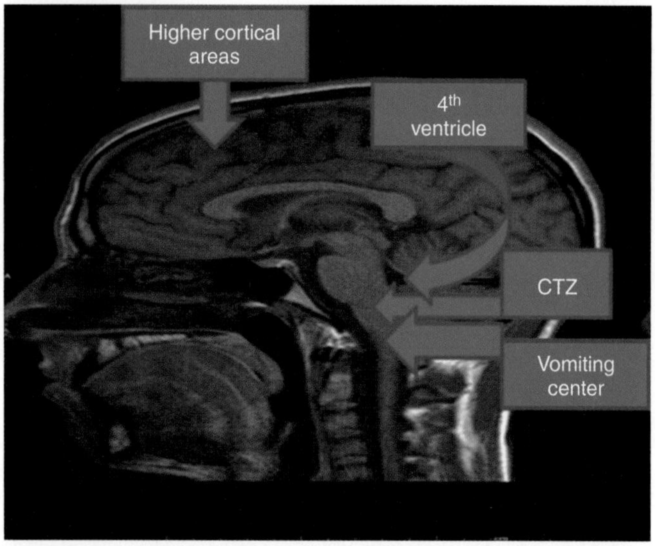

Figure 98-1 Chemical activation of the vomiting center is mediated via the chemoreceptor trigger zone (CTZ), which is sensitive to the presence of toxins and poisons in the bloodstream.

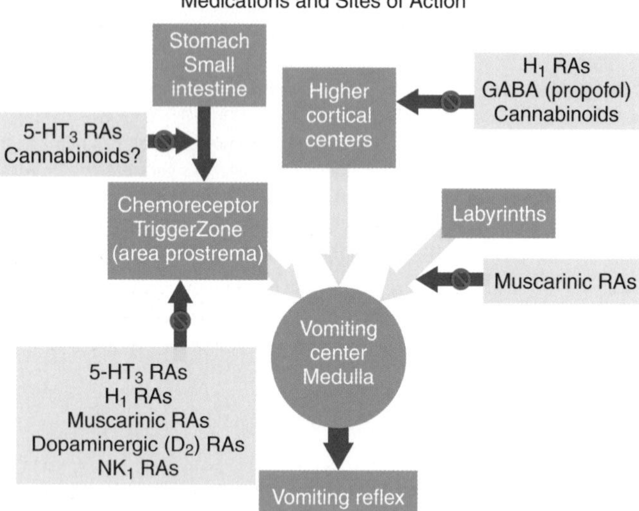

Figure 98-2 Medications used to treat nausea and vomiting and their sites of action. RAs, Receptor antagonists.

The CTZ is susceptible to stimulation from the release of dopamine and serotonin (5-HT) in the blood and cerebrospinal fluid and may also be activated by opioids and certain anesthetic agents. In addition, the release of 5-HT from the gastrointestinal tract can stimulate the CTZ. The vestibular system sends input to the vomiting center in response to changes in motion and pressure. The reflex afferent pathway from the cerebral cortex stimulates the vomiting center in response to such factors as pain, anxiety, and visual, sensory, or cognitive overload (see Figure 98-2).

Clinical scenarios in which nausea and vomiting are common include cancer chemotherapy, the postoperative period, headache syndromes, and the use of opioids. Optimization of each potentially overlapping scenario requires a tailored approach, although certain principles are worth noting. For example, factors that increase a patient's risk for developing postoperative nausea and vomiting (PONV) include increasing age, premenopausal women, obesity, previous history of motion sickness or PONV, anxiety, gastroparesis, and type and duration of the surgical procedure (e.g., laparoscopy, strabismus, middle ear procedures). Anesthesiologists have little, if any, control over these surgical factors. However, they do have control over many other factors that influence PONV (e.g., preanesthetic medication, anesthetic drugs and techniques, and postoperative pain management). PONV has an overall incidence of approximately 34% in patients receiving a general anesthetic without preoperative antiemetic therapy, with reductions of PONV by 26% with prophylactic administration of ondansetron, dexamethasone, or droperidol. Furthermore, prevention of PONV is much more effective than treatment administered after symptoms occur. Total intravenous anesthesia is preferred over inhalation agents, and the use of nonopioid analgesics—such as ketorolac, paracetamol, nonsteroidal anti inflammatory drugs, or cyclooxygenase-2 inhibitors—are often given along with morphine as part of multimodal analgesia after major operations. The use of regional anesthesia can benefit patients who are expected to have high postoperative opiate requirements.

In an attempt to reduce the risk of PONV if patients are expected to be placed on opioid therapy, current recommendations include a bowel regimen consisting of a motility agent (senna) and a stool softener (docusate) to avoid opiate-induced constipation and consequent nausea. In patients who are able to drink, psyllium and osmotic laxatives have also been suggested as beneficial.

Today, the standard of care for prevention of chemotherapy-induced nausea and vomiting (CINV) for highly and moderately emetogenic chemotherapy is a 5-HT_3-receptor antagonist, dexamethasone, with or without aprepitant or fosaprepitant.

Finally, the relatively low risk of side effects from the use of antiemetic drugs overall was confirmed in a large meta-analysis that included 737 studies involving 103,237 people and the use of eight commonly used drugs: droperidol, metoclopramide, ondansetron, tropisetron, dolasetron, dexamethasone, cyclizine, and granisetron. The authors observed that between 1 and 5 out of every 100 people experienced a mild side effect, such as sedation or headache, when given an antiemetic drug.

Antidopaminergic Drugs

Antidopaminergic drugs (D_2-receptor antagonists) include butyrophenones (haloperidol, droperidol), phenothiazines, domperidone, and metoclopramide. The D_2-receptor antagonists combined with the 5-HT_3 antagonists make up the largest number of medications currently used for treating nausea. The D_2-receptor antagonists are also the oldest class of medications used in this scenario. The D_2 receptor in the CTZ is the primary target for all drugs currently used for preventing or treating PONV and CINV; domperidone (used primarily for nausea due to gastroenteritis) is the exception owing to its inability to cross the blood-brain barrier. Olanzapine, an antipsychotic, has antagonistic properties at the D_2, acetylcholine, and 5-HT_3 receptors. The well-known antiemetic effect of propofol may be due to a D_2 antagonism, 5-HT_3 antagonism, or a cannabinoid agonism.

Latest Evidence for Efficacy

In a recent study, the dopamine antagonists and benzodiazepines were found to be more appropriately used in breakthrough and anticipatory symptoms or in preventing the delayed phase of CINV. Although less commonly used due to their boxed warning (see following discussion), recent data support the notion that droperidol, in low doses (0.75-1.5 mg), may be the most effective D_2 antagonist in a pharmacologic armamentarium to cope with PONV.

Side Effects

Antidopaminergic drugs should not be used in patients with Parkinson disease, restless leg syndrome, or any other disorder in which dopaminergic drugs are used to treat the signs and symptoms of the disease. Extrapyramidal reactions, sedation, diarrhea, and orthostatic hypotension can occur with all antidopaminergic drugs used in the treatment of PONV. Haloperidol is the drug in this class that is most likely to be implicated as the cause of excessive sedation, and prochlorperazine is responsible for most cases of orthostatic hypotension.

The U.S. Food and Drug Administration requires a boxed warning on droperidol related to the drug's propensity to prolong the QT interval;

therefore, patients who receive droperidol intraoperatively should have electrocardiographic monitoring for 4 h postoperatively.

Metoclopramide possesses the additional benefit of enhancing gastric emptying by selective peripheral cholinergic agonism, which is also the reason that this drug should be avoided in patients who have bowel obstruction. A boxed warning on metoclopramide highlights the risk for patients to develop tardive dyskinesia, but this adverse effect is seen most often with long-term use of the drug.

H_1-Receptor Agonists

H_1-receptor agonists include diphenhydramine and promethazine. Diphenhydramine is thought to have anticholinergic properties, resulting in antidyskinetic, sedative, and antiemetic effects, which likely occur at the level of the gastrointestinal tract, preventing vagally mediated transmission to the vomiting center. The antihistamine effect is thought to work at the level of the CTZ.

Latest Evidence for Efficacy

Diphenhydramine is often used prophylactically with other medications to prevent PONV. In this context, a recent study showed that a combination of metoclopramide with diphenhydramine decreased PONV more, compared with either agent alone, when added to patient-controlled analgesia with morphine. A common indication for diphenhydramine is morphine-induced pruritus.

Side Effects

Sedation is the most common side effect noted with the use of H_1-receptor agonists; dizziness, headache, hypotension, and urinary retention can occur, especially in the elderly and with high doses. The use of phenergan has decreased since the labeling has included a boxed warning of severe chemical irritation and tissue damage, including burning, thrombophlebitis, tissue necrosis, and gangrene.

Muscarinic Antagonists

Muscarinic antagonists (e.g., scopolamine) or anticholinergic agents act on the vomiting center and digestive tract and reduce gastrointestinal hyperactivity. They help in the management of motion sickness by protecting against motion-induced nausea (vestibular stimulation).

Latest Evidence for Efficacy

Morphine and synthetic opioids increase vestibular sensitivity; transdermal scopolamine provides antiemetic effects in patients treated with patient-controlled analgesia or epidural morphine for the management of postoperative pain.

Side Effects

Scopolamine is an antisialagogue approximately three times as potent as atropine. The transdermal form is less likely to cause prohibitive side effects of dry mouth, drowsiness, and blurred vision.

5-HT_3-Receptor Antagonists

The 5-HT_3-receptor agonists (ondansetron, dolasetron, and granisetron) bind to receptors in the CTZ and 5-HT_3 receptors in the gastrointestinal tract, preventing signal transmission.

Latest Evidence for Efficacy

The use of 5-HT_3-receptor antagonists has been shown to significantly decrease the cumulative incidence of postoperative emesis within 24 h, but it does not decrease nausea. The cumulative incidence of PONV increases in patients treated with both the 5-HT_3-receptor antagonists and placebo.

Ondansetron has a sublingual formulation, often used in migraineurs, and granisetron has a transdermal formulation for similar clinical situations.

Side Effects

Headache, especially in those susceptible (migraineurs), occurs in up to 10% of patients and is thought to be due to the vascular effect at the level of the cerebral vasculature. Constipation is the most common gastrointestinal side effect. Although no boxed warnings have been issued for 5-HT_3-receptor antagonists, caution is recommended when these drugs are used in patients with congenital long QT syndrome; recent data suggest lowering the recommended maximum dose for ondansetron to 16 mg.

Steroids

The exact mechanism of the anti-inflammatory action of dexamethasone is unknown; however, this drug inhibits multiple inflammatory cytokines in the central and peripheral nervous systems and stabilizes plasma membranes in central and peripheral sites.

Latest Evidence for Efficacy

Although usually administered with a 5-HT_3 antagonist, prophylactic dexamethasone administered alone has been shown to decrease the incidence of PONV after laparoscopic gynecologic operations within the first 24 h after surgery. Furthermore, dexamethasone reduces pain, PONV, bleeding, and overall postoperative complications in adults undergoing tonsillectomy.

Dexamethasone, 4 to 8 mg, is recommended in combination with a 5-HT_3-receptor antagonist, D_2 antagonist, or neurokinin (NK_1) antagonist for prevention of PONV and acute or delayed CINV.

Side Effects

The following side effects have been reported to occur with a single dose of dexmethasone: hyperglycemia (especially in obese patients, who are more likely to have insulin resistance), appetite change, insomnia, mood swings, anxiety, headache, flushing, and edema. Less common and more serious reactions include adrenal insufficiency, peptic ulcer, and steroid psychosis.

NK_1 Antagonists

The neuropeptide substance P shows a widespread distribution in both the central and peripheral nervous systems; after binding to the NK_1 receptors, substance P regulates many biologic functions in the central nervous system, such as emotional behavior, stress, depression, anxiety, emesis, migraine, alcohol addiction, and neurodegeneration. 5-HT mediates the early vomiting process that occurs within 8 to 12 h following cisplatin-based chemotherapy, after which time substance P, acting at NK_1 receptors, becomes the dominant mediator of vomiting. Aprepitant, a substance P antagonist, is typically given as a single 40-mg dose by mouth within 3 h before anesthesia. Chemotherapy regimens vary, but often consist of a 3-day course of therapy due to the risk of delayed CINV. Aprepitant is usually administered with a corticosteroid.

Latest Evidence for Efficacy

The recently revised American Society of Clinical Oncology Guidelines, as well as those from the Multinational Association for Supportive Care in Cancer, reflect the efficacy of aprepitant for prevention of delayed CINV due to highly emetogenic chemotherapy, recommending its use with a corticosteroid and against the use of 5-HT_3-receptor antagonists for this purpose.

Side Effects

Fatigue, nausea, hiccups, constipation, diarrhea, and abdominal pain can occur with the use of aprepitant; neutropenia, anaphylactic reactions, and Stevens-Johnson syndrome are more rare side effects.

Cannabinoids

The proposed effects of cannabinoids (inhaled or oral) are antagonism of dopamine receptors or 5-HT_3 receptors or activation of the cannabinoid receptors.

Latest Evidence for Efficacy

In 1985, the Food and Drug Administration approved two cannabinoid derivatives, dronabinol and nabilone, for the treatment of CINV not effectively treated by other agents. Today, the standard of care for prevention of CINV for highly and moderately emetogenic chemotherapy is a 5-HT_3-receptor antagonist and dexamethasone, with or without aprepitant or fosaprepitant. With the approval of safer and more effective agents, cannabinoids are not recommended as first-line treatment for the prevention of CINV and are reserved for patients with breakthrough nausea and vomiting.

As mentioned previously, the well-known antiemetic effect of propofol may be due to D_2 antagonism, 5-HT_3 antagonism, or a cannabinoid agonism.

Side Effects

Commonly reported side effects associated with the use of cannabinoids include dizziness, somnolence, euphoria, paranoia, abnormal thinking, ataxia, confusion, and hallucinations. Although thought to have pain-relieving properties, cannabinoids have been shown to cause abdominal pain and paradoxical cannabinoid hyperemesis syndrome.

Use of a Cooling Fan and Peribuccal Isopropyl Alcohol

The use of a cooling fan in combination with peribuccal isopropyl alcohol is thought to stimulate the V_2 distribution of the trigeminal nerve and olfactory nerve, respectively.

Latest Evidence for Efficacy

According to a recent Cochrane database review of 9 trials with a total of 402 participants, the use of isopropyl alcohol was more effective than a saline placebo for reducing PONV but less effective than standard antiemetic drugs.

Side Effects

Side effects associated with the use of a cooling fan in combination with peribuccal isopropyl alcohol are minimal.

Auricular Acupuncture and Use of the Wrist P6 Point

Many theories exist as to the mechanism of action with regard to acupuncture in treating nausea and vomiting. A popular modern theory founded in the theoretical physical sciences and attempting to consolidate previous theories is the bioelectromagnetic hypothesis. In this case, a complicated interplay between biology and electrodynamic forces—in which a somato-autonomic reflex occurs—may be responsible for the effect of acupuncture on nausea.

Latest Evidence for Efficacy

In a Cochrane review that included 40 trials involving 4858 participants, compared with sham treatment, P6 acupoint stimulation significantly reduced nausea, vomiting, and the need for rescue antiemetics. There was no evidence of difference between P6 acupoint stimulation and antiemetic drugs in the risk of nausea, vomiting, or the need for rescue antiemetics. The side effects associated with P6 acupoint stimulation were minor. There was no evidence of publication bias from contour-enhanced funnel plots.

Side Effects

Per the Dr. Helms Clinical Approach for Physicians curriculum, the psychophysiologic response to an acupuncture treatment can be lightheadedness, anxiety, agitation, or tearfulness. The sense of relaxation can sometimes evolve into a feeling of fatigue or depression, which can last for several days. Contact dermatitis to the nickel, zinc, and chromium in stainless steel needles has been documented. Syncope and retained needle are rare, and pneumothorax (the most common overall complication in acupuncture therapy) is not a concern in either the wrist P6 or auricular acupuncture therapy.

Conclusion

Nausea and vomiting represent extremely distressing and financially costly side effects of the advancements in the fields of anesthesia, surgery, and cancer chemotherapy. Many drugs are now available to treat and prevent PONV and CINV, as well as the myriad of other situations that give rise to nausea and vomiting. Major classes of drugs commonly used today include dopamine-receptor antagonists, 5-HT_3-receptor antagonists, steroids, and NK_1 antagonists. The current antiemetic efficacy rate has been unable to surpass 70% to 80% in patients treated with highly emetogenic cytotoxic drugs, the most extreme challenge for antiemetic drugs. Although much research has been focused on the development of new medications and the optimal setting and timing of medication administration, one of the potential factors explaining this suboptimal response is variability in genes encoding enzymes and proteins that play a role in metabolism, transport, and receptors related to antiemetic drugs.

Suggested Readings

Apfel CC, Korttila K, Abdalla M, et al. A factorial trial of six interventions for the prevention of postoperative nausea and vomiting. *N Engl J Med.* 2004;350: 2441-2451.

Basch E, Prestrud AA, Hesketh PJ, et al. Antiemetics: American Society of Clinical Oncology clinical practice guideline update. *J Clin Oncol.* 2011;29: 4189-4188.

Carlisle JB, Stevenson CA. Drugs for preventing postoperative nausea and vomiting. *Cochrane Database Syst Rev.* 2006;(3):CD004125.

Diakos EA, Gallos ID, El-Shunnar S, et al. Dexamethasone reduces pain, vomiting and overall complications following tonsillectomy in adults: A systematic review and meta-analysis of randomised controlled trials. *Clin Otolaryngol.* 2011;36:531-542.

Ettinger DS, Armstrong DK, Barbour S, et al. Antiemesis. *J Natl Compr Cancer Netw.* 2012;10:456-485.

Fowler CJ. Possible involvement of the endocannabinoid system in the actions of three clinically used drugs. *Trends Pharmacol Sci.* 2004;25:59-61.

Gralla RJ, de Wit R, Herrstedt J, et al. Antiemetic efficacy of the neurokinin-1 antagonist, aprepitant, plus a 5HT3 antagonist and a corticosteroid in patients receiving anthracyclines or cyclophosphamide in addition to high-dose cisplatin: Analysis of combined data from two Phase III randomized clinical trials. *Cancer.* 2005;104:864-868.

Habib AS, White WD, Eubanks S, et al. A randomized comparison of a multimodal management strategy versus combination antiemetics for the prevention of postoperative nausea and vomiting. *Anesth Analg.* 2004;99:77-81.

Helms JM. An overview of medical acupuncture. *Altern Ther Health Med.* 1998;4:35-45.

Hines S, Steels E, Chang A, Gibbons K. Aromatherapy for treatment of postoperative nausea and vomiting. *Cochrane Database Syst Rev.* 2012;4:CD007598.

Lee A, Fan LT. Stimulation of the wrist acupuncture point P6 for preventing postoperative nausea and vomiting. *Cochrane Database Syst Rev.* 2009;2: CD003281.

Lu CW, Jean WH, Wu CC, et al. Antiemetic efficacy of metoclopramide and diphenhydramine added to patient-controlled morphine analgesia: A randomised controlled trial. *Eur J Anaesthesiol.* 2010;27:1052-1057.

Merker M, Kranke P, Morin AM, et al. Prophylaxis of nausea and vomiting in the postoperative phase: Relative effectiveness of droperidol and metoclopramide. *Anaesthesist.* 2011;60:432-440 [in German].

Neufeld SM, Newburn-Cook CV. The efficacy of 5-HT3 receptor antagonists for the prevention of postoperative nausea and vomiting after craniotomy: A meta-analysis. *J Neurosurg Anesthesiol.* 2007;19:10-17.

CHAPTER 99

Diuretics

Thomas N. Spackman, MD, MS

Drugs that increase the excretion of sodium and water through the kidneys, termed diuretics, are classified on the basis of their site (Figure 99-1) or mechanism of action in the nephron. Diuretics are the recommended drugs for initial treatment of hypertension and are used in a variety of relative fluid-overload conditions, including heart failure, renal disease, and liver cirrhosis. Despite the lack of evidence that diuretic therapy prevents acute renal injury or improves outcome following injury or that diuretics reduce morbidity or mortality risk when used in chronic heart failure, they do provide symptomatic relief from fluid-overload syndromes.

Thiazide Diuretics

Thiazides inhibit Na^+ transport in the distal convoluted tubule and also in part of the cortical ascending limb of the loop of Henle. Water follows the salt that is not reabsorbed, causing the diuresis. Because the distal convoluted tubule accounts for only 5% or less of the total Na^+ reabsorption, the diuretic effect is much weaker than that of loop diuretics. Because the Na^+-Cl^- transporter is located on the luminal side of the tubule, thiazide diuretics are not effective at glomerular filtration rates of less than 30 mL/min.

Thiazides are rapidly and effectively absorbed from the gastrointestinal tract. They reach their peak action within a few hours and exert a diuretic effect for up to 12 h. Thiazides are most commonly used as initial treatment for hypertension. The early reduction in blood pressure is due to a reduction in blood volume. Chronic treatment results in blood pressure control through reduced vascular resistance despite return of fluid volumes to pretreatment levels.

The most common adverse effects of thiazides are dehydration and hypokalemia with metabolic alkalosis. Adverse effects unique to the use of thiazides include hypercalcemia and hyperuricemia from decreased renal excretion of Ca^{2+} and uric acid. Other adverse effects include hyperglycemia, hyponatremia, hypomagnesemia, fatigue, lethargy, hypersensitivity reactions, purpura, and dermatitis with photosensitivity.

Loop Diuretics

Furosemide, bumetanide, torsemide, and ethacrynic acid are classified as loop diuretics because of their action in inhibiting the reabsorption of electrolytes in the thick ascending loop of Henle. They also exert a direct effect on electrolyte transport in the proximal tubule and cause renal cortical vasodilation and increased renal blood flow. The potent diuresis results in enhanced excretion of Na^+, Cl^-, K^+, H^+, Ca^{2+}, Mg^{2+}, NH_4^-, and HCO_3^-. Cl^- excretion exceeds Na^+ excretion. Excessive losses of K^+, H^-, NH_4^-, and Cl^-, as well as rapid contraction of extracellular fluid volume, may result in metabolic alkalosis.

A temporary but substantial decrease in glomerular filtration rate, along with decreased pulmonary vascular resistance and increased peripheral venous capacitance, occurs after intravenous administration of furosemide in patients with congestive heart failure. This decreases left ventricular filling pressures, an acute action occurring before the onset of diuresis.

All four drugs are rapidly absorbed from the gastrointestinal tract and are highly protein bound. Their effectiveness depends on active secretion into the proximal tubule and, therefore, on renal plasma flow. After intravenous administration of furosemide, diuresis usually occurs within 5 min, reaches a maximum within 20 to 60 min, and persists for approximately 2 h.

Too vigorous a diuresis may induce an acute hypotensive episode. Potassium depletion in patients receiving nondepolarizing neuromuscular blocking agents can predispose these individuals to prolonged neuromuscular blockade. Hyperuricemia is common. Gastrointestinal disturbance (including bleeding), marrow depression, hepatic dysfunction, rashes, and decreased carbohydrate tolerance (furosemide may interfere with the hypoglycemic effect of insulin) also have been reported. There is one recent study suggesting that in hypotensive patients the use of furosemide decreases O_2 levels in the kidney to a critical level—presumably because O_2 supply to the kidney is inadequate to meet the increased metabolic rate caused by the furosemide.

The use of ethacrynic acid and bumetanide has been associated with hearing loss, and the use of ethacrynic acid is associated with a higher incidence of gastrointestinal disturbance, as compared with furosemide. Patients receiving chronic anticonvulsant therapy have a reduced diuretic response, and it is postulated that renal sensitivity to furosemide is diminished by these drugs. Allergic interstitial nephritis leading to reversible renal failure has been attributed to furosemide. Competition for binding sites on albumin may lead to an increased effect of drugs such as warfarin and clofibrate.

Osmotic Diuretics

Mannitol, the prototype of the osmotic diuretics, is relatively inert and draws water from tissues to the intravascular space. It is excreted unchanged in the urine and produces a greater flow rate through the lumen of the nephron, resulting in reduced efficiency of Na^+ reabsorption and significant diuresis. The osmotic diuresis can lead to volume depletion and electrolyte imbalances, especially of Na^+, K^+ and Mg^{2+}. Oral absorption is unreliable. The intravenous dose range is 0.25 to 1.0 g/kg infused over 15 to 30 min.

In patients with elevated intracranial pressure, mannitol can decrease intracranial pressure within 30 min, with maximum effect within 1 to 2 h and duration of effect of approximately 6 h. Despite its role as a free radical scavenger and proven effectiveness at reducing intracranial pressure, mannitol has not been shown to improve outcomes in brain-injured patients with cerebral edema. Mannitol has also not been shown to be effective in prevention of acute renal failure, and some studies have shown a greater risk of renal injury from mannitol compared with saline alone in patients with moderate renal dysfunction.

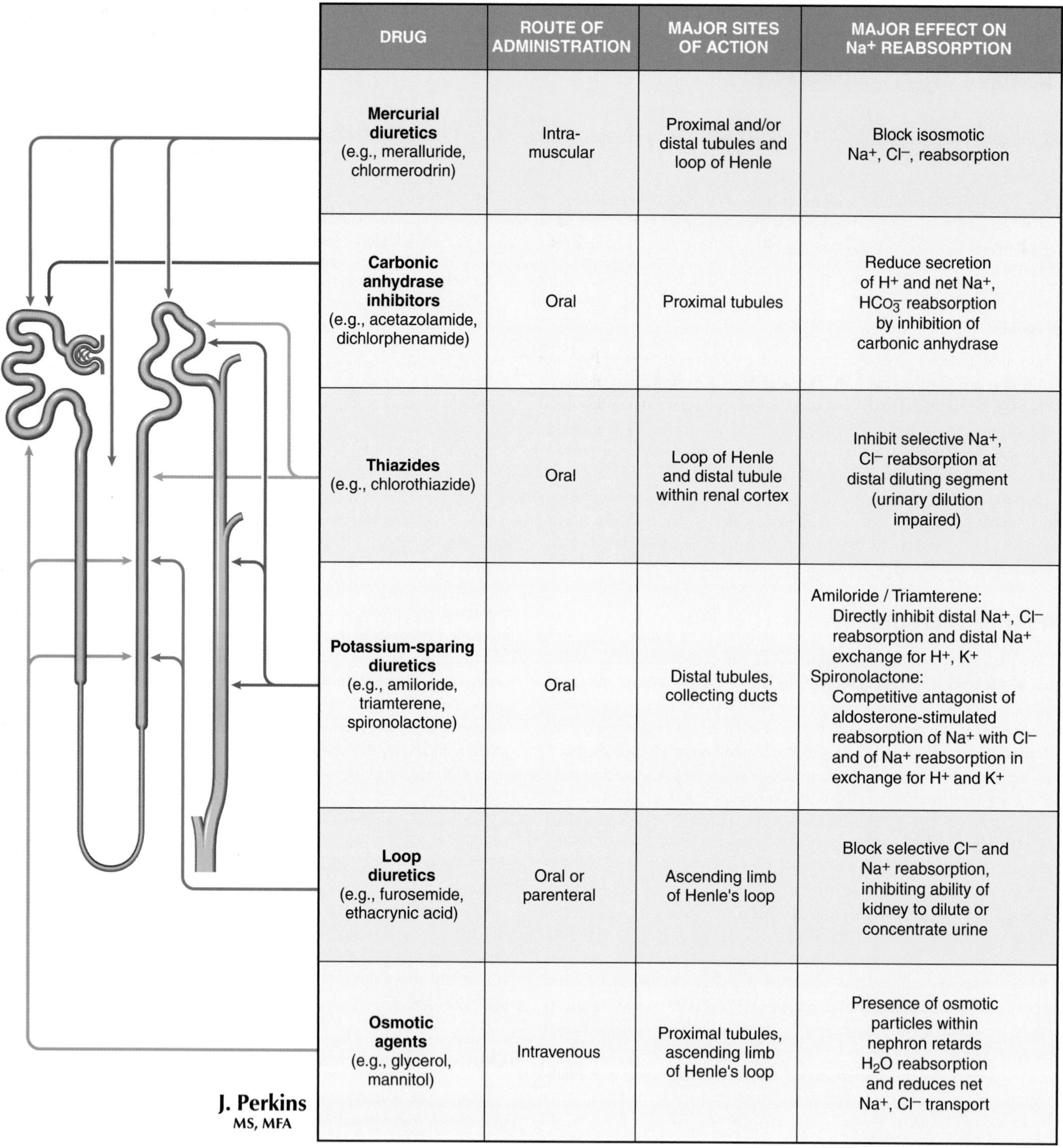

DRUG	ROUTE OF ADMINISTRATION	MAJOR SITES OF ACTION	MAJOR EFFECT ON Na^+ REABSORPTION
Mercurial diuretics (e.g., meralluride, chlormerodrin)	Intra-muscular	Proximal and/or distal tubules and loop of Henle	Block isosmotic Na^+, Cl^-, reabsorption
Carbonic anhydrase inhibitors (e.g., acetazolamide, dichlorphenamide)	Oral	Proximal tubules	Reduce secretion of H^+ and net Na^+, HCO_3^- reabsorption by inhibition of carbonic anhydrase
Thiazides (e.g., chlorothiazide)	Oral	Loop of Henle and distal tubule within renal cortex	Inhibit selective Na^+, Cl^- reabsorption at distal diluting segment (urinary dilution impaired)
Potassium-sparing diuretics (e.g., amiloride, triamterene, spironolactone)	Oral	Distal tubules, collecting ducts	Amiloride / Triamterene: Directly inhibit distal Na^+, Cl^- reabsorption and distal Na^+ exchange for H^+, K^+ Spironolactone: Competitive antagonist of aldosterone-stimulated reabsorption of Na^+ with Cl^- and of Na^+ reabsorption in exchange for H^+ and K^+
Loop diuretics (e.g., furosemide, ethacrynic acid)	Oral or parenteral	Ascending limb of Henle's loop	Block selective Cl^- and Na^+ reabsorption, inhibiting ability of kidney to dilute or concentrate urine
Osmotic agents (e.g., glycerol, mannitol)	Intravenous	Proximal tubules, ascending limb of Henle's loop	Presence of osmotic particles within nephron retards H_2O reabsorption and reduces net Na^+, Cl^- transport

Figure 99-1 Renal tubules showing the primary sites of diuretic action. (Netter illustration from www.netterimages.com.)

Carbonic Anhydrase Inhibitors

Acetazolamide acts in the proximal tubule as a potent inhibitor of carbonic anhydrase, which reduces the supply of H^+ ions in the proximal and distal tubules. More than 90% of filtered HCO_3^- is reabsorbed in the proximal tubule via an exchange with H^+. Because Na^+ is normally reabsorbed in exchange for H^+, more Na^+ and HCO_3^- remain within the tubules. A diuresis is produced by the Na^+ excretion, and the urine is alkaline from the retained HCO_3^-. Acetazolamide is a weak diuretic because its main action is in the proximal tubule, where only a small percentage of the total filtered Na^+ is absorbed.

Acetazolamide can be administered orally or intravenously. Peak plasma levels occur within a few hours when taken orally. There is no appreciable metabolism, and elimination is usually complete in 24 h.

Acetazolamide is used to induce an alkaline urine in certain drug overdoses (e.g., salicylates). It is also used to treat glaucoma, acute altitude sickness, and significant metabolic alkalosis.

Adverse effects common to other diuretics are infrequent because acetazolamide is a weaker diuretic. Patients on chronic therapy for glaucoma can present with a metabolic acidosis. Large doses can lead to paresthesias and drowsiness.

K^+-Sparing Diuretics

Triamterene and amiloride block the exchange between Na^+ and both K^+ and H^+ in the late distal tubule and collecting duct. Excessive loss of K^+ is prevented. Both of these relatively weak diuretics are more effective when used with a thiazide or loop diuretic, which act more proximally in the nephron.

Aldosterone Antagonists

Spironolactone and eplerenone act on the distal nephron to inhibit Na^+ and K^+ excretion. They can cause clinically significant hyperkalemia. Eplerenone has greater specificity for the aldosterone receptor and a lower incidence of gynecomastia and impotence in men and menstrual irregularities in women. Both are weak diuretics and are used in low doses more for their beneficial antagonism of aldosterone in patients with heart failure. Spironolactone is frequently used in patients with edema secondary to liver failure.

Suggested Readings

Reilly RF, Jackson EK. Regulation of renal function and vascular volume. in: Brunton LL, Chabner B, Knollman B, eds. ed. *Goodman and Gilman's The Pharmacological Basis of Therapeutiucs*. 12th ed. New York: McGraw Hill; 2011: 671-720.

Stoelting RK, Hilier SC. *Pharmacology and Physiology in Anesthetic Practice*. 4th ed. Philadelphia: Lippincott, Williams & Wilkins; 2006.

Textor SC, Glockner JF, Lerman LO, et al. The use of magnetic resonance to evaluate tissue oxygenation in renal artery stenosis. *J Am Soc Nephrol*. 2008;19:80-88.

Venkataraman R, Kellum J. Prevention of acute renal failure. *Chest*. 2007;131: 300-308.

Wilcox CX. Diuretics. In: *Brenner and Rector's The Kidney*. 7th ed. Philadelphia: WB Saunders; 2004.

Wang DJ, Gottlieb SS. Diuretics: Still the mainstay of treatment. *Crit Care Med*. 2008;36:S89-94.

CHAPTER 100

Albumin, Hetastarch, and Pentastarch

Edwin H. Rho, MD

The Colloid Controversy

For decades, medical debate has continued over the value of colloid infusion in the perioperative setting. It is important to note, however, that in patients who are bleeding and who require intravascular volume expansion—especially patients with trauma—first-line therapy is the use of blood products. Early colloid advocates argued that it was important to maintain normal colloid osmotic pressure to keep intravascular fluid from passing into the tissues and thereby contributing to pulmonary, cerebral, subcutaneous edema or ascites. Albumin was the most widely used colloid until hydroxyethyl starch, and pentastarch were developed, and it still is commonly used.

Albumin

Albumin is available in 5% and 25% concentrations, the latter being most useful in patients who are unable to tolerate large volumes of fluid. Albumin is a heat-stable tightly wound protein molecule derived from human whole blood. It is heated to 60°C for 10 h to eradicate infectious organisms (both bacterial and viral). Transmission of Creutzfeldt-Jakob disease has not been reported with the use of albumin.

Hetastarch and Pentastarch

Both hetastarch and pentastarch are composed of chains of glucose molecules to which hydroxyethyl ether groups have been added to retard degradation. The glucose chains are highly branched, being derived from the starch amylopectin. One in twenty glucose monomers branches. Starch chains of various lengths are present in hetastarch, giving it an average molecular weight of 450 kD. Its number-average molecular weight is 69 kD; this term describes a simple average of the individual molecular weights and is more closely related to oncotic pressure. About 80% of hetastarch polymers have molecular weights in the range of 30 to 2400 kD. Hetastarch is available as a 6% solution in 0.9% sodium chloride or a lactated electrolyte solution. The chemical and pharmacokinetic properties of hetastarch and pentastarch are listed in Table 100-1.

Hetastarch and pentastarch do not interfere with blood typing or cross-matching, are stable with fluctuating temperatures, and rarely cause allergic reactions. Both have been used successfully as an adjunct in leukapheresis by increasing the erythrocyte sedimentation rate to enhance granulocyte yield.

Table 100-1 Chemical and Pharmacokinetic Properties of Hetastarch* and Pentastarch

Property	6% Hetastarch	10% Pentastarch
pH	5.5	5.0
MW_W (kDa)	450 (range, 10-1000)	264 (range, 150-350)
MW_N (kDa)	69	63
Calculated osmolar concentration (mosmol/L)	310	326
Molar substitution ratio	0.7	0.45
Intravascular half-life (h)	25.5	2.5
Renal elimination	Molecules smaller than 50 kDa are rapidly excreted; <10% detected intravascularly at 2 weeks	Molecules smaller than 50 kDa are rapidly excreted; undetectable intravascularly at 1 week
Coagulation effects	↑ in PT, aPTT, and clotting time; may interfere with platelet function	↑ in PT, aPTT, and clotting time; may interfere with platelet function
Other miscellaneous effects	↑ in indirect serum bilirubin levels; temporary ↑ in serum amylase concentration	Temporary ↑ in serum amylase concentration

*In 2010-2011, several medical journals retracted articles describing studies examining the use of hetastarch. However, the data presented here are accurate.

aPTT, Activated partial thromboplastin time; MW_N, number-average molecular weight; MW_W, weight-average molecular weight; PT, prothrombin time.

Pharmacokinetics and Pharmacodynamics of Hetastarch and Pentastarch

The colloidal properties of both hetastarch and pentastarch resemble those of 5% human albumin. Distribution is throughout the intravascular space. The principal effect following intravenous administration of any colloidal solution is plasma volume expansion secondary to the colloidal osmotic effect. In hypovolemic patients, the prolonged plasma volume expansion causes a temporary increase in arterial and venous pressures, cardiac index, left ventricular stroke work index, and pulmonary artery occlusion pressure. The effective intravascular half-life is 25.5 h for 6% hetastarch and 2.5 h for 10% pentastarch. Both substances are eliminated by the kidney. The hydroxyethyl group is not cleared but remains attached to glucose units when excreted. Hetastarch and pentastarch molecules less than 50,000 Da are rapidly eliminated by the kidneys. However, only 33% of an initial dose of hetastarch is eliminated within 24 h of administration, compared with approximately 70% of an initial dose of pentastarch. Up to 10% of administered hetastarch can be detected intravascularly after 2 weeks. Pentastarch is undetectable intravascularly 1 week after administration.

As a result of a lower molar substitution ratio (i.e., the number of hydroxyethyl groups per glucose unit), pentastarch is more rapidly and completely degraded by circulating amylase than is hetastarch. Hetastarch has a very long tissue-retention time (a half-life of 10 to 15 days) because the larger molecules are stored in the liver and spleen, where they are slowly degraded enzymatically by amylase. There is a theoretical concern of impaired reticuloendothelial function caused by hetastarch. Accordingly, a lower molecular weight pentastarch was developed to minimize this theoretical risk.

Adverse Effects of Hetastarch and Pentastarch

Both hetastarch and pentastarch prolong prothrombin time, partial thromboplastin time, and bleeding times when given in large doses, most likely secondary to hemodilution. There is some evidence to suggest that platelet function may also be altered by both products. For this reason, the maximum recommended dose is 15 to 20 mL/kg. Although there are case reports of neurosurgical patients developing coagulopathies after large (2 L) doses of hetastarch, the effects of hetastarch on the coagulation system seem clinically insignificant when maximum dose recommendations are not exceeded. More recently, tetrastarches have been developed to enhance degradation and minimize retention in the blood and tissues. This may be beneficial, as the effects on coagulation and platelets may be decreased.

Both hetastarch and pentastarch have been reported to produce rare hypersensitivity reactions, such as wheezing and urticaria. However, neither substance has been shown to stimulate antibody formation.

Transient increases in serum amylase and indirect bilirubin levels have occurred following hetastarch and pentastarch administration. However, no association with pancreatitis or biliary injury has been reported.

Clinical Usefulness of Colloids

Multiple authors have studied the importance of colloids in perioperative fluid therapy and tried to determine the value of colloid solutions in comparison with inexpensive crystalloid solutions. The theory that albumin and other colloids would enable the body to keep more fluid in the intravascular space has never held water, figuratively speaking. Colloids have not been proved to prevent the extravascular accumulations that lead to edema in the lungs, pleura, brain, abdomen, and soft tissues of critically injured and ill patients. In the past, clinical trials failed to show a difference in outcome for patients receiving colloid versus crystalloid solutions. More recent studies have suggested that hetastarch and pentastarch may be associated with an increased risk of mortality, acute kidney injury, renal replacement therapy or a combination, compared with crystalloid solutions. Nonetheless, colloids may be useful in patients who are intolerant of receiving large volumes of intravenous fluids yet are in need of preload expansion.

Contraindications to the Use of Colloid Solutions

Hetastarch and pentastarch are contraindicated in patients with known hypersensitivity to hydroxyethyl starch, coagulopathy, congestive heart failure in which volume overload may pose a problem, or renal disease associated with oliguria or anuria.

Acknowledgment

The author and editors would like to thank Ronald J. Faust, MD, for his work on this chapter in previous editions.

Suggested Readings

Barron M, Wilkes M, Nvickis R. A systematic review of the comparative safety of colloids. *Arch Surg*. 2004;139:552-563.

Bellomo R, Morimatsu H, Presneill J, et al. Effects of saline or albumin resuscitation on standard coagulation tests. *Crit Care Resusc*. 2009;11:250-256.

Finfer S, Bellomo R, Boyce N, et al. A comparison of albumin and saline for fluid resuscitation in the intensive care unit. *N Engl J Med*. 2004;350:2247-2256.

Myburgh JA, Finfer S, Bellomo R, et al. Hydroxyethyl starch or saline for fluid resuscitation in intensive care. *N Engl J Med*. 2012;367:1901-1911.

SAFE Study Investigators; Australian and New Zealand Intensive Care Society Clinical Trials Group; Australian Red Cross Blood Service; et al. Saline or albumin for fluid resuscitation in patients with traumatic brain injury. *N Engl J Med*. 2007;357:874-884.

Soni N. British consensus guidelines on intravenous fluid therapy for adult surgical patients (GIFTASUP): Cassandra's view. *Anaesthesia*. 2009;64:235-238.

Westphal M, James M, Kozek-Langenecker S, et al. Hydroxyethyl starches. *Anesthesiology*. 2009;111:187-202.

Zarychanski R, Abou-Setta AM, Turgeon AF, et al. Association of hydroxyethyl starch administration with mortality and acute kidney injury in critically ill patients requiring volume resuscitation: A systematic review and meta-analysis. *JAMA*. 2013:309:678-688.

CHAPTER 101

Type, Screen, and Crossmatch of Red Blood Cells

Jerry L. Epps, MD, and Robert M. Craft, MD

An ABO-incompatible red blood cell (RBC) transfusion (i.e., transfusion of RBCs with A or B antigens to a recipient with the corresponding antibodies) is fatal in 10% of cases and is the second most common cause of death from transfusion. Therefore, all blood banks routinely type, screen, and crossmatch RBCs (Table 101-1) to attenuate, if not eliminate, transfusion reactions.

Type

The type (group) test determines whether the A, B, and RhD antigens are present on the patient's RBCs. The type test is divided into two steps. In the first step, commercially available antibodies that react with A, B, or RhD antigens are mixed with the patient's RBCs to check for agglutination. A reverse test is then performed by mixing commercially available cells

Table 101-1 Purposes and Preparation of Blood/Blood Product for Transfusion

Procedure	Purpose	Time Required (min)*	Description
Type	ABO RhD determination	5	Patient's RBCs are mixed with commercial anti-A, anti-B, and anti-D antibodies
Screen	Detection of unexpected antibodies	45	Patient's serum is mixed with commercial O RBCs with known antigen panel
Crossmatch	Determination of compatibility between recipient serum and actual blood unit to be transfused	45	Trial transfusion

RBCs, Red blood cells.
*For preparation of 1 unit of blood/blood product.

Table 101-2 Blood Types and Their Frequency in U.S. White Population

Blood Type	Frequency (%)
O Rh$^+$	37
A Rh$^+$	36
B Rh$^+$	9
O Rh$^-$	7
A Rh$^-$	6
AB Rh$^+$	3
B Rh$^-$	2
AB Rh$^-$	1

containing the A or B antigen with the recipient's serum to test for the presence of antibodies to the A or B antigen. This reverse test is based upon the fact that naturally occurring antibodies to the missing ABO antigens are present in virtually everyone. Thus, a type-specific blood designation of AB denotes the presence of both the A and B antigens and the absence of antibodies to these antigens. O Rh$^-$ indicates the absence of the A, B, and RhD antigens, but the likelihood of the presence of the naturally occurring IgM antibodies, anti-A and anti-B, is very high. The anti-D antibody is formed only after exposure to RhD-positive RBCs (during pregnancy and previous blood transfusion). Thus, O Rh$^-$ blood has been called the universal donor type, whereas AB Rh$^+$ is considered to be the universal recipient (Table 101-2).

Screen

The screen test is done to determine whether the recipient has "unexpected" RBC antibodies to the approximately 20 clinically significant RBC antigens found in various groups, such as Rh (C, E, c, e), Diego (Di^a, Di^b, Wr^a), Duffy (Fy^a, Fy^b), MNS (S, s), Kell (K, k, Ku), and Kidd (Jk^a, Jk^b, Jk3). Most unexpected RBC antibodies discovered at screening are either IgG alloantibodies, which develop as the result of previous transfusion of blood products or pregnancy, or naturally occurring clinically cold-reactive IgM antibodies, which are usually clinically insignificant. Commercially available type O cells with the antigens from the blood groups capable of causing hemolytic transfusion reactions are mixed with the plasma from the potential recipient to check for agglutination. If agglutination takes place, then the presence of unexpected antibodies in the recipient's plasma is known and will require additional testing (sometimes several hours in duration) to identify and then locate antigen-negative RBC units for transfusion.

Crossmatch

A crossmatch is performed by computer or serologically to ensure compatibility between the donor's RBCs and the recipient's plasma. If the recipient has not formed unexpected antibodies (i.e., negative antibody screen), then a computer program can be used to electronically match the ABO-RhD type of the recipient with a compatible donor unit, provided the ABO-RhD type has been confirmed twice (on the current sample, by comparison with previous records, on a second current sample, or a second time on the same sample). The computer program must have the inherent logic to issue an RBC unit if the ABO-RhD match between a donor and a recipient is compatible and to reject an incompatible unit. Advantages of computerized crossmatching include more rapid availability of blood for transfusion, decreased workload in the blood bank, increased flexibility in managing blood stores, and decreased waste of blood product.

A serologic crossmatch is required to ensure ABO compatibility if unexpected antibodies are present or in the absence of computer crossmatch technology. The serologic crossmatch is essentially a trial transfusion of the potential donor's RBC unit with the recipient's plasma. This consists of three phases: immediate-spin, incubation, and antiglobulin test. The immediate-spin or first phase rechecks for ABO incompatibility as well as the presence of antibodies to MNS and Lewis group antigens and requires 1 to 5 min to complete. During this incomplete crossmatch, the patient's serum is mixed with the donor's RBCs at room temperature, centrifuged, and then assessed for macroscopic agglutination. In the incubation stage, salt solution or albumin is added to the mixture of recipient plasma and donor RBCs, which are then incubated at 37° C for 10 or 45 min (for salt solution or albumin, respectively). In the incubation stage, antibodies to certain RBC antigens will attach to the specific antigen but will lack the strength to cause agglutination. However, in the third part of the crossmatch (antiglobulin phase), the addition of antiglobulin allows the incomplete recipient antibodies attached to the donor RBC antigens to cause agglutination and, thus, detect recipient antibodies to antigens found in groups such as Duffy, Kell, and Kidd.

Incompatibility Risk and Emergency Transfusion

The most common cause of a fatal hemolytic transfusion reaction (with an occurrence rate of 5.9 to 8.5 per 10 million RBC units in the United States) is a misidentification error in which the wrong unit is given to the patient. The overall incompatibility risk of immediate-spin type-specific blood (ABO compatibility checked twice) is 1 in 1000 if the recipient has never received a transfusion. This risk rises to 1 in 100 if the recipient has previously received a transfusion. Individuals with O Rh$^-$ blood represent only 7% of the population. With blood availability often scarce, the so-called universal donor, O Rh$^-$ blood, is often reserved for RhD-negative women of childbearing age, and O Rh$^-$ packed RBCs are routinely used as the first choice for emergency transfusions.

Because approximately 85% of the population in the United States is RhD$^+$, the use of O Rh$^+$ packed RBCs as an alternative to the traditional O Rh$^-$ "universal donor" blood is appropriate in emergency transfusion if the recipient is not a woman of childbearing age. Packed RBCs are preferred to whole blood to decrease the transfusion of IgM anti-A and anti-B antibodies commonly found in type O serum.

Suggested Readings

Carson J. Red blood cell transfusion: a clinical practice guideline from the AABB*. *Ann Int Med.* 2012;157:49-60

Francini M. Errors in transfusion: Causes and measures to avoid them. *Clin Chem Lab Med.* 2010;48:1075-1077.

Gorgas DL. Transfusion therapy: Blood and blood products. In: Roberts JR, ed. *Clinical Procedures in Emergency Medicine.* 4th ed. Philadelphia: WB Saunders; 2004:513-529.

Wong KF. Virtual blood banking. *Am J Clin Pathol.* 2005;124:124-128.

Yazer MH. The blood bank "black box" debunked: Pretransfusion testing explained. *Can Med Assoc J.* 2006;174:29-32.

CHAPTER 102
Red Blood Cell and Platelet Transfusion

Brian S. Donahue, MD, PhD

Red Blood Cells

Collection, Storage, and Administration

Whole blood is collected as 450-mL aliquots to which 150 mL of an anticoagulant preservative containing citrate, phosphate, and dextrose is added. Red blood cells (RBCs) are then isolated by centrifugation and preserved with 100 mL of a solution consisting of adenine, dextrose, saline, and mannitol. Adenine and dextrose are substrates, respectively, for adenosine triphosphate formation and glycolysis. Adding a phosphate buffer prolongs the viability of the unit to 42 days; the U.S. Food and Drug Administration defines a viable unit as one from which 70% of transfused RBCs are present in the recipient's circulation after 24 h.

During RBC storage, progressive intracellular acidosis, extracellular hyperkalemia, and decreased concentration of intracellular 2,3-diphosphoglycerate (2,3-DPG) levels are observed. Intracellular K^+ levels rise in RBCs shortly after the RBCs are transfused, but intracellular 2,3-DPG levels remain below normal for at least 24 h.

Rare RBC phenotypes are frozen and are stored in glycerol to prevent lysis, better preserving RBC 2,3-DPG levels. Upon thawing, the RBCs are washed in saline to remove the glycerol, which also decreases the leukocyte count and the incidence of febrile reactions. Disadvantages include cost and a short (24-h) expiration time after thawing.

In the past, RBCs were infused through 40-μm to 60-μm line filters to remove microaggregates of RBCs, fibrin, and platelets because these components were thought to cause TRALI (transfusion-related acute lung injury). Filters are not routinely used now because we have a better understanding of the cause of TRALI and because of the use of leukocyte-reduced RBC products, which have fewer microaggregates.

Autologous Blood Transfusion and Directed Transfusion

Autologous donation before a scheduled surgical procedure and transfusion to the patient during surgery has been shown to decrease allogeneic exposure in routine cardiac and orthopedic surgery, but predonation does not always eliminate the need for allogeneic blood. Predonation of autologous blood is not necessarily less expensive than collection and transfusion of allogeneic blood, nor does it completely eliminate the risks of transfusion reactions.

It is controversial as to whether autotransfusion at the site of care, also known as cell salvage, reduces allogeneic transfusions or reduces costs. Typically, allogeneic transfusion requirements are reduced, but the cost of equipment and personnel far exceeds the cost of collecting and transfusing allogeneic RBCs.

Directed donation is the process in which a patient or patient's family selects blood that comes from an identified donor, often a relative of the patient. Interestingly, directed donation may be associated with an increased infection risk because the donor who responds to a request to donate for a specific individual is no longer a volunteer; the individual may feel coerced into donating. Directed donation does not eliminate the risk of alloimmunization or immunomodulation, because this blood is allogeneic, and blood from related donors actually increases the risk of graft-versus-host disease.

Synthetic Hemoglobins

The use of hemoglobin-based O_2 carriers (HBOCs) has been hampered by difficulty in defining meaningful clinical end points, safety parameters, and risk/benefit ratios. All HBOCs rapidly bind nitric oxide, resulting in increased vascular resistance as well as interference with other functions of nitric oxide. Increased levels of inflammatory cytokines, increased platelet reactivity, and decreased organ blood flow are thought to be responsible for the pancreatitis, esophageal spasm, myocardial injury, pulmonary hypertension, and acute lung injury associated with the use of HBOCs. Reactive O_2 species, resulting from free iron release, may mediate renal and central nervous system injury. A recent meta-analysis found a statistically significant increase in death and myocardial infarction associated with the use of HBOC.

Recombinant hemoglobin-based products have the advantages of O_2-binding characteristics more similar to those of native hemoglobin but are unstable in solution, scavenge nitric oxide, and also release free iron into the bloodstream.

Red Blood Cell Transfusion

The sole reason to transfuse RBCs is to increase the content of O_2 in the blood, thereby increasing O_2 delivery ($\dot{D}O_2$), which is a product of hemoglobin concentration, arterial O_2 saturation, and cardiac output (CO, which itself is a product of stroke volume and heart rate). A specific hematocrit value may sustain adequate $\dot{D}O_2$ if CO is adequate but may be insufficient when cardiac output is limited or when arterial saturation is impaired by the presence of a transpulmonary shunt. Therefore, despite the widely accepted hemoglobin trigger of 7 g/dL, the decision to transfuse should take into consideration the current hemoglobin level, estimated blood loss, cardiac reserve, vital signs, the likelihood of ongoing hemorrhage, and the risk of tissue ischemia. The dynamic nature of surgical hemorrhage requires a more aggressive approach to blood replacement in the operating room, compared with sites elsewhere in the hospital. In patients with chronic anemia, increased 2,3-DPG levels make O_2 transport (see Chapter 21) more efficient; in acute anemia, cardiovascular mechanisms of compensation (e.g., increased CO, heart rate, myocardial O_2 consumption) are more important.

Indications for Transfusion of Red Blood Cells

The binding of O_2 to hemoglobin is represented by a sinusoidal relationship known as the oxyhemoglobin dissociation curve, (see Chapter 21), which facilitates efficient O_2 loading of hemoglobin in the lungs (where P_{O_2} is high) and unloading of hemoglobin in the tissues (where P_{O_2} is low). Because the vast majority of O_2 carried in the blood is noncovalently bound to hemoglobin, $\dot{D}O_2$ is the product of CO and O_2 content:

$$\dot{D}O_2 = CO \times C_{aO_2}$$

where O_2 content is calculated as follows:

$$C_{aO_2} = (1.365[Hb] = S_{aO_2}) + (0.0031 \times P_{aO_2})$$

Although otherwise healthy patients can make extraordinary adaptations to maintain $\dot{D}O_2$ and consumption in the face of severe anemia, there is evidence that those with cardiovascular and cerebrovascular disease have limited ability to compensate for acute anemia below hemoglobin levels of 7 to 10 g/dL. Myocardial ischemia is often silent and is not always related to the heart rate and blood pressure. Although medical management (β blockade) is important for most of these patients, anemia could add to their risk of infarction. Furthermore, although serial hemoglobin determinations are helpful intraoperatively, they do not reflect acute changes in intravascular volume and can be misleading. Overexpansion of intravascular volume with colloid or crystalloid can produce a lower hemoglobin level in a hypervolemic patient. Alternatively, inadequate administration of crystalloids or excessive diuresis can lead to a normal or high hemoglobin level in a hypovolemic patient.

A study that examined outcomes in adult patients in the intensive care unit who were randomly assigned to a restrictive transfusion strategy (target hemoglobin 7 g/dL) or a liberal strategy (target hemoglobin 9 g/dL) found no difference in overall mortality rate between the groups and a lower in-hospital mortality rate for the restrictive group in a subgroup of patients with lower APACHE (Acute Physiology, Age, and Chronic Health Evaluation) scores. In addition, myocardial infarction and pulmonary edema were also more frequent in the liberal-strategy group. In patients with coronary disease, transfusion was not associated with improved survival nor were mechanically ventilated patients more likely to be weaned from the ventilator. Similar results have been confirmed in preterm infants.

Platelet Transfusions

Platelet Preparation and Storage

Platelet concentrate is prepared by centrifuging freshly drawn donor blood to separate RBCs from platelet-rich plasma (PRP). The PRP is then transferred to a satellite bag and is recentrifuged at higher revolutions to separate the platelets from the plasma. Each unit of platelet concentrate contains about 50 mL of plasma and approximately 5.5×10^{10} platelets. Platelet concentrate is the preferred source of platelets for transfusion because these platelets provide a more rapid therapeutic effect with less volume, as compared with fresh whole blood or PRP. The platelet count of an adult should increase 5000 to 10,000/μL for each unit of platelet concentrate transfused. Multiple units of platelets can be drawn from a single donor using pheresis techniques. A continuous-flow centrifuge is used to separate platelets from plasma and RBCs. These elements are then returned to the donor. Although this technique is more costly, its advantages include decreased infectious risk and the capability of selecting compatible platelet donors for patients with multiple antiplatelet antibodies. A standard 170-μm filter is recommended for platelet administration to remove microaggregates.

Platelets are stored at room temperature with gentle agitation to minimize aggregation and increase mixing of the platelet concentrate with O_2 passing through the wall of the platelet pack. New plastics introduced in the mid-1980s increased the shelf life of platelet concentrate by allowing better gas transfer to the contained cells. Platelets infused within 24 h of being drawn are viable in the blood for 5 to 7 days. Two time-dependent processes limit the duration of storage for platelets. The first is the increased risk for bacterial contamination. The second is a functional artifact of handling and storage, known as the platelet storage lesion. During their short duration of storage, platelets gradually become activated and lose their ability to aggregate and to adhere to the extracellular matrix in laboratory assays.

Platelet Matching

Platelets are not routinely matched for ABO compatibility because expression of the A and B antigens on platelets is believed to be of either minimal or no significance. However, recent evidence indicates that ABO-incompatible platelet transfusions have decreased efficacy, as compared with those that are ABO-matched. Although platelets do not express Rh antigens, platelet transfusions are matched for Rh compatibility. That is, Rh-positive platelets are administered only to Rh-positive recipients because a small number of RBCs are almost invariably present in platelet concentrates and could, theoretically, alloimmunize an Rh-negative recipient. Despite this theoretical concern, recent studies of Rh-incompatible platelet transfusions have shown that this is probably not a significant risk.

Box 102-1 Indications for Platelet Transfusion

- Prophylactic platelet transfusion is ineffective when thrombocytopenia is due to increased platelet destruction.
- Platelet transfusion is rarely indicated in surgical patients when the platelet count is ≥ 100 × 10^9/L.
- Platelet transfusion is usually indicated when the platelet count is ≤ 50 × 10^9/L.
- The determination of whether patients with intermediate platelet counts (50 to 100 × 10^9/L) require therapy should be based on the risk of bleeding.
- Vaginal deliveries or operative procedures ordinarily associated with insignificant blood loss may be undertaken in patients with platelet counts ≤ 50 × 10^9/L.
- Platelet transfusion may be indicated despite an apparently adequate platelet count if there is known platelet dysfunction and microvascular bleeding.

Indications for Platelet Transfusion

Box 102-1 summarizes the indications for platelet concentrate transfusion listed in the American Society of Anesthesiologists' Guidelines for Perioperative Transfusion Therapy. Patients with abnormal platelet function or thrombocytopenia are likely to benefit from administration of platelet transfusions if the platelet disorder is thought to induce or exacerbate their bleeding. Platelet counts of less than 10 × 10^9/L often occur in patients receiving chemotherapeutic agents. Platelet transfusions are used to prevent spontaneous intracranial and gastrointestinal hemorrhages in these patients.

For major surgical procedures in thrombocytopenic patients, it is desirable to increase the platelet count to 50 × 10^9/L to 100 × 10^9/L, and prophylactic administration of platelet transfusions is indicated. Platelet transfusion is not indicated simply to increase platelet counts in patients who are neither bleeding nor about to undergo interventional procedures. Patients with immune thrombocytopenic purpura should not receive platelet transfusions unless they have life-threatening bleeding. These patients produce autoantibodies that react against all human platelets, and, thus, they derive little to no benefit from a platelet transfusion.

Following cardiopulmonary bypass, most patients develop both thrombocytopenia and a functional platelet impairment. Although the correlation between platelet counts and the extent of bleeding in these patients is poor, transfusing based on algorithms using platelet count as an indication for platelet transfusion reduces the number of platelets actually used.

Functional platelet disorders are encountered less frequently than is thrombocytopenia. In addition to cardiopulmonary bypass, uremia, liver disease, myeloproliferative disorders, and dysproteinemias can cause acquired functional platelet disorders. Drugs that affect cyclooxygenase (aspirin, nonsteroidal anti-inflammatory drugs), theophyllines, tricyclic antidepressants, anesthetic agents (especially halothane), and some antibiotics cause functional platelet disorders that may or may not become clinically significant. Inherited functional platelet disorders include Glanzmann thrombasthenia, Bernard-Soulier syndrome, gray platelet syndrome, and dense granule deficiency syndrome.

Risks of Platelet Transfusion

Platelet Alloimmunization and Platelet Refractoriness

Platelets have dozens of known proteins on their surfaces, and polymorphic variants have been identified in almost all of these proteins. Platelets also express HLA antigens. As a result, platelets from nonidentical donors are antigenic, and 24 immunologic platelet-specific antigens have been defined serologically. Sensitization to platelet antigens is common in patients who have received multiple platelet transfusions. Patients who are sensitized to these antigens or to HLA antigens will rapidly destroy transfused platelets, decreasing the therapeutic effectiveness of the platelet transfusion. In sensitized patients, only type-specific matched platelets are effective. Leukodepletion has been shown to be effective in reducing the incidence of platelet alloimmunization.

Other Risks of Platelet Transfusion

The other major risks associated with platelet transfusion overlap with the risks associated with the transfusion of RBCs: febrile transfusion reactions, allergic reactions, and transmission of infectious disease. Although platelet concentrates are drawn from single donors, many units are usually given at a time, increasing the risk of complications. Platelet transfusions also contain more donor plasma and are more likely to cause lung injury. Bacteria can proliferate in platelet concentrates because they are stored at room temperature; they are often implicated in septic transfusion reactions (see Chapter 104).

Suggested Readings

American Society of Anesthesiologists Task Force on Perioperative Blood Transfusion and Adjuvant Therapies. Practice guidelines for perioperative blood transfusion and adjuvant therapies: An updated report by the American Society of Anesthesiologists Task Force on Perioperative Blood Transfusion and Adjuvant Therapies. *Anesthesiology*. 2006;105:198-208.

Chockalingam P, Sacher RA. Management of patients refractory to platelet transfusion. *J Infus Nurs*. 2007;30:220-225.

Davies L, Brown TJ, Haynes S, et al. Cost-effectiveness of cell salvage and alternative methods of minimizing perioperative allogeneic blood transfusion: A systematic review and economic model. *Health Technol Assess*. 2006;10:1-210.

McMillan D, Dando H, Potger K, et al. Intra-operative autologous blood management. *Transfusion Apheresis Sci*. 2002;27:73-81.

Slichter SJ. Evidence-based platelet transfusion guidelines. *Hematol Am Soc Hematol Educ Program*. 2007:172-178.

Stafford-Smith M, Waters J, et al. The International consortium for evidence based perfusion. 2011 the update to the Society of Thoracic Surgeons and the Society of Cardiovascular Anesthesiologists blood conservation clinical practice guidelines. *Ann Thorac Surg*. 2011;91:944-982.

CHAPTER 103
Massive Transfusion

Wolf H. Stapelfeldt, MD

Transfusion of the equivalent of more than 10 to 12 units of blood may be necessary to maintain a patient's hemoglobin concentration within the guidelines promulgated by the American Society of Anesthesiologists. Accordingly, red blood cell (RBC) transfusion is almost always advocated if the patient's hemoglobin concentration is less than 6 g/dL and is recommended if the hemoglobin concentration is less than 10 g/dL if a patient's compensatory capacity for maintaining O_2 delivery may be compromised (such as in the presence of coronary artery disease) and causes a diminished ability to increase cardiac output and affect blood flow redistribution sufficient to meet metabolic needs. Ongoing blood loss may be due to surgical bleeding, disease-induced or drug-induced coagulopathy, or very often a combination of these factors. Causes for bleeding diatheses include inherited coagulopathies (hemophilias A, B, and C; platelet disorders such as idiopathic thrombocytopenic purpura, Glanzmann thrombasthenia, von Willebrand disease, or Bernard-Soulier syndrome; or vascular disorders such as Ehlers-Danlos syndrome); comorbid conditions (liver disease, disseminated intravascular coagulopathy, or uremia); the effects of anticoagulant drugs (warfarin, heparin, fibrinolytic or antiplatelet medications); drug-induced thrombocytopenia (heparin-induced thrombocytopenia [in 5% of patients this occurs within 5 days of institution of treatment]); or platelet dysfunction. Lastly, coagulopathy commonly develops over the course of massive transfusions. Although some patients may fare well and may be extubated as early as in the operating room—providing that homeostasis has been effectively maintained (hemodynamic stability, adequate oxygenation and hemoglobin concentration, normal acid-base status, electrolyte balance, normal coagulation status, good urine output, stable core temperature) and the underlying problem successfully addressed (such as in liver transplantation), patients requiring massive transfusion are typically at an increased risk of morbidity and mortality due to a variety of intraoperative and postoperative complications.

Intraoperative Complications

Transfusion reactions range from minor allergic or febrile responses, which occur in approximately 1% of blood product transfusions, to often lethal acute hemolytic reactions caused by the administration of ABO incompatible RBCs or fresh frozen plasma (FFP) in up to 1 in 12,000 transfusions, the major cause of intraoperative death. Ten times less frequent are delayed hemolytic responses, which only become apparent postoperatively (after days to weeks). Hemolytic reactions need to be expected in approximately 1 of every 1000 emergency transfusions of RBCs or FFP that have not been crossmatched and in 1 of every 100 transfusions in patients who have been pregnant or have been previously transfused. Other reactions include anaphylactic (in patients with hereditary IgA deficiency) or anaphylactoid reactions, which are another rare cause of intraoperative

Box 103-1 Causes of Disseminated Intravascular Coagulopathy

Sepsis (gram-positive or gram-negative organisms)
Viremias
Obstetric conditions
- Amniotic fluid embolism
- Fetal death in utero
- Abruptio placentae
- Preeclampsia

Extensive tissue damage
- Burns
- Trauma

Liver failure
Extensive cerebral injury
- Head injury
- Cerebrovascular injury

Extensive endothelial damage
- Vasculitis

Hemolytic transfusion reaction
Metastatic malignancies
Leukemia
Snake venoms

death (1 in 25,000 to 1 in 50,000). More common, and the most important cause of postoperative death, is transfusion-related acute lung injury (TRALI) in response to RBC, FFP, or platelet transfusion, presumably due to antibodies contained in the donor plasma. The treatment of acute transfusion reactions includes immediate discontinuation of the transfusion, pharmacologic support of the circulation if necessary, and alkalinization of the urine to prevent the precipitation of hematin and red blood cell stroma in renal tubules, depending on the degree of hemolysis. Coagulopathy often ensues, either as part of the primary underlying pathophysiology or iatrogenically as a consequence of volume resuscitation. The former includes hepatic disease (clotting factor deficiency, thrombocytopenia, primary fibrinolysis) or clinical conditions associated with disseminated intravascular coagulopathy and resulting secondary fibrinolysis (Box 103-1), including hypotension and tissue hypoxia. Dilutional coagulopathy may result from iatrogenic dilution of circulating clotting factors to less than 20% to 30% of normal (usually after loss of approximately 1.5 blood volumes) or thrombocytopenia (after loss of 2-3 blood volumes). Hypothermic coagulopathy may be manifested by an approximately 50% prolongation of the actual temperature-adjusted prothrombin time (PT), partial thromboplastin time (PTT), or thromboelastogram (TEG) reaction times, as well as hypothermic thrombocytopenia. Treatment of coagulopathy should not be prophylactic but, instead, should be specifically directed as indicated by results of coagulation tests in patients exhibiting clinically significant coagulopathy (continuous oozing lack of clot formation severe hemorrhage). The therapeutic options are discussed later.

Hypotension may result from intravascular hypovolemia, decreased blood viscosity (low hematocrit), or diminished vascular tone caused by vasodilatory mediators, such as bradykinin (particularly in the presence of angiotensin-converting enzyme inhibitors) or ionized hypocalcemia (see following discussion). The treatment goals include maintenance of intravascular normovolemia, normal cardiac output, and a sufficient systemic vascular resistance to maintain a mean arterial pressure adequate to preserve vital organ perfusion. The latter may require the use of α-adrenergic agonists, vasopressin, calcium chloride, or a combination thereof.

Hypothermia predictably develops if fluids (room temperature) or blood products (4°C) are administered without being warmed. Other contributing conditions may include hepatic failure or severe splanchnic hypoperfusion, compromising the approximate 20% contribution of hepatic metabolic activity to normal heat production. Preventive (and corrective) means to treat severe hypothermia include the use of fluid warmers, convective heating blankets, warm irrigation of open body cavities (abdomen), and raising the ambient temperature in the operating room.

Tissue hypoxia may be caused by hemorrhagic or septic shock and may be further exacerbated by a left shift of the oxyhemoglobin dissociation curve due to the decreased 2,3-phosphodiglycerate (DPG) content of transfused RBCs, subnormal (core or regional tissue) temperature, or both. Therapeutic goals are to maintain tissue oxygenation by supporting the circulation (normovolemia, normal to increased cardiac output) while maintaining an adequate blood O_2 content (hematocrit and O_2 saturation) and preventing or treating severe hypothermia.

Metabolic acidemia may progressively develop as a consequence of tissue hypoxia in conjunction with the continued exogenous administration of fluids and blood components with a less than physiologic pH (normal saline, pH 5.5; packed RBCs, pH 6.5), particularly in the presence of abnormal hepatic (liver disease, splanchnic hypoperfusion) or renal function. Treatment options are identical to those aimed at correcting tissue hypoxia. Severe acidemia (pH < 7.1) may require the administration of sodium bicarbonate to maintain or restore sufficient efficacy of endogenously released or exogenously administrated catecholamines.

Hyperkalemia may occur with rapid infusion of packed RBCs (K^+ > 20 mEq/L) if infused at a rate exceeding 90 to 120 mL/min, especially in the context of worsening metabolic acidemia and less than normal renal function (chronic renal insufficiency, acute renal failure, hepatorenal syndrome). It may manifest itself as a prolonged PR interval, widened QRS complex, and peaked T waves on the electrocardiogram and warrant treatment with hyperventilation; administration of calcium chloride, sodium bicarbonate, β-adrenergic agonists, glucose, or insulin; or a combination of several of these therapies. Refractory hyperkalemia may require venovenous hemofiltration or intraoperative hemodialysis.

Hypocalcemia may result from the reaction of the patient's ionized calcium with sodium citrate contained in whole blood, packed RBCs, or FFP (if transfused at a rate exceeding 1 unit every 5 min). Clinical signs include hypotension and narrow pulse pressure, as well as elevated left ventricular end-diastolic pressure and central venous pressure. The electrocardiogram may exhibit a widened QRS complex, prolonged QT interval, or flattened T wave. Hypomagnesemia may cause ectopic rhythms and pose an increased risk for the development of ventricular tachycardia or fibrillation, including torsades de pointes. Both electrolyte abnormalities are treated by correcting their plasma concentrations with the administration of calcium chloride or magnesium chloride, respectively.

Postoperative Complications

Patients receiving massive transfusions are at an elevated risk for developing a number of complications attributable to the administration of blood products. Major causes of postoperative death include sepsis due to bacterial infection of blood products, particularly of platelets, which are stored at room temperature prior to transfusion. This risk is greatly diminished by the routine use of leukocyte reduction filters, a use that is becoming the recommended standard. Millipore filters (40 μm) are used to prevent microaggregate injury caused by cell-saver blood. TRALI may be diagnosed in the postoperative period as a cause of persisting noncardiogenic pulmonary edema and may be associated with 5% to 8% mortality rate, the leading cause of transfusion-related death. The age of donor erythrocytes greater than 2 weeks has been inculpated as a possible cause for increased risk of postoperative morbidity and death. Lastly, despite significant risk reductions due to improved testing and donor selection, viral infection remains a small but persistent threat following the transfusion of blood products (hepatitis B in 1:350,000; hepatitis C in 1:2 million; human immunodeficiency virus in 1:2 million; human T-lymphotropic virus type I in 1:2.9 million). The risk of transmission of cytomegalovirus (present in donor leukocytes) to cytomegalovirus-negative immune-compromised recipients is reduced by the use of leukocyte-reduction filters, single-donor apheresis, or platelet irradiation.

Treatment of Coagulopathy

In an effort to minimize transfusion risks, the administration of blood products should not be prophylactic but only as specifically indicated by the results of coagulation tests in symptomatic patients. Commonly used tests include PT, PTT, activated coagulation time, platelet count, fibrinogen, fibrin split products, D-dimers (elevated in disseminated intravascular coagulation [DIC], not primary fibrinolysis), and the TEG. Additional tests are available for special circumstances, such as platelet function tests (platelet dysfunction), reptilase time (patients on heparin), ecarin clotting time (patients on direct thrombin inhibitors), or specific clotting factor assays (isolated factor deficiencies).

FFP (increased PT, TEG reaction [R] time), platelets (low platelet count; TEG maximum amplitude [MA] < 50), or cryoprecipitate (low fibrinogen; low factor VIII, factor XIII, or von Willebrand factor [vWF]) may be administered as specifically indicated. Available adjunct treatment modalities not associated with the risk of blood product transfusions include desmopressin (DDAVP) (to treat von Willebrand disease types 1 and 2A; platelet dysfunction due to antiplatelet medications, ethanol, or uremia; mild hemophilia A); recombinant factor VIIa (to treat factor VII deficiency and to promote thrombin formation independent of the intrinsic pathway boost and in the absence of disseminated intravascular coagulopathy or antifibrinolytic treatment); serine protease enzyme inhibitors (to treat primary, but not secondary, fibrinolysis; to prevent cardiopulmonary bypass–induced platelet dysfunction) and protamine (to treat heparin-caused increase in activated coagulation time, PTT, or heparinase-sensitive TEG R time). An example of a diagnostic and treatment algorithm used for the management of coagulopathy encountered during liver transplantation in over 1200 patients is shown in Figure 103-1.

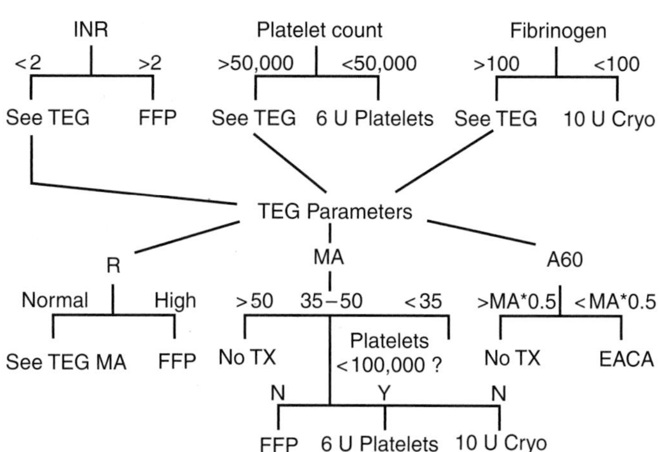

Figure 103-1 Algorithm for the perioperative assessment and treatment of coagulation abnormalities in patients undergoing orthotopic liver transplantation. A60, TEG amplitude 60 min after the time of MA; Cryo, cryoprecipitate; EACA, ϵ-aminocaproic acid; FFP, fresh frozen plasma; MA, TEG maximal amplitude; R, TEG reaction time; TEG, thromboelastrogram; TX, treatment. (Adapted from Stapelfeldt WH. Liver, kidney and pancreas transplantation. In: Murray MJ, Coursin DB, Pearl RG, Prough DS, eds. Critical Care Medicine: Perioperative Management. 2nd ed. Philadelphia, Lippincott, Williams & Wilkins, 2002.)

Suggested Readings

American Society of Anesthesiologists Task Force on Perioperative Blood Transfusion and Adjuvant Therapies. Practice guidelines for perioperative blood transfusion and adjuvant therapies: an updated report by the American Society of Anesthesiologists Task Force on Perioperative Blood Transfusion and Adjuvant Therapies. *Anesthesiology*. 2006;105:198-208.

Cohen B, Matot I. Aged erythrocytes: a fine wine or sour grapes? *Br J Anaesth*. 2013;111:i62-i70.

Koch CG, Li L, Sessler DI, et al. Duration of red-cell storage and complications after cardiac surgery. *N Engl J Med*. 2008;20:1229-1239.

Pham HP, Shaz BH. Update on massive transfusion. *Br J Anaesth*. 2013;111: i71-i82.

Sihler KC, Napolitano LM. Massive transfusion: new insights. *Chest*. 2009; 136:1654-1667.

Spahn DR, Ganter MT. Towards early individual goal-directed coagulation management in trauma patients. *Br J Anaesth*. 2010;105:103-105.

CHAPTER 104
Hemolytic Transfusion Reactions

Kip D. Robinson, MD, and Robert M. Craft, MD

Allogeneic blood transfusions are associated with well-known risks. Over the past decade, nucleic acid testing of blood products has significantly reduced the risk of transfusion-transmitted infections. Therefore, noninfectious serious hazards of transfusions have become a more prominent concern (Box 104-1). In a 10-year study in New York, the U.S. Food and Drug Administration (FDA) reported that death rates due to hemolytic transfusion reactions were more than double the rate of all combined infectious transmissions. Hemolytic transfusion reaction, transfusion-related lung injury, and transfusion-associated sepsis make up the majority of transfusion-related deaths. Of the transfusion-related deaths in the United States reported to the FDA between 2005 and 2007, 55% were attributed to transfusion-related lung injury, 21% to hemolytic transfusion reactions, and 8% to transfusion-associated

Box 104-1 Noninfectious Serious Hazards of Transfusion

Immune-Mediated Hazards	Non–Immune-Mediated Hazards
Hemolytic transfusion reaction*	Septic transfusion reaction
Febrile nonhemolytic transfusion reaction	Nonimmune hemolysis
Allergic/urticarial/anaphylactic transfusion reaction	Mistransfusion
TRALI	Transfusion-associated circulatory overload
TA-GVHD	Metabolic derangements
Microchimerism	Coagulopathic complications from massive transfusion
Alloimmunization	Complications from red cell storage lesions
	Overtransfusion
	Undertransfusion
	Iron overload

*Acute or delayed.
TA-GVHD, Transfusion-associated graft versus host disease; TRALI, transfusion-related acute lung injury.

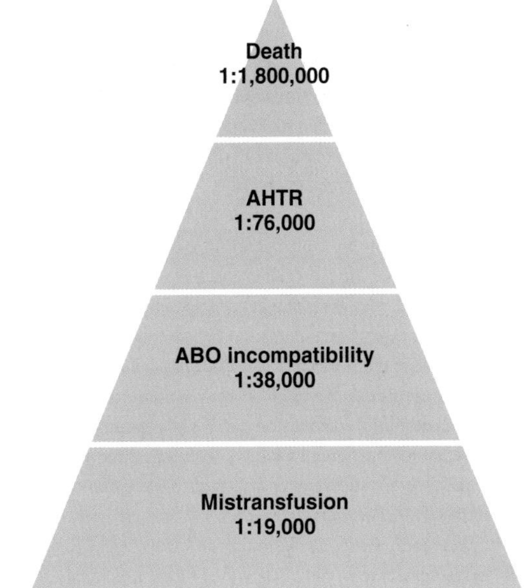

Figure 104-1 The risk of mistransfusion and the subsequent risks of ABO incompatibility, acute hemolytic transfusion reaction (AHTR), and death from the mistransfusion, as reported in the results of a 10-year study in New York State (Linden and associates, 2000). The risk is consistent with data from European hemovigilance databases.

sepsis. Whereas transfusion-related lung injury carries its greatest risk with the transfusion of products containing plasma (most commonly, fresh frozen plasma), the risk of developing transfusion-associated sepsis is highest during the transfusion of platelets (since March 2004, deaths from transfusion-associated sepsis have been cut in half by introduction of bacterial detection methods of apheresis platelets). Hemolytic transfusion reactions are most often seen in patients receiving red blood cells (RBCs).

Pathophysiology

Hemolytic transfusion reactions can be classified as acute hemolytic transfusion reactions (AHTRs) and delayed hemolytic transfusion reactions. An immune-mediated response to transfusion of blood products incompatible with the recipient's blood is the mechanism for the hemolytic transfusion reaction. The sequelae of incorrect blood component transfusion can be innocuous, mildly symptomatic, life threatening, or fatal (Figure 104-1). The severity of the reaction depends on the amount of the antigen transfused and the intensity of complement activation and cytokine release in response to the transfused antigen.

AHTRs occur primarily with mistransfusion or incorrect blood component transfusion. This mistake is typically a clerical or administrative error and, when found, suggests the importance of tracking the error. Because patients and blood components are often matched in pairs, a mismatched unit should suggest the possibility of a second patient at risk for also developing an AHTR. An overwhelming majority of these reactions have been due to incompatible RBC transfusion. There are reported cases, however, of hemolysis due to incompatible plasma. These rare cases usually involve the administration of group O platelets to patients who are not group O.

Antibodies present in the recipient recognize foreign antigens on the surface of donor cells. Most often this is due to ABO incompatibility (preformed IgM anti-A, anti-B), but complement-fixing IgG alloantibodies, such as anti-P, anti-Vel, Lewis, Kidd (anti-Jk^a, anti-Jk^b) and Kell (anti-K1), have also been implicated. Activation of complement causes rapid destruction of the transfused cells. Intravascular hemolysis is a distinctive characteristic of ABO-incompatible transfusion. Complement activation also promotes production and release of inflammatory cytokines, interleukins, anaphylatoxins, histamine, bradykinin, and vasoactive amines.

Delayed hemolytic transfusion reactions occur between 3 and 10 days after the transfusion. They can occur as a slower developing primary immune response but are typically an anamnestic response after reexposure to antigens previously encountered during prior transfusion, pregnancy, or transplantation. These circulating antibodies are at undetectable levels and rapidly increase after antigen reexposure. Antigens frequently implicated include anti-D (Rh), Duffy (Fy^a), and Kidd (Jk^a). IgG antibody-coated cells are marked for destruction by phagocytic cells in the spleen and other areas of the reticuloendothelial system. This extravascular hemolysis results in mild jaundice (elevated unconjugated bilirubin levels), increased reticulocytosis, and spherocytosis. Patients such as those with sickle cell disease who require frequent transfusions are at particular risk for developing delayed hemolytic transfusion reactions. A hemolytic transfusion reaction can often precipitate sickle cell crisis. Additional measures, including extended RBC antigen phenotyping prior to initiating transfusion therapy, can significantly reduce this risk.

Signs and Symptoms

Signs and symptoms of AHTR can be seen in Box 104-2. The classic triad of fever, flank pain, and red-brown urine is rarely seen. Unfortunately, signs and symptoms are nonspecific, and many are masked by general anesthesia, leaving a definitive diagnosis difficult to make in a timely manner. During general anesthesia, fever, hypotension, tachycardia, hemoglobinuria, and diffuse bleeding are the best clues. If these signs occur after a blood transfusion has been initiated, AHTR should be suspected.

Complications

Inflammatory cytokines, histamines, bradykinin, vasoactive amines, and anaphylatoxins are generated during the complement activation process. Fever, wheezing, hypotension, and disseminated intravascular coagulation

Box 104-2 Signs and Symptoms of Acute Hemolytic Transfusion Reaction

Chest, back, or abdominal pain	Hypotension
Chills or rigors	Nausea/vomiting
Diffuse bleeding	Pain at infusion site
Dyspnea	Oliguria or anuria
Fever	Sense of impending doom
Hemoglobinuria	

(DIC) can occur as a result, leading to shock, renal failure, respiratory failure, and death. Renal failure is a result of acute tubular necrosis, initially thought to be predominantly due to tubular damage from circulating free hemoglobin. Both free hemoglobin and antibody-coated RBC stroma have renal vasoconstricting properties. Ischemic renal failure is a result of renal vasoconstriction and systemic hypotension. Tissue factor released from hemolyzed RBCs can be a trigger for DIC.

Prevention

Primary prevention of hemolytic transfusion reactions begins with avoiding unnecessary allogeneic blood transfusion. Use of cell-salvaging devices and avoidance of unnecessary transfusion will reduce patient risk. Information systems and transfusion protocols have significantly reduced clerical error, thereby reducing mistransfusion and ABO-incompatible allogeneic blood transfusion. Machine-readable blood component containers and multiple patient identifiers, including a unique blood-band number attached to the patient, further reduce the risk of clerical error. Between 1976 and 1985, there were 158 AHTR-related deaths reported to the FDA. Mortality risk from AHTR was estimated at 1:250,000 units transfused. With current preventive measures, the risk of death is now estimated to be approximately 1:1.8 million units transfused.

Treatment

The treatment of hemolytic transfusion reactions is supportive. Due to nonspecific signs and symptoms, vigilance and a high index of suspicion are critical in identifying an AHRT. Treatment for AHTR is outlined in Box 104-3. Transfusion should immediately cease. Supportive care should target the goals of maintaining systemic perfusion, preserving renal function, and preventing DIC. Appropriate component therapy should be given if DIC manifests. The patient and blood-product containers should be reidentified, and remaining blood product should be returned to the blood bank. Blood and urine samples should be sent to the laboratory for analysis, to include repeat crossmatch. Hemoglobinuria, hemoglobinemia, and elevated indirect bilirubin concentration are evidence of hemolysis but are nonspecific and can be seen with nonimmune mechanisms of hemolysis (mechanical, thermal, osmotic, drug related). The direct antiglobin test, also known as the direct Coombs test, is the definitive test to verify an immune-mediated hemolytic process.

Box 104-3 Treatment for Acute Hemolytic Transfusion Reaction

1. Stop blood transfusion
2. Identify patient and blood labeling for error in compatibility
3. Return any unused blood product to blood bank
4. Maintain systemic blood pressure
   a. Maintain volume
   b. Administer vasopressor as needed
   c. Administer inotropes; consider using mannitol, furosemide, or both
5. Preserve renal function
   a. Promote urine output >1 mL·kg^{-1}·h^{-1}
   b. Maintain renal perfusion
   c. Maintain volume
   d. Administer diuretics
   e. Consider alkalizing urine; administer sodium bicarbonate
6. Prevent DIC
   a. Maintain cardiac output
   b. Prevent hypotension
   c. Administer appropriate component therapy if DIC manifests
7. Obtain blood and urine samples
   a. Repeat blood type and crossmatch
   b. Perform DAT
   c. Measure serum haptoglobin concentration
   d. Measure plasma and urine concentrations of free hemoglobin
   e. Measure bilirubin concentration
   f. Perform baseline coagulation tests (prothrombin time, partial thromboplastin time, and fibrinogen and fibrinogen split products concentrations) and monitor for change
   g. Briefly centrifuge the blood sample, a simple rapid test to detect hemolysis
   h. Monitor renal function; studies include blood urea nitrogen and creatinine concentrations

DAT, Direct antiglobin test, also known as the direct Coombs test; DIC, disseminated intravascular coagulopathy.

Suggested Readings

Eder AF, Chambers LA. Noninfectious complications of blood transfusion. *Arch Pathol Lab Med*. 2007;131:708-718.

Hendrickson JE, Hillyer CD. Noninfectious serious hazards of transfusion. *Anesth Analg*. 2009;108:759-769.

Linden JV, Wagner K, Voytovich AE, et al. Transfusion errors in New York state: An analysis of 10 years' experience. *Transfusion*. 2000;40:1207-1213.

Stainsby D, Jones H, Asher D, et al. Serious hazards of transfusion: A decade of hemovigilance in the UK. *Transfusion Med Rev*. 2006;20:273-282.

Stainsby D, Jones H, Wells AW, et al. Adverse outcomes of blood transfusion in children: Analysis of UK reports to the serious hazards of transfusion scheme 1996-2005. *Br J Haematol*. 2008;141:73-79.

Vamvakas EC, Blajchman MA. Transfusion-related mortality: The ongoing risks of allogeneic blood transfusion and the available strategies for their prevention. *Blood*. 2009;113:3406-3417.

Wu YY, Mantha S, Snyder EL. Transfusion reactions. In: Hoffman R, Benz E, Shattli S, et al, eds. *Hematology: Basic Principles and Practice*. 5th ed. Philadelphia: Churchill Livingstone; 2008:2267-2276.

CHAPTER 105

Nonhemolytic Transfusion Reactions

C. Thomas Wass, MD

Febrile Reactions

Nonhemolytic transfusion reactions (NHTRs) often occur in patients receiving blood product transfusions. Fever is the most common NHTR, with a median frequency of 4%. Fever, defined as an increase in body temperature of 1°C or more during or within several hours of transfusion, usually persists for less than 12 h, is most often associated with transfusion of cellular components (e.g., red blood cells, platelets, and granulocytes), but has also been observed with transfusion of noncellular components (e.g., fresh frozen plasma or cryoprecipitate). Although the etiology has yet to be fully elucidated, it is hypothesized that recipient *alloimmunization* (i.e., antibody production in response to a previous transfusion or pregnancy) toward donor white blood cells or platelets triggers release of leukocyte-derived or platelet-derived pyrogenic cytokines (e.g., IL-1β, IL-6, IL-8, TNF-α, CD40L) that increase the hypothalamic thermoregulatory set point. Alternatively, fever may occur in response to direct transfusion of pyrogenic cytokines or other inflammatory mediators that accumulate during storage of blood products such that the greater the interval between collection and transfusion, the higher the frequency of febrile NHTR. However, prestorage leukocyte reduction (e.g., using leukocyte filtration techniques) mitigates transfusion-related fever.

Should the patient develop a fever while receiving a transfusion, the transfusion must be discontinued or slowed. Bacterial contamination (diagnosed via Gram stain and cultures) and hemolytic transfusion reaction (diagnosed via repeat crossmatch and direct Coombs test, which detects antibody to transfused donor red blood cells) should be ruled out. Antipyretic drugs (e.g., acetaminophen) may be used prophylactically or to treat febrile NHTRs; however, these medications may not prevent associated symptoms (e.g., chills, rigor, soreness at the transfusion site, headache, nausea, myalgia, chest tightness).

Mild Allergic Reactions

Mild allergic reactions are the second most common NHTR, occurring with a frequency of 0.5%. Signs and symptoms are usually mild and include urticarial rash and generalized pruritus as a result of IgE-mediated histamine release from degranulated mast cells and basophils in response to foreign substances (e.g., transfused plasma proteins) found in any plasma-containing blood products (especially platelets and fresh frozen plasma). Patients who do not show signs of having an anaphylactic reaction should be treated symptomatically with diphenhydramine, and the transfusion may be continued.

Anaphylactic Reactions

Anaphylaxis, which represents the most severe form of NHTR, occurs in 1 in 20,000 to 1 in 50,000 transfusions. Patients experiencing these reactions typically have hereditary IgA deficiency, which is relatively common (1 in 700 persons). During exposure to "foreign" IgA from a previous transfusion or pregnancy, patients become alloimmunized (i.e., recipients develop IgE directed against donor IgA). IgE elicits an immune response by binding to Fc receptors on the surface of mast cells and basophils, resulting in degranulation and release of vasoactive mediators (e.g., histamine, leukotrienes, and prostaglandins). Transfusion of any plasma-containing blood product may result in an anaphylactic response. Signs, symptoms, and treatment do not differ from those of other anaphylactic reactions.

The diagnosis of an anaphylactic transfusion reaction requires quantitative confirmation of IgA deficiency and the presence of anti-IgA in recipient plasma. Levels of serum β-tryptase, a marker for mast cell degranulation, may be measured. However, these laboratory studies are often time consuming and may not be readily available. Thus, once a diagnosis of anaphylactic transfusion reaction is suspected, the transfusion should be stopped immediately. If blood transfusion must be continued, IgA-deficient blood products (e.g., blood from donors known to be IgA deficient or washed or deglycerolized red blood cells) should be used.

Both mild allergic and IgA anaphylactic reactions usually begin within 45 min after blood transfusion is started but may be delayed for as long as 1 to 3 h. Shorter onset times tend to be associated with more severe reactions.

Transfusion-Related Acute Lung Injury

Pulmonary edema following blood transfusion is often attributed to intravascular volume overload that overwhelms myocardial Frank-Starling forces (i.e., cardiogenic pulmonary edema). In contrast, transfusion-related acute lung injury (TRALI) is a noncardiogenic form of pulmonary edema that is difficult to distinguish from acute respiratory distress syndrome or other causes of acute lung injury. TRALI, a diagnosis of exclusion, usually occurs within 1 to 6 h of blood product transfusion and is characterized by acute respiratory distress, radiograph evidence of bilateral pulmonary edema, severe hypoxemia ($Pa_{O_2}/F_{I_{O_2}} < 300$ mm Hg), and no evidence of a cardiogenic cause. TRALI is likely underdiagnosed and underreported; however, it is estimated to occur in 1 in 5000 patients who receive a transfusion.

The pathogenesis of TRALI is incompletely understood but is likely multifactorial. In 65% to 90% of patients who develop TRALI, white blood cell (including class I and II HLA or neutrophil-specific) antibodies that bind recipient white blood cell antigens can be identified in donor plasma. When white blood cell antibodies are not present in the donor's serum, another explanation for the development of TRALI may be the two-hit theory—an initial insult (e.g., infection, surgery, or trauma) attracts and "primes" neutrophils that adhere to pulmonary vascular endothelium. A subsequent "activating stimulus" (e.g., transfusion of plasma containing biologically active mediators) causes these marginated neutrophils to release oxidases, O_2 free-radical species, and proteases, resulting in endothelial damage and extravasation of intravascular fluid into lung parenchyma.

Transfusion of any blood product containing plasma can cause TRALI. Interestingly, the vast majority of implicated donors are multiparous women who have been alloimmunized to paternal HLA antigens (reported to occur in up to 25% women with more than three pregnancies). Thus, some centers restrict the use of fresh frozen plasma donated by multiparous women. Treatment is supportive, and depending on the severity of TRALI, the patient may require tracheal intubation, oxygenation, and mechanical ventilation.

With a mortality rate approaching 10%, TRALI is the leading cause of transfusion-related death in the United States. However, most patients with TRALI improve clinically, physiologically, and radiographically within 48 to 96 h.

Immunomodulation

Blood transfusion can significantly improve (in a dose-dependent manner) allograft survival following renal transplantation, yet it worsens tumor recurrence and mortality rate following resection of many cancers (e.g., breast, colorectal, gastric, head and neck, hepatocellular, lung, prostate, renal, soft tissue sarcoma) when compared with patients who do not receive transfusions or individuals who receive leukocyte-reduced blood transfusions. In either case, alterations in patient outcome have been attributed to transfusion-mediated immunomodulation, referred to as a "tolerogenic effect." Such an effect may be due to upregulation of humoral immunity (i.e., B-cell function and antibody production), down regulation of cell-mediated immunity (i.e., T-cell function), or both.

Despite improved renal allograft survival in transfused transplant recipients, routine perioperative blood transfusion is not indicated because of the effectiveness and safety of immunosuppressant drugs (e.g., cyclosporine) and concerns about transfusion-related infection.

Suggested Readings

Blumberg N, Heal JM. Immunomodulation by transfusion. In: Speiss BD, ed. *Perioperative Transfusion Medicine*. 2nd ed. Philadelphia: Lippincott, Williams & Wilkins, 2006:151-167.

Pomper GJ. Febrile, allergic, and nonimmune transfusion reactions. In: Simon TL, ed. *Rossi's Principles of Transfusion Medicine*. Oxford, UK: Wiley-Blackwell, 2009:826-846.

Shulman IA, Shander A. Serious acute transfusion reactions. In: Speiss BD, ed. *Perioperative Transfusion Medicine*. Philadelphia: Lippincott, Williams & Wilkins, 2006:169-175.

Vamvakas EC, Blajchman MA. Transfusion-related mortality: The ongoing risks of allogeneic blood transfusion and the available strategies for their prevention. *Blood*. 2009;113:3406-3417.

SECTION VIII Preoperative and Postoperative Issues

CHAPTER 106

Preoperative Evaluation of the Patient with Cardiac Disease for Noncardiac Operations

Harish Ramakrishna, MD, FASE

Cardiovascular disease is one of the leading causes of death worldwide and the chief cause of death in the United States. Cardiac complications following noncardiac operations account for the majority of the morbidity and mortality risks in the perioperative period, with incidences ranging from 1.5% in the unselected population to 4% in patients at risk for, or with cardiovascular disease, to as high as 11% in patients with multiple risk factors. The key role of the anesthesiologist as perioperative physician when confronted with the patient with cardiovascular disease for a noncardiac operation is to effectively identify patients with modifiable conditions and those at risk for experiencing cardiac events in the perioperative period. The risk stratification that follows is the basis for safe perioperative management of patients with cardiovascular disease. The key issues that need to be addressed are based on the American College of Cardiology/American Heart Association (ACC/AHA) Guidelines on Perioperative Cardiovascular Evaluation for Noncardiac Surgery. The revised guidelines also include recommendations for the management of patients with coronary artery stents and the perioperative use of β-adrenergic receptor blocking agents.

Defining Comorbid Conditions

The clinician needs to identify any active cardiac conditions (Table 106-1) or clinical risk factors that have been associated with adverse outcomes. Active cardiac conditions are defined as unstable coronary syndromes, decompensated systolic or diastolic heart failure, significant arrhythmias, and severe valvular heart disease. Clinical risk factors are independent risk factors that are associated with poor outcomes and include history of ischemic heart disease (suggestive history, symptoms, or Q waves on electrocardiogram), history of prior or compensated heart failure (suggestive history, symptoms, or examination findings), history of stroke or transient ischemic attack, insulin-dependent diabetes mellitus, and renal insufficiency (serum creatinine concentration >2 mg/dL).

Assessing Surgical Risk

Evaluation of surgical risk is crucial. Surgical procedures have been classified as low-risk, intermediate-risk, and high-risk vascular operations (Table 106-2). Understandably, procedures with differing levels of stress (alterations in heart rate, blood pressure, intravascular volume, blood loss, and pain) are associated with differing levels of morbidity and mortality risks. Ophthalmologic and superficial procedures represent the lowest risk and very rarely result in morbidity and death. The intermediate-risk category (includes endovascular abdominal aortic aneurysm repair and carotid endarterectomy) represents procedures with associated morbidity and mortality risks that vary depending upon the surgical location and extent of procedure. Major vascular procedures are the highest risk procedures and mandate further investigation. In the revised ACC/AHA guidelines, vascular surgery is now the only surgical category

Table 106-1 Active Cardiac Conditions That Mandate Preoperative* Evaluation and Treatment

Condition	Examples
Unstable coronary syndromes	Unstable or severe angina† (CCS class III or IV)‡ Recent MI§
Decompensated HF (NYHA functional class IV; worsening or new-onset HF)	
Significant arrhythmias	High-grade AV block Mobitz type II AV block Third-degree AV block Symptomatic ventricular arrhythmias Supraventricular arrhythmias, including AF, with uncontrolled ventricular rate (HR >100 beats/min at rest) Symptomatic bradycardia Newly recognized ventricular tachycardia
Severe valvular disease	Severe aortic stenosis (mean pressure gradient >40 mm Hg, aortic valve area <1.0 cm^2, or symptomatic Symptomatic mitral stenosis (progressive dyspnea on exertion, exertional presyncope, or HF)

*Before noncardiac operations.

†According to Campeau L. Letter: Grading of angina pectoris. Circulation. 1976;54:522-523.

‡May include "stable" angina in patients who are sedentary.

§The American College of Cardiology (ACC) National Database Library defines "recent" myocardial infarction (MI) as occurring >7 days but ≤30 days previously.

AF, Atrial fibrillation; AV, atrioventricular; CCS, Canadian Cardiovascular Society; HF, heart failure; HR, heart rate; NYHA, New York Heart Association.

Reprinted, with permission, from Fleisher L, Beckman J, Brown K, et al. ACC/AHA 2007 guidelines on perioperative cardiovascular evaluation and care for noncardiac surgery: A report of the American College of Cardiology/American Heart Association Task Force on Practice Guidelines. J Am Coll Cardiol. 2007;50:e159-241.

Table 106-2 Surgical Risk* Stratification for Patients with Preexisting Cardiac Disease

Level of Risk	Procedure Examples
High (vascular procedures)†	Aortic and other vascular operations Peripheral vascular operations
Intermediate‡	Intraperitoneal and intrathoracic operations Carotid endarterectomy Head and neck operation Orthopedic operations Prostate operations
Low§	Endoscopic procedures Superficial procedures Cataract operations Breast operations Ambulatory operations

*Combined incidence of cardiac death and nonfatal myocardial infarction.
†Reported cardiac risk often >5%.
‡Reported cardiac risk generally 1%-5%.
§Reported cardiac risk generally <1%. These procedures do not generally require further preoperative cardiac testing.

listed as high risk or generally associated with a greater than 5% risk of perioperative cardiac complications.

Evaluating Functional Status

Assessment of functional status in the patient with cardiovascular and pulmonary disease is critical, because O_2 uptake is considered to be the best measure of cardiovascular reserve and exercise capacity. Functional status is measured using metabolic equivalents (METS) (Table 106-3). One MET represents the O_2 consumption of a person at rest (3-5 $mL{\cdot}kg^{-1}{\cdot}min^{-1}$). A functional capacity of 4 METs is considered the minimum requirement for a patient undergoing a major surgical procedure. Consequently, patients who are unable to meet a minimum 4-MET demand during daily activities are at higher risk for developing perioperative cardiovascular and pulmonary complications. Those patients with multiple medical comorbid conditions that limit activity will need to be formally tested to objectively determine cardiopulmonary reserve.

Table 106-3 Energy Requirement for Various Activities

Energy Expenditure	Can You . . .
1 MET ↓	Take care of yourself? Eat, dress, or use the toilet? Walk indoors around the house? Walk a block or two on level ground at 2 to 3 mph (3.2 to 4.8 kph)?
4 METs ↓	Do light work around the house, like dusting or doing dishes? Climb a flight of stairs or walk up a hill? Walk on level ground at 4 mph (6.4 kph)? Run a short distance? Do heavy work around the house, like scrubbing floors or lifting or moving heavy furniture?
>10 METs	Participate in moderate recreational activities, like golf, bowling, dancing, doubles tennis, or throwing a football or baseball?

kph, Kilometers per hour; MET, metabolic equivalent; mph, miles per hour.
Reprinted, with permission, from Fleisher L, Beckman J, Brown K, et al. ACC/AHA 2007 guidelines on perioperative cardiovascular evaluation and care for noncardiac surgery: A report of the American College of Cardiology/American Heart Association Task Force on Practice Guidelines. J Am Coll Cardiol. 2007;50:e159-241.

Applying the Revised American College of Cardiology/American Heart Association Guidelines

Once the clinician has performed a history and examination, the new 5-step ACC/AHA approach can then be utilized for risk stratification and determination of the need for additional cardiac testing (Figure 106-1).

Step 1. Is the noncardiac operation emergent? If so, the patient is taken to the operating room without delay, with the focus being appropriate intraoperative and postoperative cardiac surveillance.

Step 2. Is an active cardiac condition identified? If so, this mandates cardiology consultation and further diagnostic testing.

Step 3. Is the operation low risk? Recognizing that the risk for perioperative cardiac complications in low-risk operations is less than 1% even in high-risk patients, the guidelines state that the patient may proceed to surgery without further testing.

Step 4. If the patient demonstrates good functional capacity (being able to perform >4 METS of activity without cardiopulmonary symptoms) the patient may proceed to surgery.

Step 5. Patients with poor or indeterminate functional capacity for intermediate-risk or high-risk procedures must undergo an additional evaluation. The key issue here is the number of clinical predictors (derived from the Revised Cardiac Risk Index): patients with no clinical risk factors may proceed to surgery. Patients with one or two risk factors may proceed to surgery with heart rate control; noninvasive testing may be considered only if it will change management. Patients with three or more clinical risk factors warrant more scrutiny. These patients scheduled for vascular operations should be considered for noninvasive testing—if it will change management. On the other hand, even those with three or more risk factors scheduled for intermediate-risk operations should proceed to surgery with perioperative heart rate control. Noninvasive testing for this group should, again, be considered only if it will change management.

Perioperative β-Adrenergic Receptor Blockade

The issue of the use of β-adrenergic receptor blocking agents in the perioperative period is controversial, largely because of limited and conflicting data from studies performed in the surgical setting, particularly determinations of the ideal target population, type of β-adrenergic receptor blocking agent, route of administration, and duration of preoperative drug titration. Nevertheless, the latest guidelines state that perioperative β-adrenergic receptor blockade is indicated for patients already on β-adrenergic receptor blocking agents for the treatment of angina, hypertension, symptomatic arrhythmias, or congestive heart failure or for patients undergoing vascular operations who are at high cardiac risk because of ischemia (as was shown on preoperative testing).

β-Adrenergic receptor blocking agents are probably recommended for patients with coronary artery disease who are undergoing vascular or intermediate-risk to high-risk operations. They may be considered for any patient undergoing a vascular operation or those at intermediate to high cardiac risk who are undergoing intermediate-risk to high-risk operations. Their usefulness is uncertain in patients undergoing either intermediate-risk procedures or vascular operations with one or no clinical risk factors. Patients with absolute or relative contraindications to the use of β-adrenergic receptor blocking agents—such as decompensated heart failure, nonischemic cardiomyopathy, and severe valvular heart disease in the absence of flow-limiting coronary disease or severe bronchospastic disease—should not receive them. Statins should be continued, however, throughout the perioperative period in all patients.

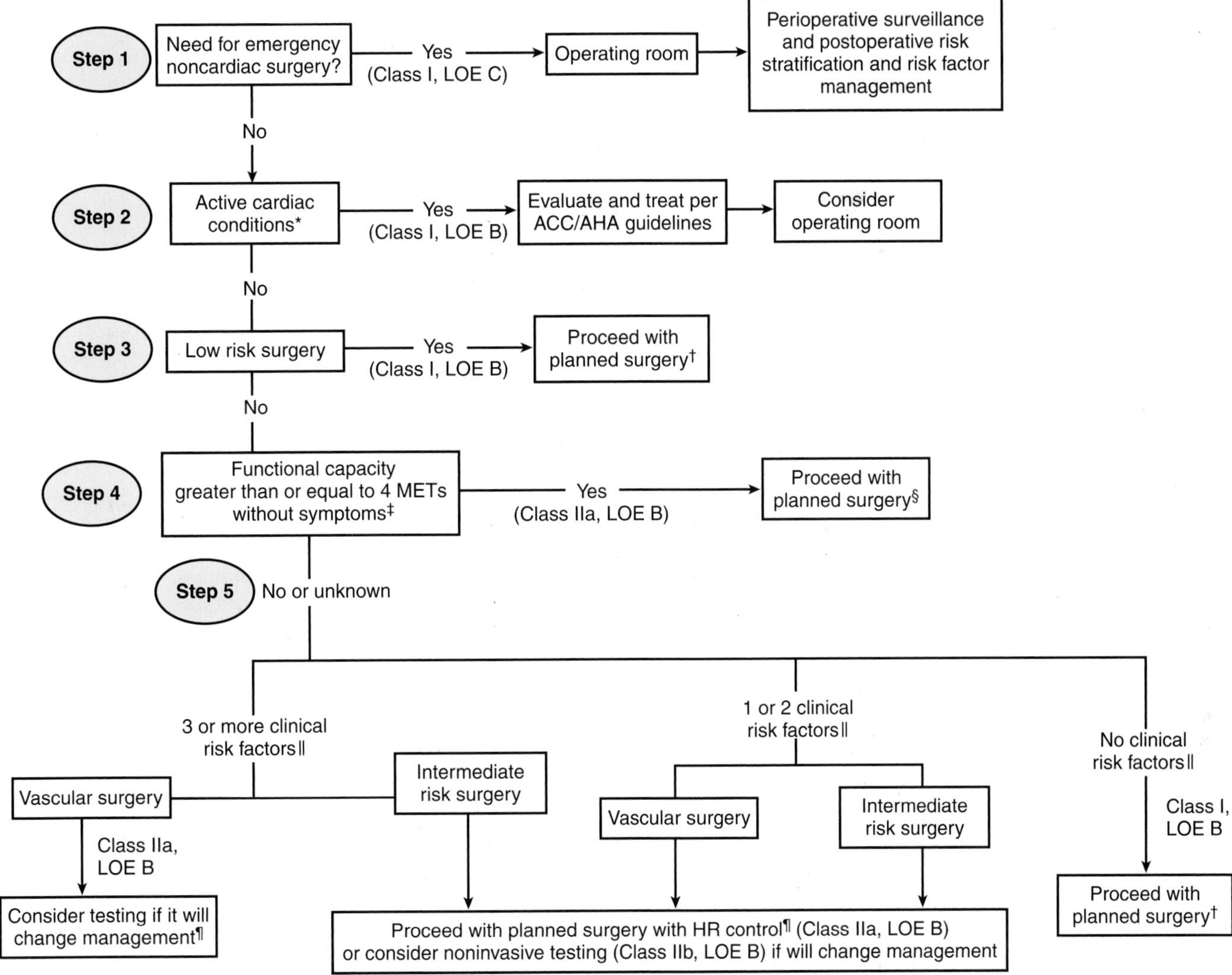

Figure 106-1 The Revised American College of Cardiology/American Heart Association (ACC/AHA) Guidelines Step by Step. An algorithm for evaluation of patients older than 50 years of age undergoing noncardiac operations. *Active clinical conditions include patients with unstable coronary syndromes such as a myocardial infarction within 7 days or unstable angina, decompensated congestive heart failure, significant arrhythmia, or severe valvular disease. †Consider performing noninvasive stress testing. ‡The metabolic equivalents (METs) should be greater than 4. §Noninvasive testing may be considered before surgery in specific patients with risk factors if it will change management. ‖Clinical risk factors include ischemic heart disease, compensated or prior heart failure, diabetes mellitus, renal insufficiency, and cerebrovascular disease. ¶Consider administering perioperative β-adrenergic receptor blockade for patient populations in which this has been shown to reduce cardiac morbidity or mortality risk. HR, Heart rate; LOE, level of evidence. (From Fleisher L, Beckman J, Brown K, et al. ACC/AHA 2007 guidelines on perioperative cardiovascular evaluation and care for noncardiac surgery: a report of the American College of Cardiology/American Heart Association Task Force on Practice Guidelines. J Am Coll Cardiol. 2007;116:418-500.)

Patients with Prior Percutaneous Coronary Interventions

Nonelective operations in patients who have undergone percutaneous coronary interventions (PCIs), with or without coronary artery stenting, present significant risks in the perioperative period. An increasing number of these patients require noncardiac operations within a year of stenting, and this puts them at high risk of developing stent thrombosis, which is associated with significant morbidity and mortality risks (significantly higher with drug-eluting stents as compared with bare metal stents). The reasons for the perioperative hypercoagulability of these patients is multifactorial and include the prothrombotic state associated with surgery, incomplete stent re-endothelialization, and premature discontinuation of dual-antiplatelet therapy. As per the revised ACC/AHA guidelines, patients who have undergone PCIs without stent placement should have elective operations delayed for at least 2 weeks to allow for healing of vessel injury at the balloon inflation site. Patients who have had bare metal stents implanted should have elective operations delayed for at least 4 to 6 weeks while being on dual-antiplatelet therapy to reduce the incidence of stent thrombosis. Lastly, drug-eluting stents pose a particular challenge due to the highly delayed re-endothelialization that is a hallmark of these stents, markedly increasing the risk of early and late stent thrombosis in patients in whom drug-eluting stents have been placed. The key factor that has been associated with this issue is the premature discontinuation of dual-antiplatelet therapy. For this reason, the guidelines mandate that elective noncardiac operations be delayed for at least 12 months while the patient is on dual-antiplatelet therapy to reduce the risk of catastrophic stent thrombosis occurring, which has a mortality rate ranging from 20% to 45%. For those patients who must undergo operations during the recommended time period for dual-antiplatelet therapy, serious consideration should be given to performing the procedure without dual-antiplatelet therapy. For certain procedures in which the surgical bleeding risk is unacceptably high with these drugs (neurosurgery, posterior chamber eye surgery, prostate resections), the dual therapy may have to be discontinued preoperatively and restarted as soon as possible in the postoperative period. Alternatively, if acceptable, monotherapy with only aspirin may be continued perioperatively to mitigate thrombotic risk.

Patients with Cardiac-Rhythm Management Devices

Patients with cardiac-rhythm management devices (pacemakers and implantable cardioverter-defibrillators [ICDs]) are another group of high-risk patients who need special attention. These patients should have their devices interrogated within 3 to 6 months after undergoing an operation. The risk of device malfunction is high perioperatively owing to electromagnetic interference. Reliance on a magnet is not recommended, except for emergencies. Preoperatively, the pacemaker should be reprogrammed to asynchronous mode. In the case of ICDs, the antitachyarrhythmia function should be turned off by reprogramming or by use of a magnet in an emergency. Postoperatively, the function of the device should be interrogated, especially if an electrosurgical unit has been used, and in the case of ICDs, tachyarrhythmia function must be restored.

Suggested Readings

Auerbach A, Goldman L. Assessing and reducing the cardiac risk of noncardiac surgery. *Circulation*. 2006;113:1361-1376.

Bonow R, Carabello B, Kanu C, et al. ACC/AHA 2006 guidelines for the management of patients with valvular heart disease: A report of the American College of Cardiology/American Heart Association Task Force on Practice Guidelines. *Circulation*. 2006;114:e84-231.

Devereaux P, Goldman L, Cook D, et al. Perioperative cardiac events in patients undergoing noncardiac surgery: A review of the magnitude of the problem, the pathophysiology of the events and methods to estimate and communicate risk. *Can Med Assoc J*. 2005;173:627-634.

Feringa H, Bax J, Boersma E, et al. High-dose beta-blockers and tight heart rate control reduce myocardial ischemia and troponin T release in vascular surgery patients. *Circulation*. 2006;114(1 Suppl):s344-349.

Fleisher L, Beckman J, Brown K, et al. ACC/AHA 2007 guidelines on perioperative cardiovascular evaluation and care for noncardiac surgery: A report of the American College of Cardiology/American Heart Association Task Force on Practice Guidelines. *J Am Coll Cardiol*. 2007;50:e159-241.

Grines C, Bonow R, Casey D Jr, et al. Prevention of premature discontinuation of dual antiplatelet therapy in patients with coronary artery stents: A science advisory from the American Heart Association, American College of Cardiology, Society for Cardiovascular Angiography and Interventions, American College of Surgeons, and American Dental Association, with representation from the American College of Physicians. *Circulation*. 2007;115:813-818.

Lee TH, Marcantonio ER, Mangione CM, et al. Derivation and prospective validation of a simple index of cardiac risk for major noncardiac surgery. *Circulation*. 1999;100;1043-1049.

POISE Study Group. Effects of extended release metoprolol succinate in patients undergoing noncardiac surgery (POISE Trial). *Lancet*. 2008;371:1839-1847.

Poldermans D, Bax J, Schouten O, et al. Should major vascular surgery be delayed because of preoperative cardiac testing in intermediate-risk patients receiving beta-blocker therapy with tight heart rate control? *J Am Coll Cardiol*. 2006;48:964-969.

Spertus J, Kettelkamp R, Vance C, et al. Prevalence, predictors, and outcomes of premature discontinuation of thienopyridine therapy after drug-eluting stent placement: Results from the PREMIER registry. *Circulation*. 2006;113:2803-2809.

Vincenzi M, Meslitzer T, Heitzinger B, et al. Coronary artery stenting and noncardiac surgery: A prospective outcome study. *Br J Anaesth*. 2006;96:686-693.

Xu-Cai YO, Brotman DJ, Phillips CO, et al. Outcomes of patients with stable heart failure undergoing elective noncardiac surgery. *Mayo Clin Proc*. 2008;83:280-288.

CHAPTER **107**

Tobacco Use in Surgical Patients

Yu Shi, MD, MPH, and David O. Warner, MD

Approximately 20% of adults in the United States smoke cigarettes, and each year an estimated 10 million smokers undergo surgical procedures. Chronic and acute exposures to cigarette smoke cause profound changes in physiology that increase the perioperative risk of cardiovascular, pulmonary, and wound-related complications occurring (Figure 107-1). Thus, the knowledge of how smoking and abstinence from cigarettes affect perioperative physiology is of practical importance. This chapter will review (1) why smokers should maintain perioperative abstinence from smoking for as long as possible, (2) why surgery provides a good opportunity to quit smoking permanently, and (3) how anesthesiologists can help their patients quit smoking.

Smoking Abstinence and Perioperative Outcomes

Although some of the effects of smoking are irreversible (e.g., airway damage in chronic obstructive pulmonary disease), abstinence from smoking can improve the function of many organ systems and reduce the risk of perioperative complications. The amount of time needed for the body to recover from the reversible effects of smoking varies widely. However, the effects of many smoke constituents are transient. For example, nicotine has a short half-life (~1-2 h), so that plasma nicotine levels are very low after 8 to 12 h of abstinence.

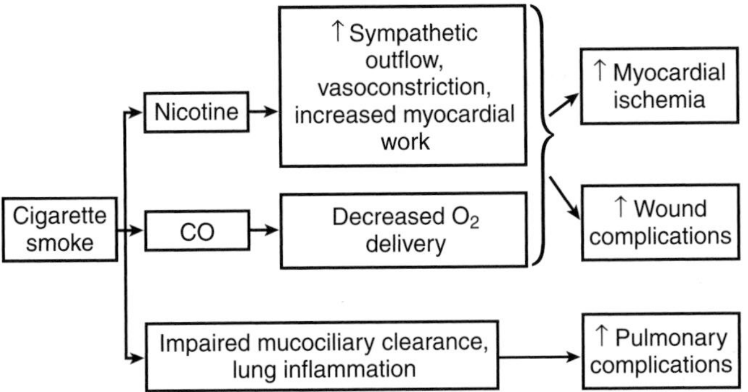

Figure 107-1 Mechanisms of how cigarette smoking increases perioperative risk. CO, Carbon monoxide.

Cardiovascular Outcomes

Smoking is a major risk factor for cardiovascular diseases. In the long term, abstinence from smoking decreases the risk for all-cause death in smokers with coronary artery disease by approximately one third. Smoking a cigarette acutely increases myocardial O_2 consumption by increasing heart rate, blood pressure, and myocardial contractility. These effects are likely mediated primarily by nicotine, which both increases sympathetic outflow and directly contracts some (but not all) peripheral vessels. The carbon monoxide in cigarette smoke binds to hemoglobin and shifts the oxyhemoglobin dissociation curve to the left, interfering with O_2 release. These effects all contribute to an increased risk of myocardial ischemia. During anesthesia, the frequency of ischemia, as assessed by the electrocardiogram, is well correlated with exhaled carbon monoxide levels. This suggests that smoking in the immediate preoperative period increases acute cardiovascular risk and that even brief preoperative abstinence may benefit the heart because carbon monoxide values fall rapidly after abstinence from smoking (within about 12 h). As the effects of nicotine and carbon monoxide dissipate, the risks of acute ischemia may also quickly decrease as myocardial O_2 demand decreases and O_2 supply increases. After 12 h of abstinence, maximum exercise capacity, a measure of overall cardiovascular function, is significantly increased.

Respiratory Outcomes

Smoking is a major cause of pulmonary diseases. For example, chronic obstructive pulmonary disease develops in about 15% of smokers. Even those smokers who do not develop clinical lung disease show acceleration in the normal age-related declines in pulmonary function. Smoking induces an inflammatory state in the lung, causing goblet cell hyperplasia, smooth muscle hyperplasia, fibrosis, and structural epithelial abnormalities. Smoking affects both the volume and composition of mucus and decreases mucociliary clearance. All of these abnormalities predispose smokers to a greater frequency of pulmonary infections and reactive airway disease. Smoking status is a consistent risk factor for several perioperative pulmonary complications, including bronchospasm and pneumonia. Even relatively low-level exposure to smoke has clinical consequences; for example, children exposed to secondhand smoke have an increased rate of upper airway complications.

Despite the inflammatory response induced by cigarette smoke, important elements of lung defenses against infection are impaired during anesthesia to a greater degree in smokers compared with nonsmokers. Lung recovery from chronic smoke exposure is a complex process. Symptoms of cough and wheezing decrease within weeks of abstinence. Goblet cell hyperplasia, mucus production, and mucociliary clearance also improve. As a result of this recovery, abstinence decreases the risk of perioperative pulmonary complications, but it appears that several months of abstinence are required for maximal benefit. However, it is *not* true that brief abstinence from smoking prior to surgery increases the risk of pulmonary complications. This belief was based on the idea that quitting smoking produces a transient increase in cough and mucus production, which is also not true. Thus, although the longer the duration of preoperative abstinence the better, smokers should never be discouraged from quitting at any time, even if only briefly before surgery.

Wound-Healing and Bone-Healing Outcomes

Smokers are more likely to develop postoperative wound-related complications, such as dehiscence and infection, especially in procedures that require undermining of the skin, such as plastic surgery. This is likely caused in part by smoking-induced decreases in tissue oxygenation, which is an important determinant of wound healing. Cigarette smoke may also directly affect the function of fibroblasts and immune cells, which play important roles in the healing process. Microvascular disease caused by smoking may also interfere with angiogenesis via impaired release of substances, such as nitric oxide, that are important for wound repair. For this reason, some surgical specialists (especially plastic surgeons) refuse to perform cosmetic procedures unless their patients at least temporarily stop smoking. Smoking has significant effects on bone metabolism and is a major risk factor for osteoporosis. Smoking increases the risk for nonunion of spinal fusions, and the healing of fractures and ligaments may also be impaired in smokers. There is now strong evidence that abstinence can reduce wound-related complications, such as wound infections. The duration of preoperative abstinence required for benefit is not known. However, because tissue oxygenation is a primary determinant of risk, and because tissue oxygenation improves quickly with the cessation of smoking, there is good reason to believe that even brief periods of abstinence would be beneficial. It is important for patients to maintain postoperative abstinence for the first week after surgery to allow for the initial stages of the healing process to occur.

Surgery Represents an Excellent Opportunity for Smoking Cessation

As discussed previously, even a brief abstinence from smoking before surgery may decrease the risk for perioperative complications. The results of a recent meta-analysis suggest that preoperative intervention on smoking cessation reduces postoperative complications (risk ratio: 0.70, 95% confidence interval 0.56, 0.88). Another reason that patients should try to quit smoking around the time of surgery is that surgery is a "teachable moment" that motivates individuals to change smoking behavior—undergoing a major surgical procedure doubles the rate of spontaneous quitting. Also, studies suggest that symptoms of nicotine withdrawal do not consistently occur in the perioperative period. For example, smokers do not report greater increases in stress over the perioperative period, compared with nonsmokers. Regardless of whether the lack of increased stress occurs because of opioids given postoperatively or the fact that patients are out of their normal environments that usually provide cues for smoking, patients can be encouraged to maintain perioperative abstinence from cigarettes without fearing that this will contribute to the stress caused by the surgical experience itself. Because smoking is the most common preventable cause of premature death, surgery is, thus, an excellent opportunity to promote the long-term health of surgical patients.

Helping Patients Quit Smoking

Treatment of tobacco dependence involves both behavioral counseling (to address the habit of smoking) and pharmacotherapy (to address nicotine addiction) (Figure 107-2). Even brief advice to stop smoking offered by physicians increases quit rates. More intensive counseling further increases quit rates. It may not be practical for anesthesiologists to deliver intensive behavioral interventions, as most are not trained to do so and time is limited in busy clinical practices; however, anesthesiologists can refer patients to other existing services, such as telephone quitlines, which are available in all states (1-800-QUIT-NOW) and can provide assistance and follow-up at

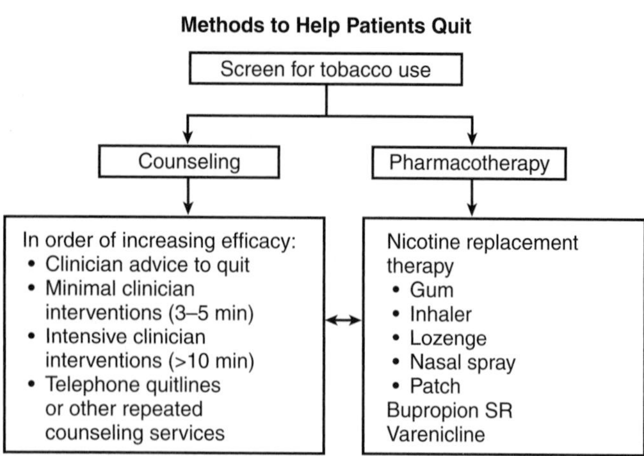
Methods to Help Patients Quit
Screen for tobacco use
Counseling
Pharmacotherapy
In order of increasing efficacy:
• Clinician advice to quit
• Minimal clinician interventions (3–5 min)
• Intensive clinician interventions (>10 min)
• Telephone quitlines or other repeated counseling services
Nicotine replacement therapy
• Gum
• Inhaler
• Lozenge
• Nasal spray
• Patch
Bupropion SR
Varenicline

Figure 107-2 Summary of methods to help patients quit smoking. (Modified from Warner DO. Helping surgical patients quit smoking: Why, when, and how. Anesth Analg. 2005;101:481-487.)

low or no cost to smokers attempting to quit. Pharmacotherapy helps smokers treat symptoms of nicotine withdrawal, including cravings for cigarettes. Nicotine replacement therapy (NRT) in the forms of gum, inhaler, patch, and lozenges is effective in promoting abstinence, with many forms available without prescription. NRT does not produce adverse cardiac effects in healthy smokers and is safe in patients with cardiovascular diseases. There is no evidence that therapeutic doses of NRT in humans affect wound healing; therefore, current evidence supports the safety of NRT for surgical patients. Good success in maintaining abstinence has been reported with a combination of pharmacotherapy (bupropion SR or varenicline tartrate) and psychotherapy (e.g., individual, group, or telephone-based therapy).

Summary

Smoking increases the risk of perioperative complications. Although patients should stop smoking for as long as possible both before and after surgery, even brief preoperative abstinence may be beneficial (and is not harmful). Anesthesiologists should consistently ask their patients about tobacco use, advise them to quit smoking, and refer them to resources, such as telephone quitlines, that can provide support for quit attempts (1-800-QUIT-NOW).

Suggested Readings

American Society of Anesthesiologists. *ASA stop smoking initiative for providers.* http://www.asahq.org/For-Members/Clinical-Information/ASA-Stop-Smoking-Initiative.aspx. Accessed November 8, 2010.

Shi Y, Warner DO. Surgery as a teachable moment for smoking cessation. *Anesthesiology*. 2010;112:102-107.

Thomsen T, Villebro N, Moller AM. Interventions for preoperative smoking cessation. *Cochrane Database Syst Rev*. 2010;7:CD002294.

Warner DO. Perioperative abstinence from cigarettes: Physiologic and clinical consequences. *Anesthesiology*. 2006;104:356-367.

CHAPTER 108 Obstructive Sleep Apnea

Melinda A. King, MD

Obstructive sleep apnea, or OSA, is sleep-disordered breathing characterized by repeated episodes of partial or complete upper airway obstruction leading to frequent nocturnal arousals. Patients may also experience episodes of hypercarbia and arterial O_2 desaturation.

Epidemiology

The prevalence of OSA is estimated at 3% to 7% of adult men and 2% to 5% of adult women. Some groups of people have a higher disease prevalence, including older adults and those who are overweight (Figure 108-1). Most OSA remains undiagnosed and, as the population ages and the obesity epidemic explodes, a surge in disease prevalence is expected.

Pathophysiology

The upper airway from the hard palate to the larynx has evolved as a multipurpose complex structure. Its ability to collapse and change shape is essential for the functions of breathing, swallowing, and speaking. The airways of patients with OSA are narrow and more prone to collapse (Figure 108-2). These individuals are more dependent on increased tone of the airway dilator muscles during wakefulness to maintain airway patency. Decreased tone at the onset of sleep in healthy patients and those with OSA causes breathing instability. Patients who are highly dependent on increased muscle tone during wakefulness are much more vulnerable to airway obstruction during the transition from wakefulness

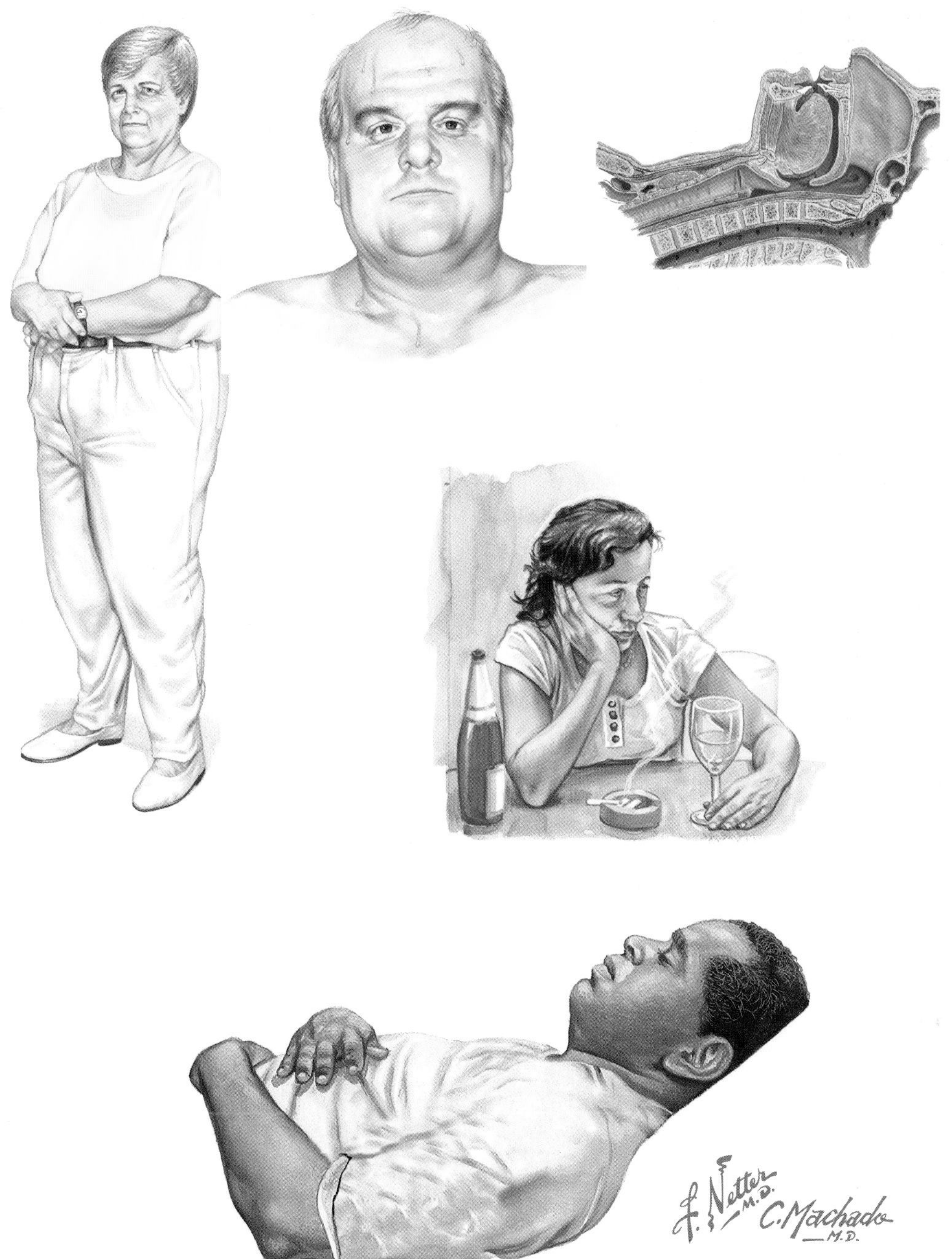

Figure 108-1 Risk factors for obstructive sleep apnea (OSA) include age (higher prevalence in older population), sex (more common in men), obesity (OSA risk increases with rising body mass index), upper airway abnormalities, smoking, alcohol consumption, and the use of certain medications. (Netter illustration from www.netterimages.com.)

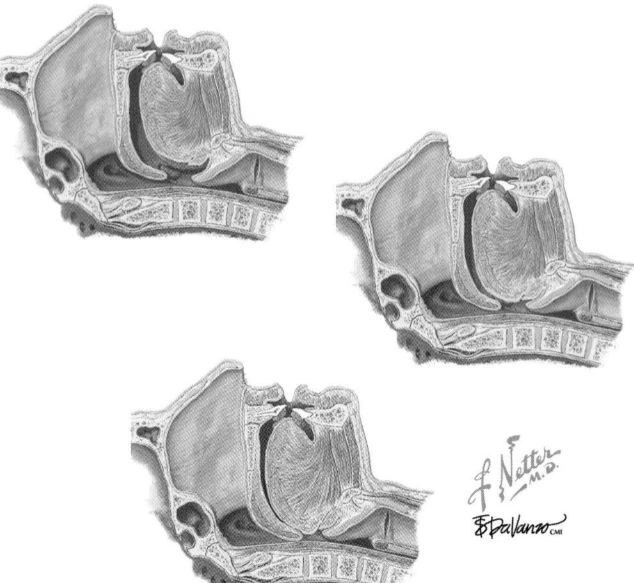

Figure 108-2 Anatomic representation of sleep apnea. (Netter illustration from www.netterimages.com. © Elsevier Inc. All rights reserved.)

Table 108-1 Severity of Obstructive Sleep Apnea	
Severity Category	**AHI***
None	0-5
Mild	6-20
Moderate	21-40
Severe	>40

*The apnea-hypopnea index (AHI) is number of apneas plus hypopneas per hour of sleep.

to sleep. Arousal from sleep helps the patient restore normal respiratory patterns, but the end result is poor-quality fragmented sleep.

Obstructive Sleep Apnea, Obesity, Cardiovascular Risk, and Metabolic Syndrome

The patient with OSA who presents to the operating room has more than a single condition. These patients have multiple intertwined comorbid conditions that make their care complicated to manage. Obesity, often an accompaniment to OSA, presents the anesthesia provider's first set of challenges. Deposition of fat in the pharyngeal tissues exacerbates the underlying narrowness and collapsibility of the pharyngeal airway. Obese patients also accumulate more visceral fat, which appears to affect the severity of the OSA. Symptom severity correlates with weight loss and gain. In the Wisconsin Sleep Cohort Study, the authors demonstrated that a 10% gain in weight in patients with OSA led to a 32% increase in the number of apneas and hypopneas experienced per hour of sleep (i.e., the apnea-hypopnea index, or AHI; Table 108-1). A modest 10% decrease in weight led to a 26% improvement in the AHI. Weight loss results in a dose-dependent decrease in the severity of the syndrome.

OSA and obesity also play a significant role in cardiovascular morbidity. Obesity increases the risk of hypertension, heart failure, stroke, and coronary heart disease (Figure 108-3). OSA independently increases the risk of cardiovascular disease regardless of age, sex, or comorbid conditions such as tobacco use, alcohol use, diabetes, and obesity. The Sleep Heart Health Study data indicate that the odds ratios of atrial fibrillation, coronary heart disease, and tachycardia are all elevated in patients with OSA. The mechanism of increased cardiovascular risk in patients with OSA has not been entirely delineated but appears to involve the sustained sympathetic activation, oxidative stress, and resulting vascular inflammation that occur with the repetitive episodes of hypercarbia and hypoxia. These patients have higher levels of inflammatory mediators such as C-reactive protein and interleukin 6 in conjunction with elevated levels of endothelin and decreased levels of nitric oxide. Treatment of OSA with continuous positive airway pressure (CPAP) improves hypertension, decreases levels of inflammatory mediators, and in some patients with dyslipidemia, promotes regression of atherogenic plaque.

Another common comorbid condition in patients with OSA is metabolic syndrome. This disorder is characterized by the clustering of concurrent metabolic conditions. Typically, the patient has central obesity, hypertension, diabetes, and dyslipidemia. Although a direct link has yet to be made between metabolic syndrome and OSA, about 60% of patients with OSA have metabolic syndrome (versus 40% of their counterparts without OSA). In addition to managing the consequences of OSA and cardiovascular morbidity, the anesthesia provider must also be cognizant of the end-organ damage that can result from metabolic syndrome.

Anesthetic Management of Patients with Obstructive Sleep Apnea

The patient with OSA presents a number of anesthetic challenges. The first critical step is identification of the disease. Upward of 80% to 90% of patients with OSA have not had the syndrome diagnosed. Any patient who presents with obesity, hypertension, or any of the components of metabolic syndrome should be considered at risk for having OSA, and, therefore, the anesthesia provider should perform a detailed history, including questioning of the sleep partner, using the STOP acronym to identify patients with OSA (Snoring, Tiredness, Observed apnea, high blood Pressure). Often, patients are completely unaware of the disease and require education. A simple identification questionnaire and scoring system can help identify at-risk patients, assess perioperative risk, and guide clinical decision making (Box 108-1 and Table 108-2).

Patients with OSA should be identified preoperatively and begun on CPAP therapy, and the medical conditions associated with OSA should be optimized. The patient should have well-controlled hypertension and glucose homeostasis, and any dyslipidemia or gastroesophageal reflux should be treated. Unfortunately, these patients with complex conditions often present the day of surgery. Management of these patients consists of two elements: optimizing the medical conditions often seen in conjunction with OSA and developing the least invasive anesthetic plan. The anesthetic goals should be to provide a quiet working field for the surgeon while minimizing patient risk and optimizing comfort.

The safest anesthetic is local anesthesia with minimal or no sedation. Given the nature of the disease, and the overall poor health of many of these patients, they usually present for procedures requiring a more invasive technique. If local anesthesia is not feasible, the anesthesia provider should consider using regional anesthesia. Peripheral nerve block and neuraxial anesthesia are excellent choices and may be successfully employed with minimal sedation. The habitus of the patient may make placement of peripheral nerve blocks difficult. However, the increasing use of ultrasound technology may significantly decrease the difficulty while improving the quality of the block. Neuraxial opioids should be avoided in patients with

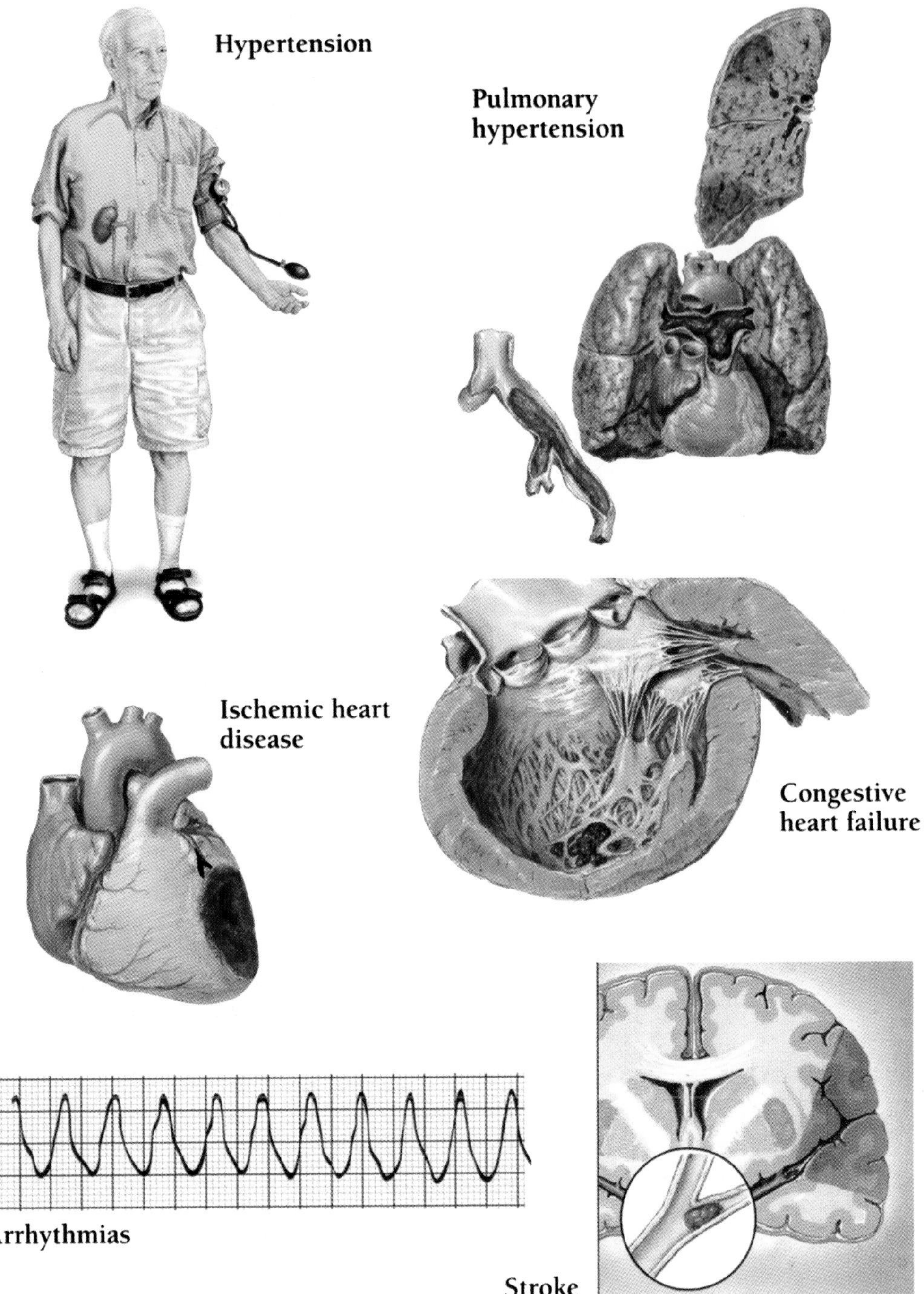

Figure 108-3 Conditions associated with obstructive sleep apnea include systemic hypertension, pulmonary hypertension, ischemic heart disease, congestive heart failure, arrhythmias, and stroke. (Netter illustration from www.netterimages.com.)

OSA because these patients are exquisitely sensitive to the respiratory-depressant effects of these drugs.

When general anesthesia is chosen, many issues should be considered. The underlying pathophysiology of OSA also makes these patients at high risk for having difficult airway management. Patients older than 55 years, who have a body mass index of more than 35 kg/m^2, or who snore are at risk for having difficult mask ventilation. Patients with a Mallampati score of 3 or 4, whose neck circumference is greater than 17 inches, who are unable to protrude the jaw, or who have significant submandibular tissue are at risk for experiencing a difficult intubation (Figure 108-4). These patients are also prone to developing rapid and severe desaturations resulting from higher metabolic demand, decreased functional reserve capacity, and increased collapsibility and obstruction of the pharyngeal airway.

Proper patient position is the first essential step in airway management. The patient should be positioned on an elevation pillow or ramp with the head in the sniffing position. Oxygen should be delivered at 100% with a tight-fitting mask for 3 to 4 min before induction. Rapid

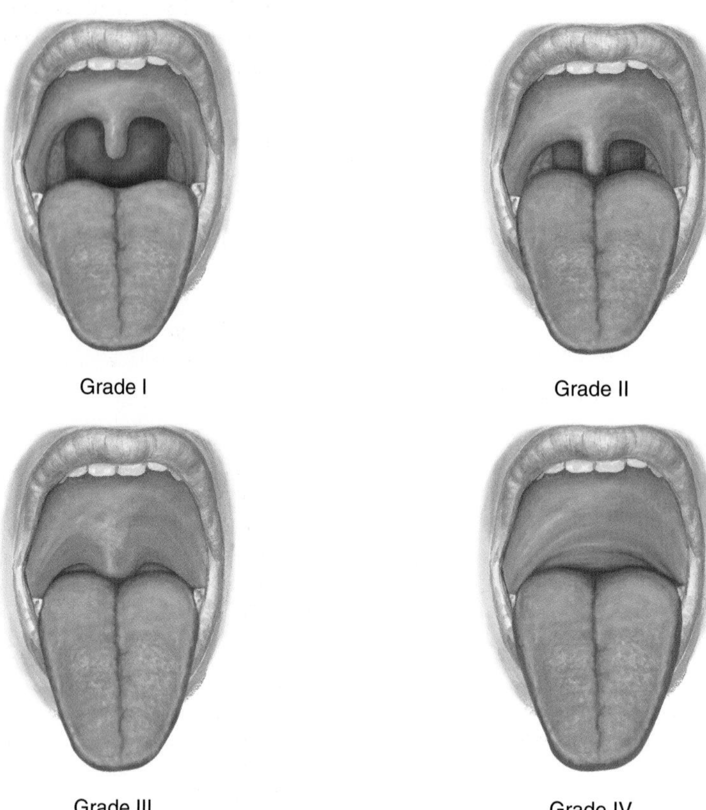

Figure 108-4 Evaluation of the oral cavity is an important component of the physical examination. A Mallampati score of 3 or 4 is often found in patients with obstructive sleep apnea. (Netter illustration from www.netterimages.com. © Elsevier Inc. All rights reserved.)

Box 108-1 Identification of Obstructive Sleep Apnea

Clinical signs and symptoms of OSA
Predisposing physical characteristics
- BMI >35 kg/m²
- Neck circumference >16" in women and 17" in men
- Craniofacial abnormalities affecting the airway
- Nasal obstruction (anatomic)

History of apparent airway obstruction during sleep (two factors if patient lives with someone who corroborates symptoms, one factor if patient lives alone)
- Loud snoring
- Observed pauses in breathing
- Awakening with a choking sensation
- Frequent arousals from sleep

Somnolence
- Frequent somnolence or fatigue despite adequate sleep
- Falls asleep easily in a nonstimulating environment (e.g., while watching television)
- Sleep study results

BMI, Body mass index; OSA, obstructive sleep apnea.

sequence induction with cricoid pressure is optimal. If the patient requires ventilation during rapid sequence induction, use of airway adjuncts such as an oral airway, nasal trumpet, or two-person bag-mask ventilation may be required. In addition to proper position, good denitrogenation, and the availability of an assistant, the anesthesia provider should have additional difficult-airway equipment at hand, as indicated. At a minimum, an appropriately sized laryngeal mask airway, several different laryngoscope blades, and a short handle should be available. More advanced management devices, such as a video laryngoscope or fiberoptic bronchoscope, should also be readily available. The anesthesia provider must be skilled in the use of these devices and advanced techniques of airway management. Occasionally, an awake fiberoptic intubation may be performed as the first-line technique.

The anesthetic plan must also take into account the significant morbidity and possible fatality associated with OSA. Patients who score a 5 or higher using the criteria listed in Table 108-2 may be at significant risk of developing postoperative airway obstruction or apnea or of dying. If the anesthetic cannot be managed with local anesthesia or regional anesthesia

Table 108-2 Obstructive Sleep Apnea Scoring System*

Scoring Factor	Points
Severity Category†	
None	0
Mild	1
Moderate	2
Severe	3
Invasiveness of the Operation	
Superficial with local or nerve block	0
Superficial with moderate sedation or general anesthesia	1
Peripheral with neuraxial anesthesia and mild to moderate sedation	2
Major operation with general anesthesia	3
Airway operation with general anesthesia	3
Use of Opioids	
No requirement for postoperative opioids	0
Low-dose oral opioids	1
High-dose oral, parenteral, or neuraxial opioids	3

*Patients with a score of 5 or higher may be at significantly increased risk for developing perioperative complications associated with obstructive sleep apnea.
†Subtract 1 point if the patient has been fitted for and uses continuous positive airway pressure via a mask.

with minimal sedation, the risk of postoperative complications is higher. Patients who have been treated with CPAP should resume therapy in the postanesthesia care unit. Some patients will require initiation of CPAP while in the hospital. This can be accomplished in consultation with the respiratory therapy department. Patients with OSA, particularly those at high risk, should be observed overnight with continuous pulse oximetry and capnometry. The use of opioids should be minimized, and nonopioid adjuncts should be utilized, including a continuous peripheral nerve block via a catheter, an epidural infusion of a local anesthetic agent, nonsteroidal anti-inflammatory drugs, and acetaminophen.

Summary

OSA is a common disease and its prevalence is ever increasing. Patients with OSA present a serious challenge to the skills of the anesthesia provider, but with careful management, they usually do well in the operating room. Anesthesia-related fatality can occur postoperatively—often due to a failure to recognize the disease and treat it as a life threat. Many of these patients will require overnight stays in the hospital with continuous oximetry and capnometry, even when the operation is an "outpatient" procedure.

Suggested Readings

Chung F, Subramanyam R, Liao P, et al. High STOP-Bang score indicates a high probability of obstructive sleep apnoea. *Br J Anaesth*. 2012;108:768-775.

Dhanda Patil R, Patil YJ. Perioperative management of obstructive sleep apnea: A survey of Veterans Affairs health care providers. *Otolaryngol Head Neck Surg*. 2012;146:156-161.

Gregoretti C, Corso RM, Insalaco G, et al. Anesthesiologists and obstructive sleep apnea: Simple things may still work. *Chest*. 2011;140:1097-1098.

Isono S. Obstructive sleep apnea of obese adults: Pathophysiology and perioperative management. *Anesthesiology*. 2009;110:908-921.

Kaw R, Gali B, Collop NA. Perioperative care of patients with obstructive sleep apnea. *Curr Treat Options Neurol*. 2011;13:496-507.

Porhomayon J, El-Solh A, Chhangani S, Nader ND. The management of surgical patients with obstructive sleep apnea. *Lung*. 2011;189:359-367.

Practice guidelines for the perioperative management of patients with obstructive sleep apnea: an updated report by the American Society of Anesthesiologists task force on perioperative management of patients with obstructive sleep apnea. *Anesthesiology*. 2013 Dec 16. [Epub ahead of print].

Punjabi, NM. The epidemiology of adult obstructive sleep apnea. *Proc Am Thor Soc*. 2008;5:136-143.

Vasu TS, Grewal R, Doghramji K. Obstructive sleep apnea syndrome and perioperative complications: A systematic review of the literature. *J Clin Sleep Med*. 2012;8:199-207.

CHAPTER 109

Postoperative Nausea and Vomiting

John M. VanErdewyk, MD

Postoperative nausea and vomiting (PONV) is the most frequent side effect that occurs after exposure to anesthetic agents, occurring in 20% to 30% of the general surgical population and up to 80% in high-risk patients. Although PONV is self-limiting, it increases patients' dissatisfaction and can be associated with significant morbidity (Box 109-1). PONV also results in higher costs from treatment, delayed discharge from the postanesthesia care unit or the hospital, and unplanned hospitalization.

Physiology

The vomiting center of the brain, in the reticular formation, receives input from the chemotactic trigger zone, gastrointestinal tract, vestibular portion of the eighth cranial nerve, and pharynx. Important neurotransmitter receptor sites documented, or suspected, to be associated with PONV include serotonin, dopamine, histamine, neurokinin-1, opioid, acetylcholine, and muscarinic receptor sites (see Chapter 98).

Risk Factors

Identification of independent risk factors for PONV is complicated because of limitations in study designs and the wide array of variables influencing PONV, including patient-related, surgery-related, and anesthesia-related factors. Some risk factors appear to be well established (Box 109-2). Other factors may be associated with PONV, but confirmation of these factors will require additional investigation. Factors that are unlikely to increase the incidence of PONV include obesity, higher intraoperative inspired fraction of O_2 (50%-80% vs. 30%), and early stage of the menstrual cycle (Figure 109-1).

Several risk-scoring systems have been developed; they combine various established risk factors in an attempt to simplify and predict the likelihood of PONV occurring (see Box 109-2). Identification of high-risk patients will allow a more effective and cost-efficient prophylactic treatment program to be established, whereas low-risk patients (i.e., most general surgical patients) would be spared the added expense and possible side effects of treatment.

Box 109-1 Conditions Associated with an Increased Prevalence of Postoperative Nausea and Vomiting

- Airway compromise
- Aspiration pneumonitis
- Dehydration
- Electrolyte changes
- Esophageal rupture
- ↑ Central venous pressure
- ↑ Intracranial pressure
- Suture or mesh disruption
- Venous hypertension and bleeding
- Wound dehiscence

Box 109-2 Risk Factors for PONV in Adults

Patient-Related Factors

- Female sex
- Nonsmoking status
- History of PONV or motion sickness

Anesthetic-Related Factors

- Use of inhalation anesthetic agents
- Use of nitrous oxide
- Use of intraoperative and postoperative opioids

Surgery-Related Factors

- Duration of the operation
- Type of operation
  - Abdominal
  - Breast
  - Gynecologic
  - Laparoscopy
  - Laparotomy
  - Maxillofacial
  - Neurologic
  - Ophthalmologic
  - Plastic surgery
  - Strabismus
  - Urologic

PONV, Postoperative nausea and vomiting.

Treatment

The first step in treating PONV is to prevent it. Some risk factors are fixed (e.g., sex, surgical procedure); however, some factors are variable and may be influenced by the anesthesiologist. A lower incidence of PONV is associated with (1) the use of regional anesthesia as compared with general anesthesia, (2) using propofol for induction or maintenance of anesthesia, (3) avoiding the use of nitrous oxide, (4) using opioid-sparing drugs (e.g., nonsteroidal anti-inflammatory drugs and cyclooxygenase-2 inhibitors), and (5) providing adequate hydration.

The next steps in preventing PONV are to identify high-risk patients and administer an effective prophylactic program to them. Next, any underlying causes of hypotension or cerebral hypoxia should be identified and corrected. For patients who develop PONV, treatment options include nonpharmacologic measures, such as acupuncture, acupressure, and transcutaneous electrical nerve stimulation, and the administration of antiemetic agents, either individually or in combination from the various classes (see Chapter 98).

Sample Adult PONV Prophylaxis and Treatment

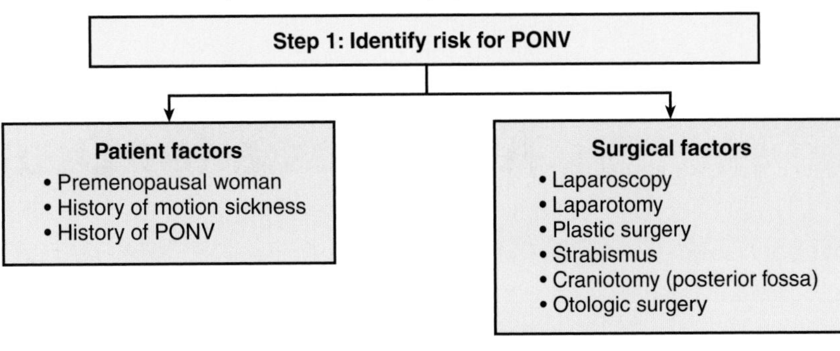

Step 1: Identify risk for PONV
Patient factors
• Premenopausal woman
• History of motion sickness
• History of PONV
Surgical factors
• Laparoscopy
• Laparotomy
• Plastic surgery
• Strabismus
• Craniotomy (posterior fossa)
• Otologic surgery

Step 2: Rate Risk and Administer Antiemetic Prophylaxis

Number of risk factors present	2	2-4	>4
Risk level	Mild to Moderate	Moderate to High	High
Before the procedure	Droperidol or dexamethasone or scopolamine	Droperidol or dexamethasone or scopolamine	Combination of antiemetic agents (>1)
During the procedure			TIVA
At the end of the procedure	5-HT_3- receptor antagonist	Higher dose of 5-HT_3- receptor antagonist	

Note: Prophylaxis is not warranted for patients at low risk for developing PONV or for patients undergoing regional anesthesia or monitored anesthesia care. TIVA refers to total intravenous anesthesia. Dexamethasone may cause glucose intolerance in some patients.

Step 3: Treat PONV

The treatment of PONV is based upon the dose and timing of previously administered antiemetic agents. If not previously administered, the use of 5-HT_3- receptor antagonists represents first-line therapy. The following drugs can also be used for the treatment of PONV.

Drug	**Intravenously administered dose**	**Frequency of administration**
Promethazine	12.5 mg or 25 mg	Every 4–6 h as needed
Prochlorperazine*	5 mg or 10 mg	As needed
Propofol	10–20 mg	As needed

*If available.

Figure 109-1 An example of an algorithm for the prevention and treatment of postoperative nausea and vomiting (PONV).

Conclusion

Further investigation is required to ultimately eliminate the problem of PONV; however, advances have been made to significantly lower the incidence of PONV through preoperatively identifying high-risk patients and providing appropriate treatment.

Suggested Readings

Gan TJ. Risk factors for postoperative nausea and vomiting. *Anesth Analg.* 2006;102:1884-1898.

Gan TJ, Meyer TA, Apfel CC, et al. Society for Ambulatory Anesthesia Guidelines for the Management of Postoperative Nausea and Vomiting. *Anesth Analg.* 2007;105:1615-1628.

CHAPTER 110
Anesthesia for Drug Abusers

Daniel J. Janik, MD

Illicit drug use is a major problem in the United States. Patients often abuse more than one substance simultaneously (polydrug abuse) and can present to the hospital requiring care because of the consequences of either acute intoxication (such as vehicular trauma) or chronic abuse (because of deterioration of major organ systems). Chronic illicit drug use can cause physical dependence (a condition in which withdrawal symptoms occur when the abused drug is withheld) and tolerance (the need for progressively larger doses to achieve the desired effect). Abuse potential correlates closely with euphoric potential. It is generally accepted that the perioperative period is not an appropriate time to attempt withdrawal. Rather, the clinician should prescribe or administer appropriate medication to substitute for the patient's maintenance dosing preoperatively and delay withdrawal until the stress of surgery has abated.

Illicit drugs that are frequently abused, as well as drugs to which a patient may become addicted after chronic prescribed use, and information pertinent to anesthesia providers are described in Table 110-1. General principles should be considered when dealing with a patient who is acutely intoxicated, has chronic tolerance, is going through withdrawal, or is "recovering."

- Tolerance is extremely common, especially to drugs that are within the same chemical class that the patient has been using.
- Patients with acute intoxication, those with chronic abuse (but not intoxicated), and the recovering addict present with different issues that can have significantly different anesthetic implications.
- Withdrawal from central nervous system depressants can be dangerous, so care should be taken to minimize the potential for withdrawal to occur during the perioperative period.

The decision on type of anesthetic agent for an acutely intoxicated individual will often depend on both the physiologic and psychological or emotional state of the patient at the time of surgery.

Suggested Readings

Caldwell TB. Anesthesia for patients with environmental and behavioral disorders. In: Katz J, Benumof JL, Kadis LB, eds. *Anesthesia and Uncommon Diseases*. 3rd ed. Philadelphia: WB Saunders; 1990:792-822.

Hall AP, Henry JA. Acute toxic effects of "Ecstasy" (MDMA) and related compounds: Overview of pathophysiology and clinical management. *Br J Anaesth*. 2006;96:678-685.

Hines RL, Marschall KE. Psychiatric disease/substance abuse/drug overdose. In: Hines RL, Marschall KE, eds. *Stoelting's Anesthesia and Co-Existing Disease*. 5th ed. Philadelphia: Churchill Livingstone; 2008:533-555.

O'Brien CP. Drug addiction and drug abuse. In: Brunton LL, Lazo JS, Parker KL, eds. *Goodman & Gillman's Pharmacological Basis of Therapeutics*. 11th ed. New York: McGraw-Hill; 2006:607-627.

Wilson Wl, Goskowitz R. Uncommon poisoning, envenomization, and intoxication. In: Benumof JL, ed. *Anesthesia and Uncommon Diseases*. 4th ed. Philadelphia: WB Saunders; 1998:561-633.

Table 110-1 Common Illicit Drugs – Physiologic Effects and Anesthetic Considerations

Drug	Class	Route	Mechanism of Action	Psychic Effects	Physical Effects	Anesthetic Effects	Anesthetic Concerns	Dependence	Abstinence Syndrome	Anesthetic Choice	Recommendations
Heroin Morphine Meperidine	Opioid	PO IV IM SQ	Activates opioid receptors throughout the nervous system Receptor μ_2 modulates euphoria and physical dependence	Stupor/coma Euphoria Hallucinations	Respiratory depression Endocarditis Pulmonary infarcts Adrenal suppression Glomerulonephritis Tetanus Myelitis	Analgesia Euphoria	Stupor/coma Respiratory depression Depressed reflexes Seizures or tremor Sudden death	Psychic Physical	Diaphoresis Mydriasis Tremor Lacrimation Seizures	GTA Regional Local	Avoid opioid antagonists Avoid opioid premedication Avoid halothane Continue opioids perioperatively Tendency toward hypotension
Secobarbital Pentobarbital Phenobarbital	Depressant	PO IV IM PR	Potentiates GABA inhibition of neurotransmitter release throughout CNS, including RAS Hepatic microsomal enzyme induction	Stupor Coma	Phlebitis/sclerosis of veins Slurred speech Ataxia Loss of gag reflex Depressed ventilation Myocardial depression	Sedation	Increased fluoride metabolism Prolonged excitement phase Hypotension from central vasomotor or myocardial depression Altered metabolic profile of medications (warfarin, phenytoin, digitalis)	Psychic Physical	Anxiety Hypotension Tachycardia Cramping/ nausea Hyperreflexia Tremor Fever Seizures	GTA Regional Local	Watch for hypovolemia Premedicate with barbiturate to prevent abstinence syndrome Chronic abusers require higher doses of sedatives and hypnotics Acute intoxication will reduce need for sedatives, hypnotics, and maintenance agents
Cocaine	Stimulant	Nasal Inhaled IV	Stimulates dopaminergic neurons in CNS Inhibits presynaptic reuptake of norepinephrine	Euphoria Excitement Hallucinations Aggression Tactile hallucinations	Hyperpyrexia Tachycardia Hypertension Arrhythmias Intracerebral hemorrhage Subarachnoid hemorrhage Cerebral infarction Seizures	Local Anesthetic	Sympathetic hyperactivity Increased myocardial O_2 demand Coronary spasm/ thrombus Myocardial depression Psychosis May increase MAC	Mild physical	Craving Occasional seizures	GTA (usually)	Control anxiety/ psychosis Avoid using pancuronium Control cardiovascular effects Control seizures with barbiturate or benzodiazepine
LSD Psilocybin Mescaline	Hallucinogen	PO IV Inhaled	Binds to dopamine and serotonin (5-HT_{2A}) receptors in CNS	CNS excitation Delusions Sensory distortion Depersonalization Hallucinations Euphoria	Mild tachycardia Mild hypertension Fever Salivation/ lacrimation Mydriasis Rare bronchoconstriction Occasional seizures	Analgesia Anticholinergic	May last 6-12 h Stress may initiate flashback Use succinylcholine cautiously Avoid ester local anesthetic agents LSD prolongs analgesic and respiratory effects of opioids	Psychic	None	GTA Regional Local	Control anxiety Little need for opioids Avoid atropine/ scopolamine

(Continued)

Table 110-1 Common Illicit Drugs – Physiologic Effects and Anesthetic Considerations—cont'd

Drug	Class	Route	Mechanism of Action	Psychic Effects	Physical Effects	Anesthetic Effects	Anesthetic Concerns	Dependence	Abstinence Syndrome	Anesthetic Choice	Recommendations
d-Amphetamine Methamphetamine	Stimulant	IV PO	Stimulate α- and β-adrenergic receptors in CNS and periphery Release catecholamines from storage sites Inhibit reuptake of catecholamines	Euphoria Hallucinations "Rush" Increased performance and power Increased interest in sex	Tachycardia Hypertension Palpitation Ketosis Increased reflexes Seizures Arrhythmias Angina/ cardiomyopathy	Augments opioid analgesia Acute intoxication increases MAC Chronic use decreases MAC	Toxic delirium Chronic depletion of norepinephrine and dopamine Metabolized to false transmitter which accumulates	Physical Psychic	Apathy Depression	GTA	Treat hypotension with direct-acting vasopressors Treat toxicity May present with hypovolemia
Phencyclidine	Stimulant	IV Inhaled Nasal	NMDA receptor antagonist Inhibits reuptake of norepinephrine and serotonin	Euphoria Amnesia Paresthesia Distorted body image Psychosis/ agitated delirium Cataleptic state Numbness of limbs	Tachycardia Hypertension Cerebral hemorrhage Rhabdomyolysis Renal failure Seizures Tremor/posturing	May inhibit pseudocholin-esterase Catalepsy Cross tolerance to ketamine	Laryngeal and gag reflexes intact but may have laryngospasm	Psychic	None	GTA	Control seizures Cataleptic state may obviate need for anesthesia, but patient will need airway control Propensity for violent behavior Avoid ketamine
Mephedrone 3,4-Methylenedioxypy-rovalerone (MDPV), ("Bath Salts; Ivory Wave; Bliss")	Stimulant (4x potency of methylphenidate)	IV Inhaled Rectal	Norepinephrine-dopamine reuptake inhibitor	Euphoria Arousal Agitation Psychosis Prolonged panic attacks Hallucinations	Tachycardia Hypertension Diaphoresis Vasoconstriction Trismus Bruxism	Similar to amphetamines, but limited data	Similar to amphetamines, but limited data	Psychic	Limited data	GTA (due to propensity for agitation)	Control cardiovascular effects as necessary Control psychosis and agitation with benzodiazepines Limited data available
Glue/paint (solvents/ propellants including Freon, toluene, benzene, xylene, carbon tetrachloride, other fluorocarbons) Lighter fluid	Depressant	Inhaled	Variety of theories, including NMDA antagonism and GABA agonist	Excitation Euphoria Vertigo Hallucinations	Stupor/coma Seizures Hepatic necrosis Renal failure/RTA Hematopoietic changes Rhabdomyolysis Pulmonary edema Encephalopathy	None	Hyperchloremia Hypokalemia Hypophosphatemia Arrhythmia Peripheral neuropathy Sensitize myocardium to effects of catecholamines	Psychic	None	Regional (if patient is cooperative) GTA (isoflurane, desflurane, balanced)	Choose anesthetic agent that avoids renal or hepatic toxicity Use reduced doses of sedatives, hypnotics, opioids, and NMBAs Avoid halothane, cocaine, ketamine, and hypercarbia especially if using epinephrine Monitor ECG
Marijuana	Euphoriant	PO Inhaled	Active ingredient THC binds to cannabinoid receptors in CNS (CB_1) and immune system (CB_2)	Tranquility Altered visual perception Loose association Memory impairment Hallucinations Depersonalization	Tachycardia Hypertension Xerostomia Tachypnea (mild) Hyperthermia (mild) Bronchitis	Mild anticho-linesterase activity Decreases MAC Prolongs sleep time of intermediate-acting barbiturates Analgesia	THC may increase narcotic respiratory depression Tachycardia may persist postoperatively Intermediate barbiturates may intensify hallucinations	Psychic	None	GTA (inhalation or balanced)	Avoid atropine Treat hallucinations with benzodiazepine Treat bronchospasm with inhalation anesthetic agent or bronchodilators

Spice; K2 1-pentyl-3-(1-naphthoyl)indole	Euphoriant	PO Inhaled	Synthetic cannabinoid 10x more active at CB_1 receptors than THC	Psychosis Anxiety Agitation Hallucinations Catalepsy Hypomotility	Tachycardia Hypertension Vomiting Tremors Pallor Hypokalemia Analgesia Hypothermia	Analgesia	Similar to marijuana but with addition of hypokalemia	Psychic	None documented	GTA	Treat hallucinations and agitation with benzodiazepines Control cardiovascular effects Watch for hypokalemia
Diazepam Lorazepam Midazolam Chlordiazepoxide Clorazepate Oxazepam	Tranquilizer	PO IV	Potentiates GABA inhibition of neurotransmitter release in cerebral cortex, cerebellum, and limbic system	Sedation Amnesia Anxiolysis Produces "high" when combined with other drugs	Decreased ventilation Decreased peripheral vascular resistance Skeletal muscle relaxation Depressed swallowing reflex	Sedation Amnesia	Moderate ventilatory depression Potentiate opioids Additive with volatile agents	Psychic Physical	Seizures Tremor Cramping/ nausea Anxiety Insomnia (generally later than with barbiturates due to long half-life)	GTA Regional Local	Acute intoxication may obviate need for preoperative sedation or will reduce dose of sedatives and hypnotics Chronic abusers require higher doses of sedatives and hypnotics
3,4- Methylenedioxy-*N*-methamphetamine (MDMA) ("ecstasy")	Empathogen; substituted amphetamine	PO	Stimulates release of serotonin, dopamine, and norepinephrine in CNS Inhibits reuptake of neurotransmitters	Energy Empathy Euphoria Elevated mood Hypersexuality (the "love drug") Panic disorder Confusion	Tachycardia Hypertension Mydriasis Sweating Hyperthermia Hyponatremia Rhabdomyolysis Dysrhythmias and sudden death Increased ADH secretion	Euphoria Mild analgesia Effects last 4-6 h	Exertional hyperpyrexia with rhabdomyolysis and multiorgan system failure Serotonin syndrome Cerebral edema (from hyponatremia) Liver failure Sympathetic nervous system hyperactivity Trismus Stroke Dehydration (possible)	Psychic	Anxiety Irritability/ anger Agitation Dizziness Headache Insomnia Panic attacks Residual feelings of empathy	GTA Regional Local (Depending on patient physiologic or psycho-logical condition)	Control anxiety Correct hyponatremia if present Control hypertension (mixed α- and β-blocker such as labetalol) Correct metabolic acidosis Treat hyperthermia with cooling, or dantrolene if temperature >39°C) Replace fluids to enable normal thermoregulation Promote diuresis if rhabdomyolysis suspected

ADH, antidiuretic hormone; CNS, central nervous system; ECG, electrocardiogram; GABA, γ-aminobutyric acid; GTA, general tracheal anesthesia; HT, hydroxytryptamine; IM, intramuscular; IV, intravenous; LSD, lysergic acid diethylamide; MAC, minimum anesthetic concentration; NMBAs, neuromuscular blocking agents; NMDA, *N*-methyl-D-aspartate; PO, per os (by mouth); PR, per rectum; RAS, reticular activating system; RTA, renal tubular acidosis; SQ, subcutaneous; THC, tetrahydrocannabinol.

CHAPTER 111
Acute and Chronic Alcoholism and Anesthesia

Frank D. Crowl, MD

Ethyl alcohol (ethanol, ETOH) is an addictive central nervous system depressant. Chronic and acute exposure to alcohol can affect multiple organ systems. Alcohol-related deaths have been attributed to trauma, cardiac arrhythmias, cardiomyopathy, cirrhosis, bleeding from gastritis or esophageal varices, hepatitis, malnutrition, pancreatitis, and psychiatric disorders.

Alcohol use disorders (AUDs) have a significant impact on all aspects of health care worldwide. The latest data from the National Institute of Alcohol Abuse and Alcoholism indicate that, in the United States in 2001, almost 10 million Americans or 4.65% of adults were abusing alcohol and an additional almost 8 million (or 3.8%) were dependent upon alcohol. In 2008, a study conducted in Germany suggested that anesthesiologists do a poor job of preoperatively identifying patients with AUDs, particularly among women and younger patients, as compared with among older men. The traditional prevalence of AUDs is higher in men than in women; however, that gap is narrowing, especially among younger women.

Metabolism

ETOH is quickly absorbed through the gastrointestinal tract. It is highly diffusible, with rapid distribution to all aqueous compartments. Because women, as compared with men, have a smaller aqueous compartment, they may have a higher blood alcohol concentration after consuming the same quantity of ETOH as do men of similar height and weight. Ninety percent of alcohol ingested is metabolized in the liver via the alcohol dehydrogenase pathway. The remaining 10% is eliminated by direct pulmonary diffusion or through perspiration and urine. Twelve ounces of beer, 1.5 ounces of spirits, or 5 ounces of wine all contain approximately the same amount of alcohol. Alcohol is metabolized in the body at a rate of approximately 15% of the blood alcohol concentration per hour. ETOH is metabolized as follows:

$$(C_2H_2O)\ \text{ethanol}\ \xrightarrow[\text{NAD}\rightarrow\text{NDH}]{\text{alchohol dehydrogenase}}$$

$$(C_2H_4O)\ \text{acetaldehyde}\ \xrightarrow[\text{NAD}\rightarrow\text{NADH}]{\text{acetaldehyde dehydrogenase}}\ CO_2 + H_2O + \text{acetate}$$

Acute Central Nervous System Effects

At low to moderate blood alcohol concentrations, ETOH binds to γ-aminobutyric acid type A ($GABA_A$) receptors, resulting in relaxation, decreased anxiety, sedation, ataxia, increased appetite, and decreased inhibition, which is occasionally manifested as violent behavior. As blood alcohol levels rise, ETOH begins to act as an antagonist to *N*-methyl-D-aspartic acid (NMDA) receptors, decreasing learning ability and memory. Opioid, dopamine, and cannabinoid receptors are also influenced by ETOH. Progressive central nervous system effects are seen as blood alcohol concentrations increase (Table 111-1); 80 mg/dL is the typical legal limit for intoxication.

Table 111-1 Central Nervous System Effects Related to Blood Alcohol Concentration

BAC (mg/dL)	Effects
50	Decreased mental activity Depression of higher cortical centers Disinhibition Impaired judgment Increased emotional excitability
150	Ataxia Emotional imbalance Slurred speech
>350	Coma Lethargy Stupor
>400	Potentially death*

*Death may result from cardiac or respiratory depression or aspiration-related asphyxia.
BAC, Blood alcohol concentration

Chronic Alcoholism

Alcoholic liver disease progresses in stages. Initially, elevated liver transaminases (e.g., Aspartate aminotransferase [SGOT], alanine aminotransferase [SGPT]) and increased mean red blood cell volume may be the only clues to the presence of parenchymal damage. Fatty liver disease (manifesting as hepatomegaly) is an early finding that will resolve if ETOH ingestion is stopped. With continued ETOH intake, however, alcoholic hepatitis (steatohepatitis)—a combination of a fatty liver, diffuse inflammation, and liver necrosis—ensues. Up to 35% of people with AUDs develop steatohepatitis, which carries an increased nonsurgical mortality rate between 25% and 60% per year, and 10% develop alcoholic cirrhosis; cirrhosis and portal hypertension are the final sequelae of alcoholic liver disease (with a 40% 5-year mortality rate). There is no good test, other than liver biopsy, for confirming early hepatic fibrosis. A blood test identifying early fibrosis could allow for earlier intervention and possible prevention of progression to cirrhosis. An investigational breath test that measures levels of carbon methacetin has been shown to reflect functional reserve in the liver and may, in the future, help identify patients with early fibrosis. Nutritional, cardiovascular, pulmonary, gastrointestinal, central nervous system, hematologic, renal, and immunologic abnormalities may be associated with alcoholic cirrhosis (Table 111-2).

Anesthetic Management of Patients with Alcohol Use Disorders

Patients with alcoholic cirrhosis may exhibit an unpredictable response to the induction of general anesthesia. For example, cross-tolerance with barbiturates

Table 111-2 Abnormalities Associated with Alcoholic Cirrhosis

System or Function	Abnormalities
Cardiovascular	Hyperdynamic state*
Central nervous system	Asterixis Encephalopathy
Gastrointestinal	Cholelithiasis Fetor hepaticus Gastroesophageal varices ↓ Gastroesophageal sphincter tone Pancreatitis Peptic ulcer disease Portal vein hypertension Splenomegaly
Hematologic	Anemia Coagulopathy†
Immunologic	Suppressed immune-defense mechanisms
Nutrition	↓ Albumin concentration Megaloblastic anemia‡ ↓ Vitamin K absorption Hypoglycemia§
Pulmonary	Hypoxia‖ Intrapulmonary arteriovenous shunting Right-to-left shunting# Pneumonia**
Renal††	↑ Aldosterone secretion ↑ Angiotensin production ↓ Glomerular filtration rate ↓ Renal blood flow ↑ Renin production

*Characterized by increased cardiac output, arteriovenous (AV) shunting, increased intravascular volume, decreased blood viscosity secondary to anemia, cardiomyopathy, and congestive heart failure.
†Secondary to decreased synthesis of clotting factors (except factor VIII), resulting in increased prothrombin time and activated partial thromboplastin time; ethyl alcohol suppresses platelet function and survival (splenic sequestration) and enhances fibrinolysis.
‡Requires vitamin B_{12} and folate replacement.
§Caused by decreased gluconeogenesis or decreased glycogen stores.
‖Secondary to extrinsic restrictive lung disease resulting from ascites-induced cephalad displacement of the diaphragm.
#Secondary to portal vein hypertension.
**Secondary to decreased pulmonary phagocytic activity or aspiration of gastric contents.
††Abrupt oliguria with concomitant cirrhosis (hepatorenal syndrome) is associated with a 60% mortality rate.

has been reported. Accordingly, barbiturate dose may need to be increased. However, if the patient's nutrition status is poor, a decrease in serum albumin may increase the amount of free drug and potentiate the myocardial-depressant effect of the drug. Patients with chronic alcoholism are at risk for aspirating gastric contents for the following reasons: increased gastric acid secretion, decreased gastric motility, ascites-induced changes in the angle of the gastroesophageal junction, and increased intragastric pressure.

The minimum alveolar concentration (MAC) of an anesthetic agent is decreased in patients following acute ETOH ingestion. In contrast, MAC is increased in patients with chronic alcoholism. Patients with alcoholic cardiomyopathy may be exquisitely sensitive to the myocardial-depressant effects of anesthetic drugs. Opioids and benzodiazepines may have prolonged half-lives because patients with chronic alcoholism may have impaired hepatic biotransformation.

Patients with alcoholism may appear to be resistant to the effects of nondepolarizing neuromuscular blocking agents (NMBAs). For example, pancuronium has been shown to bind to both albumin and gamma globulin at a ratio of 1:1.5. Gamma globulin production is markedly increased in patients with cirrhosis, which results in decreased free fraction of drug, necessitating increased initial doses of NMBAs. Increased volume of distribution is also reflected in the prolonged elimination half-lives of the long-acting nondepolarizing NMBAs. Elimination half-lives of vecuronium (in doses < 0.1 mg/kg), atracurium, and cisatracurium are unaffected by hepatic disease. Atracurium and cisatracurium have a theoretic advantage in these patients because it has a pathway for nonmetabolic elimination (Hofmann elimination). All NMBAs should be titrated to effect using transcutaneous nerve stimulation.

Plasma cholinesterase synthesis may be decreased in patients with cirrhosis, although prolongation of apnea after succinylcholine administration would usually not be clinically noticeable. Regional anesthesia may be used in patients with chronic alcoholism. Relative contraindications to the use of regional anesthesia include coagulopathy, peripheral neuropathy, and decreased intravascular volume. Monitoring should include periodic monitoring of neuromuscular blockade, measurement of urine output, and periodic measurement of serum glucose and electrolyte concentrations. Postoperative complications may include poor wound healing, bleeding, infection, and hepatic dysfunction.

Delirium Tremens

Patients with AUDs may show signs of withdrawal 6 to 8 h after their last drink. Onset of delirium tremens typically occurs 24 to 72 h after cessation of drinking. Mortality rate can be as high as 10%. Signs and symptoms of delirium tremens include tremulousness, disorientation, hallucinations, autonomic hyperactivity (diaphoresis, hyperpyrexia, tachycardia, and hypertension), hypotension, and grand mal seizures. Laboratory findings include hypomagnesemia, hypokalemia, and respiratory alkalosis. Treatment includes the use of benzodiazepines, β-adrenergic antagonists (propranolol or esmolol), protection of the patient's airway, supplemental thiamine (for the treatment of Wernicke encephalopathy), and correction of electrolyte abnormalities (especially magnesium and potassium).

Alcoholic Abstinence

Patients may present to the operating room on medications designed to promote abstinence.

Disulfiram

Disulfiram (Antabuse) blocks the conversion of acetaldehyde by acetaldehyde dehydrogenase. With alcohol ingestion, acetaldehyde levels increase rapidly and cause nausea, vomiting, tearing, and potential bronchoconstriction and cardiac arrhythmias. The half-life of disulfiram is 1 to 2 weeks. Disulfiram can inhibit the enzyme necessary for conversion of dopamine to norepinephrine (dopamine β-hydroxylase), resulting in perioperative hypotension (decreased cardiovascular response to indirect-acting sympathomimetic amines), potentiation of benzodiazepines (decreased clearance), and drowsiness. If possible, disulfiram should be discontinued 10 days before surgery.

Acamprosate

Acamprosate (Campral) is an amino acid derivative that improves treatment efficacy (abstinence). Decreased drug craving with acamprosate may be a result of reduced neural hyperexcitablity caused by chronic alcohol abuse. The mechanism of action of acamprosate may be the result of the drug blocking glutamatergic NMDA receptors while activating $GABA_A$ receptors. The anesthetic implications are unknown.

Naltrexone

Naltrexone is a μ-opioid receptor antagonist that has been shown to reduce alcohol ideation. In some situations, the use of naltrexone has decreased the incidence of relapse in recovering patients with alcoholism. Naltrexone should be stopped 3 days prior to elective operations.

Suggested Readings

Grameniz A, Caputo F, Bisselli M, et al. Alcoholic liver disease—Pathophysiological aspects and risk factors. *Aliment Pharmacol Ther*. 2006;24:1151-1161.

Kip MJ, Neumann T, Jugel, et al. New stategies to detect alcohol use disorders in the preoperative assessment clinic of a German university hospital. *Anesthesiology*. 2008;209:171-179.

May JA, White HC, Leonard-White A, et al. The patient recovering from alcohol or drug addiction: Special issues for the anesthesiologist. *Anesth Analg*. 2001;92:1601-1608.

Spies CD, Rommelspacher H. Alcohol withdrawal in the surgical patient: Prevention and treatment. *Anesth Analg*. 1999;88:946-954.

CHAPTER 112 Latex Allergy

Beth A. Elliott, MD

Equipment and materials containing natural rubber latex (NRL) were once ubiquitous in the modern health care environment. Following the recommendation by the Centers for Disease Control and Prevention for universal precautions in 1987, the use of latex gloves increased dramatically (from 800 million to 20 billion annually). Subsequently, in the 1990s, NRL emerged as a significant cause of allergic reactions in both patients and health care workers. It remains unclear whether this escalation in reactions was the result of increased NRL glove use or abnormally high levels of residual latex antigens in the gloves. Manufacturers, hospitals, and clinics have taken steps to replace NRL with nonallergenic materials wherever possible. However, NRL gloves continue to be used in many operating suites due to their superior tactile properties and fit and a desire for reliable protection against blood-borne pathogens.

What Is Latex?

Latex is derived from the milky sap of the rubber tree, *Hevea brasiliensis*, harvested primarily in Malaysia, Indonesia, and Thailand. Approximately 90% of latex is used in the production of "dry" rubber for tires; the remaining 10% is used in the manufacture of "dipped" products, such as gloves, condoms, and balloons. During the manufacturing process, a variety of chemicals are added (e.g., stabilizers, antioxidants, accelerators) to give the rubber the desired characteristics. Once formed, the rubber products are then vulcanized (i.e., cured with heat and sulfur at a temperature of 130°C for 5 to 30 min). For latex gloves, a series of leaching baths are used to rid the gloves of residual water-soluble proteins and excess additives.

Antigenic proteins constitute up to 3% of the final latex product. Antigen levels are typically much higher in dipped latex products than in dry ones, but the levels can vary as much as 1000-fold among lots of gloves by the same manufacturer and as much as 3000-fold among manufacturers. These latex proteins (allergens) are water soluble and can be eluted during contact with moist surfaces (mucous membranes, peritoneal surfaces, and normal skin moisture). Latex allergens also adsorb onto the powder inside gloves. When gloves are donned or discarded, these powders disperse into the air and are inhaled by people nearby.

Clinical Manifestations of Latex Allergy

Irritant contact dermatitis produces a dry scaly irritation of the skin, typically on the hands. This problem is the most common work-related reaction to rubber products (80%). The reaction results from direct irritation by latex and residual chemicals used in the manufacturing process and is exacerbated by frequent handwashing and use of irritant surgical soaps. This reaction is not immune mediated and can be prevented with simple barrier protection or use of a nonlatex alternative.

Allergic contact dermatitis is another common problem associated with exposure to latex products. A red vesicular rash typically appears within 6 to 72 h after contact. The reaction is a type IV cell-mediated immune response to low-molecular-weight accelerators and antioxidants in the rubber product. Antibodies are not involved in type IV reactions. The diagnosis is based on clinical history and on the morphology and distribution of skin lesions. Patch testing confirms the diagnosis. Use of a glove liner or nonlatex alternative should be preventive.

The first case of type I IgE-mediated immediate hypersensitivity reaction to latex was reported in the German literature in 1927. The second case was not reported until 1979. By the 1990s, type I allergy to NRL reached epidemic proportions, with numerous reports of anaphylaxis and death.

Contact urticaria (hives) is the most common manifestation of IgE-mediated latex allergy. Symptoms appear within 10 to 15 min after contact and include itching, redness, and wheal and flare reactions at the site of contact.

Rhinitis and asthma may follow airborne exposure. One study of latex-sensitive individuals found that 51% had experienced rhinitis and 31% dyspnea. Another study found a 73% prevalence of rhinoconjunctivitis and a 27% prevalence of asthma. Most latex-sensitive people have atopic dermatitis and may have a history of seasonal allergic asthma, which may delay the diagnosis.

Anaphylaxis is a life-threatening condition triggered by the interaction between allergen and IgE antibodies attached to mast cells and basophils. Antibodies are formed after the initial exposure. On subsequent exposure, the allergen cross-links two IgE molecules, resulting in degranulation of the mast cell and the release of a host of factors (e.g., histamine, leukotrienes, and prostaglandins) responsible for the anaphylactic response. Capillary dilation, increased vascular permeability, hypotension, edema, clotting defects, bronchoconstriction, and hypoxemia are common manifestations of anaphylaxis. Anaphylactic reactions to latex may be delayed for as long as 60 min after exposure. This delay is thought to be related to the time needed for sufficient antigen to be eluted from surgical gloves and absorbed into the body. When anaphylactic reaction to latex is recognized and treated early, the prognosis is good. Persistent hypotension and bronchospasm may require continued treatment. Intensive care monitoring is warranted for 24 to 48 h because up to 20% of people have relapses, which may occur every 1 to 8 h.

Risk Factors for Latex Allergy

Anyone with frequent exposure to NRL-containing materials is at risk for developing latex allergy. The prevalence in the mid-1990s was estimated to be as high as 3% to 9.5% of the general population and as high as 12% of health care workers. With adoption of NRL-avoidance strategies and reduced exposure to NRL, these numbers have fallen to less than 1% and 4%, respectively.

Although latex allergy was originally associated with spina bifida (in whom the incidence approaches 28% to 67%), it has recently come to light that any patient with congenital abnormalities (particularly neuraxial or urogenital) requiring multiple surgical procedures, indwelling catheters, or personal care using latex gloves is at high risk for developing significant latex allergies. There is an established association between latex allergy and allergy to various fruits and nuts, most commonly bananas, avocados, kiwi fruit, chestnuts, papaya, potatoes, and tomatoes.

Treatment of Latex Allergy

Individuals with contact dermatitis should avoid unnecessary exposure to latex products. Vinyl and neoprene gloves are available in sterile and nonsterile packaging. Barrier creams and cotton glove liners are alternative methods to limit further exposure. It should be noted that chronic open sores on the hands are a potential site of exposure and sensitization, which can lead to later type I (immediate) hypersensitivity reactions. As many as 79% of individuals with type I hypersensitivity previously had type IV skin eruptions.

IgE-mediated allergic reactions extend across a spectrum from rhinoconjunctivitis to severe life-threatening anaphylaxis. Elimination of further exposure to the antigen should be one of the first steps when responding to an acute problem. Airway management and support, volume resuscitation, and catecholamine therapy (epinephrine) remain mainstays of therapy for anaphylaxis.

Tracheal intubation and mechanical ventilation may be required in cases of significant laryngeal edema, bronchospasm, pulmonary edema, and ventilation/perfusion mismatch. As much as 20% to 40% of the intravascular volume may be lost from acute transcapillary leakage during anaphylactic reactions. Combined with peripheral vasodilation, this can result in severe hypotension. Fulminant noncardiogenic pulmonary edema, pulmonary hypertension, and right-sided heart failure frequently complicate the clinical picture.

Pharmacologic therapy for anaphylaxis is aimed at inhibiting further mediator release, providing competitive blockade of receptors interacting with mediators already released, reversing the end-organ effects of physiologically active substances, and inhibiting the recruitment and migration of other inflammatory cells.

Antihistamines and steroids probably have little effect in acute management but may help attenuate late-phase reactions and secondary inflammatory responses.

Prevention of Latex Allergy

Unlike pretreatment for anaphylactoid reactions to intravenously administered contrast dye, pretreatment of latex-sensitive patients with antihistamines, steroids, and catecholamines will not prevent IgE-mediated anaphylaxis.

Careful preoperative questioning of those patients in groups that are at high risk for having latex sensitivity should be done routinely. Patients with spina bifida and congenital urogenital abnormalities are at such high risk for latex allergy that they should completely avoid latex exposure from birth.

A totally latex-free environment is ideal but is achieved only in some hospitals. Recent efforts have focused on creating "latex-safe" environments. Medical equipment and supplies that contain NRL should have a mandated label on the packaging that warns the user of the latex material contained within.

If possible, surgical procedures involving latex-sensitive patients should be scheduled as "first cases" with all latex-containing materials removed the preceding night. Airborne particles containing latex allergens can remain suspended in air for up to 5 h. A readily available supply of nonlatex alternative equipment and supplies should be available in all health care facilities. Regardless of precautions taken to prevent latex exposure, operating personnel should be prepared to treat anaphylaxis in all latex-sensitive patients.

Work environments in which latex gloves are still used should make an effort to eliminate high-allergen products from their inventory to decrease the likelihood of sensitization of employees. Elimination of powdered latex gloves can significantly reduce both sensitization and allergic reactions to latex.

Suggested Readings

Slater JE. Latex allergy. *J Allergy Clin Immunol*. 1994;94:139-149.

Yunginger JW. Natural rubber latex allergy. In: Middleton E, ed. *Allergy: Principles & Practice*. 5th ed. St. Louis: Mosby; 1998.

Hepner DL, Castells MC. Latex allergy: An update. *Anesth Analg*. 2003;96:1219-1229.

Bousquet J, Flahault A, Vandenplas O, et al. Natural rubber latex allergy among health care workers: A systemic review of the evidence. *J Allergy Clin Immunol*. 2006;118:447-454.

Mertes PM, Tajima K, Regnier-Kimmoun MA, et al. Perioperative anaphylaxis. *Med Clin North Am*. 2010;94:761-789.

Vandenplas O, Larbanois A, Vanassche F, et al. Latex-induced occupational asthma: Time trend in incidence and relationship with hospital glove policies. *Allergy*. 2009;64:415-420.

CHAPTER 113

The Evaluation and Management of Prolonged Emergence from Anesthesia

Mary M. Rajala, MS, MD

Recovery from anesthesia occurs on a continuum: the patient initially responds to noxious stimuli and then to oral command, though the patient remains amnestic; motor control returns gradually; finally, in 15 to 45 min, the patient is able to converse rationally. Wakefulness requires diffuse cortical activation (arousal) elicited by afferent stimuli from the reticular formation in the brainstem. Within 15 min of admission to the postanesthesia care unit, 90% of patients regain consciousness. Delayed awakening after general anesthesia (i.e., >45-60 min after admission to the postanesthesia care unit) is secondary to a diverse number of causes and can be broadly classified as pharmacologic, metabolic, or neurologic (Box 113-1).

The anesthesia provider should systematically evaluate the patient with delayed emergence from anesthesia (Box 113-2) while simultaneously managing the patient's preoperative comorbid conditions and medications. This includes taking into consideration the type of operation, the type and doses of anesthetic drugs, drugs administered by the surgical team, and the duration and complications of anesthesia. Importantly, delayed emergence may be associated with the patient's inability to protect his or her airway, airway obstruction, and respiratory failure. Many of the causes of delayed emergence are overlapping and may coexist.

Box 113-1 Causes of Delayed Postoperative Arousal

Pharmacologic Causes

- Residual drugs, overdose
  - Medications administered during the perioperative period by personnel other than anesthesia providers
  - Benzodiazepines
  - Opioids
  - Anesthetic agents—induction, inhalation or intravenous
  - Neuromuscular blockade
  - Decreased metabolism, excretion, or protein binding of drugs
- Pharmacokinetic factors
  - Age
  - Malnutrition
  - Drug interactions
  - Underlying renal, hepatic, CNS, or pulmonary disease
  - Biologic variability
  - Hypothermia
  - Decreased cardiac output-hypoperfusion, hypovolemia

Metabolic Causes

- Hypothyroidism
- Adrenal insufficiency
- Hypoxemia
- Hypoglycemia
- Hyperosmolar hyperglycemic nonketotic coma
- Hyponatremia, SIADH, TURP syndrome
- Sepsis

Neurologic Causes

- Hypoperfusion
  - Low cardiac output, occlusive cerebrovascular disease
  - Embolism
    - Thrombus
    - Air-venous, paradoxical
- Intraoperative retraction, resection
  - Thrombus-atrial fibrillation
- Hypertension
  - Hyperperfusion
  - Intracerebral hemorrhage
- Elevated intracranial pressure
  - Subdural or epidural hematoma
  - Cerebral edema
  - Malfunctioning shunt
  - Pneumocephalus
- Psychogenic unconsciousness
- Head injury

CNS, Central nervous system; SIADH, syndrome of inappropriate secretion of antidiuretic hormone; TURP, transurethral resection of the prostate.

Pharmacologic Causes of Delayed Emergence

Anesthetic Agents

The rate of emergence from general anesthesia correlates with the timing, half-life, and total dose of anesthetic agents used, as well as an individual's biovariability. Residual effects of drugs administered during the perioperative period are the most frequently cited cause for delayed awakening. The cumulative effects of multiple drugs, some of which may be synergistic, may result in a relative drug overdose. Nonanesthetic medications may potentiate anesthetic effects, such as in the case of a lidocaine infusion used to treat cardiac arrhythmia. Patients given scopolamine or atropine may develop central anticholinergic syndrome. The highly soluble inhalation agents may be implicated when high concentrations are delivered for long periods of time or when hypoventilation slows emergence, prolonging recovery.

Opioids decrease the response to hypercarbia, resulting in hypoventilation and subsequent decreased clearance of inhalation agents. Benzodiazepines, droperidol, scopolamine, and ketamine—when given as premedication or as part of the anesthetic—may potentiate other general anesthetic agents, delaying arousal. Awakening may be delayed because of the timing of drug administration (e.g., agents administered shortly before emergence) or the route of administration (e.g., oral, rectal, or intramuscular have delayed absorption). Large doses of barbiturates or benzodiazepines may overwhelm lean tissue distribution and subsequent liver metabolism, thereby prolonging drug effects. Monoamine oxidase inhibitors potentiate the effects of opioids, barbiturates, and benzodiazepines.

Box 113-2 Management of Delayed Emergence

I. Airway, Breathing, Circulation

a. Maintain and protect airway; reintubate if necessary
b. Ventilate to maintain normal arterial CO_2
c. Assess heart rate, blood pressure, perfusion, and urine output

II. Drugs

a. Review all medication that the patient has received perioperatively
b. Persistent neuromuscular blockade
   i. Assess train-of-four with a peripheral nerve stimulator
   ii. Assess for phase II block in patients who received succinylcholine
c. Opioids
   i. Check for pinpoint pupils and slow respiratory rate
   ii. Administer naloxone in 40-μg increments, titrating to effect
   iii. Reexamine the patient on a regular basis; the duration of intravenously administered naloxone is approximately 17 min
d. Benzodiazepine
   i. Provide supportive management
   ii. Consider administering a benzodiazepine antagonist, flumazenil, in 0.1- to 0.2-mg increments (maximal dose, 1 mg); arrhythmias, hypertension, and convulsions are potential side effects
e. Provide active warming if necessary

III. Electrolytes

a. Check blood glucose concentration
b. Check serum sodium concentration
c. Check magnesium, calcium, and phosphate concentrations

IV. Failure to Find Cause of Delayed Emergence

a. Consider the potential for a neurologic event to have occurred
b. Order neurologic imaging studies

Neuromuscular Blockade

Muscle weakness, whether from inadequately reversed neuromuscular blocking agents or pseudocholinesterase deficiency, may result in hypoventilation, hypercarbia, and incomplete washout of inhalation anesthetic agents. Acidosis, hypermagnesemia, or certain drugs (clindamycin, gentamicin, neomycin, furosemide) accentuate the effects of neuromuscular blocking agents and may interfere with reversal of these agents. Patients may be conscious but may be unable to mount a motor response to noxious stimuli when they have muscle weakness and, therefore, appear as though they are still anesthetized.

Pharmacokinetic and Pharmacodynamic Factors

Low cardiac output can reduce perfusion to the lungs, kidneys, and liver, thus reducing metabolism and excretion of anesthetic agents. Decreased protein binding of anesthetic agents from hypoproteinemia or competition of binding sites with other drugs (e.g., intravenously administered contrast dyes, sodium acetrizoate, sulfadimethoxine) results in higher blood levels of active drug.

Liver metabolism of anesthetic agents is decreased in malnourished patients, in patients at extremes of age (through immature or decreased enzyme activity), in the presence of hypothermia (below 33°C-34°C), or during simultaneous administration of drugs dependent on liver microsomal detoxification (e.g., ethanol or barbiturates). Ketamine administration in patients with liver dysfunction delays anesthetic emergence. Patients with liver disease and a history of hepatic coma develop central nervous system (CNS) depression following the administration of small amounts of opioids; cimetidine may also cause mental-status changes in such patients. Although increased sensitivity to barbiturates has been reported in animals with hepatectomy or liver damage, such sensitivity has not been demonstrated in humans with these same conditions.

Renal failure and azotemia are associated with altered acid-base status, decreased protein binding (more likely due to hypoproteinemia than to acidosis), delayed or reduced excretion of drugs or their metabolites, and electrolyte changes, all of which contribute to delayed emergence. It is hypothesized that changes in permeability of the blood-brain barrier may increase sensitivity to hypnotics in patients with renal failure or azotemia.

Hypothermia not only reduces the metabolism of drugs by the liver, but also directly depresses CNS activity (cold narcosis) and increases the solubility of inhalation anesthetic agents, which, in turn, slows their transfer from blood into alveoli. Central respiratory depression and increased sensitivity to anesthetic agents are diagnoses of exclusion. Any anesthetic agent may cause central respiratory depression. Biologic variability in sensitivity to anesthetic drugs follows a bell-shaped gaussian distribution; sensitivity in older adults, compared with younger adults, is not equally distributed on such a curve. Anesthetic requirements diminish with age and in patients who are hypothermic or hypothyroid.

Metabolic Disturbances of Delayed Emergence

Acid-Base Disorders

Mental-status changes occur with a cerebrospinal fluid pH of less than 7.25. During acute hypercapnia, CNS activity is depressed because hydrogen ions cross the blood-brain barrier more quickly than do bicarbonate ions. Hypoxia and hypercapnia accentuate residual anesthetic effects and the effects of preexisting conditions (e.g., hepatic encephalopathy). Metabolic encephalopathies, per se, sensitize patients to the effects of CNS depressants.

Endocrine Disorders

Certain endocrine disorders (e.g., hypothyroidism, adrenal insufficiency) are associated with prolonged anesthetic emergence. The stress of anesthesia and surgery generally increases blood glucose concentrations. Sepsis, SIRS (systemic inflammatory response syndrome), uremia, pancreatitis, pneumonia, burns, and administration of hypertonic solutions or mannitol can trigger hyperosmolar hyperglycemic nonketotic coma, which can cause delayed anesthetic emergence. Hypoglycemia can occur secondary to perioperative administration of antiglycemic drugs, following manipulation of insulin-producing tumors and retroperitoneal carcinomas, or in patients with severe liver disease who have decreased gluconeogenesis. Hypoglycemia is associated with several CNS side effects, ranging from irritability to seizures and coma.

Electrolyte Abnormalities

Electrolyte disorders—such as hypo-osmolality and hyponatremia due to absorption of large volumes of hypotonic fluids (e.g., during transurethral resection of the prostate) or from the syndrome of inappropriate antidiuretic hormone secretion—may delay emergence. Other electrolyte abnormalities to consider when evaluating a patient with delayed emergence include hypercalcemia, hypocalcemia, hypermagnesemia, and hypomagnesemia.

Neurologic Causes of Delayed Emergence

Delayed arousal after anesthesia may be due to global or regional ischemia from cerebral hypoperfusion or hyperperfusion, hypoxia, elevated intracranial pressure, cerebral hemorrhage, or traumatic brain injury. Certain neurosurgical procedures and cerebral hypoperfusion from reduced cardiac output, obstruction to flow, or decreased systemic vascular resistance (systemic shock) have the potential to delay emergence from anesthesia. Arterial compression from retraction or improper positioning of the head and neck are other causes of hypoperfusion.

Hypotension occurring perioperatively may result in cerebral ischemia and stroke and occurs most often in patients with preexisting cerebrovascular disease. Thromboembolic events may be observed in patients undergoing cardiac, vascular, and invasive neck procedures or in patients with atrial fibrillation or hypercoagulable states. Venous air embolism can occur in cases in which the surgical site is higher than the heart; if patients have a patent foramen ovale, they are at increased risk for developing a paradoxical venous air embolism from even small amounts of entrained air. Stage II hypertension or a cerebrovascular accident from hemorrhage or hematoma can precipitate cerebral hyperperfusion, which can delay emergence. Intracranial pressure may increase from hyperperfusion or from intracerebral or subdural hemorrhage or hematoma. Cerebral edema, pneumocephalus, or a malfunctioning shunt or drain are also causes. Delayed emergence due to regional ischemia is manifested by hemiplegia or other focal signs, also known as differential awakening. In theory, focal areas of underperfused or previously injured brain tissue may have trapping or increased sensitivity to anesthetic agents.

Psychogenic unconsciousness, a diagnosis of exclusion, is a dissociative psychiatric disorder with sustained amnesia and unexplainable delayed emergence from anesthesia.

Suggested Readings

Karzai W, Schmidt J, Jung A, et al. Delayed emergence and acute renal failure after pneumonectomy: Tumor emboli complicating postoperative course. *J Cardiothorac Vasc*. 2009;23:219-222.

Licker M, Diaper J, Robert J, Ellenberger C. Effects of methylene blue on propofol requirement during anaesthesia induction and surgery. *Anaesthesia*. 2008; 63(4):352-357.

Sinclair R, Faleiro RJ. Delayed recovery of consciousness after anaesthesia. *Contin Educ Anaesth Crit Care Pain*. 2006;3:114-118.

Weingarten TN, Dingli M, Hall BA, Sprung J. Repeated episodes of difficulty with arousal following general anesthesia in a patient with ulnar neuropathy. *J Anesth*. 2009;1:119-122.

CHAPTER 114

Delirium in the Postanesthesia Care Unit

Carla L. Dormer, MD

Postoperative delirium is an acute onset of altered or fluctuating mental status combined with significant inattention that can present in multiple ways. Although often thought to include one or more of the following manifestations—hyperarousal, agitation, hyperactivity, and even frank psychosis—postoperative delirium more often exhibits as hypoactivity, which may include flat affect, withdrawal, and lethargy.

Postoperative delirium occurs more frequently at the extremes of age, as well as following certain operations. In children, delirium is relatively common (with a reported incidence of approximately 30%), manifesting as emergence excitement or agitation (e.g., inconsolable crying or disorientation) occurring within the first 10 min of arrival in the postanesthesia care unit (PACU) and resolving within an hour. If children are still asleep when brought to the PACU, they can nonetheless experience agitation, but it will occur later in their PACU stay.

Predisposing and Perioperative Risk Factors

Risk factors for postoperative delirium are summarized in Box 114-1. Patients with no risk factors have a 9% chance of developing postoperative delirium. For those with one or two risk factors, the chance increases to 23%, and for those with three or four risk factors, it's up to 83%. Multiple hypotheses have been proposed as to why certain individuals are at risk for developing delirium. In elderly patients, contributing factors include smaller brain mass (atrophy) and a decreased number of neurons, as well as decreased neurotransmitter (acetylcholine, serotonin, and dopamine) production and receptor density. Accordingly, the elderly appear to have limited "cognitive reserve." Therefore, even minor disturbances can lead to postoperative delirium. Specifically, severe illness, cognitive impairment with and without dementia, dehydration, and substance abuse have been shown to be predisposing risk factors. Preexisting diminished executive function and depression are independent predictors of postoperative delirium.

Perioperative risk factors also include high-risk surgical procedures (cardiac, thoracic aortic, noncardiac thoracic, orthopedic), breast and abdominal procedures, as well as prolonged operations. Many of these high-risk operations are associated with embolic phenomenon (e.g., air, thrombus, cement), large fluid shifts, and substantial rates of blood transfusion. Inflammation may also be involved; cytokines are released in response to surgical stress and have been associated with neuronal death. Given this information, one could conclude that regional anesthesia might be associated with less postoperative delirium than is general anesthesia because fewer sedatives and opioids are used with the former. However, this conclusion has yet to be substantiated.

Acetylcholine is important for maintenance of arousal, attention, and memory, whereas dopamine has an opposing effect. Thus, perioperatively administered medications that decrease levels of acetylcholine or increase levels of dopamine can lead to delirium (Figure 114-1). Central anticholinergic syndrome, caused by blockade of muscarinic cholinergic receptors in the central nervous system, manifests as decreased heart rate and contractility, bronchial constriction, decreased salivary secretions, intestinal and bladder contraction, relaxation of sphincters, and delirium. Sedatives, such as benzodiazepines, as well as opioids (especially meperidine because it is structurally similar to the anticholinergic, atropine) are prime contenders.

Box 114-1 Predisposing and Perioperative Factors Associated with Increased Risk for Delirium in Postanesthesia Care Unit

Predisposing Factors	Perioperative Factors
Abnormal glycemic control	Airway obstruction
Age >65 y	Bladder distention
ASA score ≥3	Duration of operation >1 h
BUN/Cr >18	Duration of preoperative fluid fasting*
Cognitive dysfunction or dementia†	Electrolyte imbalance
Depression	Emergent versus elective procedure
Excessive alcohol use	High-risk operation
Illicit drug use or use of ≥3 prescription drugs	Hypoxia or hypercapnia
Immobility	Orthopedic operation
Intracranial injury	Pain
Male sex	Prolonged mechanical ventilation
Neurologic disease‡	Sensory overload
Sensory impairment, particularly visual	Use of specific drugs for anesthesia and analgesia§
Sepsis	
Use of β-adrenergic receptor blocking agents	
Metabolic derangements	

ASA, American Society of Anesthesiologists; BUN/Cr, blood urea nitrogen/creatinine ratio.
*Duration of preoperative fluid fasting ≥6 h, as compared with 2-6 h, increases the risk for development of postoperative delirium.
†Particularly impairment in executive function.
‡Alzheimer disease and Parkinson disease.
§Drugs administered perioperatively that have been associated with an increased risk for development of postoperative delirium include anticonvulsants, atropine, benzodiazepines, corticosteroids, droperidol, fentanyl (larger doses), H2 receptor antagonists, ketamine, meperidine, metoclopramide, and scopolamine.

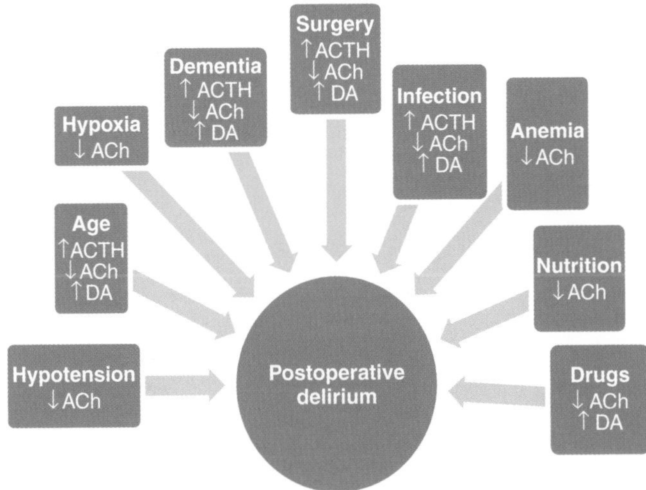

Figure 114-1 Decreased levels of acetylcholine (ACh) and increased levels of dopamine (DA) or cortisol (ACTH) can lead to postoperative delirium.

Corticosteroids, H_2-receptor antagonists, and anticonvulsants have also been implicated. Renal and hepatic dysfunction compromise clearance of these medications, resulting in further exacerbation of delirium.

In children, the highest incidence of postoperative delirium occurs in those too young (i.e., aged 2-4 years) to communicate in words when awakening from anesthesia, thereby making the differentiation between delirium and pain more difficult. Treating preoperative anxiety has some beneficial effect. When compared with the use of other inhaled anesthetics, sevoflurane and desflurane use is associated with a higher incidence of postoperative delirium in children. Using desflurane for maintenance of anesthesia after a sevoflurane induction reduces the severity of emergence delirium, when compared with sevoflurane induction and maintenance.

Table 114-1 Tools Used to Score Delirium in Postanesthesia Care Unit

Feature	CAM	DDS	Nu-DESC
Number of questions	4	5	5
Responses	Yes/No	0-2 scale	Weighted score for each of 4 possible responses
Domains measured	Acute onset or fluctuating course, inattention, disorganized thinking, altered level of consciousness	Disorientation, inappropriate behavior, inappropriate communication, illusions or hallucinations, psychomotor retardation	Orientation, hallucinations, agitation, anxiety, paroxysmal sweating

CAM, Confusion Assessment Method; DDS, Delirium Detection Score; Nu-DESC, Nursing Delirium Screening Scale.

Diagnosis

Screening tools have been developed and adapted for use in the PACU to assess patients for the presence of delirium (Table 114-1). The Nursing Delirium Screening Scale appears to be the most sensitive in detecting postoperative delirium, which is largely a diagnosis of exclusion. Common metabolic derangements that are associated with delirium include hyponatremia, hypoglycemia or hyperglycemia, hypokalemia or hyperkalemia, hypercalcemia, hypermagnesemia, lactic acidemia, hypothermia, hypothyroidism, and adrenal insufficiency. Arterial hypoxemia and alveolar hypoventilation are potential respiratory-associated causes of delirium. Postoperative nausea and vomiting and infection (e.g., urinary tract infection, pneumonia, or septicemia) should also be considered in patients who exhibit signs of postoperative delirium.

Prevention

Because the treatment of postoperative delirium is symptomatic, the best approach is prevention. A Cochrane Database review evaluated six randomized clinical trials regarding interventions to prevent delirium and concluded that evidence to support pharmacologic prevention is inadequate. However, identifying high-risk patients by means of a thorough preoperative assessment, including administration of tests that measure depression and cognitive flexibility or executive function, may be helpful in planning the anesthetic and analgesic management. The preoperative assessment should also seek to discern and address potentially modifiable risk factors (see Box 114-1).

Treatment

The goal of treatment is ensuring patient safety, which, for violent or severely agitated patients, may include the use of restraints. The initial intervention—verbal support to provide reassurance and reorientation—includes voicing the patient's name and current location, the surgeon's name, and the time of day. Physiologic causes of delirium should be considered, including distended bladder, nausea, uncomfortable positioning, or the possibility of the patient lying on a foreign object. Thereafter, treatment becomes more aggressive, beginning with the reversal of any reversible anesthetic agents via intravenous administration of flumazenil (0.2 mg increments), naloxone (0.04 mg increments), or physostigmine (1-2 mg). The use of physostigmine remains controversial but is currently indicated for the treatment of central anticholinergic syndrome. Haloperidol (2.5-5 mg every 5 min) has been reported to decrease the severity—but not the incidence—of delirium.

A multitude of drugs have been used in children undergoing surgical procedures in an attempt to prevent or treat emergence delirium. The most commonly used agents include clonidine, propofol, opioids, and dexmedetomidine. A 2 μg/kg dose of clonidine administered after induction of anesthesia has been shown to reduce the severity of emergence delirium but prolongs the PACU stay due to somnolence. Dexmedetomidine, 0.5 μg/kg, administered 5 min before the end of the surgical procedure; ketamine, 0.25 mg/kg; or nalbuphine, 0.1 mg/kg, administered at the end of anesthesia also attenuates the incidence of emergence delirium.

Outcomes and Long-Term Consequences

Emergence delirium, especially if it leads to postoperative delirium, can be costly in terms of human resources and increased length of hospital stay, as well as increased morbidity (self-extubation, pulling out tubes, lines, drains) and mortality risks. Delirious patients can also harm others should they become physically violent. If delirium in the PACU progresses to prolonged delirium, the likelihood of the patient being discharged to a skilled care facility is increased.

Suggested Readings

Ansaloni L, Catena F, Chattat R, et al. Risk factors and incidence of postoperative delirium in elderly patients after elective and emergency surgery. *Br J Surg*. 2010;97:273-280.

Bagri AS, Rico A, Ruiz JG. Evaluation and management of the elderly patient at risk for postoperative delirium. *Thorac Surg Clin*. 2009;19:363-376.

Lepousé C, Lautner CA, Liu L, et al. Emergence delirium in adults in the post-anaesthesia care unit. *Br J Anaesth*. 2006;96:747-753.

Noimark D. Predicting the onset of delirium in the post-operative patient. *Age Ageing*. 2009;38:368-373.

Radtke FM, Franck M, Macguill M, et al. Duration of fluid fasting and choice of analgesic are modifiable factors for early postoperative delirium. *Eur J Anaesthesiol*. 2010;27:411-416.

Radtke FM, Franck M, Schneider M, et al. Comparison of three scores to screen for delirium in the recovery room. *Br J Anaesth*. 2008;101:338-343.

Warshaw G, Mechlin M. Prevention and management of postoperative delirium. *Int Anesthesiol Clin*. 2009;47:137-149.

CHAPTER 115

Local Anesthetic Agents: Mechanism of Action

Steven R. Clendenen, MD

The mechanism of action of local anesthetic agents is to prevent the transmission of nerve impulses generated by a chemical, mechanical, or electrical stimulus that triggers an action potential.

Anatomy of a Nerve Cell

Nerve cells communicate with each other through axons, which are elongations of the cell body, and by dendrites. The cell membrane is a hydrophobic lipid bilayer that incorporates ion channels composed of lipoproteins. In contrast to the nerve cells of the central nervous system, many peripheral nerves are enveloped in myelin that is produced by Schwann cells. Gaps known as nodes of Ranvier, located approximately 1 mm apart in the myelin sheath have a high concentration of Na^+ channels, facilitating saltatory transmission between sequential nodes and increasing the speed of electrical conduction along the axon.

Nerve Cell Membrane and Depolarization

The cell membrane creates a barrier between the Na^+-rich extracellular fluid and the K^+-rich intracellular fluid, creating a resting membrane potential of −60 to −90 mV (Figure 115-1). There is constant movement of Na^+ ions through Na^+ channels that spontaneously open and close; active transport of Na^+ out of the cell maintains the resting membrane potential. When an appropriate stimulus of adequate magnitude opens a sufficient number of Na^+ channels, the surrounding membrane depolarizes (becomes less negative), recruiting additional channel openings—a cascade of open channels allows more Na^+ to enter the cell, with K^+ diffusing out of the cell through K^+ channels to the point that the entire membrane depolarizes, producing an all-or-nothing electrical signal (action potential) that is propagated along the axon. Once the action potential passes, an energy-dependent mechanism reestablishes the concentrations of Na^+ and of K^+, restoring the resting membrane potential.

Structure of Local Anesthetic Agents

Molecules of local anesthetic agents contain an aromatic lipophilic end, which is connected by an intermediate chain to a hydrophilic tertiary amine (weak base). The intermediate chain is either an amide or an ester linkage; this linkage is the basis for the two different classes of local anesthetic agents (esters and amides), which have similar mechanisms of action but different metabolic pathways. Because the nonionized form of the molecule crosses the cell membrane, compounds that are more lipophilic have a faster onset of blockade. And, because local anesthetic agents are weak bases, compounds with a pK_a close to physiologic pH will have a faster onset of blockade as more molecules remain in the nonionized state. Clearance of the drug from the site of injection and protein binding of local anesthetic agents by α_1-acid glycoprotein also affect the duration of action because it is the concentration of free drug that is available to diffuse across the membrane that determines blockade (Figure 115-2, Table 115-1).

Action of Local Anesthetic Agents

Intracellular pH is typically less than 7; therefore, once molecules of the local anesthetic agent cross the cell membrane, many molecules will dissociate into the ionized form of the molecule. These ions have affinity for the α subunits of the Na^+ channels. The ionized molecule of the local anesthetic agent enters a Na^+ channel from within the cell, binding with the α subunit and ultimately rendering the Na^+ channel inactive. If Na^+ cannot traverse the membrane, the cell cannot depolarize, and an action potential would not be generated. Myelinated nerves require blockade of three consecutive nodes of Ranvier to ensure impulse extinction.

Suggested Readings

Scholz A. Mechanism of (local) anaesthetics on voltage-gated sodium and other ion channels. *Br J Anaesth*. 2002;89:52-61.

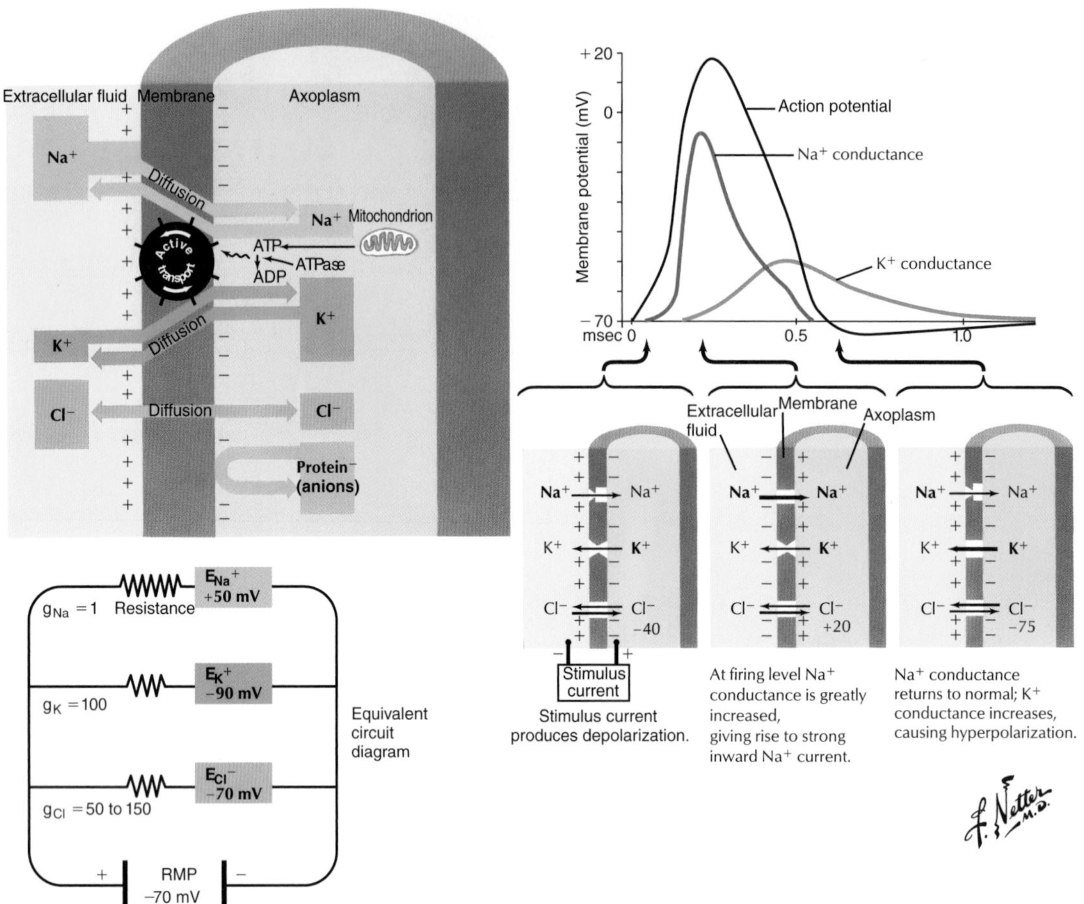

Figure 115-1 Resting membrane and action potentials. (Netter illustration from www.netterimages.com. © Elsevier Inc. All rights reserved.)

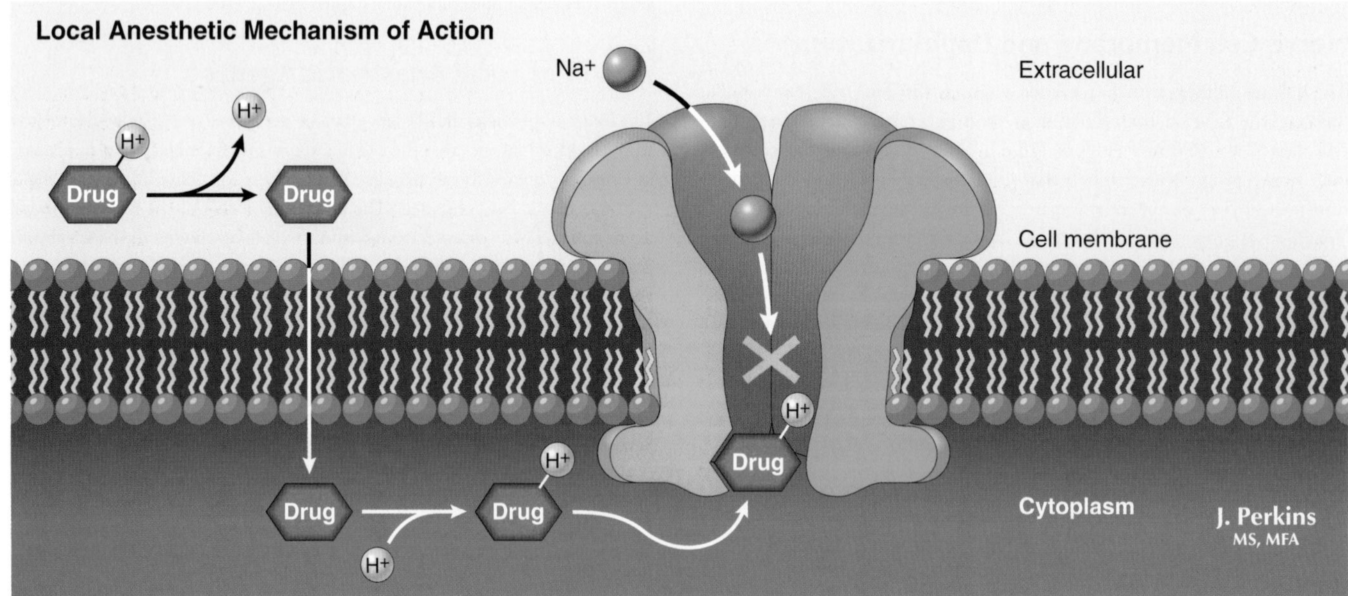

Figure 115-2 Mechanism of action of local anesthetic agents. (Netter illustration from www.netterimages.com. © Elsevier Inc. All rights reserved.)

Table 115-1 Chemical and Physical Properties of the Most Commonly Used Local Anesthetic Drugs

Property	Lidocaine	Mepivacaine	Bupivacaine	Ropivacaine	Levobupivacaine
Molecular weight	234	246	288	274	288
pK_a	7.7	7.6	8.1	8.1	8.1
Liposolubility*	4	1	30	2.8	30
Partition coefficient	2.9	0.8	28	9	28
Protein binding (%)	65	75	95	94	95
Equipotency (%)	2	1.5	0.5	0.75	0.5

*Liposolubility of each of the local anesthetic agents, as compared with mepivacaine, (e.g., lidocaine is four times more lipid soluble than mepivacaine).

CHAPTER 116

Local Anesthetic Agents: Pharmacology

Terese T. Horlocker, MD

Local anesthetic agents consist of three major chemical moieties (Figure 116-1): a lipophilic aromatic ring, a hydrophilic tertiary amine, and an ester or amide linkage. Changes in the amine or ring chemical structure result in marked alterations in lipid/aqueous solubility, potency, and protein binding. Local anesthetics are classified into two major groups based on the linkage between the lipophilic and hydrophilic components: amino esters and amino amides. Though they exert their effect by the same mechanism, they are metabolized differently (esters in the blood by pseudocholinesterase; amides by normal hepatic pathways) and have different allergic potential (ester greater than amide).

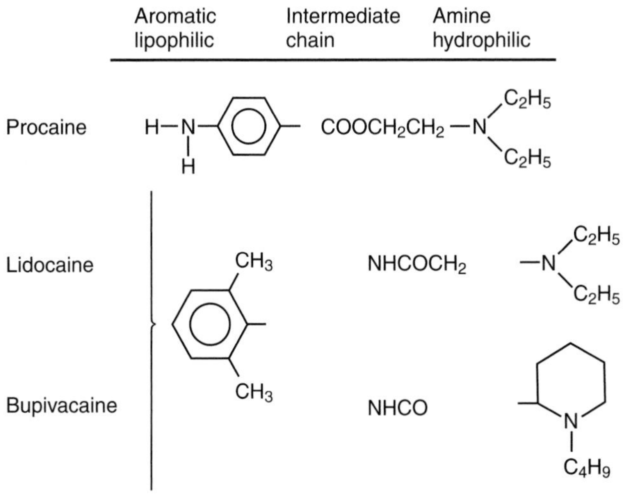

Aromatic lipophilic | Intermediate chain | Amine hydrophilic

Procaine: H–N(H)–C_6H_4– $COOCH_2CH_2$ –N(C_2H_5)(C_2H_5)

Lidocaine: CH_3 / CH_3 ring – $NHCOCH_2$ –N(C_2H_5)(C_2H_5)

Bupivacaine: $NHCO$ – piperidine N–C_4H_9

Figure 116-1 Chemical configuration of procaine, lidocaine, and bupivacaine.

The most commonly used local anesthetic agents and their physiochemical properties are described in Table 116-1.

Physiochemical Properties

Local anesthetics are weak bases with pK_a values greater than 7.4. Because the free bases are poorly water soluble, local anesthetics are dispensed as hydrochloride salts. The resulting solutions are acidic with pH values of 4 to 7.

In solution, the local anesthetics exist in equilibrium as ionized and nonionized forms (Figure 116-2). The nonionized (lipid-soluble) base crosses the axonal membrane and, once intracellular, in a more acidic environment, ionizes. The ionized (water-soluble) cation is responsible for neural blockade.

Potency is related to lipid solubility—the more lipid soluble the agent is, the more drug enters the axon. Speed of onset is related to pK_a as the pK_a affects how rapidly the drug ionizes. (Note, however, that the onset of procaine and 2-chloroprocaine blockade [$pK_a \approx 9$] is rapid because of a high solution concentration and, thus, a greater diffusion gradient.) Duration of action is related to protein binding, which influences blood concentrations and, therefore, how quickly drug is taken up at the site of injection into the blood.

Physiologic Disposition

The local anesthetic drugs are absorbed after injection of the local anesthetic agent at the site of administration. Very little metabolism of the ester compounds occurs at the site of injection, but once absorbed, they are metabolized in the blood, and the amides, in the liver. Only small amounts of either are excreted unchanged in the urine.

Table 116-1 Physicochemical/Biologic Properties of Local Anesthetic Agents

	Physicochemical Properties			Biologic Properties				
Agent	pK_a* (25° C)	Protein Binding (%)	pH, Plain Solutions†	Equieffective‡ Anesthetic Concentration	Approximate Anesthetic Duration (min)	Site of Metabolism	Onset‡	Recommended Maximum Single Dose (mg)
Procaine	9.05	6	5-6.5	2	50	Plasma, liver	Fast	500
Chloroprocaine	8.97	?	2.7-4	2	45	Plasma, liver	Fast	800 (1000 with epinephrine)
Tetracaine	8.46	75.6	4.5-6.5	0.25	175	Plasma, liver	Fast (spinal anesthesia)	20
Lidocaine	7.91	64	6.5	1	100	Liver	Intermediate	300 (500 with epinephrine)
Mepivacaine	7.76	77	4.5	1	100	Liver	Intermediate	400 (500 with epinephrine)
Prilocaine	7.9	55				Liver, extrahepatic tissue	Intermediate	400 (600 with epinephrine)
Etidocaine	7.7	94	4.5	0.25	200	Liver	Fast	400 with epinephrine
Bupivacaine (and levobupivacaine)	8.16	96	4.5-6	0.25	175	Liver	Slow	175 (225 with epinephrine)
Ropivacaine	8.2	95	4.5-6	0.5	175	Liver	Slow	225 (300 with epinephrine)

*pH corresponds with 50% ionization.
†Epinephrine-containing solutions have a pH that is 1-1.5 units lower than the pH of plain solutions.
‡When used for a brachial plexus block.
Adapted from Mather LE, Tucker GT. Properties, absorption, and disposition of local anesthetic agents. In: Cousins MJ, Carr DB, Horlocker TT, Bridenbaugh PO, eds. Neural Blockade in Clinical Anesthesia and Management of Pain. 4th ed. Philadelphia, Lippincott Williams & Williams, 2009:48-95; and Rosenberg PH, Veering BT, Urmey WF. Recommended doses of local anesthetics: A multifactorial concept. Reg Anesth Pain Med. 2004;29:264-275.

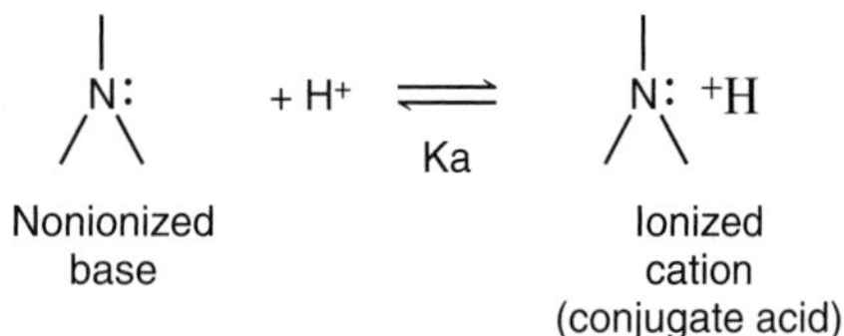

Figure 116-2 Local anesthetic substructure. (From O'Brien JE, Abbey V, Hinsvark O, et al. Metabolism and measurement of chloroprocaine, an ester-type anesthetic. J Pharm Sci. 1979;68:75-78.)

Table 116-2 Half-life of Chloroprocaine

Study Population/ Sample	No. of Patients/ Specimens	Half-life (sec)*
Mothers	7	20.9 ± 5.8
Umbilical cords	7	42.6 ± 11.2
Male control subjects	6	20.6 ± 4.1
Female control subjects	5	25.2 ± 3.7
Homozygous–atypical cholinesterase carriers	10	106.0 ± 45.0

*Data are presented as means ± SD.
Results are from O'Brien JE, Abbey V, Hinsvark O, et al. Metabolism and measurement of chloroprocaine, an ester-type anesthetic. J Pharm Sci. 1979;68:75-78.

Esters

Ester local anesthetic agents are metabolized by pseudocholinesterase (plasma cholinesterase) and partially by red blood cell esterases. Hydrolysis occurs at the ester linkage and yields an alcohol and para-aminobenzoic acid (or a PABA) derivative. Because ester local anesthetics are metabolized by pseudocholinesterase, toxicity and duration of blockade may be prolonged in patients with liver disease, in neonates, or in atypical cholinesterase carriers (Table 116-2).

Chloroprocaine is hydrolyzed four times faster than procaine, and procaine is hydrolyzed four times faster than tetracaine.

Amides

Amide local anesthetic agents are metabolized by the liver. (Prilocaine is also metabolized by extrahepatic tissues.) Three main routes of biotransformation have been identified: aromatic hydroxylation, *N*-dealkylation, and amide hydrolysis. Clearance of these agents varies in the following order: levobupivacaine < bupivacaine < ropivacaine < mepivacaine < lidocaine < etidocaine < prilocaine.

Liver disease affects metabolism of amide local anesthetic agents while having minimal effects on ester-linked compounds. In patients with severe cirrhosis, the half-life and volume of distribution of lidocaine are increased, whereas clearance is decreased because of decreased enzyme activity and shunting. Liver enzyme–inducing agents, such as barbiturates, increase the systemic clearance of amide local anesthetic agents.

Because these drugs have neurologic and cardiac toxicity, which is related to blood concentration, epinephrine in concentrations of 2.5 to 5 μg/mL should be added to the local anesthetic solution when large doses are administered, providing there are no contraindications to the use of epinephrine. The vasoconstriction caused by epinephrine decreases perfusion at the site of injection, thereby slowing systemic uptake and decreasing toxicity but also prolonging the duration of action. As a rule, conditions

Table 116-3 Lidocaine Disposition in Healthy Patients and Those With Various Diseases

Clinical Condition	Half-life (h)	V_{ss} (L/kg)	Clearance ($mL \cdot min^{-1} \cdot kg^{-1}$)
Normal	1.8	1.32	10.0
Heart failure	1.9	0.88*	6.3*
Liver cirrhosis	4.9*	2.31*	6.0*
Renal disease	1.3	1.2	13.7

*Values differ significantly in comparison with normal subjects.

V_{ss}, the volume of distribution at steady state.

From Thompson P, Melmon KL, Richardson JA, Rowland M. Lidocaine pharmacokinetics in advanced heart failure, liver disease and renal failure in humans. Ann Intern Med. 1973; 78:499-508.

(e.g., end-stage pregnancy, increased age for epidural or spinal anesthesia or analgesia) or diseases (uremia) that may increase the rate of the initial uptake of the local anesthetic agent are indications to reduce the dose in comparison to the dose used for young, healthy, and nonpregnant adults. On the other hand, the reduced clearance of local anesthetic agents associated with renal, hepatic, and cardiac diseases is the most important reason to reduce the dose for repeated or continuous administration (Table 116-3). The magnitude of the reduction should be related to the expected influence of the pharmacodynamic or pharmacokinetic change.

Clinical Use of Local Anesthetic Agents

Esters

Benzocaine

Benzocaine is almost insoluble in water. Its use is limited to topical applications, as in orotracheal administration. Methemoglobinemia is an adverse effect associated with the use of benzocaine.

Procaine

Procaine is used primarily for skin infiltration and spinal blocks because of its low potency, slow onset, and short duration of action in spinal and peripheral nerve blocks.

Chloroprocaine

The rapid onset and low toxicity of chloroprocaine make it ideal for use in labor and delivery. It is primarily used for infiltration and axillary and epidural blocks; intrathecal injection may be contraindicated because of the possibility of neurotoxicity.

Tetracaine

The most common application of tetracaine is for spinal anesthesia because of its rapid onset, dense block, and long duration of effect (4-6 h with epinephrine). Tetracaine may be used topically, although toxic reactions have been reported because of the rapid uptake.

Amides

Prilocaine

The most common application of prilocaine in North America is topical (as a component of EMLA cream [eutectic mixture of lidocaine and prilocaine]). Prilocaine is the least toxic of the amides due to its extrahepatic metabolism, but its use has been associated with methemoglobinemia.

Lidocaine

Lidocaine is the most commonly used local anesthetic agent because of its potency, rapid onset, moderate duration of action, and versatility. It can be used for infiltration as well as peripheral and central nerve blocks in concentrations ranging from 0.5% to 2.0%.

Mepivacaine

Mepivacaine is used in circumstances similar to those in which lidocaine is used; however, its duration of action is somewhat longer than that of lidocaine.

Etidocaine

Although it has a duration of action similar to that of bupivacaine, etidocaine has a much shorter onset of anesthesia due to its greater lipid solubility. The degree of motor block is also more profound than the block that is engendered with bupivacaine, producing a block more suited to prolonged surgical procedures requiring muscle relaxation. However, motor block may outlast sensory block.

Bupivacaine

Valued for its long duration in peripheral nerve and epidural blockade, bupivacaine may produce a differential sensory/motor blockade with lower concentrations. Bupivacaine is the most commonly used spinal anesthetic agent for longer procedures.

Pure Isomeric Agents

Because cardiopulmonary collapse has been reported following inadvertent intravascular injection of bupivacaine, scientists sought to identify an alternative amide with less cardiac toxicity (though one that would produce similar neural blockade). Importantly, although local anesthetic agents are typically racemic mixtures of two isomers (enantiomers), animal studies have demonstrated that the (S)− isomer is less cardiotoxic than the (R)− isomer. Consequently, more recently developed long-acting amides (ropivacaine and levobupivacaine) have been marketed as a pure isomeric solution.

Levobupivacaine The use of the (S)− isomer of bupivacaine, levobupivacaine, is associated with slightly less cardiac toxicity, as compared with bupivacaine.

Ropivacaine Provided as the (S)− racemate only, ropivacaine has less cardiac toxicity but also has a decreased potency, as compared with bupivacaine.

Suggested Readings

Butterworth JF. Clinical pharmacology of local anesthetics. In: Cousins MJ, Carr DB, Horlocker TT, Bridenbaugh PO, eds. *Neural Blockade in Clinical Anesthesia and Management of Pain*. 4th ed. Philadelphia: Lippincott, Williams & Williams; 2009:48-95.

Drasner K, Bromage PR. Choice of local anesthetics in obstetrics. In: Hughes SC, Levinson G, Rosen MA, eds. *Shnider and Levinson's Anesthesia for Obstetrics*. 4th ed. Philadelphia: Lippincott, Williams & Wilkins; 2002:73-94.

Mather LE, Tucker GT. Properties, absorption, and disposition of local anesthetic agents. In: Cousins MJ, Carr DB, Horlocker TT, Bridenbaugh PO, eds. *Neural Blockade in Clinical Anesthesia and Management of Pain*. 4th ed. Philadelphia: Lippincott, Williams & Williams; 2009:48-95.

O'Brien JE, Abbey V, Hinsvark O, et al. Metabolism and measurement of chloroprocaine, an ester-type anesthetic. *J Pharm Sci*. 1979;68:75-78.

CHAPTER 117

Toxicity of Local Anesthetic Agents

MAJ Ali Akber Turabi, MD

High blood levels of local anesthetic (LA) agents—caused by either accidental intravascular injection or increased uptake from perivascular areas—affect organs that are dependent on sodium channels to function properly. Central nervous system (CNS) abnormalities are the first manifestation of LA toxicity, whereas cardiac abnormalities result from higher concentrations of LA agents.

Prevention of LA toxicity is dependent on the injection of an appropriate volume and concentration of an LA agent, knowledge of the pharmacologic properties of these drugs, and increased vigilance for the early detection of reactions.

Factors Influencing Blood Levels of Local Anesthetic Agents

The site of and route of injection (Table 117-1), the specific drug, the dose of the drug used, the coadministration of vasoconstricting agents with the LA agent, and pathways involved in the metabolism of the drug determine blood levels of an LA agent and affect not only the speed with which blood levels of LA agents rise, but also the duration of the effect and the likelihood that toxicity will develop.

Site of Injection

Absorption of LA agents is dependent on the blood supply at the site of injection. Highly vascular areas are at greatest risk for uptake.

Choice of Local Anesthetic Agent

Injection of LA agents with a high degree of tissue binding (etidocaine and bupivacaine) or a large volume of distribution (prilocaine) result in lower blood levels, but toxicity can also be seen with the use of these agents.

Dose of Local Anesthetic Agent

The higher the concentration of the LA agent, the more likely that toxicity will occur (Table 117-2).

Table 117-1 Rapidity of Absorption of Local Anesthetic Agents, Based on Route of Administration

Route of Administration	Rapidity of Absorption
Intravenous	*Fastest*
Intercostal	↑
Caudal epidural	↑
Lumbar epidural	↑
Brachial plexus	↑
Subcutaneous	*Slowest*

Table 117-2 Maximum Dose and Duration of Commonly Used Local Anesthetic Agents

Agent	Maximum Dose (mg/kg)	Duration of Effect (h)
Esters		
Chloroprocaine	12	0.5-1
Procaine	12	0.5-1
Cocaine	3	0.5-1
Tetracaine	3	1.5-6
Amides		
Lidocaine	4.5*	0.75-1.5
Mepivacaine	4.5*	1-2
Prilocaine	8	0.5-1
Bupivacaine	3	1.5-8
Ropivacaine	3	1.5-8

*Maximum is 7 mg/kg if administered with epinephrine.

Coadministration of Vasoconstrictors

The effect of the addition of epinephrine or phenylephrine to the LA agent depends on the local blood supply at the injection site and the vasoconstrictive or dilating properties of the specific LA agent. In general, the addition of vasoconstricting agents lowers the peak blood level and increases the time to achieve the peak blood levels of LA agents.

Metabolism

Absorption and delivery to the site of metabolism (for amides, the liver; for esters, the plasma) is necessary for LA metabolism to occur.

Systemic Toxicity

Most toxic reactions to LA agents involve the CNS. More severe reactions that also involve the cardiovascular system are more difficult to treat.

Central Nervous System Toxicity

The amount of CNS toxicity is proportional to the potency of the LA agent. More potent, longer-acting drugs tend to be more toxic. The initial symptoms and signs of LA-induced CNS toxicity are tinnitus, blurred vision, dizziness, tongue paresthesias, and circumoral numbness. Excitatory phenomena (nervousness, restlessness, agitation, and muscle twitching) result from selective blockade of inhibitory pathways and often precede CNS depression, tonic-clonic seizures, and cardiopulmonary collapse. The presence of hypercarbia (secondary to CNS depression and decreased ventilatory drive) lowers the seizure threshold because the hypercarbia increases cerebral blood flow, and the associated respiratory acidosis decreases protein binding, making more free drug available.

Cardiovascular System Toxicity

All LA agents cause a dose-dependent depression in myocardial contractility and also exhibit vasodilating properties (with the exception of cocaine, a vasoconstrictor). Similar to CNS toxicity, myocardial depression is proportional to the potency of the LA agent. The use of bupivacaine has also been associated with a higher-risk profile for cardiac toxicity. When compared with lidocaine, bupivacaine is more cardiotoxic because it binds more strongly to resting or inactivated sodium channels, and bupivacaine dissociates from sodium channels during diastole more slowly than does lidocaine.

Allergy to Local Anesthetic Agents

True allergies to amide LA agents are extremely rare. Metabolism of ester LA yields para-aminobenzoic acid (PABA), which is a known allergen. A patient who is allergic to PABA should be assumed to be allergic to ester LA agents. Methylparaben, a preservative in both ester and amide LA solutions, is also metabolized to PABA and may cause allergic reactions.

Neural Toxicity

The use of chloroprocaine has been implicated in prolonged sensory and motor deficits in some patients. Studies have shown that although chloroprocaine itself is not neurotoxic, large amounts of chloroprocaine in the presence of sodium bisulfite and a low pH may cause neurotoxicity. Lidocaine and other LA agents also may cause neurotoxicity when administered in high doses.

Methemoglobinemia

Prilocaine is metabolized in the liver to *o*-toluidine, which oxidizes hemoglobin to methemoglobin. In general, doses of about 600 mg of prilocaine are required before clinically significant methemoglobinemia occurs. Methemoglobinemia makes pulse oximetry inaccurate, with a plateau occurring such that the O_2 saturation does not decrease below 84% to 86%, regardless of true oxygenation and even if methemoglobin comprises > 35% of the total hemoglobin. Methemoglobinemia may be treated by intravenous administration of methylene blue, 1 mg/kg.

Diagnosis, Prevention, and Treatment of Toxic Reactions

Most toxic reactions to LA agents can be prevented through safe performance of neural blockade, including careful selection of the dose and concentration of the LA agent. Use of a test dose and incremental injections with intermittent aspiration decrease the risk of systemic toxicity. Patients should be closely monitored for signs of intravascular injection (i.e., increased blood pressure and heart rate in the presence of epinephrine) or signs of CNS toxicity. The use of a benzodiazepine will raise the seizure threshold.

Treatment of toxic reactions due to LA agents is similar to the management of other medical emergencies, focusing on ensuring adequate airway, breathing, and circulation. Once an airway is established, 100% O_2 should be administered. Hypoxia and hypercarbia must be avoided. If convulsions occur, a small amount of a benzodiazepine or propofol will rapidly terminate the seizure without causing cardiovascular compromise. Should intubation be required to secure the airway, succinylcholine may be administered. Although the tonic-clonic motions are inhibited in a patient given a neuromuscular blocking agent, seizure activity will still be present on an electroencephalographic tracing.

Additionally, a 20% lipid emulsion should be administered (1.5-4 mL/kg bolus followed by a continuous infusion at 0.25-0.5 $mL \cdot kg^{-1} \cdot min^{-1}$ for 10-60 min) because lipid emulsions have been associated with rapid recovery from LA toxicity. Although propofol is formulated in a lipid emulsion, the formulation is only 10% lipid; therefore, propofol should not be used as a substitute for lipid emulsion in this circumstance because the lipid content is too low to provide benefit and the cardiovascular suppression associated with the use of propofol may worsen the ability to resuscitate the patient. In some cases, patients have been placed on cardiopulmonary bypass until cardiac toxicity resolves.

Though most patients require only sustained cardiopulmonary resuscitation, repeated cardioversion may be necessary and high doses of epinephrine are often required for circulatory support. Ventricular arrhythmias should be treated with bretylium instead of lidocaine.

Cauda Equina Syndrome

Prolonged neurologic injury with motor paralysis and sensory changes (including pain) is a rare complication that occurs when LA agents are used to induce spinal anesthesia. Although preservatives or other contaminants administered with the LA agent have been cited as the cause of this complication, neural toxicity has been described following injection of high concentrations and doses of certain LA agents, including chloroprocaine and lidocaine, independent of the preservative used. A number of cases were reported in the 1990s after the use of microcatheters for continuous spinal anesthesia with high-dose lidocaine, presumably because this catheter placement allowed a high concentration of the drug to accumulate near sacral nerve roots.

Transient Neurologic Symptoms

Lidocaine is not often used in spinal anesthesia due to its association with transient neurologic symptoms. Severe pain radiating down both legs is the most commonly described symptom. Associated factors include surgical position (specifically lithotomy), early ambulation, and obesity. This poses a special problem when spinal anesthesia is chosen for short procedures because there are few alternatives for outpatient regional anesthesia. Alternatives to lidocaine include procaine, mepivacaine (which has also been associated with transient neurologic syndrome), very low dose lidocaine (25 mg) with fentanyl (25 μg), and very low dose bupivacaine (4-7 mg) with fentanyl (10-25 μg).

Special Populations

Liposuction

When liposuction is performed, large amounts of dilute LA agent are used, and, therefore, the total dose of LA agent administered may be quite high. The American Academy of Dermatology has published guidelines for the performance of liposuction that recommend a maximum safe dose of lidocaine of 55 mg/kg. Because the absorption of lidocaine can be delayed in adipose tissue, toxicity is more likely to occur between 6 and 12 h after the procedure, rather than immediately after the procedure.

Suggested Readings

French J, Sharp LM. Local anaesthetics. *Ann R Coll Surg Engl*. 2012;94:76-80.

Neal JM, Mulroy MF, Weinberg GL, American Society of Regional Anesthesia and Pain Medicine. American Society of Regional Anesthesia and Pain Medicine checklist for managing local anesthetic systemic toxicity: 2012 version. *Reg Anesth Pain Med*. 2012;37:16-18.

Parry A. Management and treatment of local anaesthetic toxicity. *J Perioper Pract*. 2011;21:404-409.

Sites BD, Taenzer AH, Herrick MD, et al. Incidence of local anesthetic systemic toxicity and postoperative neurologic symptoms associated with 12,668 ultrasound-guided nerve blocks: An analysis from a prospective clinical registry. *Reg Anesth Pain Med*. 2012;37(5):478-482.

CHAPTER 118

Preservatives in Local Anesthetic Solutions

Beth L. Ladlie, MD, MPH

Although allergies to local anesthetic agents are rare, they do exist, and allergic reactions to aminoester local anesthetic agents are more common than are reactions to aminoamide local anesthetic agents. Regardless of the subclass of the agent, local anesthetic preparations often contain additives that are intended to prolong their shelf life. Some adverse reactions after administration of local anesthetic agents may be caused by these additives (Table 118-1).

Sulfites

Sulfites are antioxidants used to stabilize vasoconstricting agents (e.g. epinephrine) that are often added to local anesthetic solutions. Common sulfites include bisulfite and metabisulfite. Sulfites are capable of inducing anaphylactoid reactions, which can include angioedema, urticaria, seizures, bronchospasm, and even death. Sulfites are present as preservatives in foods and beverages, so patients will likely have had multiple exposures to sulfites prior to receiving a local anesthetic solution that contains a sulfite.

Sodium bisulfite, which is the preservative in 2-chloroprocaine, has been implicated in the development of arachnoiditis. Multiple cases have been reported of healthy patients (i.e., American Society of Anesthesiologists category 1) who have experienced bilateral lower extremity paralysis and loss of sphincter control after receiving local anesthetic agents that contain sodium bisulfite; some of these patients have only partially recovered. Many of these patients had an unintentional dural puncture and injection of a large intrathecal volume of low-pH 2-chloroprocaine–containing sodium bisulfate. Because animal studies have shown that 2-chloroprocaine is neurotoxic, it may be that the bisulfite was not the culprit; however, this issue has not been well studied, leading some to speculate that there may have been synergistic effects.

Disodium Ethylenediaminetetraacetate

Disodium ethylenediaminetetraacetate (EDTA) is a preservative added to local anesthetic agents to prolong shelf life and to enable the manufacturer to use an autoclave to sterilize the glass vials that contain the anesthetic agent. EDTA functions as a chelating agent and was originally introduced into local anesthetic agents to replace metabisulfite in 2-chloroprocaine. Large volumes (>40 mL) of epidurally injected 2-chloroprocaine formulated with EDTA have been implicated as the cause of severe pain at the injection site. The severity of EDTA-associated lumbar paraspinal muscle spasm and pain may be increased when patients are acidemic. There is no evidence of neurotoxicity resulting from EDTA.

Table 118-1 Function and Possible Toxicity of Preservatives Used in Local Anesthetic Agents

Preservative Class	Function	Possible Toxicity
Sulfites	Antioxidant	Anaphylactoid reaction Arachnoiditis
EDTA	Chelating agent	Low back pain at epidural injection site
Methylparaben	Antimicrobial	Anaphylactoid reaction

EDTA, Disodium ethylenediaminetetraacetate.

Parabens

Parabens, most commonly methylparaben, is a bacteriostatic agent often present in multiuse vials of local anesthetic agents. It has antimicrobial activity against gram-positive bacteria and fungi. Its chemical structure is similar to that of para-aminobenzoic acid (PABA), which is a known potential allergen and structurally similar to the ester local anesthetic agents. Sensitive patients may experience anaphylactoid signs and symptoms. The use of methylparaben at clinically relevant doses has not been associated with neurotoxicity.

Substitution of Preservative-Containing Solutions for Preservative-Free Solutions

Sulfites and parabens have been associated with neurotoxicity, but because all preservatives are potentially neurotoxic, anesthesiologists commonly administer only preservative-free solutions into the epidural or intrathecal space. However, according to the Orange Book published by the U.S. Food and Drug Administration, preservative-free and preservative-containing medications are considered therapeutically equivalent, and manufacturers may substitute one type for the other without notifying physicians. At least one case of cauda equina syndrome has been reported after the patient received a formulation of chloroprocaine that had been changed to a generic agent containing sodium bisulfite.

Despite the toxicity of the substances discussed here, local anesthetic agents are widely used and well tolerated. Most of the preservatives seem to be safe for human use, but when a high volume of local anesthetic agent is to be used (as with peripheral nerve blockade), the anesthesia provider should take into account the potential toxicity of the preservative.

Suggested Readings

Drolet P, Veillette Y. Back pain following epidural anesthesia with 2-chloroprocaine (EDTA-free) or lidocaine. *Reg Anesth*. 1997;22:303-307.

Eisenach JC, Hood DD, Curry R. Phase I human safety assessment of intrathecal neostigmine containing methyl- and propylparabens. *Anesth Analg*. 1997; 85:842-846.

Phillips JF, Yates AB, Deshazo RD. Approach to patients with suspected hypersensitivity to local anesthetics. *Am J Med Sci*. 2007;334:190-196.

Taniguchi M, Bollen AW, Drasner K. Sodium bisulfite: Scapegoat for chloroprocaine neurotoxicity? *Anesthesiology*. 2004;100:85-91.

Wang BC, Hillman, DE, Spielholz NI, Turndorf H. Chronic neurological deficits and Nesacaine-CE—An effect of the anesthetic, 2-chloroprocaine, or the antioxidant, sodium bisulfite? *Anesth Analg*. 1984;63:445-447.

Winnie AP, Nader AM. Santayana's prophecy fulfilled. *Reg Anesth Pain Med*. 2001;26:558-564.

CHAPTER 119
Cocaine Pharmacology

Christopher B. Robards, MD

The cocaine alkaloid (also known as benzoylmethylecgonine) is found in the leaves of the plant *Erythroxylum coca*. South American people have used it for over a millennium during social, mystical, medicinal, and religious practices. The Spanish conquistadors, upon traveling to the New World, learned of the enormous importance that the Incan civilization attached to the leaves of the coca plant. Although evidence for its use as a local anesthetic is lacking, some believe that the saliva generated from chewing of coca leaves was used as an analgesic during an operation historically performed in Peru and Bolivia known as skull trepanation. Centuries later, the German chemist Friedrich Gaedcke isolated the cocaine alkaloid. Albert Niemann improved the purification process of alkaloid isolation, publishing *On a New Organic Base in the Coca Leaves* in 1860. However, it was not until 1884 that Carl Koller realized the link between the observed anesthetic effect of cocaine and clinical application when he successfully performed ophthalmologic operations using cocaine as a local anesthetic. In the northern German city of Kiel, August Bier used a fine hollow needle to inject 5% cocaine into the lumbar subarachnoid space in a patient undergoing amputation of the foot, essentially launching the study and use of regional anesthesia. The dangers of cocaine were quickly recognized. By the end of the nineteenth century, hundreds of reports of systemic cocaine intoxication and multiple fatalities had been published.

Pharmacology

Cocaine, an ester of benzoic acid, is similar to other ester-type local anesthetic agents in that it contains an aromatic residue and a tertiary amine connected by an ester linkage (Figure 119-1). Commercially, the coca alkaloids are hydrolyzed to ecgonine and then benzoylated and methylated to the base cocaine. The hydrochloride salt results in a powdery white crystalline substance with a pK_a of 8.6 that is water soluble. One percent to 10% solutions are available; a 4% solution is used most commonly for topical application. The maximum recommended dose is 1 to 3 mg/kg. Cocaine, which is readily absorbed across mucous membranes and into the systemic circulation, has a half-life of approximately 0.5 to 1.5 h.

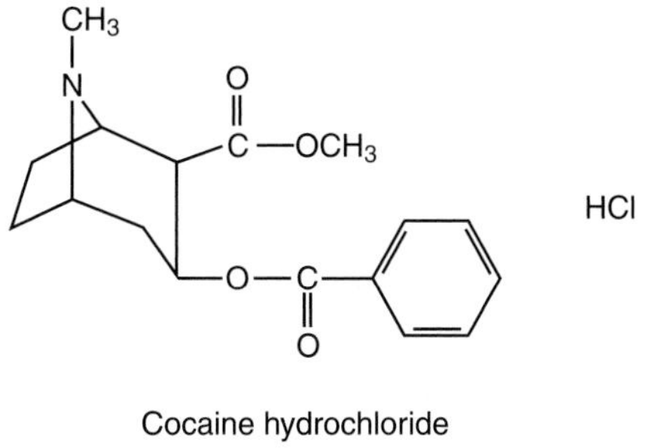

CH_3 N O C —OCH_3 HCl O—C O

Cocaine hydrochloride

Figure 119-1 Cocaine hydrochloride.

Because its metabolism is dependent on liver and plasma cholinesterases, its half-life can be prolonged in patients with impaired hepatic function and those with atypical cholinesterase (including homozygous, heterozygous, and acquired states).

Actions

Local Anesthetic Actions

Similar to that of other local anesthetic agents, the action of cocaine is mediated by its ability to reversibly block the flux of sodium ions across neuronal cell membranes.

Sympathomimetic Actions

Systemically, cocaine acts as a norepinephrine reuptake inhibitor, causing sympathetic nervous system stimulation, manifested by mydriasis, hyperglycemia, and hyperthermia. It has effects on behavior and catecholamine metabolism that are not seen with other norepinephrine reuptake inhibitors, suggesting other mechanisms of action.

Central Nervous System Actions

The initial effects of cocaine are stimulatory, causing euphoria and arousal; cocaine is thus a potent behavior reinforcer. It has a biphasic action on seizure threshold, exerting anticonvulsant effects at low doses and convulsant effects at higher doses.

Cardiovascular Actions

At low doses, cocaine exerts primarily vagal effects, characterized by bradycardia. Moderate doses can lead to elevations in blood pressure, tachycardia, cardiac arrhythmias, and even myocardial ischemia. Cocaine may cause accelerated coronary artery disease, induce coronary spasm, and reduce coronary blood flow. If inhaled into the lungs, cocaine may result in alveolar hemorrhage and pulmonary edema. Cocaine use has been associated with ruptured aortic aneurysm, infective endocarditis, vascular thrombosis, myocarditis, dilated cardiomyopathy, ruptured cerebral aneurysm, and subarachnoid hemorrhage.

Anesthetic Uses and Considerations

In current practice, cocaine is primarily used topically to anesthetize and vasoconstrict the mucous membranes of the nasal cavity and nasopharynx during nasal procedures. Two milliliters of a 10% solution on cotton pledgets is applied to contact branches of the anterior ethmoidal nerve and sphenopalatine ganglion (Figure 119-2). Alternatively, a 5% spray or a 10% paste can be applied in a similar fashion. Because of the potential for toxic side effects, the use of other drugs has been advocated; 1% lidocaine and 0.5% phenylephrine are as efficacious in dilating the nasal passage as is 5% cocaine. Ocular use is limited because of corneal damage that can result

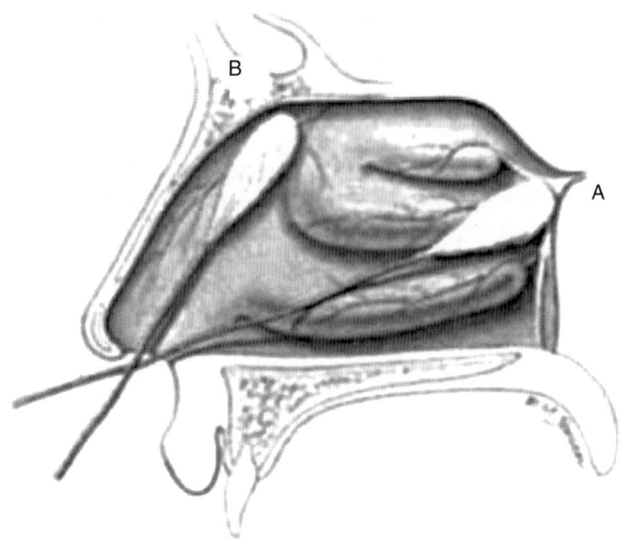

Figure 119-2 Cotton pledgets applied to contact branches of sphenopalatine ganglion (*A*) and ethmoidal nerve (*B*). (From DeWeese DD, Saunders WH, Schuller DE, Schleuning AJ II, eds. Otolaryngology—Head and Neck Surgery. 7th ed. St. Louis, Mosby, 1988.)

from vasoconstriction. Cocaine may potentiate neuromuscular blockade, either by reducing acetylcholine release or by decreasing postjunctional membrane sensitivity. The use of cocaine is contraindicated in patients with hypertension and in those taking tricyclic antidepressants or monoamine oxidase inhibitors.

Cocaine abuse by parturients can lead to multiple obstetric complications, including preterm labor, placental abruption, and stillbirth. Cocaine-induced thrombocytopenia has been reported and may increase the risks associated with the use of regional anesthesia, particularly neuraxial blockade. Ester-type local anesthetic agents may compete with cocaine for metabolism by plasma cholinesterase, prolonging the effects of both.

Management of Toxic Side Effects

Systemic toxicity with the use of cocaine is primarily managed with airway protection, maintenance of adequate ventilation, control of cardiac rhythm and hemodynamic function, suppression of seizures, and maintenance of normothermia. Propranolol has been used to treat the β-adrenergic effects of cocaine, but unopposed α-adrenergic stimulation may accentuate hypertension and constrict coronary arteries. Labetalol may offer a better choice for managing side effects by blocking both α-receptors and β-receptors. Benzodiazepines are the most appropriate therapy for cocaine-induced seizure activity. Chlorpromazine may be helpful in treating hyperthermia but does so at the cost of lowering seizure threshold.

Suggested Readings

Cheng D. Perioperative care of the cocaine-abusing patient. *Can J Anaesth*. 1994; 41:883-887.

DeWeese DD, Saunders WH, Schuller DE, Schleuning AJ II, eds. *Otolaryngology—Head and Neck Surgery*. 7th ed. St. Louis: Mosby; 1988.

Deschner B, Robards C, Somasundaram L, Harrop-Griffiths W. The history of local anesthesia. In: Hadzic A, ed. *Textbook of Regional Anesthesia and Acute Pain Management*. New York: McGraw-Hill; 2007.

Lange RA, Cigarroa RG, Yancy CW Jr, et al. Cocaine-induced coronary-artery vasoconstriction. *N Engl J Med*. 1989;321:1557-1562.

CHAPTER 120

Multimodal Analgesia

Roy A. Greengrass, MD

Traditionally, perioperative pain has been treated with systemic opioids as the only analgesic drug (monomodal therapy); unfortunately, this approach often resulted in inadequate analgesia because the dose of opioids necessary to completely attenuate the pain was associated with unacceptable side effects. Poorly treated pain has significant physiologic and psychological consequences that adversely affect patient satisfaction and convalescence and is associated with increased costs. To address this problem, the concept of multimodal analgesia, which incorporates the use of different analgesic agents acting, often times synergistically, at specific sites along nociceptive pathways to decrease or eliminate the need for administration of systemic opioids, has developed. It is generally agreed that it is better to prevent, rather than treat, pain; thus, these multimodal strategies should be initiated prior to surgery. Medications should be administered at scheduled times rather than on an as-needed basis. Agents utilized for multimodal analgesia include nonselective and cyclooxygenase-2 (COX-2) selective nonsteroidal antiinflammatory drugs (NSAIDs), acetaminophen, steroids, local anesthetic agents (e.g., for regional anesthesia), α_2-receptor agonists, ketamine, opioids, and $\alpha_2\delta$ ligands.

The Nonsteroidal Antiinflammatory Drugs

Surgical injury causes activation of COX-2 receptors, which enhance prostaglandin production, resulting in hyperalgesia at the site of injury (primary hyperalgesia). Central release of prostaglandins results in secondary hyperalgesia. The use of NSAIDs, thus, presents an opportunity to block these components of the nociceptive pathway. NSAIDs are considered to be the drugs of choice for mild to moderate postoperative pain. NSAIDs have a ceiling effect for analgesia but not for side effects.

Nonselective NSAIDs may result in gastrointestinal erosions, particularly in the elderly. COX-2 NSAIDS decrease, but do not eliminate, gastrointestinal erosion. All NSAIDs decrease renal blood flow and may result in sodium retention and edema. Nonselective NSAIDs also impair platelet function and have been associated with increased blood loss in some surgical procedures.

Acetaminophen

Acetaminophen has no antiinflammatory or peripheral activity. Its antipyretic and analgesic properties are thought to emanate via two possible mechanisms: stimulation of descending central inhibitory pathways or inhibition of central COX-3 (COX-3 being a variant of COX-2) pathways.

Published trials evaluating acetaminophen have demonstrated opioid-sparing effects in the range of 20%, less than that of NSAIDs. Acetaminophen, when administered orally, has a bioavailability of 80% to 90%; however, important variation in individual absorption of acetaminophen occurs in the early postoperative period as a result of delayed gastric emptying. Rectal administration of acetaminophen results in poor and unpredictable absorption. Intravenous acetaminophen is now approved for use in the Unites States.

Steroids

Steroids have potent antiinflammatory and immunosuppressive effects, which decrease the inflammatory response at the site of surgery, thereby decreasing nociceptive input into the spinal cord. A direct effect of steroids of decreasing signal transmission in nociceptive C fibers has also been demonstrated. A single dose of glucocorticoids has been demonstrated to inhibit the synthesis and release of proinflammatory and antiinflammatory mediators in major abdominal and cardiovascular operations. Among the steroids, glucocorticoids are preferred for perioperative antiinflammatory use due to enhanced efficiency and avoidance of mineralocorticoid effects of fluid retention and edema. Suppression of the hypothalamic-pituitary-adrenal axis after single-dose steroid therapy is not an issue. Additionally, there is no evidence in the literature that single-dose steroid administration will increase the risk of wound infection, though a single dose administered to obese patients has been associated with hyperglycemia during the perioperative period.

Regional Anesthesia

Central and peripheral nerve blocks attenuate or prevent nociceptive signals from reaching central processing centers, thus minimizing the occurrence of secondary hyperalgesia and windup. Local anesthetic agents directly depress central and peripheral neuronal excitability after systemic absorption, independent of a nerve block. Local anesthetic agents administered intravenously will suppress gastrointestinal reflexes and bowel wall inflammation.

α_2-Receptor Agonists

α_2-Receptor agonists have effects at peripheral, spinal, and brainstem loci. Prototypes, such as clonidine, appear to work by hyperpolarizing neurocircuits, both peripherally and centrally, rather than by an α_2-receptor block. Combinations of a local anesthetic agent plus clonidine or an opioid plus clonidine have been found to result in superior analgesia following total joint arthroplasty. Clonidine has also been demonstrated to enhance analgesia in peripheral nerve blocks, particularly with intermediate-duration local anesthetic agents. The ability of clonidine to enhance the quality of analgesia with long-acting local anesthetic agents is controversial.

Ketamine

Because ketamine has been shown to be a noncompetitive *N*-methyl-D-aspartate (NMDA) antagonist, the use of subanesthetic or low-dose ($<$1 mg/kg) ketamine has been demonstrated to have significant analgesia without the dysphoric effects of traditional high-dose methods.

Opioids

When used preoperatively, opioids have been demonstrated to result in prolonged postoperative analgesia. Because it has been demonstrated that opioids activate NMDA and COX prenociceptive systems leading to hyperalgesia, multimodal analgesia using NMDA and COX antagonists with opioids may reduce opioid-induced hyperalgesia and acute tolerance.

$\alpha_2\delta$ Ligands

$\alpha_2\delta$ Ligands, such as gabapentin, gabapentin enacarbil, and pregabalin, bind to the $\alpha_2\delta$ subunit of voltage-gated calcium channels, preventing release of nociceptive neurotransmitters. Sites of action include peripheral sites, primary afferent neurons, spinal neurons, and supraspinal sites. As part of multimodal therapy, these agents enhance analgesia provided by opioids, NSAIDs, and COX-2 inhibitors. Side effects of $\alpha_2\delta$ ligands include sedation, dizziness, and nausea.

Suggested Readings

Joshi GP. Multimodal analgesia techniques and postoperative rehabilitation. *Anesth Clin North Am.* 2005;23:185-202.

Schug SA, Manopas A. Update on the role of non-opioids for postoperative pain treatment. *Best Pract Res Clin Anaesth.* 2007;21:15-30.

White PF, Kehlet H, Neal JM, et al, for the Fast-Track Surgery Study Group. The role of the anesthesiologist in fast-track surgery: From multimodal analgesia to perioperative medical care. *Anesth Analg.* 2007;104:1380-1396.

CHAPTER 121

Needle Blocks of the Eye

Michael P. Hosking, MD

In most cases, anesthesia for cataract surgery is performed using regional techniques; in the United States, 50% of patients have retrobulbar blocks, 25% have peribulbar blocks, and the remaining patients receive topically applied anesthetic agents, sub-Tenon blocks, or inhalation agents. Increasingly, these regional blocks are performed by the ophthalmologist; however, whether the block is performed by the surgeon or the anesthesiologist, anesthesiologists must be cognizant of the technique and its side effects.

Anatomy

The ciliary ganglion, a parasympathetic ganglion that is 1 to 2 mm in diameter, is located approximately 1 cm anterior to the posterior wall of the orbit between the lateral surface of the optic nerve and the ophthalmic artery (Figure 121-1). Parasympathetic fibers originating in the oculomotor nerve and postganglionic fibers supply the ciliary body and sphincter pupillae muscles. The nasociliary nerve, a branch of the ophthalmic nerve, supplies the sensory innervation of the cornea, iris, and ciliary body via the short ciliary nerves, which are 6 to 10 small filaments accompanying the ciliary arteries.

Terminology

Although the terms *retrobulbar* and *peribulbar* identify types of block used in ophthalmologic operations, the terms are often confused and imprecise. Indeed, technically, all orbital blocks are retrobulbar, simply meaning that the block takes place behind the orbit. The more precise and anatomically correct terms are intraconal and extraconal, for retrobulbar and peribulbar, respectively.

Local Anesthetic Agents

The most commonly used agents are a 1:1 mixture of 2% lidocaine and 0.5% or 0.75% bupivacaine. Adding hyaluronidase to the anesthetic agent, in a typical dose of 3.5 units/mL, ostensibly shortens the time to onset of effect and improves the quality of the block; however, not all clinicians are convinced of the efficacy of hyaluronidase. The addition of epinephrine to the anesthetic agent improves the quality and duration of the block; again, however, its use is controversial in that it may lead to problems related to the retinal vasculature.

Types of Eye Blocks

Intraconal Block

An intraconal block primarily involves the ciliary ganglion, ciliary nerves, and cranial nerves II, III, and VI. The classic Atkinson technique (described in Box 121-1, Figure 121-2, *A* to *C*) typically uses a 35-mm, 25-gauge, blunt needle inserted to a depth of one third of the distance medially from the outer lower orbital margin. It requires not only deep injection of a local anesthetic agent into the orbit, but also a separate block of the seventh cranial nerve to provide akinesia and anesthesia to the surgical field.

In the past 2 decades, major changes have taken place in the performance of intraconal blocks. The position of the eye in Atkinson blocks has been supplanted by a forward-looking position. Based on cadaver and other data, the length, bevel, position, and size of the needle, as well as the amount of anesthetic agent injected, have all been revised. To reduce the incidence of needle-related complications, the current recommended needle sizes for performing either an intraconal or extraconal block are no longer than 2.5 cm, and as short as 1.5 cm, and 25 gauge. More often than not, sharp, beveled, narrow-gauge needles have replaced the blunt dull needles used more commonly in the past.

Extraconal Block

An extraconal block involves injections above and below the orbit, with local anesthetic deposited in and behind the *orbicularis oculi* muscle and beneath, above, and behind the globe. The potential for intraocular or intradural injection is decreased because the anesthetic is deposited outside the muscle cone. The risk of intraconal hemorrhage and direct optic nerve injury is also decreased. A 2008 Cochrane Database Review found no significant differences in success rate or complications between peribulbar and retrobulbar blocks.

Sub-Tenon Block

The sub-Tenon block involves the peribulbar insertion of a flexible curved cannula and infusion of an anesthetic agent into the sub-Tenon space. Because this technique does not use a sharp needle, it obviates the risk of globe penetration, retrobulbar hemorrhage, and trauma to the optic nerve.

Contraindications

Eye blocks are not used in procedures that are anticipated to last longer than 90 min, nor in patients younger than 15 years of age. Any factor that precludes the patient from following commands or lying still during the procedure or increases the patient's bleeding risk is also a contraindication to the use of an eye block (Box 121-2).

Complications

Retrobulbar Hemorrhage

The most common complication, retrobulbar hemorrhage, occurs secondary to puncture of the vessels within the retrobulbar space. It is characterized by simultaneous appearance of an excellent motor block of the globe, closing of the upper lid, proptosis, and a palpable increase in intraocular pressure. Many retrobulbar hemorrhages are minimal or even subclinical, and, on rare occasion, surgery may be continued; however, because of the significant risk

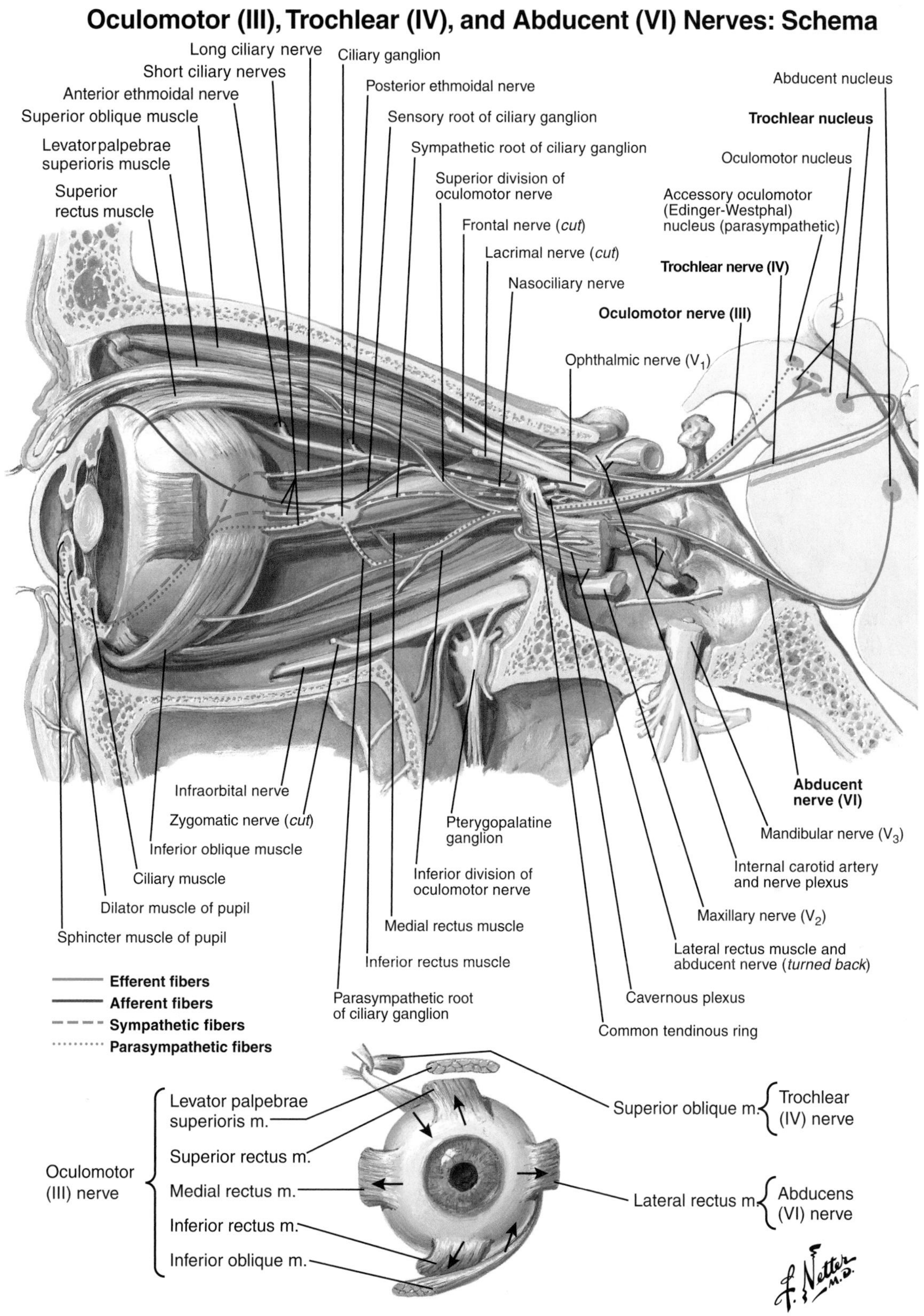

Oculomotor (III), Trochlear (IV), and Abducent (VI) Nerves: Schema

Long ciliary nerve
Ciliary ganglion
Short ciliary nerves
Anterior ethmoidal nerve
Posterior ethmoidal nerve
Superior oblique muscle
Sensory root of ciliary ganglion
Levator palpebrae superioris muscle
Sympathetic root of ciliary ganglion
Superior rectus muscle
Superior division of oculomotor nerve
Frontal nerve (*cut*)
Lacrimal nerve (*cut*)
Nasociliary nerve
Abducent nucleus
Trochlear nucleus
Oculomotor nucleus
Accessory oculomotor (Edinger-Westphal) nucleus (parasympathetic)
Trochlear nerve (IV)
Oculomotor nerve (III)
Ophthalmic nerve (V_1)
Infraorbital nerve
Zygomatic nerve (*cut*)
Inferior oblique muscle
Ciliary muscle
Dilator muscle of pupil
Sphincter muscle of pupil
Pterygopalatine ganglion
Inferior division of oculomotor nerve
Medial rectus muscle
Inferior rectus muscle
Parasympathetic root of ciliary ganglion
Abducent nerve (VI)
Mandibular nerve (V_3)
Internal carotid artery and nerve plexus
Maxillary nerve (V_2)
Lateral rectus muscle and abducent nerve (*turned back*)
Cavernous plexus
Common tendinous ring

Efferent fibers
Afferent fibers
Sympathetic fibers
Parasympathetic fibers

Oculomotor (III) nerve: Levator palpebrae superioris m.; Superior rectus m.; Medial rectus m.; Inferior rectus m.; Inferior oblique m.
Superior oblique m. — Trochlear (IV) nerve
Lateral rectus m. — Abducens (VI) nerve

F. Netter M.D.

Figure 121-1 Orbital anatomy as seen from the lateral approach. (Netter illustration from www.netterimages.com. © Elsevier Inc. All rights reserved.)

Box 121-1 Technique Commonly Employed to Perform an Intraconal Block

Clean the lower eyelid with an alcohol wipe.
Palpate the inferolateral margin of the orbit and make a skin wheal.
Ask the patient to look straight ahead.*
Using a 5-mL syringe attached to a 23-gauge, 1.5-inch, flat-grind needle, insert the needle through the skin at the junction of the lateral and middle thirds of the inferior orbital rim (see Figure 121-2, *A*).
Advance the needle slowly. The needle should penetrate only the retrobulbar fat and intermuscular septum.
Advance the needle to 35 mm. In patients with shallow ocular orbits, a shorter needle and less advancement of the needle may be necessary.
Aspirate; if no blood returns, slowly inject 2 to 4 mL of local anesthetic solution over 20 to 30 sec (see Figure 121-2, *B* and *C*).
Ask the patient to close the eye.
Withdraw the needle.
Provide firm pressure for 90 to 120 sec.
Observe the eye for proptosis or blood in lower fornix, which indicates retrobulbar hemorrhage.
If hemorrhage occurs, treat it with firm pressure and massage; this complication may necessitate cancellation of the operation.

*Recently, ophthalmologists have cautioned against the conventional upward and inward positioning of the eye because this places the routine needle path in close proximity to the optic nerve and the ophthalmic artery and vein.

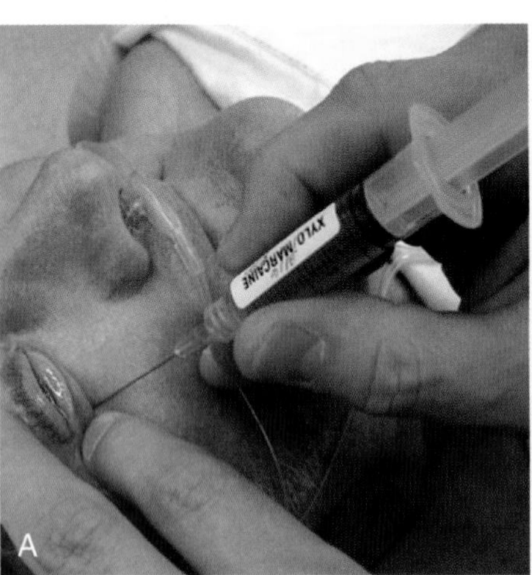

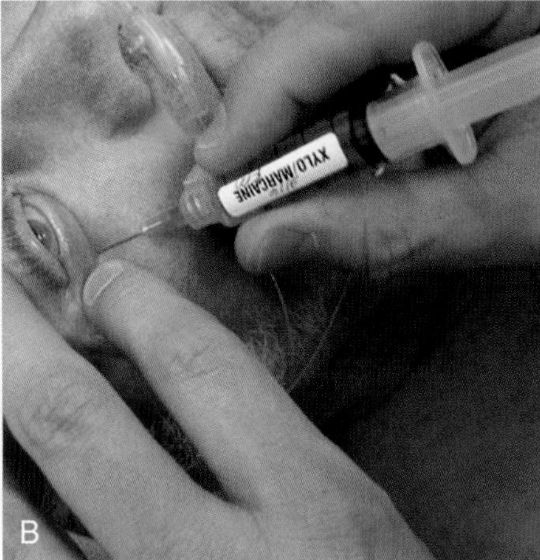

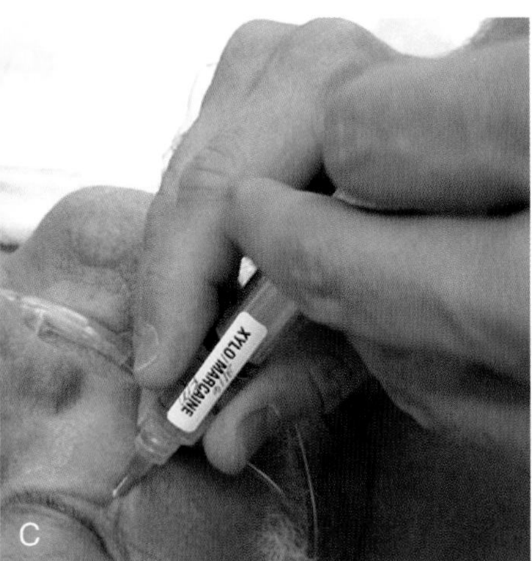

Figures 121-2 **A** to **C**, Administering the intraconal block. See Box 121-1 for further explanation of technique shown. (Images courtesy of eyerounds.org.)

Box 121-2 Contraindications to the Use of an Eye Block

Procedure is anticipated to last > 90 min
Patient has
- Uncontrolled cough, tremor, or convulsive disorder
- Excessive anxiety or claustrophobia
- Bleeding or coagulation disorder

Perforated globe
Language barrier
Patient is
- Deaf
- Disoriented
- Cognitively impaired
- Unable to lie flat
- Younger than 15 years old

of repeat hemorrhage, with its devastating complications, surgery often must be postponed.

Oculocardiac Reflex

An oculocardiac reflex (see Chapter 38) manifested by bradycardia, arrhythmias, and even periods of cardiac asystole—may occur acutely with block placement or expanding retrobulbar hemorrhage. The latter may happen some hours after a retrobulbar hemorrhage as additional blood extravasates. The reflex is trigeminal-vagal via the ciliary branch of the ophthalmic division of the trigeminal nerve. If an arrhythmia develops, surgical manipulation should be stopped and intravenous atropine (0.007 mg/kg) given.

Diplopia

The incidence of diplopia following retrobulbar block for cataract surgery is reported to be between 0.1% and 4%, depending upon the experience of the clinician performing the block. The cause of diplopia is multifactorial, but intramuscular injection of a local anesthetic agent into the small intraocular muscles with subsequent hemorrhage and scarring may be enough to disturb the exquisite balance that is normally maintained among the intraocular muscles. These patients may subsequently present for repair of their resultant strabismus.

Central Retinal Artery Occlusion

Retrobulbar hemorrhage can result in central retinal artery occlusion that, if not treated promptly and sufficiently, may result in total loss of vision. This potentially blinding complication can also occur if the dura around the optic nerve is penetrated and local anesthetic is accidentally injected into the subarachnoid space.

Puncture of Posterior Globe

Perforation of the globe can occur during retrobulbar injection despite the use of a blunted needle in this procedure. The patient experiences immediate ocular pain and restlessness after perforation. Intraocular hemorrhage and retinal detachment may result from this complication.

Penetration of the Optic Nerve

Optic atrophy and permanent loss of vision may occur even in the absence of retrobulbar hemorrhage. The postulated mechanisms include direct injury to the optic nerve, injection into the nerve sheath with compressive ischemia, and intramural sheath hemorrhage.

Inadvertent Brainstem Anesthesia

Accidental access to the cerebrospinal fluid can occur during performance of retrobulbar block secondary to perforation of the meningeal sheaths surrounding the optic nerve. The patient may experience disorientation, amaurosis fugax, aphasia, hemiplegia, unconsciousness, convulsions, and respiratory or cardiac arrest. In one large series, the incidence of central nervous system spread was shown to be 0.13%.

Direct intravascular injection via the optic nerve sheath or local anesthetic carried via the ophthalmic and internal carotid artery by retrograde flow to the thalamus and midbrain can also precipitate sudden obtundation, convulsions, and cardiopulmonary arrest. Prompt recognition and treatment necessitate careful patient monitoring.

Epinephrine Toxicity

In patients with hypertension, angina, or arrhythmias, the amount of exogenous epinephrine injected with the local anesthetic agent should be reduced. A total injection of 0.05 mg (10 mL of 1:200,000) epinephrine does not contribute significantly to problems in these patients. In fact, the release of endogenous catecholamines secondary to a patient experiencing anxiety with suboptimal analgesia may greatly exceed the relatively minute amount of exogenous catecholamine.

Suggested Readings

Alhassan MB, Kyari F, Ejere HQ. Peribulbar versus retrobulbar anaethesia for cataract surgery. *Cochrane Database Syst Rev*. 2008;(3):CD004083.

Eichel R, Goldberg I. Anaesthesia techniques for cataract surgery: A survey of delegates to the Congress of the International Council of Ophthalmology, 2002. *Clin Exp Ophthalmol*. 2005;33:469-472.

Kumar CM. Needle-based blocks for the 21st century ophthalmology. *Acta Ophthalmol*. 2011;89:5-9.

Kumar CM, Dodds C. Ophthalmic regional block. *Ann Acad Med Singapore*. 2006;35:158-167.

CHAPTER 122 Spinal Anesthesia

Lopa Misra, DO

The use of spinal anesthesia gained popularity in the United States in the 1940s. However, due to reports of adverse neurologic effects, the number of spinal anesthetics administered declined until a large study demonstrated the relative rarity of such complications, leading to a resurgence in the use of spinal blocks.

When spinal anesthetics are used in appropriately selected patients, their advantages include a decreased incidence of thromboembolism, cardiac morbidity and death, and bleeding, the latter resulting in a decreased need for transfusion. In addition, the use of subarachnoid blocks decreases the incidence of lower extremity vascular graft occlusion and of postoperative pneumonia. The advantages of subarachnoid blocks are probably due to multiple factors, including a decreased hypercoagulable state, increased tissue blood flow (because of vasodilation below the level of the block), increased oxygenation (because of maintenance of normal ventilation), increased peristalsis (related to the need for lower doses of opioids), and decreased stress response (because of the blockade of afferent activity at the spinal cord level as opposed to blockade at the level of the reticular activating center/cortex).

The mechanism of action of spinal anesthesia is due to the effect of local anesthetic agents on the individual nerve roots, effects that depend on the size and myelin content of nerve fibers, concentration of the local anesthetic agent, and duration of contact between the nerve root and the local anesthetic agent. The loss of conductivity of impulses through the fibrils follows a fixed sequence—first, sympathetic and parasympathetic activity are lost, and then sensation in the C, B, and A fibers is lost. C—fibers quit firing first, progressing finally to loss of activity in the Aα fibers, which accounts for the loss of motor function lastly. Heavy myelinated fibers present in motor nerves are most resistant to the effects of local anesthetic agents; hence, loss of activity in these nerves is the last group of nerves to be blocked. Because of the increased sensitivity of autonomic nerve fibers, blockade of these nerves extends for two or more dermatomes above the level of skin anesthesia, and blockade of motor fibers is seen two or more levels below the level of skin anesthesia (Box 122-1, Table 122-1).

Box 122-1 Factors Affecting the Level of Spinal Anesthesia
Most Important Factors
Baricity* of the solution
Patient position
During the injection
Immediately following the injection
Drug dose
Injection site
Other Factors
Patient-related factors
Age
Height
Intra-abdominal pressure
Spinal curvature
Volume of cerebrospinal fluid†
Injectate volume
Needle direction

*Baricity is defined as the density of the local anesthetic agent in relation to the density of the cerebrospinal fluid.

†Factors such as venous engorgement (as occurs during the third trimester of pregnancy) or spinal stenosis impinge on the intrathecal space and decrease the volume of cerebrospinal fluid.

Table 122-1 Dose and Duration of Effect for Local Anesthetic Agents Commonly Administered Intrathecally

		Dose (mg)			Duration of Effect (min)	
Drug	**Preparation**	**Perineum**	**Lower Abdomen**	**Upper Abdomen**	**Plain**	**With Epinephrine**
Bupivacaine	0.75% in 8.25% dextrose	4-10	12-14	12-18	90-120	100-150
Procaine	10% solution	75	125	200	45	60
Ropivacaine*	0.2-1% solution	8-12	12-16	16-18	90-120	90-120
Tetracaine	1% solution in 10% glucose	4-8	10-12	10-16	90-120	120-240

*Intrathecal injection is an off-label use for ropivacaine.

Other Factors Affecting the Level of Blockade

The most important factors affecting the level of blockade are the baricity of the local anesthetic (density of a local anesthetic compared to the density of cerebrospinal fluid [~ 1.0003]), patient positioning during and after placement, and local anesthetic dose. Hyperbaric solutions (often created by mixing the local anesthetic with 5% to 8% dextrose) are impacted by gravity and move to dependent portions of the intrathecal space, whereas hypobaric solutions (created by mixing the local anesthetic with distilled water) rise in the intrathecal space. Isobaric solutions remain at the site of the injection.

Spinal Anesthetic Agents

The most commonly used local anesthetic solutions are hyperbaric bupivacaine and hyperbaric tetracaine. Lidocaine has been used in the past but is rarely used in current practice because of its association with the development of transient neurologic symptoms and cauda equina syndrome. The quality and duration of blocks can be enhanced by adding a vasoconstrictor, such as epinephrine, or an opioid to the local anesthetic solution. Clonidine and neostigmine also have some analgesic properties when administered intrathecally.

Cardiovascular Effects

The loss of sympathetic activity that accompanies a spinal anesthetic results in vasodilation below the level of blockade, decreasing systemic vascular resistance, and the associated venodilation decreases cardiac preload and, therefore, cardiac output. If the level of blockade is sufficiently cephalad, loss of activity occurs in the cardiac accelerator nerves, which is manifested by bradycardia. The net effect of these physiologic changes can manifest as a profound decrease in systemic blood pressure. The most effective approach to the sympathectomy is (1) to provide prophylaxis by administering a bolus of intravenous fluids to the patient before the intrathecal administration of the local anesthetic agent and (2) to have a vagolytic drug and a vasopressor readily available to administer intravenously to treat the bradycardia and hypotension. Risks for the development of bradycardia (<50 beats/min) following a spinal anesthetic include (1) a baseline heart rate below 60 beats/min, (2) the use of β-adrenergic receptor blocking agents prior to presentation for a spinal anesthetic, (3) prolonged PR interval on the electrocardiogram (4) sensory level above T6, (5) age younger than 50 years and (6) American Society of Anesthesiologists I physical status.

Pulmonary Effects

Pulmonary effects seen with subarachnoid blocks are usually minimal because the diaphragm is innervated by motor fibers in the phrenic nerves that exit the spinal column at C3-C5. However, if spinal blockade is sufficiently high, in the midthoracic to upper thoracic region, vital capacity decreases because of loss of abdominal muscle activity, but tidal volume remains unchanged.

In patients with severe chronic lung disease, a high thoracic spinal anesthetic may lead to loss of accessory muscle function. Many patients with chronic lung disease depend on the accessory muscles for maintenance of ventilation.

As a general rule all patients should receive supplemental O_2 because acute airway closure, atelectasis, and hypoxia have been observed in patients with otherwise normal pulmonary function. The apnea seen with a high spinal block is more commonly due to hypoperfusion of the brainstem because of hypotension and not necessarily from the activity of the local anesthetic agents on the C3 to C5 nerve roots. When a high spinal block is identified, the patient should be placed in the Trendelenburg position to increase cardiac preload, cardiac output, and perfusion of the brainstem; if pulmonary ventilation remains compromised, tracheal intubation, assisted ventilation, or both may be necessary.

Gastrointestinal Effects

The sympathectomy associated with a spinal anesthetic maintains peristalsis, leading to a small contracted gastrointestinal tract. Hepatic blood flow may be reduced secondary to the decreased mean arterial pressure.

Genitourinary Effects

Spinal blockade has minimal effect on renal blood flow because renal blood flow is autoregulated. With spinal blockade at the lumbar or sacral level, autonomic control of bladder function can be lost, leading to urinary retention, which resolves when the blockade wears off.

Cerebral Blood Flow

Cerebral blood flow is maintained during spinal anesthesia. However, if mean arterial pressure is less than 60 mm Hg, cerebral blood flow can decrease, manifested by nausea and vomiting and, if sufficiently low, by apnea and hypoxia.

Contraindications to Spinal Anesthesia

Absolute contraindications include patient refusal, coagulation abnormalities, severe hypovolemia, increased intracranial pressure, infection, and severe stenotic aortic and mitral valvular heart disease (Box 122-2). Other relative and controversial contraindications are also listed in Box 122-2.

Box 122-2 Contraindications to Neuraxial Blockade

Absolute

Infection at the site of injection
Patient refusal
Coagulopathy or other bleeding diathesis
Severe hypovolemia
Increased intracranial pressure
Severe aortic stenosis
Severe mitral stenosis

Relative

Sepsis
Uncooperative patient*
Preexisting neurologic deficits
Demyelinating lesions
Stenotic valvular heart lesions
Severe spinal deformity

Controversial

Prior back surgery at the site of injection
Inability to communicate with the patient
Complicated operation
    Prolonged operation
    Major blood loss anticipated
    Maneuvers that compromise respiration

*Neuraxial blockade may be performed in conjunction with general anesthesia.

Suggested Readings

Arzola C, Wieczorek PM. Efficacy of low-dose bupivacaine in spinal anaesthesia for Caesarean delivery: Systematic review and meta-analysis. *Br J Anaesth.* 2011;107:308-318.

Cooper DW. Caesarean delivery vasopressor management. *Curr Opin Anaesthesiol.* 2012;25:300-308.

Harned ME, Dority J, Hatton KW. Transient neurologic syndrome: A benign but confusing clinical problem. *Adv Emerg Nurs J.* 2011;33:232-236.

Horlocker TT. Regional anaesthesia in the patient receiving antithrombotic and antiplatelet therapy. *Br J Anaesth.* 2011;107:i96-106.

Langesæter E, Dyer RA. Maternal haemodynamic changes during spinal anaesthesia for caesarean section. *Curr Opin Anaesthesiol.* 2011;24: 242-248.

Loubert C. Fluid and vasopressor management for Cesarean delivery under spinal anesthesia: Continuing professional development. *Can J Anaesth.* 2012;59:604-619.

Prats-Galino A, Reina M, Puigdellívol-Sánchez A, et al. Cerebrospinal fluid volume and nerve root vulnerability during lumbar puncture or spinal anaesthesia at different vertebral levels. *Anaesth Intensive Care.* 2012;40(4): 643-647.

Vercauteren M, Waets P, Pitkänen M, Förster J. Neuraxial techniques in patients with pre-existing back impairment or prior spine interventions: A topical review with special reference to obstetrics. *Acta Anaesthesiol Scand.* 2011;55:910-917.

CHAPTER 123

Epidural Anesthesia

Terese T. Horlocker, MD

Epidural anesthesia has clinical applications in three main areas: surgery, obstetrics, and chronic pain relief.

Applied Anatomy of the Epidural Space

The epidural space, a potential space surrounding the spinal meninges, contains fat, nerve roots, and vascular plexuses. The anatomy of the spine, ligaments, meninges, and blood flow throughout the spinal cord are described in detail in Chapter 57. Knowledge of surface anatomy (Figure 123-1) and key anatomic features of the cervical, thoracic, and lumbar spinal regions (Box 123-1) are critical to the performance of safe and reliable epidural needle placement.

All segments of the spinal canal from the base of the skull to the sacral hiatus are accessible to epidural injection. Epidural anesthesia, provided either alone or in combination with general anesthesia, may be adapted to almost any surgical procedure that takes place below the level of the patient's chin. Ideally, needle and catheter placement should occur at the level of the surgical incision (e.g., lumbar placement for lower extremity operations and thoracic placement for thoracic/abdominal operations) to allow for block of only the parts of the body that fall within the surgical field. However, a lumbar technique may be used for even upper abdominal procedures, although it would result in a complete sympathectomy, including potentially blocking the cardiac accelerator fibers. Assessment of the dermatomal sensory level enables the anesthesiologist to determine approximate level of sympathectomy and anticipate the resulting hemodynamic effects (Table 123-1).

Identification of the Epidural Space

The epidural space may be approached using a midline or a paramedian needle insertion (Figure 123-2). The epidural space is identified by the passage of the needle from an area of high resistance (*ligamentum flavum*) to an area of low resistance (epidural space). After the needle is positioned in the *ligamentum*

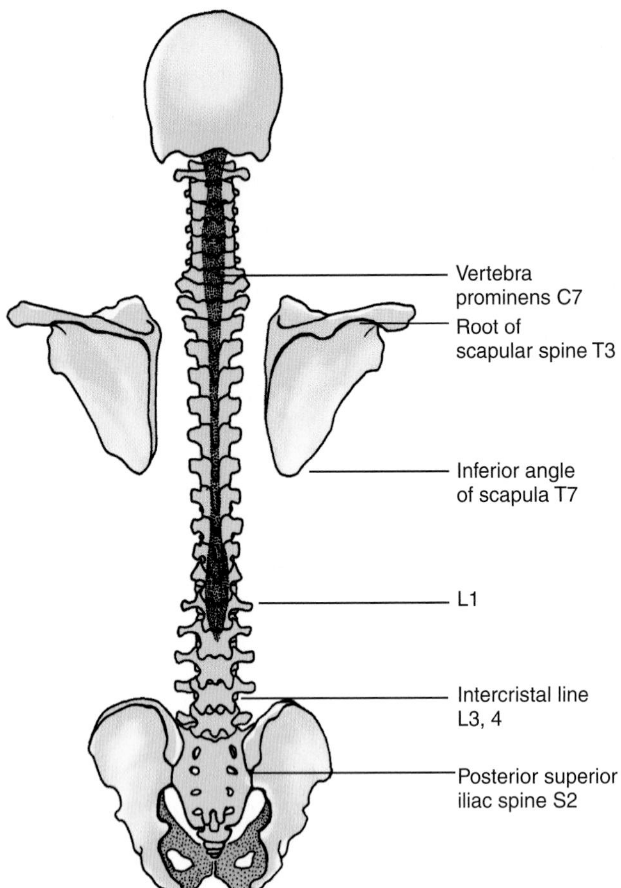

Figure 123-1 Surface anatomy and landmarks for epidural blockade. Termination of the spinal cord is at L1 in adults. The dural sac terminates at S2. Needle placement between C7 and T1 is different because of the narrow epidural space. Between T1 and T7, a paramedian approach is recommended to bypass angled spinous processes. Below T7, needle placement becomes progressively similar to that for L2-L3. (Modified from Bromage PR. Epidural Analgesia. Philadelphia: WB Saunders; 1978:8.)

Table 123-1 Sensory Level of Epidural Blockade Required for Surgical Procedures

Cutaneous Landmark	Segmental Level	Type of Operation	Significance
Fifth finger	C8		All cardioaccelerator fibers (T1-T4) blocked
Nipple line	T4-T5	Upper abdominal	Possibility of cardioaccelerator blockade
Tip of xiphoid	T6	Lower abdominal	Splanchnics (T5-L1) blocked
Umbilicus	T10	Hip	Sympathetic blockade to lower extremities
Lateral aspect of foot	S1	Leg and foot	No lumbar sympathectomy
Perineum	S2-S4	Hemorrhoidectomy	

Box 123-1 Anatomic Features of Cervical, Thoracic, and Lumbar Spine Regions

Lumbar Spine

The epidural space is widest, i.e., 5-6 mm.
Needle insertion below L1 (in adults) avoids the spinal cord.
The *ligamentum flavum* is thickest in the midline in the lumbar area.
The spinous processes have only slight downward angulation.
The epidural veins are prominent in the lateral portion of the epidural space.

Thoracic Spine

The epidural space is 3-5 mm in the midline, narrow laterally.
The *ligamentum flavum* is thick but less so than in the midlumbar region.
The spinous processes have extreme downward angulation; the paramedian approach is recommended.

Cervical Spine

The epidural space is narrow, only 2 mm at C3-6.
The *ligamentum flavum* is thin.
The spinous process at C7 is almost horizontal.

flavum, a syringe with a freely movable plunger is attached, and continuous pressure is applied to the plunger. If the needle is positioned correctly in the ligament, the syringe should not inject when pressure is applied to the plunger. As the needle passes into the epidural space, a sudden loss of resistance in the plunger will be felt, and the air or fluid will easily inject. At this point, a flexible nylon catheter may be advanced 3 to 4 cm through the needle into the epidural space to allow repeated and incremental injections. Preinsertion ultrasound imaging has been demonstrated to accurately identify the level of the vertebrae as well as to estimate the depth of the epidural space (Figure 123-3).

A test dose of 3 mL of local anesthetic solution (typically lidocaine, 1.5%) containing 1:200,000 epinephrine is then injected, and the patient is observed for signs of intravascular, subdural, or subarachnoid injection. An increase in systolic blood pressure of at least 15 mm Hg or an increase in heart rate of at least 10 beats/min represents intravascular injection, whereas a change in lower extremity sensation (with or without a decrease in blood pressure) denotes subdural or subarachnoid injection.

Selection and Dose of Local Anesthetic Agent

The major sites of action of epidurally injected local anesthetics are the spinal nerve roots, where the dura is relatively thin. Only a small amount of local anesthetic agent actually diffuses across the dura into the subarachnoid space. A local anesthetic agent should be selected on the basis of speed of onset, degree of motor blockade required, and duration of the surgical procedure (Table 123-2).

Local anesthetic dose may be calculated by the following formula: dose equals 1 to 1.5 mL of local anesthetic agent per segment blocked. The dose may need to be significantly reduced in parturients and in obese and elderly patients. In these situations, incremental doses are advised. A second dose of approximately 50% of the initial dose will maintain the original level of anesthesia if injected when the blockade has regressed 1 or 2 dermatomes (see Table 123-2).

The addition of epinephrine can prolong the duration of lidocaine nerve block by up to 50%. Less dramatic results are usually observed when bupivacaine or etidocaine is used. The addition of vasoconstricting agents reduces blood flow in the richly vascularized epidural space, reducing systemic absorption; because more of the drug remains in proximity to the nerve, the onset of block is quicker and the duration of action is longer. Confirmation of this concept comes from studies demonstrating that the peak plasma levels of various agents are lower when epinephrine is present. Epinephrine also acts on α-adrenergic receptors located in the central nervous system, modulating central pain processing at those sites.

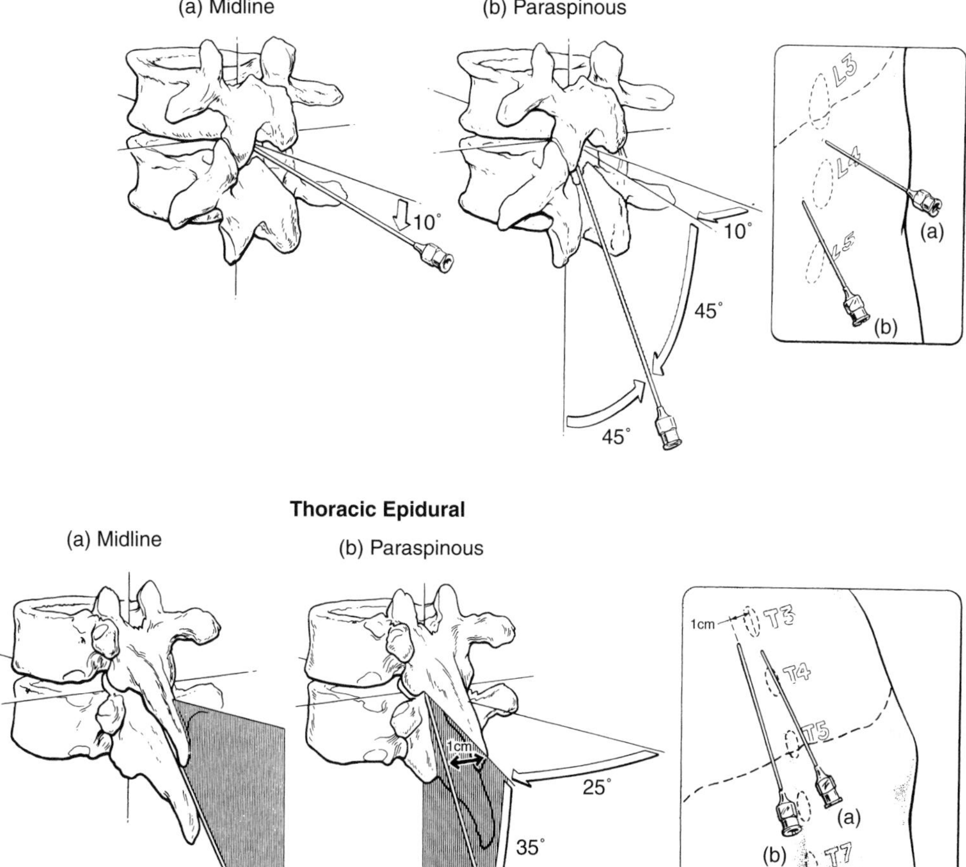

Figure 123-2 Epidural block: sites of needle insertion. *Upper panel*: Lumbar epidural: *(a)* midline—note insertion closer to the superior spinous process and with a slight upward angulation; *(b)* paraspinous (paramedian)—note insertion beside caudad edge of "inferior" spinous process, with 45° angulation to long axis of spine below. *Lower panel*: Thoracic epidural: *(a)* midline—note extreme upward angulation required in midthoracic region—paramedian approach may be technically easier; *(b)* paramedian—note needle insertion next to caudad tip of the spinous process above interspace of intended level of entry through *ligamentum flavum*—upward angulation is 55° to long axis of spine below and inward angulation is 10-15°.

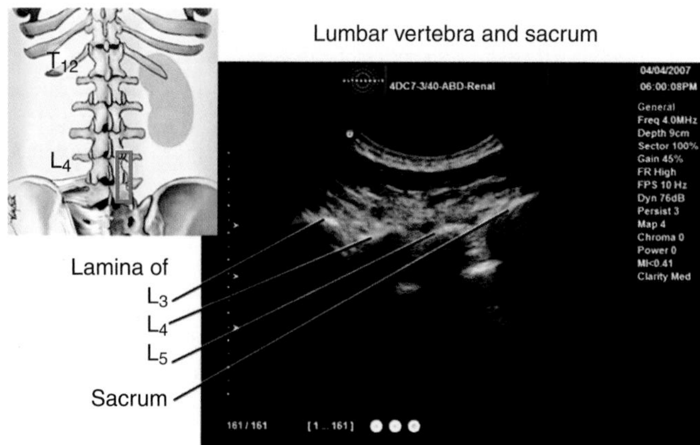

Figure 123-3 Preinsertion ultrasound of the sacrum and lumbar spine. The red rectangle shows the transducer position. (From Tran D, Kamani AA, Lessoway VA, et al. Preinsertion paramedian ultrasound guidance for epidural anesthesia. Anesth Analg. 2009;109:661-667.)

Complications

Although severe or disabling neurologic complications are rare with the use of epidural anesthesia, the results of recently conducted surveys suggest that the frequency of some serious complications, including spinal hematoma and central nervous system infections, is increasing. An epidemiologic study evaluating severe neurologic complications after neuraxial block conducted in Sweden between 1990 and 1999 reported some disturbing trends. During the 10-year study period, approximately 1,260,000 spinal and 450,000 epidural (including 200,000 epidural blocks for labor analgesia) were performed. A total of 127 serious complications were noted, including spinal hematoma (33), cauda equina (32), meningitis (29), and epidural abscess (13). The nerve damage was permanent in 85 patients. Complications occurred more often after epidural than after spinal blockade and were different in character, with cauda equina syndrome, spinal hematoma, and epidural abscess more likely to occur after epidural block and meningitis more often associated with a spinal technique. Undiagnosed spinal stenosis (detected during evaluation of the new neurologic deficits) was a risk factor for cauda equina

Table 123-2 Clinical Effects of Local Anesthetic Solutions Commonly Used for Epidural Blockade

Drug	Time Spread to ± 4 Segments ± 1 SD (min)	Approximate Time to 2-Segment Regression ± 2 SD* (min)	Recommended Top-up Time from Initial Dose* (min)
Lidocaine, 2%	25 ± 5	100 ± 40	60
Prilocaine, 2%-3%	15 ± 4	100 ± 40	60
Chloroprocaine, 2%-3%	12 ± 5	60 ± 15	45
Mepivacaine, 2%	15 ± 5	120 ± 150	60
Bupivacaine, 0.5%-0.75%	18 ± 10	200 ± 80	120
Ropivicaine, 0.75%-1%	20.5 ± 7.9	177 ± 49	120
Levobupivacaine, 0.5%-0.75%	20 ± 9	200 ± 80	120

*Note that top-up time is based on duration +/− 2 SD, which encompasses the likely duration in 95% of the population. In a conscious cooperative patient, an alternative is to use frequent checks of segmental level to indicate the need to top-up. All solutions contain 1:200,000 epinephrine.

Reprinted, with permission, from Veering BT, Cousins MJ. Epidural neural blockade. In: Cousins MJ, Carr DB, Horlocker TT, Bridenbaugh PO, eds. Neural Blockade in Clinical Anesthesia and Management of Pain, 4th ed. Philadelphia: Lippincott Williams & Williams; 2009:241-295.

syndrome and paraparesis. The results of this large series suggest that the incidence of severe anesthesia-related complications is not as low as previously reported.

Suggested Readings

Bromage PR. *Epidural Analgesia*. Philadelphia: WB Saunders; 1978:8.

Guay J. The epidural test dose: A review. *Anesth Analg*. 2009;108:1232-1242.

Moen V, Dahlgren N, Irestedt L. Severe neurological complications after central neuraxial blockades in Sweden 1990-1999. *Anesthesiology*. 2004;101:950-959.

Tran D, Kamani AA, Lessoway VA, et al. Preinsertion paramedian ultrasound guidance for epidural anesthesia. *Anesth Analg*. 2009;109:661-667.

Veering BT, Cousins MJ. Epidural neural blockade. In: Cousins MJ, Carr DB, Horlocker TT, Bridenbaugh PO, eds. *Neural Blockade in Clinical Anesthesia and Management of Pain*. 4th ed. Philadelphia: Lippincott, Williams & Williams; 2009:241-295.

CHAPTER 124 Combined Spinal-Epidural Blockade

Katherine W. Arendt, MD

Combined spinal-epidural (CSE) blockade was first described in 1937 but was not commonly used until the early 1980s. Combining the advantages of each of its component techniques, CSE blockade combines the rapid onset, reliability, and minimal drug toxicity associated with subarachnoid blocks with the flexibility of the dosing, duration, and analgesic-level control of an indwelling epidural catheter. CSE block is used primarily for obstetric analgesia and anesthesia, but its use has been described for a variety of applications, including general surgery, orthopedic and trauma surgery of the lower limb, urologic surgery, and gynecologic surgery.

Applied Anatomy

The essence of a CSE block is single-shot administration of intrathecal anesthetic or analgesic agents along with placement of a catheter into the epidural space. The applied anatomy of a CSE block is the same as that for subarachnoid and epidural blockade (see Chapter 123, Epidural Anesthesia, Figure 123-1).

Indications

CSE blockade can be utilized in patients in whom a neuraxial technique is indicated and for whom it is necessary to combine the rapid onset of analgesia or anesthesia achieved with spinal anesthesia with the ability to provide prolonged analgesia, as is usually done with a continuous infusion of medication through an epidural catheter.

Contraindications

Contraindications for CSE block are the same as those for all neuraxial blocks (Table 124-1).

Table 124-1 Absolute and Relative Contraindications to Neuraxial Anesthesia/Analgesia

Absolute	Relative
Patient refusal	Preexisting neurologic disease
Bacteremia/sepsis	Severe psychiatric disease or dementia
Increased intracranial pressure	Aortic stenosis
Infection at needle insertion site	Left ventricular outflow tract obstruction
Shock or severe hypovolemia	Various congenital heart conditions (absolute contraindication if severe)
Coagulopathy or therapeutic anticoagulation*	Deformities or previous surgery of the spinal column

*See Chapter 125.

Advantages

A systematic review comparing CSE and epidural labor analgesia found no evidence for differences in maternal satisfaction, mode of delivery, incidence of hypotension, or the ability to ambulate. However, the advantages of using a CSE technique (as opposed to an epidural technique alone) do exist and may include the following:

- The onset of anesthesia or analgesia is faster.
- The total dose of local anesthetic agent required to achieve analgesia/anesthesia is smaller than the dose necessary with an epidural-only technique, thus reducing the risk of local anesthetic toxicity. This may ultimately result in lower systemic and fetal (if used for labor and delivery) concentrations of local anesthetic agents.
- For obstetric cases, intrathecal opioids can be administered as the sole agent, without the addition of local anesthetic drugs, providing analgesia for the first stage of labor with no motor block.
- Epidural catheters placed during a CSE technique are less likely to fail than are epidural catheters placed during an epidural-only technique. This is likely because the epidural space is verified by the return of cerebrospinal fluid through the spinal needle.
- Subsequent epidural dosing may provide greater sacral nerve root coverage when a prior dural hole has been made during a CSE technique. This likely occurs from translocation of epidural drugs into the intrathecal space. In obstetric anesthesia, this may decrease the incidence of sacral sparing during the second stage of labor even if the dose of the intrathecally administered local anesthetic agent has worn off before the onset of the second stage of labor.
- During labor, more rapid cervical dilation *may* be associated with the use of a CSE block.
- In anesthesia for cesarean delivery, a CSE (with a full surgical intrathecal dose) results in less intraoperative discomfort, better muscle relaxation, less shivering, and less vomiting than with an epidural-only technique and, if the epidural catheter is left in place, an option for providing continued postoperative analgesia.

Disadvantages

Possible disadvantages of using a CSE technique, in comparison with an epidural technique, include the following:

- Determining the adequacy of the epidural catheter for surgical anesthesia may be delayed.
- Intrathecally administered opioids can cause pruritus.
- Theoretically, the risk of infection may be increased because the subarachnoid space is accessed.
- When used for labor analgesia, intrathecally administered opioid medications may increase the incidence of post analgesia fetal heart rate decelerations; however, this disadvantage is controversial, and the complex discussion is beyond the scope of this chapter.

Equipment and Technique

CSE blockades are typically performed via a needle-through-needle technique with traditional epidural and spinal needles (Figure 124-1). When the needle-through-needle technique is performed, a sterile field is created at the procedure site, the skin and subcutaneous tissue are infiltrated with a local anesthetic agent, and an epidural needle is inserted into the *ligamentum flavum*. Loss of resistance with air or saline is used to identify the epidural space. A spinal needle is then advanced through the epidural needle into the subarachnoid space. The spinal needle must be longer than the epidural needle to allow dural puncture, projecting 13 to 17 mm beyond the tip of the epidural needle. Following the appearance of cerebrospinal fluid, the intrathecal anesthetic or analgesic agent is injected, and the spinal needle is removed. Finally, a catheter is advanced through the epidural needle into the epidural space, and the epidural needle is removed.

Other CSE techniques include the use of specially designed CSE epidural needles that include a guide for the spinal needle alongside the outer wall of the epidural needle or a guide incorporated into the epidural needle wall (Figure 124-1). These guided needles make it possible to place an epidural catheter before intrathecally administering drugs. However, many anesthesiologists believe that these specially designed needles offer little advantage.

Another CSE technique involves performing separate passes, either in the same or different interspaces, with a spinal followed by an epidural. This technique requires two needle passes instead of one. If the spinal portion is performed first, then the patient may be exposed to the risks associated with performing a neuraxial technique on nerves surrounded by local anesthetic agent. If the epidural catheter is inserted first, then there may be the very remote risk of damaging the epidural catheter with the spinal needle.

Epidural Test Doses

The timing of the epidural test dose is controversial. If a local anesthetic agent has been injected into the intrathecal space, detecting an intrathecal catheter with injection of a test dose of local anesthetic agent through the catheter may be difficult. Furthermore, a successful test dose does not guarantee a properly placed epidural catheter because the catheter could conceivably migrate after the test dose is administered but before the catheter is loaded. However, it

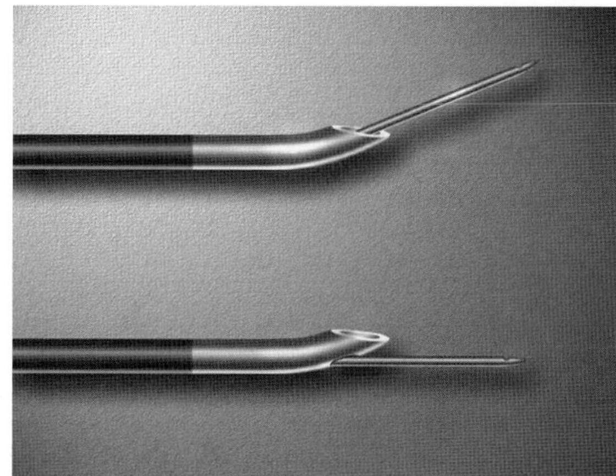

Figure 124-1 *Top:* Traditional epidural and spinal needles in a needle-through-needle technique. *Bottom:* Specially designed combined spinal-epidural needles with a guide for the spinal needle incorporated into the wall of the epidural needle. (From Wong CA, Nathan N, Brown DL. Spinal, epidural, and caudal anesthesia: Anatomy, physiology, and technique. In: Chestnut DH, Polley LS, Tsen LC, Wong CA, eds. Chestnut's Obstetric Anesthesia. 4th ed. Philadelphia, Mosby Elsevier, 2009:223-245.)

may not be convenient to wait until the spinal block from the initial intrathecal injection of drug has worn off before administering a test dose through the catheter. Many anesthesiologists recommend the early use of test doses of local anesthetic agents with epinephrine to confirm catheter position.

Complications

In comparison with an epidural technique alone, the CSE technique is not associated with an increased frequency of anesthetic complications, including postdural puncture headache. Potential complications of the CSE technique are the same as those for spinal and epidural techniques and include postdural puncture headache, total spinal anesthesia, hypotension, bradycardia, meningitis, spinal abscess and hematoma, intravascular injection, intrathecal catheter migration, and nerve injury and, when used for labor analgesia, fetal bradycardia.

Suggested Readings

Cappiello E, O'Rourke N, Segal B, Tsen L. A randomized trial of dural puncture epidural technique compared with the standard epidural technique for labor analgesia. *Anesth Analg*. 2008;107:1646-1651.

Choi DH, Kim JA, Chung IS. Comparison of combined spinal epidural anesthesia and epidural anesthesia for cesarean section. *Acta Anaesthesiol Scand*. 2000;44:214-219.

Norris MC, Fogel ST, Conway-Long C. Combined spinal-epidural versus epidural labor analgesia. *Anesthesiology*. 2001;95:913-910.

Pan PH, Bogard TD, Owen MD. Incidence and characteristics of failures in obstetric neuraxial analgesia and anesthesia: A retrospective analysis of 19,259 deliveries. *Int J Obstet Anesth*. 2004;13:227-233.

Simmons S, Cyna A, Dennis A, Hughes D. Combined spinal-epidural versus epidural analgesia in labour. *Cochrane Database Syst Rev*. 2007;(3): CD003401.

Skupski DW, Abramovitz S, Samuels J, et al. Adverse effects of combined spinal-epidural versus traditional epidural analgesia during labor. *Int J Gynaecol Obstet*. 2009;106:242-245.

Tsen LC, Thue B, Datta S, et al. Is combined spinal-epidural analgesia associated with more rapid cervical dilation in nulliparous patients when compared with conventional epidural analgesia? *Anesthesiology*. 1999;91:920-925.

Wong CA, Nathan N, Brown DL. Spinal, epidural, and caudal anesthesia: Anatomy, physiology, and technique. In: Chestnut DH, Polley LS, Tsen LC, Wong CA, eds. *Chestnut's Obstetric Anesthesia*. 4th ed. Philadelphia: Mosby Elsevier; 2009:223-245.

CHAPTER 125

Neuraxial Anesthesia and Anticoagulation

Terese T. Horlocker, MD

The actual incidence of neurologic dysfunction resulting from hemorrhagic complications associated with neuraxial blockade is unknown; however, the incidence cited in the literature is estimated to be less than 1 in 150,000 epidural anesthetics and less than 1 in 220,000 spinal anesthetics. In 57 of 61 (87%) cases of spinal hematoma associated with epidural or spinal anesthesia, a hemostatic abnormality or traumatic or difficult needle placement was present. More than one of these risk factors was present in 20 of 61 cases. Neurologic dysfunction tended to be reversible in patients who underwent laminectomy within 8 h of onset of neurologic dysfunction.

The American Society of Anesthesiologists Closed Claims project noted that spinal cord injuries were the leading cause of claims in the 1990s. Spinal hematomas accounted for nearly half of the claims related to spinal cord injuries. The primary risk factor for spinal hematoma was epidural anesthesia in the presence of intravenously administered heparin during a vascular surgical or diagnostic procedure. Importantly, the presence of postoperative numbness or weakness was typically initially attributed to the effect of the local anesthetic agent rather than to spinal cord ischemia, which delayed the diagnosis. Patient care was rarely judged to have met standards (12 of 13 cases did not meet standards), and the median payment for the claim was very high.

In a review of nearly 2 million neuraxial blocks, there were 33 spinal hematomas, with the risk associated with epidural analgesia in women undergoing childbirth significantly less (1 in 200,000) than that in elderly women undergoing knee arthroplasty (1 in 3600, $p < 0.0001$). Likewise, women undergoing operations under spinal anesthesia to repair a hip fracture had an increased risk of developing a spinal hematoma (1 in 22,000) compared with all patients undergoing spinal anesthesia (1 in 480,000).

Overall, these series suggest that the risk of clinically significant bleeding varies with age (and associated abnormalities of the spinal cord or vertebral column), the presence of an underlying coagulopathy, difficulty during needle placement, and an indwelling neuraxial catheter during sustained anticoagulation (particularly with standard heparin or low-molecular-weight heparin [LMWH]). Prompt diagnosis and intervention are critical to prevent or attenuate permanent neurologic dysfunction.

Intravenously and Subcutaneously Administered Standard Heparin

Several large studies have documented the safety of short-term intravenously administered heparinization in patients undergoing neuraxial anesthesia, provided that the heparin activity is closely monitored, indwelling catheters are removed at a time when circulating heparin levels are relatively low, and patients with a preexisting coagulation disorder are not included in the study. Conversely, traumatic needle placement, initiation of anticoagulation within

1 h of needle insertion, or concomitant aspirin therapy have been identified as risk factors in the development of spinal hematoma in patients receiving anticoagulant therapy.

Intravenous heparin administration should be delayed for 1 h after needle placement. Indwelling catheters should be removed 1 h before a subsequent heparin administration or 2 to 4 h after the last heparin dose. Evaluation of the patient's coagulation status may be appropriate before catheter removal if the patient has demonstrated enhanced response to heparin or is receiving high doses of heparin. Although a bloody or difficult needle placement may increase risk, no data support mandatory cancellation of a case should this occur. Prolonged therapeutic anticoagulation appears to increase the risk of spinal hematoma formation, especially if combined with other anticoagulants or thrombolytic agents. Therefore, neuraxial blocks should be avoided in this clinical setting. If systematic anticoagulation therapy is begun with an epidural catheter in place, catheter removal should be delayed for 2 to 4 h after discontinuation of heparin and after evaluation of coagulation status (Table 125-1).

Table 125-1 Recommendations for Management of Patients Receiving Neuraxial Blockade and Anticoagulant Drugs

Drug	Recommendations
Warfarin	Discontinue chronic warfarin therapy 4-5 days before spinal procedure and evaluate INR. INR should be within the normal range at time of procedure to ensure adequate levels of all vitamin K-dependent factors. Postoperatively, INR should be assessed daily with catheter removal occurring with an INR <1.5.
Antiplatelet medications	No contraindications with aspirin or other NSAIDs. Thienopyridine derivatives (clopidogrel and ticlopidine) should be discontinued 7 days and 14 days, respectively, before procedure. GP IIb/IIIa inhibitors should be discontinued to allow recovery of platelet function before procedure (8 h for tirofiban and eptifibatide, 24-48 h for abciximab).
Thrombolytics/ fibrinolytics	There are no available data to suggest a safe interval between procedure and initiation or discontinuation of these medications. Follow fibrinogen level and observe the patient for signs of neural compression.
LMWH	Delay procedure at least 12 h from the last dose of thromboprophylaxis LMWH dose. For "treatment" dosing of LMWH, at least 24 h should elapse before initiation of procedure. LMWH should not be administered within 24 h after the procedure. Indwelling epidural catheters should be maintained with caution and only with once-daily dosing of LMWH and strict avoidance of additional hemostasis-altering medications, including ketorolac.
Unfractionated SQ heparin	There are no contraindications to neuraxial procedure if total daily dose is less than 10,000 units. For higher dosing regimens, manage according to intravenous heparin guidelines.
Unfractionated IV heparin	Delay needle/catheter placement 2-4 h after last dose; document normal aPTT. Heparin may be restarted 1 h after procedure. Sustained heparinization with an indwelling neuraxial catheter is associated with increased risk; monitor the patient's neurologic status aggressively.

aPTT, Activated partial thromboplastin time; GP IIb/IIIa, platelet glycoprotein receptor IIb/IIIa; INR, international normalized ratio; IV, intravenous; LMWH, low-molecular-weight heparin; NSAIDs, nonsteroidal anti-inflammatory drugs; SQ, subcutaneous.
Adapted from Horlocker TT, Wedel DJ. Anticoagulation and neuraxial block: Historical perspective, anesthetic implications, and risk management. Reg Anesth Pain Med. 1998; 23:129-134.

Low-dose standard (unfractionated) heparin is subcutaneously administered for thromboprophylaxis in patients undergoing major thoracoabdominal operations. Despite the widespread use of thromboprophylaxis with subcutaneously administered heparin, only a few cases of spinal hematoma have been associated with neuraxial blockade in the presence of low-dose heparin. It is important to note that, although the American College of Chest Physicians' guidelines for prevention of thromboembolism more often recommend thrice daily administration of subcutaneous heparin (due to patient comorbid conditions and increased risk of thromboembolism), the safety of neuraxial block in these patients is unknown.

There is no contradiction to the use of neuraxial techniques along with standard heparin therapy administered subcutaneously in a twice-daily (5000 units) regimen. However, more frequent administration or higher doses may be associated with an increased risk of neuraxial bleeding. Regardless of dosing regimen, the risk of neuraxial bleeding may be reduced by delaying the heparin injection until after the block is performed and may be increased in debilitated patients or after prolonged therapy.

The concurrent use of medications that affect other components of the clotting mechanisms may increase the risk of bleeding complications for patients receiving intravenously or subcutaneously administered standard heparin. These medications include antiplatelet medications, LMWH, and oral anticoagulants.

Low-Molecular-Weight Heparin

LMWH was introduced for thromboprophylaxis following knee or hip arthroplasty. Extensive clinical testing and use of LMWH in Europe over the last 10 years has suggested that no increased risk of spinal hematoma exists in patients undergoing neuraxial anesthesia while perioperatively receiving LMWH thromboprophylaxis. However, in the first 5 years after LMWH was released for general use in the United States in May 1993, more than 60 cases of spinal hematoma associated with neuraxial anesthesia administered in the presence of perioperative LMWH prophylaxis were reported. Many of these events occurred when LMWH was administered intraoperatively or early postoperatively to patients undergoing continuous epidural anesthesia and analgesia. Concomitant antiplatelet therapy was present in several cases (Box 125-1). Timing of catheter removal may also have an impact. Although the actual frequency of spinal hematoma in patients receiving LMWH while undergoing spinal or epidural anesthesia is difficult to determine, the incidence has been estimated to be 1 in 3100 continuous epidural anesthetics and 1 in 41,000 spinal anesthetics. This frequency of spinal

Box 125-1 Patient, Anesthetic, and Low-Molecular-Weight Heparin Dosing Variables Associated with Spinal Hematoma

Patient Factors

Female sex
Increased age

Anesthetic Factors

Traumatic needle/catheter placement
Epidural (compared with spinal) technique
Indwelling epidural catheter during LMWH administration

LMWH Dosing Factors

Immediate preoperative (or intraoperative) LMWH administration
Early postoperative LMWH administration
Concomitant antiplatelet or anticoagulant medications
Twice-daily LMWH administration

LMWH, low-molecular-weight heparin.
Reprinted, with permission, from Horlocker TT, Wedel DJ. Neuraxial block and low-molecular-weight heparin: Balancing perioperative analgesia and thromboprophylaxis. Reg Anesth Pain Med. 1998;23:164-177.

hematoma is similar to that reported for women undergoing total knee replacement with epidural analgesia.

The indications and labeled uses for LMWH continue to evolve. Indications for thromboprophylaxis as well as treatment of thromboembolism or myocardial infarction have been introduced. Several off-label applications of LMWH are of special interest to the anesthesia provider. LMWH has been demonstrated to be efficacious as a "bridge therapy" for patients chronically anticoagulated with warfarin, including parturients and patients with prosthetic cardiac valves, a history of atrial fibrillation, or a preexisting hypercoagulable condition. The doses of LMWH are those associated with thromboembolism treatment, not prophylaxis, and are much higher. An interval of at least 24 h is required for the anticoagulant activity to resolve.

Using an antifactor Xa assay to measure patients' levels of heparin, low molecular weight heparin, danaparoid, etc., is not predictive of the risk of bleeding and, thus, is not helpful in the management of patients undergoing neuraxial blocks. Antiplatelet or orally administered anticoagulant medications in combination with LMWH may increase the risk of spinal hematoma.

A single-dose spinal anesthetic may be the safest neuraxial technique in patients preoperatively receiving LMWH. In these patients, needle placement should be done at least 10 to 12 h after the last dose of LMWH. Patients receiving higher "treatment" doses of LMWH (e.g., enoxaparin 1 mg/kg twice daily) will require longer delays (24 h). Neuraxial techniques should be avoided in patients receiving a dose of LMWH within 2 h preoperatively (i.e., patients undergoing general surgery) because needle placement occurs during peak anticoagulant activity; ideally, at least 12 h should elapse after the last dose of LMWH is administered before proceeding with a neuraxial technique (see Table 125-1).

Patients with postoperative initiation of LMWH thromboprophylaxis may safely undergo single-dose and continuous catheter techniques. The first dose of LMWH should be administered no earlier than 24 h postoperatively. In addition, it is recommended that indwelling catheters be removed before initiation of LMWH thromboprophylaxis. The decision to implement LMWH therapy in the presence of an indwelling catheter must be made with care, and this therapy should occur only (1) with once-daily dosing of LMWH *and* (2) all other medications that affect hemostasis should be avoided. Extreme vigilance of the patient's neurologic status is warranted.

For any LMWH prophylaxis regimen, timing of catheter removal is of paramount importance. Catheter removal should be delayed for at least 10 to 12 h after a dose of LMWH is administered. Subsequent dosing should be withheld for at least 2 h after catheter removal.

Oral Anticoagulants

Little data exist regarding the risk of spinal hematoma in patients with indwelling epidural catheters receiving anticoagulation with warfarin. Importantly, most clinicians recommend that, except in extraordinary circumstances, spinal or epidural needle/catheter placement and removal should not be performed in fully anticoagulated patients. Although neuraxial anesthesia, including postoperative epidural analgesia, may be safely performed in patients who are anticoagulated perioperatively with warfarin, the optimal duration of indwelling catheter use and the timing of its removal remain controversial. Variable patient response to warfarin anticoagulation is also well documented; a prothrombin time (PT) and corresponding international normalized ratio (INR) must be assessed daily to guide therapy.

Anesthetic management of patients who are anticoagulated perioperatively with warfarin depends on the dose and timing of initiation of therapy. PT and INR values in patients on chronic oral anticoagulation therapy will take 3 to 5 days to normalize after discontinuation of anticoagulant therapy. It is recommended that the patient's normal coagulation status be documented before implementation of the neuraxial block.

Often, the first dose of warfarin is administered the night before surgery. For these patients, the PT and INR should be checked before the neuraxial block is placed if the first dose of warfarin was given more than 24 h earlier, or if a second dose of oral anticoagulant was administered. Patients receiving low-dose warfarin therapy during epidural analgesia should have their PT and INR monitored on a daily basis, and these values should be checked before catheter removal if the initial dose of warfarin was administered more than 36 h beforehand. Initial studies evaluating the safety of epidural analgesia in association with oral anticoagulation used low-dose warfarin, with mean daily doses of approximately 5 mg. Higher-dose warfarin therapy may require more intensive monitoring of coagulation status. Reduced doses of warfarin should be given to patients who are likely to have an enhanced response to the drug. There is no definitive recommendation for removal of neuraxial catheters in patients with an INR greater than 1.5 and less than 3. Caution must be exercised in making decisions about removing or maintaining these catheters (see Table 125-1).

Antiplatelet Medications

Antiplatelet medications are seldom used as primary agents of thromboprophylaxis. Several large studies have demonstrated the relative safety of neuraxial blockade in both obstetric and surgical patients receiving nonsteroidal anti-inflammatory drugs (NSAIDs). The use of NSAIDs does not appear to represent a significant risk for the development of spinal hematoma in patients having epidural or spinal anesthesia. However, the concurrent use of medications that affect other components of clotting mechanisms—such as oral anticoagulants, standard heparin, and LMWH—may increase the risk of bleeding complications for patients receiving antiplatelet agents (see Box 125-1).

Ticlopidine (Ticlid) and clopidogrel (Plavix) are also platelet-aggregation inhibitors. These agents interfere with platelet-fibrinogen binding and subsequent platelet-platelet interactions. The effect is irreversible for the life of the platelet. Ticlopidine and clopidogrel have no effect on platelet cyclooxygenase, acting independently of aspirin. Platelet dysfunction is present for 5 to 7 days after discontinuation of clopidogrel and 10 to 14 days with ticlopidine. Platelet glycoprotein IIb/IIIa receptor antagonists—including abciximab (ReoPro), eptifibatide (Integrilin), and tirofiban (Aggrastat)—inhibit platelet aggregation by interfering with platelet-fibrinogen binding and subsequent platelet-platelet interactions. Time to normal platelet aggregation following discontinuation of therapy ranges from 8 h (eptifibatide, tirofiban) to 48 h (abciximab). Increased perioperative bleeding in patients undergoing cardiac and vascular operations after receiving ticlopidine, clopidogrel, or glycoprotein IIb/IIIa antagonists warrants concern regarding the risk of anesthesia-related hemorrhagic complications. It is recommended that platelet function be allowed to recover prior to neuraxial block in patients receiving ticlopidine, clopidogrel, or platelet glycoprotein IIb/IIIa inhibitors.

Conclusion

The decision to perform spinal or epidural anesthesia or analgesia and the timing of catheter removal in a patient receiving anticoagulants perioperatively should be made on an individual basis, weighing the definite (albeit small) risk of spinal hematoma with the benefits of regional anesthesia for a specific patient. The patient's coagulation status should be optimized at the time of spinal or epidural needle or catheter placement, and the level of anticoagulation must be carefully monitored during the period of epidural catheterization (see Table 125-1). Patients should be closely monitored in the perioperative period for early signs of cord compression, such as severe back pain, progression of numbness or weakness, and bowel and bladder dysfunction. A delay in diagnosis may lead to irreversible cord ischemia. Significant neurologic recovery is unlikely if surgery is postponed more than 8 h.

Suggested Readings

Cheney FW, Domino KB, Caplan RA, Posner KL. Nerve injury associated with anesthesia: A closed claims analysis. *Anesthesiology*. 1999;90:1062-1069.

Geerts WH, Bergqvist D, Pineo GF, et al. Prevention of venous thromboembolism: American College of Chest Physicians Evidence-Based Clinical Practice Guidelines, 8th ed. *Chest*. 2008;133:381S-453S.

Horlocker TT, Wedel DJ. Anticoagulation and neuraxial block: Historical perspective, anesthetic implications, and risk management. *Reg Anesth Pain Med*. 1998;23:129-134.

Horlocker TT, Wedel DJ. Neuraxial block and low-molecular-weight heparin: Balancing perioperative analgesia and thromboprophylaxis. *Reg Anesth Pain Med*. 1998;23:164-177.

Horlocker TT, Wedel DJ, Rowlingson JC, et al. Regional anesthesia in the patient receiving antithrombotic or thrombolytic therapy: American Society of Regional Anesthesia and Pain Medicine Evidence-Based Guidelines, 3rd ed. *Reg Anesth Pain Med*. 2010;35:64-101.

Moen V, Dahlgren N, Irestedt L. Severe neurological complications after central neuraxial blockades in Sweden 1990-1999. *Anesthesiology*. 2004;101:950-959.

CHAPTER 126

Paravertebral Nerve Blocks

Roy A. Greengrass, MD

Paravertebral nerve blocks (PVBs) provide an opportunity to block multiple mixed nerve roots soon after they emanate from the intervertebral foramina. These largely somatic blocks provide anesthesia and analgesia for a multitude of surgical and medical procedures, as well as for treatment of chronic pain syndromes. A catheter can be placed in the paravertebral space, allowing for continuous infusion of local anesthetics, which offers advantages over primary central neuraxial techniques.

Indications

PVBs can be utilized to provide anesthesia and analgesia for a variety of procedures (Box 126-1). PVBs provide excellent analgesia after thoracotomy and have unique advantages in patients with anatomic abnormalities, such as kyphoscoliosis and ankylosing spondylitis, in which thoracic epidural placement may be difficult or impossible. PVBs provide better deafferentation than does a thoracic epidural technique, which may help explain why PVBs result in better preservation of pulmonary function, compared with epidural analgesia. There is also evidence that the intensive deafferentation provided by PVBs may attenuate chronic pain and, when used during surgery for resection of (breast) malignancy, may decrease the incidence of metastasis.

PVBs are particularly useful in patients with multiple rib fractures and associated spinal or cranial trauma, in which placement of a thoracic epidural catheter is contraindicated. In these clinical situations, PVBs, especially if a continuous technique is used, obviate the need for systemic analgesia or sedation, which facilitates continuous neurologic assessment.

PVBs have been documented to reverse ischemic cardiac pain and, thus, may provide a treatment option for patients who have had medical and surgical treatment but continue to have ischemic symptoms.

PVBs can be utilized for obstetric analgesia and are particularly useful in situations in which anatomic abnormalities, such as Harrington rods, preclude the use of epidural analgesia.

Box 126-1 Procedures in Which Paravertebral Nerve Blocks May Be Used

- Breast cancer operations, from simple biopsy to modified radical mastectomy and axillary dissection
- Noncancer breast operations, including augmentation and reduction mammoplasty
- Herniorrhaphy, including incisional, ventral, umbilical, inguinal
- Thoracotomy or thoracoscopy
- Abdominal wall procedures
- Endovascular aortic aneurysm surgery
- Iliac crest bone harvesting
- Upper extremity surgery, including orthopedic and general surgical procedures, such as shoulder surgery

Contraindications

Contraindications to performance of PVBs include generic contraindications to any peripheral nerve block, including infection at the site of insertion, indeterminate neuropathy, major coagulopathy, and patient refusal. The need for subsequent anticoagulation is a relative contraindication to the use of a continuous technique.

Regional Anatomy

The paravertebral space is a wedge-shaped anatomic compartment adjacent to the vertebral bodies. The space is defined anterolaterally by the parietal pleura; posteriorly by the superior costotransverse ligament (thoracic levels); medially by the vertebra, vertebral disk, and intervertebral foramina; and superiorly and inferiorly by the heads of the ribs. Within this space, the spinal root emerges from the intervertebral foramen and divides into dorsal and ventral rami (Figure 126-1).

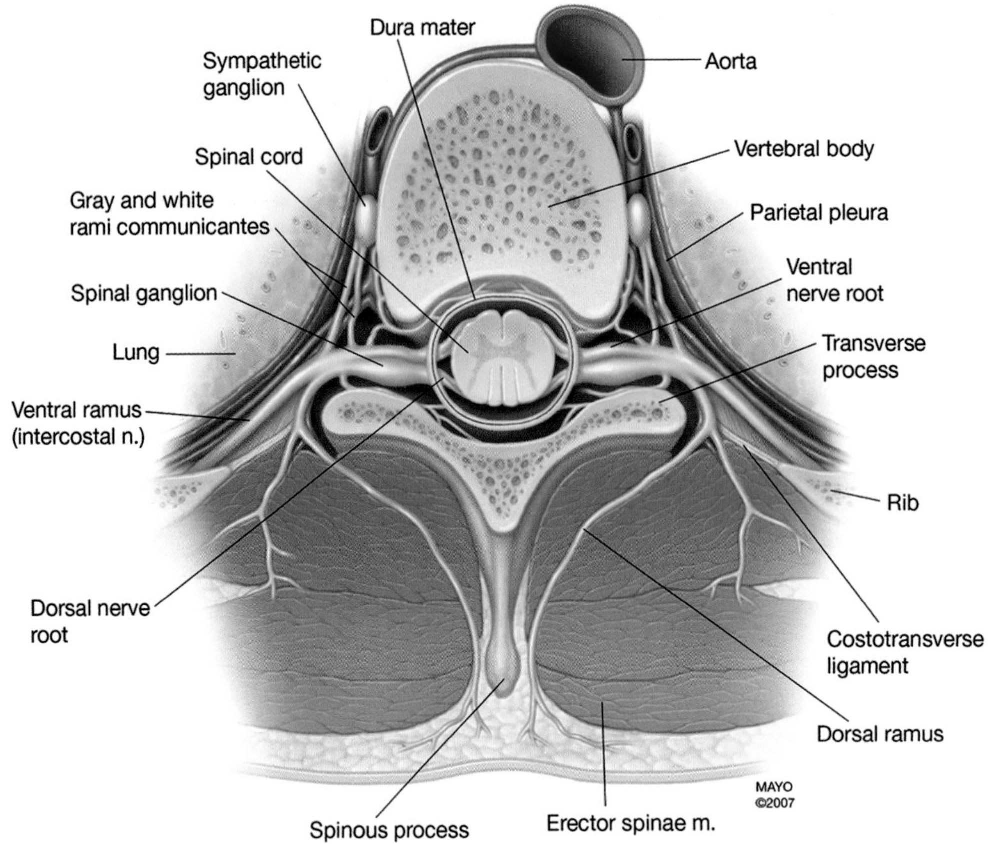

Figure 126-1 Paravertebral anatomy in the thoracic and lumbar regions. (By permission of Mayo Foundation for Medical Research and Education. All rights reserved.)

Anatomic Technique

Position

Patients are seated with the neck flexed forward with the chin to the chest, the back is arched posteriorly, and shoulders are relaxed forward (similar to performance of a thoracic epidural).

Landmarks

The spinous process of each level is identified, and a mark is placed at the most superior aspect. From the midpoint of these marks, a needle-entry site is marked 2.5 cm laterally (Figure 126-2). In the thoracic area, these marks should overlie the transverse process of the immediately caudal vertebra (because of the extreme angulation of the thoracic spinous processes). In the lumbar area, the transverse process is at the same level as the spinous process or even one level above the spinous process.

Block Performance

Employing aseptic technique, a skin wheal is placed at each mark. Using a 22G, 8.9-cm Tuohy epidural needle attached via extension tubing to a syringe, the shaft of the needle is grasped by the dominant hand of the operator. The needle is inserted through the skin wheal and advanced anteriorly in the parasagittal plane (perpendicular to the back in all planes) until it contacts the transverse process (2-6 cm, depending on the body habitus of the patient). As a safety measure, to prevent inadvertent deep placement, the needle is grasped at a point from its tip that is equal to the estimated depth from the skin to the transverse process. Inserting the needle 1 cm past this predicted depth is allowed. If the transverse process is not identified at an appropriate depth, it is assumed that the needle tip lies between adjacent transverse processes. The needle is then redirected caudad or cephalad until the transverse process is successfully contacted. This depth is noted as the estimated distance to subsequent transverse processes. The needle is then withdrawn to the subcutaneous tissue and angled to "walk off" the caudad edge of the transverse process 1 cm, following which 2 to 4 mL of local anesthetic is incrementally injected.

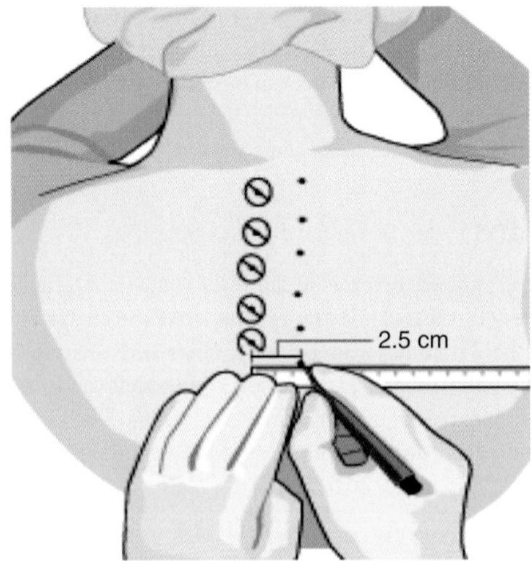

Figure 126-2 Technique for performing a paravertebral block. The spinous process of each level is identified, and a mark is placed at the most superior aspect. From the midpoint of these marks, a needle entry site is marked 2.5 cm laterally. (By permission of Mayo Foundation for Medical Research and Education. All rights reserved.)

Nerve Stimulation Technique

A nerve stimulation technique can be used, performed similarly to the anatomic technique described earlier. In the author's opinion, nerve stimulation techniques should be utilized in lumbar and lower thoracic levels only to minimize complications such as pneumothorax, which might occur secondary to the multiple needle manipulations that may be required with the nerve stimulation technique. The same anatomic landmarks as discussed in the anatomic technique are utilized.

Ultrasound Guidance

As with the practice of regional anesthesia in other applications, ultrasound-guided PVBs have proved to be useful, particularly in patients with anatomic abnormalities, such as significant scoliosis.

Choice of Local Anesthetic Agent

Similar to other peripheral nerve blocks, PVBs can be performed utilizing an intermediate agent such as lidocaine or mepivavaine with onset 5-10 minutes, time to surgical anesthesia is 20 minutes and duration is 4-6 hours. Long acting agents such as bupivacaine or ropivacaine have onset times of 10-15 minutes, time to surgical anesthesia 20-30 minutes and duration 18-24 hours (longer duration with increasing concentration). For continuous PVB, ropivacaine 0.2% is utilized.

Complications

Complications associated with PVBs include possible intraneural injection, significant epidural spread of the local anesthetic agent, pneumothorax, and local anesthetic toxicity.

Suggested Readings

Coveney E, Weltz CR, Greengrass R, et al. Use of paravertebral block anesthesia in the surgical management of breast cancer: Experience in 156 cases. *Ann Surg*. 1998;227:496-501.

Exadaktylos AK, Buggy DJ, Moriarty DC, et al. Can anesthetic technique for primary breast cancer surgery affect recurrence or metastasis? *Anesthesiology*. 2006; 105:660-664.

Greengrass R, Buckenmaier CC III. Paravertebral anaesthesia/analgesia for ambulatory surgery. *Best Pract Res Clin Anaesthesiol*. 2002;16:271-283.

Kairaluoma PM, Bachmann MS, Rosenberg PH, Pere PJ. Preincisional paravertebral block reduces the prevalence of chronic pain after breast surgery. *Anesth Analg*. 2006;103:703-708.

Richardson J, Sabanathan S, Mearns AJ, et al. Efficacy of pre-emptive analgesia and continuous extrapleural intercostal nerve block on post-thoracotomy pain and pulmonary mechanics. *J Cardiovasc Surg*. 1994;35:219-228.

Weltz CR, Klein SM, Arbo JE, Greengrass RA. Paravertebral block anesthesia for inguinal hernia repair. *World J Surg*. 2003;27:425-429.

CHAPTER 127
Upper Extremity Blocks

Sandra L. Kopp, MD, Susan M. Moeschler, MD, and Denise J. Wedel, MD

Successful neural blockade of the upper extremity requires extensive anatomic knowledge of the brachial plexus, from its origin as the roots emerge from the intervertebral foramina and of the nerves of the arm and forearm (Figure 127-1). Also important is knowledge of the side effects and complications of peripheral nerve blocks in the upper extremity, as well as the clinical application of available local anesthetic agents for these blocks. Finally, one must not underestimate the role of appropriate sedation during placement of the nerve block and during the surgical procedure (Table 127-1).

Interscalene Block

The interscalene approach to the brachial plexus, at the level of the trunks, is best suited to operations on the shoulder, when a block of the cervical plexus is also desirable. Blockade of the inferior trunk (C8-T1) is often incomplete, requiring supplementation of the ulnar nerve for adequate surgical anesthesia in that distribution. Advantages of this block include technical ease because of easily palpated landmarks and the ability to perform the block with the patient's arm in any position, which is especially important for cases involving

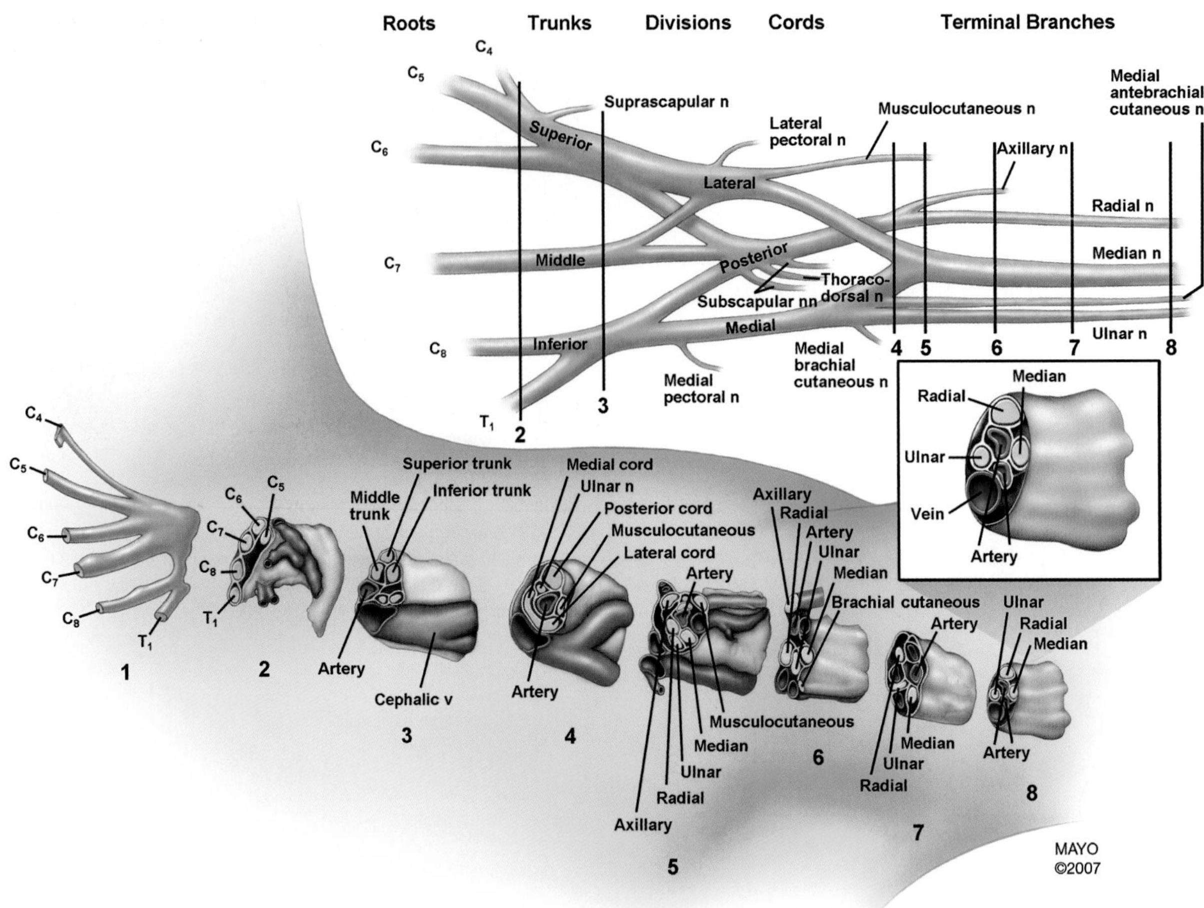

Figure 127-1 Brachial plexus anatomy. (Used with permission of Mayo Foundation for Medical Education and Research.)

Table 127-1 Regional Anesthetic Techniques for Upper Extremity Operations

Brachial Plexus Technique	Level of Blockade	Peripheral Nerves Blocked	Surgical Applications	Comments
Axillary	Peripheral nerves	Radial, ulnar, median; musculocutaneous unreliably blocked	Operations of the forearm and hand	Unsuitable for proximal humerus or shoulder surgery Requires patient to abduct the arm
Supraclavicular	Distal trunk–proximal cord	Radial, ulnar, median, musculocutaneous, axillary	Operations of the midhumerus, elbow, forearm, and hand	Risk of pneumothorax requires caution in ambulatory patients Phrenic nerve paresis in 30% of cases
Interscalene	Upper and middle trunks	Entire brachial plexus, although inferior trunk (ulnar nerve) is inconsistently blocked	Surgery to shoulder, proximal and mid humerus	Phrenic nerve paresis in 100% of patients for duration of the block Unsuitable for patients unable to tolerate a 25% reduction in pulmonary function

Adapted from Kopp SL, Horlocker TT. Regional anaesthesia in day-stay and short-stay surgery. Anaesthesia. 2010;65(Suppl 1):84-96.

upper extremity trauma or other painful conditions. Use of a nerve stimulator or ultrasound guidance is recommended with this technique to place the local anesthetic solution accurately.

Technique

With the patient in the supine position, the patient's head is turned away from the side to be anesthetized. The lateral border of the sternocleidomastoid muscle is palpated and marked; identification of the muscle is facilitated by having the patient briefly lift his or her head. The interscalene groove may be palpated by rolling the fingers posterolaterally from the muscle border, over the belly of the anterior scalene muscle. A line is extended laterally from the cricoid cartilage to intersect the vertical line of the interscalene groove; this represents the level of the C6 transverse process. The external jugular vein often crosses at this level but is not a reliable anatomic landmark (Figure 127-2).

A 22-gauge, 4-cm, short-bevel needle is inserted perpendicular to the skin with a 45-degree caudad and slightly posterior angle. The needle is advanced until the patient exhibits paresthesia or, if a nerve stimulator is being used, a motor response is observed in the forearm or hand. The brachial plexus is usually quite superficial in the interscalene area (1 to 2 cm). A "click" may be felt as the blunt needle penetrates the prevertebral fascia, giving another confirmation of accurate needle location. If the needle

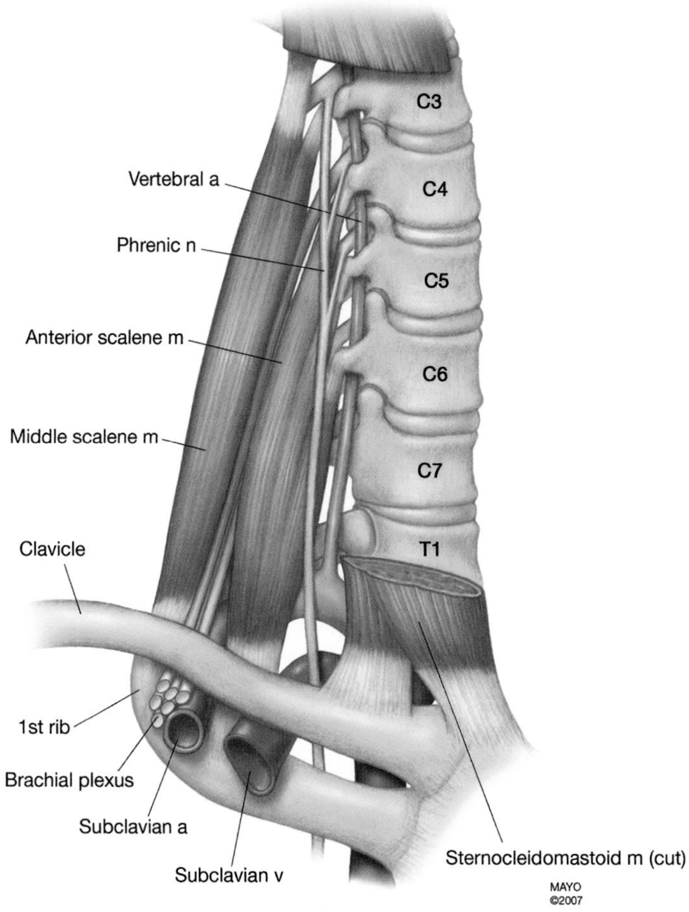

Figure 127-2 Interscalene anatomy. (Used with permission of Mayo Foundation for Medical Education and Research.)

encounters bone within 2 cm of the skin surface, this is likely the transverse process, and the needle should be gently "walked off" anteriorly. After a test dose of local anesthetic agent is given, 10 to 30 mL of the agent is injected incrementally, with frequent aspiration. Caudad spread of the local anesthetic may be facilitated by maintaining digital pressure proximal to the injection site and placing the patient in a head-up position during or following blockade.

This block is very suited to the use of ultrasound guidance. It is often easiest to obtain a supraclavicular view (see description later) of the subclavian artery and brachial plexus and then trace the plexus up the neck with the ultrasound probe until the plexus trunks are visualized as hypoechoic structures between the anterior and medial scalene muscles (Figure 127-3, *A* and *B*). The needle can then be advanced in an out-of-plane or an in-plane approach to a depth of 1 to 3 cm in most patients. After negative aspiration, a test dose is administered to confirm appropriate placement of the needle.

Side Effects and Complications

Nerve damage or neuritis can occur secondary to needle trauma or pharmacologic toxicity but is uncommon and usually self-limited. Local anesthetic toxicity as a result of intravascular injection should be guarded against by careful aspiration and incremental injection. The phrenic nerve is frequently blocked, probably because of its anatomic proximity on the anterior surface of the anterior scalene muscle. The patient may complain of subjective shortness of breath. The risk of pneumothorax is low when the needle is correctly placed at the C5 or C6 level because of the distance from the dome of the pleura. Blockade of the vagus, recurrent laryngeal, and cervical

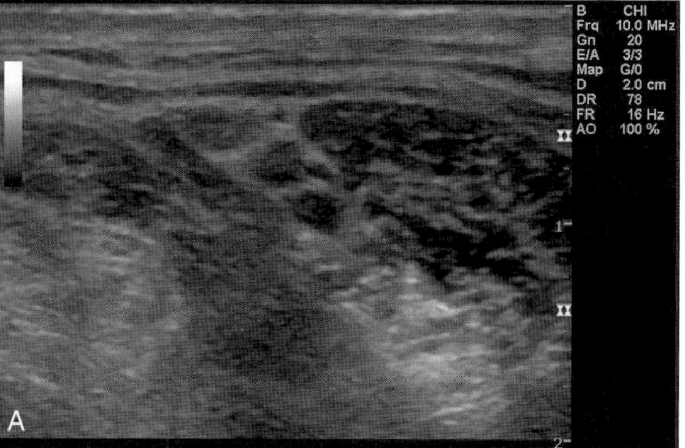

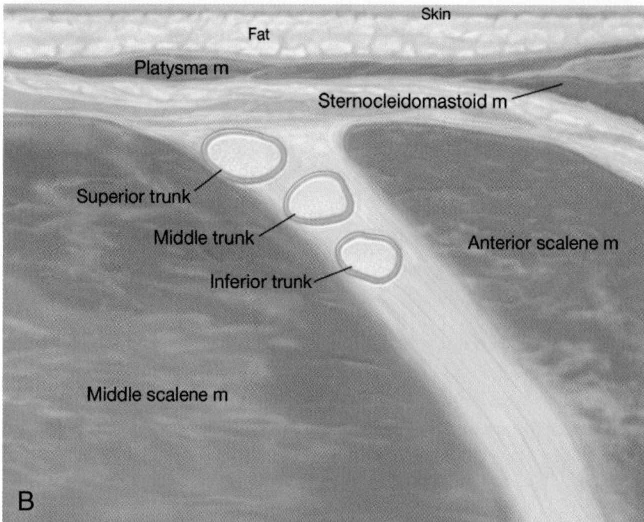

Figure 127-3 Ultrasound-guided interscalene block. **A,** Ultrasound image. **B,** Corresponding anatomy. (Used with permission of Mayo Foundation for Medical Education and Research.)

sympathetic nerves, as well as epidural and intrathecal injections, have been reported to have occurred during interscalene block. Reports of catastrophic nerve damage resulting from cord injection or high-dose spinal injections underscore that *this block should not be performed in a heavily sedated or anesthetized patient.*

Supraclavicular Block

Because of the compact arrangement of the trunks of the brachial plexus at the level of the first rib, the supraclavicular approach is extremely efficient; relatively small volumes of local anesthetic agent result in rapid and profound neural blockade when injected accurately. The supraclavicular approach provides excellent surgical anesthesia for the elbow, forearm, and hand. The use of ultrasound has led to a resurgence of this block.

Technique

The three trunks of the brachial plexus are compactly arranged cephaloposterior to and surrounding the subclavian artery at the level of the first rib, inferior to the clavicle at approximately its midpoint (Figure 127-4).

The patient is positioned in the supine position with the head turned away from the side to be blocked and the arm adducted and stretched as far as possible toward the ipsilateral knee. In the classic description, the midpoint of the clavicle is marked. The lateral border of the sternocleidomastoid muscle is identified (aided by the patient lifting the head), and the interscalene groove is palpated by rolling the fingers back from the muscle

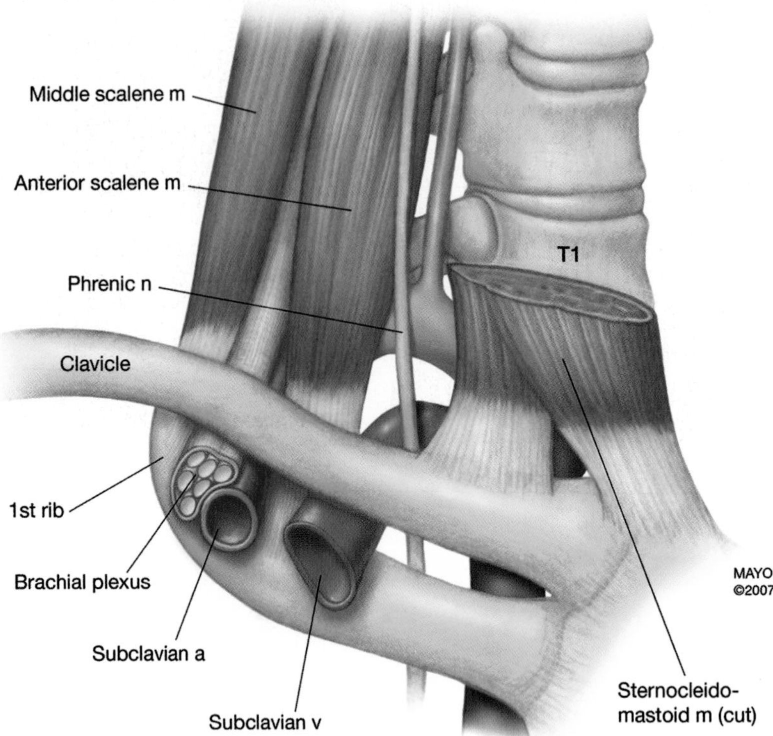

Figure 127-4 Supraclavicular anatomy. (Used with permission of Mayo Foundation for Medical Education and Research.)

border over the anterior scalene muscle. A mark is then made 1.5 to 2.0 cm posterior to the clavicle at its midpoint within the interscalene groove. Palpation of the subclavian artery, if possible, provides further verification of the correct needle placement.

A 22-gauge, 4-cm, short-bevel needle is directed in a caudad, slightly medial, and posterior direction until the patient exhibits a paresthesia or the first rib is encountered. This needle orientation lies in a plane parallel to a line joining the skin-entry site and the patient's ear. If the first rib is encountered before a paresthesia is elicited, then the needle can be walked anteriorly and posteriorly along the rib until a paresthesia is elicited or the subclavian artery is encountered. If the artery is located, the needle should be redirected in a more posterolateral direction, a maneuver that usually results in elicitation of a paresthesia. A nerve stimulator can also be used to aid needle placement.

The use of ultrasound for the supraclavicular block allows the practitioner to see the brachial plexus structures to be blocked, as well as the subclavian artery and pleura, just below the first rib, which are to be avoided. The patient is positioned as described previously, and the ultrasound probe is placed just cephalad and parallel to the clavicle. The probe is moved medially and laterally until the plexus is viewed just lateral to the subclavian artery. The needle is advanced in plane, lateral to medial, toward the plexus. Following negative aspiration, 20 to 40 mL of local anesthetic agent is injected around the plexus; spread around the neural structures can be seen on the ultrasound (Figure 127-5).

Side Effects and Complications

The major complication associated with supraclavicular blockade is pneumothorax, which usually presents in the postoperative period. The incidence ranges from 0.5% to 6%, decreasing with the experience of the practitioner. Block of the phrenic (50% to 60%), recurrent laryngeal, and cervical sympathetic nerves are minor inconveniences requiring only reassurance. Nerve damage is uncommon and usually transient. Intravascular injection is largely preventable by careful technique, including the use of test doses, aspiration, and incremental injection.

Axillary Block

The axillary approach to the brachial plexus is used because of its ease of performance, safety, and reliability, particularly for hand and forearm surgery. A variety of approaches to the axillary block have been described, including elicitation of paresthesias, transarterial injection, sheath blocks, use of a nerve stimulator, and the use of ultrasound guidance. In experienced hands, all seem to result in a reasonable success rate. Use of this technique is confined to patients who are able to abduct their arms sufficiently to allow access to the neurovascular bundle within the axilla. The musculocutaneous nerve may not always be blocked with this approach but can be supplemented either at the level of the coracobrachialis muscle or as it courses superficially above the interepicondylar line at the elbow.

Technique

For all approaches to the axillary block, the patient is positioned supine with the arm to be anesthetized abducted at right angles with the body and the elbow flexed to 90 degrees. The axillary artery is palpated as close to the axillary crease as possible, and a line is drawn tracing the course of the artery distally. The artery is fixed against the humerus at the level of the axillary crease by the index and middle fingers of the nondominant hand. Placement of the needle proximal to the fingers, along with maintenance of distal pressure, encourages proximal spread of the local anesthetic solution, increasing the likelihood of blocking the musculocutaneous nerve.

Paresthesia techniques involve elicitation of single or multiple paresthesias with a small-gauge (22G-25G), 2-cm needle. A minimum volume of 10 mL of local anesthetic agent is carefully injected at each paresthesia.

Nerve stimulators can be used with a Teflon-coated (insulated) needle or commercially available nerve stimulators. This technique avoids sensory paresthesias but requires additional equipment.

Transarterial techniques have been described involving placement of a sharp needle through the axillary artery and injecting a local anesthetic agent (40 to 50 mL) behind the artery or, in some descriptions, dividing the total volume of agent and injecting it behind and superior to the artery.

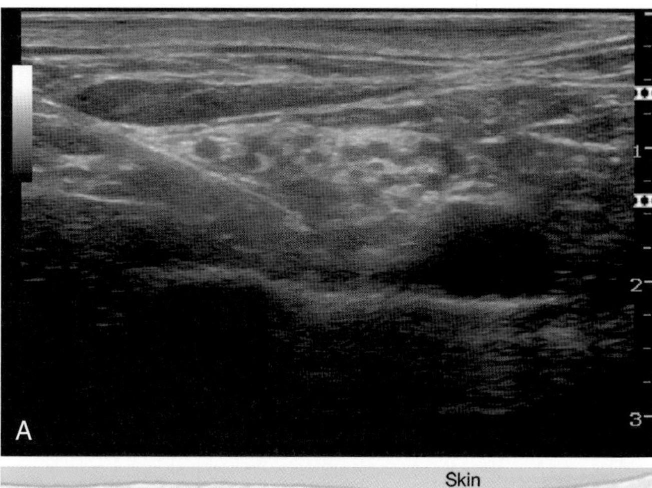

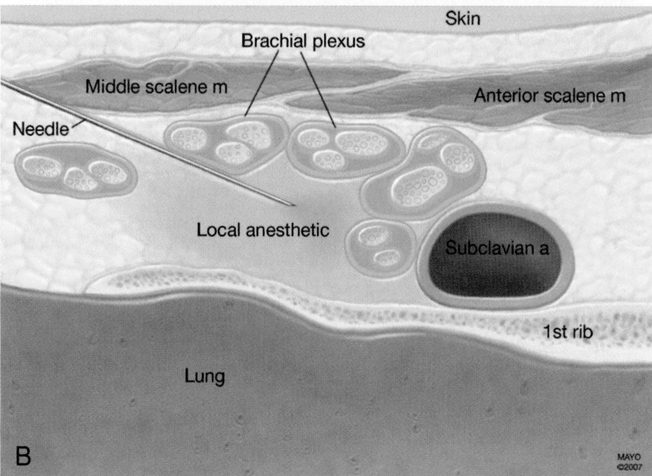

Figure 127-5 Ultrasound-guided supraclavicular block. **A,** Ultrasound image showing injection of local anesthetic around neural structures. **B,** Corresponding anatomy. (Used with permission of Mayo Foundation for Medical Education and Research.)

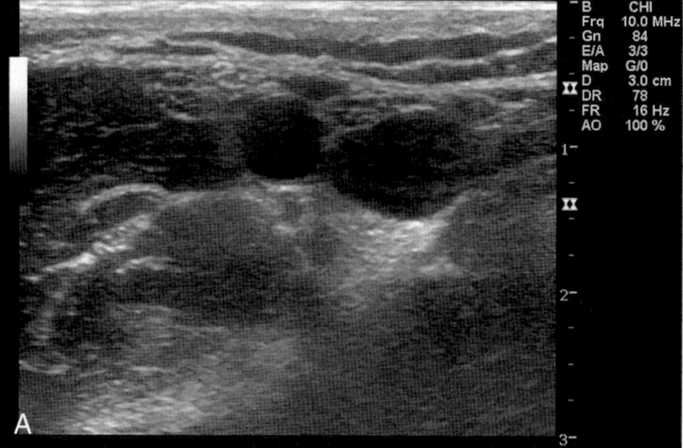

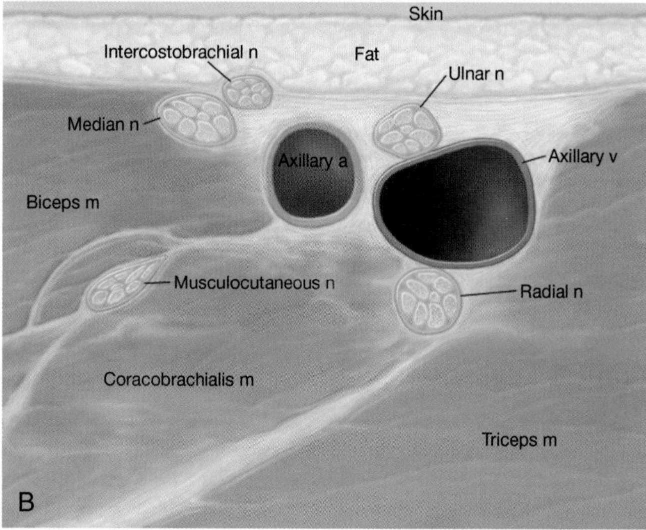

Figure 127-6 Ultrasound-guided axillary block. **A,** Ultrasound image. **B,** Corresponding anatomy. (Used with permission of Mayo Foundation for Medical Education and Research.)

Obviously, great care must be taken to avoid intravascular injection with this technique.

The ultrasound approach to the axillary block involves visualizing the axillary artery and surrounding distinct neural structures at various positions relative to the artery. The block requires several needle redirections to adequately deposit local anesthetic agent around each neural structure. The patient is positioned as described previously. The ultrasound probe is placed just distal and parallel to the axillary crease at a point that best identifies the artery in close proximity to the median, ulnar, and radial nerves (Figure 127-6). The needle is advanced in an in-plane approach to individually block each nerve. Finally, the musculocutaneous nerve can be identified by scanning further laterally within the coracobrachialis muscle. It should be blocked via a separate needle-insertion site.

Side Effects and Complications

Because of the large volumes of local anesthetic agent often recommended for axillary blocks, the proximity of large blood vessels and the popularity of "immobile" needle techniques, local anesthetic toxicity from rapid uptake or intravascular injection may be a higher risk with this technique, compared with other approaches to the brachial plexus. Frequent aspiration combined with incremental injection is an important feature of any method used in this block. Hematoma, sometimes with associated vascular compromise of the upper extremity, and infection are rare but reported complications.

Suggested Readings

Brown DL, Bridenbaugh PO. The upper extremity: somatic blockade. In: Cousins MJ, Chan V, Finucane BT, et al, eds. *Atlas of Ultrasound and Nerve Stimulation-Guided Regional Anesthesia*. New York: Springer; 2007:53-61, 68-72.

Chan V, Finucane BT, Grau T, Walji AH. Atlas of ultrasound and nerve stimulation-guided regional anesthesia. New York: Springer Science & Business Media; 2007.

Cousins MJ, Bridenbaugh PO, Carr DP, Horlocker TT, eds. *Neural Blockade in Clinical Anesthesia and Pain Management*. 4th ed. Philadelphia: Lippincott, Williams & Wilkins; 2008.

Hebl JR, Lennon RL, eds. *Mayo Clinic Atlas of Regional Anesthesia and Ultrasound-Guided Nerve Blockade*. Rochester, MN: Mayo Clinic Scientific Press; 2009.

Neal JM, Hebl JR, Gerancher JC, Hogan QH. Brachial plexus anesthesia: Essentials of our current understanding. *Reg Anesth Pain Med*. 2002;27:402-428.

CHAPTER 128

Lower Extremity Block: Psoas Compartment Block

Sandra L. Kopp, MD

The psoas compartment block (PCB) is a lumbar plexus block utilizing a posterior approach. Introduced in the 1970s in response to criticism that the femoral "3-in-1" block did not reliably block the femoral, obturator, and lateral femoral cutaneous nerves, the PCB did not gain immediate popularity owing to the unreliability of the loss-of-resistance technique. Not until the introduction of nerve stimulation techniques in 1989 did practitioners begin to commonly perform this peripheral nerve block.

Clinical Applications

The PCB allows for complete blockade of the lumbar plexus with a single injection. This technique is primarily used to provide analgesia to the upper thigh and hip, although it can be used for any procedure in which blockade of the lumbar plexus is desired. When combined with a sciatic nerve block, complete anesthesia or analgesia of the lower extremity may be achieved. This technique is most commonly used to provide postoperative analgesia for any major knee or hip operation. The main advantage of the PCB, as compared with a neuraxial technique, is unilateral lower extremity analgesia.

Relevant Anatomy

The lumbar plexus is most commonly formed from the ventral rami of L1 through L4, although frequently a branch of T12 and, occasionally, a branch from L5 are included. The plexus lies anterior to the transverse processes of the lumbar vertebrae and descends vertically with the psoas muscle. The branches of the lumbar plexus emerging from the psoas muscle are the femoral nerve (L2-L4), obturator nerve (L2-L4), lateral femoral cutaneous nerve (L2-L3), iliohypogastric nerve (L1), ilioinguinal nerve (L1), and genitofemoral nerve (L1-L2) (Figure 128-1). It provides sensory innervation to the anterior thigh and to the medial portion of the lower leg via the saphenous nerve (distal branch of the femoral nerve), as well as the majority of the femur, ischium, and ilium.

The surface anatomy consists of three main landmarks: (1) the intercristal line, the line connecting the iliac crests; (2) the midline, identified by a line connecting the spinous processes; and (3) the posterior superior iliac spine (PSIS), a projection at the posterior aspect of the ilium.

As the needle passes from posterior to anterior at the level of L4 through L5, the following structures are encountered: skin, subcutaneous adipose tissue, posterior lumbar fascia, paraspinous muscles, anterior lumbar fascia, quadratus lumborum, and the psoas muscle (Figure 128-2). The distance from skin to lumbar plexus varies greatly with sex and body mass index, whereas the distance from the transverse process of L4 to the lumbar plexus consistently ranges from 1.5 to 2.0 cm in both sexes.

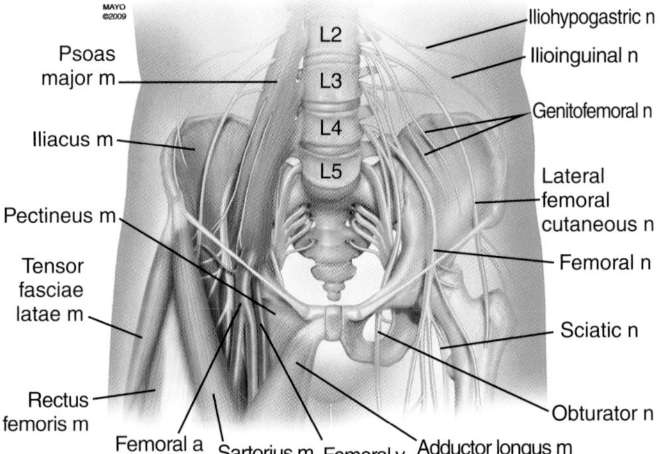

Figure 128-1 Anatomy of the lumbar plexus in situ. (From Kopp SL. Posterior lumbar plexus (psoas compartment) blockade. In: Hebl JR, Lennon RL, eds. Mayo Clinic Atlas of Regional Anesthesia and Ultrasound-Guided Nerve Blockade. Rochester, MN: Mayo Clinic Scientific Press; 2009:336. Used with permission of Mayo Foundation for Medical Education and Research.)

Technique

Patient Position

The patient is positioned laterally with the hips flexed and perpendicular to the horizontal plane (similar to the position utilized for an intrathecal injection) with the operative leg uppermost.

Needle Insertion Site

One of several needle insertion sites can be used, although the landmarks described by Capdevila and colleagues use localization of the L4 transverse process, thereby reducing the likelihood of excessive needle depth. The intercristal line is identified and drawn. A horizontal line is drawn identifying the midline. A line originating at the PSIS is drawn parallel to midline. The distance between the PSIS and midline is dissected into thirds. The needle insertion site is 1 cm cephalad to the intercristal line at the junction of the lateral one-third line and the medial two-thirds line (Figure 128-3).

With the use of a nerve stimulator, the needle is advanced perpendicular to the skin at the entry site until contact is made with the transverse process of L4. The needle is then withdrawn and "walked off" the transverse process in a caudad direction until a motor response of the lumbar plexus is elicited. A motor response of the quadriceps femoris muscle is

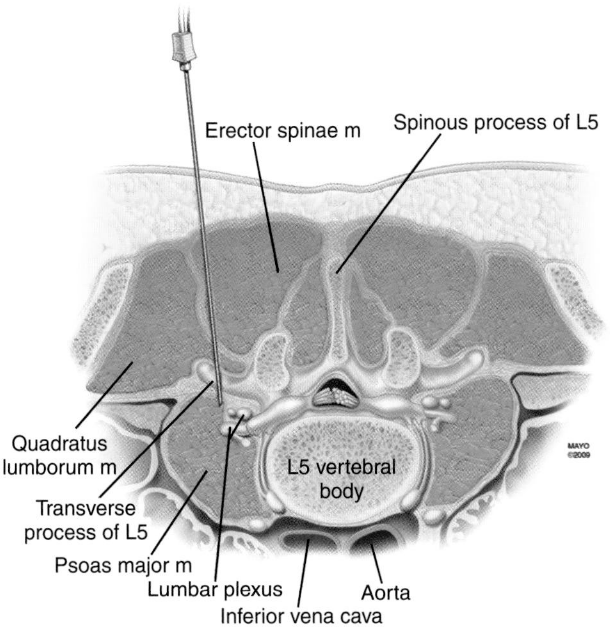

Figure 128-2 Cross-sectional anatomy of the lumbar region. (From Kopp SL. Posterior lumbar plexus (psoas compartment) blockade. In: Hebl JR, Lennon RL, eds. Mayo Clinic Atlas of Regional Anesthesia and Ultrasound-Guided Nerve Blockade. Rochester, MN: Mayo Clinic Scientific Press; 2009:339. Used with permission of Mayo Foundation for Medical Education and Research.)

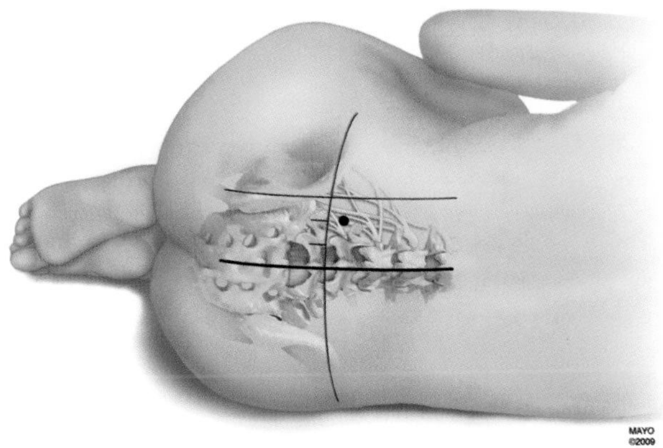

Figure 128-3 Position and surface landmarks of the lumbar region. See further discussion in Technique: Needle Insertion Site. (From Kopp SL. Posterior lumbar plexus (psoas compartment) blockade. In: Hebl JR, Lennon RL, eds. Mayo Clinic Atlas of Regional Anesthesia and Ultrasound-Guided Nerve Blockade. Rochester, MN; Mayo Clinic Scientific Press; 2009:343. Used with permission of Mayo Foundation for Medical Education and Research.)

ideal, although any motor response of the lumbar plexus may be utilized. Once the desired motor response is obtained, the local anesthetic solution is slowly administered with frequent aspiration for blood or cerebrospinal fluid. For a continuous-catheter technique, a 20G catheter is threaded through an 18G insulated needle approximately 4 to 5 cm into the psoas compartment.

Needle Redirection Cues

If contact with the transverse process is not made on the first pass, the needle is redirected, first caudad, then cephalad, searching for the transverse process. If the transverse process has not been contacted and the desired motor response has not been elicited, the needle is redirected slightly medial, and the preceding steps are repeated until a lumbar plexus motor response is obtained. Owing to an increased incidence of complications, extreme medial redirection of the needle should be avoided. Dural sleeves surround the roots of the lumbar plexus at this level; therefore, stimulation at currents less than 0.5 mA could indicate needle placement within the dural sleeve. Injection of a local anesthetic agent within a dural sleeve could cause significant epidural or subarachnoid spread. If a motor response of the hamstring muscles is obtained, the needle was inserted too caudally. The needle should be withdrawn and reinserted in a more cephalad direction. In some patients, the normal kidney may extend down to the level of the L3 vertebrae; therefore, it is important to avoid extreme cephalad redirection when the needle insertion site is at the level of L4.

Ultrasound-Guided Posterior Lumbar Plexus Block

Despite the recent popularity of the use of ultrasound guidance in regional anesthesia, there has been limited interest in utilizing ultrasound for lumbar plexus blockade. This is likely due to the depth of the plexus in relation to the skin, the increasing number of obese patients, and the need for specialized, curved-array, low-frequency probes.

Side Effects and Complications

Unlike the relatively minor complications associated with the use of other lower extremity nerve blocks, the risks associated with a PCB can be quite severe. Because of the proximity of the neuraxis, intrathecal or epidural injection of a local anesthetic agent or catheter placement is a potential complication. Epidural spread of local anesthetic agent is the most common complication, with an incidence of approximately 1.8% to 16%. The factors that may contribute to epidural spread are a medially directed needle, injection of large volumes of local anesthetic agent, and the presence of a spinal deformity (scoliosis). Less commonly, intrathecal or subarachnoid injection or catheter placement have been reported, leading to a high spinal anesthetic.

Because the PCB results in injection of a local anesthetic agent into or in close proximity to large, richly vascularized muscles (psoas, quadratus lumborum), severe retroperitoneal or renal capsular hematomas are possible. Most patients who have developed these hematomas had undergone a PCB while they were anticoagulated, or they received anticoagulation medication shortly after a PCB was placed or in the presence of a continuous psoas catheter. Although larger studies are needed, the American Society of Regional Anesthesia conservatively recommends that patients having a PCB be managed in much the same way as those patients undergoing neuraxial blockade when thromboprophylaxis is ordered.

Although nerve injury is uncommon, lumbar plexus injury has occurred following continuous psoas compartment blockade. Nerve injury during PCB may be caused by direct needle trauma to the nerve roots. Local anesthetic agents should not be injected if the patient complains of pain or paresthesia; therefore, in adults, this block should not be performed in patients who have received general anesthesia, although, because of the depth of the plexus from the skin, sedation is usually required. Hypotension is rare due to a unilateral sympathectomy, although if epidural spread or an intrathecal injection occurs, significant hypotension may be seen.

Suggested Readings

Capdevila X, Macaire P, Dadure C, et al. Continuous psoas compartment block for postoperative analgesia after total hip arthroplasty: New landmarks, technical guidelines, and clinical evaluation. *Anesth Analg.* 2002; 94:1606-1613.

De Biasi P, Lupescu R, Burgun G, et al. Continuous lumbar plexus block: Use of radiography to determine catheter tip location. *Reg Anesth Pain Med.* 2003; 28:135-139.

Farny J, Drolet P, Girard M. Anatomy of the posterior approach to the lumbar plexus block. *Can J Anaesth.* 1994;41:480-485.

Horlocker TT, Wedel DJ, Benzon H, et al. Regional anesthesia in the anticoagulated patient: Defining the risks (the second ASRA Consensus Conference on Neuraxial Anesthesia and Anticoagulation). *Reg Anesth Pain Med.* 2003; 28:172-197.

Kirchmair L, Entner T, Kapral S, Mitterschiffthaler G. Ultrasound guidance for the psoas compartment block: An imaging study. *Anesth Analg.* 2002;94: 706-710.

Weller RS, Gerancher JC, Crews JC, Wade KL. Extensive retroperitoneal hematoma without neurologic deficit in two patients who underwent lumbar plexus block and were later anticoagulated. *Anesthesiology.* 2003; 98:581-585.

Winnie AP, Radonjic R, Akkineni SR, Durrani Z. Factors influencing distribution of local anesthetic injected into the brachial plexus sheath. *Anesth Analg.* 1979;58:225-234.

CHAPTER 129 Lower Extremity Blocks: Femoral, Sciatic, Popliteal

Sandra L. Kopp, MD

Peripheral nerve blocks of the lower extremity are frequently utilized for postoperative analgesia. Patients with a peripheral nerve block as part of a multimodal pain regimen frequently have lower postoperative pain scores, improved analgesia, and better joint range of motion. Surgical anesthesia can be provided in one limb without complete sympathectomy, in contrast with neuraxial blockade. The use of anticoagulants in the surgical population may dictate which block can be performed safely, and close monitoring in these patients is essential (Table 129-1).

Femoral Nerve Block

Anatomy

The femoral nerve is formed within the psoas major muscle by the posterior divisions of L2 to L4, emerges from the lateral border of that muscle, and descends in the groove between the psoas and iliacus muscles (Figure 129-1). It enters the thigh lateral to the femoral artery and divides into anterior and posterior branches distal to the inguinal ligament. The femoral nerve supplies

Table 129-1 Regional Anesthetic Techniques for Lower Extremity Operations

Peripheral Technique	Area of Blockade	Peripheral Nerves Blocked	Duration of Blockade (h)*	Comments
Femoral	Femoral, partial lateral femoral cutaneous and obturator	Lumbar plexus L2-4	12-18	Provides anesthesia/analgesia to anteriomedial thigh, anterior knee, and medial calf Necessity for minor arthroscopy operations has not been demonstrated Decreased VAS scores when used for ACL repair and total knee arthroplasty
Psoas compartment	Femoral, partial lateral femoral cutaneous, obturator, sciatic S1	Lumbar plexus L1-5 Sciatic S1	12-18	Anesthesia/analgesia to entire lumbar plexus Owing to low pain scores associated with minor knee arthroscopy procedures, the risk profile may not justify use
Saphenous	Medial aspect of lower leg and foot	L2-4 branch of femoral nerve	4-6	Required for complete anesthesia/analgesia of foot and ankle Allows for use of calf tourniquet when combined with popliteal sciatic nerve block
Proximal sciatic	Posterior thigh and leg (except saphenous area)	Sciatic L4-5, S1-3	18-30	Superior analgesia and fewer hospital admissions when combined with a femoral block for patients undergoing ACL repair and total knee arthroplasty
Popliteal sciatic	Posterior lower leg and foot (except saphenous area)	Sciatic L4-5, S1-3	12-24	When combined with a saphenous nerve block, anesthesia/analgesia is similar to spinal anesthesia with fewer side effects for procedures below the knee
Ankle	Forefoot and midfoot	Posterior tibial, deep peroneal, superficial peroneal, sural, and saphenous	8-12	Relatively simple to perform, high success rate, few complications Little or no effect on ambulation Does not provide anesthesia for tourniquet use

*Duration of block performed with long-acting local anesthetic agent (e.g., bupivacaine, ropivacaine).
ACL, Anterior cruciate ligament; VAS, visual analog scale.

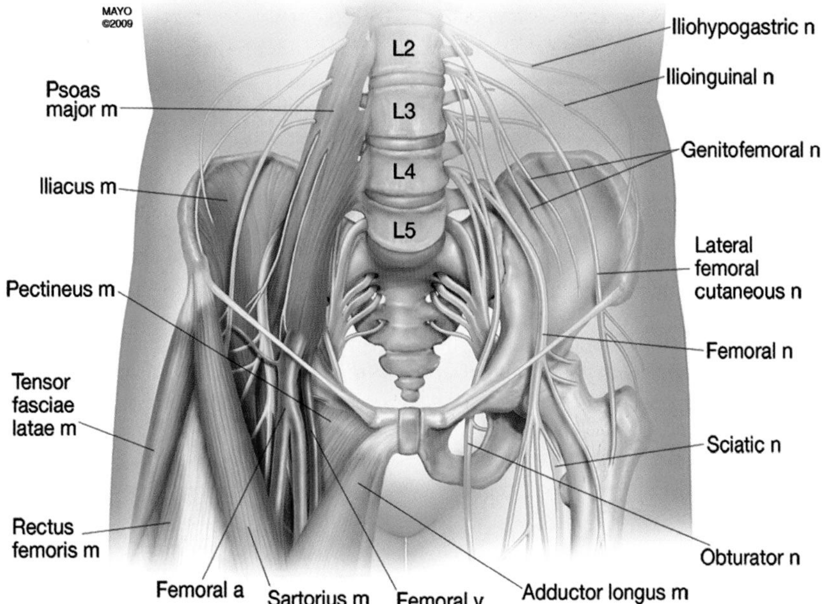

Figure 129-1 Anatomy of the lumbar plexus. (From Hebl JR, Lennon RL, eds. Mayo Clinic Atlas of Regional Anesthesia and Ultrasound-Guided Nerve Blockade. Rochester, MN: Mayo Clinic Scientific Press; 2009. Used with permission of Mayo Foundation for Medical Education and Research.)

the anterior compartment muscles of the thigh (quadriceps, sartorius) and skin of the anterior thigh from the inguinal ligament to the knee. Below the knee, it supplies sensation to the medial side of the leg, extending to the big toe in the distribution of the saphenous nerve.

Clinical Applications

Because of its limited sensory distribution, the femoral nerve block is usually combined with other peripheral blocks in clinical practice. However, it can be used alone for muscle biopsies of the quadriceps muscle or other surgical procedures limited to the anterior thigh, and its use has been described for anesthetic management of knee arthroscopy, total knee arthroplasty, and surgical repair of fractures of the midfemoral shaft.

Technique

With the patient in the supine position, a line representing the inguinal ligament is drawn between the palpated anterior superior iliac spine and the pubic tubercle. A second line is drawn representing the femoral artery (Figure 129-2). Using a nerve stimulator, the anesthesia provider advances

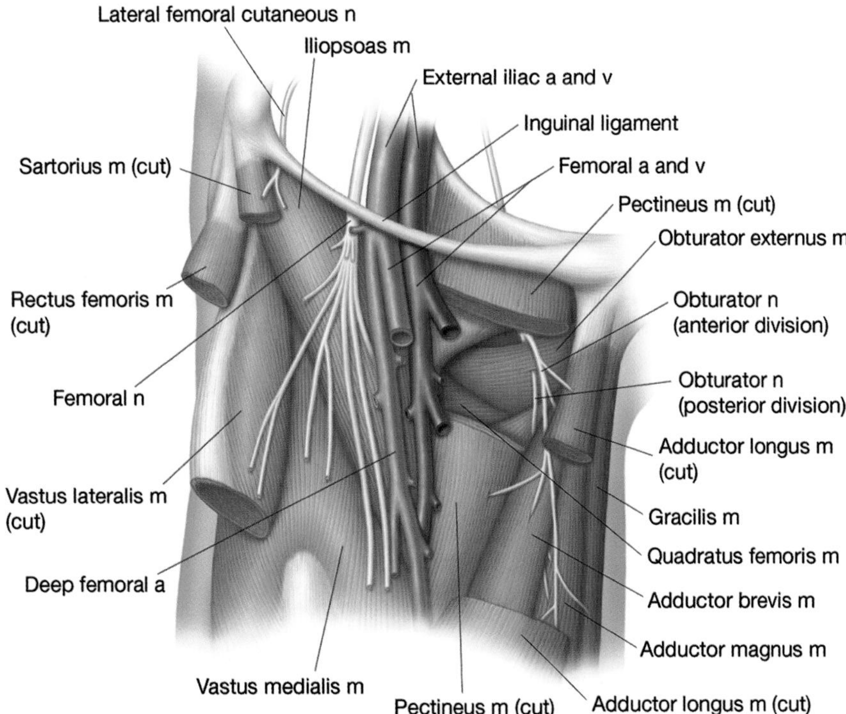

Figure 129-2 Anatomy of the femoral and obturator nerves. (From Hebl JR, Lennon RL, eds. Mayo Clinic Atlas of Regional Anesthesia and Ultrasound-Guided Nerve Blockade. Rochester, MN: Mayo Clinic Scientific Press; 2009. Used with permission of Mayo Foundation for Medical Education and Research.)

a 22G, 3-cm to 5-cm, short-bevel needle until a motor response of the quadriceps muscle is obtained (patellar snap). After negative aspiration, 10 to 30 mL of local anesthetic solution is injected incrementally through the needle. A catheter may be placed for continuous analgesia.

The use of ultrasound may be useful in patients in whom it is difficult to palpate a femoral pulse because of weight, anatomic variability, or scarring at the needle insertion site (prior radiation or surgery). The femoral nerve can be identified lateral to the artery as a triangular structure.

Adverse Effects and Complications

The proximity of the femoral artery may increase the risk of hematoma and intravascular injection. However, the nerve and artery are located anatomically in separate sheaths approximately 1 cm apart. In most patients, the femoral artery can be easily palpated, allowing safe needle positioning lateral to the pulsation. Blockade of the femoral nerve should probably be avoided in patients who have undergone femoral vascular grafts because the distorted anatomy may increase the risk of excessive bleeding. Nerve damage from needle trauma or drug toxicity is an unlikely complication from this block.

Perivascular Femoral Block

The perivascular femoral block (a "3-in-1 block") is based on the premise that injection of a large volume of local anesthetic within the femoral canal while holding distal pressure will result in proximal spread of the solution into the psoas compartment, resulting in a lumbar plexus block. The key anatomic assumption is that the fascial sheath surrounding the lumbar roots extends into the femoral canal and acts as an enclosed conduit for the spread of local anesthetic solutions.

Fascia Iliaca Nerve Block

Clinical Applications

The *fascia iliaca,* or modified femoral nerve block, is a good alternative in patients postoperatively or as a rescue block for a previously failed regional attempt for procedures on the hip and proximal lower extremity. It relies on a double-pop technique that is some distance from the femoral neurovascular structures, thus making it safe in previously anesthetized patients or those who may have already received a regional block.

Anatomy and Technique

With the patient in the supine position, a line is drawn connecting the pubic tubercle to the anterior superior iliac crest. The line is divided into thirds, with the entry point just caudad to the intersection between the medial two thirds and lateral one third on the line. An initial skin puncture should be made so that skin is not mistaken for a fascial pop. Then, a blunt needle, such as an 18G Hustead needle or bullet-tipped needle, is advanced perpendicular to the skin until two distinct pops are felt as the needle traverses the *fascia lata* and *fascia iliaca.* A volume of 20 to 40 mL of local anesthetic can be incrementally injected or, alternatively, a catheter can be threaded for continuous analgesia.

Adverse Effects and Complications

In most patients, the femoral nerve and artery will be medial to the insertion site, and, thus, nerve damage and vascular injury are unlikely. Patients who have had previous vascular grafts and radiation to the area are not good candidates for this procedure.

Obturator Nerve Block

Anatomy

The obturator nerve is derived primarily from L3 to L4, with variable minor contributions from L2. It lies deep in the obturator canal after descending from the medial psoas muscle border. It forms anterior and posterior branches as it leaves the obturator canal (see Figure 129-2). The anterior branch supplies an articular branch to the hip, the anterior adductor muscles, and a variable cutaneous branch to the lower medial thigh. The posterior branch supplies the deep adductor muscles, with a variable articular branch to the knee.

Clinical Applications

Because the obturator nerve is primarily a motor nerve, it is rarely blocked in isolation. Rather, it is usually combined with another lower extremity peripheral nerve block for knee surgery.

Technique

With the patient in the supine position, a mark is made 1 to 2 cm lateral and 1 to 2 cm caudad to the palpated pubic tubercle. Using sterile technique, a skin wheal is raised with a local-anesthetic solution, and a 22G, 8-cm to 10-cm, short-bevel needle is advanced slightly medially toward the pubic tubercle. The inferior pubic ramus will usually be encountered at a depth of 2 to 4 cm. At that point, the needle is "walked" medially and cephalad in small steps until it drops into the obturator canal. The obturator nerve is located 2 to 3 cm past the point of contact with the pubic ramus. After negative aspiration, 10 to 15 mL of local anesthetic solution is injected. A nerve stimulator is very useful for accurate location of this motor nerve; a twitch will be observed in the medial thigh adductor muscles as the needle approaches the obturator nerve.

Adverse Effects and Complications

The obturator canal contains vascular and neural structures, increasing the potential risk of intravascular injection or nerve damage. Because of the deep location of the nerve in the obturator canal, this is a difficult block to learn and perform.

Sciatic Nerve Block

Anatomy

The sciatic nerve derives from L4 to L5 and S1 to S3. It is a large peripheral nerve with a width of 2 cm. It exits the pelvis with the posterior cutaneous nerve of the thigh, passes through the sacrosciatic foramen beneath the piriformis muscle, and courses between the greater trochanter of the femur and the ischial tuberosity. At the lower border of the gluteus maximus muscle, the sciatic nerve becomes superficial as it begins its descent down the posterior thigh toward the popliteal fossa (Figure 129-3). The sciatic nerve supplies sensation to the largest area of the lower extremity, including the posterior thigh and everything below the knee, with the exception of a thin medial strip supplied by the saphenous nerve (terminal branch of the femoral nerve).

Clinical Applications

Because of its wide sensory distribution, the sciatic nerve block can be used alone for any operation below the knee that does not require a thigh tourniquet. It can also be combined with other peripheral nerve blocks to provide anesthesia for surgical procedures involving the thigh and knee. This form of anesthesia avoids the sympathectomy associated with centroneuraxial blocks, and, thus, its use may be advantageous in cases in which any shift in hemodynamics might be deleterious, such as in patients with significant aortic stenosis.

Technique

Posterior Approach of Labat

The patient is positioned laterally, with the leg to be blocked fully flexed and rolled forward so that the heel of the upper (operative) leg rests on the knee of the dependent (nonoperative) leg, which is stretched out in a straight line with the torso. A line is drawn between the palpated posterior superior iliac

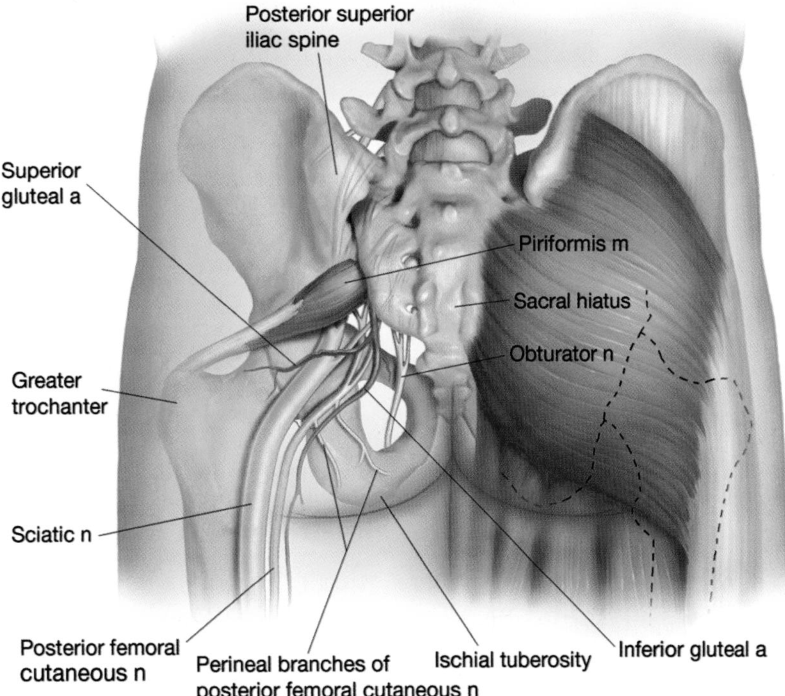

Figure 129-3 Sciatic nerve anatomy. (From Hebl JR, Lennon RL, eds. Mayo Clinic Atlas of Regional Anesthesia and Ultrasound-Guided Nerve Blockade. Rochester, MN: Mayo Clinic Scientific Press; 2009. Used with permission of Mayo Foundation for Medical Education and Research.)

spine and the greater trochanter of the femur. This line is bisected with a perpendicular line extending approximately 5 cm caudad. Now a line is drawn between the greater trochanter of the femur and the sacral hiatus, which will cross the perpendicular at a point 3 to 5 cm along the line. This represents the point of needle insertion (Figure 129-4). Using sterile technique, a 22G, 10-cm to 12-cm, short-bevel needle is advanced perpendicular to the skin until a paresthesia is elicited or bone is encountered (see Figure 129-3). If bone is contacted, the needle is redirected to systematically sweep in a lateral-medial direction until the nerve is located. The use of a nerve stimulator is helpful in ascertaining the correct needle position. When the sciatic nerve is located, 25 to 30 mL of local anesthetic solution is injected.

An alternative approach in the lateral decubitus position is the subgluteal approach, with or without ultrasound guidance. If ultrasound is used, a curvilinear probe is placed just distal to the gluteal cleft and scanned lateral to medial. The sciatic nerve can be identified as a flat hyperechoic structure medial to the greater trochanter and lateral to the hyperechoic border of the ischial tuberosity. An 8-inch 21G insulated needle is advanced in an out-of-plane approach toward the sciatic nerve (the simultaneous use of a nerve stimulator can help to confirm the location of the nerve), and, after negative aspiration, 20 to 30 mL of local anesthetic is injected around the nerve.

Anterior Approach

This technique is useful for situations in which the patient cannot be positioned for the classic posterior approach because of pain or lack of cooperation. The patient is placed in the supine position, and a line is drawn between the anterior superior iliac spine and the pubic tubercle, representing the inguinal ligament. This line is trisected, and a second parallel line is drawn from the point of the tuberosity of the greater trochanter of the hip. The intersection of this second line with the more medial of the perpendicular lines represents the point of needle entry. Using sterile technique, a 22G, 10-cm to 12-cm, short-bevel needle is advanced with a slight lateral angulation until the lesser trochanter of the femur is encountered. At this point, the needle is redirected slightly medially, "walked off" the femur, and advanced until a motor response of the distal extremity is elicited (approximately 5 cm past bone). A total of 25 to 30 mL of local anesthetic solution is injected incrementally after careful aspiration.

Adverse Effects and Complications

Performing a sciatic nerve block is technically difficult and can be quite painful for the patient. Providing adequate sedation/analgesia to the patient is an important component of this procedure, although given the patient's position for the performance of this block, sedation, if administered, may complicate airway management. Hematoma formation and nerve damage are potential risks of the procedure. Because of the large area of blockade with a sciatic nerve block, vasodilation with venous pooling will occur in the affected extremity and may result in hypotension.

Popliteal Block

Clinical Applications

This peripheral nerve block is useful for foot and ankle operations. It can be utilized as a single-shot injection, or a catheter can be placed for postoperative analgesia. A saphenous nerve block is often performed to supplement this block, depending on the surgical procedure.

Anatomy

The sciatic nerve diverges into the tibial and peroneal nerves proximal to the popliteal crease. The tibial nerve continues straight through the popliteal fossa, whereas the peroneal branch lies along the lateral border of the *biceps femoris* muscle and then wraps laterally around the head of the fibula.

Technique

Posterior Approach to the Popliteal Fossa

The patient is placed in the prone or semiprone position. The popliteal crease can be easily identified with leg flexion. The popliteal fossa, bounded

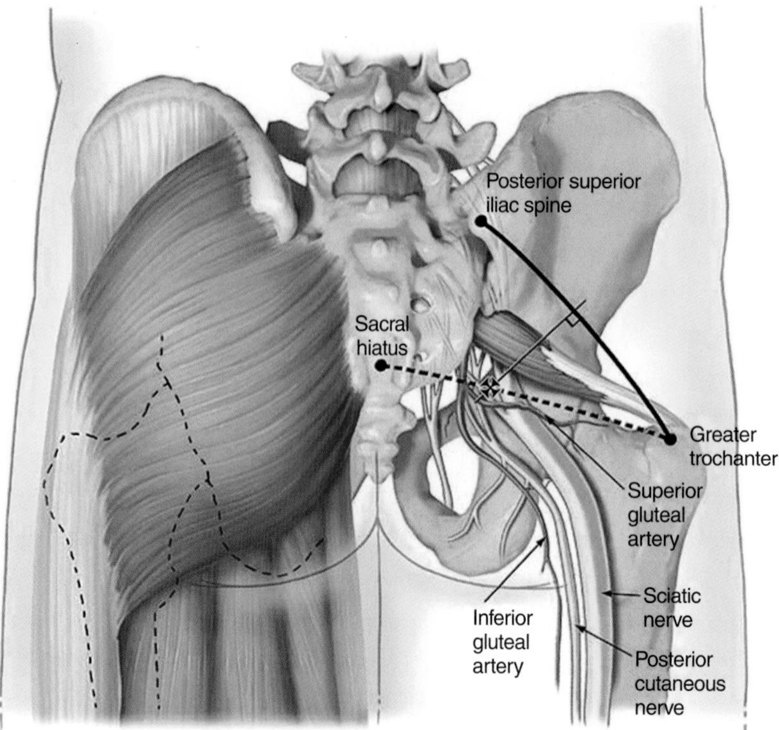

Figure 129-4 Landmarks for the posterior sciatic approach of Labat. (From Hebl JR, Lennon RL, eds. Mayo Clinic Atlas of Regional Anesthesia and Ultrasound-Guided Nerve Blockade. Rochester, MN: Mayo Clinic Scientific Press; 2009. Used with permission of Mayo Foundation for Medical Education and Research.)

by semimembranous and semitendinous muscles medially and the biceps femoris muscle laterally, is divided into medial and lateral triangles. An × is made 5 to 7 cm proximal from the crease, just lateral to midline. A 4-inch insulated needle is advanced at a 45° angle at the aforementioned insertion site until an appropriate nerve twitch is obtained. After negative aspiration, 30 to 40 mL of local anesthetic agent is incrementally injected.

The use of ultrasound can help to identify the point of divergence of the sciatic nerve into the peroneal and tibial branches. The ultrasound probe is placed parallel to the popliteal crease, and the leg is scanned in a proximal direction. It is often easiest to first identify the popliteal artery and then to locate the nerves just lateral and superficial to the artery. Using either an in-plane or out-of-plane approach, a 4-inch, 21G insulated needle is directed at the sciatic nerve at, or just before, its point of divergence. After negative aspiration and injection, local anesthetic spread can be visualized, often described as a "donut sign" around the sciatic nerve. Nerve stimulation can also be used to confirm the identity of the sciatic nerve prior to local anesthetic deposition.

Adverse Effects and Complications

Adverse effects and complications associated with a popliteal block are similar to those associated with a sciatic nerve block.

Suggested Readings

Chan V, Finucane BT, Grau T, Walji AH. *Atlas of Ultrasound and Nerve Stimulation-Guided Regional Anesthesia*. New York: Springer Science+Business Media; 2007:53-61, 68-72.

Enneking FK, Chan V, Greger J, et al. Lower-extremity peripheral nerve blockade: Essentials of our current understanding. *Reg Anesth Pain Med*. 2005;30:4-35.

Hebl JR, Lennon RL, eds. *Mayo Clinic Atlas of Regional Anesthesia and Ultrasound-Guided Nerve Blockade*. Rochester, MN: Mayo Clinic Scientific Press; 2009.

Horlocker, TT, Wedel DJ, Benzon H, et al. Regional anesthesia in the anticoagulated patient: Defining the risks (the second ASRA Consensus Conference on Neuraxial Anesthesia and Anticoagulation). *Reg Anesth Pain Med*. 2003; 28:172-197.

CHAPTER 130

Nerve Block at the Ankle

Douglas A. Dubbink, MD

Anesthesia distal to the ankle is accomplished by interrupting the five major nerves that innervate the foot: the tibial nerve and the deep peroneal nerve, which supply the deep structures of the foot, and the superficial peroneal nerve, the sural nerve, and the saphenous nerve, which supply sensory innervation to the skin. The ankle block is a relatively easy block to learn if the anatomy is well understood. Ankle blocks can be effective for nearly any surgical procedure of the foot. Major complications are rare; however, prolonged paresthesias have been reported. No epinephrine-containing local anesthetic agents should be used when performing an ankle block.

Technique

The tibial nerve supplies the sole and plantar portions of the toes up to the nails. It lies behind the posterior tibial artery anteromedial to the Achilles tendon and deep to the flexor retinaculum, which must be penetrated for a successful block (Figure 130-1).

The block is started by injecting a small amount of local anesthetic agent medial to the Achilles tendon at the level of the upper border of the medial malleolus. A 3-cm to 5-cm, 22G or 25G needle is directed at right angles to the tibia. The needle tip is slowly advanced until a paresthesia is elicited (a nerve stimulator can be used) or bone is contacted. At this point, 5 to 7 mL of local anesthetic agent is injected near the posterior aspect of the tibia, with an equal volume of local anesthetic injected during withdrawal of the needle to the skin surface if a paresthesia is not elicited.

The sural nerve is a superficial nerve that provides cutaneous sensation to the lower posterolateral ankle, lateral foot, and fifth toe. Five to 10 mL of local anesthetic agent is administered by infiltrating the solution posterior to the lateral malleolus to the Achilles tendon at the level of the upper border of the lateral malleolus.

The deep peroneal, superficial peroneal, and saphenous nerves can all be blocked using a single injection site. The deep peroneal nerve courses midway between the malleoli before assuming a position between the anterior tibial tendon and the extensor hallucis longus tendon beneath the extensor

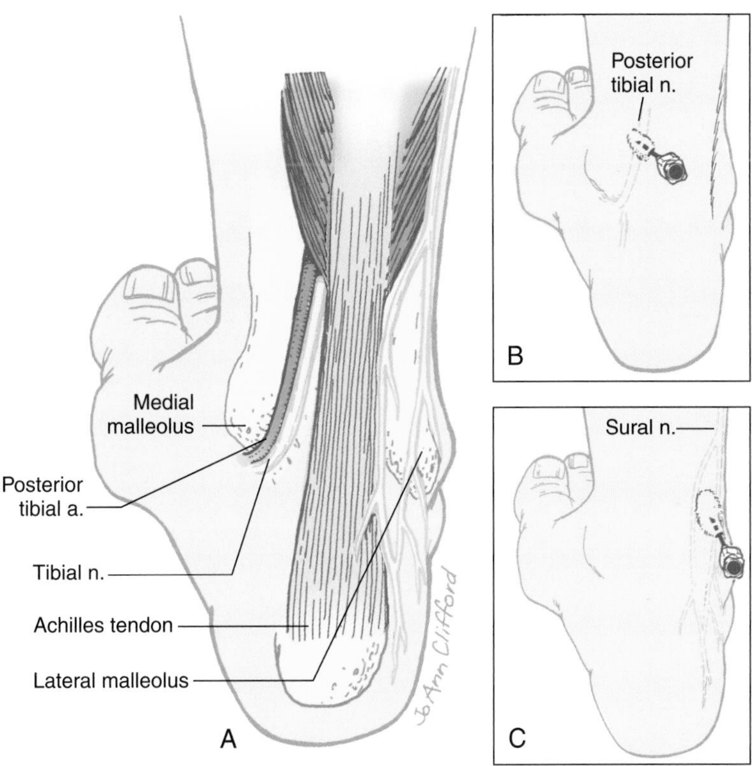

Figure 130-1 **A,** Anatomic landmarks for block of the posterior tibial and sural nerves at the ankle. **B,** Posterior tibial nerve: method of needle placement for block at the ankle. **C,** Sural nerve: method of needle placement for block at the ankle. (From Miller RD, ed. Nerve block at the ankle. In: Miller's Anesthesia. 7th ed. Philadelphia: Churchill Livingstone; 2010:1659-1661.)

retinaculum at the dorsum of the foot. It innervates the short extensors of the toes and provides skin sensation to the interdigital cleft between the great and second toes. With the patient dorsiflexing the foot, the tendons of the anterior tibial and extensor hallucis longus muscles can be readily identified at a level just above a line connecting the malleoli. The pulsation of the anterior tibial (dorsalis pedis) artery will often be felt. The nerve is lateral to the artery and deep to the extensor retinaculum. A 25G, 3-cm to 5-cm needle is inserted perpendicular to skin, as depicted in Figure 130-2. A loss of resistance will often be felt during passage through the extensor retinaculum, at which time between 3 mL and 5 mL of local anesthetic agent is injected.

The superficial peroneal nerve supplies cutaneous sensation to the dorsum of the foot and toes (except between great and second toes). Blockade of this nerve can be achieved by injecting local anesthetic agent subcutaneously laterally from the site of injection of the deep peroneal nerve toward the superior aspect of the lateral malleolus using 5 mL to 10 mL of solution.

The saphenous nerve is anterior to the medial malleolus near the long saphenous vein supplying cutaneous innervation to the anteromedial side of the lower leg and medial foot midway to the toes. The saphenous nerve is blocked with 3 mL to 5 mL of local anesthetic agent injected subcutaneously medially from the site of injection of the deep peroneal nerve toward the saphenous vein.

Position

Typically, the patient is in the supine position with the procedural leg elevated on a padded support. Patient cooperation is not essential for a successful block; thus, adequate sedation will enhance patient acceptance.

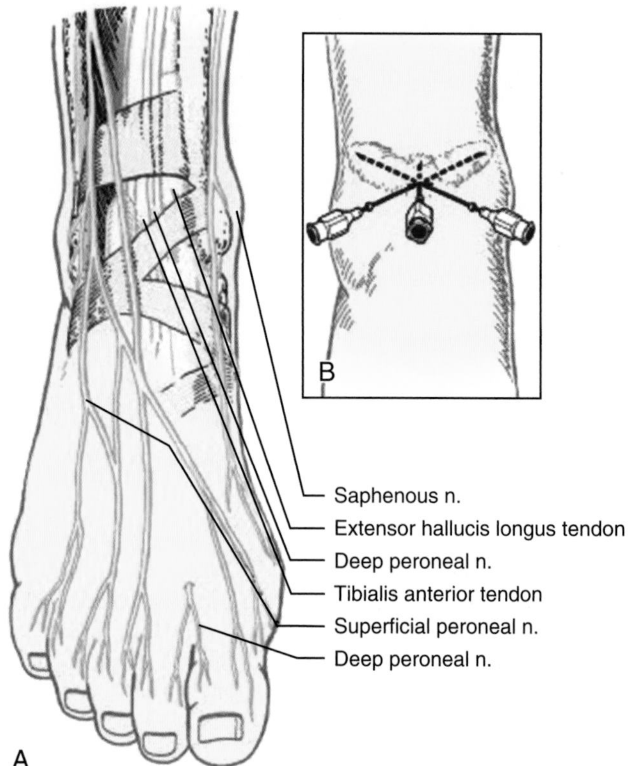

Figure 130-2 **A,** Anatomic landmarks for block of the deep peroneal, superficial peroneal, and saphenous nerves at the ankle. **B,** Method of needle placement for block of the deep peroneal, superficial peroneal, and saphenous nerves through a single needle entry site. (From Miller RD, ed. Nerve block at the ankle. In: Miller's Anesthesia. 7th ed. Philadelphia: Churchill Livingstone; 2010:1659-1661.)

Suggested Readings

Brown DL. *Atlas of Regional Anesthesia*. 3rd ed. Philadelphia: Saunders Elsevier; 2006:139-143.

Hadzic A. *Textbook of Regional Anesthesia and Acute Pain Management*. New York: McGraw-Hill; 2007.

PART B Neuroanesthesia

CHAPTER 131

Cerebral Protection

Robert E. Grady, MD

Cerebral ischemia results when the metabolic demands of cerebral tissue exceed substrate (primarily O_2) delivery. Ischemia can be categorized as either global—with interruption of substrate delivery to the entire brain, as occurs in cardiac arrest—or focal—with interruption of substrate delivery to a defined region of the brain, such as is produced by embolic cerebral artery occlusion. Cerebral protection is an attempt to prolong the ischemic tolerance of brain tissue and to reduce or abolish neuronal injury.

The traditional concept of cerebral metabolism is illustrated in Figure 131-1. Cerebral metabolism may be divided into a functional component and a cellular integrity component. The functional component comprises 60% of neuronal O_2 use. This component is responsible for generating action potentials and may be assessed by evaluating the electroencephalogram. The cellular integrity component consists of the remaining 40% of O_2 utilized for protein synthesis and other activities geared toward maintaining cellular integrity.

Anesthetic agents and hypothermia are both capable of reducing the functional component of cerebral metabolism, resulting in, at most, a 60% reduction in O_2 use. Hypothermia, however, can further reduce O_2 use by also decreasing the cellular integrity component. In this traditional and simplistic O_2 supply–metabolic demand paradigm, cerebral protection may be produced by simply altering the balance in favor of supply by increasing cerebral perfusion pressure (CPP) and O_2 delivery while depressing cerebral metabolism via anesthetic agents and hypothermia.

New evidence paints a much more complex picture of cerebral ischemia, in which an initial ischemic event may trigger a process of neuronal demise that continues long after the inciting event has resolved (Figure 131-2). Excitotoxicity is a cascade of glutamate-mediated neuronal demise that occurs shortly after the onset of neuronal ischemia. Apoptosis (programmed cell death via proteases) and inflammation are initiated by the ischemic event and continue to contribute to neuronal death for days. In this newer model of cerebral ischemia, it may be possible to limit ischemic damage by invoking cerebral protective therapies before, during, or after an ischemic event (Table 131-1). The currently available evidence in support of the use of cerebral protection is derived from a mixture of human experiments and animal data extrapolated to human subjects.

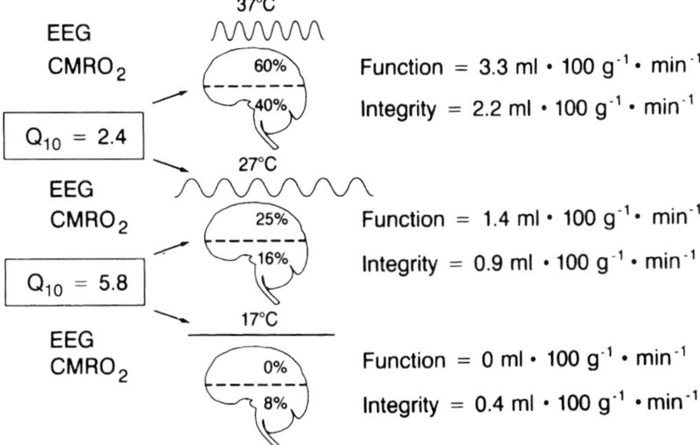

Figure 131-1 Theoretical interaction of temperature, brain function, cerebral metabolic O_2 consumption ($CMRO_2$), and calculated Q_{10} value. Q_{10} is defined as the ratio of metabolic rates at two temperatures separated by 10°C. In reducing temperature from 37° C to 27° C, function is maintained and both of the energy-consuming processes (i.e., function and integrity) are presumed to be affected equally, with a reduction of $CMRO_2$ of slightly more than 50%, thus generating a Q_{10} value of about 2.4. With a further 10° C reduction in temperature to 17° C, function is abolished, resulting in a steep decrease in $CMRO_2$ such that the calculated Q_{10} value is 5.0 or greater. At this point, the total O_2 consumed by the brain is reduced to less than 8% of the normothermic value of O_2. (Reprinted, with permission, from Michenfelder JD, ed. Anesthesia and the Brain. New York: Churchill Livingstone; 1988:14.)

Regulation of Physiologic Parameters

Temperature

Hypothermia reduces both the functional and cellular integrity components of cerebral metabolism. Deep hypothermia (18°-22° C) has long been known to be highly protective of cerebral tissue, permitting little or no

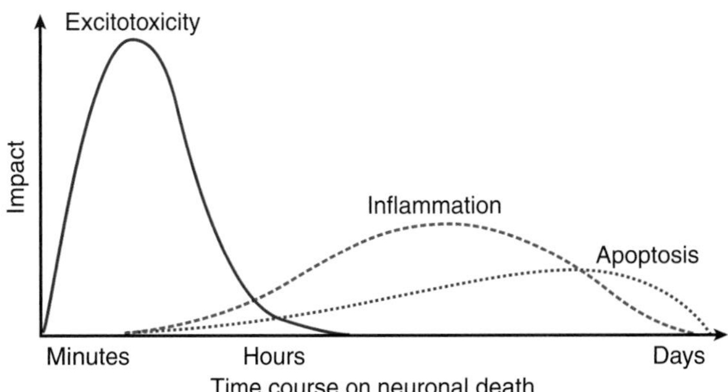

Figure 131-2 Time course of neuronal death after cerebral ischemia. Excitotoxicity rapidly leads to neuronal necrosis. Inflammation and neuronal apoptosis contribute to ongoing cell death for a period that extends from several days to weeks. (From Patel P. Cerebral ischemia and intraoperative brain protection. In: Gupta AK, Gelb AW, eds. Essentials of Neuroanesthesia and Neurointensive Care. Philadelphia: WB Saunders; 2008:36-48.)

Table 131-1 Evidence-Based Status of Plausible Interventions to Reduce Perioperative Ischemic Brain Injury

	Efficacy in Experimental Animals		Efficacy in Humans		Sustained Protection in	
Intervention	**Preischemic**	**Postischemic**	**Preischemic**	**Postischemic**	**Animals**	**Humans**
Hypothermia						
Mild	++	++	±	++*	++	++
Moderate	−−−	−−−	−−	−−	−−−	
Hyperventilation	−−	−−	−−	−−	−−	−−
Normoglycemia	++	−−	+	+	++	−−
Hyperbaric O_2	++	−−	−−	±	−−	−−
Barbiturates	++	−	+	+	++	−−
Propofol	++	+	−	−−	−−	−
Etomidate	−−−	−−	−−	−−	−−	−−
N_2O	−	−−	−−	−−	−−	−−
Isoflurane	++	−−	−−	−−	++	−−
Sevoflurane		−−	−−	−−	++	−−
Desflurane	++	−−	−−	−−	−−	−−
Lidocaine	++	−−	+	−−	−−	−−
Ketamine	++	−−	−−	−−	−−	−−
Glucocorticoids	−−−	−−	−−	−−	−−	−−

++, Supported by evidence from repeated physiologically controlled studies in animals/randomized, prospective, adequately powered clinical trials; +, consistent suggestion by case series/retrospective or prospective trials with small sample sizes or data extrapolated from other paradigms; ±, inconsistent findings in clinical trials; may be dependent on characteristics of insult; −, well-defined absence of benefit; −−, absence of evidence in physiologically controlled studies in animals/randomized, prospective adequately powered clinical trials; −−−, evidence of potential harm.
*Out-of-hospital ventricular fibrillation cardiac arrest.
(Adapted, with permission, from Fukuda S, Warner DS. Cerebral protection. Br J Anaesth. 2007;99:10-17.)

cerebral blood flow (CBF) for extended periods of time (~1 h) without neurologic sequelae. Studies of adults who have survived out-of-hospital cardiac arrest and of neonates with asphyxia have shown that mild hypothermia (32°-35° C) has beneficial cerebral protective effects; however, studies have failed to demonstrate the efficacy of mild hypothermia in patients with a ruptured cerebral aneurysm. Hyperthermia should be avoided because it will increase cerebral metabolism and worsen ischemic insults.

The Cerebral Perfusion Pressure

The CPP equals mean arterial pressure minus intracranial pressure (CPP = MAP − ICP). Under normal conditions, CBF autoregulates over a CPP range from 50 to 150 mm Hg and is shifted to the right in patients with chronic hypertension. Studies of CBF in patients with traumatic brain injury have demonstrated that CPP should be in the range of 60 to 70 mm Hg if clinically feasible. Hypotension may decrease CBF and worsen ischemia.

CO_2 Tension

Hyperventilation produces hypocapnia, which in turn vasoconstricts the cerebral vasculature. Lowered CBF caused by hypocapnic vasoconstriction may worsen neurologic outcome after traumatic brain injury.

Oxygenation

Restoration of O_2 delivery to ischemic tissues should, by definition, resolve the ischemia. However, supranormal levels of O_2 in the tissues may lead to the formation of reactive O_2 species, with a paradoxically deleterious result.

Glucose Metabolism

During ischemic conditions, glucose undergoes anaerobic metabolism, leading to intracellular acidosis and a worsening of neurologic outcome. Frequent glucose monitoring should be performed in patients at risk for developing cerebral ischemia to avoid both hypoglycemia and hyperglycemia.

Anesthetic Agents

Barbiturates

Barbiturates have been considered to be the "gold standard" neuroprotective anesthetic agent when they are administered prior to a focal ischemic event. The neuroprotective properties of barbiturates are supported by a single human study in patients undergoing cardiopulmonary bypass, and corroborative evidence in humans is lacking. Researchers initially thought that the mechanism of barbiturate cerebral protection in laboratory animals was a dose-dependent reduction in the cerebral metabolic rate. However, subsequent studies revealed that barbiturate doses resulting in electroencephalographic isoelectricity or burst suppression are equally cerebroprotective, suggesting that additional protective mechanisms are in effect. Unwanted effects of high-dose barbiturates, such as cardiovascular instability and delays in awakening and neurologic assessment, must be taken into consideration when using this class of drug.

Propofol

In laboratory animals, propofol has been shown to have cerebroprotective activity, but human confirmation is lacking.

Inhalation Anesthetic Agents

Modern inhalation anesthetic agents produce significant electroencephalographic suppression at clinically tolerated doses, with rapid reversibility. Animal studies demonstrate protection from focal ischemia, as well as transient global ischemia, with the use of inhalation anesthetic agents; however, supporting human data are lacking.

Lidocaine

In typical antiarrhythmic doses, lidocaine may inhibit apoptosis, but supratherapeutic (toxic) doses are required to provide a meaningful diminution of cerebral metabolism.

Etomidate

Etomidate will decrease cerebral metabolism to a degree similar to that of the barbiturates; however, etomidate has not been convincingly shown to have neuroprotective effects. The lack of neuroprotective effects of etomidate is postulated to be due to its inhibition of nitric oxide production, with a subsequent decrease in CBF.

Conclusion

Protection of the nervous system from ischemic insult via pharmacologic and physiologic means has been a long-sought-after goal of anesthesiology. The current cerebral protective armamentarium has few proven interventions and many speculative ones. Box 131-1 provides a reasonable framework for addressing an ischemic insult based on the current level of knowledge.

Box 131-1 Considerations When Anticipating or Managing a Perioperative Ischemic Insult

Ensure the absence of hyperthermia
Manage blood glucose concentration with insulin to induce normoglycemia
Optimize oxyhemoglobin saturation*
Establish normocapnia
Consider the use of inhalation anesthetic agents if the operation is prolonged†
Resist the use of glucocorticoids
Consider the use of postoperative sustained induced moderate hypothermia if global ischemia is present‡

*Increasing concern has arisen that hypoxemia may be adverse in global ischemia.
†Not tested by clinical trials in the perioperative environment but supported by consistent efficacy when used in out-of-hospital ventricular fibrillation cardiac arrest.
‡No evidence of efficacy; preclinical evidence of adverse effect in global ischemia.
(Adapted, with permission, from Fukuda S, Warner DS. Cerebral protection. Br J Anaesth. 2007;99:10-17.)

Suggested Readings

Brain Trauma Foundation, American Association of Neurological Surgeons, Congress of Neurological Surgeons. Guidelines for the management of severe traumatic brain injury. Cerebral perfusion thresholds. *J Neurotrauma*. 2007;24(Suppl 1):S59-64.

Coles JP, Fryer TD, Coleman MR, et al. Hyperventilation following head injury: Effect on ischemic burden and cerebral oxidative metabolism. *Crit Care Med*. 2007;35:568-578.

Fukuda S, Warner DS. Cerebral protection. *Br J Anaesth*. 2007;99:10-17.

Michenfelder JD, ed. *Anesthesia and the Brain*. New York: Churchill Livingstone; 1988:14.

Nussmeier NA, Arlund C, Slogoff S. Neuropsychiatric complications after cardiopulmonary bypass: Cerebral protection by a barbiturate. *Anesthesiology*. 1986;64:165-170.

Patel P. Cerebral ischemia and intraoperative brain protection. In: Gupta AK, Gelb AW, eds. *Essentials of Neuroanesthesia and Neurointensive Care*. Philadelphia: WB Saunders; 2008:36-48.

Shankaran S, Laptook AR, Ehrenkranz RA, et al. Whole-body hypothermia for neonates with hypoxic-ischemic encephalopathy. *N Engl J Med*. 2005;353:1574-1584.

The Hypothermia After Cardiac Arrest Study Group. Mild therapeutic hypothermia to improve neurologic outcome after cardiac arrest. *N Engl J Med*. 2002;346:549-556.

Todd MM, Hindman BJ, Clarke WR, et al. Mild intraoperative hypothermia during surgery for intracranial aneurysm. *N Engl J Med*. 2005;352:135-145.

Warner DS, Takaoka S, Wu B, et al. Electroencephalographic burst suppression is not required to elicit maximal neuroprotection from pentobarbital in a rat model of focal ischemia. *Anesthesiology*. 1996;84:1475-1484.

Wass CT, Lanier WL. Glucose modulation of ischemic brain injury: Review and clinical recommendations. *Mayo Clin Proc*. 1996;71:801-812.

CHAPTER 132 Increased Intracranial Pressure

C. Thomas Wass, MD

Intracranial pressure (ICP) is determined by the relationship of the volumes of the intracranial vault (formed by the skull) and the intracranial contents. The latter is composed of three volume compartments: brain parenchyma, cerebrospinal fluid (CSF), and blood. By definition, intracranial hypertension exists when ICP is sustained above 15 mm Hg.

Brain

The brain parenchyma is composed of cellular elements and intracellular and interstitial water. The average adult brain weighs between 1350 and 1450 g and accounts for approximately 90% of the intracranial volume. This compartment may expand because of tumor growth or cytotoxic cerebral edema.

Cerebrospinal Fluid

CSF occupies approximately 5% of the intracranial volume (i.e., 75 mL, of which approximately 25 mL is within the ventricular system). The rate of CSF production is about 0.35 to 0.40 mL/min in the normal adult. Expansion of this compartment occurs with communicating or obstructive hydrocephalus.

Blood

Intracranial blood accounts for the remaining 5% of the intracranial volume. The cerebral blood volume (CBV) is 3 to 7 mL/100 g brain weight. Elevation of the head decreases both CBV and ICP. Expansion of the blood compartment may result from cerebral hemorrhage or dilation of resistance or capacitance vessels (e.g., vasogenic cerebral edema). This compartment is most amenable to acute manipulation by the anesthesiologist (see following discussion). With few exceptions (e.g., cerebral vasospasm, profound hypotension), increases in cerebral blood flow (CBF) usually result in parallel increases in CBV and ICP.

Intracranial Elastance

Historically, the intracranial pressure-volume relationship has been termed *compliance* in the medical literature. Compliance is defined as unit or units of volume (e.g., intracranial volume) change per unit or units of pressure (e.g., ICP) change (i.e., $\Delta V/\Delta P$). However, the pressure-volume curve presented in Figure 132-1 and most other textbooks actually depicts the reciprocal of compliance, or *elastance*.

Elastance is defined as $\Delta P/\Delta V$. Under normal physiologic conditions, small volume increases in any one of the three intracranial compartments results in little or no change in ICP. The compensatory mechanisms that initially protect against an elevation in ICP are (a) translocation of intracranial CSF through the foramen magnum to the subarachnoid space surrounding the spinal cord, (b) increased CSF absorption through the arachnoid granulations, and (c) translocation of blood out of the intracranial vault. Once these mechanisms are exhausted, abrupt increases in ICP occur in association with small increases in intracranial volume (see Figure 132-1). That is, intracranial compliance is decreased, or more correctly, *intracranial elastance is increased*.

Anesthetic Considerations

The goals of managing a patient with intracranial hypertension include preventing cerebral ischemia and preventing brain herniation (Figure 132-2).

Respiratory

$Paco_2$ is the single most potent physiologic determinant of CBF (Figure 132-3) and CBV. At a $Paco_2$ between 20 and 80 mm Hg, CBF decreases 1 mL/100 g brain weight/min and CBV decreases 0.05 mL/100 g brain weight for each 1-mm Hg decrease in $Paco_2$. Decreasing $Paco_2$ to 25 to 28 mm Hg should provide near-maximal reductions in ICP, lasting up to 24 h, without adversely affecting acid-base or electrolyte status or decreasing cerebral O_2 delivery (i.e., resulting from combined cerebral vasoconstriction and leftward shift in the oxyhemoglobin dissociation curve). Accordingly, in the setting of severe traumatic brain injury, the Brain Trauma Foundation states that aggressive hyperventilation (i.e., $Paco_2 \leq 25$ mm Hg) is not recommended, as further reductions in $Paco_2$ may result in iatrogenic brain injury.

Hypoxia (Pao_2 <50 mm Hg) will increase CBF and ICP. Application of positive end-expiratory pressure may decrease venous effluent from the cranium and exacerbate intracranial hypertension.

Coughing against a closed glottis (i.e., Valsalva maneuver) will increase ICP. Intravenously administered lidocaine, esmolol, or opioids can be used to attenuate the ICP response to direct laryngoscopy, tracheal intubation, or coughing.

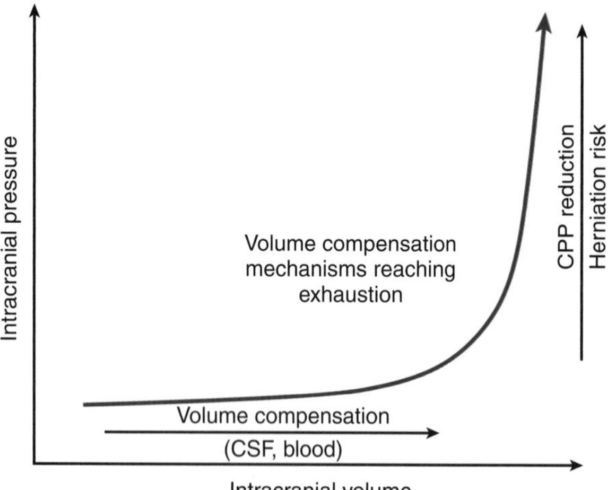

Figure 132-1 Idealized intracranial pressure-volume curve. The horizontal segment depicts maintenance of intracranial pressure (ICP) via physiologic compensatory mechanisms that respond to expanding intracranial volume (e.g., tumor, hematoma). Once these compensatory mechanisms are exhausted, elastance is increased, and small changes in intracranial volume result in large changes in ICP. CPP, Cerebral perfusion pressure; CSF, cerebrospinal fluid. (From Drummond JC, Patel PM. Neurosurgical anesthesia. In: Miller RD, ed. Miller's Anesthesia. Philadelphia: Churchill Livingstone Elsevier; 2009:2045-2087.)

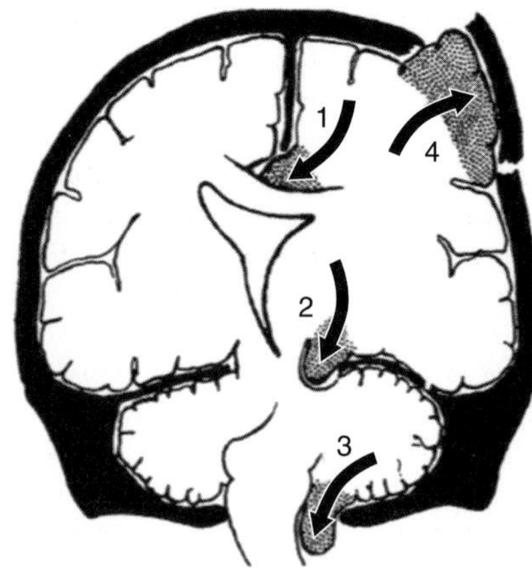

Figure 132-2 Schematic representation of various types of brain herniation: (1) cingulate gyrus, (2) temporal lobe (uncal), (3) cerebellar, and (4) transcalvarial (postoperative or traumatic). (From Drummond JC, Patel PM. Neurosurgical anesthesia. In: Miller RD, ed. Miller's Anesthesia. Philadelphia: Churchill Livingstone Elsevier; 2009:2045-2087.)

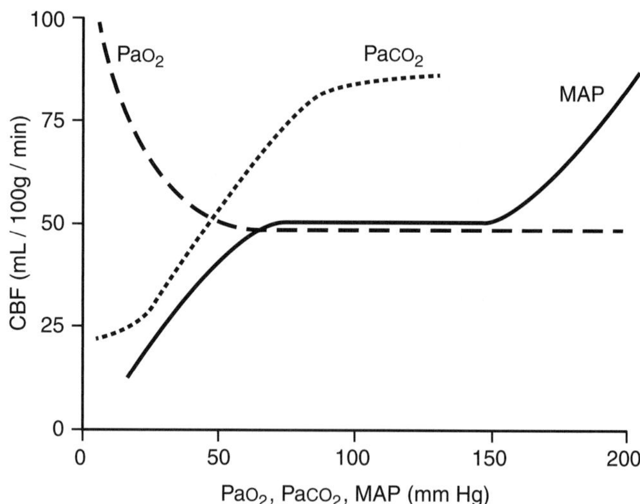

Figure 132-3 Effects of PaO_2, $PaCO_2$, and mean arterial pressure on cerebral blood flow. CBF, Cerebral blood flow; MAP, mean arterial pressure.

Cardiovascular

Mean arterial pressure (MAP) is a determinant of cerebral perfusion pressure (CPP) (i.e., CPP = MAP − ICP). The blood-brain barrier and autoregulation may be disrupted at the site of cerebral ischemic, traumatic, hemorrhagic, or osmolar insults. In these regions, it is correct to assume that CBF is passively dependent on CPP. Before the dura is opened, it is prudent to treat all hypertensive episodes by deepening the level of anesthesia, administering antihypertensive drugs that lack the ability to dilate cerebral vessels—and thus elevate ICP—(e.g., esmolol, labetalol, metoprolol), or both deepen the level of anesthesia and administer antihypertensive drugs. With respect to CPP, the critical threshold for ischemia is approximately 50 to 60 mm Hg. However, routine use of vasopressors and intravenously administered fluids to maintain the CPP greater than 70 mm Hg is not advised. Taking this information together, one can infer that maintaining the CPP near 60 to 70 mm Hg is advisable in the setting of traumatic brain injury.

Intravenous fluid administration should not be spared at the expense of hemodynamic stability. Osmolar, not oncotic, pressure is the primary determinant of fluid shifts within the brain. Therefore, maintaining intravascular isovolemia with a near-isoosmolar solution (e.g., normal saline, lactated Ringer's solution) is safe and beneficial to end-organ preservation. Hypoosmolar glucose-containing fluids (e.g., D_5W) have the ability to

(1) increase cerebral edema, (2) increase ICP, and (3) induce hyperglycemia, which exacerbates ischemic neurologic injury.

Renal

Both osmotic (e.g., mannitol 0.25-1.0 g/kg) and loop diuretics are effective in reducing the parenchymal fluid compartment and decrease CSF formation. Mannitol administration in patients with intracranial hypertension is not associated with a transient increase in ICP.

Metabolic

Cerebral metabolism decreases approximately 6% to 7% per 1 of temperature reduction. Mild hypothermia (i.e., temperature reductions of 1°C - 6°C) has been reported to improve neurologic outcome following focal or global brain ischemia in laboratory studies. Conversely, fever may worsen postischemic neurologic outcome. Proposed mechanisms for temperature modulation of postischemic neurologic outcome include alterations in cerebral metabolism, blood-brain barrier stability, membrane depolarization, ion homeostasis (e.g., calcium), neurotransmitter release (e.g., glutamate or aspartate), enzyme function (e.g., phospholipase, xanthine oxidase, or nitric oxide synthase), and free radical production or scavenging. Despite convincing laboratory data, large clinical trials have produced mixed results.

Musculoskeletal

The use of a nondepolarizing neuromuscular blocking agent without histamine-releasing properties (e.g., rocuronium, vecuronium, cisatracurium) is ideal for facilitating tracheal intubation and maintaining muscle paralysis. In the pathologic brain, pancuronium and gallamine can induce systemic and intracranial hypertension. Succinylcholine may increase ICP, possibly by increasing muscle afferent activity, but the clinical relevance is debatable.

Specific Anesthetic Agents

In general, all inhalation anesthetic agents are vasodilators that, with normocapnia, will increase CBF, CBV, and ICP. The vasodilator potency of isoflurane, sevoflurane, and desflurane is similar. Cerebral vasodilation is overcome by hyperventilating patients.

All intravenously administered anesthetic agents except ketamine cause some degree of reduction in cerebral metabolism, CBF, and ICP (provided ventilation is not depressed). Todd and colleagues were unable to demonstrate a significantly different outcome (incidence of new neurologic deficits, total hospital stay, or hospital cost) in neurosurgical patients anesthetized with a combination of propofol and fentanyl, isoflurane and N_2O, or fentanyl and N_2O.

Postoperative

Rapid and smooth emergence enables the neurosurgeon to evaluate the patient's neurologic status before discharge from the operative suite.

Suggested Readings

Brain Trauma Foundation. Guidelines for the management of severe traumatic brain injury: Cerebral perfusion thresholds. *J Neurotrauma*. 2007;24:S59-64.

Brain Trauma Foundation. Guidelines for the management of severe traumatic brain injury: Hyperventilation. *J Neurotrauma*. 2007;24:S87-90.

Kaieda R, Todd MM, Cook LN, et al. Acute effects of changing plasma osmolality and colloid oncotic pressure on the formation of brain edema after cryogenic injury. *Neurosurgery*. 1989;24:671-678.

Marion D, Bullock MR. Current and future role of therapeutic hypothermia. *J Neurotrauma*. 2009;26:455-467.

Ravussin P, Abou-Madi M, Archer D, et al. Changes in CSF pressure after mannitol in patients with and without elevated CSF pressure. *J Neurosurg*. 1988;69:869-876.

Todd MM, Warner DS, Sokoll MD, et al. A prospective, comparative trial of three anesthetics for elective supratentorial craniotomy. *Anesthesiology*. 1993; 78:1005-1020.

Wass CT, Lanier WL. Hypothermia-associated protection from ischemic brain injury: Implications for patient management. *Int Anesthesiol Clin*. 1996;34: 95-111.

CHAPTER 133

Functional Neurosurgery

Jeffrey J. Pasternak, MS, MD

Functional neurosurgery is a broad term applied to a variety of neurosurgical procedures performed to treat conditions in which the function of the brain is abnormal, typically in the context of normal gross structure and anatomy. These conditions include Parkinson disease, essential tremor, dystonia, obsessive compulsive disorder, and, possibly, Tourette syndrome, depression, refractory obesity, and epilepsy. The major challenge during functional neurosurgical procedures is to accurately and safely identify the abnormal regions of brain tissue, which is usually accomplished via neurologic assessment in an awake or partially sedated patient. Alternatively, radiographically guided or electrophysiologically guided techniques may be employed in patients having general anesthesia.

Implantation of Deep Brain Stimulators

Deep brain stimulation (DBS) involves the implantation of electrodes into select regions of the brain, allowing for electrical stimulation of the area to

Table 133-1 Disease States and Potential Anatomic Targets for Deep Brain Stimulation

Disease	Potential Deep Brain Stimulation Target(s)
Parkinson disease and essential tremor	Subthalamic nucleus Globus pallidus
Dystonia	Globus pallidus
Cerebellar tremor from multiple sclerosis	Thalamic ventral intermediate nucleus
Pantothenate kinase–associated neurodegeneration	Globus pallidus
Medically refractory depression	Subgenual cingulate region
Tourette syndrome	Anterior limb of the internal capsule Thalamic centromedian-parafascicular complex
Obsessive-compulsive disorder	Nucleus accumbens Anterior limb of the internal capsule
Central pain syndromes	Motor cortex Periaqueductal gray matter Periventricular gray matter Thalamus
Medically refractory epilepsy	Anterior nucleus of the thalamus Centromedian nucleus of the thalamus Subthalamic nucleus
Cluster headaches	Posterior hypothalamus
Obesity	Lateral hypothalamus Ventromedial hypothalamus Nucleus accumbens

Modified, with permission, from Siddiqui MS, Ellis TL, Tatter SB, Okun MS. Deep brain stimulation: Treating neurological and psychiatric disorders by modulating brain activity. NeuroRehabilitation. 2008;23:105-113.

modulate brain activity, resulting in attenuation, if not elimination, of the symptoms and signs of a number of disease states (Table 133-1). The specific site of electrode implantation depends on the disorder for which the patient requires treatment (Figure 133-1). Despite the use of DBS for many decades, the exact mechanism or mechanisms accounting for its clinical efficacy are not well understood, but the electric current is believed to somehow modulate abnormal neuronal function, either by acting directly on neuronal action potentials or altering neurotransmitter release. Use of DBS has generally replaced ablative procedures, such as pallidotomy or thalamotomy (i.e., thermal, mechanical, or electrical destruction of a region of the globus pallidus or thalamus, respectively), for the treatment of Parkinson disease. Unlike these earlier procedures, DBS is reversible.

DBS implantation is typically conducted via frame-based stereotactic techniques. In essence, a stereotactic head frame is applied, usually under monitored anesthesia care, and the neurosurgeon injects a local anesthetic agent at the sites where the pins of the head frame will be inserted to immobilize the skull within the head frame, after which the patient undergoes imaging (i.e., computed tomography or magnetic resonance imaging) to localize the deep brain target relative to the stereotactic head frame. An electrode is advanced via a burr hole to the approximate location of the target. Implantation of the electrode into the exact target nucleus is usually facilitated by single-neuron recordings and then confirmed, if possible, by the resolution of symptoms upon stimulation. The nature of various disorders, such as obesity, epilepsy, and obsessive-compulsive disorder, may not allow for immediate confirmation of symptom resolution. Following electrode implantation, the wires are tunneled under the skin to reach a generator, which is typically implanted in the pectoral region.

Generally, electrode implantation is performed with the patient in a semiseated position with monitored anesthesia care with sedatives administered to keep the patient "comfortable" but not so sedated that the surgeon cannot intraoperatively assess and optimize the efficacy of electrode placement. Providing an adequate but not excessive level of sedation can prove to be very challenging because the procedures tend to be of long duration and access to the airway is limited due to the presence of the head frame, which is rigidly fixed to the operating table. A means to rapidly secure the airway

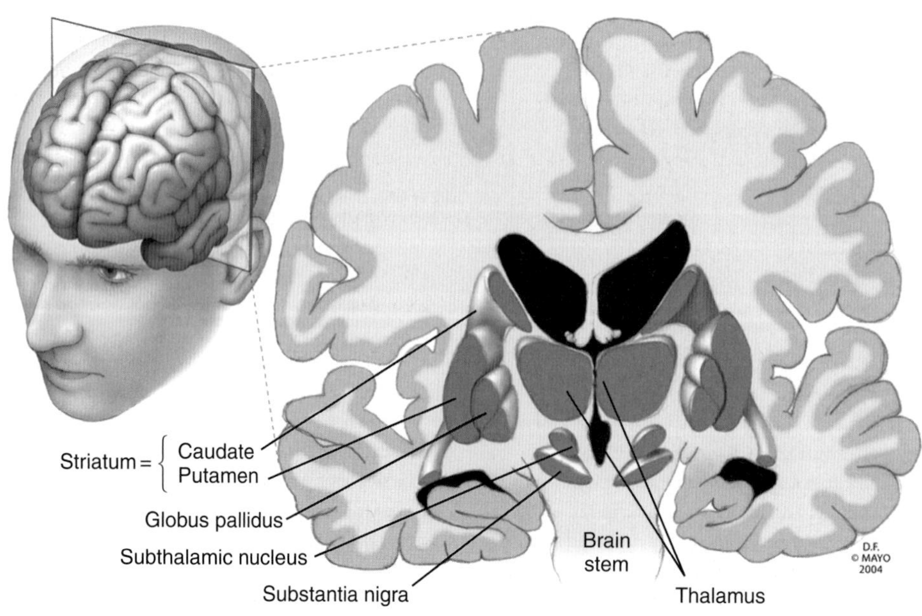

Figure 133-1 The basal ganglia are primary targets for the treatment of a variety of disorders via deep brain stimulation. (© Mayo Foundation for Medical Education and Research. All rights reserved.)

(i.e., laryngeal mask airway, fiberoptic bronchoscope) should be readily available. Some sedative drugs (i.e., propofol, benzodiazepines) can inhibit neuronal activity, thus influencing the ability to utilize single-neuron recordings to accurately identify the deep brain target. Short-acting opioids (e.g., fentanyl, remifentanil) and dexmedetomidine have been used successfully to provide sedation for these procedures.

Alternatively, in patients not able to tolerate the procedure with sedation (e.g., children or adults with impaired cognitive or intellectual abilities) implantation of a depth electrode can be conducted with general anesthesia. Drugs used to maintain general anesthesia may significantly impact the ability to identify and monitor neuronal electrical recordings. In these situations, proper placement of the depth electrode is usually dependent on imaging data referenced to the stereotactic head frame; thus, the likelihood of improper or ineffective electrode position may be greater when using general anesthesia.

Clinically consequential venous air embolism has been reported with the implantation of electrodes for deep brain stimulation, and the use of precordial Doppler sonography monitoring should be considered. Of note, electrical impedance from precordial Doppler sonography may impair neuronal electrical recording and may need to be suspended during recording of neuronal activity. Tunneling of electrode leads and implantation of the pulse generator are usually conducted during general anesthesia following removal of the stereotactic head frame.

Cervical Denervation for Dystonia

Dystonias are a group of disorders in which inappropriate and sustained muscle contractions lead to twisting movements and abnormal postures. The causes are many and types include congenital, idiopathic, trauma-induced, and drug-induced dystonias. Conservative treatment options include antiparkinsonian drugs (such as trihexyphenidyl or the combination of carbidopa and levodopa), antiepileptics, benzodiazepines, and β-adrenergic receptor blocking agents. If these medications do not produce satisfactory results, injection of botulinum toxin into the affected muscles may also provide some improvement and is the most commonly performed invasive procedure. DBS has been approved by the Food and Drug Administration in the United States for treatment of cervical dystonia and is currently under investigation, assessing efficacy compared to other treatment options, for other dystonias.

Refractory cervical dystonia may also be treated with selective peripheral muscular denervation, which involves identifying and transecting the nerves supplying the affected muscles. This procedure is usually conducted under general anesthesia with the patient in either the prone or sitting position. In either case, the surgeon will directly stimulate nerves with an electric current to identify specific musculle innervation; hence, the use of neuromuscular blocking agents is contraindicated during this segment of the procedure. In patients undergoing cervical denervation in the sitting position, techniques used to monitor for (i.e., transesophageal echocardiography, precordial Doppler sonography) and to treat (i.e., central venous catheter) air entrained into the venous system should be considered.

Epilepsy Surgery

Epilepsy, or recurrent seizure disorder, affects 50 million people worldwide and occurs in all age groups. Initial management of epilepsy is usually with the use of one or more antiepileptic drugs. Despite this, many patients either continue to experience frequent seizures despite the use of multiple antiepileptic agents or are unable to tolerate the side effects of these drugs, which include somnolence, ataxia, hepatitis, cutaneous reactions, or aplastic anemia. Active epilepsy has a major negative impact on quality of life. For example, patients are unable to drive automobiles, may have work limitations, and also suffer the embarrassment of having seizures in public. In these patients, surgical management should be considered as a treatment option. Although epilepsy surgery was long considered as a last resort, the loss of developmental milestones in children and young adults who continue to experience seizures or have unacceptable side effects with the use of antiepileptic medications has increased the number and decreased the age of those having surgery. There are two major types of epilepsy surgery: (1) resective and (2) nonresective or functional procedures.

Resective Procedures

The goal of resective procedures is to remove an abnormal region of brain that is thought to give rise to seizures (i.e., an epileptogenic focus). Preoperative identification of the epileptogenic focus is usually determined by history and physical examination, brain imaging, and video-electroencephalography. In the latter procedure, patients are admitted to a video telemetry unit, and simultaneous videotaping of the patient's activity and electroencephalography are conducted to correlate the electrical characteristics of the seizure with motor or behavioral findings. In some patients, depth electrodes may be implanted prior to video-electroencephalography to allow for characterization of epileptogenic foci in deeper regions of the brain. Because many epileptogenic foci amenable to surgery are found to exist in the anterior temporal lobe, resection of this region is common, accounting for 75% of resective procedures. In many cases, intraoperative electrocorticography may be employed to allow for accurate identification of the epileptogenic focus. Electrode-containing grids are placed directly on the brain surface and abnormal epileptiform activity (i.e., abnormal background electroencephalographic activity) generated by the epileptogenic focus is recorded, allowing for a more precise resection. In cases in which electrocorticography is employed, anesthetic drugs that suppress epileptiform activity should be avoided or minimized during mapping. These drugs include inhalation anesthetic agents, sedative and anesthetic doses of barbiturates and propofol, and benzodiazepines. Nitrous oxide, opioids, diphenhydramine, droperidol, and possibly dexmedetomidine may be used to maintain sedation or general anesthesia during this period. Additionally, low-dose methohexital (0.3-1 mg/kg), etomidate (0.1-0.3 mg/kg), or alfentanil (50 μg/kg) may be administered as a bolus to enhance epileptiform activity generated by the seizure focus. Patients requiring intraoperative electrocorticography should be counseled preoperatively on the increased risk of intraoperative awareness, given the limited choices and doses of drugs that are available. In patients undergoing resection near the language center located in the temporal lobe, the procedure may be carried out with local anesthesia and sedation (i.e., awake craniotomy) allowing for intraoperative language assessment. Given the possibility of an intraprocedural seizure, the clinician should be prepared with airway equipment to secure an airway in a situation with limited airway access. Options may include temporary mask ventilation, an intubating laryngeal mask airway, and fiberoptically guided intubation. Additionally, termination of a seizure should be accomplished with agents that cause minimal respiratory depression in the setting of an unsecured airway. Additionally, the surgeon may irrigate the brain surface with cold saline solution in an effort to terminate a seizure.

Nonresective or Functional Procedures

In patients who continue to have frequent seizures despite resective treatment or are deemed not to be candidates for resective options (e.g., those with lesions near eloquent cortex, those in whom a primary epileptogenic focus cannot be identified, and those with multiple medical comorbid conditions that increase anesthetic risk), functional surgical procedures may be considered. Functional procedures are generally palliative and are considered a means to achieve a reduction in seizure frequency, as opposed to achieving a cure of epilepsy. Functional procedures include electrical stimulation techniques (i.e., vagal nerve, cortical, DBS), multiple subpial transection, and corpus callosotomy.

Vagal nerve stimulation involves placement of an electrode in the left vagal nerve sheath in the neck and a pulse generator in the pectoral region; it is performed with general anesthesia. The left vagus nerve is the preferred target, because parasympathetic innervation of the heart is predominantly derived from the right vagus nerve. A 50% or greater reduction in seizure frequency occurs in about 30% of patients with this technique. The exact mechanism by which vagal nerve stimulation results in a reduction in seizure frequency is not currently understood. The most common side effects are cough and hoarseness. Other stimulation techniques currently under investigation for seizure control include cortical stimulation and DBS. The major advantage of stimulation-based techniques for epilepsy control is reversibility, such that, if patients are unable to tolerate side effects or experience no benefit, the pulse generator and electrode can be removed with minimal injury to brain tissue.

The treatment goal of the remaining functional procedures is to limit seizure spread to the adjacent cortex. These techniques include multiple subpial transection and corpus callosotomy, both typically performed with general anesthesia. In the former technique, multiple incisions of about 4 mm in depth are made in cerebral cortex in an effort to transect fibers that may be involved in seizure propagation. The goal is to limit seizure spread while maintaining the function of eloquent cortex. Corpus callosotomy, performed more frequently in children than in adults, involves complete or staged transection of the corpus callosum to prevent seizure propagation to the adjacent cerebral hemisphere.

Suggested Readings

Duncan JS. Epilepsy surgery. *Clin Med.* 2007;7:137-142.

Kofke WA, Tempelhoff R, Dasheiff RM. Anesthesia for epileptic patients and for epilepsy surgery. In: Cottrell JE, Smith DS, eds. *Anesthesia and Neurosurgery.* 4th ed. St. Louis: Mosby; 2001:473-500.

Siddiqui MS, Ellis TL, Tatter SB, Okun MS. Deep brain stimulation: Treating neurological and psychiatric disorders by modulating brain activity. *Neuro Rehabilitation.* 2008;23:105-113.

CHAPTER 134

Management of Cerebral Aneurysms

Eric L. Bloomfield, MD, MS, MMI, FCCM

The prevalence of cerebral aneurysms in the general population in the United States is estimated to be 4% to 6%. The incidence of subarachnoid hemorrhage (SAH) resulting from rupture of a cerebral aneurysm is about 12 per 100,000 persons per year. From another perspective, aneurysms that have not ruptured carry a 1% to 2% per year risk of hemorrhage. Incidence increases with age, and the female-male ratio is 1.6:1. Cerebral aneurysms may also be seen in women during pregnancy, with an increased incidence during 30 to 40 weeks of gestation. However, delivery is rarely associated with aneurysmal rupture.

Predisposing factors for rupture include increased aneurysm size, weak aneurysm wall, history of previous rupture, and elevated transmural pressure gradient. The transmural pressure gradient is influenced by the difference between the pressure inside the aneurysm (mean arterial pressure) and the pressure outside the aneurysm (intracranial pressure [ICP]). Sudden changes in blood pressure or ICP may lead to rupture or rebleed of an aneurysm.

Aneurysm Rupture

When an aneurysm ruptures, blood flows into the subarachnoid space. Patients may experience sudden onset of severe headache (often described as "the worst headache of my life"), altered level of consciousness, focal or global neurologic deficits, or coma, depending on the location and magnitude of the bleed. As the blood spreads in the subarachnoid space, signs of meningismus become evident. Obstructive hydrocephalus and increased ICP may occur. Categorizing the severity of rupture is achieved using the Hunt-Hess classification system, which is based on a 5-grade scoring scale. Grades 1 and 2 are associated with increasing headache, and grades 3 and 4, with increasing neurologic deficits; grade 5 signifies deep coma. Latter grades are associated with worse outcomes. Definitive diagnosis is made with imaging of the head (i.e., computed tomography or magnetic resonance imaging) or cerebral angiography.

Major causes of morbidity and death include rebleeding, cerebral vasospasm, and obstructive hydrocephalus. The worst among these causes continues to be vasospasm, the exact cause of which is unknown. If vasospasm is left untreated, permanent neurologic damage from ischemia is likely to occur. Vasospasm usually manifests at about 72 h after the rupture of the aneurysm. The initial clinical diagnosis of cerebral vasospasm is made with changes in neurologic status. Definitive diagnosis can be made with transcranial Doppler ultrasonography. Reference velocities are less than 120 cm/sec; velocities greater than this value are an indication that intracranial vessels are constricting.

Nimodipine is the standard drug used to manage vasospasm because it improves collateral blood flow (Table 134-1); however, it does not relieve the vasospasm of the main vessel. Optimal management entails the use of hypertension, hydration, and hemodilution (triple-H therapy) to overcome the vasospasm, which usually lasts for up to 14 days.

Other post-SAH problems include electrocardiographic changes, which may result from an intense sympathetic discharge. Some of these changes are benign; however, others may be indicative of myocardial damage. When these changes do occur, more intense invasive monitoring is necessary. If cardiac intervention is required, percutaneous endovascular therapy is probably the preferred treatment method.

Other problems associated with SAH include hyponatremia secondary to cerebral salt-wasting syndrome or syndrome of inappropriate antidiuretic

Table 134-1 Management of Aneurysms

Management Aspect	Aneurysm Category: Nonruptured	Ruptured
Monitoring	Standard	Standard plus ICP
Brain protection	No	Probable
Vasospasm	No	Most likely
Triple-H therapy	No	Yes
Surgical treatment	Elective	Emergent
Surgical treatment versus endovascular coil placement	Location-dependent	Location-dependent
Nimodipine	No	Yes
Outcomes	Good	Depends on Hunt-Hess classification and severity of bleed

ICP, Intracranial pressure; triple-H therapy, use of hypertension, hydration, and hemodilution.

hormone secretion (SIADH). The former results from secretion of atrial natriuretic hormone from the brain, causing a clinical triad of hyponatremia, volume contraction, and high urine sodium concentration. These patients may require fluid resuscitation. SIADH results from inappropriately excessive release of antidiuretic hormone and subsequent excessive free-water retention. In contrast with the treatment of cerebral salt-wasting syndrome, the treatment of SIADH is fluid restriction. However, because of vasospasm, restricting fluid may not be possible because fluid administration, rather than fluid restriction, is a primary component of triple-H therapy. In this situation, the administration of hypertonic saline should be considered.

Surgical Treatment

Previously, when an aneurysm ruptured and an SAH ensued, the patient was observed for 10 to 14 days to allow time for resolution of both vasospasm and cerebral edema; however, the incidence of rebleeding was extremely high, with resultant morbidity and death. Today, treatment is early surgical intervention with either a surgical clip or an endovascular coil. Placement of either of these devices makes it easier to administer triple-H therapy should vasospasm occur. These interventions also decrease the incidence of rebleeding.

Aneurysms smaller than 7 mm have a low incidence of rupture. In aneurysms of this size, the principal treatment was previously to place a clip around the neck of the aneurysm. This treatment was in use until about 15 years ago, when Guglielmi detachable coils were introduced as a minimally invasive endovascular alternative. The International Subarachnoid Aneurysm Trial was conducted to evaluate surgery versus endovascular coiling. Some patients in the trial were observed for up to 7 years. Major results showed a decreased death rate in the endovascular coiling group (23.5% vs. 30.9%; $P < 0.0001$) and less epilepsy but, compared with the surgical group, a higher incidence of rebleeding and less than optimal occlusion rate. However, as endovascular coiling techniques have improved, an increasing number of patients are treated with endovascular therapy.

Anesthetic Management

Surgical and anesthetic management go hand in hand when caring for patients with an aneurysm. When compared with individuals with a higher grade of aneurysm, patients with a Hunt-Hess grade 1 or 2 aneurysm have a lower incidence of having increased ICP. Major blood loss is a potential adverse outcome during surgery, and brain relaxation probably will be necessary. With intracranial hemorrhage, cerebral autoregulation is lost. Consequently, the anesthesia care team must closely monitor, and maintain stable, the transmural pressure gradient.

In former times, intraoperative bleeding was restrained with controlled hypotension. Now, most surgeons prefer to have the blood pressure at baseline to maintain cerebral perfusion pressure. Temporary clipping of the main feeder vessel to the aneurysm may be needed. With this clipping, it may be necessary to temporarily increase the patient's blood pressure to improve collateral circulation. Although evidence of barbiturate-mediated brain protection in humans is lacking, this technique may be requested by the surgical team. If nothing else, the barbiturates are effective in decreasing ICP and may help "relax" the brain during clip placement. If the temporary clip is removed, any dramatic increase in blood pressure that could lead to bleeding should be avoided.

During the operation, the use of standard American Society of Anesthesiologists monitors plus invasive arterial blood pressure monitoring are indicated. A central venous catheter may be helpful but is not necessary, depending on the patient's comorbid conditions. Monitoring of the electroencephalogram and sensory-evoked potentials may be used, but no human trials have shown consistent benefit. If hydrocephalus is present, the neurosurgeon may opt to place a ventriculostomy for monitoring ICP and cerebrospinal fluid drainage. Brain bulk can also be decreased with intravenously administered mannitol.

Anesthesia induction can be accomplished with propofol and maintained with an opioid, such as fentanyl citrate, and an inhalation agent, such as isoflurane. It may become necessary to avoid an anesthesia level that exceeds 1 MAC (minimum alveolar concentration) of an inhalation agent to avoid cerebral vasodilation and subsequent increases in ICP. If the brain is extremely edematous, use of a total intravenous anesthetic technique may be considered.

Aside from avoiding hyperglycemia and fever during periods when the brain is at risk for developing ischemic injury, definitive evidence for brain-protective interventions are devoid in the human literature (see Chapter 131). Despite this, many physicians use barbiturates or propofol to achieve burst suppression (4-6 bursts/min) during critical periods of aneurysm operations. The Intraoperative Hypothermia for Aneurysm Surgery Trial did not show any benefit of a mild temperature decrease (to 33° C) during operations. No other research results have been published on this topic recently.

Recovery

Regardless of whether the patient has undergone endovascular coiling or surgical clipping, smooth emergence from general anesthesia facilitates postoperative neurologic examination. Patients with a Hunt-Hess grade 3 or 4 aneurysm may benefit from continued postoperative airway and sedative management, as well as from ICP monitoring with a ventriculostomy or a Camino intracranial device. Again, vasospasm will generally not occur until about 72 h after the rupture of the aneurysm. If vasospasm is suspected, patients can be monitored with transcranial Doppler ultrasonography, and therapy can be initiated if vasospasm becomes evident. A repeat computed tomographic scan or angiography may be indicated.

Acknowledgment

The author and editors would like to thank Paul E. Stensrud, MD, for his past contributions to this chapter.

Suggested Readings

Bulsara KR, McGirt MJ, Liao L, et al. Use of the peak troponin value to differentiate myocardial infarction from reversible neurogenic left ventricular dysfunction associated with aneurysmal subarachnoid hemorrhage. *J Neurosurg*. 2003;98:524-528.

Chang HS, Hongo K, Nakagawa H. Adverse effects of limited hypotensive anesthesia on the outcome of patients with subarachnoid hemorrhage. *J Neurosurg*. 2000;92:971-975.

Colby GP, Coon AL, Tamargo RJ. Surgical management of aneurysmal subarachnoid hemorrhage. *Neurosurg Clin North Am*. 2010;21:247-261.

Dorai Z, Hynan LS, Kopitnik TA, Samson D. Factors related to hydrocephalus after aneurysmal subarachnoid hemorrhage. *Neurosurgery*. 2003;52:763-769.

Gelb AW, Wilson JX, Cechetto DF. Anesthetics and cerebral ischemia: Should we continue to dream the impossible dream? *Can J Anaesth*. 2001;48:727-731.

Molyneux AJ, Kerr RS, Yu LM, et al, International Subarachnoid Aneurysm Trial (ISAT) Collaborative Group. International Subarachnoid Aneurysm Trial (ISAT) of neurosurgical clipping versus endovascular coiling in 2143 patients with ruptured intracranial aneurysms: A randomised comparison of effects on survival, dependency, seizures, rebleeding, subgroups, and aneurysm occlusion. *Lancet*. 2005;366:809-817.

Pearl M, Gregg L, Gailloud P. Endovascular treatment of aneurysmal subarachnoid hemorrhage. *Neurosurg Clin North Am*. 2010;21:271-280.

Todd MM, Hindman BJ, Clarke WR, Torner JC, Intraoperative Hypothermia for Aneurysm Surgery Trial (IHAST) Investigators. Mild intraoperative hypothermia during surgery for intracranial aneurysm. *N Engl J Med*. 2005;352:135-145.

Yee AH, Burns JD, Wijdicks EF. Cerebral salt wasting: Pathophysiology, diagnosis, and treatment. *Neurosurg Clin North Am*. 2010;21:339-352.

CHAPTER 135

Anesthesia for Hypophysectomy

Jeffrey J. Pasternak, MS, MD

In adults, the pituitary gland has a volume of 0.5 to 1.5 mm^3 and is located inferior to the hypothalamus within the sella turcica (Figure 135-1). Despite its small size, the pituitary gland plays a crucial role in human physiology. It consists of two functionally separate regions: (1) the anterior pituitary or adenohypophysis and (2) the posterior pituitary or neurohypophysis. The pituitary gland secretes a variety of hormones that either directly affect other tissues or control the regulation of other endocrine substances. Pituitary tumors are a common cause of primary pituitary dysfunction and can manifest by hypersecretion or hyposecretion of hormones or by invasion of the structures surrounding the sella turcica.

Adenohypophysis

The adenohypophysis secretes an array of hormones under the regulation of the hypothalamus. Releasing and inhibiting factors are secreted into a capillary network within the hypothalamus (Table 135-1). Via portal vessels,

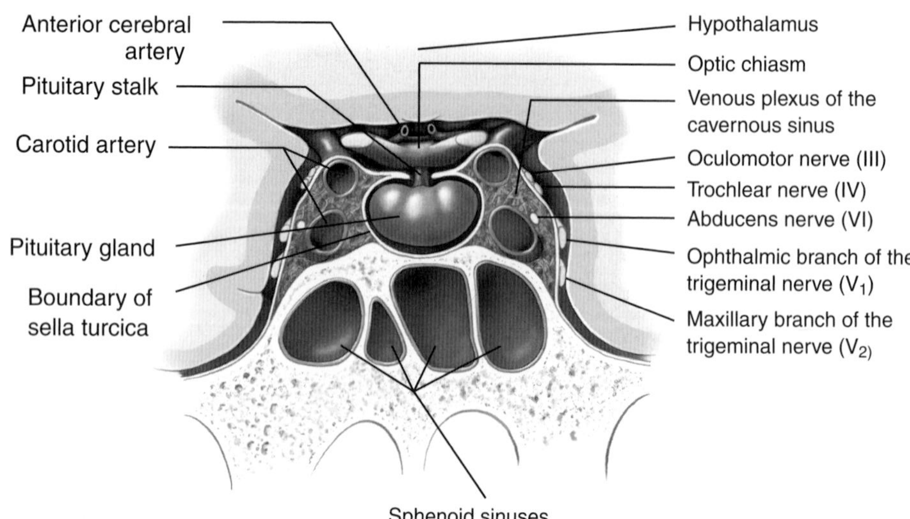

Figure 135-1 Coronal section of the sella turcica depicting the anatomic relationships among the pituitary gland, cranial nerves, carotid arteries, and cavernous and sphenoid sinuses.

Table 135-1 Hypothalamic Hormones and Adenohypophyseal Responses

Hypothalamic Hormone	Pituitary Cell Target	Pituitary Response	Overall Effect
CRH	Corticotrophs	↑ production of ACTH	↑ production of cortisol by the adrenal gland
TRH	Thyrotrophs	↑ production of TSH	↑ production of T_3 and T_4 by the thyroid gland
GnRH	Gonadotrophs	↑ production of FSH and LH	Regulates estrogen, progesterone, testosterone, and inhibin production by gonads
GHRH	Somatotrophs	↑ production of GH	↑ production of IGF
Somatostatin	Somatotrophs	↓ production of GH	↓ production of IGF
PRF	Lactotrophs	↑ production of prolactin	Promote lactation
Dopamine	Lactotrophs	↓ production of prolactin	Inhibit lactation

ACTH, Adrenocorticotropic hormone; CRH, corticotropin-releasing hormone; FSH, follicle-stimulating hormone; GH, growth hormone; GHRH, growth hormone–releasing hormone; GnRH, gonadotropin-releasing hormone; IGF, insulin-like growth factor; LH, luteinizing hormone; PRF, prolactin-releasing factor; T_3, triiodothyronine; T_4, thyroxine; TRH, thyroid-releasing hormone; TSH, thyroid-stimulating hormone.

these compounds then enter a second capillary network within the adenohypophysis, where they either enhance or inhibit secretion of adenohypophyseal hormones (Figure 135-2). Further secretion of hormones by the anterior pituitary is then regulated via feedback control of hypothalamic and adenohypophyseal secretion in response to concentrations of hormones secreted by target glands. Given the complex interactions among the hypothalamus, anterior pituitary, target endocrine glands, and end organs, disease or dysregulation at any point within these pathways can cause dysfunction of one or more hormone axes.

Cushing Disease

Adrenocorticotropic hormone (ACTH) acts upon the adrenal cortex to increase cortisol production. In patients with Cushing disease, excessive production of ACTH, usually by an ACTH-producing adenoma, results in hypercortisolemia. Cortisol has a broad range of physiologic effects, including increased gluconeogenesis, reduced systemic glucose utilization, protein catabolism, increased lipolysis, increased gastric acid production, bone reabsorption, and immune suppression. Clinical manifestations include hyperglycemia, skeletal muscle weakness, "moon facies," "buffalo hump," osteoporosis, poor wound healing, and increased infection rate. Perioperative concerns include possible difficulty with airway management, aberrant serum electrolyte or glucose concentrations, muscle weakness, and difficulty positioning due to osteoporosis or body habitus.

Acromegaly

Acromegaly results from excessive secretion of growth hormone by the adenohypophysis. Growth hormone exerts its effect either directly on target cells or via stimulating hepatic secretion of insulin-like growth factor (also known as somatomedin C). Together, excessive growth hormone and somatomedin C production result in inappropriately increased protein synthesis, gluconeogenesis, lipolysis, chondrocyte proliferation, and bone mineralization, as well as muscle sarcomeric hyperplasia. This results in organomegaly and overgrowth of bones, muscles, and connective tissues.

The impact of these changes on the respiratory and cardiac systems are of primary concern during the perioperative period. Specifically, hypertrophy of facial bones, tongue, airway soft tissues, and glottic structures render the patient susceptible to developing obstructive sleep apnea. Additionally, difficulties with mask fit, bag-mask ventilation, and direct laryngoscopy have been reported. Mandibular hypertrophy increases the distance between the lips and vocal cord. Vocal cord dysfunction, secondary to stretching of

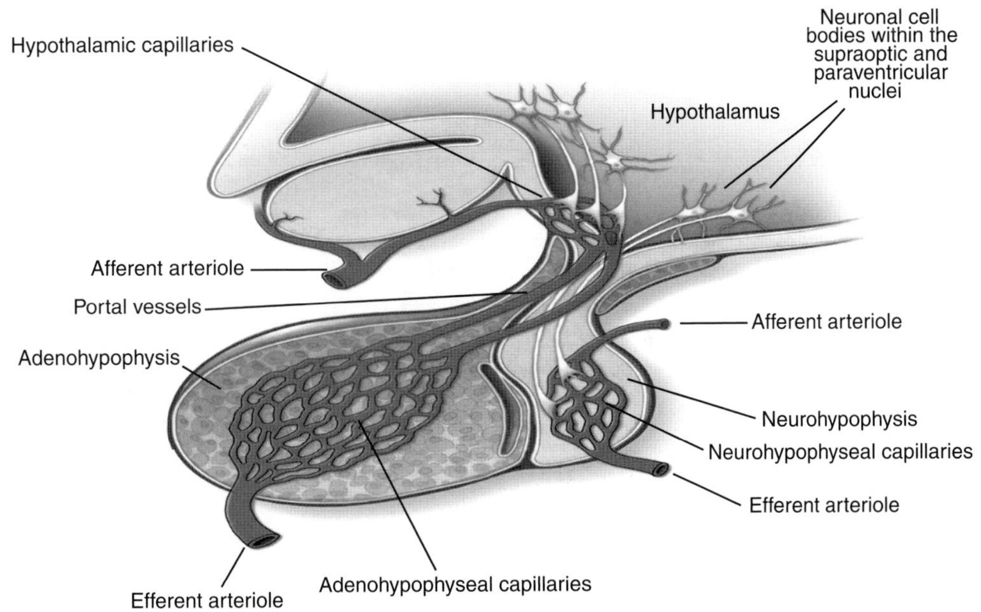

Figure 135-2 Physiology of the pituitary gland. Hormones secreted by the hypothalamus reach the adenohypophysis via the portal vessel. These hypothalamic hormones enter a second capillary network and act upon adenohypophyseal cells, thus regulating the secretion of hormones by the adenohypophysis. The neurohypophysis contains axons of neurons located in the supraoptic and paraventricular nuclei of the hypothalamus. When stimulated, these neurons secrete either oxytocin or vasopressin into the capillary network of the neurohypophysis.

the recurrent laryngeal nerve, and impaired mobility of the cricoarytenoid joints can further impact airway management. Indirect videolaryngoscopic (e.g., McGrath Series 5 video laryngoscope or GlideScope Ranger) or awake fiberoptic intubations are prudent options when managing the airway of these individuals. Intubation may be performed after the induction of anesthesia, but difficulty with mask ventilation and laryngoscopy, by any means, should be anticipated, and backup equipment should be readily available. Costal cartilage hypertrophy can lead to restrictive pulmonary physiology.

Cardiovascular manifestations of acromegaly include hypertension, cardiac hypertrophy, left ventricular diastolic dysfunction (generally with preserved systolic function at rest until late in the course of the disease), and arrhythmias. Coronary artery insufficiency can occur and is related to increased O_2 demand from a hypertrophic heart and reduced coronary blood flow due to increased cardiac filling pressures that occur with diastolic dysfunction. Despite beliefs to the contrary, hypertrophy of the transverse carpal ligament does not increase the risk of ischemic complications of the hand with cannulation of the radial artery.

Hyperprolactinemia

Signs and symptoms of increased prolactin production are more concrete in women (i.e., galactorrhea, amenorrhea, infertility) than in men (e.g., decreased libido, erectile dysfunction). As such, prolactin-secreting tumors tend to be larger, and possibly more invasive, in men at the time of surgery because of delayed diagnosis. Although the manifestations of hyperprolactinemia cause no overt concerns for anesthesia, medications used to pharmacologically manage increased serum prolactin concentration (e.g., bromocriptine or cabergoline) can be associated with nausea, orthostatic hypotension, and cardiac valvular dysfunction.

Pituitary Hyperthyroidism

Pituitary hyperthyroidism results from excessive production of thyroid-stimulating hormone by a pituitary adenoma that, in turn, causes increased triiodothyronine (T_3) and thyroxine (T_4) production (both are important metabolic regulators). These tumors are rare, and thus, many patients undergo treatment for other causes of hyperthyroidism (e.g., Graves disease) prior to detection of the pituitary disease, thereby delaying the diagnosis. Such interventions include radioactive thyroid ablation or thyroidectomy, leading to decreased thyroid hormone production and loss of negative feedback on secretion of thyroid-stimulating hormone, which, in turn, can enhance tumor growth. Delayed diagnosis and tumor growth increase the likelihood of neoplastic encroachment on surrounding structures (e.g., the cavernous sinus), which places the patient at increased risk for developing intraoperative bleeding and iatrogenic central nervous system injury during the resection. Patients may also be hyperthyroid, hypothyroid, or euthyroid at the time of surgery. Unless visual loss is acutely threatened, patients should be rendered physiologically euthyroid, using medical treatment, prior to surgery.

Hypopituitarism

Hypopituitarism, or pituitary failure, most commonly results from compression of normal gland by pituitary tumors. However, other causes are possible, such as infection, inflammation, and trauma. Signs and symptoms are often nonspecific and depend on the extent of hormone deficiency. In acute pituitary failure (i.e., apoplexy or acute pituitary infarction), decreases in serum corticotropin and cortisol levels occur quickly due to their short half-lives. As such, signs and symptoms of acute apoplexy include acute hyponatremia, profound hypotension, and shock. In this context, treatment with corticosteroids can be lifesaving. In those with chronic hypopituitarism, growth hormone deficiency is most common; deficiencies of thyroid-stimulating hormone, prolactin, and hormones produced by the neurohypophysis (i.e., oxytocin and vasopressin) are quite rare. Patients with chronic hypopituitarism will likely require perioperative corticosteroid supplementation.

Neurohypophysis

Unlike the adenohypophysis, which contains hormone-secreting cells, the neurohypophysis contains distal axons of peptidergic neurons with cell bodies located in the supraoptic and paraventricular nuclei of the hypothalamus. These neurons synthesize and secrete either oxytocin or vasopressin (i.e., antidiuretic hormone), which are released into the systemic circulation via capillaries located in the neurohypophysis (see Figure 135-2).

Oxytocin is best known for modulating labor and delivery and release of breast milk. Vasopressin is one of the principal hormones regulating water balance. Normally, the strongest stimulus for vasopressin secretion is increased serum osmolality, mediated via hypothalamic osmoreceptors. Vasopressin increases water reabsorption by the kidney and causes systemic arteriolar constriction.

The most common manifestation of the syndrome of inappropriate antidiuretic hormone secretion (SIADH) is hyponatremia. SIADH is usually asymptomatic if the syndrome is mild; however, seizures and coma can occur if the serum sodium concentration acutely decreases below 120 mEq/L. In the setting of chronic SIADH, adaptive mechanisms minimize symptoms despite very low serum sodium concentrations. Treatment usually involves fluid restriction for mild cases and, otherwise, slow ($<$1-2 $mEq \cdot L^{-1} \cdot h^{-1}$) correction of hyponatremia with hypertonic saline, as rapid correction can potentially cause central pontine myelinolysis.

Diabetes insipidus (DI) refers to inappropriate production of hypotonic urine due to either inadequate production of vasopressin (i.e., central DI) or renal unresponsiveness to vasopressin (i.e., nephrogenic DI). Initial treatment should focus on replenishing intravascular volume, which may require the use of 0.9% saline in patients with severe hypovolemia, despite hypernatremia, and correcting hypernatremia. Additionally, for central DI, vasopressin or a synthetic analog (i.e., 1-desamino-8-D-arginine vasopressin [DDAVP]) may be administered. No specific treatment exists for nephrogenic DI.

Management of Patients Having Pituitary Operations

The most common indication for pituitary surgery is tumor resection. Tumors derived from secretory cells are typically smaller at the time of diagnosis than nonsecreting tumors. As cited earlier, delayed diagnosis of pituitary neoplasia may result in tumor growth manifesting clinically as headache or visual field deficit (due to optic chiasm compression).

The pituitary gland is most commonly approached transnasally via the sphenoid sinus, whereas craniotomy is usually reserved for patients with large and invasive tumors. The preoperative evaluation should focus on the physiologic and anesthetic implications of any endocrinopathy; any preexisting neurologic deficits should be noted, and the risk of intraoperative bleeding or surgical disruption of adjacent structures (i.e., cavernous sinus, optic chiasm) should be stratified.

For transnasal operations, the hypopharynx is packed with moistened gauze following orotracheal intubation to minimize gastric accumulation of blood. The surgeon may request placement of a lumbar cerebrospinal fluid (CSF) drain. This will allow injection of air into the CSF, slightly increasing CSF volume and, thus, displacing a tumor inferiorly, or withdrawal of CSF, displacing a tumor superiorly within the sella turcica. N_2O should be used with care in patients in whom air was injected into the lumbar CSF drain. Local anesthetic agents containing epinephrine may be injected into the nasal mucosa, with or without application of topical cocaine, to reduce bleeding. This intervention may induce transient, but significant, hypertension.

Common complications following surgery include nausea and vomiting, CSF leak, and transient hypopituitarism with or without DI. Other complications include infection or injury to neural (i.e., optic chiasm, cranial nerves contained within the cavernous sinus) or vascular (i.e., carotid artery) structures.

Suggested Readings

Khan ZH, Rasouli MR. Intubation in patients with acromegaly: Experience in more than 800 patients. *Eur J Anaesthesiol*. 2009;26:354-355.

Losasso T, Dietz NM, Muzzi DA. Acromegaly and radial artery cannulation. *Anesth Analg*. 1990;71:204.

Matjasko MJ, Anesthetic considerations in patients with neuroendocrine disease. In: Cottrell JE, Smith DS. *Anesthesia and Neurosurgery*. 4th ed. St. Louis: Mosby; 2001:591-610.

Nemergut EC, Dumont AS, Barry UT, Laws ER. Perioperative management of patients undergoing transsphenoidal pituitary surgery. *Anesth Analg*. 2005; 101:1170-1181.

Nemergut EC, Zuo Z. Airway management in patients with pituitary disease: A review of 746 patients. *J Neurosurg Anesthesiol*. 2006;18:73-77.

CHAPTER 136

Anesthesia for the Sitting Position

Robert M. Craft, MD, and Daniel R. Bustamante, MD

The sitting position may be used for posterior approaches to the cervical spinal column and for operations involving the posterior cranial fossa (see Chapter 56). Alternative positions for these procedures include park bench, prone, and supine with the head turned to the side. A properly positioned patient for a sitting-position case is actually in a modified recumbent position (Figure 136-1). Patients requiring cervical spine operations should be carefully evaluated preoperatively because decreased cervical range of motion, cervical instability, or position-related neurologic symptoms may necessitate awake intubation. Positioning for patients with posterior fossa tumors should be approached with the knowledge that brainstem structures may be adversely affected by compression and that obstructive hydrocephalus may result in elevated intracranial pressure. Relative contraindications to the sitting position are listed in Box 136-1. Right-to-left intracardiac shunt may be considered an absolute contraindication to operations performed with the patient in the sitting position.

In addition to applications in neurosurgery, the sitting position ("beach chair" position) is often used in orthopedic surgery, particularly for shoulder operations. Catastrophic complications in this setting, resulting from inadequate cerebral perfusion, underscore the importance of measuring blood pressure at the level of the brain. It is essential to account for the difference between arterial blood pressure at the site of measurement and at the brain in any position in which these values may differ. Unlike patients who are undergoing neurosurgical procedures, most patients undergoing shoulder operations do not have arterial lines placed for blood pressure monitoring.

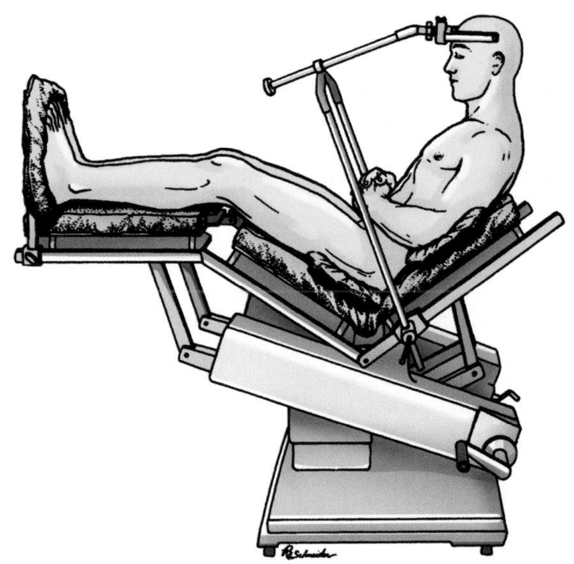

Figure 136-1 Standard sitting position. (From Milde LN. The head-elevated positions. In: Martin JT, Warner MA, eds. Positioning in Anesthesia and Surgery. 3rd ed. Philadelphia: WB Saunders: 1997:71-93.)

Potential Advantages and Complications of the Sitting Position

A variety of potential advantages (Box 136-2) are associated with the use of the sitting position. However, complications may develop (Box 136-3). Complications associated with the use of the sitting position are promoted by noncollapsible venous structures and surgical sites above the level of the heart.

Venous Air Embolism and Paradoxical Air Embolism

Although most often feared as a complication of the sitting position, venous air embolism (VAE) can occur in a variety of other settings, including cesarean section, laparoscopy, orthopedic operations, and prostate operations. A large study revealed that, although the incidence of VAE was greater in sitting patients than in horizontal patients (45% vs. 12%), there was no difference in morbidity or mortality rates. A paradoxical air embolism occurs when air crosses to the arterial circulation, usually through a patent foramen ovale. A patent foramen ovale is present in approximately 27% of adults.

Box 136-1 Relative Contraindications to the Use of the Sitting Position

Cerebral ischemia when the patient is upright and awake
LA pressure (PAOP) < RA pressure
Platypnea-orthodeoxia*
Preoperative demonstration of patent foramen ovale or right-to-left shunt
Hypotension†
Extremes of age
Ventriculoatrial shunt in place and open

*Platypnea-orthodeoxia is a condition in which there is a right-to-left shunting of the blood at the atrial level only with assumption of the upright position.
†Usually due to decreased intravascular volume; note that if the patient were to have a cardiac arrest in this position, chest compressions would be ineffective.
LA, Left atrial; PCOP, pulmonary artery occlusion pressure; RA, right atrial.
Reprinted, with permission, from Black S, Cucchiara RF. Tumor surgery. In: Cucchiara RF, Michenfelder JD, eds. Clinical Neuroanesthesia. 2nd ed. New York: Churchill Livingstone; 1998:343-365.

Box 136-2 Advantages to the Sitting Position for Surgery

↓ Blood loss
↑ Surgical exposure with less tissue retraction
↑ Access to the tracheal tube, extremities, and chest
↓ Facial swelling
↓ Intracranial pressure by ↑ drainage of both venous blood and cerebrospinal fluid

Box 136-3 Complications Associated with the Use of the Sitting Position for Surgery

Circulatory instability
Cranial nerve dysfunction
Impaired venous drainage
Paradoxical air embolism
Peripheral nerve injury
Postoperative central apnea
Quadriplegia
Tension pneumocephalus
Venous air embolism

Some authors have recommended routine screening for patent foramen ovale using echocardiography prior to utilizing the sitting position. VAE and paradoxical air embolism are further discussed in Chapter 137.

Tension Pneumocephalus

Although there is a high frequency of pneumocephalus in patients who undergo procedures while in the sitting position, symptomatic pneumocephalus is uncommon. Cerebrospinal fluid is more likely to drain through the wound in sitting patients who have cortical atrophy, allowing the entrapment of air (the inverted soda bottle phenomenon). Whether the use of N_2O has an impact on the frequency and severity of pneumocephalus has not been confirmed.

Circulatory Instability

Anesthesia in the sitting position is associated with decreased pulmonary artery occlusion pressure, stroke volume index, cardiac index, systolic blood pressure, and mean arterial pressure. Heart rate and systemic vascular resistance are increased. These changes can be minimized by providing adequate preoperative hydration, having the patient wear compression stockings, changing the patient's position slowly, and maintaining the patient's hips and knees in a flexed position. A large retrospective study failed to show a difference in the incidence of hypotension between sitting and horizontal patients.

Impaired Venous Drainage

Venous drainage may be compromised by extreme neck flexion. This can result in significant tongue and airway swelling. Compromised venous drainage may be avoided by limiting head flexion to allow two fingerbreadths between the mandible and the sternum.

Postoperative Central Apnea

Potential causes of central apnea occurring during the postoperative period include brainstem hematoma and surgical damage to the respiratory centers. Rigorous prevention and treatment of postoperative hypertension are indicated to help prevent hematoma formation.

Cranial Nerve Dysfunction

Cranial nerves V, VII, IX, X, XI, and XII may be involved (Figure 136-2). Postoperative airway protection may be impaired by dysfunction of cranial nerve IX, X, or XII.

Quadriplegia

Reported cases of quadriplegia are thought to have been caused by mechanical compression of the spinal cord or by ischemia resulting from stretching of the blood vessels of the spinal cord secondary to neck flexion. Preventive measures include preoperative examination of the cervical range of motion and radiographic determination of cervical canal dimensions, as well as prompt intraoperative treatment of hypotension and limitation of neck flexion.

Peripheral Nerve Injury

Common postoperative neuropathies include the sciatic nerve and its division, the common peroneal nerve. Peripheral nerve injury may be prevented by carefully positioning the patient and padding pressure points.

Monitoring

Frequently utilized monitors for the sitting position include electrocardiography (ECG), pulse oximetry, direct arterial monitoring (transduced at the base of the skull), expired gas analysis, right atrial catheter, precordial Doppler, and transesophageal echocardiography (TEE). Electrophysiologic monitoring, employing modalities such as brainstem auditory evoked response (BAER), somatosensory evoked potential, and electromyography (EMG), is becoming more common.

The cardiopulmonary system may be assessed with ECG, pulse oximetry, arterial line, central venous line, and perhaps TEE. The brainstem may be evaluated for signs of surgical trespass via the ECG, with potential warning signs including tachycardia, bradycardia, and arrhythmias. BAER or somatosensory evoked potential may also provide evidence of surgical transgression.

Evidence of cranial nerve stimulation may be revealed through examination of the ECG, arterial line, EMG, and BAER. Manipulation of cranial nerve V results in hypertension and bradycardia, whereas manipulation of cranial nerve X results in hypotension and bradycardia. Mechanical stimulation of cranial nerves V, VII, and XI may be revealed via EMG monitoring of the corresponding muscle groups, and insult to cranial nerve VIII will be evident on examination of BAER.

Venous Air Embolism

TEE is the most sensitive intraoperative monitor for VAE and offers the advantage of direct visualization of air in the left side of the heart (paroxysmal air embolism). Precordial Doppler is a sensitive monitor that is more easily employed than is TEE. The classic physical finding of a "mill-wheel" murmur is an insensitive sign of VAE (see Chapter 137).

Choice of Anesthetic Agents

Anesthetic concerns that may influence the choice of anesthetic agents include maintenance of cardiovascular stability, the risk of air embolism,

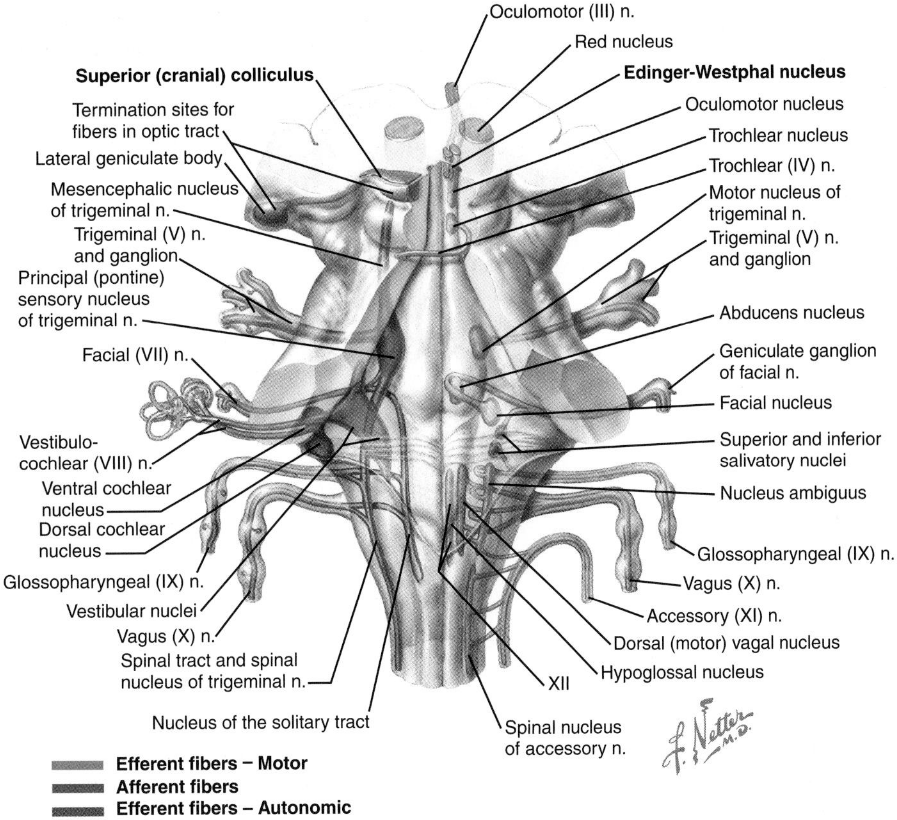

Figure 136-2 A schematic view of cranial nerves and their nuclei. (Netter illustration from www.netterimages.com. © Elsevier Inc. All rights reserved.)

possible increased intracranial pressure, and the desire for rapid emergence to allow for prompt postoperative neurologic evaluation. To these ends, no particular technique has proved to be superior. Many clinicians favor the use of sevoflurane and low-dose opioids with nondepolarizing neuromuscular blocking agents (or higher-dose inhalation anesthetic agents without nondepolarizing neuromuscular blocking agents in cases in which electromyographic monitoring is used). Combinations of inhalation anesthetic agents, N_2O, and short-acting opioids allow for easily controlled anesthetic depth, stable hemodynamic parameters, and rapid emergence. The use of N_2O must be tempered by the knowledge of its effects on intracranial pressure and VAE. Total intravenous anesthesia, utilizing propofol and opioid infusions, is another well-accepted technique, particularly when neurophysiologic monitoring is utilized.

Suggested Readings

Artru AA. Breathing nitrous oxide during closure of the dura and cranium is not indicated. *Anesthesiology*. 1987;66:719.

Black S, Cucchiara RF. Tumor surgery. In: Cucchiara RF, Michenfelder JD, eds. *Clinical Neuroanesthesia*. 2nd ed. New York: Churchill Livingstone; 1998:343-365.

Black S, Ockert DB, Oliver WC, et al. Outcome following posterior fossa craniectomy in patients in the sitting or horizontal position. *Anesthesiology*. 1988;69:49-56.

Cullen DJ, Kirby RR. Beach chair position may decrease cerebral perfusion. *APSF Newsletter*. 2007;22:25-27.

Duke DA, Lynch JJ, Harner SG, et al. Venous air embolism in sitting and supine patients undergoing vestibular schwannoma resection. *Neurosurgery*. 1998; 42:1282-1287.

Gale T, Leslie K. Anaesthesia for neurosurgery in the sitting position. *J Clin Neurosci*. 2004;11:693-696.

Hagen PT, Scholz DG, Edwards WD. Incidence and size of patent foremen ovale during the first 10 decades of life, an autopsy study of 965 normal hearts. *Mayo Clinic Proceedings* 1984;59:17-20.

Milde LN. The head-elevated positions. In: Martin JT, Warner MA, eds. *Positioning in Anesthesia and Surgery*. 3rd ed. Philadelphia: WB Saunders; 1997:71-93.

Mirski MA, Lele AV, Fitzsimmons L, Toung TJK. Diagnosis and treatment of vascular air embolism. *Anesthesiology*. 2007;106:164-177.

Porter JM, Pidgeon C, Cunningham AJ. The sitting position in neurosurgery: A critical appraisal. *Br J Anaesth*. 1999;82:117-128.

CHAPTER 137

Physiology and Treatment of Venous Air Embolism

Susan Black, MD

Etiology

Venous air embolism (VAE) can occur whenever a noncollapsible vein is opened and a pressure gradient exists favoring air entrainment rather than bleeding. VAE classically occurs when the operative site is above the level of the heart, but it may also occur when noncollapsible veins are opened in an operative field into which gas has been insufflated under pressure.

Prevalence

VAE has been reported in most neurosurgical procedures, with the highest incidence (50%) occurring during posterior fossa craniotomy with the patient in the sitting position (Table 137-1). VAE has been reported to occur in many other surgical procedures that involve an operative site above the level of the heart or using gas for insufflation or to cool surgical instruments (gas may be inadvertently injected into a cavity or a joint or directly into vascular structures).

Pathophysiology

The consequences of VAE depend on the rate of air entry. Rarely, massive VAE may create an "air lock" in the right ventricle (RV), resulting in RV outflow obstruction, RV failure, and cardiovascular collapse. More commonly, VAE is a slow entrainment of air into the venous system, right side of the heart, and the pulmonary vasculature, leading to increasing pulmonary vascular resistance via two mechanisms. Mechanical obstruction of small arteries and arterioles and release of endogenous vasoactive agents cause pulmonary vasoconstriction, leading to increasing pulmonary vascular resistance, increasing RV afterload, increased pulmonary artery pressure, and, ultimately, increased central venous pressure as the RV begins to fail. As VAE continues, hypotension develops as cardiac output falls. Acute respiratory distress syndrome may develop after large VAE episodes.

Paradoxical air embolism (PAE) or arterial air embolism may also develop. Air may pass from the right to the left side of the heart through either an intracardiac defect or the pulmonary vasculature. Once a PAE occurs, more serious complications may develop from obstruction of coronary and cerebral arteries. Arrhythmias, myocardial ischemia, and focal neurologic deficits have developed as a complication of PAE.

Morbidity and Mortality

Morbidity and mortality risks from VAE are low in procedures in which the potential for VAE is recognized and proper monitors are utilized. However, mortality from VAE continues to occur, particularly after procedures in which VAE rarely occurs (such as lumbar spine operations) when VAE is not recognized at the onset of hemodynamic instability. Of the cases of VAE that have been reported to have occurred during spine operations, mortality rate approach 50% because the diagnosis usually occurred late in the course of the event.

Diagnosis

The most sensitive monitors for VAE are transesophageal echocardiography (TEE) and Doppler echocardiography, followed by expired nitrogen, end-tidal CO_2, pulmonary artery pressure, central venous pressure, right atrial (RA) catheter, and (least sensitive) an esophageal stethoscope (Figure 137-1).

The precordial Doppler is advocated as the basic monitor because it is reasonably priced, relatively easy to use, noninvasive, and very sensitive. The Doppler probe should initially be placed at the fourth or fifth intercostal space at the right sternal border and then moved until maximal heart tones are heard (Figure 137-2). Proper position is verified by injection of agitated saline via a central or large-bore free-running peripheral intravenous catheter. A characteristic sound ("mill-wheel murmur") of turbulent flow is heard when air enters the right heart chambers. TEE is a very sensitive monitor for VAE that detects localized air in the cardiac chambers. Although TEE may be slightly more sensitive than the precordial Doppler, there are disadvantages to the use of TEE. First, it requires more experience to place and carries a rare risk for esophageal injury. Second, the image must be watched, whereas the Doppler is an audible monitor. A multiorifice RA catheter can be used to confirm a Doppler-based diagnosis of VAE and, rarely, for lifesaving aspiration of significant volumes of air during massive VAE. Proper placement of the RA catheter high in the RA by electrocardiographic control can increase the effectiveness of the catheter by placing it where the air tends to collect during neurosurgical procedures with the patient in the sitting position. Correct catheter placement may be confirmed by (1) recording of the electrocardiogram via the RA catheter and identifying large negative P waves when the catheter tip is high in the RA, (2) transducing pressure recordings obtained when the catheter enters the RV and is pulled back, or (3) chest radiograph.

Treatment

The goals of treatment are to support the cardiovascular system and to stop the influx of air at the surgical site. Flooding the field with saline should submerge the area of air entry. The application of manual jugular venous compression for about 15 sec will frequently raise the venous pressure in the wound sufficiently that the vessel will back-bleed and can be identified.

Table 137-1 Operative Incidence of Venous Air Embolism

Procedure	Reported Frequency of VAE, %
Neurosurgical	
Sitting posterior fossa craniotomy	45-55
Posterior fossa craniotomy, "horizontal" position	10-15
Sitting cervical laminectomy	5-15
Transsphenoidal pituitary resection	12
Craniosynostosis	85
Lumbar spine procedures	1-2
OB/GYN	
Cesarean section	11-44
Hysteroscopy, laser endometrial ablation	*
Orthopedic	
Total hip replacement	Up to 65
Intramedullary femur nailing, irrigation of pelvic fractures, removal of bone cyst, arthroscopy	*
General Surgery	
Laparoscopy, laser tumor resection, instillation of liquid nitrogen, insertion of peritoneovenous shunt, hepatic resection, GI endoscopy, venovenous bypass during liver transplantation	*
Plastic Surgery	
Removal of tissue expander	*
Trauma	
Head and neck trauma, penetrating lung trauma	*
Dental	
Dental implant procedures	*
Urologic	
Prostatectomy	*
ICU	
Mechanical ventilation, central line placement and removal	*

GI, Gastrointestinal; ICU, intensive care unit; OB/GYN, obstetrics and gynecology; VAE, venous air embolism.
*Case reports.

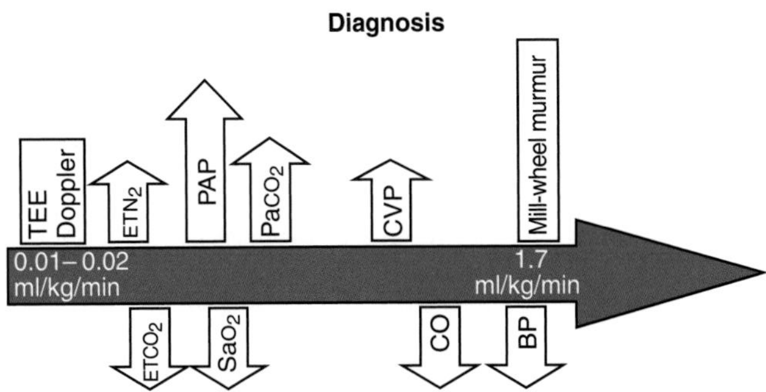

Figure 137-1 Changes in detection parameters for venous air embolism with increasing volumes of air. Data are aggregated from human and animal studies. BP, Blood pressure; CO, cardiac output; CVP, central venous pressure; $ETCO_2$, end-tidal carbon dioxide; ETN_2, end-tidal nitrogen; $PaCO_2$, partial pressure of carbon dioxide; PAP, pulmonary artery pressure; SaO_2, arterial oxygen saturation; TEE, transesophageal echocardiography. The mill-wheel murmur is the characteristic sound of turbulent flow heard on Doppler when the agitated saline (air) enters the right heart chambers.

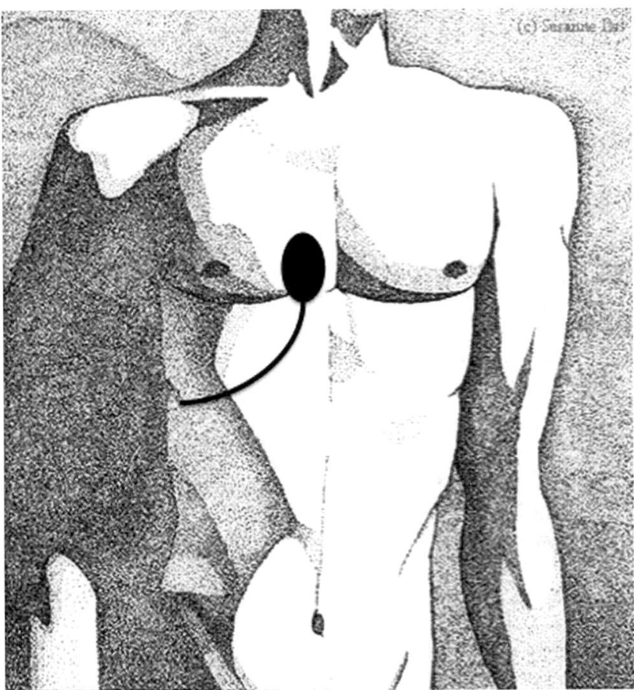

Figure 137-2 Proper position for precordial Doppler placement.

Because N_2O has low solubility, it will diffuse into the VAE, increasing the size of the VAE; therefore, the use of N_2O should be discontinued. Vasopressors and volume infusion will increase preload, increase cardiac output, and aid in moving the VAE through the heart and peripheral pulmonary circulation. Aspiration of air from the RA catheter should be attempted. To decrease VAE, some authors have recommended the use of positive end-expiratory pressure to increase central venous pressure and cerebral venous pressure, but most studies have demonstrated that the use of positive end-expiratory pressure is ineffective. Also, with the use of positive end-expiratory pressure, increased right-sided heart pressures may increase the risk of PAE. In cases of VAE-related cardiovascular compromise, the classic recommendation has been to place the patient in the Durant position (left lateral decubitus position) to relieve RV outflow obstruction. Recent studies have not proven the efficacy of this maneuver.

Initial treatment of PAE is aimed at stopping further air entry. If myocardial ischemia develops, the use of positive inotropic agents, usually epinephrine, is recommended to support the hemodynamics and increase contractility of the ventricles, causing breakup of the emboli. If symptomatic cerebral ischemia occurs, hyperbaric O_2 therapy should be considered as soon as the patient can be transported into a hyperbaric chamber.

Anesthetic Considerations

Certain conditions increase the risk of either significant VAE-related or PAE-related morbidity, should VAE develop. In the presence of these risk factors, efforts should be focused on decreasing the likelihood of VAE occurring.

The use of N_2O in procedures that carry a risk for VAE is controversial. Animal and human data suggest that, if the use of N_2O is discontinued when VAE is diagnosed with precordial Doppler, the incidence and severity of VAE are not increased. If sensitive monitors for VAE are being used, N_2O can be used safely in procedures that have an increased risk for VAE because the N_2O can be discontinued upon diagnosis of VAE. If the use of sensitive monitors is not possible, N_2O should not be used.

Suggested Readings

Mirski MA, Lele AV, Fitzsimmons L, et al. Diagnosis and treatment of vascular air embolism. *Anesthesiology*. 2007;106:164-177.

Wills J, Schwend RM, Paterson A, et al. Intraoperative visible bubbling of air may be the first sign of venous air embolism during posterior surgery for scoliosis. *Spine*. 2005;30:E629-635.

CHAPTER 138

Perioperative Implications of Caring for Patients with Epilepsy

C. Thomas Wass, MD

Epilepsy is one of the most common neurologic disorders, with a prevalence approaching 1% of the population; nearly 3 million people in the United States have a seizure disorder. Seizures are characterized based primarily on the clinical manifestation and electroencephalographic (EEG) features (Box 138-1).

Anecdotal observations and case reports suggest that the process of anesthesia and surgery is associated with increased perioperative seizure activity (frequency and duration). Proposed etiologic factors include withholding antiepileptic drugs (AEDs) because of the patient's NPO (nil per os) status prior to surgery, hypoglycemia, hyponatremia, hyperpyrexia, sleep deprivation, fatigue, stress, excessive alcohol consumption, and use of proconvulsant medications. Anesthetics (discussed in greater detail later) implicated in this response include inhalation anesthetic agents, local anesthetic agents (e.g., lidocaine, bupivacaine), opioids (e.g., fentanyl, alfentanil, sufentanil, meperidine), and some sedative-hypnotic medications (e.g., etomidate, ketamine, methohexital). Considering that these drugs are administered to most patients requiring general anesthesia, it is imperative to understand the effects of anesthetic agents on individuals with seizure disorders. Anesthesia providers must have an understanding of the implications of caring for patients with epilepsy who require anesthesia for non-neurosurgical operations, as well as the intricacies of providing anesthesia for patients with epilepsy undergoing resection of an epileptogenic focus.

Box 138-1 Classification of Seizures*

- Generalized seizures
  - Tonic-clonic (in any combination)
  - Absence
    - Typical
    - Atypical
    - Absence with special features
      - Myoclonic absence
      - Eyelid myoclonia
  - Myoclonic
    - Myoclonic
    - Myoclonicationic
    - Myoclonictonic
  - Clonic
  - Tonic
  - Atonic
- Focal seizures
- Unknown
  - Epileptic spasms

*Seizure that cannot be clearly diagnosed into one of the preceding categories should be considered unclassified until further information allows their accurate diagnosis. This is not considered a classification category. however.

Bert AT, Berkovic SF, Brodie MJ, et al. Revised terminology and concepts for organization of seizures and epilepsies: report of the ILAE Commission on Classification and Terminology, 2005-2009. Epilepsia. 2010: 51(4): 676-685.

Perioperative Seizure Frequency

The incidence of perioperative seizure activity in individuals without a history of epilepsy is unknown. In contrast, recent clinical investigations have provided information on the frequency of seizures in patients with a history of epilepsy undergoing either regional or general anesthesia. More specifically, in a study of 411 patients undergoing epidural, caudal, or peripheral nerve block, 24 (5.8%) experienced postoperative seizures. However, based on the temporal relationship (i.e., extended time interval) between local anesthetic administration and the seizure, it was unlikely that the regional anesthetic was the primary cause or a contributing factor. Similarly, Benish and colleagues observed that 6 of 297 (2%) patients with epilepsy undergoing general anesthesia experienced seizures. Of these 6 patients, only 1 (0.003%) required intravenous therapy to terminate the seizure. These studies show that, although many anesthetic medications (both regional and general) have proconvulsant properties, clinically relevant dosing was not temporally related to an escalation of perioperative seizure frequency. Rather, these authors concluded that perioperative seizure activity correlated more strongly with the patient's underlying seizure history (i.e., baseline frequency) and number of AEDs than it did with the type of anesthesia to which the patients were exposed. Further, patients with a preoperative diagnosis of epilepsy did not appear to be at increased risk of experiencing anesthesia-related perioperative morbidity or of dying.

Effect of Anesthetics on Epilepsy

Inhalation Anesthetic Agents

Inhalation anesthetic agents (e.g., enflurane > sevoflurane) have both proconvulsant and anticonvulsant properties. At low doses, these inhalation anesthetic agents have the potential to induce EEG-identified epileptiform activity in individuals with or without a history of seizures. Although the mechanism of action has yet to be fully elucidated, these changes likely result from preferential inhibition of inhibitory central nervous system neurotransmission. As a result, excitatory neurotransmission is left unchecked in cortical and subcortical brain regions. In contrast, with escalating doses of the inhalation agents, the EEG progresses through a continuum of increased beta activity followed by burst suppression and, eventually, isoelectricity. Accordingly, inhalation anesthetic agents can be administered to facilitate cortical mapping during epilepsy surgery or (at higher doses) to terminate status epilepticus in patients whose seizures are refractory to conventional therapy.

Opioids

It is well established that opioids have the potential to induce epileptiform activity in both laboratory animals and humans. Opioid-induced epileptiform activity may be used to localize the epileptogenic zone activity in patients undergoing epilepsy surgery. Alfentanil, sufentanil, and remifentanil (i.e., short-acting opioids) may be used to "activate" epileptiform loci during intraoperative electrocorticography (ECoG) at the time of focal cortical resection. The cause of opioid-induced limbic system seizures has not been fully determined. Proposed mechanisms include selective activation of limbic opioid receptors, augmented release of excitatory amino acids (e.g., glutamate), and facilitation of coupling between excitatory postsynaptic potentials and somatic spike-generating sites or suppression of inhibitory interneurons (i.e., the disinhibition hypothesis). According to the disinhibition hypothesis, opioids indirectly excite limbic system structures by inhibiting neighboring γ-aminobutyric acid–secreting inhibitory interneurons.

Local Anesthetic Agents

Local anesthetic toxicity is a potential risk for all patients (both with and without epilepsy) undergoing regional anesthesia, particularly during procedures that require a large dose of local anesthetic agent, such as an epidural or caudal anesthetic or a peripheral nerve block. Systemic local anesthetic toxicity presents as a spectrum of neurologic symptoms and signs that worsen as plasma drug levels continue to rise. Symptoms of central nervous system toxicity generally follow a progression from lightheadedness, dizziness, and perioral numbness to visual or auditory disturbances (e.g., tinnitus). These symptoms are usually followed by peripheral muscle twitching and, ultimately, generalized tonic-clonic convulsions. As discussed earlier, a preoperative diagnosis of epilepsy does not appear to escalate the likelihood of local anesthetic-induced seizures in patients undergoing regional anesthesia.

Effect of Antiepileptic Drugs on Perioperative Patient Care

The most relevant interaction between AEDs and anesthetic medications pertains to the use of nondepolarizing neuromuscular blocking agents (NMBAs) in patients chronically taking phenytoin, carbamazepine, phenobarbital. More specifically, this patient population may require a larger initial bolus dose of an NMBA to induce muscle paralysis, as well as more frequent dosing to maintain a steady-state plasma concentration. Although the cause has yet to be fully understood, the larger initial dose is —in part— related to increased plasma concentrations of α-acid glycoprotein (AAG), which is an inducible plasma protein responsible for binding basic drugs such as NMBAs. Thus, in the setting of chronic AED administration, AAG synthesis is increased, thereby decreasing the quantity of free (i.e., unbound, pharmacologically active) NMBA available to interact with nicotinic receptors at the neuromuscular junction. In regard to more frequent dosing, AEDs induce hepatic enzyme activity that, in turn, hastens metabolic inactivation of NMBAs.

Additionally, AEDs may cause hematologic perturbations (e.g., valproate can cause a dose-dependent thrombocytopenia), alter the results of liver function tests (γ-glutamyl transpeptidase, alkaline phosphatase, and alanine aminotransferase), and cause hepatotoxicity. Often, these alterations are not symptomatic and not thought to be clinically significant.

Suggested Readings

Benish SM, Cascino GD, Warner ME, et al. Effect of general anesthesia in patients with epilepsy: A population-based study. *Epilepsy Behav*. 2010;17:87-89.

Kofke WA, Templehoff R, Dasheiff R. Anesthesia for epileptic patients and for epilepsy surgery. In: Cottrell JE, Smith DS, eds. *Anesthesia and Neurosurgery*. 4th ed. St. Louis: Mosby; 2001:474.

Kopp SL, Wynd KP, Horlocker TT, et al. Regional blockade in patients with a history of a seizure disorder. *Anesth Analg*. 2009;109:272-278.

Niesen AD, Jacob AK, Aho LE, et al. Perioperative seizures in patients with a history of a seizure disorder. *Anesth Analg*. 2010;111:729-735.

Hines RL, Marschall K. *Stoelting's Anesthesia and Co-Existing Disease*. 5th ed. Philadelphia: Churchill Livingstone; 2008:232-234.

Wass CT, Grady RE, Fessler AJ, et al. The effects of remifentanil on epileptiform discharges during intraoperative electrocorticography in patients undergoing epilepsy surgery. *Epilepsia*. 2001;42;1340-1344.

CHAPTER 139
Carotid Endarterectomy

Brooke E. Albright, MD, Major USAF

Carotid artery stenosis can be repaired surgically by performing a carotid endarterectomy (CEA) or endovascularly by placing a carotid stent. For purposes of this chapter, the discussion will be limited to CEA. Indications for CEA include symptomatic patients (i.e., those who present with transient ischemic attacks of visual loss [amaurosis fugax], paresthesias, unsteadiness, speech problems, or permanent sequelae due to cerebral infarction) who have a greater than 70% stenosis of one or both carotid arteries. Only marginal benefit has been shown in symptomatic patients with 50% to 69% stenosis. Current evidence supports early operation in these patients, ideally within 2 weeks of the patient's last neurologic symptoms. Results of randomized controlled studies have shown a 17% reduction in the occurrence of ipsilateral stroke at 2 years with CEA, compared with medical management alone.

Preoperative Evaluation

A thorough preoperative evaluation, with a particular focus on cardiac history and functional status, should be performed in all patients with known carotid artery disease. CEA surgery is considered an intermediate-risk surgery for perioperative cardiac events, with myocardial ischemia representing the predominant cause of perioperative death associated with this procedure. Because of this increased risk, further workup with a cardiologist prior to surgery should be considered in those individuals with active cardiac disease (acute myocardial ischemia [<1 week], severe valvular disease, arrhythmias, or decompensated congestive heart failure) or two or more risk factors with unknown functional status if the patient is amenable to intervention and his or her health may benefit in the long term.

The Carotid Endarterectomy Procedure

The CEA can be performed under general or regional anesthesia. An international, multicentered, randomized trial comparing outcome in patients who receive general anesthesia and those who receive local anesthesia for CEA showed no differences between groups in rates of perioperative morbidity and mortality, quality of life, and longer-term outcome in terms of stroke-free survival.

Key aspects of the surgery involve making an incision in the neck at the location of the blockage, placing a carotid clamp to occlude blood flow during dissection of the plaque from the artery, and occasionally, placing a shunt to reroute blood around the clamped vessel. Not all surgeons routinely place shunts during surgical dissection because of the risk of thromboembolic events occurring during placement; instead, some first evaluate the patient's need for a shunt by assessing cerebral blood flow with one of several monitoring techniques. Each monitoring technique has its own theoretical or practical advantages and limitations, with the ultimate goal of using the results to decide on the use of a shunt to avoid decreased cerebral blood flow and changes in neurologic function and performance.

Potential Adverse Events

Complications of CEA surgery include new neurologic deficits attributed predominantly to thromboembolic events that occur intraoperatively, cerebral hyperperfusion syndrome resulting from excess blood flow to the brain due to impaired autoregulation, and poor control of blood pressure postoperatively due to carotid sinus dysfunction, with hypertension more common than hypotension. If a bilateral CEA is performed, it is possible to abolish the compensatory hyperventilation response to hypoxemia due to disruption of the carotid bodies at the level of the carotid bifurcation (Figure 139-1).

Physiologic Effects

CEA causes physiologic changes related to temporary obstruction of the blood flow through the carotid artery. Surgical technique requires temporary total occlusion of the carotid artery, thereby rendering the ipsilateral hemisphere dependent solely on collateral blood flow from the vertebral arteries and the contralateral carotid artery through the circle of Willis (Figure 139-2), which is complete in only 42% to 47% of people. During CEA surgery, an incomplete circle of Willis formation predisposes approximately one sixth of individuals to developing cerebral ischemia during carotid clamping or transient closure of the carotid artery. In those patients with coexisting contralateral internal carotid artery occlusion, the risk of cerebral ischemia rises more than threefold. Some institutions are beginning to use preoperative cerebral vasculature angiograms to assess collateral flow, predict the need for additional cerebral protection or

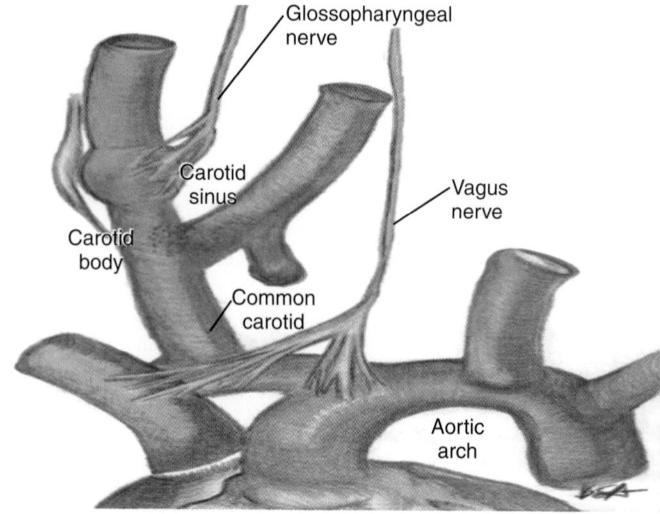

Figure 139-1 Anatomy of the right side of the neck showing the common carotid artery, demonstrating the relationship of the carotid body to the carotid sinus at the origin of the internal carotid artery. (Image © Brooke Albright, MD.)

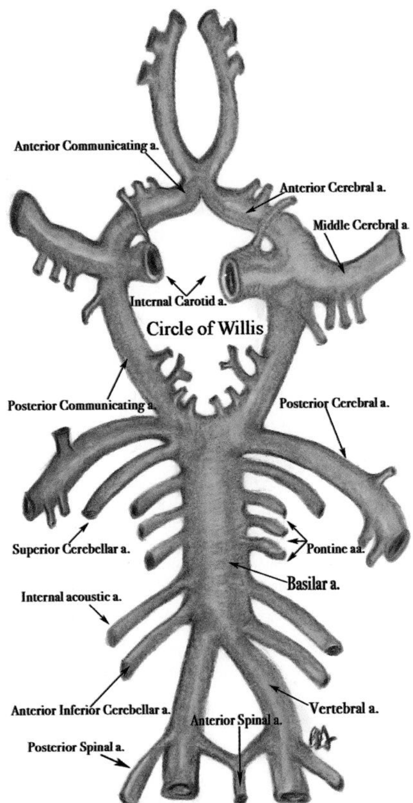

Figure 139-2 Blood supply of the circle of Willis. During cross-clamping of the internal carotid artery, blood supply to the ipsilateral cerebral hemisphere is from the contralateral internal carotid artery and from the basilar artery through the circle of Willis. (Image © Brooke Albright, MD.)

monitoring, and determine the possible need for intraluminal shunting during the procedure.

Techniques for Cerebral Monitoring

Ensuring adequate cerebral blood flow to the ipsilateral brain during clamping of the carotid artery is a critical aspect of CEA surgery. Some clinicians use cerebral monitoring to decrease the incidence of perioperative stroke by detecting thromboemboli, intraoperative hypoperfusion, and postoperative hyperperfusion syndrome. However, not all clinicians use cerebral monitoring due to concerns of actual benefit and associated high costs.

Evaluating the Awake Patient

The most sensitive and specific cerebral monitor is neurologic assessment of the awake patient. If both the patient and surgeon are comfortable with performing the operation while the patient is awake, then verbal communication and frequent examination of strength using contralateral handgrip can be used to assess level of consciousness, motor function, and cerebral perfusion. Assessment is best performed every 2 to 5 min. Adequate anesthesia for CEA in the awake patient is provided by regional blockade of the superficial and deep cervical plexus but may not be feasible in the extremely anxious or claustrophobic patient or in the patient with cardiopulmonary disease who is unable to lie flat because of dyspnea, experiences coughing spells, or is otherwise unable to lie still for a length of time. Another potential disadvantage to performing CEA in an awake patient is the anesthesia provider's inability to maintain control of the patient's airway, especially in the event cerebral blood flow is compromised, the patient loses consciousness, and emergency airway protection is required. It is also possible that the effects of the regional anesthetic may not last as long as the surgical procedure.

Electroencephalography

In the anesthetized patient, the electroencephalogram (EEG) is considered the most reliable cerebral monitor for detecting cerebral ischemia. A standard 16-channel EEG monitor utilizes 20 scalp electrodes, with 8 channels for each hemisphere, covering parasagittal and temporal brain regions. EEG changes, which are apparent within seconds of changes in cerebral blood flow occurring, are defined as ipsilateral or bilateral appearance of increased theta or delta activity, suppression of alpha or beta activity of more than 50%, or both. EEG changes occur in about 20% of patients during carotid occlusion and are considered to be indicative of potentially serious ischemia. Data show a strong correlation between persistent EEG changes of 10 min or longer and postoperative neurologic deficit; however, not all changes in electrical activity are specific for life-threatening cerebral ischemia. Nonetheless, because of the strong correlation, most surgeons consider changes in EEG activity an indication for immediate shunt placement.

Disadvantages of EEG monitoring are the need for continuous observation by a highly trained technician, the inability to detect subcortical ischemia with the use of EEG, and the decreased predictive value of EEG in the patients with preexisting neurologic deficits. Physiologic changes in temperature, $Paco_2$, and depth of anesthesia can also affect EEG monitoring reliability.

Somatosensory Evoked Potentials

Monitoring of somatosensory evoked potentials (SSEP) involves electrically stimulating a peripheral or cranial nerve and comparing the latency and amplitude of the stimulation to normal values (baseline). Latency is the time from the application of the stimulus to the peak onset of the response. The amplitude is the voltage of the recorded response. A decrease in amplitude of 50% or more from baseline or an increase in latency of more than 10% is considered clinically significant and, if the cause is uncorrected, can be associated with new postoperative neurologic deficits.

Monitoring of EEG and SSEPs has similar sensitivity and specificity for detecting cerebral ischemia. SSEP monitoring offers some potential advantage over a 16-channel EEG in that it is technically easier to perform and interpret and provides information specific to the sensory cortex, an area supplied by the middle cerebral artery, which is placed at risk during cross-clamping of the carotid artery. SSEPs may also detect ischemia in subcortical structures better than EEG does.

Carotid Stump Pressure

Systolic pressure beyond the carotid clamp can be measured by placing either a needle or intraluminal Fogerty balloon catheter in the distal carotid artery. Some studies have suggested that a carotid artery stump pressure of at least 40 mm Hg systolic may be considered as an equally reliable but more cost-effective method, compared with EEG, to predict the need for carotid shunting during CEA under general anesthesia; however, other research utilizing stump-pressure measurements of less than 40 mm Hg as an indication for selective shunt placement (compared with routine shunt placement) showed no difference in stroke rate when either stump pressure or EEG was used. Measured stump pressures may not always correlate with cerebral perfusion pressure or accurately predict cerebral ischemia because the threshold for ischemia may vary considerably from one individual to another. In some patients, stump pressures of 40 mm Hg may be high enough to ensure adequate cerebral blood flow, whereas in others, considerably higher pressures may be required.

Transcranial Doppler Ultrasound

Transcranial Doppler ultrasound utilizes the thin petrous temporal bone as an acoustic window for detecting Doppler signals and ultrasound visualization of the middle cerebral artery. Unlike other cerebral monitors, transcranial Doppler ultrasound can be used to measure blood flow velocities and detect embolic signals in real time. Because most perioperative neurologic events are embolic or thrombotic in nature, the transcranial Doppler ultrasound can prove to be a very useful monitor when performed by a trained technologist.

Three transcranial Doppler ultrasound variables have been identified as predictors of stroke after CEA: the occurrence of emboli during dissection or wound closure, a greater than 90% decrease in middle cerebral artery peak systolic velocity at cross-clamping, and a 100% or greater increase in the pulsatility index of the Doppler signal at clamp release. One limitation related to the use of transcranial Doppler ultrasound is that the location of the probe is relatively near the surgical site, which may hinder observance of the monitor by the operator and, perhaps, require continual readjustment of the monitor.

Other Considerations

Dissection of the atheromatous plaque at the level of the carotid bifurcation can disrupt the carotid sinus baroreceptor function and lead to direct and indirect hemodynamic effects. Normal-functioning carotid sinus baroreceptors sense arterial wall stretch, and, when the stretch is increased, the vasomotor center in the medulla receives increased afferent input via the glossopharyngeal nerve. In response, efferent impulses via the vagus nerve result in decreased sympathetic output and increased parasympathetic output, resulting in bradycardia and hypotension. Patients with coronary artery disease, increased age, or a low ejection fraction are most at risk of developing severe symptoms during manipulation of the carotid sinus. Discontinuation of the sinus stimulation attenuates the signs; however, if they persist, 1 to 2 mL of a local anesthetic agent can be injected into the area of the carotid bifurcation to block the impulse propagation. In certain situations, it may be necessary to intravenously administer atropine, fluid boluses, or vasopressors when manipulation of the sinus causes profound hypotension or bradycardia.

After removal of atheromatous plaques in patients who have intact functioning of the carotid sinus, postoperative hypotension may occur as a result of hyperactivity of the newly exposed carotid sinus to the perceived increased blood pressure. Hypersensitivity of the carotid sinus after CEA can eventually lead to carotid sinus syndrome, which is characterized by nausea, vomiting, dizziness, syncope, severe hypotension, and asystole. Treatment may require a pacemaker, glossopharyngeal nerve block or ablation, or surgical denervation of the glossopharyngeal nerve at the level of the carotid bifurcation. More commonly, removal of the plaque may result in denervation of the baroreceptor nerve fibers within the arterial wall, leading to sympathomimetic electrocardiographic changes and hypertension.

Suggested Readings

Aburahma AF, Stone PA, Hass SM, et al. Prospective randomized trial of routine versus selective shunting in carotid endarterectomy based on stump pressure. *J Vasc Surg*. 2010;51:1133-1138.

Ackerstaff RG, Moons KG, van de Vlasakker CJ, et al. Association of intraoperative transcranial Doppler monitoring variables with stroke from carotid endarterectomy. *Stroke*. 2000;31:1817.

Ardakani SK, Dadmehr M, Nejat F, et al. The cerebral arterial circle (circulus arteriosus cerebri): An anatomical study in fetus and infant samples. *Pediatr Neurosurg*. 2008;44:388-392.

Calligaro KD, Dougherty MJ. Correlation of carotid artery stump pressure and neurologic changes during 474 carotid endarterectomies performed in awake patients. *J Vasc Surg*. 2005;42:684-689.

Gianaros PJ, Jennings JR, Olafsson GB, et al. Greater intima-media thickness in the carotid bulb is associated with reduced baroreflex sensitivity. *Am J Hypertens*. 2002;15:486-491.

Lewis SC, Warlow CP, GALA Trial Collaborative Group. General anaesthesia versus local anaesthesia for carotid surgery (GALA): A multicentre, randomised controlled trial. *Lancet*. 2008;372:2132-2142.

Mackey WC, O'Donnell TF, Callow AD. Cardiac risk in patients undergoing carotid endarterectomy: Impact on perioperative and long-term mortality. *J Vasc Surg*. 1990;11:226-234.

Manninen H, Mäkinen K, Vanninen R. How often does an incomplete circle of Willis predispose to cerebral ischemia during closure of carotid artery? Post mortem and clinical imaging studies. *Acta Neurochir*. 2009;151:1099-1105.

Messick JM Jr, Casement B, Sharbrough FW, et al. Correlation of regional cerebral blood flow (rCBF) with EEG changes during isoflurane anesthesia for carotid endarterectomy: Critical rCBF. *Anesthesiology*. 1987;66:344-349.

North American Symptomatic Carotid Endarterectomy Trial Collaborators. Beneficial effect of carotid endarterectomy in symptomatic patients with high-grade carotid stenosis. *N Engl J Med*. 1991;325:445-453.

Toorop RJ, Scheltinga MR, Moll FL, Bleys RL. Anatomy of the carotid sinus nerve and surgical implications in carotid sinus syndrome. *J Vasc Surg*. 2009;50:177-182.

CHAPTER 140
Management of Acute Spinal Cord Injury

Eric L. Bloomfield, MD, MS, MMI, FCCM

Pathophysiologic Factors

Spinal cord injury can have catastrophic results. A typical injury to the cord results in edema, hemorrhage, and involvement of sensory, motor, and sympathetic changes that may result in spinal shock. Injuries are more likely to damage the spinal cord when they involve C3 and vertebrae below it. Injuries involving the C1 and C2 vertebrae are less likely to impinge on and damage the spinal cord; patients who survive the precipitating event have a good chance of retaining neurologic function. However, injuries severe enough to damage C1 and C2 vertebrae often have a high mortality rate, either because of associated traumatic brain injury or injury to the airway.

Respiratory Considerations

A lesion at a vertebra above T7 may alter respiratory function. Vital capacity, expiratory reserve volume, and forced expiratory volume typically are decreased. The resulting respiratory physiologic characteristics depend on three factors: intercostal muscle function, the diaphragmatic function, and the use of accessory muscles of respiration.

Neurons exiting the cord at C3, C4, and C5 provide innervation of the diaphragm, so a spinal cord injury at C3 results in paralysis of the diaphragm; if the injury is not recognized and treated immediately, patients with such lesions asphyxiate. With a C5 lesion, a patient may have signs of partial diaphragmatic paralysis. By comparison, a C6 lesion enables the patient to maintain ventilation because innervation of the diaphragm is intact. Even so, the patient will have some compromised respiratory function, with sternal retraction and paradoxical breathing. This problem of respiratory compromise is due to intercostal paralysis; the patient can still have a compromised cough and an inability to clear secretions.

Spinal cord lesions are not always static. They may be complete or incomplete, such as a Brown-Séquard syndrome. A spinal cord lesion may involve a spreading hematoma that then leads to increased edema and ischemia of the neural tissue. Ondine curse, "central" sleep apnea, can be caused by a lesion involving the anterolateral portion of C2 through C4 spinal cord segments. Patients who have traumatic injury to the spinal cord with associated neurologic deficit have an increased risk of developing deep venous thrombosis and pulmonary embolic events due to thrombus, or from a fat embolus, the latter associated with other bone-related injuries. Other pulmonary disorders associated with spinal cord injury are neurogenic pulmonary edema, aspiration pneumonia, and acute respiratory distress syndrome.

Cardiovascular Considerations

After spinal cord injury, blood pressure and heart rate increase, sometimes dramatically, because of the associated sympathetic storm. Over time, parasympathetic activity increases, manifested by bradycardia, sinus node pauses, sick sinus syndrome, supraventricular arrhythmias, ventricular ectopy, and possibly ST-segment changes, based on the individual's coronary anatomy.

Depending on the level and severity of injury, spinal shock may occur and last up to 6 weeks as a result of a loss of vascular tone and of the vasopressor reflex. Injury to the spinal cord from the level of the T1 to L2 damages the sympathetic nervous system (see Chapter 40) and may result in orthostatic hypotension and, potentially, bradycardia. The bradycardia results from the loss of cardiac acceleration fibers. Prompt treatment of spinal shock with intravascular fluids and vasoactive agents (see Chapter 88) to maintain a mean arterial pressure of 65 mm Hg to 75 mm Hg can potentially improve neurologic outcome.

Gastrointestinal Considerations

Many patients with spinal cord injury subsequently develop paralytic ileus, resulting in gastric distention impinging on diaphragmatic excursion, and decreasing functional reserve capacity of the lungs, requiring prolonged preoxygenation prior to induction of anesthesia for any surgical procedures. The gastric distention and delayed gastric emptying place these patients at increased risk of regurgitating and aspirating gastric contents during induction of anesthesia.

Metabolic Considerations

On initial presentation, patients with spinal cord injury often require emergency airway management. Succinylcholine is preferred by many in the emergency department or operating room to manage patients with acute spinal cord injury. When these same patients subsequently return to the operating room for additional surgical procedures, the use of succinylcholine can lead to a tremendous potassium release, which may cause ventricular fibrillation and cardiac arrest. With denervation of muscle, there is an increase in the number of nicotinic receptors: some from the muscle membrane where, previously, there were no nictonic receptors and also from the appearance of new isoforms of these nicotinic receptors. All of these receptors respond to succinylcholine with release of potassium from a larger area of muscle membrane than would normally occur, and hence, hyperkalemia results. The change in the number and type of receptors occurs as early as 3 days after injury and may be ongoing for up to 6 months. The marked hyperkalemic response has been reported to occur as early as 5 days after injury, but the hyperkalemia also occurs in patients who have an associated ongoing infectious process.

Patients with an injury to the spinal cord at between T1 and L2, with sufficient damage to the sympathetic nervous system, lose the ability to thermoregulate. Hypothermia can lead to vasoconstriction, metabolic acidosis from peripheral vasoconstriction and myocardial ischemia from coronary artery vasoconstriction. Conversely, patients with spinal cord lesions above C7 have an inability to sweat, which can be manifested by hyperthermia.

In patients with longstanding paralysis, bone reabsorption can lead to hypercalcemia. Patients with impaired ventilatory drive can present with respiratory acidosis, with or without a compensating alkalosis.

Anesthetic Management

Preoperative Management

Airway management mandates stabilization of the neck while intubating the trachea in an expeditious manner for the reasons mentioned previously. Chest physiotherapy, deep vein thrombosis prophylaxis (beginning 2-3 days after the injury to avoid hemorrhage at the site of injury), decompression of the stomach, administration of stress-related ulcer prophylaxis, and monitoring gas exchange are all considerations.

Airway Management

All patients with cervical spine fractures are considered to have a difficult airway. The main goal of their care is to maintain cervical stability and, at the same time, oxygenate, ventilate and protect the airway by placing a tracheal tube in a timely manner. If the patient is in immediate need of an airway, inline stabilization with direct laryngoscopy may be the best choice. If timing allows, awake intubation may be the best choice to avoid manipulation of the cervical spine. Nasal intubation should be avoided in patients with basilar skull fractures, raccoon eyes, Battle sign, Le Fort fractures, or any evidence of cerebrospinal fluid leak.

Intubation maneuvers (Table 140-1) can be gauged in accordance with the time needed and the amount of cervical neck manipulation associated with the use of a laryngoscope versus a fiberoptic bronchoscope.

Table 140-1 Comparison of Options for Anesthesia Management of Spinal Injury Procedures

Method	Cervical Spine Motion	Intubation Difficulty	Time Required
Indirect vs. conventional laryngoscope	↓	↓	↕
Intubation guides vs. fiberoptic bronchoscope	NA	0-↑	↓
Intubation guides vs. indirect laryngoscope	0	↕	↓
Miller laryngoscope vs. Macintosh laryngoscope	0	0	0
LMA and intubating LMA vs. conventional direct laryngoscope	↓	0	0-↑
Inline stabilization	↓	0-↑	↑
Rigid collar	0	↑	NA

LMA, Laryngeal mask airway; NA, not applicable.

Cardiovascular Considerations

Lesions located above T4 are associated with neurogenic shock. Restoration of an adequate perfusion pressure is paramount to preventing extension of the neurologic deficit. During surgery for spinal cord stabilization, monitoring of motor-evoked or sensory-evoked potentials, or both, is often used.

The use of corticosteroids, such as methylprednisolone (30 mg/kg bolus followed by 5.4 $mg \cdot kg^{-1} \cdot h^{-1}$ for 24-48 h), is associated with a small but statistically significant improvement in outcome—assuming that the cord is not completely transected—if the therapy is started within 8 h of injury.

The patient's hemodynamic instability from shock will stabilize after 10 to 14 days. However, patients with lesions at T4 or above are at risk of developing autonomic hyperreflexia. Despite an injured patient's lack of sensation below the site of injury, anesthesia may be necessary if the patient returns to the operating room, and precautions must be taken to attenuate if not avoid the complication.

In summary, the goals in the treatment of a patient with spine cord injury are the following:

- Maintain an adequate airway without manipulating the spine.
- Treat spinal shock promptly.
- Start corticosteroid treatment within 8 h of injury.
- Treat other multisystem involvement, including respiratory insufficiency, electrolyte abnormalities, and temperature fluctuation and assess other multiorgan-multisystem trauma.

Suggested Readings

Black S. *Anesthesia for spine surgery*. Paper presented at the annual meeting of the American Society of Anesthesiologists, Oct. 18-22, 2008, Orlando, FL: ASA Refresher Course Lecture material; No. 236.

Bracken MB, Shepard MJ, Holford TR, et al. Administration of methylprednisolone for 24 or 48 hours or tirilazad mesylate for 48 hours in the treatment of acute spinal cord injury: Results of the Third National Acute Spinal Cord Injury Randomized Controlled Trial, National Acute Spinal Cord Injury Study. *JAMA*. 1997;277:1597-1604.

Geisler FH, Coleman WP, Benzel E, et al. Spinal cord injury. *Lancet*. 2002;360:1883.

Lennarson PJ, Smith DW, Sawin PD, et al. Cervical spinal motion during intubation: Efficacy of stabilization maneuvers in the setting of complete segmental instability. *J Neurosurg*. 2001;94:265-270.

Popitz MD. Anesthetic implications of chronic disease of the cervical spine. *Anesth Analg*. 1997;84:672-683.

Todd MM. *Cervical spine motion, cervical spine injury, and the unstable neck*. Paper presented at the annual meeting of the American Society of Anesthesiologists, Oct 18-22, 2008, Orlando, FL: ASA Refresher Course Lecture material; No. 506.

PART C Cardiac Anesthesia

CHAPTER 141

Detection and Treatment of Perioperative Acute Coronary Syndromes

Guy S. Reeder, MD

The acute coronary syndromes (ACS) constitute a spectrum of myocardial ischemia and damage, including ST-segment elevation myocardial infarction (MI) (STEMI), non–ST-segment elevation MI (NSTEMI), and unstable angina pectoris. Early in the course of NSTEMI, separating NSTEMI from prolonged unstable angina may be difficult. The latter is diagnosed if cardiac enzyme markers do not become abnormal; initial management is similar.

The pathogenesis of perioperative ACS is similar to that of spontaneously developing myocardial ischemia and MI. In many cases, plaque rupture or erosion leads to formation of partially or totally occlusive intracoronary thrombus, most often at the site of a preexisting nonstenotic plaque. In cases without plaque rupture, increased O_2 demand owing to catecholamine release from surgical stress and a hypercoagulable state secondary to the surgical procedure cause ischemia in the setting of a preexisting severe coronary stenosis, (demand ischemia). Total coronary occlusion most often leads to STEMI, whereas subtotal occlusion is most commonly associated with non–ST-segment elevation coronary syndromes (although many other factors—including the degree of preexistent collateral vessels, level of O_2 demand, and coronary vasomotion—may alter this generalization).

Detection of ACS is enhanced by appropriate perioperative monitoring of high-risk patients. Intraoperative monitoring includes multilead electrocardiography (ECG) and may include trend monitoring of pulmonary artery occlusion pressure and, in some cases, transesophageal echocardiographic evaluation of regional and global left ventricular systolic function. Postoperative monitoring includes ECG and measurement of cardiac enzyme markers of necrosis, usually troponin T or I. Troponin T and I are more sensitive and specific for myocardial injury than are older markers, such as creatine kinase-MB. While elevation of troponin is sensitive for necrosis, mild elevations may occur with tachycardia (including rapid atrial fibrillation), pulmonary embolism, cardiac trauma, stress cardiomyopathy (apical ballooning syndrome), acute neurologic disease, and critical illness (e.g., respiratory or renal failure) and thus do not alone define MI. Routine postoperative troponin measurement is not recommended in low-risk patients undergoing low-risk procedures but should be considered in high-risk patients or those who develop signs or symptoms of ischemia.

The incidence of ACS peaks on the third postoperative day and declines thereafter. Although chest pain or pressure may be the major clinical symptom, patients with perioperative ACS more commonly describe vague or no symptoms. Occasionally, dyspnea because of pulmonary edema, ventricular arrhythmia, or cardiac arrest may be the first manifestation.

A general approach to the management of ACS is shown in Figure 141-1. Urgent cardiology consultation is warranted when ACS is suspected. Necessary adjustments in anesthetic and fluid management should be made to optimize oxygenation, intravascular blood volume, and hemoglobin concentrations while minimizing myocardial O_2 demand. Because the underlying problem in ACS is often platelet-rich thrombus, pharmacotherapy includes the administration of antiplatelet and antithrombotic agents. These agents greatly increase the risk of bleeding in the perioperative setting and, thus, must be used cautiously. In patients in whom the risk of postoperative hemorrhage is low, aspirin should be administered immediately, and the use of intravenously administered unfractionated heparin should be considered. Low-molecular-weight heparin has been shown to be more effective than unfractionated heparin in treating ACS; however, the effects of low-molecular-weight heparin are more difficult to monitor with the use of commonly available tests and are more difficult to reverse quickly. The use of the potent intravenously administered glycoprotein IIb/IIIa platelet antagonists is generally contraindicated in the setting of ongoing or recent surgery because of the high risk of hemorrhagic complications. Anti-ischemic therapy should include nitrates and β-adrenergic receptor blocking agents, preferably with a quickly reversible agent such as esmolol, as well as intravenously administered nitroglycerin, unless the patient is hypotensive or has hemodynamic compromise.

The treatment approach then diverges based on ECG findings. Patients with ST-segment elevation or new left bundle branch block will be considered separately from those with ST-segment depression or nonspecific ECG changes (see Figure 141-1).

ST-Segment Elevation Myocardial Infarction

ST-segment elevation is a highly specific finding indicative of acute MI. Such patients typically have occlusion of an epicardial coronary artery and are candidates for urgent reperfusion therapy, which is most beneficial if achieved early but is of some value up to 12 h after event onset. Although thrombolytic therapy is contraindicated in the immediate postoperative setting, many postoperative patients may tolerate aspirin and intravenously administered heparin with acceptable bleeding risk and are then candidates for primary angioplasty, usually with stent implantation. Emergent patient transfer may be necessary to a center providing percutaneous coronary intervention, if unavailable locally.

Complications of MI include congestive failure, ventricular arrhythmias, cardiogenic shock, and cardiac arrest. Patients must be diligently monitored for these conditions, and the complications must be corrected with appropriate pharmacologic measures. The use of intra-aortic balloon pumping or temporary left ventricular mechanical support may be helpful before patients transfer or if they develop delayed shock or heart failure. Angiotensin-converting

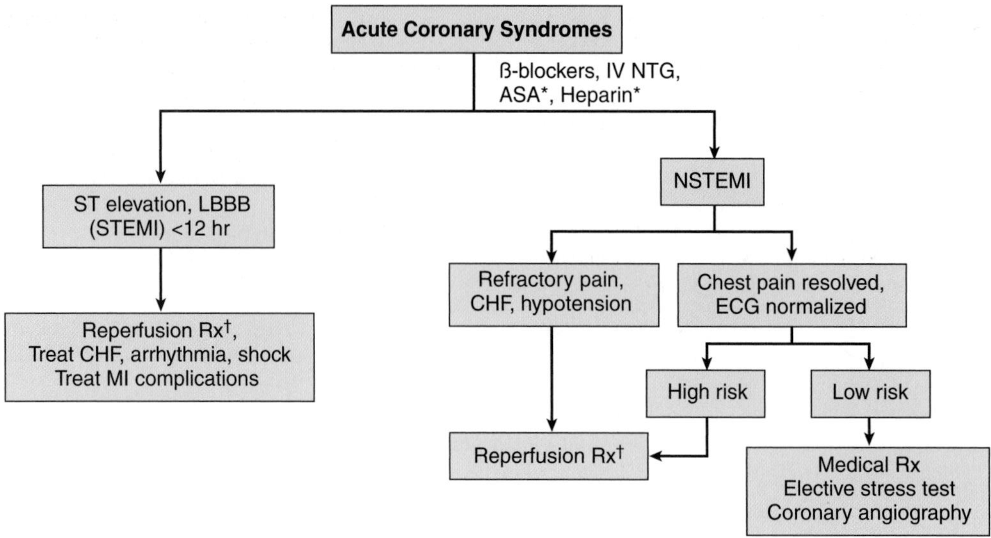

Figure 141-1 Therapy and decision making for patients with acute coronary syndromes. Reperfusion therapy includes angioplasty, thrombolysis, or both. ASA, Aspirin; CHF, congestive heart failure; ECG, electrocardiogram; IV, intravenously administered; LBBB, left bundle branch block; MI, myocardial infarction; NSTEMI, non–ST-segment elevation MI; NTG, nitroglycerin; Rx, therapy; STEMI, ST-segment elevation MI.

enzyme inhibitors, aspirin, β-adrenergic receptor blocking agents, and appropriate lipid-lowering therapy are indicated over the long term.

Non–ST-Segment Elevation Acute Coronary Syndromes

Non–ST-segment elevation ACS most commonly results from an incompletely occlusive coronary thrombus. Patients may present with chest pain or, more commonly, are found to have elevated cardiac enzyme markers postoperatively. Medical therapy with aspirin, β-adrenergic receptor blocking agents, nitrates, lipid-lowering agents, and antithrombotic agents is the mainstay of treatment. Patients at high risk for subsequent fatality and morbidity include those with persistent ST-segment depression, those with elevated cardiac serum markers such as troponin or creatine kinase-MB, and those manifesting hemodynamic instability, including hypotension, shock, pulmonary edema, right-sided heart failure, and frequent ventricular arrhythmia. These high-risk patients, as well as those with refractory ischemic pain, should be considered for coronary angiography and reperfusion therapy. The same caveats regarding assessment of bleeding risk and the use of potent platelet and thrombin inhibitors apply. For other patients who are minimally symptomatic and hemodynamically stable, urgent angiography is not necessary, as long as the patient's condition remains stable. ECG monitoring and serial assessment of cardiac enzyme markers are appropriate. Further investigation can be delayed until later in the patient's convalescence and usually includes stress imaging, angiography, or both. Guidelines for the management of preoperative risk stratification and acute MI and for the use of percutaneous coronary intervention are available.

Special Situations

For patients who are allergic to aspirin, clopidogrel, 75 mg daily, may be substituted. Heparin-induced thrombocytopenia typically does not occur during the first 5 days of therapy unless recent earlier exposure to heparin has occurred. Patients with this disorder will usually have an antibody to the heparin-platelet factor 4 complex. A direct-acting thrombin inhibitor that is structurally and functionally unrelated to heparin, such as Bivalirudin or Argatroban, may be substituted for heparin in this circumstance.

The use of β-adrenergic receptor blocking agents is contraindicated in patients with second-degree or greater atrioventricular block, shock, cardiogenic pulmonary edema, severe heart failure, or severe asthma but should not be withheld in patients with diabetes mellitus. The use of calcium channel blockers is indicated for rate control of rapid atrial fibrillation, which may accompany or precipitate ACS in some individuals. However, there is no other primary indication for these agents in ACS, and their use should generally be avoided.

For patients with refractory ventricular tachycardia or ventricular fibrillation, the current drug of choice is a 150-mg bolus of intravenously administered amiodarone followed by infusion.

For patients with an anterior wall MI, pump failure is the most serious complication and is a strong indication for reperfusion therapy as well as for inotropic support and left ventricular support. For those with an inferior wall MI, complications such as papillary muscle dysfunction or rupture, as well as hemodynamically significant right ventricular MI, are more common. The use of surface or transesophageal echocardiography allows rapid and accurate differentiation of these disorders.

Symptoms of ACS may be vague in the postoperative patient because the patient is still recovering from the effects of anesthesia. In any patient in the postanesthesia care unit who experiences sudden hemodynamic collapse, a diagnosis of ACS must be considered. The differential diagnosis should also include pulmonary embolus, aortic dissection, pneumothorax, cardiac tamponade, and sepsis.

Suggested Readings

Alpert JS, Thygesen K, Antman E, Bassand JP. Myocardial infarction redefined—A consensus document of the Joint European Society of Cardiology/American College of Cardiology Committee for the Redefinition of Myocardial Infarction. *J Am Coll Cardiol*. 2000;36:959-969.

Anderson JL, Adams CD, Antman et al. American College of Cardiology Foundation/ American HeartAssociation Task Force on Practice Guidelines. 2012 ACCF/AHA focused update incorporated into the ACCF/AHA 2007 guidelines for the management of patients with unstable angina/non-ST-elevation myocardial infarction: A report of the American College of Cardiology Foundation/American Heart Association Task Force on Practice Guidelines. *Circulation*. 2013;127:e663-e828.

Kushner FG, Hand M, Smith SC Jr, et al. American College of Cardiology Foundation/ American Heart Association Task Force on Practice Guidelines. 2009 Focused Updates: ACC/AHA Guidelines for the Management of Patients With ST-Elevation Myocardial Infarction (updating the 2004 Guideline and 2007 Focused Update) and ACC/AHA/SCAI Guidelines on Percutaneous Coronary

Intervention (updating the 2005 Guideline and 2007 Focused Update): A report of the American College of Cardiology Foundation/American Heart Association Task Force on Practice Guidelines. *Circulation*. 2009;120:2271-2306.

Berger PB, Bellot V, Bell MR, et al. An immediate invasive strategy for the treatment of acute myocardial infarction early after noncardiac surgery. *Am J Cardiol*. 2001;87:1100-1102.

Fleisher LA, Beckman JA, Brown KA, et al. ACC/AHA 2007 guidelines on perioperative cardiovascular evaluation and care for noncardiac surgery: A report of the American College of Cardiology/American Heart Association Task Force on Practice Guidelines (Writing Committee to Revise the 2002 Guidelines on Perioperative Cardiovascular Evaluation for Noncardiac Surgery) developed in collaboration with the American Society of Echocardiography, American Society of Nuclear Cardiology, Heart Rhythm Society, Society of Cardiovascular Anesthesiologists, Society for Cardiovascular Angiography and Interventions, Society for Vascular Medicine and Biology, and Society for Vascular Surgery. *J Am Coll Cardiol*. 2007;50:e159.

Jessup M, Abraham WT, Casey DE, et al. 2009 focused update: ACCF/AHA guidelines for the diagnosis and management of heart failure in adults. *Circulation*. 2009;119:1977-2016.

Rinfret S, Goldman L, Polanczyk CA, et al. Value of immediate postoperative electrocardiogram to update risk stratification after major noncardiac surgery. *Am J Cardiol*. 2004;94:1017.

CHAPTER 142

Heart Failure: Classification, Compensation, and Treatment

Christopher A. Thunberg, MD

Heart failure (HF) is a condition in which cardiac pumping function does not satisfy the metabolic needs of the body. Traditionally, HF has implied that the patient has abnormal systolic function with a reduced ejection fraction. However, diastolic dysfunction, in which filling of the left ventricle is impaired, is responsible for approximately 50% of all cases of HF. The patient with diastolic HF may have a normal ejection fraction.

Types of Heart Failure

Clinical scenarios involving HF can be broadly grouped into three categories: acute HF, chronic HF, and chronic HF with acute decompensation.

Acute Heart Failure

Patients with acute HF have no history of HF but experience a sudden cardiac injury (such as massive myocardial infarction) that severely compromises pump function. The injury presents so acutely that there isn't sufficient time for compensatory mechanisms to develop, so dyspnea, pulmonary edema, and cardiogenic shock are prominent.

Chronic Heart Failure

The typical patient with chronic HF has an underlying systemic disease such as coronary artery disease or hypertension (Box 142-1) that results in cardiac dysfunction that develops over many years; patients present with fatigue, anorexia, and peripheral edema. Compensatory mechanisms initially ameliorate some of the signs and symptoms (see following discussion).

Chronic Heart Failure with Acute Decompensation

Patients with stable chronic HF who do not adhere to dietary restrictions or comply with medical therapy or who have worsening of the underlying medical condition (myocardial ischemia) can acutely decompensate. This decompensation of cardiac function is manifested by the same symptoms and signs as mentioned previously.

Classification of Heart Failure

The New York Heart Association classification system (Table 142-1) is symptom based, whereas the newer American College of Cardiology/American Heart Association classification emphasizes disease progression (Table 142-2).

Compensatory Mechanisms in Heart Failure

A reduction in cardiac output activates neurohumoral systems (Table 142-3) that initially may be beneficial by (1) increasing perfusion of vital organs

Box 142-1 Etiology of Chronic Heart Failure

Coronary artery disease—may progress to dilated cardiomyopathy	Drugs and toxins
Hypertension—associated with diastolic dysfunction	Alcohol
Valvular heart disease—results in volume or pressure overload	Cocaine
Genetic cardiomyopathies	Doxorubicin
Hypertrophic	Endocrine disorder
Dilated	Hypothyroidism
Infection	Hyperthyroidism
Myocarditis	Nutritional deficiency
AIDS	Deficiency of thiamine, selenium, or carnitine
	Infiltrative disease
	Sarcoidosis
	Amyloidosis
	Hemochromatosis

AIDS, Acquired immunodeficiency syndrome.

Table 142-1 New York Heart Association Functional Classification of Heart Failure

Class	Description
I	No limitation—symptoms of HF only at activity levels that would limit normal individuals
II	Slight limitation—symptoms with ordinary levels of activity
III	Marked limitation—symptoms with less-than-normal levels of activity
IV	Symptoms of HF at rest—very poor prognosis

HF, Heart failure.
Adapted from Jessup M, Abraham WT, Casey DE, et al. 2009 focused update: ACCF/AHA Guidelines for the Diagnosis and Management of Heart Failure in Adults: a report of the American College of Cardiology Foundation/American Heart Association Task Force on Practice Guidelines: developed in collaboration with the International Society for Heart and Lung Transplantation. Circulation. 119: 1977-2016, 2009.

Table 142-2 American College of Cardiology/American Heart Association Classification of Chronic Heart Failure

Stage	Description	Clinical Correlation/ Presentation
A	High risk for developing HF but without structural heart disease or symptoms of HF	Hypertension, diabetes mellitus, CAD, obesity, family history of cardiomyopathy
B	Structural heart disease but without signs or symptoms of HF	Previous MI, LV dysfunction, asymptomatic valvular heart disease
C	Structural heart disease with prior or current symptoms of HF	Structural heart disease, dyspnea and fatigue, impaired exercise tolerance
D	Refractory end-stage HF	Marked symptoms at rest despite maximal medical therapy

CAD, Coronary artery disease; HF, heart failure; LV, left ventricular; MI, myocardial infarction.
Adapted from Jessup M, Abraham WT, Casey DE, et al. 2009 focused update: ACCF/AHA Guidelines for the Diagnosis and Management of Heart Failure in Adults: a report of the American College of Cardiology Foundation/American Heart Association Task Force on Practice Guidelines: developed in collaboration with the International Society for Heart and Lung Transplantation. Circulation. 119: 1977-2016, 2009.

through vasoconstriction, (2) restoring cardiac output by augmenting inotropy and chronotropy, and (3) increasing preload through expansion of the intravascular volume. However, over time, these mechanisms can result in a combination of pathologic myocardial remodeling (fibrosis and hypertrophy), worsening myocardial ischemia, and volume overload manifested by peripheral or pulmonary edema.

Management of Chronic Heart Failure

Management of chronic HF is directed at maintenance of homeostasis by fine-tuning the compensatory neurohumoral mechanisms with β-adrenergic receptor blocking agents, angiotensin-converting enzyme inhibitors, angiotensin receptor blockers, and aldosterone antagonists, all of which have been shown to reduce mortality rate and prevent disease progression.

Table 142-3 Neurohumoral Systems Activated in Patients with Heart Failure

System	Action	Negative Effects
Sympathetic nervous system	Vasoconstriction Increased inotropy Increased chronotropy	Increased afterload Ischemia Myocardial remodeling
Renin-angiotensin-aldosterone system	Vasoconstriction Increased intravascular volume	Increased afterload Ischemia Myocardial remodeling Volume overload
Antidiuretic hormone	Vasoconstriction Increased intravascular volume	Increased afterload Volume overload
Endothelin	Vasoconstriction	Ischemia Myocardial remodeling

Patients with chronic HF who have an acute decompensation are best treated with loop diuretics and venodilators (nitrates) to reduce preload. Ultrafiltration may be used to reduce circulating blood volume if resistance or intolerance to diuretic therapy occurs. Afterload is reduced with the use of angiotensin-converting enzyme inhibitors and arterial vasodilators (e.g., hydralazine or sodium nitroprusside).

To control life-threatening arrhythmias, the patient may be taking antiarrhythmic medication (β-adrenergic receptor blocking agents, amiodarone) or have an automatic implanted cardioverter-defibrillator. Many patients with advanced HF undergo cardiac resynchronization therapy in which biventricular pacing is used to restore the normal sequence of activation and contraction of the ventricles. Digoxin is reserved for use in patients with rapid atrial fibrillation and reduced ejection fraction.

Critically ill patients with HF and signs of low cardiac output may receive inotropic therapy (e.g., a catecholamine, such as dobutamine, or a phosphodiesterase inhibitor, such as milrinone) or undergo insertion of an intra-aortic balloon pump. Surgical options for end-stage HF include placement of a ventricular assist device or heart transplantation.

Suggested Readings

Abraham WT, Greenberg BH, Yancy CW. Pharmacologic therapies across the continuum of left ventricular dysfunction. *Am J Cardiol*. 2008;102:21G-28.

Groban L, Butterworth J. Perioperative management of chronic heart failure. *Anesth Analg*. 2006;103: 557-575.

Jessup M, Abraham WT, Casey DE, et al. 2009 focused update: ACCF/AHA Guidelines for the Diagnosis and Management of Heart Failure in Adults: A Report of the American College of Cardiology Foundation/American Heart Association Task Force on Practice Guidelines: Developed in collaboration with the International Society for Heart and Lung Transplantation. *Circulation*. 2009; 119:1977-2016.

McMurray JJ. Clinical practice. Systolic heart failure. *N Engl J Med*. 2010;362(3): 228-238.

CHAPTER 143

Management of End-Stage Heart Failure: Heart Transplantation and Ventricular Assist Devices

Doris B. M. Ockert, MD

End-Stage Heart Failure

Heart failure (HF) is defined as insufficient cardiac output to meet the metabolic requirements of the tissues at normal cardiac-filling pressures. Cardiogenic shock is defined as sustained hypotension and tissue hypoperfusion. HF can be systolic (impaired contractility with impaired ejection fraction) or diastolic (decreased relaxation and compliance). Activation of the compensatory neurohormone system (renin-angiotensin-aldosterone system and release of natriuretic peptides, angiotensin II, norepinephrine, and endothelin) results in fluid retention, peripheral vasoconstriction, downregulation of β-adrenergic receptors, and ventricular remodeling. Eventually, left ventricular (LV) failure leads to pulmonary hypertension and right ventricular (RV) failure.

Echocardiography is used to assess ventricular function, to identify structural and functional cardiac abnormalities, and to guide therapy. The American Heart Association classification defines four stages of HF: A through D. Stage D is end-stage HF, (Figure 143-1). Coronary artery disease is the most common cause of both systolic and diastolic failure. Other causes include dilated nonischemic, restrictive, hypertrophic, and stress-induced cardiomyopathy. The most common cause of death is ventricular arrhythmia.

Patients with coronary artery disease or valvular heart disease should have medical therapy optimized and, depending on the anatomy, revascularization performed or valves repaired or replaced as appropriate. In patients with an ejection fraction of less than 30%, placement of an implantable cardioverter defibrillator (ICD), pacemaker resynchronization therapy, or both is recommended. Routine anticoagulation is not recommended. Surgical treatment options include placement of an intra-aortic balloon pump, ventricular assist device (VAD), or total artificial heart (TAH) or orthotopic heart transplantation.

Clinical indications for the use of a mechanical device before multisystem organ failure occurs include myocardial infarction, failed percutaneous coronary intervention, acute viral myocarditis, peripartum cardiomyopathy, cardiac contusion, postcardiotomy shock, chronic cardiomyopathy with acute decompensation, and intractable ventricular arrhythmias. Early intervention improves survival.

Ventricular Assist Devices

VADs to support the left, right, or both ventricles are either pulsatile or nonpulsatile pumps, located paracorporeally or intracorporeally, and are used as a bridge to recovery (short-term), a-bridge to transplantation, or destination therapy. The first-generation VADs use pulsatile pumps with valves that displace a given volume of blood with every beat. One pulsatile pump is still marketed in the United States, a paracorporeal VAD (pVAD; Thoratec, Pleasanton, CA) for short-term to intermediate-term use in patients who require bridge to transplantation or bridge to recovery (Figure 143-2). Approximately 10% of patients recover sufficient function to be weaned completely from mechanical support. Compared with previous devices, the pVAD allows for greater patient mobility (a portable device is available for patients who leave the hospital) and longer-term use (weeks to months and, in a few cases, years); its use is associated with lower rates of morbidity. Short-term anticoagulation is provided with heparin, whereas long-term anticoagulation requires warfarin and sometimes aspirin.

Second-generation VADs are smaller, intracorporeal, nonpulsatile, axial-flow pumps without valves. Third-generation VADs are bearingless and use a combination of magnetically and hydrodynamically suspended impellers. Currently available in the United States are the Heartmate II (Thoratec), a second-generation device approved by the U.S. Food and Drug Administration (FDA) for bridge to transplantation in 2008 and for destination therapy for patients who are not candidates for heart transplantation in 2010 (Figure 143-3), and the HeartWare ventricular assist system (Framingham, MA), a third-generation device approved in 2012 by the FDA as a bridge to transplantation (Figure 143-4).

Left VADs (LVADs) drain blood from the LV through an inflow cannula to the pump and return blood via an outflow cannula into the proximal aorta. The Randomized Evaluation of Mechanical Assistance for the Treatment of Congestive Heart Failure (REMATCH) trial demonstrated that patients did better when they had a device implanted sooner rather than later (before they developed organ dysfunction, i.e., kidney failure). Long-term survival is approximately 80% at 1 year and more than 50% at 2 years after device implantation.

Total Artificial Heart

SynCardia (Tucson, AZ) produces two TAHs, each consisting of two independent pulsatile devices (ventricles) that, once the native ventricles are excised, are anastomosed to the native atria with the outflow cannulas inserted into the ascending aorta and pulmonary outflow tract, respectively. The FDA approved the 75-mL TAH (Figure 143-5) as a bridge to transplant in 2004 and designated two humanitarian use device labels for the 50-mL TAH in 2013—destination therapy and pediatric bridge to transplant.

Anesthetic Considerations for Patients with End-Stage Heart Failure Requiring Implantation of a VAD or TAH

Preoperative Considerations

The preparation of these patients is similar to that required for other patients having cardiac surgical procedures involving cardiopulmonary bypass (CPB).

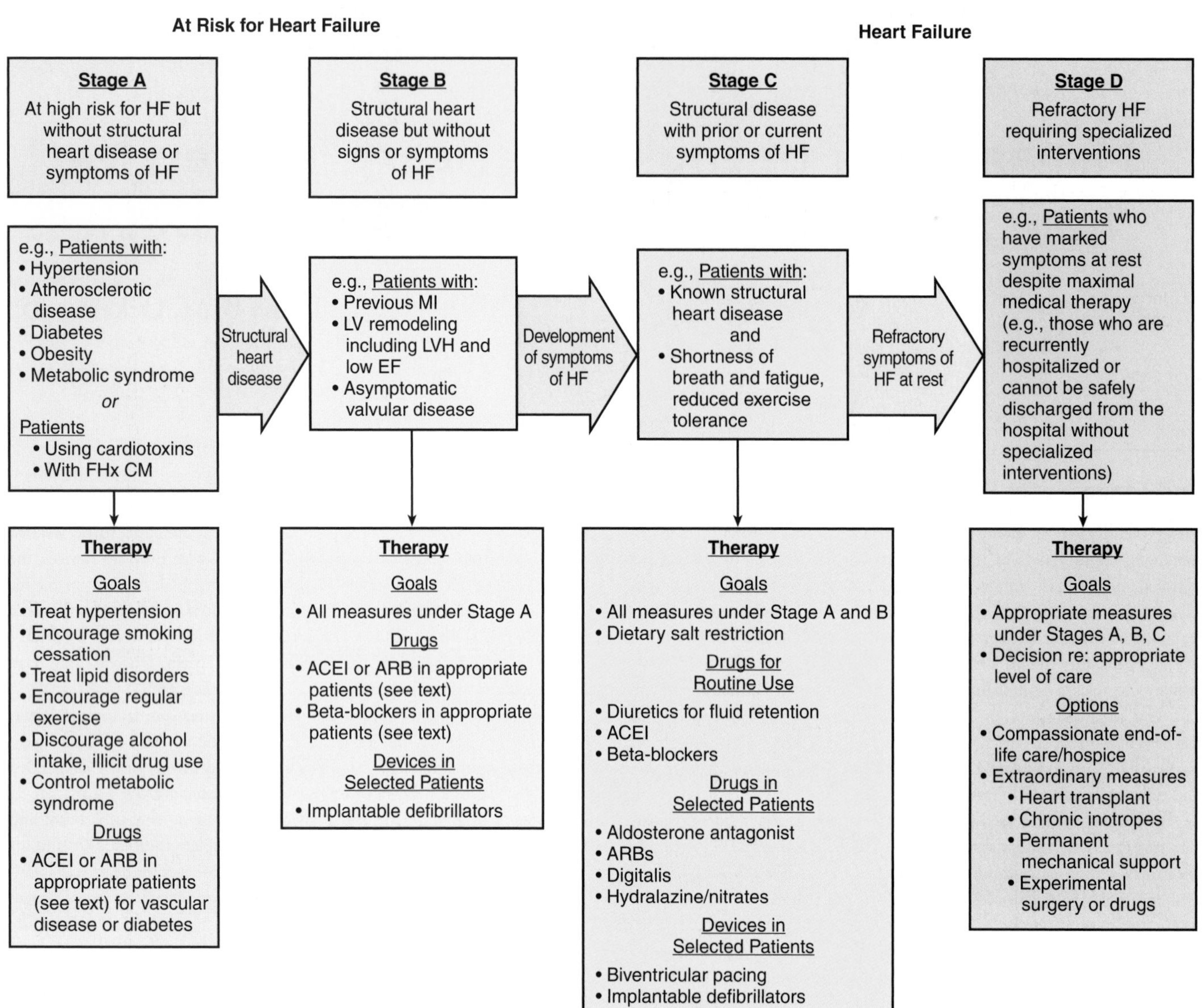

Figure 143-1 Stages in the development of heart failure and recommended therapy by stage. ACEI, Angiotensin-converting enzyme inhibitor; ARB, angiotensin II receptor blocker; EF, ejection fraction; FHx CM, family history of cardiomyopathy; HF, heart failure; LV, left ventricular; LVH, left ventricular hypertrophy; MI, myocardial infarction. (Modified from Jessup M, Abraham WT, Casey DE, et al. 2009 focused update: ACCF/AHA Guidelines for the Diagnosis and Management of Heart Failure in Adults: a report of the American College of Cardiology Foundation/American Heart Association Task Force on Practice Guidelines: developed in collaboration with the International Society for Heart and Lung Transplantation. Circulation 2009;119:1977-2016. © 2013 American Heart Association, Inc. All rights reserved.)

However, patients who are receiving VADs, a TAH, or heart transplants are at greater risk for experiencing hemorrhage and are at risk for developing systolic dysfunction, ventricular arrhythmias, and sudden death prior to CPB.

A thorough preoperative evaluation should include an extensive review of the patient's cardiac, pulmonary, renal, and metabolic history; a comprehensive examination of the patient; and a complete assessment of all laboratory results and imaging studies. All previously implanted devices such as pacemakers and ICDs should be interrogated. Packed red blood cells (cytomegalovirus free), fresh frozen plasma, and platelets must be available in the blood bank because these patients will have received anticoagulant therapy, have chronic anemia, and are at high risk of developing perioperative bleeding.

Intraoperative Management

Patients Receiving a VAD

In addition to standard American Society of Anesthesiologists monitoring devices, these patients should have a cannula placed in a radial or femoral artery prior to induction of anesthesia, if possible, for continuous measurement of arterial blood pressure. Central venous access should be achieved either with an 8.5F or 9F introducer through which a catheter may be inserted for measurement of central venous, pulmonary artery, and pulmonary artery occlusion pressures and cardiac output. Many clinicians prefer to perform these procedures prior to the induction of anesthesia because of the severity of the patient's underlying heart disease. The pharmacologic agents used for induction and maintenance of anesthesia are similar to those used for any other patient with severe cardiomyopathy. After the trachea is intubated, a transesophageal echocardiographic (TEE) probe should be inserted. Patients with preexisting coagulopathy need baseline coagulation studies and possibly thromboelastography. Defibrillation pads must be placed prior to deactivation of defibrillation therapies.

Prior to CPB, a TEE examination should be performed to assess for the presence of a patent foramen ovale (PFO), aortic or mitral insufficiency, and intracardiac thrombi. Because the LVAD will create negative pressure at the tip of the cannula in the left ventricle, it is important to repair a PFO to prevent paradoxical embolism of air bubbles and thrombi and shunting of

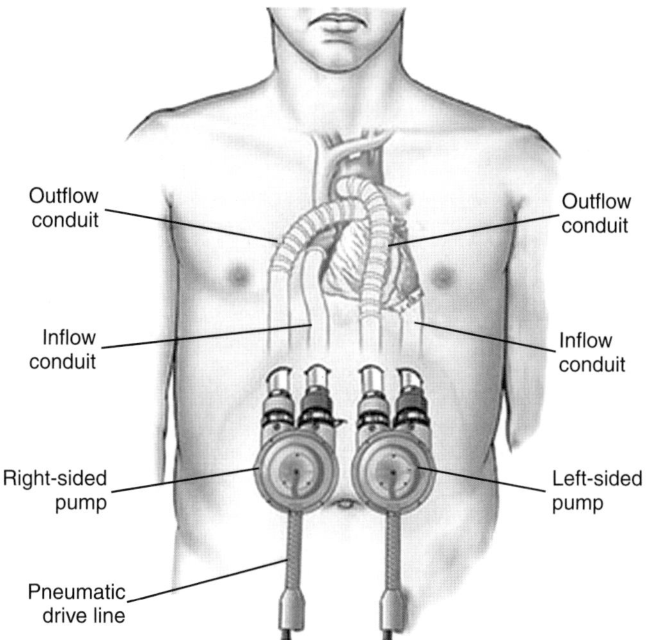

Figure 143-2 Paracorporeal ventricular assist device—a pulsatile first-generation device. (Reprinted, with permission, from Thoratec Corporation, Pleasanton, CA.)

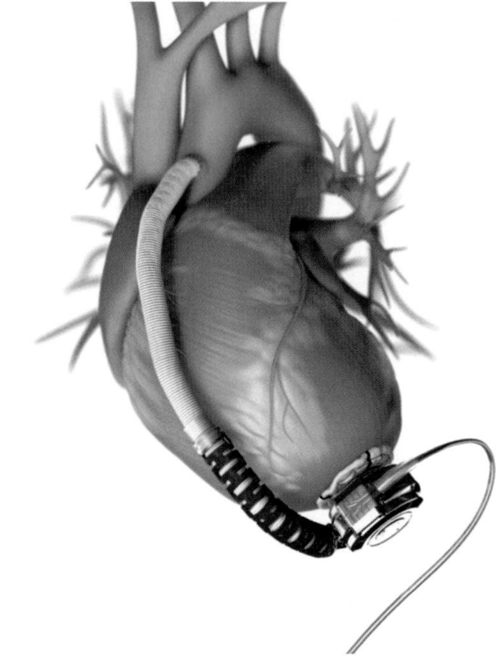

Figure 143-4 Heartware ventricular assist system, an intracorporeal ventricular assist device—a third-generation, continuous-flow, ventricular assist device. (Reprinted, with permission, from Heartware International, Framingham, MA.)

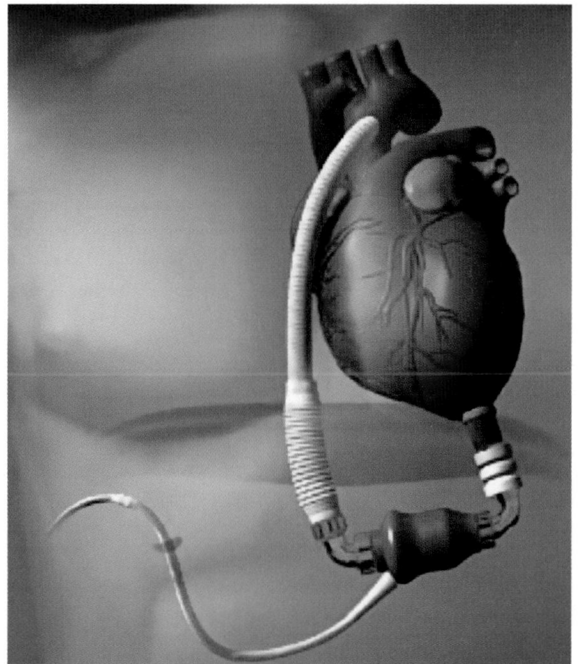

Figure 143-3 Heartmate II, an intracorporeal ventricular assist device—a second-generation, continuous-flow, ventricular assist device. (Reprinted, with permission, from Thoratec Corporation, Pleasanton, CA.)

desaturated blood from right to left. The PFO may only be detected after CPB when the left heart is decompressed. Similarly, if the patient has aortic insufficiency, the device may create a flow loop, in which blood flowing from the device into the aortic root is drawn back through the incompetent aortic valve into the device and back into the root, etc., with insufficient flow to vital organs. In addition, if the LV continues to contract with the LVAD off-loading the LV and augmenting cardiac output, significant mitral regurgitation will decrease preload to the device and limit its effectiveness. Removing cardiac thrombi is critical to avoid their entry into the pump. The results of

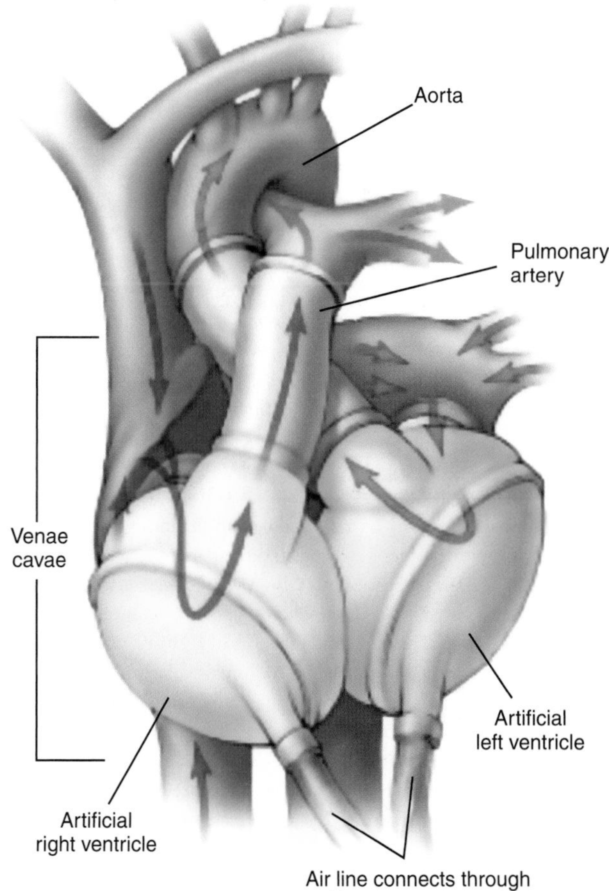

Figure 143-5 Total artificial heart. (Reprinted, with permission, from Syncardia, Tucson, AZ.)

the intraoperative TEE examination should be shared with the surgeon so that he or she can assess the situation and decide whether any deficits should be corrected surgically. The midesophageal four-chamber or two-chamber TEE view may help guide the surgeon to the potential ventriculostomy site for the inflow cannula for the device. Because of the severity of the cardiomyopathy, any reduction in preload, heart rate, or contractility prior to CPB may produce sudden cardiovascular collapse. Vasoactive drugs such as phenylephrine, ephedrine, epinephrine, norepinephrine, or vasopressin may be required to maintain hemodynamic stability.

The primary cause for failure to wean the patient from CPB is inadequate LV preload. This may be caused by decreased intravascular volume, vasodilation, or RV failure, most likely secondary to pulmonary hypertension. Therapeutic options to improve LV preload include intravascular volume replacement, vasoconstrictor therapy (vasopressin, norepinephrine, phenylephrine), appropriate inotropic support in the case of RV failure (milrinone, epinephrine, dobutamine), and primary pulmonary vasodilator therapy (nitric oxide, prostaglandins).

After implantation of the device, a TEE exam is used to assess the inflow to and outflow from the LVAD. Once the patient is weaned from CPB, the most common causes of hypotension are decreased intravascular volume and decreased systemic vascular resistance.

Patients Receiving a Total Artificial Heart

A TAH may be an option for patients who have end-stage heart disease of sufficient severity that VADs fail to provide sufficient support and who have confounding factors that make heart transplantation unlikely or contraindicated. The anesthetic management for patients undergoing TAH implantation is similar to that previously described, except for the treatment of hypotension, and special care is needed to prevent air emboli. Because the native ventricles are excised, no benefit is gained with the use of inotropes for the treatment of hypotension. In addition to infusing fluids to increase intravascular volume and therefore venous return, vasopressors may be required to increase systemic vascular resistance and venous return. Nitric oxide and prostaglandins may be required to treat pulmonary hypertension. Following anastomosis of the artificial ventricles to the native atria, the mechanical ventricles must be primed. Therefore, the patient should be placed in Trendelenburg position and a TEE examination performed to detect air and monitor its evacuation as the mechanical ventricles begin to contract and eject. Once the mechanical ventricles are functioning and the patient's hemodynamic values are satisfactory, the patient is weaned from CPB, bleeding is controlled, and the chest is closed and the patient may be transported to the intensive care unit.

Postoperative Management

Complications of all devices include bleeding, thromboembolism, infection, hemolysis, device malfunction, and multiorgan failure. The management of the patient with an LVAD or both an LVAD and an RVAD is similar to the management of patients who have had a cardiac surgical procedure for which CPB is used: postoperative bleeding and hemodynamic values must be carefully monitored and stabilized, and the patient is weaned from mechanical ventilation. The possibility of RV dysfunction must be considered in a patient with only an LVAD in whom hypotension develops. Once the patient leaves the intensive care unit, the most likely cause of hypotension is decreased preload secondary to decreased intravascular volume.

Patients with VADs frequently require other surgical procedures. For unknown reasons, but probably related to the nonpulsatile blood flow with the second-generation and third-generation devices, approximately 40% to 50% of these patients will develop gastrointestinal bleeding because of arteriovenous malformations that form in the walls of the gastrointestinal tract. These patients will often require upper gastrointestinal endoscopy. Arteriovenous malformations are also occasionally seen in the wall of the urinary bladder. Arterial pulses are very weak, if present at all, in patients with axial flow pumps, making noninvasive blood pressure monitoring difficult. Measurement of blood pressure with either Doppler or an intra-arterial cannula is often necessary.

Considerations for Patients for Heart Transplantation

Patients with end-stage heart disease are carefully screened for possible heart transplantation. They must be adherent with treatment, not abuse substances (including alcohol), have an adequate support system, be free of cancer, and have a body mass index of less than 38. Severe irreversible pulmonary hypertension is an absolute contraindication to heart transplantation (pulmonary vascular resistance > 6 Wood units or > 480 Dynes$\cdot$sec$^{-1}\cdot$cm^{-5}).

When the United Network for Organ Sharing is notified that a patient has been declared brain dead and the organs are available for transplantation, they identify potential recipients by matching the donor heart with potential recipients, based on the severity of the recipient's disease, through HLA typing, ABO blood group compatibility, and body size. Once the best candidate is found, the transplant center is notified, and, if the transplant team and patient agree, the candidate is posted for transplantation.

These cases are always performed on an emergency basis. Donor-heart ischemic time should optimally be kept at less than 4 hours. Sterile technique is imperative because the patient will be immunosuppressed and at high risk of developing infection. Immunosuppression protocols vary. Commonly, 500 mg of methylprednisolone is administered after induction and again after release of the aortic cross-clamp. Other immunosuppressant drugs may be utilized depending on the preferences of the institution's transplant service.

The surgical technique involves four major anastomoses: left and right atria and the end-to-end aortic and pulmonary anastomoses. The bicaval technique is used in some cases instead of the right atria anastomosis. Because the donor heart is denervated, only direct-acting β-adrenergic agents will increase heart rate.

RV failure is the most common cause for failure to wean from CPB after heart transplantation. Preventing hypoxia and hypercarbia are essential, and the use of pulmonary vasodilators (prostaglandin E1, nitric oxide, milrinone) and inotropes (epinephrine, dobutamine, milrinone) to support the RV may be necessary. Norepinephrine and vasopressin may be needed to support systemic vascular resistance. In the early postoperative period, patients are at risk for developing hyperacute and acute rejection, pulmonary and systemic hypertension, cardiac arrhythmias, respiratory failure, renal failure, and infection.

Allograft coronary artery disease is the major limiting factor to long-term survival following heart transplantation. This is diffuse disease that involves the vessels circumferentially. Cyclosporine and corticosteroids are the mainstays of long-term immunosuppression and may cause nephrotoxicity, hypertension, and malignant neoplastic disease. The survival rates for transplantation approach 90% for the first year and 75% at the seventh year.

Suggested Readings

Chumnanvej S, Wood MJ, MacGillivray TE, Melo MF. Perioperative echocardiographic examination for ventricular assist device implantation. *Anesth Analg*. 2007;105:583-601.

Groban L, Butterworth J. Perioperative management of chronic heart failure. *Anesth Analg*. 2006;103:557-555.

Jessup M, Abraham WT, Casey DE, et al. 2009 focused update: ACCF/AHA Guidelines for the Diagnosis and Management of Heart Failure in Adults: A report of the American College of Cardiology Foundation/American Heart Association Task Force on Practice Guidelines: Developed in collaboration with the International Society for Heart and Lung Transplantation. *Circulation*. 2009;119:1977-2016.

Shanewise J. Cardiac transplantation. *Anesthesiol Clin North Am*. 2004;22:753-765.

Slaughter MS, et al. Clinical management of continuous-flow left ventricular assist devices in advanced heart failure. *J Heart Lung Transplant*. 2010;29:S1-S29.

Vegas A. Assisting the failing heart. *Anesthesiol Clin*. 2008;26:539-564.

CHAPTER 144

Coronary Artery Stents

Amy G. Voet, DO, MS, and James A. Giacalone, BS, MEd

Coronary artery stents were first developed in the 1980s and are now placed in most percutaneous coronary interventions (PCIs). Interventional cardiologists have a wide choice of stents for implantation. The choices range from bare-metal stents (BMSs) and drug-eluting stents (DESs) (Table 144-1) that are widely used in contemporary practice to new stents, such as DESs with novel coatings, biodegradable stents, DESs with biodegradable polymers, DESs that are polymer free, dedicated bifurcation stents, and self-expanding stents. A number of DESs are currently undergoing study or are available outside the United States (Table 144-2).

Ulrich Sigwart placed the first stent in 1986. This BMS proved to be effective as a rescue device for patients who were in imminent danger of vessel closure and, thus, reduced the number of patients undergoing emergency coronary artery bypass grafting. However, the risk of subacute thrombotic coronary occlusion hindered the further development of these stents. Coronary artery stenting finally became widely accepted in 1994 after evidence showed that stenting was safe with the use of dual antiplatelet therapy (typically, aspirin and a platelet $P2Y_{12}$ receptor antagonist). By 1999, the placement of coronary artery stents made up more than 80% of PCIs. The risk of subacute thrombosis remained, and a new iatrogenic problem developed of in-stent neointimal hyperplasia, which resulted in 20% to 30% restenosis rates, stimulating the development of the DES. The risk of stent thrombosis after the placement of either a BMS or DES can be reduced by implementation of platelet $P2Y_{12}$ receptor antagonist therapy in combination with aspirin therapy. Box 144-1 lists definitions of stents, complications with their use, and related types of therapy.

Complications

Thrombosis, Hemorrhage, Myocardial Infarction, Stroke, and Contrast Nephropathy

The U.S. Food and Drug Administration's (FDA) approval for the use of DESs is currently limited to simple lesions. Sirolimus-eluting stents are approved for use in de novo lesions that are 30 mm or shorter and have a vessel diameter of 2.5 to 3.5 mm. Paclitaxel-eluting stents are approved for de novo lesions that are 28 mm or shorter and have a diameter of 2.5 to 3.75 mm. Early studies of DESs were criticized because only patients who were stable and who received a DES for an FDA-approved indication were enrolled.

Table 144-1 U.S. Food and Drug Administration–Approved Drug-Eluting Stents

Stent	Manufacturer	Drug Eluted
Cypher	J&J Cordis	Sirolimus
TAXUS Express and Liberté	Boston Scientific	Paclitaxel
Endeavor	Medtronic	Zotarolimus
Xience V	Guidant, Abbott	Everolimus

Table 144-2 Metallic Stents Available Outside the United States or Undergoing Clinical Evaluation

Stent	Drug(s) Eluted	Approved Outside U.S.	Ongoing Trials
Endeavor RESOLUTE	Zotarolimus	X	
Elixir DESyne	Novolimus		X
TAXUS Element	Paclitaxel	X	
PROMUS Element	Everolimus	X	
Supramilus	Sirolimus		X
Excel Stent	Sirolimus		X
NEVO	Sirolimus		X
BioMatrix	Biolimus A9	X	
NOBORI	Biolimus A9	X	
Axxess	Biolimus A9	X	
XTENT	Biolimus A9	X	
SYNERGY	Everolimus		X
Combo	EPC + sirolimus		X
Elixir Myolimus	Myolimus		X
Infinnium	Paclitaxel		X
JACTAX Liberté	Paclitaxel		X
AmazoniaPax	Paclitaxel	X	
BioFREEDOM	Biolimus A9		X
VESTAsync	Sirolimus		X
Tukon	Sirolimus	X	
Catania stent	Polyzene F	X	
TINOX stent	Titanium nitride-oxide	X	
Genous stent	$CD34^+$ antibody	X	

A much greater percentage of devices are implanted for off-label uses, although the results of studies conducted for off-label uses are equivocal. Some studies have determined that off-label use of the DES is associated with an increased risk of death, myocardial infarction (MI), and repeat revascularization, whereas other studies have demonstrated a significant improvement in outcome with the use of DESs. These differences have been attributed to the patient populations and lesion characteristics and not to a specific problem with DESs. Overall, the use of DESs significantly reduces the risk of

Box 144-1 Definitions

Bare metal stent (BMS): Non–drug-coated vascular stent composed of various metal alloys deployed into a coronary artery or vascular conduit to restore the luminal integrity of the vessel.
Drug-eluting stent (DES): Drug-coated vascular stent that is deployed into a coronary artery or vascular conduit to restore the luminal integrity of the vessel, designed to release the coating into the vessel wall to prevent neointimal growth and restenosis.
Early stent thrombosis (EST): Stent thrombosis occurring between 0 and 30 days after implantation: acute, <24 h; subacute, 1-30 days.
Late stent thrombosis (LST): Stent thrombosis occurring between 30 days and 1 year after implantation.
Very late stent thrombosis (VLST): Stent thrombosis occurring more than 1 year after implantation.
Aspirin effect: Aspirin irreversibly acetylates platelet cyclooxygenase-1, preventing formation of thromboxane A_2 and, thus, stimulation of platelet aggregation.
$P2Y_{12}$ receptor antagonist: A class of drugs that induce irreversible conformational change in the $P2Y_{12}$ receptor for adenosine diphosphate (ADP) and inhibit platelet aggregation and limit ADP-mediated conversion of glycoprotein IIb-IIIa to its active form.

restenosis, compared with BMSs, without increasing the overall risk of MI and death.

Stent thrombosis has surfaced as the major safety concern following the placement of coronary artery stents in practice today. A review of published data indicates no difference between DES and BMS in terms of risk of early or late stent thrombosis (0.1% and 0.9%, respectively). However, the risk for very late stent thrombosis with a DES is much higher than with a BMS (0.6-0.7% vs. 0.0-0.2%, respectively). The data also indicate that the risk of stent thrombosis is higher in patients treated with a DES for off-label use compared with patients treated for on-label use. The exact mechanism remains unclear, but several factors have been implicated. Some risk factors associated with early or late stent thrombosis include early cessation of dual antiplatelet therapy, clopidogrel unresponsiveness, complexity of lesions, multistent implantation, small lesion diameter, and lesions longer than 28 to 30 mm. Risk factors associated with very late stent thrombosis include factors such as renal failure and prior brachytherapy (Table 144-3). Other complications of PCI include hemorrhage, MI, stroke, and contrast-induced nephropathy.

Hemorrhage that results in hemodynamic instability or transfusion therapy arises in approximately 0.5% to 4% of patients who have undergone PCI and is dependent on several factors, including patient characteristics, the specifics of the procedure, and patient-specific pharmacologic variables. These factors include, but are not limited to, age and sex, location of femoral arteriotomy, and level of antithrombotic therapy. The risk of stroke is relatively low (<0.2%), whereas MI complicates 5% to 38% of PCIs, with the rate depending upon the definition used for MI. New Q-wave appearance has an incidence of 1%, whereas any elevation of creatine kinase-MB occurs in up to 38% of patients. Contrast-induced nephropathy is also dependent upon multiple variables, including age, presence of congestive heart failure, preexisting renal failure, previous exposure to contrast agents, and the presence of peripheral vascular disease and is seen in about 5% to 6% patients.

Recommendations

The American College of Cardiology/American Heart Association guidelines currently recommend antiplatelet therapy for a minimum of 1 month or 4 to 6 weeks for a BMS and a minimum of 12 months and, possibly indefinitely with DES implantation, especially in patients who are at higher risk for developing thrombosis. Premature discontinuation of antiplatelet therapy has been shown to result in an increased risk of life-threatening stent thrombosis. The guidelines also recommend that nonurgent surgical procedures be postponed until after these periods of susceptibility. If the operations cannot be delayed, they may need to be performed while the patient is on dual therapy or aspirin alone because surgery itself causes a prothrombotic state. If platelet $P2Y_{12}$ receptor antagonist must be withheld, it should be done for, optimally, 5 days preoperatively or fewer days for patients with DESs, who are at higher risk for developing thrombosis. After the procedure, platelet $P2Y_{12}$ receptor antagonist therapy should be restarted as soon as possible. Some reports have shown that 6% of patients with DESs who undergo noncardiac operations within 1 year of implantation experience a major cardiac event. Therefore, patients in need of noncardiac operations within 1 year of DES implantation or within 1 month of BMS implantation should be carefully evaluated for the risk of ischemic events and bleeding. Maximizing the success of the operation requires collaboration among the cardiologist, surgeon, and anesthesiologist and sufficient lead time (2 weeks) before the procedure that will allow for implementation of a perioperative, intraoperative, and postoperative plan. Discussion with the patient of treatment options is also necessary for the patient to make an informed decision. The operation should be performed at a facility with the ability to perform emergency PCI or cardiac surgery. Stent thrombosis typically presents as acute MI, cardiogenic shock, and sudden death; thus, immediate thrombus retrieval is essential. Finally, it is imperative to educate patients about the risks of early discontinuation of dual antiplatelet therapy and encourage compliance with their prescribed regimen.

Suggested Readings

Cohn L. Myocardial revascularization with percutaneous devices. *Cardiac Surgery in the Adult*. 3rd ed. New York: McGraw-Hill; 2008:Ch 21.
Garg S, Serruys PW. Coronary stents: Current status. *J Am Coll Cardiol*. 2010;56:S1-42.
Garg S, Serruys PW. Coronary stents: Looking forward. *J Am Coll Cardiol*. 2010;56:S43-78.
The American Society of Anesthesiologists Committee on Standards and Practice Parameters. Practice alert for the perioperative management of patients with coronary artery stents. *Anesthesiology*. 2009;110:22-23.
Savonitto S, D'Urbano M, Caracciolo M, et al. Urgent surgery in patients with a recently implanted coronary drug-eluting stent: A phase II study of "bridging" antiplatelet therapy with tirofiban during temporary withdrawal of clopidogrel. *Br J Anaesth*. 2010;104:285-291.

Table 144-3 Risk Factors for Stent Thrombosis

Lesion-Specific Factors	Patient Risk Factors	Procedural Factors	Device Factors
Bifurcation stenting	Renal failure	Inadequate stent expansion	Hypersensitivity to drug coating/polymer
Ostial stenting	Diabetes	Incomplete stent apposition	Incomplete endothelialization
Lesion/stent length	Left ventricular impairment	Stent deployment in necrotic lumen	Stent design
Vessel/stent diameter	Prior brachytherapy		
Multiple stents/vessels	Prior subacute stent thrombosis		
Left main artery stent	Premature cessation of dual antiplatelet therapy		
Bypass graft stent	Clopidogrel unresponsiveness		
Calcification of vessel	STEMI		

STEMI, ST-segment elevation myocardial infarction.

CHAPTER 145

Off-Pump Coronary Artery Bypass and Minimally Invasive Direct Coronary Artery Bypass

Roxann D. Barnes Pike, MD

Definitions and Indications

Cardiopulmonary bypass (CPB) can be avoided for coronary artery bypass grafting (CABG) by using either off-pump coronary artery bypass (OPCAB) or minimally invasive direct coronary artery bypass (MIDCAB). OPCAB involves CABG of one or more vessels accessed via a median sternotomy on the beating heart. MIDCAB consists of CABG done through a lateral anterior thoracotomy on the beating heart. The initial indication for MIDCAB was to treat patients with single-vessel disease that was not amenable to percutaneous transluminal coronary angioplasty and who wanted to avoid the deleterious effects of CPB.

In both techniques, each diseased artery is identified and immobilized, often using a specialized stabilization device. Improved results and more reliable and reproducible coronary anastomoses are achieved when mechanical stabilization devices are used (Figure 145-1). The stenotic segments are bypassed without the use of CPB or the need for cardioplegia or hypothermia.

Advantages and Disadvantages of Minimally Invasive Direct Coronary Artery Bypass and Off-Pump Coronary Artery Bypass

Advantages

The purported advantages of MIDCAB over the tradional approach for CPB include the avoidance of a median sternotomy with its associated risk of sternal wound infection and reduced musculoskeletal injury. OPCAB and MIDCAB can be used either as primary operations or as reoperations, and both avoid the adverse effects associated with the systemic inflammatory response syndrome in response to CPB and its deleterious effects, such as coagulation derangements, microvascular thromboembolism and endothelial dysfunction, arrhythmias, and multiorgan dysfunction. Cannulation, with manipulation and cross-clamping of the ascending aorta, required with CPB increases the risk of aortic dissection and of neurologic sequelae, such as neurocognitive dysfunction and stroke. A recent meta-analysis showed a significant reduction in perioperative stroke after OPCAB versus on-pump coronary revascularization. Other purported advantages of MIDCAB and OPCAB over conventional CPB include decreased surgical time, decreased need for transfusion, less atrial fibrillation, shorter hospital lengths of stay, and possibly decreased cost.

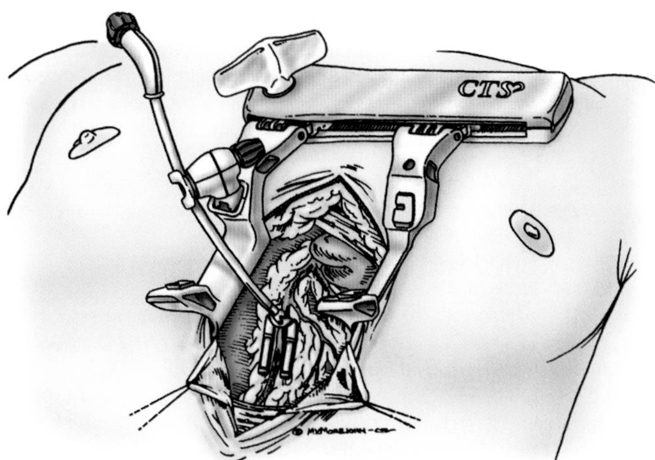

Figure 145-1 Example of an off-pump coronary artery bypass stabilization device.

Disadvantages

The main disadvantage associated with the use of MIDCAB and OPCAB, compared with conventional CABG, is lack of optimal exposure of coronary vessels. MIDCAB allows the most limited exposure; therefore, fewer vessels can be grafted—often only the internal thoracic artery to the left anterior descending artery. Other vessels must be treated with angioplasty. OPCAB, however, allows grafting of multiple vessels. MIDCAB is also associated with more trauma to costal cartilages (with or without removal of rib segments) and more postoperative pain. Both procedures are associated with more hemodynamic instability (especially during displacement of the heart with OPCAB), which may pressure the surgeon to perform the procedure more quickly and, along with limited exposure, result in questionable anastomotic quality and completeness of revascularization. Patients will benefit from on-pump CABG if they have multiple lesions and their anatomy is complex. Patients who are not at increased risk for developing the complications associated with CPB have more effective revascularization if an on-pump CABG is performed. Overall, graft patency rate is higher and mortality is likely lower after on-pump CABG, compared with OPCAB.

Anesthetic Technique

Preparation and Monitoring

Large-bore intravenous cannulas are needed for volume resuscitation, if and when it is necessary. Crossmatched blood should be available, and intraoperative collection and reinfusion of shed autologous blood is recommended. A CPB machine with the circuit setup should be available with a perfusionist on standby.

Patients are typically hemodynamically unstable, and, thus, extensive invasive monitoring is indicated. Placement of an arterial cannula for continuous monitoring of arterial pressure is critical, with careful site selection if harvesting of the radial artery is planned. A pulmonary artery catheter is useful for assessing volume status and serial cardiac output measurement and for placement of electrical leads for transvenous pacing; a pulmonary artery catheter with the capability of measuring cardiac output and mixed venous O_2 saturation is especially useful. A pulmonary artery catheter with multiple central ports allows concomitant instillation of various vasoactive drugs.

With MIDCAB, access is limited should the need arise to defibrillate or pace the heart; therefore, external defibrillator and pacing pads are used. Transesophageal echocardiography is used to assess global ventricular function, regional wall motion abnormalities, and volume status.

Induction and Maintenance

To avoid prolonged intubation, a "fast-track" anesthetic approach is used, limiting opioids to 2 μg/kg of sufentanil, 10 μg/kg of fentanyl, or an infusion of remifentanil. Any anesthetic technique that facilitates early extubation and provides hemodynamic stability is acceptable.

Some surgeons prefer one-lung ventilation during the procedure for improved exposure. For MIDCAB, one-lung ventilation is particularly useful if the internal thoracic artery pedicle is harvested thoracoscopically. The use of one-lung ventilation is not necessary with OPCAB.

The use of antifibrolytic agents is not indicated for these procedures because of the concern that their use might contribute to graft thrombosis.

Induced bradycardia facilitates surgical success, especially with MIDCAB. Besides optimizing the surgical field, bradycardia reduces myocardial O_2 demand until revascularization is complete. Bradycardia may be facilitated by the choice of anesthetic agent (Box 145-1). Induced bradycardia is less critical with OPCAB since the advent of newer stabilization devices, such as the CTS retractor, the Octopus, and the Cohn stabilizer (see Figure 145-1). These devices hold a segment of the diseased coronary artery immobile while the heart is beating so that the anastomoses can be performed.

Surgery on the beating heart readily precipitates arrhythmia—from ischemia, manipulation, and reperfusion—that must be treated aggressively. Lidocaine and magnesium are used routinely; other antiarrhythmic agents must be readily available, and antiarrhythmic strategies may be used (Box 145-2).

Box 145-1 Agents Used in Off-Pump Coronary Artery Bypass Grafting That Decrease the Risk of Patients Developing Bradycardia

β-Adrenergic receptor blocking agents such as esmolol, as a bolus or infusion, or labetalol
Calcium channel blocking agents
Neuromuscular blocking agents that do not induce tachycardia
Opioids such as fentanyl, sufentanil, and remifentanil

Box 145-2 Strategies to Minimize the Risk of or to Treat Arrhythmias Associated with the Use of Off-Pump Coronary Artery Bypass Grafting

Continuing antiarrhythmic medication
Correcting electrolyte and acid-base abnormalities
Ensuring that defibrillation pads are placed preoperatively
Having lidocaine and magnesium boluses and/or infusions, as well as other antiarrhythmic medications, readily available
Having the surgeon temporarily stop manipulation
Preventing myocardial ischemia
Treating excessive bradycardia pharmacologically or with epicardial or transvenous pacing

Surgical Considerations

After anesthesia induction, saphenous vein, radial artery, or both saphenous vein and radial artery harvesting is accomplished. A median sternotomy (OPCAB) or anterior thoracotomy (MIDCAB) is used. One half to two thirds of a full heparinizing dose for CPB (150-200 units/kg) is given. The internal thoracic artery is dissected. The activated clotting time is checked every 30 min, and additional heparin doses of 3000 to 5000 units are given as necessary to maintain an activated clotting time of 300-350 sec. Antiarrhythmic agents are given before vessel occlusion is done. Baseline cardiac output pulmonary artery pressures, and ST-segment analyses are assessed before and after vessel occlusion to guide interventions.

To facilitate surgical exposure, the heart must be lifted and rotated. When the heart is repositioned, venous return is compromised, causing insufficient preload and a possibly precipitous drop in cardiac output. Fluid resuscitation, inotropic medications, and peripheral vasoconstricting agents (e.g., phenylephrine) are used. Mean arterial pressures must be maintained at or above preoperative pressures to ensure adequate coronary perfusion.

Once the internal thoracic artery is anastomosed to the left anterior descending artery, hemodynamics improve. If necessary, vein grafts or radial artery grafts are then grafted to other coronary arteries. For OPCAB proximal anastomoses, a side-biting C-clamp is placed on the aorta while the blood pressure is temporarily reduced. Nitroglycerin causes vasodilation of the coronary arteries, prevents vasospasm of the radial artery, and reduces wall stress during ischemic periods. Sodium nitroprusside can also be used for rapid titratable control of blood pressure.

If the patient's heart cannot tolerate the ischemia from vessel occlusion, options include stenting of the artery via an arteriotomy or emergent institution of CPB. Although the stented vessel provides blood flow to distal ischemic myocardium, there is a risk of intimal dissection.

Postoperative Considerations

The incision is closed after all anastomoses are completed. Heparin is not routinely reversed, or only partially reversed. The patient may be extubated in the operating room. Infiltration of a local anesthetic agent into the anterior thoracotomy wound reduces postoperative pain.

Suggested Readings

Abu-Omar Y, Taggert DP. The present status of off-pump coronary artery bypass grafting. *Eur J Cardiothorac Surg*. 2009;36:312-321.

Baincridge D, Cheng DC. Minimally invasive direct coronary artery bypass and off-pump coronary artery bypass surgery: anesthetic considerations. *Anesthesiol Clin*. 2008;26:437-452.

Couture P, Denault A, Limoges P, et al. Mechanisms of hemodynamic changes during off-pump coronary artery bypass surgery. *Can J Anaesth*. 2002;49: 835-849.

Gayes JM. The minimally invasive cardiac surgery voyage. *J Cardiothorac Vasc Anesth*. 1999;13:119-122.

Hu S, Zheng Z, Yuan X, et al. Increasing long-term major vascular events and resource consumption in patients receiving off-pump coronary artery bypass: a single-center prospective observational study. *Circulation*. 2010;121: 1800-1808.

Kuss O, von Salviati B, Borgermann J. Off-pump versus on-pump coronary artery bypass grafting: a systematic review and meta-analysis of propensity score analyses. *J Thorac Cardiovasc Surg*. 2010;140:829-835.

Lytle BW. On-pump and off-pump coronary bypass surgery. *Circulation*. 2007; 116:1108-1109.

Marasco SF, Sharwood LN, Abramson MJ. No improvement in neurocognitive outcomes after off-pump versus on-pump coronary revascularisation: A meta-analysis. *Eur J Cardiothorac Surg*. 2008;33:961-970.

Møller CH, Perko MJ, Lund JT, et al. No major differences in 30-day outcomes in high-risk patients randomized to off-pump versus on-pump coronary bypass surgery: The Best Bypass Surgery Trial. *Circulation*. 2010;121;498-504.

Nierich AP, Diephuis J, Jansen EW, et al. Heart displacement during off-pump CABG: How well is it tolerated? *Ann Thorac Surg*. 2000;70:466-472.

Pillai JB, Suri RM. Coronary artery surgery and extracorporeal circulation: The search for a new standard. *J Cardiothorac Vasc Anesth*. 2008;22:594-610.
Selke FW, Chu LM, Cohn WE. Current state of surgical myocardial revascularization. *Circ J*. 2010;74:1031-1037.
Sharony R, Bizekis CS, Kanchuger M, et al. Off-pump coronary artery bypass grafting reduces mortality and stroke in patients with atheromatous aortas: a case control study. *Circulation*. 2003;108:II15-20.
Shroyer AL, Grover FL, Hattler B, et al. On-pump versus off-pump coronary bypass surgery. *N Engl J Med*. 2009;361:1827-1837.
Takagi H, Matsui M, Umemoto T. Lower graft patency after off-pump than on-pump coronary artery bypass grafting: an updated meta-analysis of randomized trials. *J Thorac Cardiovasc Surg*. 2010;140:e45-e47.
Takagi H, Matsui M, Umemoto T. Off-pump coronary artery bypass may increase late mortality: a meta-analysis of randomized trials. *Ann Thorac Surg*. 2010;89:1881-1888.

CHAPTER 146

Cardiopulmonary Bypass

David J. Cook, MD, and Eduardo S. Rodrigues, MD

Cardiopulmonary bypass (CPB) replaces heart and lung function during cardiopulmonary arrest. The basic features of the circuit are a pump, an oxygenator, and venous return and arterial inflow lines. A heat exchanger and a blood reservoir are also essential elements.

Cardiopulmonary Bypass Circuit Structure

A right atrial or bicaval cannula is the source for drainage of blood into the venous reservoir. Blood exits the reservoir, goes to a pump (roller or centrifugal), and is pumped through an oxygenator (typically hollow fiber), most of which have integrated heat exchangers. For hollow-fiber oxygenators, the Pao_2 is determined by the Fio_2 of the fresh-gas flow passing countercurrent through the hollow fibers; the $Paco_2$ is determined by the total gas flow rate though the oxygenator. The pressurized oxygenated blood then typically passes through an arterial line filter before entering the aortic cannula (usually placed in the proximal aorta).

Additional features of the CPB circuit include several monitors of temperature and oxygenation, a cardioplegia delivery system, and a means for cardiotomy suctioning and ventricular venting.

Control of Systemic Oxygenation During Cardiopulmonary Bypass

The factors that control systemic oxygenation during non-CPB conditions also control oxygenation during CPB. Oxygen requirements are most profoundly affected by body temperature, whereas O_2 delivery $\dot{D}o_2$ is determined by pump flow and hematocrit.

The Basic Relationships

$$\text{Arterial } O_2 \text{ content } (Cao_2) = 1.34\,(\text{hemoglobin})\,(O_2\text{sat\%}) + 0.003\,(Pao_2)$$

$$\text{Arteriovenous } O_2 \text{ content difference } (Cao_2 - C\overline{v}o_2) = Cao_2 - C\overline{v}o_2$$

$$\text{Systemic } \dot{D}o_2 = \text{cardiac output or CPB pump flow} \times Cao_2$$

$$\text{Systemic } O_2 \text{ consumption } (\dot{V}o_2) = \text{cardiac output} \times (Cao_2 - C\overline{v}o_2)$$

The temperature coefficient (Q_{10}) describes the ratio of metabolic rates at two temperatures separated by 10° C. In humans, the Q10 is approximately 2 (i.e., when a patient's temperature rises from 27° C to 37° C, the metabolic rate doubles. Conversely, every 10° C decrease in body temperature decreases the $\dot{V}o_2$ by about 50%.

The General Practice of Cardiopulmonary Bypass

Nonpulsatile flow (2.0-2.5 $L \cdot min^{-1} \cdot m^{-2}$) is based on the cardiac index under anesthesia in non-CPB conditions. The flow rate may also be expressed as $mL \cdot kg^{-1} \cdot min^{-1}$. The most recent literature suggests that mild to moderate hypothermia more close to the normal range (i.e., 28° C-35° C) reduces the incidence of low cardiac output syndromes without an attendant increase in neurologic complications.

Moderate normovolemic hemodilution should be maintained. The literature, comprising primarily retrospective data, suggests that increased complication rates (neurologic, cardiovascular, and renal) occur when the hematocrit is less than 20% to 23%. However, other data suggest that "treating" this anemia with transfusion of red blood cells may worsen outcomes. It is likely that CPB-related anemia is a function of the prebypass period and, therefore, primarily a marker of greater comorbidity instead of being an independent determinant of adverse outcome.

A mean arterial pressure (MAP) of 60 to 80 mm Hg should be maintained. Even with moderate hypothermia, cerebral autoregulation begins to fail below a cerebral perfusion pressure of 50 to 55 mm Hg. In patients with a history of hypertension or peripheral vascular disease, keeping the MAP at a minimum of 70 mm Hg reduces the incidence of adverse cardiac and neurologic outcomes. A practical way to calculate the goal MAP during CPB is to use the patient's age as a goal for MAP in patients older than 60 years of age.

Cardiopulmonary Bypass Hemodynamics and Hemodilution

Under non-CPB conditions, moderate hemodilution decreases Cao_2 but may not decrease $\dot{D}o_2$ because hemodilution is associated with increases in cardiac output. However, during CPB, pump flow is typically less than the cardiac output that would be seen with equivalent hemodilution under non-CPB conditions, resulting in a decrease in whole body $\dot{D}o_2$ during CPB, which is approximately equivalent to the degree of hemodilution. Additionally, in the absence of increases in compensatory flow, MAP during CPB is typically reduced because the lower blood viscosity associated with hemodilution reduces systemic vascular resistance (SVR).

Effect of Temperature Change on Systemic Oxygenation

Hypothermia to 27°C reduces systemic O_2 requirements by approximately 60%. Because O_2 demand decreases so dramatically with hypothermia, adequate oxygenation can be maintained with reduced flows, greater degrees of hemodilution, or a combination thereof. However, during the early and late CPB period, when patients approximate normothermia, the margin between systemic O_2 supply and demand is narrowed. A beneficial effect of hypothermia is that the associated increases in SVR may offset the reductions in SVR associated with hemodilution alone.

Effect of Anesthetic Depth on Systemic Oxygenation

Anesthetic depth has less influence than does hypothermia on $\dot{V}o_2$ during CPB. However, anesthetic depth is of greater relative importance at body temperatures above 32°C. Plasma levels of anesthetic agents decrease with the onset of CPB secondary to dilution from an increased circulatory volume. Therefore, intravenous infusion techniques or the use of inhalation agents during CPB helps ensure adequate anesthesia.

Monitoring the Adequacy of Perfusion During Cardiopulmonary Bypass

Systemic O_2 Saturation

Mixed venous O_2 saturation ($S\bar{v}o_2$) reflects venous O_2 content, i.e., the amount of O_2 left in the venous blood after systemic O_2 requirements are met. Although $S\bar{v}o_2$ does not measure either $\dot{V}o_2$ or $\dot{D}o_2$, it does provide an index of the adequacy of their matching. As such, $S\bar{v}o_2$ monitoring conveys extremely valuable information as to the interaction among systemic O_2 requirements, pump flow, arterial O_2 content, hematocrit level, and temperature. An $S\bar{v}o_2$ above 65% generally indicates a satisfactory margin of safety for systemic oxygenation. A higher saturation is indicated during hypothermia given that hypothermia increases the O_2 affinity of hemoglobin.

In-line hemoglobin or hematocrit monitors are available and are usually coupled to the $S\bar{v}o_2$ detector. Temperature monitoring is performed in three areas: the venous line (reflecting the adequacy of whole body cooling or warming), the arterial inflow line, and the heat exchanger, where temperature should not exceed 38.5°C. Optional arterial in-flow line-monitoring devices are available to monitor gases (Pao_2, pH, $Paco_2$, base deficit, and temperature).

Difficulties in Maintaining Systemic Oxygenation During Cardiopulmonary Bypass

During stable hypothermia, systemic oxygenation is easy to maintain, but the transitions to and from hypothermia can be a problem. Initiation of CPB is associated with nearly instantaneous hemodilution and decreased SVR. In the absence of increased flow, hypotension commonly occurs until cooling is initiated, SVR is increased pharmacologically, or volume resuscitation occurs.

During rewarming from CPB, SVR and MAP will fall as vasodilation occurs and blood viscosity decreases. This occurs at a time when systemic O_2 demand may double (27° C-37° C).

Cardioplegia

Cardioplegia with a high-K^+ solution results in depolarization and diastolic arrest. This induces electromechanical silence and reduces myocardial O_2 demand by more than 80%. The use of cardioplegia is indicated when the aortic cross-clamp is in place because there is no coronary blood flow at this time. Cardioplegia may consist of an oxygenated blood–high-K^+ mixture (blood cardioplegia) or high-K^+ solution alone (crystalloid cardioplegia). Cardioplegia is usually given intermittently into the aorta proximal to the cross-clamp (antegrade) or directly into the coronary ostia. Retrograde cardioplegia via the coronary sinus is also used. Left ventricular hypertrophy and coronary artery disease make myocardial protection more difficult to achieve.

Suggested Readings

Cook DJ. Changing temperature management for cardiopulmonary bypass. *Anesth Analg*. 1999;88:1254-1271.

Cook DJ. Optimal conditions for cardiopulmonary bypass. *Semin Cardiothorac Vasc Anesth*. 2001;5:265-272.

DiNardo JA. *Anesthesia for Cardiac Surgery*. Norwalk, CT: Appleton & Lange; 1998.

Gravlee GP, Davis RF, Kurusz M, et al. *Cardiopulmonary Bypass: Principles and Practice*. Baltimore: Lippincott, Williams & Wilkins; 2000.

Mangano CM, Hill L, Cartwright CR, et al. Cardiopulmonary bypass and the anesthesiologist. In: Kaplan JA, ed. *Cardiac Anesthesia*. 4th ed. Philadelphia: WB Saunders; 1999:1061.

Murphy GS, Hessel EA, Groom RC. Optimal perfusion during cardiopulmonary bypass: An evidence-based approach. *Anesth Analg*. 2009;108:1394-1417.

Shanewise JS, Hug CC Jr. Anesthesia for adult cardiac surgery. In: Miller RD, ed. *Anesthesia*. 5th ed. Philadelphia: Churchill Livingstone; 2000:1753.

CHAPTER 147

Evaluation of the Coagulation System

Craig M. Combs, MD, and Robert M. Craft, MD

Evaluation of the coagulation system may be useful for the preoperative assessment of coagulation status and measurement of anticoagulation therapy, as well as the diagnosis and management of intraoperative coagulopathy. The dual-cascade concept of coagulation, which involves the intrinsic and extrinsic pathways, is now understood to be an inadequate and incomplete representation of in vivo coagulation. The three-stage process of actual in vivo coagulation (activation, amplification, and propagation) involves complex interactions among the vascular endothelium, tissue factor, platelets, and soluble clotting factors. However, the classic dual-cascade view may still be beneficial in providing a reasonable model of in vitro coagulation tests, that is, the activated partial thromboplastin time (aPTT) and prothrombin time (PT) (Figure 147-1).

Preoperative Assessment

The best method to screen patients preoperatively for bleeding disorders remains a thorough clinical history. Routine coagulation testing is not warranted without indications. Clinical indications for testing include congenital or acquired bleeding disorders, excessive bleeding during previous operations, liver disease, and the use of drugs or supplements with anticoagulant properties. Table 147-1 summarizes the most common preoperative coagulation studies used for assessing the coagulation status of patients.

Common Point-of-Care Tests of Coagulation

Point-of-care (POC) testing, or testing at the bedside, has become more frequently used in the perioperative period due to the technologic advancement and miniaturization of monitoring devices. The benefits of POC tests, compared with conventional laboratory-based tests, include faster turnaround times and the ability to assess the coagulation status of whole blood. POC monitors that are currently available can be used to measure the ability of blood to generate clot, heparin concentrations, the viscoelastic properties of whole blood, and platelet function.

Functional Measures of Coagulation

Activated Clotting Time

The activated clotting time (ACT) measures the adequacy of the intrinsic and common pathways. Fresh whole blood is added to a contact activation initiator, such as celite or kaolin, that initiates and accelerates clot formation, and the time to clot formation is measured. Two commercial ACT monitors currently in use, the Hemochron (International Technidyne, Inc., Edison, NJ) and the Hepcon and ACT II (Medtronic Blood Management, Parker, CO) automate clot detection by different mechanisms.

Clinically, the ACT is commonly used in the operating room to monitor heparin therapy. Advantages of the ACT are its low cost, simplicity of use, speed, and linear response even at high heparin concentrations. However, the utility of the ACT is affected by poor reproducibility of results and low sensitivity to low heparin concentrations. Factors that can prolong the ACT are hypothermia, hemodilution, thrombocytopenia, and platelet dysfunction.

Heparin Concentration Measurement

The most common method for assessing heparin concentration in the perioperative period is protamine titration. Protamine titration is capable of measuring heparin concentrations due to the fact that every 1 mg of protamine will inhibit approximately 100 units of heparin (1 mg). Thus, if a blood sample is divided and analyzed with several doses of protamine, the portion with the closest heparin and protamine concentrations will clot most rapidly. The appropriate heparin dose to obtain a specific plasma heparin concentration can be determined, as well as the amount of protamine needed to reverse a specific heparin concentration. Advantages of the protamine titration method include relative resistance to the effects of hypothermia and hemodilution, as well as sensitivity at low heparin concentrations. POC monitors currently in use, such as Hepcon HMS (Medtronic Blood Management), use automated measurement techniques.

Viscoelastic Measures of Coagulation

Thromboelastography and the Sonoclot

The thromboelastograph (TEG) (Haemascope, Niles, IL), like other viscoelastic measures of coagulation, is capable of measuring the complete coagulation process, from initial fibrin formation through fibrinolysis. The changes in viscoelasticity at all stages are both measured and displayed graphically. Even though the various TEG parameters do not directly correlate with other laboratory-based coagulation tests, they do correlate with specific abnormalities throughout the coagulation process. Figure 147-2 displays the variables measured by the TEG, as well as common abnormalities. Although the TEG is occasionally used in cardiac and trauma surgery, it is most frequently utilized during liver transplantation. The amounts of packed red blood cells and fresh frozen plasma that are transfused are lower when the TEG is used to guide transfusion, compared with transfusing based on routine coagulation tests.

The Sonoclot Analyzer (Sienco, Inc., Arvada, CO) is another device used to monitor the viscoelastic properties of blood. It provides information on the entire hemostatic process in both a qualitative and quantitative fashion. The qualitative graph is known as the Sonoclot Signature (Figure 147-3), and the quantitative results measured are the ACT, the clot rate, and platelet function.

Platelet Function Monitors

Optical platelet aggregometry is considered by many to be the reference standard for platelet function monitoring, although the method suffers from a lack of standardization, as well as the cost of the test itself and the amount

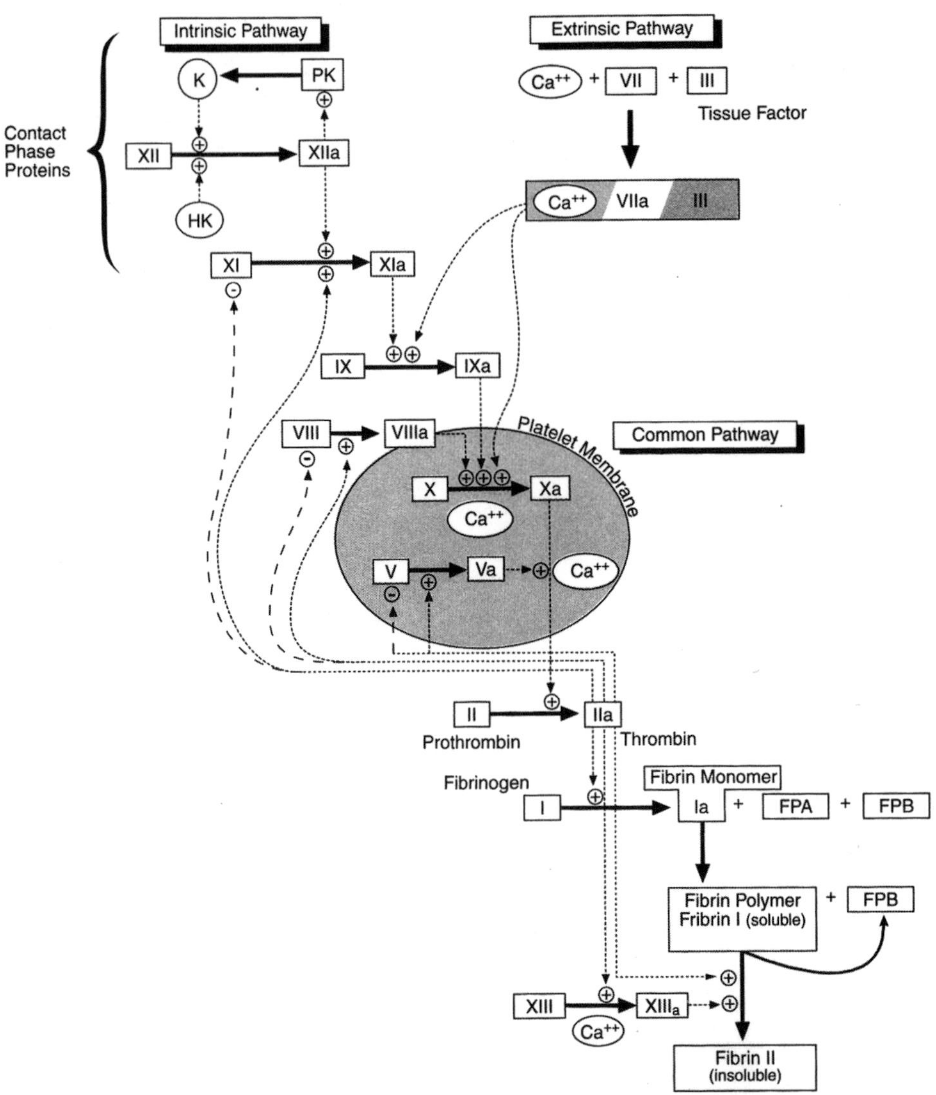

Figure 147-1 Activation of proteins leading to blood coagulation. A positive-feedback system (amplification) magnifies initial pathway reactions. A negative-feedback system (inhibition) serves as a countervailing force and limits coagulation. Dotted arrows and + signs indicate facilitation of the process; dashed arrows and − signs indicate inhibition of the process. The intrinsic pathway is initiated by the action of kallikrein (K) and high-molecular-weight kininogen (HK) and prekallikrein (PK) cofactors on factor XII. Fibrinopeptide A (FPA) and fibrinopeptide B (FPB) are two peptides released when the fibrin monomer is formed. (From Carvalho ACA. Hemostasis and thrombosis. In: Schiffman FJ, ed. Hematologic pathophysiology. Philadelphia: Lippincott-Raven; 1998:161-243.)

of labor required to perform the test. As mentioned previously, viscoelastic coagulation tests (TEG and Sonoclot) reflect platelet dysfunction, but without significant modification (such as the platelet mapping [Haemascope] paradigm), they have limited sensitivity and specificity. Several platelet function monitors have recently been marketed as POC devices, including the PFA-100 (Platelet Function Analyzer; Dade International Inc., Miami, FL) and Plateletworks (Helena Laboratories, Beaumont, TX). The PFA-100 simulates injury via a membrane with an aperture that contains platelet activators (adenosine diphosphate or epinephrine) and has been shown to be capable of identifying congenital and acquired platelet dysfunction. Plateletworks measures the percentage of aggregation of platelets in the presence and absence of collagen or adenosine diphosphate and correlates with optical platelet aggregometry. Unfortunately, there remains a remarkable variability of results when all of these methods are compared.

Table 147-1 Studies Commonly Used Preoperatively for Assessing Patients' Coagulation Status

Test	Measured Aspect	Comments
PT	Extrinsic pathway and common pathway	The PT is prolonged if any of factors VII, X, V, II, and I are deficient, abnormal, or inhibited. The coagulant activity of these factors must be <30% of normal and the fibrinogen concentration must be <100 mg/dL for the PT to be prolonged. The PT may be used as a screening test for patients on oral anticoagulant therapy. The PT may be used to assess the synthetic function of the liver.
aPTT	Intrinsic pathway and common pathway	The aPTT is prolonged when any of factors XII, XI, IX, VIII, X, V, II, and I are deficient, abnormal, or inhibited. The coagulant activity of these factors must be <30% of normal and the fibrinogen concentration must be <100 mg/dL for the PT to be prolonged. The aPTT is prolonged by heparin therapy. The aPTT is prolonged in hemophiliacs and, usually, in people with von Willebrand disease.
Fibrinogen	Fibrinogen level; common pathway	Levels <100 mg/dL may be associated with the inability to form a clot and severe bleeding.
Platelet count	Quantitative platelet assessment	The platelet count does not provide information regarding platelet function. Thrombocytopenia is defined as a platelet count <150,000/μL. Bleeding during surgery may be severe in patients with platelet counts of 40,000-70,000/μL. Spontaneous bleeding is unlikely to occur if the platelet count is >10,000-20,000/μL.
Bleeding time	Platelet function assessed by evaluating the time for a platelet plug to form after vascular injury	Bleeding times are prolonged in patients with platelet dysfunction (e.g., patients on aspirin therapy or those who are uremic). Owing to the techniques used for the test, reproducibility is poor, and results are imprecise. The bleeding time is not useful for routine screening.
Platelet aggregometry	Assesses the ability of platelets to aggregate after exposure to ADP, epinephrine, collagen, or ristocetin	Only qualitative results (clot retraction versus no clot retraction) are reported. Quantitative results are difficult to obtain.

ADP, Adenosine diphosphate; aPTT, activated partial thromboplastin time; PT, prothrombin time.

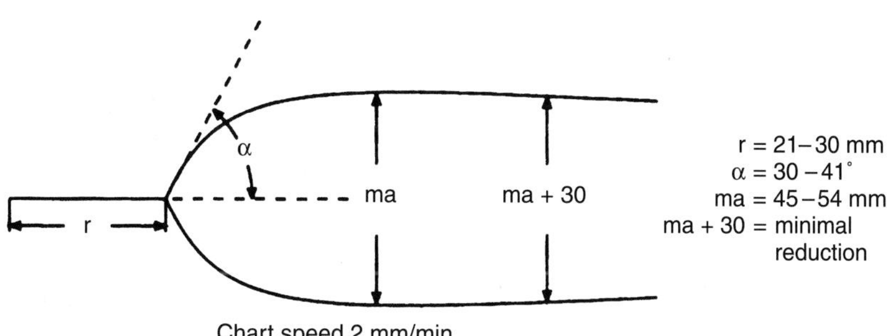

Variable	Measures	Abnormality		Example
r reaction time	thromboplastin generation via the intrinsic pathway	↑ r	Factor deficiency Heparin Severe thrombocytopenia	Factor deficiency
α angle of divergence	rate of clot formation	↓ α	Hypofibrinogenemia Thrombocytopenia Thrombocytopathy	Hypofibrinogenemia
ma maximum amplitude	maximum clot strength/elasticity	↓ ma	Thrombocytopenia Thrombocytopathy Hypofibrinogenemia Factor XIII deficiency	Thrombocytopenia
ma + 30	clot retraction after 30 minutes	↓ ma + 30	Fibrinolysis	Fibrinolysis

Figure 147-2 Typical thromboelastograph pattern and variables measured, normal values, and examples of some abnormal tracings.

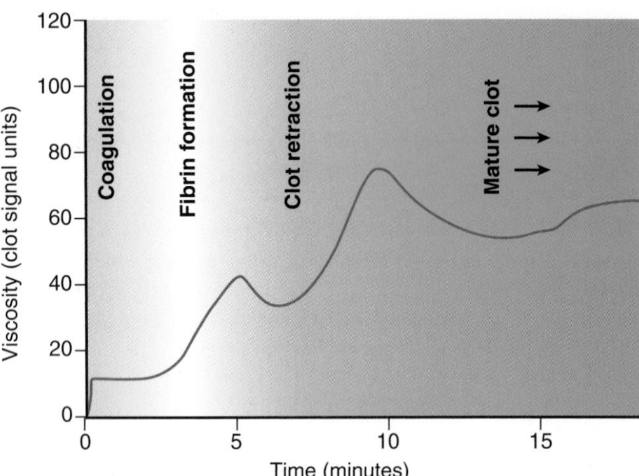

Figure 147-3 As the blood sample clots, a variety of hemostasis-related mechanical changes occur that alter the signal value of the clot. A typical Sonoclot Signature is shown.

Suggested Readings

Carvalho ACA. Hemostasis and thrombosis. In: Schiffman FJ, ed. *Hematologic Pathophysiology*. Philadelphia: Lippincott-Raven; 1998:161-243.

Ganter MT, Hofer CK. Coagulation monitoring: Current techniques and clinical use of viscoelastic point-of-care coagulation devices. *Anesth Analg*. 2008;106:1366-1375.

Kozek-Langenecker SA. Perioperative coagulation monitoring. *Best Pract Res Clin Anaesthesiol*. 2010;24:27-40.

Levy JH, Key NS, Azran MS. Novel oral anticoagulants: Implications in the perioperative setting. *Anesthesiology*. 2010;113(3):726-745.

Shore-Lesserson L. Evidence based coagulation monitors: heparin monitoring, thromboelastography, and platelet function. *Semin Cardiothorac Vasc Anesth*. 2005;9:41-52.

CHAPTER 148

Anticoagulation and Reversal for Cardiopulmonary Bypass

Brian S. Donahue, MD, PhD

Anticoagulation During Cardiopulmonary Bypass

The surfaces of the cardiopulmonary bypass (CPB) circuit are highly thrombogenic and readily activate the coagulation cascade when blood comes in contact with them. To prevent thrombus formation, thrombin generation, and coagulation factor consumption, anticoagulation must be initiated prior to, and sustained during, CPB.

Heparin

Heparin (MW 750-1000 kDa) is a glycosaminoglycan, or mucopolysaccharide, composed of alternating D-glucuronic *N*-acetyl-D-glucosamine acid residues. Heparin has one of the highest negative charge-to-size ratios of any known biologic compound. Heparan sulfate is a related biologic compound that has fewer sulfate groups than heparin and, therefore, has less potency. Heparin inhibits coagulation by serving as a catalyst—antithrombin III (AT) binds to its surface, inducing a conformational change in AT, making its active site more accessible to any of several proteases involved in the intrinsic and common coagulation pathways (thrombin [IIa], factor Xa, factor XIa, factor XIIa, and factor IXa). However, the anticoagulant effects of heparin are primarily mediated by the inhibition of thrombin and factor Xa that occurs when thrombin and factor Xa are bound by AT. Once these covalent bonds are established, the heparin moiety is released and available to bind to another molecule of AT. Heparin also induces the release of tissue factor pathway inhibitor from intravascular endothelium. Fragments of tissue factor pathway inhibitor may contribute to post-CPB coagulopathy.

Administration and Monitoring of Heparin During Cardiopulmonary Bypass

Heparin is administered intravenously as a bolus dose of 300 to 400 units/kg. Traditionally, the extent of inhibition of coagulation has been monitored using the whole-blood activated clotting time (ACT). With this technique, the patient's blood is mixed in a test tube with an activator (e.g., diatomite or kaolin), and the time until clot forms is recorded as the ACT. Although practice varies markedly, most surgeons require an ACT of 400 to 450 sec before they will allow initiation of CPB; however, these limits were established with very little data. The ACT is widely used because it has several advantages: the prolongation of the ACT is generally linear with the heparin level, and the test is widely available, is inexpensive, is easy to perform, and has stood the test of time. However, the ACT has many drawbacks—there is wide variability not only between tests of blood run on different instruments, but also between aliquots of the same blood run on the same instrument. Other methods of anticoagulation monitoring include the measurement of heparin concentration by protamine titration, high-dose thrombin time, and the heparin concentration test. The most popular of these non-ACT methods is the heparin-concentration test, which has been compared with the ACT in efforts to arrive at the most optimal evidence-based management. In a few randomized trials, the heparin-concentration test, compared with the ACT, was found to be associated with greater suppression of the coagulation pathway, decreased perioperative transfusion requirements, and greater total heparin dosing. Overall, a 2006 best-evidence review of point-of-care coagulation testing during CPB concluded that using the heparin-concentration test results in higher heparin and lower protamine dosing, with possible sparing of coagulation system activation and decreased transfusion requirements.

Problems Associated with the Use of Heparin

Heparin-Induced Thrombocytopenia

The occasional patient with heparin-induced thrombocytopenia presents a challenge to the cardiac surgical team. Heparin-induced thrombocytopenia is caused by IgG antibodies that bind to heparin–platelet factor (PF) 4 complexes on platelets, thus activating the platelets and leading to microaggregate formation, thrombocytopenia, and vascular thrombosis (usually arterial). Even without the existence of thrombocytopenia, the very presence of antibodies directed against heparin-PF4 complexes is a risk factor for the occurrence of major adverse events in patients with cardiovascular disease. Currently, many patients with acute heparin-induced thrombocytopenia will undergo plasmapheresis before surgery to effectively reduce antibody levels to zero; however, if plasmapheresis is not available or an emergency arises that does not allow time to perform plasmapheresis, the use of thrombin inhibitors is indicated to anticoagulate the patient.

Heparin Resistance

Up to 20% of patients have heparin resistance, i.e., an inadequate response to an acceptable dose of heparin (as measured via the ACT). When heparin resistance occurs, common practice is to give another dose of heparin from a different vial and lot and, if the ACT is still inadequate, to then replace AT because a decreased level of AT is the usual cause. In the past, fresh frozen plasma was administered, but, increasingly, physicians are administering concentrates of AT.

Nonhemorrhagic Side Effects

As many as 80% of patients receiving heparin will have a transient increase in aminotransferase levels. Approximately 5% to 10% of patients who have received heparin will develop hyperkalemia secondary to heparin-induced aldosterone suppression. The hyperkalemia may appear hours to days after the infusion of heparin.

Problems Associated with Heparin Manufacture

In 2007, lots of heparin were removed from the market because several syringes were found to be contaminated with *Serratia marcescens.* In 2008, Baxter withdrew all of its heparin from the market after more than 80 deaths were associated with its use. The heparin, imported from China, had a contaminant—oversulfated derivatives of chondroitin sulfate, a shellfish-derived supplement.

In 2009, the U.S. Food and Drug Administration notified physicians of a new reference standard to measure the potency of heparin so as to bring the U.S. pharmacopeia unit dose in compliance with the World Health Organization international standard unit dose. This change resulted in an approximately 10% reduction in the potency of the heparin sold in the United States.

Heparin Alternatives for Cardiopulmonary Bypass

Alternatives to the use of heparin in CPB include direct thrombin inhibitors, such as lepirudin and bivalirudin; platelet glycoprotein inhibitors; danaparoid and other heparinoids; and ancrod. Because a specific reversal agent, such as protamine, is lacking for these agents, bivalirudin is the most commonly used heparin alternative because it has the shortest duration of action. The ACT is typically not sensitive enough to the effects of thrombin antagonists to be useful during CPB; therefore, a similar test, the ecarin clotting time, has been developed. In medical institutions in which the ecarin clotting time is not available, success has been reported with the use of a modified ACT.

In two open-label safety trials of bivalirudin in patients with heparin-induced thrombocytopenia who were undergoing either on-pump or off-pump cardiac procedures, the authors reported procedural success rates equivalent to those from cases in which heparin was used. Investigators of the EVOLUTION study—a randomized, open-label, multicenter trial comparing heparin and bivalirudin—reported similar procedural success rates and hemostatic outcomes in patients undergoing either on-pump or off-pump cardiac operations. Koster and colleagues reported acceptable hemostatic results with the use of bivalirudin as an anticoagulant in a series of 141 patients undergoing on-pump or off-pump operations.

Reversal of Heparin Following Cardiopulmonary Bypass

Protamine is a polyanionic peptide that binds rapidly and noncovalently to circulating heparin to inactivate the anticoagulant effect. Although protamine is the chief heparin-reversal agent used in clinical practice, other agents—such as heparinase and heparin-ecarin clotting time 4—have been used.

Excess protamine impairs postoperative platelet function, increases ACT, and may contribute to coagulopathy following CPB. Insufficient protamine results in residual circulating heparin that is too low in concentration to be detected by ACT, yet is high enough to impair coagulation. Ideally, the dose of protamine should be determined by measuring residual heparin concentration or by titrating the protamine dose response. If these techniques are not an option, most clinicians use weight-based dosing as opposed to a fixed dose.

Protamine administration has been associated with a range of systemic cardiovascular reactions, such as vasodilation, pulmonary hypertension, bronchospasm, anaphylaxis, myocardial depression, and circulatory collapse. These reactions may range from mild and clinically inconsequential to severe and ultimately fatal. The immunologic mechanism responsible for protamine reactions is complex and probably involves release of anaphylatoxins and eicosanoids, complement activation, histamine, and preformed antiprotamine or antiprotamine–heparin-complex antibodies. Fish or shellfish allergy, prior use of NPH insulin, and previous vasectomy have been classically taught as risk factors for protamine reactions, although the evidence supporting these associations is weak or anecdotal. Previous exposure to protamine appears to increase the incidence of protamine-induced pulmonary vasoconstriction, whereas preoperative aspirin use seems to decrease it. Treatment of protamine reactions is generally supportive and aimed at restoring normal hemodynamics. The use of inhaled nitric oxide to manage pulmonary hypertension and right-sided heart failure associated with protamine use has been reported.

Suggested Readings

De Somer F, Van Belleghem Y, Caes F, et al. Tissue factor as the main activator of the coagulation system during cardiopulmonary bypass. *J Thorac Cardiovasc Surg*. 2002;123:951-958.

Despotis GJ, Gravlee G, Filos K, Levy J. Anticoagulation monitoring during cardiac surgery: A review of current and emerging techniques. *Anesthesiology*. 1999;91:1122-1151.

Donahue BS, Gailani D, Mast AE. Disposition of tissue factor pathway inhibitor during cardiopulmonary bypass. *J Thromb Haemost*. 2006;4:1011-1016.

Dyke CM, Smedira NG, Koster A, et al. A comparison of bivalirudin to heparin with protamine reversal in patients undergoing cardiac surgery with cardiopulmonary bypass: The EVOLUTION-ON study. *J Thorac Cardiovasc Surg*. 2006;131:533-539.

Fischer T, Kuppe H, Koster A. Impact of heparin management on release of tissue factor pathway inhibitor during cardiopulmonary bypass. *Anesthesiology*. 2004;100:1040.

Greinacher A, Warkentin TE. The direct thrombin inhibitor hirudin. *Thromb Haemost*. 2008;99:819-829.

Koster A, Dyke CM, Aldea G, et al. Bivalirudin during cardiopulmonary bypass in patients with previous or acute heparin-induced thrombocytopenia and heparin antibodies: Results of the CHOOSE-ON trial. *Ann Thorac Surg*. 2007;83:572-577.

Merry AF. Focus on thrombin: Alternative anticoagulants. *Semin Cardiothorac Vasc Anesth*. 2007;11:256-260.

Owings JT, Pollock ME, Gosselin RC, et al. Anticoagulation of children undergoing cardiopulmonary bypass is overestimated by current monitoring techniques. *Arch Surg*. 2000;135:1042-1047.

Spiess BD. Treating heparin resistance with antithrombin or fresh frozen plasma. *Ann Thorac Surg*. 2008;85:2153-2160.

CHAPTER 149
Aortic Stenosis

Martin L. De Ruyter, MD

Clinical Features

Aortic stenosis (AS), the most common cardiac valve lesion among people living in the United States, is found in one fourth of all patients with chronic valve disease. Left ventricular outflow tract obstruction can occur in the subvalvular, valvular, and supravalvular regions. Stenosis of the aortic valve itself is most common, occurring in 75% of patients with outflow tract obstruction. The three major types of AS are (1) a congenital malformation (bicuspid instead of the normal tricuspid valve) that becomes stenotic over decades, (2) calcification or degeneration in a previously normal tricuspid aortic valve, and (3) rheumatic aortic valve disease, which usually occurs in conjunction with mitral valve abnormalities. In developed countries, the number of people with rheumatic AS has declined significantly, so that congenital stenosis (a bicuspid valve that later calcifies) and calcific stenosis of a tricuspid valve have emerged as the more common causes of AS. Between 1% and 2% of the population has a bicuspid aortic valve, which is thought to be inherited as an autosomal-dominant trait with variable penetrance. Flow through a bicuspid valve is turbulent, creating abnormal pressures on the leaflets that lead to thickening of the leaflets and, eventually, stenosis.

The risk factors for calcific degenerative AS are similar to those for atherosclerosis (e.g., older age, male sex, hypertension, hyperlipidemia with evidence of inflammation at the site of disease). However, systemic hypertension occurs in only about half of all patients with AS; a systolic pressure above 200 mm Hg is thought to generally exclude severe narrowing of the valve.

Eighty percent of patients with symptomatic AS are men, approximately 50% will have coronary artery disease, and most of these patients will be at least 70 years old (AS due to a bicuspid valve tends to occur in patients younger than 70 years of age [Figure 149-1]). Overall, however, AS is a disease of the elderly, with a prevalence of more than 4% in North American adults older than 75 years. In a study of 5201 men and women over the age of 65 years, 26% had aortic sclerosis (a thickening of the valve without hemodynamic sequelae), and 2% had AS. The prevalence of aortic sclerosis

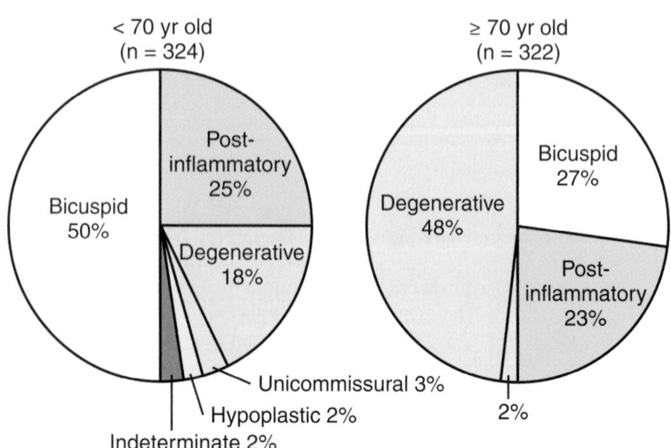

Figure 149-1 Distribution of aortic valve disease based on age. (Adapted from Fuster V, O'Rourke RA, Walsh RA, Poole-Wilson P. Hurst's The Heart. 13th ed. Chapter 76. Available at: http://www.accessmedicine.com.)

increased with age in this study: 20% in patients aged 65 to 75 years, 35% in those aged 75 to 85 years, and 48% in patients older than 85 years (AS rates were 1.3%, 2.4%, and 4%, respectively, in these groups).

Natural History

Patients with AS are at increased risk of dying suddenly (likely from cardiac arrhythmia due to ischemia from mismatching of O_2 supply and demand), yet the typical natural history of AS is a gradual onset of symptoms manifesting in the fifth to seventh decades of life. Aortic sclerosis is not an uncommon finding in patients older than 65 years, but about 16% of patients with sclerosis develop AS within 7 years. Patients with aortic sclerosis are asymptomatic, but once the pressure gradient across the valve exceeds the upper limits of normal, exertional dyspnea, angina, and syncope–the cardinal symptoms of AS–can appear within 5 years. The mortality rate is approximately 25% per year among symptomatic patients (Figure 149-2), with three quarters of those whose AS is untreated dying within 3 years of the onset of symptoms (Figure 149-3). Asymptomatic patients, on the other hand, even those with severe disease, have a more favorable outlook (risk of death <1% per year).

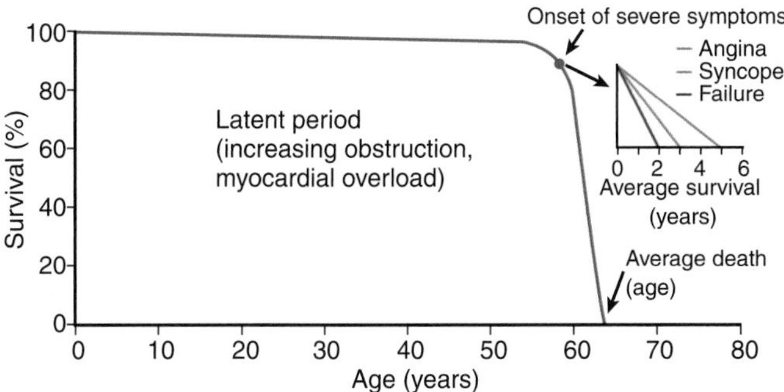

Figure 149-2 Survival of patients with aortic stenosis over time.

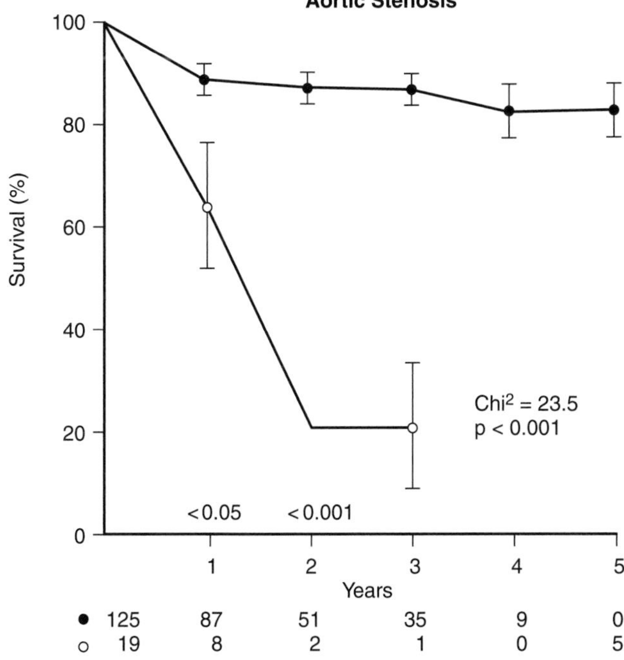

Figure 149-3 Impact of medical intervention on mortality risk in patients with aortic stenosis. (Adapted from Fuster V, O'Rourke RA, Walsh RA, Poole-Wilson P. Hurst's The Heart. 13th ed. Chapter 76. Available at: http://www.accessmedicine.com.)

The typical timeframes from the onset of symptoms until death are 4.5 years for patients with angina, 2.6 years for patients with syncope, 2 years for patients with dyspnea, and 1 year for patients with congestive heart failure, with the latter being the cause of death in one half to two thirds of patients with untreated AS.

Anatomic Considerations

The internal cross-sectional area of a normal aortic valve during systole is 3.0 to 4.0 cm^2; significant hemodynamic obstruction does not occur until the valve area is less than 1.5 cm^2. Based upon measurements of valve area, peak blood flow velocity across the valve (AoVmax), mean pressure gradient, and effective orifice area, the degree of AS is categorized as mild, moderate, severe, or critical and is most commonly assessed with echocardiography (Table 149-1). The measurement of pressure gradients is accurate less than 50% of the time because the pressure gradients are flow dependent. Measuring the valve area is the most reliable method of assessing severity of AS because it depends less on ventricular contractility than do pressure gradients, but measuring valve area using two-dimensional echocardiography has several factors that may limit its usefulness, including the difficulty in obtaining the correct short-axis view, the presence of calcifications that create shadowing on the image, and the inability with a "pinhole" valve to identify the orifice during systole. Therefore, the effective valve area or the effective orifice area is calculated using the following continuity equation:

$$\text{Aortic Valve Area} = \frac{\text{LVOT}_{\text{Area}} \times \text{LVOT}_{\text{VTI}}}{\text{Aortic Valve}_{\text{VTI}}}$$

where LVOT is the left ventricular outflow tract and VTI is the velocity time integral. Critical AS is defined as a valve area smaller than 0.8 cm^2 and an outflow gradient exceeding 50 mm Hg.

Surgical Correction

Each year, approximately 50,000 aortic valve replacements secondary to calcific AS are performed in the United States. The timing of the operation is based on the type, duration, and severity of symptoms and the degree of valve narrowing. Bioprosthetic (tissue) valves and mechanical valves can be used to replace a diseased valve. Valve selection depends on balancing the risks associated with the use of chronic anticoagulation, the likelihood of structural failure of a bioprosthetic valve (and hence the need for subsequent replacement), and the patient's expected longevity and functional status. An 11-year follow-up study of patients who were randomly assigned to receive either a bioprosthetic valve or a mechanical valve found no difference in survival rates between the two groups. Structural valve failure was observed in the bioprosthetic group, but this was offset by increased bleeding complications in the patients who were anticoagulated because they had a mechanical valve. In general, 10-year survival rate after aortic valve replacement is approximately 67%.

Table 149-1 Aortic Stenosis: Measurements and Severity of Disease

Stenotic Lesion Characteristic	Clinical Status/Disease Severity			
	Normal	**Mild**	**Moderate**	**Severe**
Valve area (cm^2)	3.0-4.0	>1.5	1.0-1.5	<1.0
AoVmax (m/sec)	<1.5	2.5-3.0	3.0-4.0	>4.0
MPG (mm Hg)	0	<20	20-40	>40
EOA (cm^2)	3.0-4.0	>1.5	1.0-1.5	<1.0

AoVmax, Peak blood flow velocity across the valve; EOA, effective orifice area; MPG, mean pressure gradient.

Clinical experience has quelled the initial enthusiasm that developed for the use of percutaneous transluminal aortic valvuloplasty because the associated postoperative improvements in pressure gradients across the valve and in symptoms were often only temporary and the operation did not lead to improved overall mortality rates. More recently, many centers have begun using percutaneous aortic valve replacement, otherwise known as transcatheter aortic valve replacement, in which a prosthetic valve is placed via either a transfemoral arterial approach (placing a valve retrograde across the native valve) or a transapical approach (via a thoracotomy, instrumentation of the left ventricle apex, and placement of the valve antegrade across the native valve). Patients who are poor candidates for conventional operations are considered to be the best candidates for this procedure, but choice of appropriate candidates remains to be determined once further experience is gained with this procedure.

Concomitant Diseases

Patients with AS often have additional medical problems, including coronary artery disease, as mentioned earlier, with even asymptomatic patients having an incidence of coronary artery disease of up to 33%. The manifestations of Heyde syndrome, which occurs in the elderly, include AS, acquired coagulopathy, and anemia due to bleeding from intestinal angiodysplasia.

Anesthetic Considerations for Aortic Valve Replacement

Many clinicians prefer using an opioid-based technique when anesthetizing patients who require aortic valve replacement. Opioids preserve systemic vascular resistance and left ventricular contractility better than do the inhalation anesthetic agents. However, many of the concerns vis-à-vis inhalation anesthetic agents are theoretical and of little clinical consequence. In practice, most clinicians use a combination of an opioid and either an inhalation agent or an intravenously administered hypnotic to produce optimal hemodynamics and early weaning from mechanical ventilation and tracheal extubation in the intensive care unit.

In addition to routine American Society of Anesthesiologists recommended monitors, arterial and pulmonary artery catheters (the latter often inserted more for postoperative care than intraoperative care) and a transesophageal echocardiographic probe are used. Echocardiography permits assessment of preload, left ventricular function, valve gradients, and prosthetic valve function and provides real-time information to the surgical team. Arrhythmias and hypotension should be treated aggressively. Anesthetic goals are summarized in Box 149-1.

Box 149-1 Anesthetic Goals for Aortic Valve Replacement

- Avoid hypotension
- Maintain sinus rhythm, avoiding both bradycardia and tachycardia
- Optimize intravascular volume to maintain venous return and left ventricular filling
- Avoid sudden increases or decreases in systemic vascular resistance
- Identify and treat myocardial ischemia

Anesthesia for Patients with Aortic Stenosis Undergoing Noncardiac Operations

Patients with AS who undergo noncardiac operations are also at increased risk of developing perioperative myocardial infarction, congestive heart failure, and arrhythmia. An adequate history for symptoms should be obtained and appropriate diagnostic testing should be performed before patients with AS undergo elective operations. Anesthetic goals for noncardiac operations are similar to those for aortic valve replacement (see Table 149-1). Given the potential for deleterious effects of a reduced systemic vascular resistance and reduced coronary perfusion, the use of spinal or epidural anesthesia is relatively contraindicated.

Suggested Readings

Billings FT, Kodali SK, Shanewise JS. Transcatheter aortic valve implantation: Anesthetic concerns. *Anesth Analg*. 2009;108:1453-1462.

Carabello BA, Paulus WJ. Aortic stenosis. *Lancet*. 2009;373:956-966.

Chambers JB. Aortic stenosis. *Eur J Echocardiogr*. 2009;10:i11-19.

Cosmi JE, Tunik PA, Rosenzweig BP, et al. The risk of development of aortic stenosis in patients with "benign" aortic valve thickening. *Arch Intern Med*. 2002;162:2345-2347.

Huang G, Rahimtoola SH. Prosthetic heart valve. *Circulation*. 2011;123:2602-2605.

Massyn MW, Khan SA. Heyde syndrome: A common diagnosis in older patients with severe aortic stenosis. *Age Ageing*. 2009;38:267-270.

Nkomo VT, Gardin JM, Skelton TN, et al. Burden of valvular heart disease: A population-based study. *Lancet*. 2006;368:1005.

Patel JH, Matthew ST, Hennebry TA. Transcatheter aortic valve replacement: A potential option for the nonsurgical patient. *Clin Cardiol*. 2009;32:296-301.

Rosamond W, Flegal K, Friday G, et al. Heart disease and stroke statistics—2007 update: A report from the American Heart Association Statistics Committee and Stroke Statistics Subcommittee. *Circulation*. 2007;115:e69-171.

Supino PG, Borer JS, Preibisz J, et al. The epidemiology of valvular heart disease: A growing public health problem. *Heart Fail Clin*. 2006;2:379-393.

CHAPTER 150

Mitral Regurgitation

Joshua D. Stearns, MD, and Michael J. Murray, MD, PhD

Anatomy of the Mitral Valve

The approach to repair of mitral valve incompetency continues to evolve, but regardless of the changes in technology, the successful anesthetic management of a patient with mitral regurgitation (MR) undergoing any surgical procedure is dependent on the anesthesia care provider understanding the anatomy and physiology of the mitral valve.

The mitral valve, so named because it resembles a bishop's miter, is composed of a fibrous annulus and anterior and posterior leaflets. The combined area of the two leaflets being more than twice the area of the annulus itself. The two leaflets are connected to the anterolateral and posteromedial papillary muscles by first-order (primary), second-order (secondary), and third-order (tertiary) chordae tendineae. The anterior leaflet attaches to approximately one third of the annulus, and the ratio of its height to its base is greater than that of the posterior leaflet, which attaches to the other two thirds of the annulus. The two leaflets are connected at the sides of the annulus to comprise the anterolateral and posteromedial commissures. The posterior mitral valve has three components, the P1, P2, and P3 "scallops," with corresponding segments on the anterior valve denoted as A1, A2, and A3. The P1 and A1 segments are attached at the anterolateral commissure, whereas the A3 and P3 segments adjoin at the posteromedial commissure.

Pathophysiology of Mitral Regurgitation

Incompetence of the mitral valve with regurgitation of blood from the left ventricle (LV) into the left atrium (LA) during systole is common (Figure 150-1). Although MR has a number of different causes, in most cases, MR occurs as a result of senescence of the mitral leaflets, and its prevalence increases with age. Degenerative MR is second only to calcific aortic stenosis as the most common valvular cardiac disorder in high-income countries. Mitral valve incompetence usually develops over many years, but incompetence of the valve can develop acutely for reasons other than degenerative disease (e.g., rupture of chordae tendineae from ischemic heart disease). Furthermore, acute MR can superimpose on chronic mitral insufficiency. Barlow disease of the mitral valve is another common condition resulting in MR, characterized by myxoid degeneration of the leaflets leading to thickened and redundant leaflets, mitral annular dilation, and chordal elongation.

Acute MR is usually quite symptomatic (Figure 150-2) and requires surgical intervention. However, the management of chronic regurgitation of the mitral valve is controversial; patients who are symptomatic or who have a decreased ejection fraction are at increased risk of developing complications and are usually considered candidates for surgery. Surgical repair or replacement of the valve not only relieves symptoms, but has increasingly been shown to improve long-term outcome, with reductions in morbidity and mortality rates. Patients who have MR and who have a decreased ejection fraction, an increased LV end-diastolic volume (LVEDV; i.e., dilated LV), chronic atrial fibrillation, or pulmonary hypertension have better long-term outcomes when the valve incompetence is surgically corrected earlier in the course of the disease. Increasing evidence indicates that life expectancy is improved in patients with MR who have surgery before the previously mentioned morbidities develop. Fortunately, the success of valve repair (compared with replacement) and the low morbidity and mortality rates associated with surgical intervention favor early elective surgery. In an effort to prevent progression to worsening disease and subsequent increase in morbidity and mortality rates, current efforts focus on identifying patients with asymptomatic mitral valve disease whose long-term outcome may be favorably impacted if their MR is corrected at an early stage.

Natural History of Mitral Regurgitation

Three-dimensional echocardiography has significantly changed the approach to evaluating MR. In the past, the mitral annulus was believed to be a fixed cartilaginous structure to which the anterior and posterior leaflets were attached. We now recognize that the annulus undergoes significant conformational changes throughout the cardiac cycle. During systole, the annulus "contracts," or narrows, allowing the edges of the anterior and posterior leaflets to coapt, thereby preventing regurgitation of blood into the atrium during ventricular systole. The opposite occurs during diastole: the annulus "widens," increasing the cross-sectional area of the mitral valve orifice, thereby facilitating inflow into the LV during diastole.

MR can be classified as acute, chronic compensated, or chronic decompensated. Acute MR (as might be caused by rupture of a chorda tendinea) leads to a large volume of blood being ejected retrograde into the LA during LV systole because LA pressure is considerably lower than aortic root pressure. In turn, increased LA blood volume leads to increased LA pressure, which is ultimately transmitted retrograde into the pulmonary vasculature. As a result, pulmonary artery pressure, pulmonary artery occlusion pressure (PAOP), and pulmonary capillary wedge pressure increase acutely. As described by Starling, the increase in end capillary hydrostatic pressure leads to transudation of fluid into the alveoli, which is manifested clinically by dyspnea, orthopnea, paroxysmal nocturnal dyspnea, and rales (as can be heard on auscultation of the lungs) as well as pulmonary edema (as can be seen on chest radiograph).

In patients in whom incompetence of the valve develops over time (i.e., changes due to senescence), the volume of blood that regurgitates into the LA is initially small; therefore, cardiac output can be maintained by an equivalent increase in LVEDV, and stroke volume ejected into the aorta remains unaffected. The regurgitant volume in the left atrium is not large enough to increase PAOP and end capillary hydrostatic pressure. Consequently, there is no transudation of fluid into the alveoli. However, as the regurgitant volume increases, the LV hypertrophies to reduce the wall stress that accompanies the rise in total stroke volume (total stroke volume equals LA regurgitant volume plus stroke volume into the aorta). Over time, as the

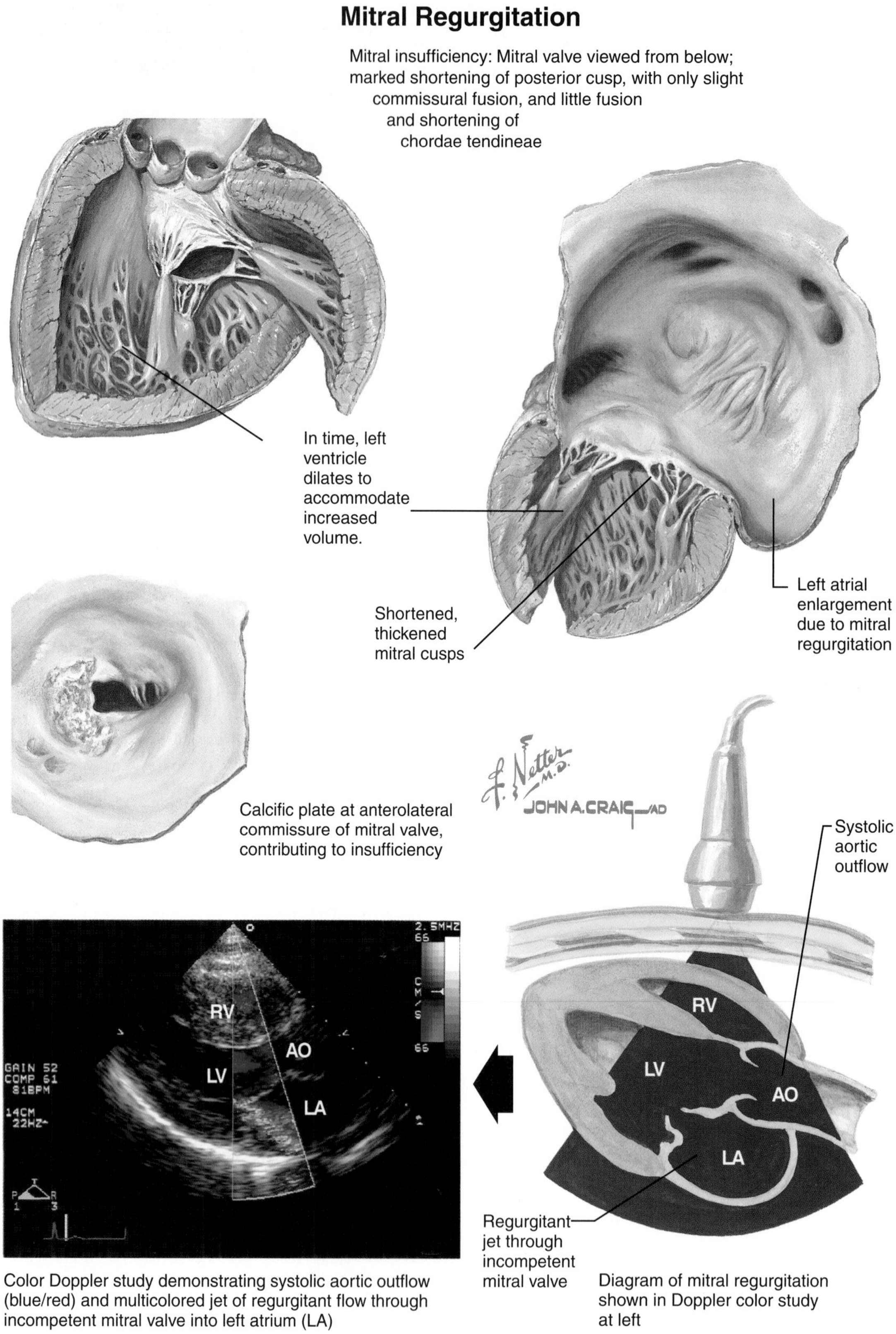

Figure 150-1 Pathophysiology of mitral regurgitation. (Netter illustration from www.netterimages.com. © Elsevier Inc. All rights reserved.)

valve becomes more incompetent, the increasing volume of regurgitant into the LA dilates the LA while maintaining a relatively "normal" LA pressure. These compensatory changes allow cardiac output to be maintained and minimize the effects of increasing regurgitant volume on the pulmonary vasculature. The compensatory phase of MR may last for many years but, eventually, will manifest by LV dysfunction, the sine qua non of decompensated MR. It is not completely clear why or when a patient transitions from the compensated to the decompensated phase of MR, but, as mentioned previously, it is important to intervene surgically before the patient's condition decompensates. Once LV dysfunction develops, it is difficult if not impossible to reverse, and life expectancy is considerably reduced.

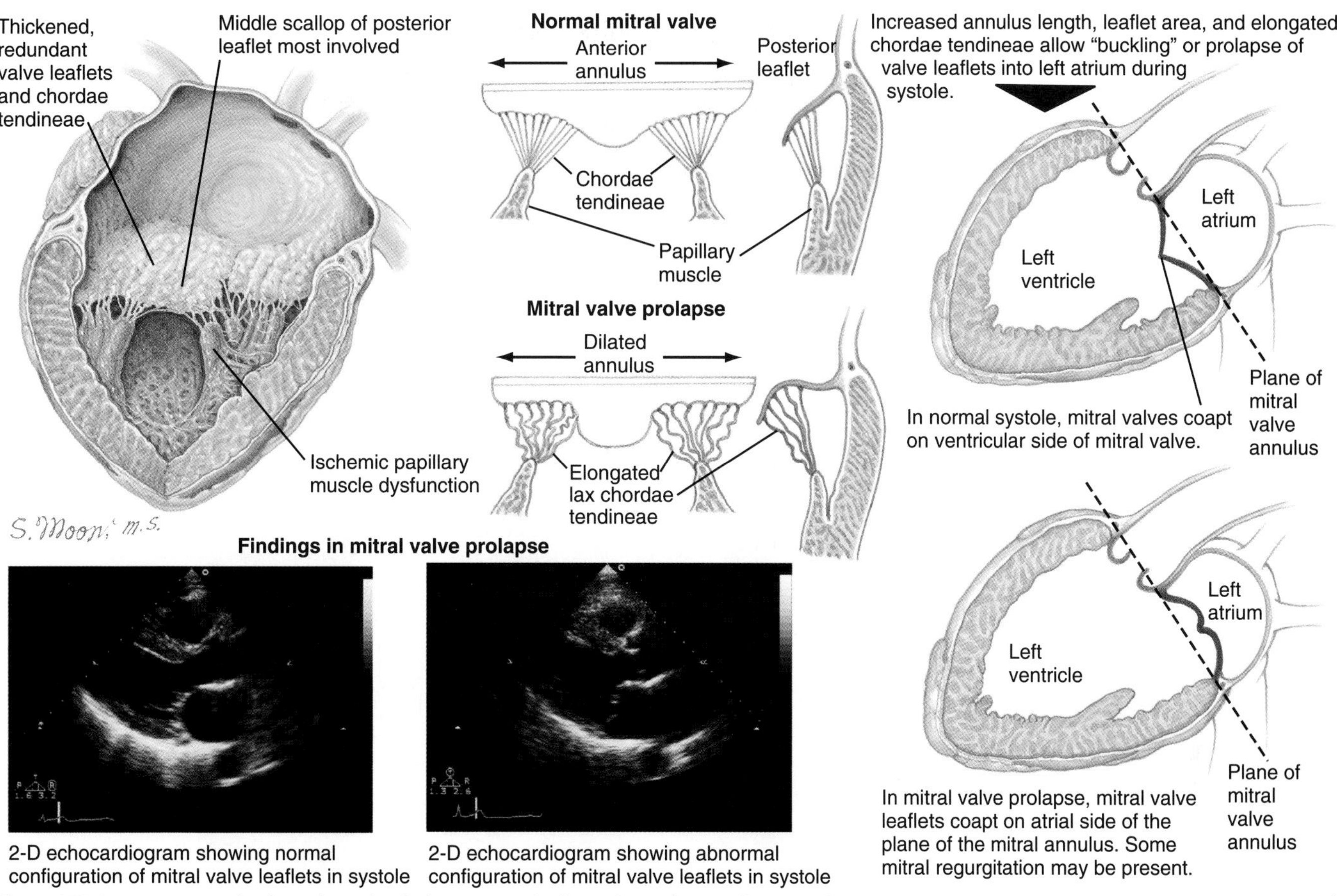

Figure 150-2 Anatomic and echocardiographic findings in mitral valve prolapse. (Netter illustration from www.netterimages.com. © Elsevier Inc. All rights reserved.)

Chronic compensated MR transitions to decompensated chronic MR when the LV begins to dilate to accommodate the LVEDV necessary to accommodate both the LA regurgitant fraction and the stroke volume ejected to the aorta (i.e., the total volume ejected from the LV). As the LV dilates, the myocardiocytes are no longer able to contract adequately to compensate for the volume overload, and stroke volume begins to decrease. The reduced stroke volume decreases cardiac output, and LV end-systolic volume subsequently increases. A vicious cycle ensues: an increase in end-systolic volume in the LV increases LVEDV, LA pressure, and PAOP. As the PAOP increases, alveoli begin to fill with fluid, leading to the symptoms and signs of pulmonary edema and congestive heart failure. Mild MR is associated with few, if any, complications. However, severe MR may lead to the development of a variety of sequelae (Box 150-1).

Box 150-1 Sequelae of Prolonged Mitral Regurgitation

- Atrial fibrillation
- Endocarditis
- Cardiogenic shock
- Pulmonary edema
- Pulmonary hypertension
- Right-sided heart failure
- Thromboembolic disease

Concomitant Disease

As was discussed earlier, the clinical manifestations of MR are due to dilation of the LA. This dilatation can lead to atrial fibrillation (with increased risk for thromboembolic events), an increased LA pressure manifested by pulmonary hypertension, and heart failure. Although these sequelae of MR can initially be managed medically, as soon as there is any evidence of end-diastolic enlargement of the LV, the mitral valve incompetence must be surgically corrected.

MR, per se, does not lead to coronary artery disease (CAD); however, CAD can lead to MR in two ways: myocardial ischemia and infarction can lead to necrosis and rupture of a papillary muscle, resulting in the acute onset of severe MR. Likewise, CAD resulting in regional wall motion abnormalities can lead to papillary dysfunction, as well as annular architectural changes, which both contribute to MR. Nevertheless, the principal etiology of MR in high-income countries is senescence of the mitral valve apparatus and valve leaflets. Because the incidence of CAD likewise increases with age, older patients often present for treatment of CAD and are found to have some degree of MR. If the MR is due to ischemia (e.g., as a result of regional wall motion abnormalities such as hypokinesis or akinesis in the subvalvular LV) the management can be challenging because none of the options for correcting these abnormalities is ideal. In such patients, depending on a variety of factors, the surgeon may chose to replace the valve rather than attempt to repair it because the success rate of repair in patients with MR due to ischemia is much lower than the rate in patients with MR because of degenerative changes.

Surgical Correction of Mitral Regurgitation

Carpentier revolutionized the treatment of MR when, more than 30 years ago, he published his experience with repairing the mitral valve as opposed to replacing it. His findings, as well as those of others, have led to mitral valve repair being the preferred technique for correcting MR. Approximately 50,000 patients have mitral valve repair annually in the United States. The most common technique to repair the valve is annuloplasty, with or without surgical correction of any defects in the leaflets themselves, or repair of dysfunctional chordae tendineae or reattachment of a ruptured chorda tendinea (Figures 150-3 and 150-4).

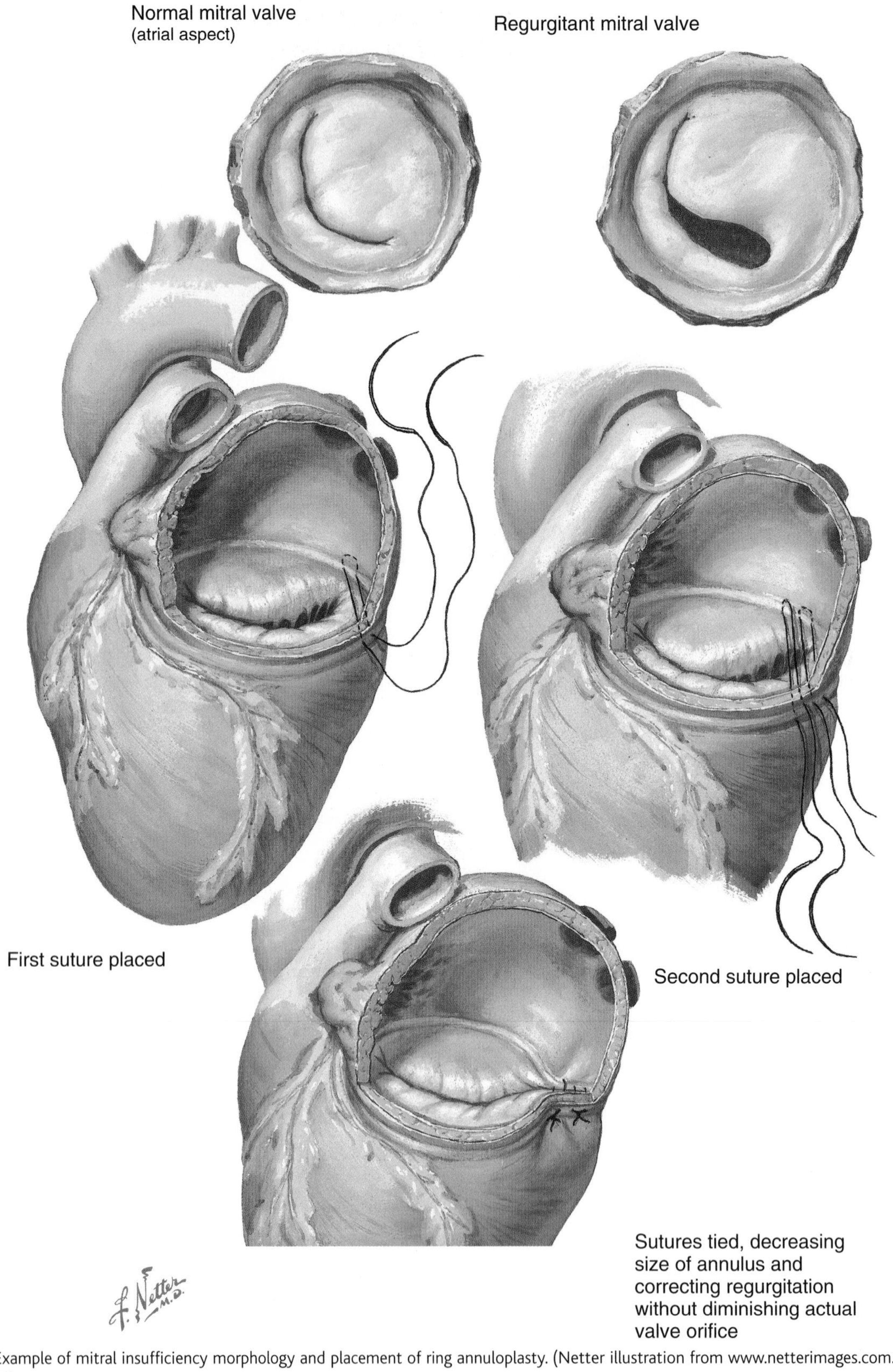

Normal mitral valve
(atrial aspect)

Regurgitant mitral valve

First suture placed

Second suture placed

Sutures tied, decreasing size of annulus and correcting regurgitation without diminishing actual valve orifice

F. Netter M.D.

Figure 150-3 Example of mitral insufficiency morphology and placement of ring annuloplasty. (Netter illustration from www.netterimages.com. © Elsevier Inc. All rights reserved.)

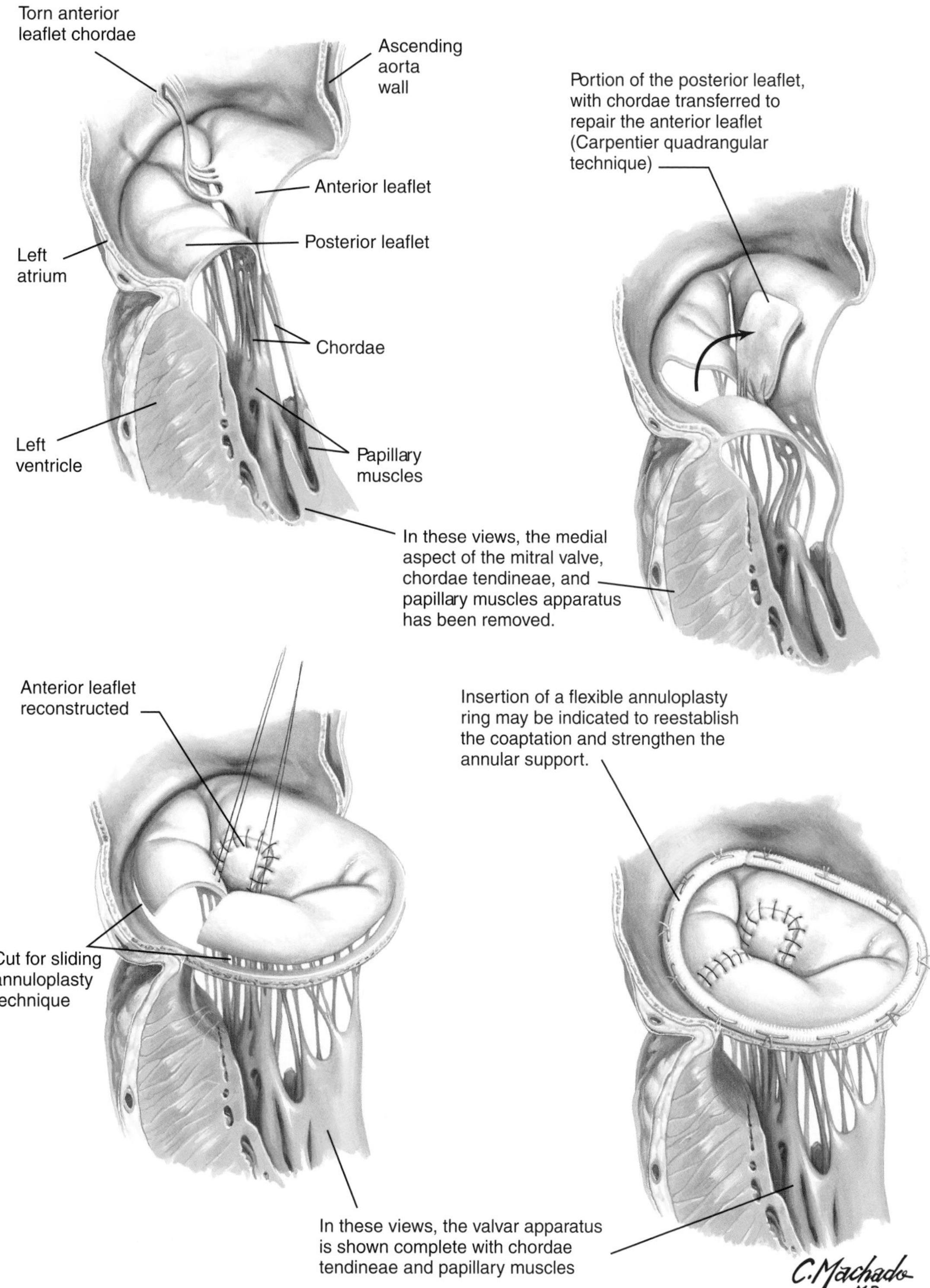
Chordal Transfer, Sliding Annuloplasty, and Ring Annuloplasty
Torn anterior leaflet chordae
Ascending aorta wall
Anterior leaflet
Posterior leaflet
Left atrium
Chordae
Left ventricle
Papillary muscles
Portion of the posterior leaflet, with chordae transferred to repair the anterior leaflet (Carpentier quadrangular technique)
In these views, the medial aspect of the mitral valve, chordae tendineae, and papillary muscles apparatus has been removed.
Anterior leaflet reconstructed
Insertion of a flexible annuloplasty ring may be indicated to reestablish the coaptation and strengthen the annular support.
Cut for sliding annuloplasty technique
In these views, the valvar apparatus is shown complete with chordae tendineae and papillary muscles
C. Machado M.D.

Figure 150-4 Surgical approaches and techniques for mitral valve repair. (Netter illustration from www.netterimages.com. © Elsevier Inc. All rights reserved.)

The goal of annuloplasty is to implant an annuloplasty "device"—commonly referred to as a "ring"—onto the annulus to restore its structural integrity and function. The cardiac surgeon has multiple options from which to choose when selecting a ring to perform the annuloplasty: the plastic rings can be complete 360-degree rings or incomplete rings; rigid, semirigid or flexible; adjustable or nonadjustable; or either flat or saddle-shaped. The goal is to restore the annulus in such a way that the anterior and posterior leaflets coapt during ventricular systole. If there is redundancy or prolapse of one of the components of the valve leaflets, then the redundant tissue can be resected, or, alternately, if there is incompetence between subcomponents of the leaflets (e.g., between P2 and P3), such an area of the valve can be plicated. If there is incompetence of the valve leaflets because of abnormalities of the chordae, the surgeon can shorten them or reattach them if they are ruptured. Increasingly, in as many as 20% of institutions, mitral valve repair is being performed with minimally invasive techniques that involve mini right-sided thoracotomies with or without robotic assistance.

As the field has advanced, cardiologists are using a variety of new devices and advances in technology to repair incompetent valves in the cardiac catheterization suite using percutaneous techniques. The efficacy of percutaneous repair has been demonstrated in patients with MR who underwent repair using the MitraClip (Abbott Laboratories, Santa Clara, CA). At 12 months following MitraClip repair, mitral valve function and LV ejection fraction had improved. In addition, when compared with a control group, the MitraClip cohort demonstrated greater reduction in diastolic and systolic LV dimensions and volumes, LV mass, and peak wall stress.

Anesthetic Considerations in the Patient with Mitral Regurgitation

Understanding the nature and etiology of the patient's MR is critical to formulating an anesthetic plan for patients undergoing mitral valve procedures. During the preoperative visit, in addition to the customary history and examination conducted on all patients about to undergo an anesthetic, the anesthesia provider must determine the etiology of the MR. Although senescence of the mitral valve is the most common cause of MR, patients may also have MR as a consequence of rheumatic fever, ischemic cardiomyopathy, or other less common causes. The anesthesia provider must also determine whether the patient has mild symptomatic chronic MR or acute regurgitation imposed on chronic MR. Any concomitant disease processes must be elucidated and medical therapies (e.g., the use of anticoagulants or β-adrenergic receptor blocking agents) must be considered.

In the operating room, the monitoring requirements and management of patients undergoing a midline sternotomy and atriotomy are the same as for other patients having cardiopulmonary bypass. Minimally invasive techniques may require special considerations and should be discussed with the surgeon, the cardiologist, or both in advance. Often, minimally invasive approaches to mitral valve repair require lung isolation, groin cannulation, and the placement of a cannula in the superior vena cava. In addition, surgeons may request that a coronary sinus catheter be placed via the jugular vein cannula site for retrograde perfusion.

The maxim for managing patients with MR is to maintain or decrease systemic vascular resistance during induction and maintenance of anesthesia because any increase in systemic vascular resistance will decrease LV output into the aorta, along with a corresponding increase in the severity of MR. Equal emphasis should be placed on avoiding tachycardia because of the adverse effects of decreased diastolic time on LVEDV, which, in turn, will limit cardiac output.

Intraoperative transesophageal echocardiography (TEE) is an integral part of the mitral valve repair process. Following induction of anesthesia and tracheal intubation, an orogastric tube should be inserted, the stomach suctioned (in this case, primarily to remove air), the gastric tube removed, and, unless the patient has a condition in which the use of TEE is absolutely contraindicated, an echocardiographic probe should be inserted into the esophagus. A preprocedural intraoperative examination using TEE should be performed, noting the patient's systemic blood pressure and central venous pressure (or pulmonary artery pressure, if available) and to describe the anatomy of the mitral valve and the relative size of the cardiac chambers, with particular attention paid to the size of the LA. This baseline information is important because it provides the surgeon with valuable information about the nature and etiology of the MR and can help direct the repair. Hemodynamic conditions should be noted during the echocardiographic examination, with the goal of reproducing similar hemodynamics (i.e., systemic blood pressure) that a patient has while not under general anesthesia. The reduction of systemic vascular resistance that often accompanies the maintenance of a general anesthetic can significantly alter the severity of MR and may not highlight all areas of regurgitation. Volume loading, the use of vasopressors, or a combination thereof may be necessary to reproduce preoperative hemodynamic values.

Before the patient is separated from cardiopulmonary bypass, a second, postprocedural echocardiographic examination should be performed to assess the adequacy of the repair and to identify any concerns about the repair. One common concern (incidence 2%-16%) following a mitral valve repair with annuloplasty is that of systolic anterior motion (SAM) of the mitral valve and the LV outflow tract obstruction that it may, in turn, create. Likewise, the preprocedural intraoperative TEE may also help identify patients at high risk of developing SAM after repair and help surgeons modify their repair to reduce the likelihood of SAM. Often, with mild SAM, medical management, including volume loading, heart rate control, and increasing system vascular resistance may resolve the obstruction of the LV outflow tract. However, if obstruction of the LV outflow tract persists despite these maneuvers, the mitral valve repair may need to be revised, often by using a larger size annuloplasty and, at times, employing an Alfieri repair to reduce leaflet excursion during diastole.

Once the repair is determined to be successful, separation from cardiopulmonary bypass may ensue, anticoagulation (heparinization) can be reversed, the heart and vessels can be decannulated, and the patient managed as any other patient would be who has undergone cardiopulmonary bypass.

The care of patients having a minimally invasive technique is less complicated, but, in these patients, because of the concern about the adequacy of the repair of the mitral valve using minimally invasive techniques, the echocardiographic examination must be conducted more thoroughly. The degree of residual MR must be documented, and, because the use of these techniques has not been fully established, care must be taken to examine for and document any unanticipated sequelae.

Suggested Readings

American Society of Anesthesiologists and Society of Cardiovascular Anesthesiologists Task Force on Transesophageal Echocardiography. Practice guidelines for perioperative transesophageal echocardiography. An updated report by the American Society of Anesthesiologists and the Society of Cardiovascular Anesthesiologists Task Force on Transesophageal Echocardiography. *Anesthesiology*. 2010;112:1084-1096.

Cheea T, Hastona R, Togoa A, Rajab SG. Is a flexible mitral annuloplasty ring superior to a semi-rigid or rigid ring in terms of improvement in symptoms and survival? *Interactive Cardiovasc Thorac Surg*. 2008;7:477-484.

Deja MA, Grayburn PA, Sun B, et al. Influence of mitral regurgitation repair on survival in the surgical treatment for ischemic heart failure trial. *Circulation*. 2012;125:2639-2648.

El Oakley R, Kleine P, Bach DS. Choice of prosthetic heart valve in today's practice. *Circulation*. 2008;117:253-256.

Enriquez-Sarano M, Schaff HV, Frye RL. Mitral regurgitation: What causes the leakage is fundamental to the outcome of valve repair. *Circulation*. 2001; 108:253-256.

Maslow AD, Regan MM, Haering JM, et al. Echocardiographic predictors of left ventricular outflow tract obstruction and systolic anterior motion of the mitral valve after mitral valve reconstruction for myxomatous valve disease. *J Am Coll Cardiol*. 1999;34:2096-2104.

Rosenhek R, Rader F, Klaar U, et al. Outcome of watchful waiting in asymptomatic severe mitral regurgitation. *Circulation*. 2006;113:2238-2244.

Varghese R, Anyanwu AC, Itagaki S, et al. Management of systolic anterior motion after mitral valve repair: An algorithm. *J Thorac Cardiovasc Surg*. 2012;143:S2-7.

CHAPTER 151 Pacemakers

Efrain Israel Cubillo, IV, MD

Overview

The high prevalence of cardiac disease in patients presenting for noncardiac operations poses a considerable challenge to the anesthesia provider. Many of these patients have pacemakers, which are being used with increasing frequency to treat conduction problems, arrhythmias, and ventricular dysfunction. More than 500,000 people in the United States have pacemakers, and nearly 115,000 new devices are implanted each year.

Early pacing systems consisted of a single-lead asynchronous pacemaker, which paced the heart at a fixed rate. Over the years, technologic advances have revolutionized pacemakers; today's sophisticated multiprogrammable devices have dramatically increased the number of indications for the use of pacing. Care of the patient with a pacemaker during surgery, therefore, requires an understanding of the pacemaker and of the associated anesthetic and surgical implications.

Generic Codes of Pacemaker

Developed originally by the International Conference on Heart Disease and subsequently modified by the NASPE/BPEG (North American Society of Pacing and Electrophysiology/British Pacing and Electrophysiology Group) alliance, the NASPE/BPEG code consists of five letters of the alphabet that describe the five programmable functions of the pacing system (Box 151-1). The first letter of the code indicates the chamber being paced; the second, the chamber being sensed; and the third, the response to sensing (I and T indicate inhibited or triggered responses, respectively). An R in the fourth position indicates that the pacemaker incorporates a sensor to modulate the rate independently of intrinsic cardiac activity, such as with activity or respiration. A P in the fifth position, for example, indicates that the pacemaker "paces" to treat a tachyarrhythmia. However, letters in the fourth and fifth positions are uncommonly used. Table 151-1 summarizes commonly used configurations.

Box 151-1 North American Society of Pacing and Electrophysiology/British Pacing and Electrophysiology Group (NASPE/BPEG) Generic Pacemaker Code

Position 1 (chamber paced): V, A, D, S, O *
Position 2 (chamber sensed): V, A, D, S, O *
Position 3 (mode of response): T, I, D, O †
Position 4 (programmability, rate modulation): P, M, C, R, O ‡
Position 5 (antitachyarrhythmia functions): P, S, D, O §

*V, Ventricular; A, atrial; D, dual-chamber (i.e., ventricle and atrium); S, single-chamber (i.e., ventricle or atrium); O, none.
†T, Triggered; I, inhibited; D, dual-chamber (atrial-triggered and ventricular-inhibited); O, none.
‡P, Programmable (rate and/or output); M, multiprogrammable; C, communicating; R, Rate-modulated; O, none.
§P, Pacing (antitachyarrhythmia functions); S, shock; D, dual (pacing and shock); O, none.

Preoperative Evaluation

Preoperative (and postoperative, if electrocautery was used) evaluation of the patient and the pacemaker is an important aspect of the anesthetic management of a patient with a permanent pacemaker who is undergoing a noncardiac operation. The patient should be asked about the initial indication for the pacemaker and preimplantation symptoms. The location of the pulse generator should be noted. Generally, the generator for endocardial electrodes is placed subcutaneously in the left lateral subclavicular region, and the generator for epicardial electrodes is placed subcutaneously in the abdomen.

Routine biochemical and hematologic investigations should be performed as indicated on an individual basis. A 12-lead electrocardiogram, chest radiograph (for visualization of continuity of leads), and measurement of serum electrolytes (especially K^+) should be performed.

The current standard is to have the pacemaker evaluated by a qualified technician in the preoperative period if it has not been evaluated in the past 6 weeks. The technician places an interrogator over the pacemaker, which then sends stored data to the interrogator. This information is vital to ensuring that the pacemaker is operating effectively and under the right settings. Most of the information about the pacemaker, such as type (fixed rate or demand rate), time since implantation, rate at the time of implantation, and half-life of the pacemaker battery can be found in the manufacturer's book, which the patient should have brought to the preoperative area. A 10% decrease in the rate that was set at the time that the pacemaker was implanted indicates power-source depletion. In patients with a VVI generator in whom the intrinsic heart rate is greater than the set rate of the pacemaker, pacemaker function can be evaluated by slowing the patient's heart rate. Slowing can be accomplished by massaging the patient's carotid sinus while continuously monitoring the patient's electrocardiogram, having the patient perform the Valsalva maneuver, or administering edrophonium (5-10 mg).

If the patient has an implanted cardioverter-defibrillator, it should be disabled before induction of anesthesia and before surgical procedures are performed in which electrocautery is to be used. If the risk of electromagnetic interference (EMI) is high, such as when electrocautery is used in close proximity to the generator, an alternative temporary cardiac pacing device should be available. A magnet can be used to reprogram the pacemaker to a fixed rate in patients who are pacemaker dependent and should be placed over the pacemaker in patients in whom electrocautery is to be used.

Effect of a Magnet on Pacemaker Function

Magnets are used in the operating room to protect the pacemaker-dependent patient from the effects of EMI. A magnet placed over the pulse generator triggers the reed switch present in the pulse generator, which deactivates the demand function, deactivates the sensing function, and activates asynchronous pacing at a fixed rate. However, not all pacemakers switch to an asynchronous mode with application of a magnet. The response varies with the model and the manufacturer and may be in the form of no apparent change

Table 151-1 Common Permanent Pacemaker Modes

Pacing Mode	Indication	Function	Perioperative Management
VVI	Bradycardia without the need for preserved AV conduction	Demand ventricular pacing	Magnet use may be helpful and converts to asynchronous pacing, usually at 72 beats/min
VVIR	Bradycardia without the need for preserved AV conduction; chronotropic incompetence	Allows a somewhat physiologic response to exercise	Pacemaker may sense perioperative changes (e.g., temperature, respiratory rate) as related to exercise or unpredictable response to magnet placement; suggest postoperative interrogation
DDD	Bradycardia when AV synchrony can be preserved	Provides more physiologic response; maintains AV concordance	Unpredictable response to magnet placement; suggest postoperative interrogation
DDDR	Patients requiring physiologic response of heart rate (i.e., chronotropic incompetence).	Provides increased physiologic response to exercise; maintains AV concordance	Pacemaker may sense perioperative changes (e.g., temperature, respiratory rate) as related to exercise or unpredictable response to magnet placement; suggest postoperative interrogation

AV, Atrioventricular.

in rate or rhythm, brief asynchronous pacing, continuous or transient loss of pacing, or asynchronous pacing without rate response. Thus, it is advisable to have the pacemaker interrogated by a qualified technician and to consult with the manufacturer, if necessary. The routine use of a magnet during surgery is not without risk, however, and, at times, may not be justified. Switching to asynchronous pacing may trigger ventricular asynchrony in patients with myocardial ischemia, hypoxia, or electrolyte imbalance. The new generation pacemakers are relatively immune to magnet application, and placement of a magnet may not convert a pacemaker to an asynchronous mode. Constant magnet application over the pacemaker may alter its programming, leading to either inhibited or triggered pacing, or may cause continuous or transient loss of pacing. Magnets placed over programmable pacemakers, in the presence of EMI, have been known to reprogram the pulse generator. This new "surprise" program may not be evident until after the magnet is removed. A further problem with magnetic application is the variability of response between devices, as there is no universal standard. Thus, a magnet may be safe for use with nonprogrammable pacemakers; however, the newest devices should be considered programmable unless otherwise indicated.

Intraoperative Management

Intraoperative monitoring should be based on the patient's underlying disease and the type of operation to be undertaken. Depending on the pacemaker and type of operation, mechanical evidence of cardiac output should be monitored by manual palpation of the pulse, the use of pulse oximetry and a precordial stethoscope, and a blood pressure tracing from an arterial line, if indicated.

The presence of a pacemaker should not affect the choice of anesthetic agent; both intravenous (with the exception of ketamine and etomidate) and inhalation agent–based techniques can be used because they do not alter the current and voltage thresholds of the pacemaker. Skeletal myopotentials, electroconvulsive therapy, succinylcholine fasciculation, myoclonic movements, and direct muscle stimulation can inappropriately inhibit or trigger pacemaker stimulation, depending on the programmed pacing modes. Case reports have indicated that myoclonus associated with the use of etomidate and ketamine may affect pacemaker function. In patients with rate-responsive pacemakers, the rate-responsive mode should be deactivated before surgery. If this is not possible, the mode of rate response must be known so that conditions causing changes in paced heart rate can be avoided. For example, shivering and fasciculations should be avoided if the pacemaker is "activity" rate responsive, ventilation (respiratory rate and tidal volume) should be controlled in case of "minute ventilation" rate responsive, and temperature must be kept constant in "temperature" rate responsive pacemakers.

Electromagnetic Interference

Among the various sources of EMI, electrocautery is the most important. Electrocautery involves the use of radiofrequency currents of 300 to 500 kHz. Fatal arrhythmias and deaths have been reported with the use of electrocautery leading to failure of pacemakers. Between 1984 and 1997, the U.S. Food and Drug Administration was notified of 456 adverse events with the use of pulse generators—255 from electrocautery—with a significant number of device failures. The following measures may decrease the possibility of adverse effects due to electrocautery:

- Bipolar cautery should be used as much as possible because it causes less EMI.
- If unipolar cautery is to be used during the operation, the grounding plate should be placed close to the operative site and as far away as possible from the site of pacemaker, usually on the patient's thigh.
- Electrocautery should not be used within 15 cm of a pacemaker.
- The use of electrocautery should be limited to 1-sec bursts in every 10 sec to prevent asystole.
- During the use of cautery, the magnet should not be placed on the pulse generator because it may cause pacemaker malfunction.
- Drugs, such as isoproterenol and atropine, should be available.
- If defibrillation is required in a patient with a pacemaker, paddles should be positioned as far away as possible from the pacemaker generator. If possible, the paddles should be placed anterior to posterior.
- Careful monitoring of pulse (by pulse oximetry or direct arterial pressure measurement) is necessary during electrocautery because electrocardiograph monitoring can also be affected by interference.
- The lead from nerve stimulators should not overlay the generator.
- The device should always be rechecked after the operation if electrocautery was used during the procedure.

Summary

Patients with implanted pacemakers can be managed safely for surgery and other nonsurgical procedures, but to do so requires a thorough understanding of the indication for and the programming of the pacemaker. Anesthetic management should be planned preoperatively according to patient's medical status, and for those patients who are pacemaker dependent, intraoperative monitoring of a pulse is recommended. Precautions should be taken to minimize EMI while using electrocautery. The magnet should not be placed over the pacemaker in the operating room while electrocautery is in use. Rate-responsive pacemakers should have the rate-responsive mode disabled before the operation begins. Provision of temporary pacing should be available in the operating room to deal with pacemaker malfunction (Table 151-2).

Table 151-2 Pacemaker Malfunctions: Mechanisms and Potential Causes

Malfunction	Description/Manifestation	Potential Causes
Failure to output	No pacing artifact is present despite an indication to pace.	Battery failure Lead fracture Fractured lead insulation Oversensing (inhibiting pacer output) Poor lead connection at the takeoff from the pacer "Cross-talk" (i.e., a phenomenon occurring when atrial output is sensed by a ventricular lead in a dual-chamber pacer)
Failure to capture	Pacing artifact is not followed by an atrial or a ventricular complex.	Lead fracture Lead dislodgement Fracture lead insulation Elevated pacing threshold Myocardial infarction at the lead tip Drugs (e.g., flecainide) Metabolic abnormalities (e.g., hyperkalemia, acidosis, alkalosis) Cardiac perforation Poor lead connection at the takeoff from the generator Improper amplitude or pulse width settings
Oversensing*	A pacer senses noncardiac electrical activity and is inhibited, resulting in a heart rate lower than the present rate.	Muscle activity—particularly of the diaphragm or pectoralis muscles Electromagnetic interference Fractured lead insulation
Undersensing†	A pacer misses intrinsic depolarization and paces despite intrinsic activity, resulting in the pacemaker's operating in an asynchronous mode.	Poor lead positioning Lead dislodgement Magnet application Low battery Myocardial infarction
Pacemaker-mediated tachycardia*	A PVC occurs in a patient with a dual-chamber pacemaker.	If a PVC is transmitted in a retrograde manner through the AV node, it may in turn depolarize the atria. The depolarization is detected by the atrial sensor, which then stimulates the ventricular leads to fire, thereby creating an endless loop. Although the maximum rate is limited by the programmed upper limit of the pacemaker, ischemia may develop in susceptible patients.
Runaway pacemaker	A malfunction of the pacemaker generator resulting in life-threatening rapid tachycardia (up to 200 beats/min).	Battery failure External damage to the generator
Pacemaker syndrome	Patient feels worse after pacemaker placement and presents with progressively worsening CHF.	Loss of AV synchrony, whereby the pathway is reversed and now has a ventricular origin
Twiddler syndrome‡	Chest radiograph reveals twisting, coiling, fracture, dislodgement, or migration of the leads.	Patient persistently disturbs or manipulates the generator, resulting in malfunction.
Cardiac monitor pseudomalfunction§	Cardiac monitor reports incorrect heart rate.	No malfunction is present; the monitor inappropriately interprets pacing artifacts.
Pacemaker pseudomalfunction¶	Pacing system appears to malfunction.	No malfunction is present; the "malfunction" is a normal programmed pacer function, primarily due to new algorithms that preserve intrinsic conduction and more physiologic pacing.

*This condition is diagnosable and treatable with magnet application.
†Management is similar to that for other types of failures.
‡Requires surgical correction and patient counseling and education.
§Clinicians faced with this issue should first palpate the patient's pulse and correlate this finding with the results of a pulse oximeter plethysmogram to verify the findings on the cardiac monitor. New monitors have settings to adapt for patients with pacemakers and provide more accurate heart rates.
¶ Correction may involve changing the programming or changing the device.
AV, Atrioventricular; CHF, congestive heart failure; PVC, premature ventricular contraction.

Suggested Readings

Allen M. Pacemakers and implantable cardioverter defibrillators. *Anaesthesia*. 2006;61:883-890.

Anand NK, Maguire DP. Anesthetic implications for patients with rate-responsive pacemakers. *Semin Cardiothorac Vasc Anesth*. 2005;9:251-259.

MacPherson RD, Loo CK, Barrett N. Electroconvulsive therapy in patients with cardiac pacemakers. *Anaesth Intensive Care*. 2006;34:470-474.

Mattingly E. Arrhythmia management devices and electromagnetic interference. *AANA J*. 2005;73:129-136.

Rastogi S, Goel S, Tempe DK, Virmani S. Anaesthetic management of patients with cardiac pacemakers and defibrillators for noncardiac surgery. *Ann Card Anaesth*. 2005;8:21-32.

Rozner MA. The patient with a cardiac pacemaker or implanted defibrillator and management during anaesthesia. *Curr Opin Anaesthesiol*. 2007;20:261-268.

Salukhe TV, Dob D, Sutton R. Pacemakers and defibrillators: Anaesthetic implications. *Br J Anaesth*. 2004;93:95-104.

Senthuran S, Toff WD, Vuylsteke A, et al. Implanted cardiac pacemakers and defibrillators in anaesthetic practice. *Br J Anaesth*. 2002;88:627-631.

Vijayakumar E. Anesthetic considerations in patients with cardiac arrhythmias, pacemakers, and AICDs. *Int Anesthesiol Clin*. 2001;39:21-42.

CHAPTER 152

Implantable Cardioverter-Defibrillators

Efrain Israel Cubillo, IV, MD

Overview

Approximately 300,000 Americans die each year from sudden cardiac arrest, many of whom were taking antiarrhythmic drugs, but drugs alone were insufficient to prevent ventricular tachycardia and fibrillation. The implantable cardioverter-defibrillator (ICD) has revolutionized the treatment of patients at risk for experiencing sudden cardiac death due to these ventricular tachyarrhythmias. The superiority of the ICD device over antiarrhythmic therapy has been confirmed in several randomized trials. Expanding clinical indications for the implantation of these devices arose with the publication of the MADIT (Multi-center Autonomic Defibrillator Implantation Trial), the results of which have been validated by the MUSTT (Multicenter UnSustained Tachycardia Trial). Both studies demonstrated a survival benefit of ICDs over antiarrhythmic medication and placebo in patients with nonsustained ventricular tachycardia. The number of ICD implants continues to increase, with the United States leading the world in both total number and rate per population (434 new implants per 1 million people). In 2009 alone, based on industry statistics, 133,262 ICDs were implanted in the United States. ICD technology has progressed exponentially since its introduction by Michel Mirowski and colleagues in the early 1980s. Early devices were true "shock boxes," capable of detecting a tachycardia and delivering a shock without the ability to pace.

The ICD System

The ICD system comprises a microprocessor/pulse generator, a battery, and a conducting lead system. The lead system is required for sensing, pacing, and the delivery of therapy. Earlier systems required that the pulse generators be placed abdominally because of their large size. Defibrillation was delivered via two epicardial patches positioned anteriorly and posteriorly. Occasionally, a transvenous spring electrode in the superior vena cava was utilized with an epicardial patch. Sensing was achieved through separate epicardial screw-in electrodes. Initial lead placement required a sternotomy, lateral thoracotomy, or a subxiphoid incision, making early implants quite cumbersome. ICD implantation has evolved quite rapidly due to advancements in lead technology, generator technology, and the development of biphasic defibrillation electric impulses, which lowered the energy requirements necessary for successful defibrillation. The creation of a bipolar lead combining pacing and sensing capabilities with a high-voltage electrode coil allowed for nonthoracotomy system implants, which reduced surgical morbidity and mortality rates. The leads were positioned transvenously via the subclavian vein and fixed to the inside of the right ventricle. However, the leads still had to be tunneled subcutaneously to the abdomen, as the generators remained fairly large. In current practice, generators are fairly small—the smallest commercially available devices today are approximately 7 cm × 5 cm × 1 cm and weigh well under 100 g—allowing for subcutaneous pectoral implantation and simplification of the implantation process. The ICD generator houses the batteries, high-voltage capacitors, and microprocessors necessary to process sensed intrinsic cardiac electrical activity. In essence, the generator is a minicomputer within a hermetically sealed titanium box, which is capable of storing an electric charge that can be delivered, "shocking" the atria and ventricles back to a sinus rhythm. Typically, ICDs deliver no more than 6 shocks per event, although some can deliver as many as 18. Within an event, each successive therapy must be at equal or greater energy than the previous attempt. Once a shock is delivered, no further antitachycardia pacing can take place.

Typical ICDs contain lithium silver vanadium oxide cells that store between 2 and 7 volts. The high voltages necessary for defibrillation are generated with the aid of high-voltage capacitors that are able to generate 700 to 800 volts of defibrillation energy in under 20 sec.

Current devices allow extensive programmability for tiered antitachycardia pacing, tiered high-voltage therapies, bradycardia pacing, supraventricular tachycardia discrimination algorithms, and detailed diagnostics of tachycardic and bradycardic episodes. They also allow physicians to conduct completely noninvasive programmed stimulation. The most recent iterations provide dedicated dual-chamber and antitachycardia pacing as well as options for atrial defibrillation. Diagnostic functions, including stored electrocardiograms, allow for verification of shock appropriateness. Device battery longevity has also increased; early devices lasted 2 years or less, whereas current devices are expected to last 6 years or longer.

ICD Placement

Transvenous placement is performed by cardiologists to place ICDs, usually in the left or right infraclavicular area, with the leads tunneled transvenously while the patient receives intravenous sedation using monitored anesthesia care. A deeper level of anesthesia, which most would consider general anesthesia, is provided to the patient for the discomfort that occurs when the unit is tested (i.e., discharged) and an electric shock is delivered to the patient. Defibrillation can lead to prolonged periods of asystole that can result in significant myocardial and cerebral ischemia. Enough time should be allowed between tests to ensure reperfusion and restoration of hemodynamic stability. The anesthesia provider must monitor the duration and frequency of testing and ischemic periods. Vasoactive drugs are often used to stabilize these patients during and immediately after the testing period. Minimum monitoring includes standard American Society of Anesthesiologists monitors and continuous arterial pressure measurement, usually through an arterial cannula placed by the cardiologist.

Function of Pacemakers with an ICD

Single-chamber and dual-chamber pacemakers can function in the presence of an ICD as long as the pacing electrodes are bipolar. An ICD with a built-in capability for pacing will begin pacing when the RR interval is greater than previously set limits. Beginning about 1993, most ICDs incorporated backup VVI pacing to protect the patient from the common occurrence of postshock bradycardia. In July 1997, the U.S. Food and Drug Administration approved devices with sophisticated dual-chamber pacing modes and rate-responsive behavior for patients with ICDs who needed permanent pacing (about 20% of patients with ICDs). If a patient with an ICD requires temporary pacing, bipolar leads, the lowest possible amplitude for capture, and the slowest rate associated with adequate hemodynamic status should be used. It is possible for a pacing spike followed by a QRS complex to be interpreted as ventricular tachycardia, causing discharge of the unit. Inactivation of the ICD may be required during temporary pacing if interference occurs. Cardioverter units for atrial fibrillation are presently under investigation. The perioperative management of these devices is unknown, but they will most likely behave similar to ICDs.

Indications for Cardiodefibrillator Implantation

The American College of Cardiology (ACC) and American Heart Association (AHA), in collaboration with the American Association for Thoracic Surgery and the Society of Thoracic Surgeons, have developed an extensive set of guidelines for cardiodefibrillator implantation. These guidelines represent a consensus statement that is largely evidence based and that summarizes the available clinical evidence as of the time of its initial publication in May 2008 and further revision in October 2012. The latest update emphasizes the role that left bundle branch block with a QRS complex of 150 ms or greater has in sudden death and now considers this to be an indication for implantation of a cardiodefibrillator if the patient's status is New York Heart Association classification II or higher.

Electromagnetic Interference and ICDs

The ability of ICDs to function is dependent on their ability to sense intrinsic cardiac electrical activity. Hermetic shielding, filtering, interference rejection circuits, and bipolar sensing have safeguarded ICDs (and pacemakers) against the effects of common electromagnetic sources. However, exposure to electromagnetic interference (EMI) may still result in oversensing, asynchronous pacing, ventricular inhibition, and spurious ICD discharges. EMI may also lead to loss of output, increased pacing thresholds, and decreased R-wave amplitude. Common sources of EMI include cellular phones, electronic article surveillance (antitheft) devices, and metal detectors. Occupational sources of EMI include high-voltage power lines, electrical transformers, and arc welding. Interference of concern to anesthesia providers can occur during procedures, such as magnetic resonance imaging, or from electrocautery, spinal cord stimulators, transcutaneous electrical nerve stimulator units, radiofrequency catheter ablation, therapeutic diathermy, and lithotripsy.

Inappropriate ICD Shocks

One of the risks associated with an ICD is that of inappropriate ICD shocks, which can occur from EMI, as mentioned previously, or from inaccurate detection of other arrhythmias. An inappropriate ICD shock is one that is not precipitated by accurate detection of a malignant ventricular arrhythmia, ventricular tachycardia, or ventricular fibrillation. Typically, inappropriate ICD shocks result when atrial arrhythmias, such as atrial fibrillation, atrial tachycardia, or atrial flutter, accelerate the ventricular rate beyond the set limit for delivery of ICD shock therapy. Analysis of the MADIT II trial data revealed that 11.5% of the patients with an ICD received inappropriate ICD shocks and that 31.2% of all ICD shocks were deemed inappropriate. Inappropriate ICD shocks due to arrhythmias were attributed to atrial fibrillation (44%), supraventricular tachycardia (36%), and abnormal sensing (20%). Patients with inappropriate shocks had greater all-cause mortality rate (hazard ratio 2.29, $P = 0.025$).

ICD Magnets

As with pacemakers, ICDs can be altered by magnets. Antitachycardia therapy in some Guidant/CPI devices can be permanently disabled by magnet placement for 30 sec. The application of a magnet overlying the ICD pulse generator forms a magnetic field that trips a reed switch in the ICD generator circuit, resulting in a suspension of tachycardia detection and therapy delivery. The magnet response of an ICD varies from manufacturer to manufacturer. In Medtronic devices, the application of a magnet temporarily disables tachycardia detection and therapy with no effect on bradycardia pacing. Removal of the magnet will resume arrhythmia detection. When activated, newer Medtronic devices (Gem II DR, patient alert function) will elicit a continuous beep lasting for 15 sec if a magnet is placed directly over the ICD. A magnet applied over Guidant/CPI defibrillators also inhibits tachycardia therapy with no effect on bradycardic pacing. These devices also generate beeping tones, which, if they change to a continuous tone, indicate that the device is off and will not deliver antitachycardia therapy; the device can be turned on by reapplying the magnet for 30 sec. Tones will now change from continuous to beeping synchronous with R waves, signifying that the device is on again. To ensure correct magnet placement on their devices, Medtronic plans to market a "smart magnet" that maintains communication with the device and reports on the device's status during the magnet session. Newer generation Guidant ICDs (Prism II) have a built-in electrocautery feature that can be activated by use of the Guidant programmer. This will suspend tachyarrhythmia therapies and pace in the DOO (dual pacing, no sensing, no inhibition) mode. Regular functioning of the ICD is restored by turning this feature off. Interrogating the device by a trained technician or by calling the manufacturer remain the most reliable ways to determine response to a magnet.

Preoperative Evaluation

All ICDs should have the antitachycardia therapy disabled before induction of anesthesia and commencement of the procedure if electrocautery is to be used. As with pacing devices, monopolar electrosurgical cautery has been reported to "confuse" an ICD into delivering inappropriate therapy. Also, many ICDs have no noise reversion behavior, so electrosurgical cautery-induced ventricular oversensing might cause nonpacing in a patient who depends on an ICD for pacing.

Intraoperative Management

No special monitoring or anesthetic technique is required for the patient with an ICD. However, the Heart Rhythm Society and American Society of Anesthesiologists have developed guidelines and recommendations for how the patient with an ICD coming to the operating room for an elective procedure (Box 152-1) or an emergent procedure (Box 152-2) should be managed. Electrocardiographic monitoring and the ability to deliver prompt external cardioversion or defibrillation must be present if the ICD is being disabled, are recommended whether or not the device is used for pacing, and are recommended whether or not the patient is pacemaker dependent (Box 152-3). Should external defibrillation become necessary, device manufacturers recommend using the lowest possible energy, placing the paddles perpendicular to the path of the implanted leads, and keeping the paddles away from the implanted generator, the same as with a

Box 152-1 General Principles of ICD Management

The perioperative management of ICDs must be individualized to the patient, the type of ICD, and the procedure being performed.
An ICD team is defined as the physicians and physician extenders who monitor the ICD function of the patient.
The anesthesia team should communicate the type of procedure and likely risk of EMI with the ICD team.
The ICD team should communicate with the anesthesia team to deliver a prescription for the perioperative management of patients with ICDs:

1. Manufacturer and model
2. Indication for device
3. Battery longevity documented as >3 months
4. Are any of the leads <3 months old?
5. What is the response of this device to magnet placement?
6. Will ICD detection resume automatically with removal of the magnet?

Note: Inactivation of ICD detection is not a universal requirement for all procedures.
EMI, Electromagnetic interference; ICD, implantable cardioverter-defibrillator.
Modified from Crossley GH, Poole JE, Rozner MA, et al. The Heart Rhythm Society (HRS)/American Society of Anesthesiologists (ASA) Expert Consensus Statement on the perioperative management of patients with implantable defibrillators, pacemakers and arrhythmia monitors: Facilities and patient management. Heart Rhythm. 2011;8:1114-1154.

Box 152-2 Approach to Emergent/Urgent Procedures

Identify the type of device:
Evaluate the medical record
Examine the patient registration card
Telephone the company to clarify device type
Examine the chest radiograph
Determine if the patient is pacing:
Obtain a 12-lead electrocardiogram or rhythm strip documentation
If there are pacemaker spikes in front of all or most P waves or QRS complexes, assume pacemaker dependency*
Whether or not the patient is pacemaker dependent, place magnet† over ICD to suspend tachyarrhythmia detection, use short electrosurgical bursts‡
Monitor patient with plethysmography or arterial line
Place transcutaneous pacing and defibrillation pads anterior/posterior
Evaluate the ICD before leaving a cardiac-monitored environment

*Pacemaker (PM) dependency is defined as absence of a life-sustaining rhythm without the pacing system.
†A magnet placed over an implantable cardioverter-defibrillator (ICD) (or cardiac resynchronization therapy-ICD [CRT-ICD]) will not result in asynchronous pacemaker function. This can only be accomplished by reprogramming of ICDs (or CRT-ICDs) capable of this feature (majority of newer devices implanted).
‡Long electrosurgery application (>5 sec or frequent close-spaced bursts) may result in PM inhibition, causing hemodynamic risk in a PM-dependent patient. Long electrosurgery application in close proximity to the device generator may rarely result in power on reset or Safety Core programming.
Modified from Crossley GH, Poole JE, Rozner MA, et al. The Heart Rhythm Society (HRS)/American Society of Anesthesiologists (ASA) Expert Consensus Statement on the perioperative management of patients with implantable defibrillators, pacemakers and arrhythmia monitors: Facilities and patient management. Heart Rhythm. 2011;8:1114-1154.

Box 152-3 Problems That Can Occur During Procedures in Patients with ICDs

Bipolar electrosurgery does not cause EMI unless it is applied directly to an ICD.
EMI from monopolar electrosurgery is the most common problem incurred during surgical procedures.
ICDs with antitachycardia function may be inhibited or may falsely detect arrhythmias when exposed to EMI.
Pulse generator damage from electrosurgery can occur, but is uncommon.
Impedance-based rate-responsive systems may go to upper rate behavior with electrosurgery exposure.
Risk mitigation strategies can be effective.
Keeping the current path away from ICDs diminishes the potential for adverse interaction with the device.
Use bipolar electrosurgery whenever possible.
Minimize the length of monopolar electrosurgery bursts to ≤5 sec.
Radiofrequency ablation can cause all of the interactions that monopolar electrosurgery can cause but may have a more significant risk profile because of the prolonged exposure to current.
TENS units can result in EMI.

EMI, Electromagnetic interference; ICD, implantable cardioverter-defibrillator; PM, pacemaker; TENS, transcutaneous electrical nerve stimulation.
Modified from Crossley GH, Poole JE, Rozner MA, et al. The Heart Rhythm Society (HRS)/American Society of Anesthesiologists (ASA) Expert Consensus Statement on the perioperative management of patients with implantable defibrillators, pacemakers and arrhythmia monitors: Facilities and patient management. Heart Rhythm. 2011;8:1114-1154.

Box 152-4 Indications for the Interrogation of ICDs Prior to Patient Discharge or Transfer from a Cardiac Telemetry Environment

Patients with ICD reprogrammed prior to the procedure that left the device nonfunctional such as disabling tachycardia detection in an ICD
Patients with ICDs who underwent hemodynamically challenging surgeries such as cardiac surgery or significant vascular surgery (e.g., abdominal aortic aneurysm repair)*
Patients with ICDs who experienced significant intraoperative events including cardiac arrest requiring temporary pacing or cardiopulmonary resuscitation and those who required external electrical cardioversion*
Emergent operations in which the site of EMI exposure was above the umbilicus
Cardiothoracic operations
Patients with ICDs who underwent certain types of procedures that emit EMI with a greater probability of affecting device function
Patients with ICDs who have logistic limitations that would prevent reliable device evaluation within 1 month from their procedure*

*The general purpose of this interrogation is to ensure that reset did not occur. In these cases, a full evaluation, including threshold evaluations, is suggested.
EMI, Electromagnetic interference; ICD, implantable cardioverter-defibrillator.
Modified from Crossley GH, Poole JE, Rozner MA, et al. The Heart Rhythm Society (HRS)/American Society of Anesthesiologists (ASA) Expert Consensus Statement on the perioperative management of patients with implantable defibrillators, pacemakers and arrhythmia monitors: Facilities and patient management. Heart Rhythm. 2011;8:1114-1154.

standard pacemaker device. The guidelines outline when and how the ICD must be reinterrogated and reenabled postoperatively (Box 152-4).

Complications

Implantation of an ICD has an intraoperative and perioperative risk of approximately 1% to 3%, including a death rate of 1% or less, perforation and cardiac tamponade of 1% or less, and acute lead dysfunction. Postimplantation pocket infection is a major complication, which generally requires the removal of the complete system. It is reported to occur in 1% to 2% of patients. The most frequently identified organism in patients with a postimplantation pocket infection is *Staphylococcus aureus*. Infection risk seems to be a little higher at the time of battery or lead replacement than at the time of initial implantation. Lead dislodgement can occur shortly after implantation or at any time thereafter. In patients in whom the lead is completely dislodged, monitoring and timely removal of the lead is mandatory to avoid mechanically induced arrhythmias. Lead dysfunction from insulation breakage or insulation erosion is most frequently preceded by inappropriate ICD discharge caused by electrical noise on the rate electrocardiogram. It usually displays high, frequent, irregular signals with pseudo-RR intervals at the resolution boundary of the device. Some newer devices provide a counter for these specific signals to detect the problems early and avoid inappropriate discharges.

Suggested Readings

Aliot E, Chauvin M, Daubert JC, et al. Indications for implantable automatic ventricular defibrillators. *Arch Dis Heart Vessels*. 2006;99:141-154.

Anand NK, Maguire DP. Anesthetic implications for patients with rate-responsive pacemakers. *Semin Cardiothorac Vasc Anesth*. 2005;9:251-259.

Angelilli A, Katz ES, Goldenberg RM. Cardiac arrest following anaesthetic induction in a world-class bodybuilder. *Acta Cardiol*. 2005;60:443-444.

Crossley GH, Poole JE, Rozner MA, et al. The Heart Rhythm Society (HRS)/American Society of Anesthesiologists (ASA) Expert Consensus Statement on the perioperative management of patients with implantable defibrillators, pacemakers and arrhythmia monitors: Facilities and patient management. *Heart Rhythm*. 2011;8:1114-1154.

Epstein AE, Dunbar D, DiMarco JP, et al. 2012 ACCF/AHA/HRS focused update of the 2008 guidelines for device-based therapy of cardiac rhythm abnormalities. A Report of the American College of Cardiology Foundation/American Heart Association Task Force on Practice Guidelines. *J Am Coll Cardiol*. 2012;60:1297-1313.

Fox DJ, Davidson NC, Royle M, et al. Safety and acceptability of implantation of internal cardioverter-defibrillators under local anesthetic and conscious sedation. *Pacing Clin Electrophysiol*. 2007;30:992-997.

Graf D, Pruvot E. Inappropriate AICD shocks. *Heart*. 2007;93:1532.

Haas S, Richter HP, Kubitz JC. Anesthesia during cardiologic procedures. *Curr Opin Anaesthesiol*. 2009;22:519-523.

Huschak G, Schmidt-Runke H, Rüffert H. Anaesthesia and cardiac contractility modulation. *Eur J Anaesthesiol*. 2007;24:819-825.

Jinnouchi Y, Kawahito S, Kitahata H, et al. Anesthetic management of a patient undergoing cardioverter defibrillator implantation: Usefulness of transesophageal echocardiography and near infrared spectroscopy. *J Anesth*. 2004;18:220-223.

Joshi GP. Perioperative management of outpatients with implantable cardioverter defibrillators. *Curr Opin Anaesthesiol*. 2009;22:701-704.

Marquié C, Duchemin A, Klug D, et al. Can we implant cardioverter defibrillator under minimal sedation? *Europace*. 2007;9:545-550.

Mattingly E. AANA Journal Course: Update for nurse anesthetists. Arrhythmia management devices and electromagnetic interference. *AANA J*. 2005;73:129-136.

Ozin B, Borman H, Bozbaş H, et al. Implantation of submammary implantable cardioverter defibrillators. *Pacing Clin Electrophysiol*. 2004;27:779-782.

Rozner MA. The patient with a cardiac pacemaker or implanted defibrillator and management during anaesthesia. *Curr Opin Anaesthesiol*. 2007;20:261-268.

Salukhe TV, Dob D, Sutton R. Pacemakers and defibrillators: Anaesthetic implications. *Br J Anaesth*. 2004;93:95-104.

Senthuran S, Toff WD, Vuylsteke A, et al. Implanted cardiac pacemakers and defibrillators in anaesthetic practice. *Br J Anaesth*. 2002;88:627-631.

Stevenson WG, Chaitman BR, Ellenbogen KA, et al. Clinical assessment and management of patients with implanted cardioverter-defibrillators presenting to nonelectrophysiologists. *Circulation*. 2004;110:3866-3869.

Stone ME, Apinis A. Current perioperative management of the patient with a cardiac rhythm management device. *Semin Cardiothorac Vasc Anesth*. 2009;13:31-43.

Vijayakumar E. Anesthetic considerations in patients with cardiac arrhythmias, pacemakers, and AAICDs. *Int Anesthesiol Clin*. 2001;39:21-42.

CHAPTER 153
Intraaortic Balloon Pump

David J. Cook, MD, and Eduardo S. Rodrigues, MD

The intraaortic balloon pump (IABP) is a mechanical device used to provide temporary circulatory support during a period of acute cardiac failure.

Equipment

Historically, the adult IABP consisted of an 8.5F to 12F catheter, the distal 30 cm of which was covered with a polyurethane balloon. For adult patients, 7F catheters also with 25-mL to 50-mL balloons are currently most commonly used, with the size of the balloon dependent upon the patient's height. The pediatric catheter is 4.5F to 7F with a 2.5-mL to 12-mL balloon.

The catheter is inserted into the common femoral artery percutaneously by the Seldinger technique or by an open surgical procedure. It is then threaded proximally so that the balloon lies high in the descending thoracic aorta, just distal to the origin of the left subclavian artery.

The catheter is connected to a drive console that has a pneumatic pump that uses helium to rapidly inflate the balloon and, just as quickly, deflate the balloon after a brief period of time. Balloon cycling is triggered either from the electrocardiogram R wave, inflating with diastole and deflating with onset of systole (Figure 153-1), or from the aortic pressure waveform. It should be adjusted to inflate when the dicrotic notch occurs in the pressure cycle (Figure 153-2). The balloon can be set to trigger with every beat, every other beat, or some other pattern.

Hemodynamic Effects

With balloon deflation at onset of systole, the peak aortic systolic pressure falls 10% to 15% (systolic unloading) and inflates immediately with appearance of the dicrotic notch. Balloon inflation can increase intraaortic diastolic pressure by approximately 70%. The cardiac index increases 10% to 15%, whereas the pulmonary artery occlusion pressure falls by a similar amount. Coronary blood flow increases as a result of increased diastolic pressure.

As the balloon deflates, a decrease occurs in the pressure in the aorta in proximity to the balloon, reducing the systemic vascular resistance, which, in turn, reduces myocardial O_2 demand and a shift of the Starling curve to

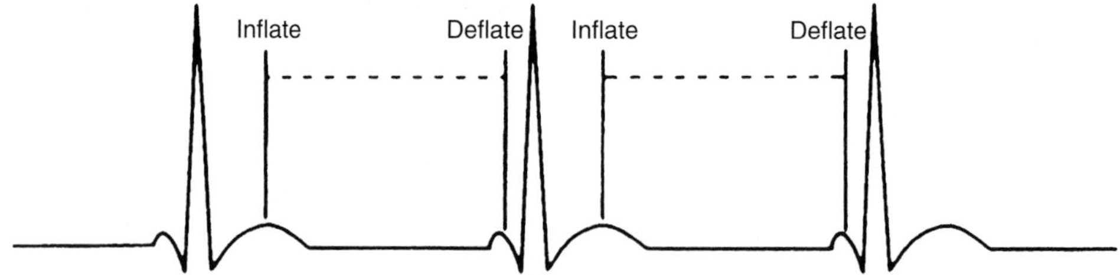

Figure 153-1 Inflation/deflation timing of an intraaortic balloon correlated with the electrocardiogram. (Modified from Gray JR, Faust RJ. Intraaortic balloon counterpulsation and ventricular assist devices. In: Tarhan S, ed. Cardiovascular Anesthesia and Postoperative Care. 2nd ed. Chicago, Year Book Medical, 1989:513.)

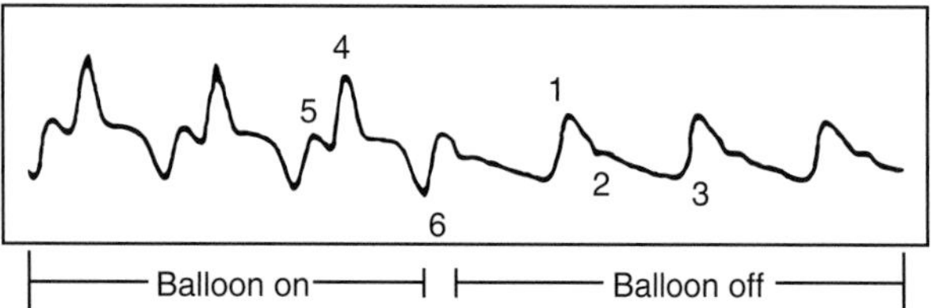

Figure 153-2 Arterial pressure tracing (balloon on 1:1 and balloon off). Note diastolic peak (4) balloon augmentation and systolic peak (1), dicrotic notch (2), diastolic low (3), diastolic peak (4), systolic peak (5), and end-diastolic dip (6). (Modified from Gray JR, Faust RJ. Intraaortic balloon counterpulsation and ventricular assist devices. In: Tarhan S, ed. Cardiovascular Anesthesia and Postoperative Care. 2nd ed. Chicago, Year Book Medical, 1989:513.)

Box 153-1 Criteria for Emergency Use of Intraaortic Balloon Pump After Cardiac Surgery

Relative

Requirement for large doses of vaso pressor agents
Malignant arrhythmia with evidence of intraoperative infarction not well controlled with drug therapy

Definite

Difficulty in weaning from cardiopulmonary bypass after 30 to 45 min (or 3 attempts) at flow rates above 500 mL/min
Hypotension (<60 mm Hg mean) and low cardiac index ($<1.8\ L \cdot min^{-1} \cdot m^{-2}$) with high pulmonary artery occlusion pressure (>25 mm Hg) despite pressor agents and afterload reduction
Continued postoperative use (if intraaortic balloon pump was initiated before surgery)

the right. These effects can last as long as 48 to 72 h after initiation of the balloon counterpulsation.

Indications

The IABP is used primarily for treatment of acute cardiac failure refractory to pharmacologic intervention. Most commonly, it is used for low-output states associated with acute coronary syndromes and after cardiopulmonary bypass. The pump can also be placed preoperatively when the surgical stress is anticipated to exceed the functional capacity of a diseased heart. In very high-risk heart operations, the elective preoperative placement of an intraaortic balloon and initiation of counterpulsation can improve the patient's prognosis. In recent years, the IABP has also found use as a temporary bridge to cardiac transplantation, to placement of a left ventricular assist device, or to placement of a total artificial heart.

Approximately 3% to 4% of patients undergoing cardiopulmonary bypass need IABP support. If the patient is not hypovolemic and the heart rhythm is suitable for IABP use, the criteria listed in Box 153-1 can be used to determine appropriate initiation of IABP support.

Contraindications

The classic contraindications to the use of intraaortic counterpulsation are severe aortic insufficiency, severe peripheral vascular disease, thrombocytopenia (platelet count <50,000), contraindication to anticoagulation, acute stroke, and active bleeding.

Weaning from Intraaortic Balloon Pump Support

Following resolution of the problem for which the intraaortic balloon was placed, patients have traditionally been weaned from IABP support by a gradual reduction in augmentation rate (1:1, then 1:2, then 1:3, etc.). Most hemodynamic changes occur while going from 1:1 to 1:2 augmentation. To institute a more gradual reduction in circulatory assist and to reduce the risk of thrombus formation around a static balloon, an alternate weaning approach is to maintain a 1:1 augmentation rate but gradually reduce the degree of balloon inflation because the rate and degree of deflation are determined by changes in the intraaortic diastolic pressure.

Complications

Previously reported complication rates with the use of IABP were 5% to 27%, but more recent reviews suggest a complication rate around 3% to 4%. Placement of a large catheter in the common femoral artery can occlude the artery, which is manifested by a loss of distal pulses; the aortotomy site can bleed; or the site can become infected. The relative frequency of each of these complications varies widely among reports, and the literature is inconsistent as to the impact of chronic placement on complication rates. Nevertheless, it may be reasonable to expect up to a 9% incidence of bleeding or vascular compromise in these patients. These complications may readily become life threatening.

Outcome

Clinicians have evaluated immediate and long-term prognosis following IABP support with the aim of identifying reliable determinants of survival but have made their assessments using nonrandomized groups. The primary determinant of survival after use of an IABP is early recovery (within 24 h) of cardiac function with maintenance of vital organ perfusion. Conversely, the use of inotropes, direct current cardioversion, chronic left ventricular failure, and the functional severity of the patient's heart disease have been associated with poor outcome.

Theoretically, the predicted improvement in the O_2 demand-supply ratio offered by IABP support can benefit patients with acute cardiac decompensation. Nevertheless, it remains to be determined to what extent IABP will improve survival and for whom this technology is best used.

Suggested Readings

Basra SS, Loyalka P, Kar B. Current status of percutaneous ventricular assist devices for cardiogenic shock. *Curr Opin Cardiol*. 2011;26:548-554.

Hanlon-Pena PM, Quaal SJ. Intra-aortic balloon pump timing: Review of evidence supporting current practice. *Am J Crit Care*. 2011;20:323-333.

Hashemzadeh K, Hashemzadeh S. Early outcomes of intra-aortic balloon pump in cardiac surgery. *J Cardiovasc Surg*. 2012;53:387-392.

Moulopoulos SD. Intra-aortic balloon counterpulsation 50 years later: Initial conception and consequent ideas. *Artif Organs*. 2011;35:843-848.

Parissis H, Soo A, Al-Alao B. Intra aortic balloon pump: Literature review of risk factors related to complications of the intraaortic balloon pump. *J Cardiothorac Surg*. 2011;6:147.

Theologou T, Bashir M, Rengarajan A, et al. Preoperative intra aortic balloon pumps in patients undergoing coronary artery bypass grafting. *Cochrane Database Syst Rev*. 2011:CD004472.

Zaky SS, Hanna AH, Sakr Esa WA, et al. An 11-year, single-institution analysis of intra-aortic balloon pump use in cardiac surgery. *J Cardiothorac Vasc Anesth*. 2009;23:479-483.

PART D Thoracic Anesthesia

CHAPTER 154

Intraoperative Wheezing: Etiology and Treatment

Mary M. Rajala, MS, MD

Wheezing or rhonchi, lung sounds detected by auscultation, are produced when gas flows through a narrowed or obstructed upper or lower airway. The lung sounds are caused by turbulence or resistance to flow. The obstruction can be extrinsic to the airway, intrinsic (within the airway wall), or within the lumen (Box 154-1). For a patient who is intubated and ventilated, an increase in peak airway pressure, a decrease in tidal volume, or a decrease in the slope of the expiratory CO_2 curve may indicate airway narrowing or increased airway resistance. Persistent and severe airway obstruction may be followed by O_2 desaturation, hypercapnia, and hypotension secondary to increased intrathoracic pressure. Most (80%) of the resistance to flow in airways occurs in the large central airways, leaving 20% of airway resistance from the peripheral bronchioles. Thus, large changes in the caliber of small airways may result in small changes in resistance, making the small airways a clinically silent area. In the American Society of Anesthesiologists closed claims analysis, respiratory events that lead to death or permanent brain damage, 56 (11%) were associated with bronchospasm.

Box 154-1 Causes of Ventilatory Obstruction

Airway Disease

- Asthma
- Bronchitis
- Chronic obstructive pulmonary disease
- Cystic fibrosis
- Tumors of the larynx or pharynx
- Foreign body
- Bronchiectasis
- Tracheomalacia
- Laryngeal edema or infection

Bronchoconstriction during Anesthesia

- Airway manipulation
- Tracheal intubation
- Bronchial intubation
- Carinal pressure from the tracheal tube
- Light anesthesia
- Secretions in large airways
- Aspiration of stomach contents
- Infection, pneumonia
- Pulmonary edema
- Pulmonary or amniotic fluid embolus
- Pneumothorax
- Allergens
- Anaphylaxis, anaphylactoid reactions
- Drug reactions from histamine release, antagonism
- Carcinoid tumors

Mechanical Obstruction

- Kinked tracheal tube
- Secretions in tracheal tube
- Obstructed tracheal tube
- High intra-abdominal pressure (laparoscopy)

Reversible and Irreversible Airway Disease

Wheezing may indicate the presence of obstructive lung disease—asthma, chronic obstructive pulmonary disease, chronic bronchitis, or cystic fibrosis. Asthma, a reactive airway disease, is manifest by reversible airway obstruction. Resting bronchial tone is regulated primarily by the parasympathetic nervous system via vagal nerve fibers and muscarinic acetylcholine receptors, of which 3 types exist, M_1 and M_3, which enhance the parasympathetic effects, and M_2, which is inhibitory. Numerous factors—including exercise, cold air, allergens, respiratory infections, emotional factors, β-adrenergic blockade, and the use of a prostaglandin inhibitor, such as aspirin—may override the baseline bronchial tone, provoking an attack in patients with bronchospastic disease. Cross-sensitivity between aspirin and other nonsteroidal antiinflammatory drugs is common and needs to be considered as a cause for bronchospasm, especially in patients with the triad of asthma, nasal polyps, and aspirin-induced asthma. The immunologic component to asthma is well recognized and includes immunoglobulin-E antibody fixed to mast cells and basophils, which release immune mediators in response to challenge with specific antigens. In adults, irritant reflexes are a more important cause, whereas, in children, allergy is an important component in reactive airway disease. The immune mediators include serotonin, eicosanoids, prostaglandins (PGD_2, PGF_2), thromboxane A_2 and leukotrienes (LTC_4, LTD_4, LTE_4), kinin, and perhaps histamine (H_1). Prostaglandins are produced from arachidonic acid by the cyclooxygenase pathway and are potent mast-cell mediators that cause bronchospasm. Leukotrienes are synthesized after mast-cell activation from the metabolism of arachidonic acid via the lipooxygenase pathway. Kinin, produced by mast cells and basophils, can cause bronchoconstriction. In addition, thromboxane A_2, and its metabolite B_2, produced in polymorphonuclear leukocytes and mast cells by the action of cyclooxygenase on arachidonic acid, also constrict pulmonary blood vessels and can lead to pulmonary hypertension.

Perioperative Bronchospasm

Airway Manipulation

Manipulation of the airway can cause reflex bronchoconstriction. Wheezing can be a sign of airway irritation from stimulation of the cholinergic system and subsequent bronchiolar constriction, which occurs when intubation is undertaken in a hyperreflexic airway or if the depth of anesthesia is inadequate at the time of intubation.

Anesthesia and Associated Drugs

The use of either propofol or ketamine offers advantages in patients with a history of bronchospasm. Propofol reduces airway resistance in patients with asthma and chronic obstructive disease. Ketamine helps protect against irritant reflexes, although it increases secretions from salivary and tracheobronchial mucus glands (which can be prevented pharmacologically). Ketamine also stimulates the sympathetic system and attenuates vagal reflexes, leading to smooth muscle relaxation. The newer S-stereoisomer form of ketamine has fewer psychomimetic effects but is also less effective in relaxing smooth muscles. The use of methohexital is associated with wheezing if other drugs are not used to blunt the effect or if adequate depth of anesthesia is not achieved before airway manipulation.

Inhalation anesthetic agents can be used to deepen the level of anesthesia prior to airway manipulation or surgical stimulation or when bronchospasm is mild. In true bronchospasm, the administration of inhalation anesthetic agents will depress airway reactivity and bronchoconstriction by blunting parasympathetic constrictive reflexes and directly relaxing bronchiolar smooth muscle.

Histamine release may occur with administration of anesthetic drugs, including atracurium, cis-atracurium meperidine, and morphine. When administered rapidly or in large doses (as occurs during induction and subsequent airway manipulation), these drugs are more likely to increase the risk of bronchoconstriction. The muscarinic action of cholinesterase inhibitors used for reversal of an anesthetic agent may precipitate bronchospasm. In these situations, prudence suggests using larger than usual doses of atropine (>1.0 mg), or glycopyrrolate (>0.5 mg) to minimize potential bronchospasm in patients who are actively wheezing.

The use of β_2-adrenergic receptor antagonists (labetolol, esmolol) may increase the risk of bronchoconstriction. Although they have been used without untoward effect in the treatment of hypertension in patients with stable chronic obstructive pulmonary disease, the American College of Chest Physicians recommends that these agents be used with extreme caution if at all in patients with reactive airways diseases.

Anaphylactic Reactions

Bronchospasm may result from an anaphylactic or anaphylactoid reaction. Antibiotic drugs, blood products, or intravenously administered contrast agents may be the trigger, with an initial manifestation of wheezing accompanied by hypotension, periorbital and airway edema, urticaria, tachycardia, and arrhythmias.

Carcinoid Syndrome

Rarely, carcinoid tumors may cause bronchospasm. Serotonin (5-hydroxytryptamine [5-HT]) secreted by carcinoid tumors causes bronchoconstriction, which can accompany the hypotension, diarrhea, flushing, and valvular heart disease of carcinoid syndrome. Conventional treatment for bronchospasm is not helpful and may actually provoke bronchospasm in these patients. Therefore, most recommendations are targeted toward preventing release of tumor substances. Anesthetic care involves avoiding histamine-releasing agents (morphine, atracurium), succinylcholine, indirect-acting or direct-acting catecholamines, and extremes of blood pressure to decrease the release of 5-HT from carcinoid tumors. Succinylcholine is thought to provoke release by increasing abdominal pressure and compressing the tumor, and not by intrinsic releasing properties. In addition to avoiding or treating bronchospasm, the anesthesia provider must be ready to intraoperatively deal with decreased peripheral resistance, hypotension, and hypertension in patients with carcinoid tumors. Somatostatin analog (Sandostatin) (100 μg - 600 μg, intravenously) should be administered prophylactically and, if a crisis occurs, rebolused. In addition to blocking the release of pituitary growth hormone and thyrotropin, somatostatin analog, which reduces hormone and exocrine secretions from the gut, has become the therapy of choice for preoperative, intraoperative, and postoperative management of carcinoid crises.

Miscellaneous Pulmonary Diseases

Aspiration pneumonitis, pulmonary edema, or pneumothorax may also trigger bronchospasm.

Treating Perioperative Bronchospasm

Preoperative/Prevention

Patients with reversible airway obstruction or bronchial reactivity are at increased risk of developing bronchospasm. A history of recent upper respiratory infection (within 3 weeks, especially in patients with obstructive airway disease), recent smoking, cough, dyspnea, fever, chronic bronchitis, asthma, or intolerance to cold air, dust, or smoke and prior tolerance of general anesthesia with tracheal intubation are all pertinent in predicting intra operative wheezing. Management should be aimed at identifying these patients through preoperative evaluation and treating them with β_2-adrenergic receptor agonists or inhaled or orally administered corticosteroids. Consideration should be given to using a regional anesthetic technique. Because bronchospasm in children is more frequently due to allergens, the use of mediator inhibitors and anti inflammatory medications is important in prevention. In adults, reducing or reversing irritant reflexes should be the goal. Adequate anxiolysis plays a role in prevention. Treatment should be directed toward the cause of bronchospasm. Antimuscarinic drugs—such as atropine, ipratropium, and glycopyrrolate—have been used to treat bronchoconstriction. However, they are nonselective and, at low doses, may block the beneficial effects of M_2 more than M_1 and M_3, thereby worsening bronchoconstriction. At higher doses, antimuscarinic drugs block all three receptors, resulting in bronchodilation. Anesthetic depth should be adequate prior to intubation or airway manipulation. Lidocaine (1-2 mg/kg), administered topically through a tracheal tube or intravenously (1-3 min prior to intubation), is effective in preventing bronchoconstriction during airway manipulation or in treating acute intraoperative bronchoconstriction.

Intraoperative Bronchospasm—Crisis Management

When intraoperative bronchospasm occurs and causes O_2 desaturation or inadequate ventilation, the following must occur almost simultaneously: administer 100% O_2, deepen anesthesia, cease stimulation or surgery, and immediately call for help. Next, remove the patient's breathing system from the ventilator, hand ventilate, and listen for breath sounds over the chest and central epigastrium. These actions will exclude anesthesia machine and ventilator malfunction as potential causes and help exclude esophageal or bronchial intubation as the cause of desaturation or inadequate ventilation and will allow for assessment of airway resistance. If, while passing a suction catheter down the tracheal tube, the anesthesia provider encounters an obstruction or is able to aspirate secretions (analyzing pH to assess for gastric contents), the tracheal tube may be misplaced, kinked, or blocked. A β_2-adrenergic receptor agonist (e.g., 4-8 puffs of albuterol initially followed by 2 puffs every 10 min) should be administered via the tracheal tube, timed with patient inhalation, through a connector into the tracheal tube. Ipratropium (6 puffs, followed by 2 puffs every 10 min) can also be given in this manner. Once the initial assessment has been completed, corticosteroids (e.g., methylprednisolone 1-2 mg/kg) can be given.

For bronchospasm that does not resolve, an intravenously administered bronchodilator may need to be added to the regimen (e.g., magnesium, 2-4 mg; lidocaine, 1.5-2 mg/kg; or epinephrine, 0.1μg/kg bolus followed by 10-25 $\mu g \cdot kg^{-1} \cdot min^{-1}$ titrated to vital signs and response). Changing from an anesthesia machine ventilator to a higher performance intensive care unit ventilator and stopping the operation as quickly as possible may be necessary. The administration of inhalation anesthetic agents increases anesthetic depth, but doing so may be difficult in patients with acute bronchospasm because of ventilation/perfusion mismatch. Aminophylline and theophylline have less of a role in treating acute bronchospasm, as compared with β_2-adrenergic receptor agonists.

Postoperative Management of a Patient with Intraoperative Bronchospasm

Extubating a wheezing patient who is under deep anesthesia is not typically safe. Although deep extubation will likely reduce bronchospasm, it exposes the patient to residual anesthetic effects, including ventilation/perfusion mismatch, hypercapnia, narcosis, and aspiration of gastric contents.

Suggested Readings

Cheney FW, Posner KL, Lee LA, et al. Trends in anesthesia-related death and brain damage: A closed claims analysis. *Anesthesiology*. 2006;105:1081-1086.

Fanta CH. Asthma. *N Engl J Med*. 2009;360:1002-1014.

Groeben H. Strategies in the patient with compromised respiratory function. *Best Pract Res Clin Anesthesiol*. 2004;18:4:579-574.

Westhorpe RN, Ludbrook GL, Helps SC. Crisis management during anesthesia: Bronchospasm. *Qual Saf Health Care*. 2005;1:e7.

CHAPTER 155

Anesthesia for Laryngeal Operations

Gurinder M. S. Vasdev, MD, MBBS, and Barry A. Harrison, MD

In operations involving the larynx, both the surgeon and the anesthesiologist must share the patient's airway, making an understanding of the operative and anesthesia requirements and ongoing communication among team members essential. Indications for laryngeal operations include congenital (Box 155-1) and acquired conditions. The main acquired conditions include trauma, inflammatory conditions, and tumor (benign and malignant). Laryngeal signs and symptoms vary from a sore throat and hoarseness to difficulty in breathing, stridor, and, if severe, complete upper airway obstruction. The main types of laryngeal operations that necessitate anesthesia, including management of the airway, are direct laryngoscopy, thyroplasty, laryngectomy, and importantly, trauma to the larynx.

Airway Anatomy and Physiology

The human larynx has three basic functions: inspiration, tracheobronchial protection, and phonation. These tasks are achieved through a complex system of neuronal innervation to intrinsic and extrinsic laryngeal musculature suspended on cartilaginous structures. The vagus nerve (cranial nerve X), via the superior and recurrent laryngeal nerve, is responsible for the sensory and motor innervation of the larynx. The internal branch of the superior laryngeal nerve provides ipsilateral sensation to the supraglottic (i.e., above the true vocal folds) larynx. Below the vocal cords, ipsilateral sensation is supplied by the recurrent laryngeal nerve. The posterior half of the vocal cords has the highest density of touch receptors. This is important to remember during fiberoptic intubation when regional or topical anesthesia is used. Stimulation of epiglottic water-sensitive chemoreceptors causes slowed respiration with increased tidal volume, resulting in increased laryngeal airflow. This centrally mediated response appears to be more active in children and is a mechanism by which humidification improves breathing during partial airway obstruction (i.e., slow, large-tidal-volume breathing decreases turbulent airflow).

The recurrent laryngeal nerve provides the motor supply to all intrinsic laryngeal muscles except the cricothyroid muscle. The cricothyroid muscle receives motor innervation from the external branch of the superior laryngeal nerve. The actions of each muscle are summarized in Figure 155-1. There is little chance of effective reinnervation with good laryngeal function when trauma to these nerves occurs.

Phonation is produced by fundamental tone formation in the larynx. This is modified by the resonating chambers of the upper airway. Frequency is determined by isotonic contraction of the cricothyroid muscle. Pitch is determined by changes in the length of the cords and subglottic pressure.

This knowledge is applied in thyroid and parathyroid operations, during which recurrent laryngeal nerve injury may occur. To minimize the possibility of nerve injury, surgeons monitor recurrent laryngeal nerve function by stimulating this nerve via a tracheal tube positioned at the level of the larynx, with the stimulation occurring at the level of the larynx and the recording electrodes positioned at the level of the vocal cords.

Box 155-1 Congenital Laryngeal Pathologic Conditions

- Atresia
- Congenital hemangioma
- Congenital laryngeal paralysis
- Congenital subglottic stenosis
- Laryngomalacia
- Laryngotracheoesophageal cleft
- Laryngeal web
- Lymphangiomas

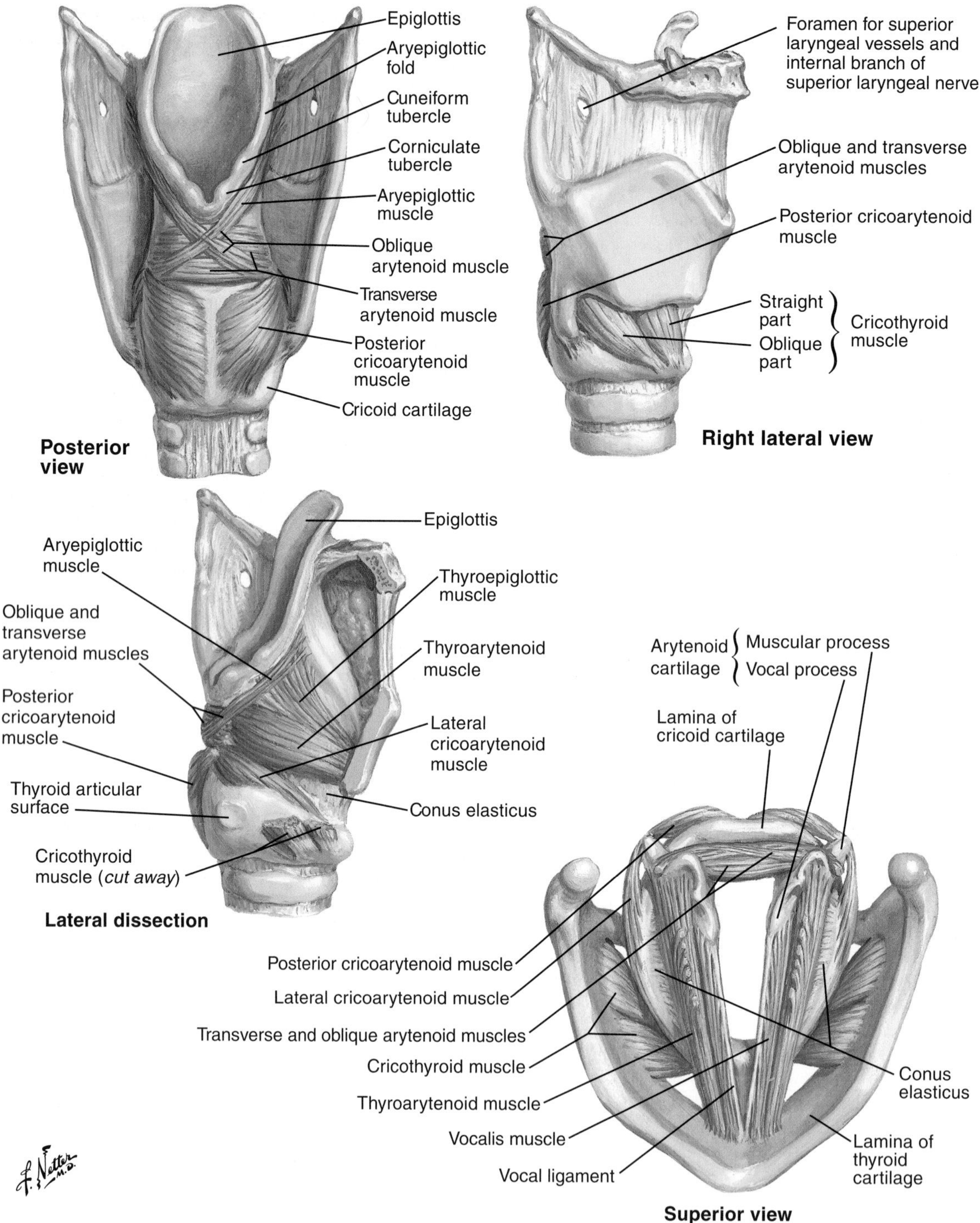

Figure 155-1 The intrinsic muscles of the larynx. (Netter illustration from www.netterimages.com. © Elsevier Inc. All rights reserved.)

Direct Laryngoscopy

Direct laryngoscopy is used for supraglottic, glottic, subglottic, and tracheal examinations for diagnostic, therapeutic, or both diagnostic and therapeutic purposes. Because preexisting cardiac disease accounts for 1.5% to 4% of perioperative deaths in this patient population, preoperative cardiac assessment is important. Preoperative airway assessment is equally important and includes a physical examination, either direct or indirect laryngoscopy, computed tomography, and magnetic resonance imaging. If airway patency is questionable, then awake fiberoptic intubation, tracheotomy, or tracheostomy should be performed under local anesthesia. Premedication with an antisialagogue is beneficial. In surgical procedures requiring general anesthesia, induction can be achieved with either spontaneous ventilation (using a nonirritating inhalation anesthetic) or intravenously administered medications. Topical application of local anesthetic on the vocal cords and adjacent mucosa can decrease the requirements for inhalational anesthesia. Oxygenation is maintained with the use of insufflation in a spontaneously breathing patient with or without the use of a tracheal tube.

Regardless of the technique used, dental injury can occur. Patients with difficult airways are at particular risk for incurring a dental injury. Otorhinolaryngologic surgeons often use dental guards in patients to reduce the risk of injury during direct laryngoscopy. Postsurgical hemoptysis, obstruction, laryngeal edema, and laryngospasm are major risks associated with direct laryngoscopy. As modern technology evolves, direct laryngoscopy may be replaced by indirect methods.

Without a Tracheal Tube

Apneic Oxygenation

During apneic oxygenation, patients are hyperventilated with 100% O_2 and an inhalation anesthetic agent. The surgeon is then allowed airway access in 3-min to 5-min epochs or until desaturation occurs. CO_2 monitoring is not possible with this technique; accordingly, hypercapnia is a potential problem.

Jet Ventilation

In jet ventilation, air is entrained by the Venturi effect when a 30-psi to 50-psi blast from the jet ventilator insufflates O_2 into the airway. A properly placed jet allows visualization of chest wall movement. During jet ventilation, inhalation anesthesia is not possible; intravenously administered anesthesia is best suited for this oxygenation technique.

With a Tracheal Tube

Microlaryngeal Tubes

Microlaryngeal tubes are tracheal tubes with a 3.5-mm to 4-mm external diameter that require stylet-guided placement. General anesthesia should be maintained with short-acting medications because emergence can be challenging. If a laser is being used, a tracheal tube that is laser compatible must be used.

Thyroplasty

Vocal cord operations requiring injection of Teflon, gelatin, botulinum neurotoxin, or steroid can be performed with conscious sedation but may require general anesthesia. The typical patient undergoing a thyroplasty has paralysis of a vocal cord secondary to injury to the recurrent laryngeal nerve. The use of a supraglottic airway is important for the patient who has previously had a thyroplasty and who now requires a general anesthetic.

Laryngectomy

Laryngeal carcinoma accounts for 2% to 3% of all malignancies. Tobacco or alcohol use, radiotherapy, and herpes simplex infection have been implicated as risk factors for the development of laryngeal carcinoma. Patients are predominantly men over the age of 50 years. Laryngeal carcinoma occurs in supraglottic (30%), glottic (60%), and subglottic (10%) forms.

Careful preoperative patient assessment is vital because these patients often have significant comorbid disease (e.g., chronic obstructive pulmonary disease, coronary artery disease, congestive heart failure, hypertension, nicotine dependence, and alcohol abuse). Liver function should be evaluated in patients with a significant history of alcohol intake.

The airway is often secured using awake techniques with conscious sedation (e.g., fiberoptic intubation or tracheotomy). The type of anesthesia (i.e., awake vs. general) is determined by airway anatomy, severity of comorbid diseases, patient preference, and health care team preference. Continuous monitoring of arterial pressure via an indwelling arterial cannula is helpful, particularly when the neck dissection involves the area around the carotid sinus. Additionally, an arterial catheter provides access for obtaining blood for laboratory studies (e.g., obtaining serial hemoglobin concentrations), which is essential during surgical procedures associated with large blood loss (e.g., total laryngectomy with neck dissection). If the use of a central venous catheter is indicated, the catheter can be placed via the subclavian route or a long line can be inserted from the antecubital space or via the femoral vein. Potential perioperative complications include air embolism, hypertension, parathyroid and cranial nerve dysfunction, and facial edema. The use of a nasogastric tube is helpful in the postoperative period for both gastric drainage and postoperative feeding. Preliminary experience with transoral robotic surgery for head and neck cancer is encouraging, suggesting that this modality will be used more frequently in the future.

Laryngeal and Tracheal Trauma

Laryngeal or tracheal trauma is seen in approximately 1 in 43,000 emergency department admissions. Clinical signs include hoarseness, tenderness, subcutaneous emphysema, respiratory distress (e.g., stridor), dysphagia, and hemoptysis. The best outcomes are observed when an otolaryngologist is involved in managing the patient's airway and any treatment is performed in the operating room. If the patient's airway is stable, oral intubation under general anesthesia, with either rapid sequence or inhaled induction, may be used. If the patient's airway is unstable, if the laryngeal mucosa is disrupted, or if the patient has a laryngoskeletal fracture (confirmed with computed tomography), awake fiberoptic intubation or awake tracheotomy under local anesthesia should be performed. Inhaled induction of anesthesia followed by orotracheal intubation may be necessary in confused or uncooperative patients, even in the presence of a risk for aspiration.

Suggested Readings

Barakate M, Maver E, Wotherspoon G, Havas T. Anaesthesia for microlaryngeal and laser laryngeal surgery: Impact of subglottic jet ventilation. *J Laryngol Otol*. 2010;124:641-645.

Irwin E, Lonnée H. Management of near fatal blunt laryngeal trauma. *Acta Anaesthesiol Scand*. 2006;50:766-767.

Kochilas X, Bibas A, Xenellis J, Anagnostopoulou S. Surgical anatomy of the external branch of the superior laryngeal nerve and its clinical significance in head and neck surgery. *Clin Anat*. 2008;21:99-105.

Lin HW, Bhattacharyya N. Incidence of perioperative airway complications in patients with previous medialization thyroplasty. *Laryngoscope*. 2009; 119:675-678.

Ramachandran SK, Cosnowski A, Shanks A, Turner CR. Apneic oxygenation during prolonged laryngoscopy in obese patients: A randomized, controlled trial of nasal oxygen administration. *J Clin Anesth*. 2010;22:164-168.

Sasaki CT, Weaver EM. Physiology of the larynx. *Am J Med*. 1997;103:9S-18.

CHAPTER 156

Anesthesia for Bronchoscopy

Barry A. Harrison, MD, and Gurinder M. S. Vasdev, MD, MBBS

Bronchoscopy allows for direct visualization of the tracheobronchial tree utilizing either a rigid metallic tube with an attached light source (rigid bronchoscope) or a flexible tube with a bundle of optical fibers running through the tube (flexible bronchoscope). Because of its size and rigidity, the rigid bronchoscope is used primarily in the central airways, where it is used for removing endobronchial tumor, inserting stents to dilate major bronchi, removing foreign bodies, and aspirating blood. Gustav Killian first described the use of the bronchoscope in 1897, and in 1963, optical fibers were first used to make a flexible bronchoscope. The fiberoptic bronchoscope (FOB) provides excellent visualization of, and access to, the tracheobronchial tree and is used in more than 90% of all bronchoscopic procedures. In the past, the size of the bronchoscope limited its use, but as technology has advanced, the FOB is used more often, along with laser therapy and stents, to relieve central airway obstruction due to tumor or stenosis following lung transplantation.

Clinical Aspects of Bronchoscopy

The indications for bronchoscopy are outlined in Box 156-1. A complete history and physical examination are necessary for all patients undergoing bronchoscopy for whom an anesthesia provider has been asked to assist.

Box 156-1 Indications for Bronchoscopy

Therapeutic	Diagnostic

Removal of
  Foreign body
  Secretions
Control of hemorrhage
Treat endobronchial obstruction with
  Thermal lasers
  Photodynamic therapy
  Brachytherapy
Dilate airway with
  Rigid scope
  Stent
  Balloon
Close bronchopleural fistula
	Identify source of
	  Hemorrhage in a patient with hemoptysis
	  Unexplained cough
	Assess
	  Airway anatomy
	  Airway function
	  Tracheobronchial mucosa
	  Peribronchial structures
	Brush
	  Mucosa, lung parenchyma, cytology
	  Protective brush for quantitative bacteriologic culture
	Biopsy
	  Bronchial wall
	  Transbronchial lung biopsy
	  Transbronchial lymph node biopsy
	Lavage
	  Qualitative for inflammatory cells, neutrophils
	  Quantitative for bacteria

Concurrent medical problems increase the risks associated with the procedure; for example, patients who have a history of lung disease have an increased incidence of bronchospasm during bronchoscopy. Similarly, patients with restrictive ventilatory defects (e.g., interstitial lung disease) with or without preexisting hypoxia may have significant hypoxia during the procedure. Patients with lung cancer undergoing bronchoscopy may have other comorbid conditions (e.g., central airway obstruction, superior vena cava obstruction, metastatic lesions [bone, brain, liver] and electrolyte imbalance [hyponatremia and hypercalcemia]). Patients with pulmonary hypertension, elevated blood urea nitrogen (>30 mg/dL), chronic renal disease, and aspirin ingestion have an increased risk of postoperative bleeding. Interestingly, patients with recent myocardial infarction, unstable angina, or refractory arrhythmias often undergo bronchoscopy without significant complications.

A preoperative chest radiograph is mandatory; other investigations (e.g., complete blood count, electrolyte panel, and coagulation studies) are performed as indicated. Resting pulse oximetry prior to the procedure is essential in providing baseline information. Pulmonary function testing establishes the presence and severity of restrictive versus obstructive disease and the degree of reversibility, if any, with treatment. If respiratory failure is suspected or if the patient is on domiciliary oxygen, a preoperative arterial blood gas analysis is indicated.

Aims of Anesthesia for Bronchoscopy

During bronchoscopy, it is important to suppress the patient's cough reflex and the hemodynamic response associated with bronchoscopy. Anesthesia may vary from no sedation, to mild to deep sedation, to general anesthesia. The type of anesthesia depends on the type of bronchoscope used—(FOB or rigid). The use of a topical anesthetic agent with or without sedation is used in most flexible FOB procedures. General anesthesia is usually required for rigid bronchoscopy and often in patients undergoing relief of a central obstruction with a FOB: however, sedation and local anesthesia may also be successfully used in both of these scenarios.

Preoperative Preparation

After anesthesia and risks are discussed with a fasting (>6 h) patient, an antisialagogue (either atropine, 0.4-0.8 mg, or glycopyrrolate, 0.1-0.2 mg) is administered intramuscularly or intravenously 40 min prior to the procedure. Aerosolized bronchodilators, β_2-adrenergic receptor agonists, and anticholinergic agents are administered to patients with reactive airway disease before they undergo bronchoscopy. Corticosteroids are indicated during an exacerbation of reactive airway disease. The American Heart Association recommends subacute bacterial endocarditis prophylaxis for rigid bronchoscopy but not for bronchoscopy using a FOB unless the patient has a prosthetic heart valve, a surgically corrected intracardiac defect, or a history of endocarditis. Depending on the situation, patients on intravenous heparin should have the heparin discontinued 4 to 6 h before the procedure, and platelets should be transfused to maintain platelet levels greater than 50,000/mL. For patients undergoing any type of anesthesia, the American Society of Anesthesiology guidelines for monitoring should be followed.

Sedation

Without sedation, bronchoscopy is associated with increased cough, increased sense of asphyxiation, less amnesia for the procedure, and a significant increase in heart rate and blood pressure. Conscious sedation is usually achieved with intravenously administered incremental doses of midazolam (0.5-1.0 mg) or diazepam (1-2 mg). Intravenously administered opioids act synergistically with benzodiazepines to provide sedation and suppress airway reflexes but at the expense of potentiating respiratory depression. Fentanyl, sufentanil, alfentanil, and remifentanil are suitable opioid choices. Propofol can be used as a sedative agent, titrated in 10-mg doses, to provide conscious sedation and suppression of cough reflexes; however, significant hypotension and even apnea may result from excess drug administration. Intravenously administered dexmedetomidine has also been used to provide sedation for flexible bronchoscopy with a FOB.

Topical Anesthesia for Bronchoscopy

The sensory innervation of the upper airway is described in Table 156-1. Topical anesthetic agents, administered topically or via peripheral nerve blocks, can be used to anesthetize the upper airway. Two percent lidocaine (liquid or gel) is commonly used for topical airway anesthesia due to its margin of safety, rapid onset, and short duration of action. The maximum safe dose of lidocaine is 4 mg/kg. Toxicity depends on the rate of absorption and the resulting blood levels. Two percent lidocaine sprayed into or 4% viscous lidocaine-soaked pledgets placed in the nares (along with phenylephrine or cocaine to vasoconstrict the mucosal surfaces) can be used to anesthetize the nasopharynx. Oropharyngeal anesthesia can be achieved by one of several means (Box 156-2). These techniques provide satisfactory anesthesia of the upper airway. If persistent gag reflex prevents bronchoscopy, then the use of bilateral glossopharyngeal nerve blocks is indicated. Using a tonsillar needle, 3 mL of 2% lidocaine is injected into the midpoint of both posterior tonsillar pillars to a depth of 1 cm. This will effectively block the submucosa pressor receptors at the posterior aspect of the tongue. These blocks should always be performed following superior laryngeal nerve blocks because, without them, significant pharyngeal muscle and tongue relaxation may result, obstructing the airway.

Table 156-1 Sensory Innervation of the Upper Airway

Anatomic Structure	Nerve Supply
Nose	Trigeminal V—ophthalmic V_1, maxillary V_2
Tongue	
Anterior	Trigeminal V—lingual V_3
Posterior	Glossopharyngeal IX
Pharynx	
Nasal	Trigeminal V—maxillary branch V_2
Oral	Glossopharyngeal IX
Larynx	Vagus X—internal laryngeal branch
Vocal cords	Vagus X—internal laryngeal branch
Trachea	Vagus X—internal laryngeal branch

Box 156-2 Methods to Achieve Oropharyngeal Anesthesia During Bronchoscopy

Mouth and pharynx—gargle and rinse with 2% viscous lidocaine
Nebulized 2% lidocaine solution (95% effective when nebulized for 10 min)
Superior laryngeal nerve blocks
Transcricothyroid membrane injection
Topicalization through suction port of the FOB
Application of 4 mL of EMLA cream to the posterior one third of the tongue

EMLA, Eutectic mixture of local anesthetics (lidocaine and prilocaine); FOB, fiberoptic bronchoscope.

Treatment of Hypoxemia for Bronchoscopy with a Fiberoptic Bronchoscope Under Sedation and Topical Anesthesia

Hypoxemia during bronchoscopy may occur because of a decreased inspired fraction of O_2 (FIO_2), hypoventilation due to excess sedation or upper airway obstruction, ventilation-perfusion mismatch due to pneumothorax secondary to transbronchial biopsy or excessive bleeding or from pulmonary lavage. Pulse oximetry is essential for monitoring, with a goal of maintaining an O_2 saturation (SpO_2) of at least 90%. Administration of supplemental O_2 (4-6 L/min) via nasal prongs or mask may help achieve this goal. If hypoxia persists, a nasopharyngeal tube should be inserted and O_2 administered via this route. If the SpO_2 saturation remains below 90%, the next step is to administer O_2 via a catheter passed nasally that is placed either above the larynx or in the proximal trachea. If O_2 desaturation continues, the bronchoscope should be withdrawn, an arterial blood gas should be measured, the sedation reversed, and an anesthesia bag and mask used to ventilate the patient. In such circumstances, tracheal intubation and ventilation with a high FIO_2 may be necessary.

General Anesthesia

Rigid Bronchoscopy

An awake intubation should be planned for an anticipated difficult airway. If awake intubation is not feasible, an inhalation induction technique is a safe alternative. An intravenous induction technique is used if no airway difficulty is anticipated. Anesthesia can be maintained with either an inhalation or intravenous technique.

Propofol is an ideal choice to maintain anesthesia if a total intravenous anesthetic technique is used because of its rapid onset and offset plus its suppression of airway reflexes. The administration of a potent opioid is often necessary because bronchoscopy can increase mean arterial pressure, heart rate, cardiac output, and pulmonary artery occlusion pressure to unacceptable levels. Fentanyl and sufentanil can be administered intermittently, or alfentanil and remifentanil can be given as a continuous infusion following a loading dose.

Neuromuscular blockade, which is often required, can be achieved with the use of a nondepolarizing agent with rapid onset and intermediate duration of action (e.g., rocuronium) or, alternatively, with a succinylcholine drip. Lambert-Eaton syndrome, a neuromuscular disorder associated with small cell lung neoplasms, increases the sensitivity of patients who have the syndrome to the effects of both depolarizing and nondepolarizing neuromuscular blocking agents.

If the duration of the procedure is short, apneic oxygenation with intermittent ventilation is both easy and effective. Following induction of anesthesia and neuromuscular blockade, the patient is denitrogenated with 100% O_2, and then O_2 at 6 L/min is insufflated through a catheter passed through the vocal cords to lie just above the main carina. Although it may be possible to maintain SaO_2, the $PaCO_2$ tension will increase approximately 4 to 6 mm Hg the first minute and 2 to 4 mm Hg per minute thereafter. Intermittent periods of ventilation may be necessary to attenuate the associated respiratory acidosis.

Sealing the open end of a rigid bronchoscope with the attached magnifying glass and attaching the breathing circuit from an anesthesia machine to the side arm of the rigid bronchoscope allows the anesthesia provider to better oxygenate and ventilate the patient, with the added benefit of permitting the provider to maintain anesthesia using an inhaled anesthetic agent. When this technique is used for prolonged procedures, hypoxemia and hypercapnia may develop during times that the proximal end of the bronchoscope is open for instrumentation of the airway.

The Sanders jet injector technique, with is now frequently employed, makes use of the Venturi principle, in which gas ($FIO_2 \geq 0.21$) under high pressure (50 psi) flows through a long metal tube with a small orifice entraining air from the open outlet, maintaining ventilation. This technique works well except in patients with decreased lung compliance in whom ventilation and oxygenation may be difficult to maintain. Because the gas is injected under high pressure, care must be taken to avoid barotrauma.

Bronchoscopy with a Fiberoptic Bronchoscope

A 7.5-ID or larger tracheal tube is necessary to allow passage of an FOB of sufficient size to perform any planned procedures. The decrease in cross-sectional area of the tracheal tube once the FOB is inserted often requires assisted ventilation and supplemental O_2. A closed system is achieved with a self-sealing rubber diaphragm in the connector to the breathing circuit of the anesthesia machine. As with rigid bronchoscopy, bronchoscopy with an FOB can be performed with either a total intravenous technique or an inhalation technique. The topical administration of a local anesthetic agent to the airway prior to the induction of general anesthesia decreases anesthetic requirements.

Removal of a Foreign Body

The typical patient having a foreign body removed is a young, distressed, nonfasted child who has aspirated a peanut. Atropine is typically administered for its vagolytic and antisialagogue effects. Induction is aimed at reducing patient distress, which has the potential to disrupt the foreign body and cause asphyxia. Either systemic ketamine or a gradual inhalation technique with sevoflurane can be used. Following induction, the aim is to keep the patient spontaneously breathing to prevent further dislodgement of the foreign body. If neuromuscular blockade is necessary, then adequate expiratory time is important to prevent barotrauma from a ball-valve effect of the foreign body. The peanut usually lodges in the right main bronchus; adequate oxygenation and ventilation are maintained via the left lung; when the peanut is being removed, however, it may detach from the forceps and obstruct the lumen of the trachea. If the peanut is not readily retrieved and the patient becomes increasingly hypoxic, the solution is to push the peanut distally back into the bronchus to relieve the tracheal obstruction. When significant manipulation takes place, postprocedural obstruction due to mucosal edema may occur; therefore, corticosteroids are often administered prophylactically.

Management of Massive Hemoptysis

Massive hemoptysis (>600 mL of blood/24 h) is a rare but life-threatening crisis. The immediate therapy involves correcting the hypoxia by placing a tracheal tube (preferably a double-lumen tracheal tube if the bleeding is from either the right or left lung) and administering 100% O_2. Intravenous fluid resuscitation is indicated to correct hypovolemia, if present. If the bleeding is from the trachea or proximal main bronchi, the tracheal tube can be withdrawn and replaced with a rigid ventilating bronchoscope to locate the source of bleeding, aspirate blood and clots, instill iced saline and vasoconstrictors, and, if necessary, place a bronchial blocker into the bronchus from which the blood is emanating. A jet ventilation technique would be inappropriate in this situation because dry gas under pressure will cause the blood to solidify, thus exacerbating the obstruction and hypoxemia.

Bronchoscopy Management of Central Airway Obstruction

Until recently, central airway obstruction was usually caused by a foreign body or massive hemoptysis. Now, intrinsic processes (intraluminal malignancy and strictures related to lung transplantation or intubation) or extrinsic processes (external compression by tumors) are providing challenging cases for therapeutic bronchoscopy. For urgent obstruction relief, laser ablation, electrocautery, argon plasma coagulation, and placement of airway stents (metal, silicone, and hybrid) are used. Cryotherapy, brachytherapy, and photodynamic therapy provide delayed relief of central airway obstruction. A FOB or a rigid bronchoscope can be used, depending on the planned procedure and skill and experience of the bronchoscopist. With the use of a rigid bronchoscope for relief of an obstruction of the trachea or major bronchi, an inhalation induction technique should be attempted, with a trial of positive-pressure ventilation used once the patient has been adequately anesthetized. The rigid bronchoscope is then introduced, and the patient's nose and mouth packed. Obstruction of the airway due to necrotic tissue and excessive bleeding during treatment of the obstruction, most often with laser therapy, can precipitate hypoxia, requiring cessation of the procedure, administration of 100% O_2, and vigorous suction. During laser therapy, it is important to decrease the FIO_2 to 0.3 or less to minimize the possibility of airway fires. The anesthesia provider must communicate with the bronchoscopist if unable to maintain an SpO_2 of at least 90% with an FIO_2 to 0.3 or less; in this situation, the bronchoscopist should stop using the laser until oxygenation is improved and the FIO_2 is again decreased to 0.3 or less.

Both lasers and argon plasma coagulation technology involve the use of gas flow, which has the potential to lead to gas embolism, exacerbating hypoxemia and, in some instances, causing cardiac arrest. A review of patients undergoing rigid bronchoscopy under general anesthesia for airway-stent placement found a complication incidence of 19.8% and a 30-day mortality rate of 7.8%, which was correlated with the patients' underlying health status and the urgency of the procedure.

Complications Associated with Bronchoscopy

A mortality rate of less than 0.1%, a rate of major complications of less than 1.5%, and a rate of minor complications of less than 6.5% have been reported with the use of bronchoscopy (Box 156-3). Significantly, 50% of complications are due to the premedication, the general anesthetic, or the local anesthetic agent used for the procedure. Because rigid bronchoscopy is usually carried out under total intravenous anesthesia, awareness is a recognized complication.

Box 156-3 Complications of Bronchoscopy

General	Local
Hypoxemia	Dental and facial trauma
Sedation/anesthesia	Hemorrhage
Methemoglobinemia	Bronchospasm
Hypercarbia	Pneumothorax
Sedation/anesthesia	Central airway obstruction
Inadequate ventilation	caused by
Cardiac arrhythmias	Tumor
Awareness and recall	Blood
Neurologic—seizures	Secretions
Cardiac arrest and death	Peripheral airway obstruction
	due to
	Asthma
	Chronic bronchitis
	Emphysema
	Airway trauma

Bronchoscopy-induced hemodynamic changes increase myocardial O_2 demand in patients at risk of developing myocardial ischemia. Hypoxemia predisposes the patients to developing cardiac arrhythmias and ST-segment changes, whereas coronary artery disease, per se, does not increase the risk for developing arrhythmias. Hypoxemia and hypercarbia contribute greatly to the cardiovascular complications associated with bronchoscopy. Severe hypoxemia and hypercarbia may also result in seizures, but these are usually associated with local anesthetic toxicity.

Summary

The anesthesia provider is challenged during a bronchoscopic procedure because she or he must share the airway with the bronchoscopist. During bronchoscopy, the airway is always at risk for obstruction so the provider must remember, "A FOB is never an airway, whereas a rigid bronchoscope may be." Complications of bronchoscopy, such as hypoxemia and hypercarbia, are common and can result in cardiovascular complications, even cardiopulmonary arrest. Because the airway is shared, so too are the complications shared between the anesthesia provider and the bronchoscopist. Communication, cooperation, vigilance, and attention to detail—especially to O_2 saturation and minute ventilation—improve outcomes.

Suggested Readings

Kaplan JA, Slinger PD. *Thoracic Anesthesia*. Philadelphia: Churchill Livingstone; 2003.

Ross AF, Ferguson JS. Advances in interventional pulmonology. *Curr Opin Anaesth*. 2009;*22*:11-17.

Wang K-P, Mehat AC, Turner F. *Flexible Bronchoscopy*. Hoboken, NJ: Wiley-Blackwell; 2012.

CHAPTER 157
Double-Lumen Tracheal Tubes

David J. Cook, MD, and Eduardo S. Rodrigues, MD

Double-lumen tracheal tubes enable functional separation of the lungs. This separation can prevent spillage or contamination of blood and pus from one lung to the other and can control the distribution of ventilation. The most common indication for single-lung ventilation is to improve surgical exposure; this is a relative indication (Box 157-1). Although single-lung ventilation can also be achieved with single-lumen tubes and bronchial blockers, double-lumen tubes have several advantages (Box 157-2).

Lung separation can be lifesaving, but its initiation can produce sudden and dramatic impairment of O_2 exchange. Other disadvantages particular to the use of double-lumen tubes are that they increase airway resistance and can make clearance of secretions difficult. Relative contraindications must also be considered when contemplating placement of these tubes (Box 157-3).

Box 157-1 Indications for Separation of the Two Lungs (Double-Lumen Tube Intubation) or One-Lung Ventilation

Absolute Indication	Relative Indication
Isolation of one lung from the other to avoid spillage or contamination because of	Surgical exposure (high priority) for
Infection	Thoracic aortic aneurysm
Massive hemorrhage	Pneumonectomy
Control of the distribution of ventilation due to	Upper lobectomy
Bronchopleural fistula	Mediastinal exposure
Bronchopleural cutaneous fistula	Thoracoscopy
Surgical opening of a major conducting airway	Surgical exposure (medium [lower] priority) for
Giant unilateral lung cyst or bulla	Middle and lower lobectomies and subsegmental resections
Tracheobronchial tree disruption	Esophageal resection
Life-threatening hypoxemia due to unilateral lung disease	Procedures on the thoracic spine
Unilateral bronchopulmonary lavage for pulmonary alveolar proteinosis	Postcardiopulmonary bypass status after removal of totally occluding chronic unilateral pulmonary emboli
Video-assisted thoracic surgery	Severe hypoxemia due to unilateral lung disease
Minimally invasive cardiac surgery	

Reprinted, with permission, from Benumof JL. Anesthesia for Thoracic Surgery. 2nd ed. Philadelphia: WB Saunders; 1995.

Box 157-2 Advantages to the Use of Double-Lumen Tracheal Tubes

Relative ease of placement
Rapid conversion from one-lung to two-lung ventilation
Provision for suctioning from both lungs
Application of CPAP to the nonventilated lung

CPAP, Continuous positive airway pressure.

Box 157-3 Relative Contraindications to the Use of a Double-Lumen Tracheal Tube

Presence of a lesion along the pathway of the double-lumen tube
Difficult or impossible conventional direct-vision intubation
Critically ill patients with single-lumen tube in situ who cannot tolerate even a short time without mechanical ventilation
Full stomach or high risk of aspiration

Modified, with permission, from Benumof JL. Anesthesia for Thoracic Surgery. 2nd ed. Philadelphia: WB Saunders; 1995.

Tube Selection

Double lumen tubes include Carlens, White, Bryce-Smith, and Robertshaw which all share common features: they have two lumina, one terminating in the trachea and the other in the right or left main bronchus; have two cuffs; and are molded to conform to the oropharynx and main bronchus. The Carlens is a left-sided tube with a carinal hook. The White is essentially a right-sided Carlens; the Bryce-Smith lacks a carinal hook and has a slotted cuff on its right-sided version to allow right upper lobe ventilation.

Other than the modern Robertshaw, none of these double-lumen tubes are available any longer. The Robertshaw clear plastic and disposable, with left-sided and right-sided versions. It lacks a carinal hook and generally has a lower resistance to airflow than do other designs. The tubes are available in sizes 41F, 39F, 37F, 35F, 32F (left only), and 28F (with an internal diameter of each lumen of approximately 6.5, 6.0, 5.5, 5.0, 4.5 and 4.0 mm, respectively). Both cuffs are high-volume, low-pressure type, with the bronchial cuff colored bright blue; this bronchial cuff is also slanted in the right-sided version to improve right upper lobe ventilation. Finally, this version has a radiopaque line at the end of each lumen to allow for radiographic detection of placement.

The left-sided double-lumen tube can be used for most thoracic procedures requiring one-lung ventilation, regardless of the operative side. It should be used for right thoracotomies requiring right-lung collapse and can also be used for left thoracotomies with left-lung collapse. In left-sided operations, the bronchial portion of the left-sided tube can be withdrawn into the trachea at the time of left main bronchus clamping and continue to be used for right-lung ventilation through both lumens.

Conversely, use of the right-sided tube can be problematic. To ventilate the right upper lobe, the slot of the bronchial portion of the right-sided tube must be closely opposed to the orifice of the right upper lobe. Because the length of the right main bronchus is shorter and more variable than that of the left main bronchus, right-sided bronchial intubation poses a significant risk for right upper lobe collapse and hypoventilation. Generally, the left main bronchus is 5.0 cm long until the bifurcation of the left upper lobe occurs. On the right side, the upper lobe will depart after 2 cm in most people, but in 10% of patients, this could be shorter, and in 3% of patients, it comes from the trachea. This gives a margin of safety on the positioning as short as 1 mm, and dislocation during surgery is more common, making adequate ventilation of the right upper lobe a challenge.

The contraindications to left-sided placement are carinal or proximal left main bronchus lesions that could be traumatized by a left-sided tube. Except for these contraindications, a left-sided tube is preferred when possible.

Double-Lumen Tube Placement Technique

To place the double-lumen tube, the following steps are performed.

- Choose the correct tube size using preoperative chest radiographs and computed tomography to measure the patient's trachea and left main bronchi. In the past, the largest tube possible was chosen; however, it has now been established that airway trauma is related to the size of the tube.

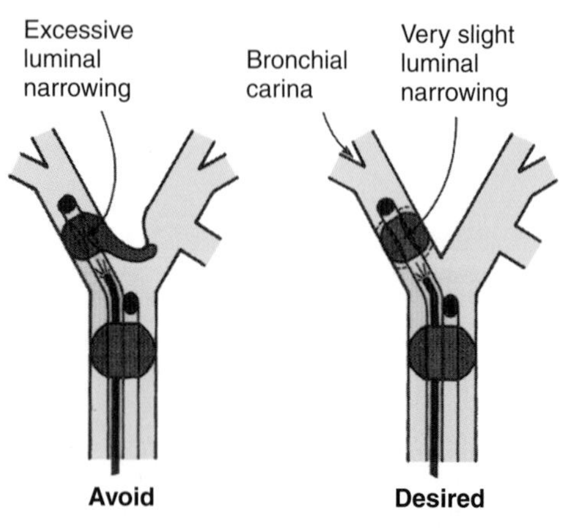

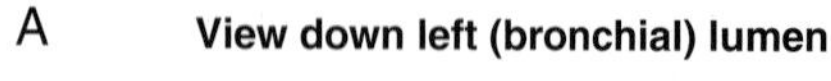

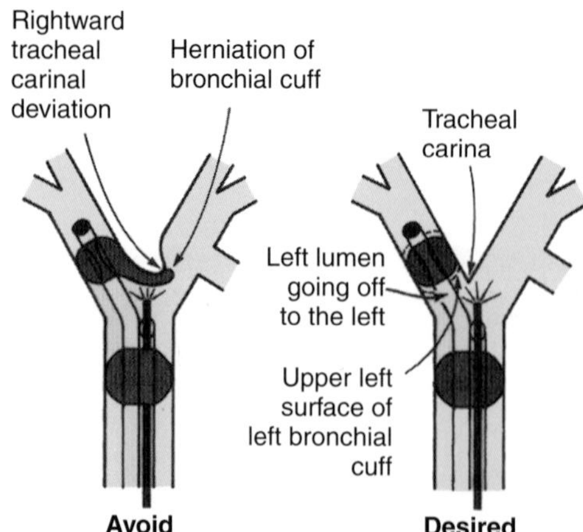

Figure 157-1 This schematic diagram depicts the complete fiberoptic bronchoscopy picture of left-sided double-lumen tracheal tubes (both the desired view and the view to be avoided from both of the lumina). **A,** When the bronchoscope is passed down the left lumen of the left-sided tube, the endoscopist should see a very slight left luminal narrowing and a clear straight-ahead view of the bronchial carina off in the distance. Excessive left luminal narrowing should be avoided. **B,** When the bronchoscope is passed down the right lumen of the left-sided tube, the endoscopist should see a clear straight-ahead view of the tracheal carina and the upper surface of the blue left endobronchial cuff just below the tracheal carina. Excessive pressure in the endobronchial cuff, as manifested by tracheal carinal deviation to the right and herniation of the endobronchial cuff over the carina, should be avoided. (Adapted from Benumof JL. Anesthesia for Thoracic Surgery. 2nd ed. Philadelphia: WB Saunders; 1995.)

A 37F tracheal tube is appropriate for use in most women and a 39F for men. Amar and associates showed that a 35F tube is appropriate for most patients and does not increase the risk of hypoxia. The amount of airway hygiene that will be required during surgery needs to be taken into account when selecting the correct tube size.

- Review the patient's history and examine the patient for conditions that may affect tube choice or require special intubation techniques.
- Check both cuffs (the bronchial cuff usually requires less than 3 mL of air); cuffs can be protected at intubation with a tooth guard.
- In most cases, use a Macintosh blade for intubation because this blade approximates the curvature of the tracheal tube.
- Pass the tip of the tube through the larynx, with the distal curvature concave anteriorly.
- Once the tip is through the larynx, remove the stylette, and rotate the tube 90 degrees toward the appropriate side.
- After intubation, the anesthesia provider must use an established routine to verify tube placement; this method can comprise clinical signs or fiberoptic visualization. Clinical signs alone may miss malpositioning 48% of the time. For this reason, fiberoptic bronchoscopy is routinely used to confirm proper positioning (Figure 157-1).
- Tube position must be reconfirmed after repositioning the patient. Head flexion may cause tube advancement, bronchial placement of the tracheal lumen, or upper lobe obstruction if a right-sided tube is used. Head extension can cause bronchial decannulation. In addition, intraoperative surgical manipulation may displace the tube.
- Most of the complications associated with the placement of double-lumen tracheal tubes (Box 157-4) involve the use of older Carlens tubes and can be avoided by checking tube position multiple times, selecting an appropriately sized tube, paying attention to cuff inflation, using extreme care in repositioning patients, and using caution in patients with bronchial wall abnormalities.

Box 157-4 Complications of the Use of Double-Lumen Tracheal Tubes

Malpositioning
Tracheobronchial tree disruption
Traumatic laryngitis
Suturing of the double-lumen tracheal tube to the intrathoracic structure

Reprinted, with permission, from Benumof JL. Anesthesia for Thoracic Surgery. 2nd ed. Philadelphia: WB Saunders; 1995.

Suggested Readings

Amar D, Desiderio D, Heerdt PM, et al. Practice patterns in choice of left double-lumen tube size for thoracic surgery. *Anesth Analg*. 2008;106:379-383.

Benumof JL, Alfery DD. Anesthesia for thoracic surgery. In: Miller RD, ed. *Anesthesia*. 5th ed. Philadelphia: Churchill Livingstone; 2000:1665-1752.

CHAPTER 158

One-Lung Ventilation and Methods of Improving Oxygenation

Michael J. Murray, MD, PhD, and Sarang S. Koushik, MD

One-lung ventilation (OLV) is achieved through a double-lumen tracheal tube, through a single-lumen tracheal tube advanced into either the right or left mainstem bronchus, or by advancing a bronchial blocker though a single-lumen tracheal tube into one of the mainstem bronchi. Multiple indications for OLV are noted in Table 158-1.

Table 158-1 Indications for One-Lung Ventilation

Absolute	Relative
Video-assisted thoracoscopy	Surgery on thoracic aorta or esophagus
Protective isolation (infection, hemorrhage)	
Differential ventilation (bronchopleural fistula)	Pneumonectomy or lobar resection*
Pulmonary alveolar lavage	

*If one-lung ventilation is used, the surgical incision can be smaller because the deflation of the nondependent lung enables the surgeon to have better surgical access without a large thoracotomy incision.

Mechanism of Hypoxia

The lateral decubitus position is often necessary to perform various thoracic operations and for some cardiac surgical procedures. When patients are in the lateral position, their dependent lung is often underventilated because it is compressed by the abdominal contents and by the mediastinum. The nondependent lung is relatively overventilated because its compliance is increased, particularly when the corresponding hemithorax is opened. Conversely, because of gravity, the dependent lung is well perfused, whereas the nondependent lung is underperfused. Because of the mismatch of perfusion to ventilation, hypoxemia is common in patients operated upon in the lateral decubitus position. Once ventilation to the nondependent lung ceases and the dependent lung is the only lung being ventilated (as occurs with OLV), the nondependent lung becomes atelectatic and the ventilation-perfusion ratio approaches 0, creating a transpulmonary shunt through the upper lung. The degree of hypoxemia correlates with the degree of the shunt. Because CO_2 is 20 times more diffusible than O_2 in the lung, ventilation through the dependent lung removes sufficient CO_2 so that hypercarbia is rarely seen.

Factors Affecting Oxygenation During One-Lung Ventilation

Many factors may affect oxygenation during OLV. Normally, when part of a lung is not ventilated (e.g., atelectasis, edema), "hypoxic" pulmonary vasoconstriction (HPV) restricts flow to the affected alveoli. HPV is of greatest benefit when 30% to 70% of the alveoli in a region contain a hypoxic gas mixture or are collapsed. Many factors blunt HPV and contribute to the development of hypoxemia, even when the patient is ventilated with 100% O_2. Most systemic vasodilators (e.g., nitroglycerin, nitroprusside, calcium channel blockers, and many β_2-receptor agonists) inhibit HPV. With the exception of N_2O, the inhalation anesthetic agents also inhibit HPV but not to such an extent as to be clinically relevant. Anything that increases pulmonary arterial pressure—volume overload, elevated left atrial pressure, pulmonary embolism, vasoconstriction in the pulmonary vasculature caused by drugs (dopamine, epinephrine, phenylephrine, and other vasoconstrictors that preferentially constrict normoxic lung vessels and defeat the HPV mechanism), or hypocarbia—will decrease flow through the dependent lung and increase the shunt through the nondependent lung. Hypocapnia directly inhibits HPV, but during OLV this can be achieved only through hyperventilation of the dependent lung, leading to increased airway pressure and increased pulmonary vascular resistance (PVR) in the ventilated lung, which redirects blood flow into the nondependent lung, thereby worsening the shunt.

Although HPV is responsible for most of the redistribution of blood flow away from the nonventilated lung, compression of the nonventilated lung may further reduce blood flow in the nonventilated lung.

Preoperative and Intraoperative Condition of the Dependent Lung

The PVR of the dependent lung determines the ability of that lung to accept redistributed blood flow from the nondependent lung. Preexisting pulmonary hypertension (i.e., high PVR in the dependent lung) interferes with the ability of HPV to redistribute flow to the dependent lung. Clinical conditions that may increase PVR in the dependent lung include low inspired O_2 tension and hypothermia. Maintaining the patient in the lateral decubitus position for long periods of time may cause a pericapillary transudate in the dependent lung, collapsing alveoli and increasing PVR in the dependent lung.

Methods to Attenuate Hypoxemia During One-Lung Ventilation

An FIO_2 of 1.0 protects against hypoxemia and has been associated with PaO_2 values between 150 and 250 mm Hg during OLV. A high FIO_2 also promotes vasodilation in the dependent lung to accept blood flow redistribution from the hypoxic nondependent lung. However, a high FIO_2 may lead to absorption atelectasis or O_2 toxicity, and in patients who have been previously treated with bleomycin, a high FIO_2 may induce lung injury. The risks and benefits of high FIO_2 should be assessed on a case-by-case basis.

The dependent lung should initially be ventilated with a tidal volume of 6 to 8 mL/kg at a rate sufficient to maintain the $PaCO_2$ at 40 mm Hg or less. Tidal volumes below 6 mL/kg may lead to increased atelectasis in the dependent lung. The patient's respiratory rate should be adjusted to maintain the $PaCO_2$ at approximately 40 mm Hg.

Despite these efforts, patients may still develop hypoxemia, and, when hypoxemia occurs, routine issues and problems such as an FIO_2 of less than 1.0, a kinked or occluded (with secretions or blood) tracheal tube, or malposition of the tracheal tube must be addressed. If the hypoxemia is thought to be secondary to OLV, the treatment is controversial, evidenced by a letter sent to program directors of anesthesia residencies by the American Board of Anesthesiology (ABA) stating that individuals taking the written examination for ABA certification were marking the incorrect answer for treating hypoxemia during OLV. Examinees were choosing continuous positive airway pressure (CPAP) to the nondependent lung first and then applying positive end-expiratory pressure (PEEP) to the dependent lung if CPAP failed to correct the hypoxemia. The ABA, presumably based on the Seventh Edition of *Miller's Anesthesia* (the previous six editions advised using CPAP first, followed by PEEP), had scored the correct answer as PEEP to the dependent lung first, followed by CPAP to the nondependent lung second. However, animal studies from the early 1990s and clinical experience have validated the concept that, in patients who develop hypoxemia during OLV, CPAP to the nondependent lung is the most effective way to increase PaO_2. CPAP at 5 to 10 cm H_2O maintains the patency of alveoli that have not already collapsed in the nondependent lung, drawing blood flow from already collapsed alveoli, allowing some gas exchange to occur in the nondependent lung.

If CPAP to the nondependent lung fails to reverse the hypoxemia, then PEEP of 5 to 10 cm H_2O to the dependent lung should be applied. PEEP to the dependent lung should not be tried first because it may compress small interalveolar vessels, increasing PVR, shunting more blood to the nondependent lung, and ultimately decreasing PaO_2 even more.

The only circumstance in which CPAP to the nondependent lung does not work is if the nondependent lung is *completely* collapsed (a very uncommon situation; i.e., *all* alveoli in the nondependent lung are collapsed); in this case, 5 to 10 cm H_2O pressure will not expand these alveoli (it takes ~30 cm H_2O pressure to open alveoli if all are collapsed), and the hypoxia will persist. PEEP applied to the lower lung, by increasing functional residual capacity in that lung, may, to the extent that it optimizes the ventilation-perfusion ratio in the lower (dependent) lung, attenuate some of the hypoxemia.

If neither CPAP nor PEEP improves the hypoxemia, then the anesthesia provider should communicate with the surgeon to advise him or her of the degree of the patient's desaturation and what has been tried to resolve the problem. If the surgical procedure involves removal of a lobe of lung—or is a pneumonectomy—and the surgeon is in a position to ligate the pulmonary vessels supplying the lung tissue to be resected, the surgeon might decide to do so expeditiously because this will decrease the shunt. If ligation of the pulmonary vasculature is not an option for whatever reason, then the surgeon should pause while the anesthesia provider ventilates both lungs, applying enough CPAP to the nondependent lung to reexpand that lung; the hypoxia should resolve. The nondependent lung is again allowed to collapse, and the operation continues until the hypoxemia progresses to the point that the upper lung must again be reexpanded and ventilated.

Miscellaneous Causes of Hypoxemia

As mentioned previously, various other causes of hypoxemia during OLV must be considered and ruled out when one is implementing the algorithm outlined earlier, including failure of the O_2 supply, or malfunction of the tracheal tube in the dependent lung because of malposition or blockage of the lumen by secretions or blood.

Suggested Readings

Kim SH, Choi YS, Lee JG, et al. Effects of a 1:1 inspiratory to expiratory ratio on respiratory mechanics and oxygenation during one-lung ventilation in the lateral decubitus position. *Anaesth Intensive Care*. 2012;40:1016-1022.

Ueda K, Goetzinger C, Gauger EH, et al. Use of bronchial blockers: A retrospective review of 302 cases. *J Anesth*. 2012;26:115-117.

CHAPTER 159

Bronchopleural Fistula

Glenn E. Woodworth, MD

A bronchopleural fistula is a connection between the bronchi or lung parenchyma and the pleural space. If the fistula communicates with the surface of the chest, it is a bronchopleural cutaneous fistula. Communication between the airways and the pleural space substantially increases the risk of infection and can make ventilation difficult, accounting for the high morbidity associated with this condition. Anesthesia providers may encounter patients with bronchopleural fistulas when these patients present for surgical repair of the fistula or in the intensive care unit when the patients require ventilator management of the condition. In rare cases, a patient may present to the operating room for surgery in which the fistula is an incidental condition.

Etiology

Common causes of bronchopleural fistula include trauma and infection; fistulas may also occur as a postoperative complication of lung surgery. The mechanism is usually rupture or erosion of a lung abscess, bronchus, bulla, cyst, suture line, or parenchymal tissue into the pleural space; however, by far the most common cause is a complication of thoracic surgery. The incidence of postoperative formation of a bronchopleural fistula has been reported to be 2% to 40% after pulmonary resection. Persistent air leak, sepsis, empyema, purulent sputum, and respiratory distress characterize such fistulas. Predisposing factors include perioperative radiation or chemotherapy, residual neoplasm, age greater than 60 years, infection at the resection site, and an avascular bronchial stump.

Treatment

Treatment of bronchopleural fistulas is highly dependent on the cause and nature of the fistula. In general, attempts are made to reduce the pleural space and seal the fistula by either placing a chest tube or performing pleurodesis. In those patients who are intubated, ventilator management is critical to give the fistula the best chance of healing. If the fistula is large (e.g., disruption of a postpneumonectomy bronchial stump), conservative management is often not effective, and surgical intervention will be necessary.

Anesthetic Considerations

The primary clinical concern when caring for patients undergoing surgical repair of bronchopleural fistulas relates to providing adequate alveolar gas exchange during positive-pressure ventilation. The following must be considered.

- Tidal volume is preferentially delivered into the pleural space through the low-resistance fistula.
- Air leak into the pleural space can produce a tension pneumothorax.
- Healthy lung tissue should be protected from contamination by the infected lung.
- Differences in compliance and gas exchange between healthy lung and diseased lung or diseased lung and the fistula can exacerbate the difficulty in delivering an adequate tidal volume through the fistula.

Tension pneumothorax is prevented or treated by placement of a chest tube. If an empyema or lung abscess is present, drainage under local anesthesia or bronchoscopy should be considered. Because the use of positive-pressure ventilation may exacerbate difficulties in providing adequate gas exchange, alternative anesthetic techniques—including maintenance of spontaneous ventilation and the use of regional anesthesia (e.g., thoracic epidural anesthesia)—have been used. Unfortunately, most procedures to repair or treat bronchopulmonary fistulas will require general anesthesia and the use of positive-pressure ventilation.

Mechanical Ventilation

In general, the goal of positive-pressure ventilation in patients with bronchopleural fistulas is to minimize tidal volume loss to the pleura or atmosphere by isolating the fistula, e.g., by using double-lumen tracheal tubes or bronchial blockers. If this is not possible, the goal is to keep airway pressures and tidal volumes to a minimum. In addition, the differing physiology and mechanics of varying regions of diseased and nondiseased lung may require different ventilation strategies for different portions of the lung (Table 159-1). In patients with bronchopleural fistulas, delivering adequate ventilation with conventional mechanical ventilators and single-lumen tracheal tubes may be difficult unless the fistula is small.

Suggested Readings

Ha DV, Johnson D. High frequency oscillatory ventilation in the management of a high output bronchopleural fistula: A case report. *Can J Anesth.* 2004: 51:1;78-83.

Konstantinov IE, Saxena P. Independent lung ventilation in the postoperative management of large bronchopleural fistula. *J Thorac Cardiovasc Surg.* 2010;139:e21-22.

Lois M, Noppen M. Bronchopleural fistulas. *Chest.* 2005:128:3955-3965.

Shekar K, Foot C, Fraser J, et al. Bronchopleural fistula: An update for intensivists. *J Crit Care.* 2010;25:47-55.

Williams A, Kay J. Thoracic epidural anesthesia for thoracoscopy, rib resection, and thoracotomy in a patient with bronchopleural fistual postpneumonectomy. *Anesthesiology.* 2000:92:1;1482-1484.

Table 159-1 Approaches to Positive-Pressure Ventilation for Reducing Trans-Fistula Gas Flow

Technique	Pro	Con
Single-lumen tracheal tube Pressure- or volume-controlled ventilation with increased respiratory rate, low tidal volumes, increased inspiratory time, and minimal, if any, PEEP	Simple to perform	Effective only with very small air leak Difficult to keep airway pressures low enough
Timed occlusion of chest tubes during inspiration	Increases pleural pressure during inspiration to decrease trans-fistula pressure gradient Can be added to other techniques	Requires specialized equipment
Single-lumen tracheal tube with intubation of contralateral lung	Simple to perform Protects contralateral lung from infection	Underlying pulmonary disease may make one-lung ventilation difficult
Double-lumen tracheal tube	Relatively simple to perform Protects contralateral lung from infection Can be positioned with bronchoscope Allows for addition of CPAP with 100% O_2 to nonventilated lung	Underlying pulmonary disease may make one-lung ventilation difficult even with the addition of CPAP with 100% O_2
Double-lumen tracheal tube with different ventilation of each lung	Protects contralateral lung from infection Can be positioned with bronchoscope Allows for use of optimal ventilatory mode for each lung Can be combined with a bronchial blocker or HFO technique	Complex to perform Still may be difficult to ventilate diseased lung while minimizing tidal volume loss
Bronchial blockers	Can provide for highly selective isolation (level of the individual bronchus) of the leak, thereby maximizing amount of lung that can be ventilated Can be combined with other techniques	Requires skillful placement with a bronchoscope Blockers can become dislodged during surgery
HFO ventilation	Can be combined with other techniques Airway pressures are decreased Allows for humidification and warming of gases Gas trapping on expiration is decreased Can be used for prolonged ventilation in the ICU	Requires specialized equipment and knowledge
High-frequency jet ventilation	Can be combined with other techniques	Requires specialized equipment and knowledge Control of tidal volume and agent delivery may be difficult Warming and humidification may be difficult Ventilation may be complicated by gas trapping

CPAP, Continuous positive airway pressure; HFO, high-frequency oscillation; ICU, intensive care unit; PEEP, positive end-expiratory pressure.

CHAPTER 160

High-Frequency Ventilation

Joshua Horowitz, DO, and Keith A. Jones, MD

High-frequency ventilation (HFV) is the delivery of small tidal volumes (equal to or less than the anatomic dead space) at rates of 60 to 900 or more cycles per minute. The nomenclature for HFV includes high-frequency positive-pressure ventilation (HFPPV), high-frequency jet ventilation (HFJV), and high-frequency oscillation (HFO). High-frequency chest wall compression is occasionally discussed in the literature under the heading of HFV, but high-frequency chest wall compression is not used to ventilate patients; it is a chest physiotherapy technique used primarily on patients with cystic fibrosis to help them clear secretions.

Table 160-1 compares the major types of HFV. HFPPV can be delivered by a standard mechanical ventilator, though most are not designed to achieve rates greater than 60 to 100/min.

Physiology

Gas transport (i.e., O_2 insufflation and CO_2 elimination) at ventilation rates greater than 170 breaths/min depends on convection, diffusion, and other complex mechanisms that are very different from those that occur during conventional mechanical ventilation (CMV) and are not well understood. CO_2 elimination can and does occur at tidal volumes that are much lower than the volume of air contained in the anatomic dead space. The decrease in airway resistance associated with HFV somehow facilitates penetration of gas to alveoli, alveolar minute ventilation, and CO_2 elimination. However, CO_2 elimination increases linearly as ventilation rate increases up to only a certain point (3-6 Hz; 180-360 breaths/min); at higher rates, dead-space to tidal volume ratio and alveolar minute ventilation are constant.

HFV does not substantially improve oxygenation, compared with CMV; in both situations, oxygenation correlates with mean airway pressure. However, the ability to maintain lower peak and mean airway pressures with HFV is beneficial for other reasons (e.g., hemodynamic stability). The magnitude of the hemodynamic effects is related to the amount of positive pressure applied to the airway. At lower peak and mean airway pressures, the adverse effects should be fewer; however, the lower levels of adverse effects have not been shown to be consistent. Fluctuations in intracranial pressure with the use of HFV, compared with CMV, are typically lower, but the mean intracranial pressure does not decrease.

Table 160-1 General Comparison of the Major Types of High-Frequency Ventilation

Feature	HFPPV	HFJV	HFO
Frequency (Hz)	1-2	2-6	10-20
Breaths/min	60-120	120-400	600-1200
Tidal volume (mL/kg)	3-5	1-1.5	?*

*Actual value unknown because of entrainment.
HFJV, High-frequency jet ventilation; HFO, high-frequency oscillation; HFPPV, high-frequency positive-pressure ventilation.

Clinical Applications

High-Frequency Jet Ventilation

HFJV has several clinical applications. HFJV is often used in laryngeal and tracheal operations because it can be delivered with a cannula or catheter much smaller than a traditional tracheal tube. The use of such a catheter minimizes the intra-airway space occupied by the tracheal tube, thereby increasing the working space available to the otolaryngologic or thoracic surgeon. HFJV also decreases ventilatory excursion, which also improves operating conditions for the surgeon.

Percutaneous transtracheal HFJV can be used to manage the difficult airway in an emergency by inserting a small cannula through the cricothyroid membrane. The cannula can be connected to any of several jet ventilators or to a hand-held flush valve connected to an adequate pressure source—the O_2 flush valve on a Dräger anesthesia machine has been found to provide sufficient pressure. Pressing the valve briefly ($\leq$0.3 sec) delivers a pulse of O_2 at high pressure that dissipates quickly into the airway—slight expansion of the chest may be observed. If the valve is held open too long ($\geq$0.5 sec), the volume of O_2 fills the airway and pressure rises; the high pressure can be communicated directly to the airway and lung, leading to barotrauma.

High-Frequency Oscillation

HFO has been used for decades, mostly in newborn and premature infants with respiratory distress syndrome. Unlike in HFJV, in which "inspiration" is active and "exhalation" is passive, in HFO, both inspiration and expiration are active processes. As mentioned previously, the mean airway pressure can be increased to improve oxygenation levels. Increasing the amplitude of the gas wave generated by the oscillator increases the rate of CO_2 elimination. Several randomized studies and meta-analyses have not demonstrated clear-cut benefits of HFO, as compared with CMV; in most centers with a neonatal intensive care unit, HFO is used as rescue therapy to treat patients with respiratory distress syndrome who do not respond to treatment with CMV. If neonates or infants are not fully supported with HFO or their condition deteriorates further, the use of extracorporeal membrane oxygenation is often considered as the next step.

There are few recent studies of the use of HFO in adults, largely because the ARDS Network has demonstrated that low-volume, pressure-targeted ventilation strategies, compared with CMV strategies, significantly reduce mortality rates in patients with acute lung injury/acute respiratory distress syndrome. In 2006, however, Derdak and colleagues published the results of a large randomized controlled trial comparing HFO with CMV in patients with acute respiratory distress syndrome and showed that the 30-day mortality rate was reduced from 52% in the CMV group to 37% in the HFO group.

Box 160-1 General Potential Risks and Benefits Associated with Use of High-Frequency Ventilation

Risks or Drawbacks	Benefits
Barotrauma	↓ Chest wall and tracheobronchial movement
Inability to monitor:	↓ Intrathoracic pressures
Tidal volume	↓ Intracranial pressures
$ETCO_2$	↑ Improved hemodynamics
Necrotizing tracheobronchitis	
Auto-PEEP	
Poor humidification	
High gas usage	
Insufficient alarms	

$ETCO_2$, End-tidal CO_2, PEEP, positive end-expiratory pressure.

Potential Risks and Benefits

Box 160-1 provides the potential risks and benefits associated with the use of HFV.

Suggested Readings

Cools F, Askie LM, Offringa M, et al, on behalf of the PreVILIG collaboration. Elective high-frequency oscillatory versus conventional ventilation in preterm infants: A systematic review and meta-analysis of individual patients' data. *Lancet*. 2010;375:2082-2091.

Derdak S, Mehta S, Stewart TE, et al. High-frequency oscillatory ventilation for acute respiratory distress syndrome in adults: A randomized, controlled trial. *Am J Respir Crit Care Med*. 2002;166:801-808.

Fan E, Needham D, Stewart T. Ventilatory management of acute lung injury and acute respiratory distress syndrome. *JAMA*. 2005;294:22:2889-2896.

Fassl J, Jenny U, Nikiforov S, et al. Pressures available for transtracheal jet ventilation from anesthesia machines and wall-mounted oxygen flowmeters. *Anesth Analg*. 2010;110:94-100.

Henderson-Smart DJ, De Paoli AG, Clark RH, Bhuta T. High frequency oscillatory ventilation versus conventional ventilation for infants with severe pulmonary dysfunction born at or near term. *Cochrane Database Syst Rev*. 2009: CD002974.

Louise R. Clinical application of ventilator modes: Ventilatory strategies for lung protection. *Aust Crit Care*. 2010;23:71-80.

PART E General/Urologic/ENT

CHAPTER 161

Thermoregulation and Perioperative Hypothermia

C. Thomas Wass, MD

Heat Balance and Thermoregulation

Body heat is unevenly distributed, with a typical core-to-peripheral temperature gradient of 2° C to 4° C. As with any other neurally mediated physiologic process, thermoregulation involves afferent thermal sensing, central processing, and efferent responses. Thermal receptors are distributed throughout the body (e.g., skin, abdominal and thoracic tissues, spinal cord, hypothalamus), with impulses in response to hypothermia and hyperthermia transmitted to the central nervous system via Aδ and C fibers, respectively. Central processing (primarily in the hypothalamus) results in voluntary (e.g., wearing appropriate attire, adjusting ambient temperature) and involuntary (autonomic) efferent responses. The slope of the efferent response intensity (e.g., magnitude of vasomotor changes) versus core temperature defines the gain.

In unanesthetized patients, cold-induced autonomic defenses follow a hierarchical pattern that progresses from vasoconstriction to nonshivering thermogenesis and, finally, shivering thermogenesis (Figure 161-1). Vasoconstriction decreases cutaneous blood flow and heat loss, primarily in the fingers and toes. Although its effects are minimal in adults, nonshivering thermogenesis can double metabolic heat production in the mitochondria-rich brown fat of neonates and infants. Shivering thermogenesis results from involuntary skeletal muscle activity that increases metabolic rate and heat production.

The threshold for warmth-induced autonomic responses, such as active vasodilation and sweating, is similar. Each gram of evaporated sweat dissipates approximately 540 calories of heat to the environment.

Core temperatures between the first cold-induced (i.e., vasoconstriction) and warmth-induced (i.e., vasodilation) responses define the interthreshold range (ITR). Temperatures within this 0.2° C range do not trigger thermoregulatory defense mechanisms.

Effects of Anesthesia on Thermoregulation

General Anesthesia

Intravenously administered and inhaled anesthetic agents inhibit thermoregulation in a dose-dependent manner. That is, general anesthetic agents increase the thresholds for warmth-induced thermoregulatory responses and decrease the thresholds for cold-induced defenses. Accordingly, there is a 20-fold increase (i.e., from 0.2° C to 4.0° C) in the ITR. As a result, anesthetized patients are poikilothermic over this 4° C range, which renders them susceptible to developing heat loss and hypothermia.

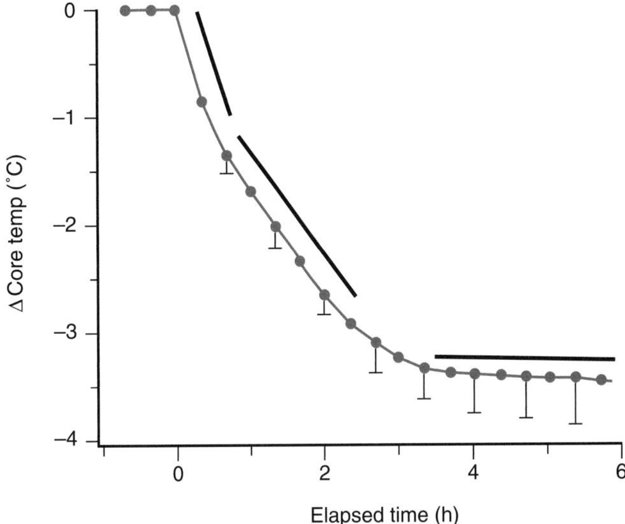

Figure 161-1 Heat loss during anesthesia. Almost all anesthetics are vasodilators; core temperature decreases 1.0° C to 1.5° C during the first hour of anesthesia owing to heat redistribution from the core to the periphery. Subsequent decreases occur less precipitously for the next 2 to 3 h. This drop results from heat loss exceeding metabolic heat production. During this phase, heat is lost via skin surfaces, with radiant and convective losses contributing far more than evaporative or conductive losses. After 3 to 5 h of anesthesia, the core temperature plateaus in a thermal steady state, with heat loss equaling heat production.

Regional Anesthetic Agents

As discussed earlier, thermoregulatory defenses are neurally mediated. Nerve blocks disrupt these neural pathways and interfere with thermoregulation. Neuraxial anesthesia inhibits central thermoregulatory control by an amount that depends on the level of the block. Because thermoregulation remains intact above the level of the neuraxial block, increases in the ITR (e.g., from 0.2° C to 0.8° C) are not as dramatic as those observed during general anesthesia.

Systemic Side Effects of Perioperative Hypothermia

Central Nervous System

A large amount of experimental evidence indicates that hypothermia may protect the brain from ischemic and traumatic injury. In contrast, fever has been reported to worsen outcomes following cerebral ischemia or head trauma. Hypothermia decreases brain activity, as measured by electroencephalography, and increases latency in the somatosensory evoked potential. Changes in the amplitude of the somatosensory evoked potential are less clearly defined. Mild intraoperative hypothermia has also been reported to prolong postoperative recovery.

Cardiovascular

Decreased core temperature can slow intracardiac conduction, predispose patients to developing lethal cardiac arrhythmias, increase pulmonary and systemic vascular resistance, decrease myocardial contractility, decrease cardiac output, induce myocardial ischemia, and interfere with platelet function and the coagulation cascade (e.g., decreased thrombin production). Interestingly, myocardial ischemia is not entirely due to shivering-induced increases in whole-body metabolism. That is, other contributory mechanisms include increased myocardial work resulting from catecholamine-induced increases in systemic vascular resistance, blood pressure, and heart rate. In patients who have been successfully resuscitated after cardiac arrest due to ventricular fibrillation, two large prospective studies have shown that therapeutic mild hypothermia has been shown increases the rate of a favorable neurologic outcome and reduces chances of a fatal outcome. However, a more recent prospective study did not find any benefit to mild hypothermia (34° C vs. 37° C) in patients following a cardiac arrest.

Wound Infections

Decreased cutaneous blood flow impairs regional tissue O_2 delivery, neutrophil function (e.g., impaired leukocyte mitogenesis, motility, and phagocytosis, resulting in impaired oxidative bacterial killing), and delivery of systemic antibiotics to the wound site. Collectively, these hypothermia-mediated perturbations have been shown to increase the risk of wound infection and the duration of hospitalization (up to 20%).

Miscellaneous

Systemic hypothermia also causes a leftward shift of the oxyhemoglobin dissociation curve, decreases O_2 consumption and CO_2 production, slows metabolism of anesthetic drugs, and predisposes patients to developing citrate toxicity.

Mechanisms and Prevention of Perioperative Hypothermia

Perioperative hypothermia occurs via several heat-loss mechanisms: redistribution, convection, radiation, conduction, and evaporation. Although all of these mechanisms are important to some extent, the initial drop in core temperature—and the most important cause of perioperative hypothermia—is predominantly due to redistribution (i.e., transfer) of heat from the core to peripheral tissues (see Figure 161-1). Rapid core-to-peripheral heat transfer produces hypothermia in nearly all patients regardless of the type of anesthesia delivered (e.g., general or regional).

Prevention and treatment of hypothermia may be achieved using passive techniques (e.g., applying cotton blankets, sterile drapes, reflective "space" blankets) or active techniques (e.g., using forced-air convective warmers, resistive-heating blankets, conductive circulating water mattresses, intravenous fluid warmers, radiant infrared lamps, and airway heating and humidification). Of these techniques, heat conservation is most effectively achieved using forced-air convective surface warming or carbon-fiber resistive heating blankets.

Suggested Readings

Frank SM, Fleisher LA, Breslow MJ, et al. Perioperative maintenance of normothermia reduces the incidence of morbid cardiac events. *JAMA*. 1997;277:1127-1134.

Kurz A. Thermal care in the perioperative period. *Best Pract Res Clin Anaesthesiol*. 2008;22:39-62.

Negishi C, Hasegawa K, Mukai S, et al. Resistive-heating and forced-air warming are comparably effective. *Anesth Analg*. 2003;96:1683-1687.

Nielsen N, Wetterslev J, Cronberg T, et al. Targeted temperature management at 33° C versus 36° C after cardiac arrest. *N Engl J Med*. 2013;369:2197-2206.

Sessler DI. Perioperative thermoregulation and heat balance. *Ann N Y Acad Sci*. 1997;813:757-777.

Sessler DI. Temperature monitoring and perioperative thermoregulation. *Anesthesiology*. 2008;109:318-338.

The Hypothermia After Cardiac Arrest Study Group. Mild therapeutic hypothermia to improve the neurologic outcome after cardiac arrest. *N Engl J Med*. 2002;346:549-556.

Wass CT, Lanier WL. Hypothermia-associated protection from ischemic brain injury: implications for patient management. *Int Anesthesiol Clin*. 1996;34:95-111.

CHAPTER 162

The Anesthesia Provider's Role in the Prevention of Surgical Site Infections

William J. Mauermann, MD

Surgical site infections (SSIs) continue to be a substantial source of patient morbidity and fatality after surgical procedures. They are the second most common cause of nosocomial infections, lead to increased length of stay in the hospital and increased mortality rate, and contribute significantly to health care costs. More recently, SSIs have become a marker of quality of care in the United States. Regulatory agencies have deemed that some SSIs are avoidable; in the United States, Medicare will no longer reimburse institutions for certain SSIs, including mediastinitis after cardiac surgery and SSIs following bariatric surgery and some orthopedic operations. This chapter will focus on the pathophysiology of SSIs as well as the anesthesia provider's role in the prevention of these complications.

Pathophysiology of Surgical Site Infections

Even with strict aseptic technique and a clean surgical wound, some degree of bacterial contamination undoubtedly occurs in every operation. It has been well documented that the first 4 to 6 h after contamination determine whether the body will clear the bacteria or an established infection will occur. Thus, preventing SSIs relies in large part on optimizing the immune system during the perioperative period.

The body's first defense against bacterial contamination is the neutrophil. Neutrophils are critically dependent on adequate O_2 stores to maintain their oxidative killing capacity. In one study, subcutaneous O_2 tension was measured in operative patients considered at elevated risk for developing SSI. In patients with subcutaneous O_2 tensions greater than 90 mm Hg, no SSIs developed, whereas patients with a subcutaneous O_2 tension of 40 to 50 mm Hg had an infection rate of 43%. As will be detailed in the following discussion, anesthesiologists may play an important role in the maintenance of immune and, in particular, neutrophil function.

Hypothermia

Without active efforts to warm patients, mild perioperative hypothermia (core body temperature 34° C-36° C) is commonly observed. In a landmark study, 200 patients undergoing colorectal operations were randomly assigned to a mild hypothermia group (34.4° C ± 0.4° C) or a normothermia group (37° C ± 0.3° C). This trial was stopped early because of the high rates of SSIs in the hypothermia group; the incidence of SSIs in the hypothermia group was 18.8%, versus 5.8% in the normothermia group. Patients who developed SSIs stayed nearly 1 week longer in the hospital. In addition, patients who were maintained at normothermia had evidence of increased wound healing and tolerated oral intake sooner. In a subgroup analysis, 74% of the hypothermic patients had evidence of intraoperative vasoconstriction, versus 6% of the normothermic patients.

The effect of hypothermia on SSIs is multifactorial. In the aforementioned study, the high incidence of vasoconstriction in the hypothermic group likely means a decrease in blood flow and O_2 delivery to the surgical site and, thus, impairment in the oxidative killing capacity of neutrophils. In addition, animal models have shown that hypothermia induces an anti inflammatory T-cell cytokine profile similar to that seen in patients with thermal injuries. Lastly, irrespective of the effect on blood flow and O_2 delivery to the surgical wound, hypothermia decreases the neutrophils' production of superoxide radicals for any given O_2 tension. Indeed, bacterial killing by neutrophils is reduced in the face of hypothermia. With all that is known regarding the complications from mild perioperative hypothermia, including an increased risk of SSIs, it should be every clinician's goal to maintain patients' normothermia unless contraindicated.

Hyperoxia

In most clinical scenarios, O_2 delivery to end organs is vastly more dependent on the amount of O_2 bound to hemoglobin than the amount of O_2 dissolved in the blood. However, the subcutaneous tissue uses very little O_2, compared with the rest of the body. In addition, the mean partial pressure of O_2 in the subcutaneous tissue is approximately 60 mm Hg, a level above the range in which O_2 readily dissociates from hemoglobin. Lastly, when the microvasculature is traumatized at the site of the wound, the diffusion distance for O_2 is increased. These facts likely combine to decrease the importance of hemoglobin-bound O_2 on O_2 tension at the site of the wound and increase the importance of O_2 dissolved in the bloodstream (Figure 162-1).

To date, two randomized trials involving 800 patients undergoing colorectal operations have evaluated the effects of 80% inspired O_2 versus 30% inspired O_2 administered intraoperatively and for 2 h (500 patients) or 6 h (300 patients) postoperatively. Both studies found significantly decreased rates of SSIs in the patients receiving 80% inspired O_2. When data from the two studies are pooled, the relative risk reduction for developing an SSI is 45% ($p = 0.02$) in patients treated with hyperoxia. A subgroup analysis did not show any detrimental effects of 80% inspired O_2 during the study period when patients were evaluated with computed tomography scanning and pulmonary function tests.

Providing 80% O_2 in the operating suite is likely helpful in preventing SSIs and does not seem to be associated with any significant risk, but the continuation of 80% O_2 for 2 to 6 h postoperatively does present some potential procedural complications. It remains to be seen whether or not hyperoxia in the operating room without continuation in the postoperative period decreases SSIs.

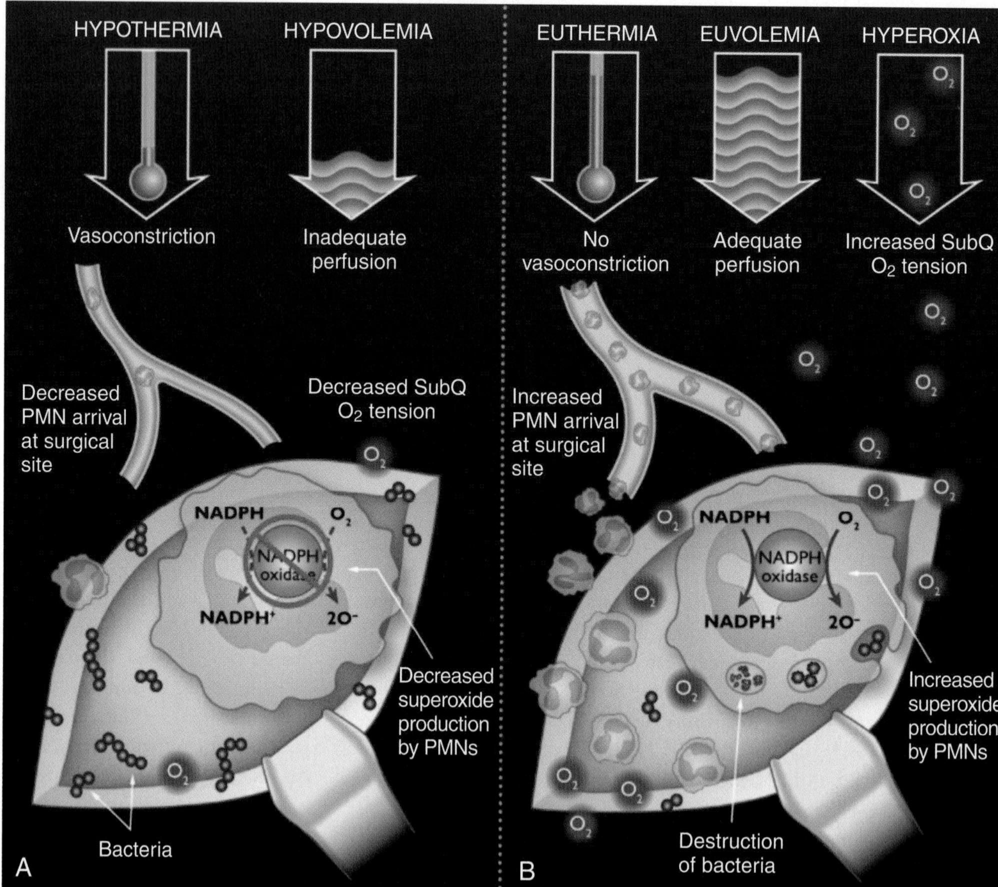

Figure 162-1 Conditions leading to decreased (**A**) and increased (**B**) O_2 tension. Decreases in subcutaneous (SubQ) O_2 tension increase the incidence of surgical site infection. NADPH, Nicotinamide adenine dinucleotide phosphate; PMN, polymorphonuclear cell. (Reprinted, with permission, from Mauermann WJ, Nemergut EC. The anesthesiologist's role in the prevention of surgical site infections. Anesthesiology. 2006;105:413-421.)

Hyperglycemia

Hyperglycemia has been shown to have numerous deleterious effects on immune function in both in vitro and human models (Figure 162-2). A glucose challenge in healthy subjects induces a transient reduction in leukocyte counts. Hyperglycemia also deactivates immunoglobulins by nonenzymatic glycosylation and glycosylation of the C3 component of complement blocks binding to bacterial surfaces. The importance of neutrophils in preventing SSIs has already been emphasized, and the neutrophils of diabetic patients have numerous functional deficits, including impaired chemotaxis, decreased phagocytic ability, and lower bactericidal capacity. If these dysfunctional neutrophils are placed in a normoglycemic environment, their function can be at least partially restored in a short period of time. Lastly, it has been shown that, in patients undergoing cardiac surgery, glucose control with continuous insulin infusions improves the phagocytic function of neutrophils when compared with the use of intermittent insulin boluses to treat hyperglycemia.

What does the preceding discussion mean for the management of perioperative hyperglycemia with the goal of preventing SSIs? Surprisingly few studies have been performed with the goal of answering this question. In a frequently cited retrospective study of diabetic patients undergoing cardiac operations, it was shown that continuous insulin infusions to maintain blood glucose levels between 150 and 200 mg/dL decreased the incidence of sternal wound infections by 66% versus historical control subjects who were treated with sliding-scale insulin with the goal of maintaining blood glucose levels less than 200 mg/dL. To date, only one study has evaluated tight glycemic control (goal 80-110 mg/dL) in the operating room. In patients undergoing cardiac operations, tight glucose control has not been shown to improve outcomes but did lead to a higher incidence of stroke.

There is certainly significant in vitro data to suggest that hyperglycemia adversely affects the immune system, but the optimal goal for blood glucose levels is currently unknown. It appears that the historical threshold for treating blood glucose levels greater than 200 mg/dL is too high. However, very tight glycemic control is currently not supported by the literature and may, in fact, be dangerous.

Antibiotic Prophylaxis

A detailed discussion of perioperative antimicrobial prophylaxis is beyond the scope of this chapter, but some salient points warrant discussion. The goal of perioperative antibiotic administration is to obtain blood and tissue drug levels that exceed the minimum inhibitory concentration of the organisms likely to be encountered. Adequate blood and tissue levels of the antibiotic must be obtained before incision, and current recommendations state that the infusion should begin within 60 min of incision. This period can be lengthened to 120 min for drugs, such as vancomycin, in which rapid administration may have adverse effects.

The choice of antibiotic is as important as the timing. Prophylaxis should target the most commonly encountered organisms and should not be administered with the goal of covering all possible pathogens. For most operations that do not violate chronically colonized organs, such as the bowel, the most common pathogens will be skin flora microbes, specifically *Streptococcus* and *Staphylococcus*. A first-generation cephalosporin (cefazolin) adequately covers these organisms. Procedures involving the bowel necessitate gram-negative coverage as well. Recently there has been discussion that vancomycin may be the antibiotic of choice for prophylaxis in institutions with a high incidence of methicillin-resistant *Staphylococcus* infections. It should be noted that there is no evidence to support this practice, and it is not recommended by any national organization. First-generation cephalosporins have a wider spectrum of coverage and are superior bactericidal agents, as compared with vancomycin, and they should be considered the first-line agents for surgical prophylaxis.

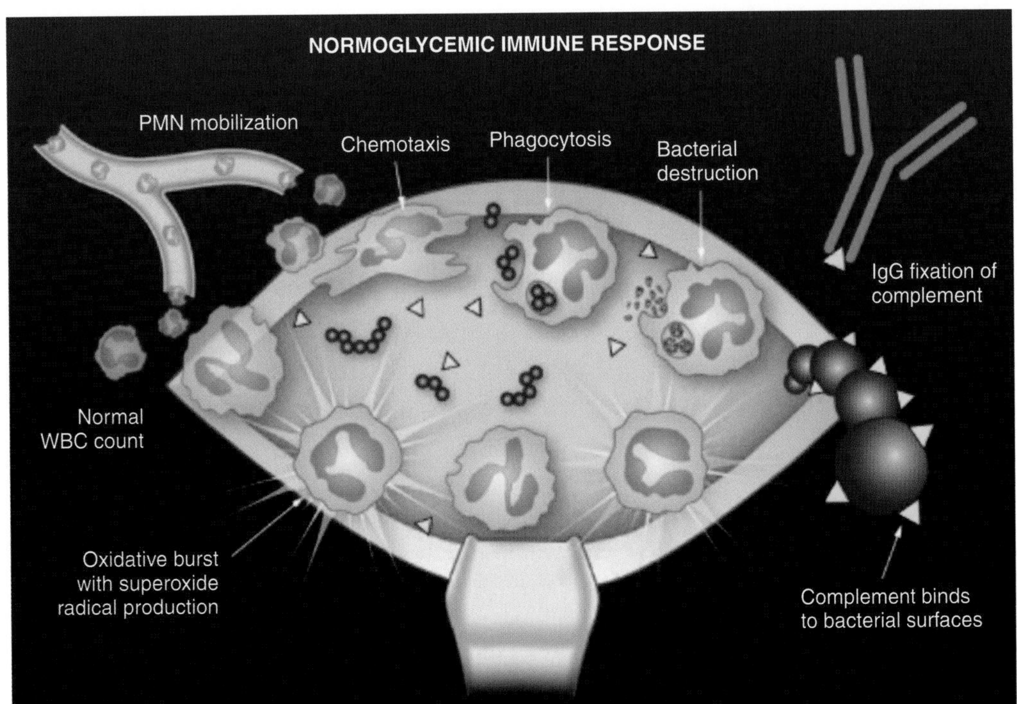

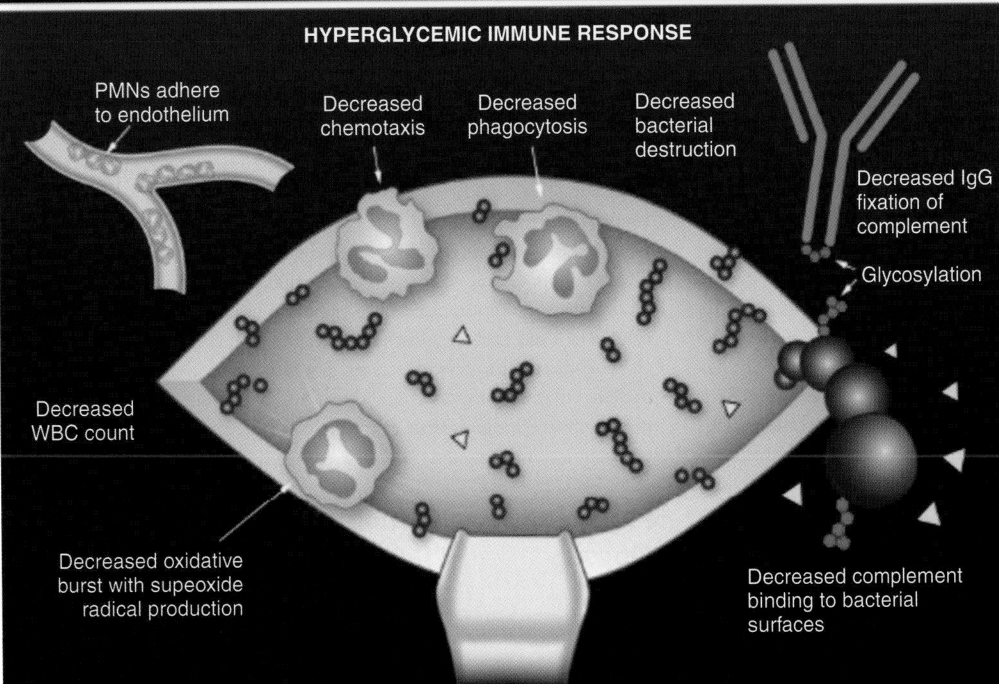

Figure 162-2 Normoglycemic (*top*) and hyperglycemic (*bottom*) immune responses are compared. Hyperglycemia induces a host of negative effects on the normal immune response in surgical wounds. IgG, Immunoglobulin G; PMN, polymorphonuclear cell; WBC, white blood cell. (Reprinted, with permission, from Mauermann WJ, Nemergut EC. The anesthesiologist's role in the prevention of surgical site infections. Anesthesiology. 2006;105: 413-421.)

Conclusions

SSIs continue to be a major source of morbidity and death after surgical procedures. The critical window for preventing SSIs is the first few hours after the inevitable bacterial contamination; during this time, the anesthesiologist has the opportunity to help optimize the patient's immune function so that these infections can be prevented.

Suggested Readings

Bratzler DW, Houck PM. Antimicrobial prophylaxis for surgery: An advisory statement from the National Surgical Infection Prevention Project. *Clin Infect Dis.* 2004;38:1706-1715.

Esnaola NF, Cole DJ. Perioperative normothermia during major surgery: is it important? *Adv Surg.* 2011;45:249-263.

Kavanagh T, Buggy DJ. Can anaesthetic technique effect postoperative outcome? *Curr Opin Anaesthesiol.* 2012;25:185-198.

Kurz A, Sessler DI, Lenhardt R. Perioperative normothermia to reduce the incidence of surgical-wound infection and shorten hospitalization. Study of Wound Infection and Temperature Group. *N Engl J Med.* 1996;334:1209-1215.

Mauermann WJ, Nemergut EC. The anesthesiologist's role in the prevention of surgical site infections. *Anesthesiology.* 2006;105:413-421.

Reynolds L, Beckmann J, Kurz A. Perioperative complications of hypothermia. *Best Pract Res Clin Anaesthesiol.* 2008;22:645-57.

Togioka B, Galvagno S, Sumida S, et al. The role of perioperative high inspired oxygen therapy in reducing surgical site infection: A meta-analysis. *Anesth Analg.* 2012;114:334-342.

Zerr KJ, Furnary AP, Grunkemeier GL, et al. Glucose control lowers the risk of wound infection in diabetics after open heart operations. *Ann Thorac Surg.* 1997;63:356-361.

CHAPTER 163

Anesthesia in the Patient with Extreme Obesity

James P. Conterato, MD

General

Obesity has rapidly become an endemic disorder of Western society. Its presentation is now a daily phenomenon for the practicing anesthesia provider. Obesity is a condition of excess body fat, its derivation coming from the Latin word *obesus*, meaning *fattened by eating*. Body fat is a relative state, but in healthy Western societies, body fat averages for women are 20% to 30%, for men 18% to 25%, and for ultrafit marathoners approximately 7%. Obesity is a disorder that has genetic, socioeconomic, and endocrine causes. In developing countries, it correlates with a higher socioeconomic status, whereas in Western society, it more frequently occurs in lower socioeconomic classes. The original definitions of obesity are derived from the concept of ideal body weight calculations, developed by insurance companies to describe those population groups with the lowest mortality rates for age, and calculated as follows:

$$\text{Ideal body weight (kg)} = \text{height (cm)} - x$$

where x equals 105 for women and 100 for men. Body mass index (BMI) is a more relevant measure of height-weight relationships and is the currently accepted standard used to stratify obesity, although evidence has accumulated that the distribution of fat (central and intra-abdominal vs. peripheral) may best correlate with morbidity and mortality rates, recognizing that central intra-abdominal fat is a more metabolically active, proinflammatory substrate. BMI is calculated as body weight (in kilograms) divided by height (in meters) squared. The World Health Organization and the Centers for Disease Control and Prevention have defined levels of obesity (Table 163-1). Obesity can be further subdivided into *morbid obesity* (defined as a BMI >35 and <54.9) and *super* or *extreme morbid obesity* (BMI >55).

The inflection point for risk is a BMI greater than 30, at which point an exponential increase occurs in multiple risks for morbidity and mortality.

Table 163-1 Classification of Weight by Body Mass Index (BMI)

Category	BMI (kg/m²)	Obesity Class
Underweight	<18.5	
Normal weight	18.5-24.9	
Overweight	25.0-29.9	
Obesity	30.0-34.9	Obesity class I
	35.0-39.9	Obesity class II
Extreme obesity	≥40	Obesity class III

Adapted from Obesity: Preventing and Managing the Global Epidemic. Geneva, Switzerland, World Health Organization; 1997. Report No. 894.

Fat-distribution analyses suggest that the waist-to-hip ratio may correlate best with risk and dramatically increases at values of greater than 1 for women and greater than 0.8 for men.

The literature is replete with documentation that the morbidly obese are at increased risk for developing a wide variety of comorbid conditions, including a threefold to fourfold increased incidence of the age-related risks for diabetes, hypertension, cerebrovascular disease, and ischemic heart disease. Obesity predisposes an individual to develop the now well-recognized metabolic syndrome, consisting of hypertension, insulin resistance with adult-onset diabetes (type 2), and hyperlipidemia. It represents a proinflammatory and prothrombotic state associated with vascular endothelial dysfunction, which dramatically increases one's risk of developing atherosclerotic disease. Additionally, meta-analyses demonstrate increased incidences of essentially all solid-tissue cancers except esophageal cancer, and of deep venous thrombosis and thromboembolism, osteoarthritis, gout, chronic back pain, asthma, infertility, impotence, and gallbladder disease in obese people. Other potentially key considerations are the cardiorespiratory complications of obstructive sleep apnea, apnea-hypoventilation syndrome (pickwickian syndrome), and cardiomyopathy of obesity.

The anesthesia provider faces potential issues in caring for obese patients that encompass these comorbid conditions and impact airway management, cardiorespiratory physiology, pharmacokinetics and pharmacodynamics of drugs, and positioning concerns, to name a few.

Physiology and Pathophysiology of Morbid Obesity

Cardiovascular Effects

Each kilogram of fat develops approximately 3000 m of blood vessels and requires a progressive increase in cardiac output that averages 100 mL/min. As a result, circulating blood volumes in the systemic and pulmonary circuits increase, resulting in increased cardiac preload and afterload. Ventricular dilatation and increased stroke volume develop, which eventually elicit ventricular hypertrophy, all of which increase cardiac work. The systemic hypertension and cardiomegaly seen are a result of increases in circulating blood volumes and cardiac output, as are the development of hyperinsulinemia-induced sympathetic activity and tone and progressive peripheral insulin resistance eliciting increased pressor effects of renin and angiotensin II. The development of pulmonary hypertension is a result of increased circulating blood volume, increased sympathetic tone, and chronic arterial hypoxemia (see following discussion under "Airway and Pulmonary Effects").

The constellation of events that lead to hypertrophy-induced diastolic dysfunction can eventually result in the failure of hypertrophy compensating for ventricular dilatation, resulting in eventual systolic dysfunction—what is described as obesity-induced cardiomyopathy. Patients lose the ability to compensate for additional work stress on the cardiovascular system, relying more on increases in heart rate than stroke volume. Studies have documented an impaired response to exercise in the morbidly obese, with $\dot{V}O_2$ max rarely reaching above 25 mL of O_2 per kilogram per minute, indicating that levels of work that are submaximal in normal patients can only be met by an increased anaerobic debt in morbidly obese individuals.

Airway and Pulmonary Effects

Obesity imposes a restrictive ventilatory defect on the patient because of weight gain involving the chest wall and because of excessive diaphragmatic loading from abdominal fat, impeding the normal excursion of the diaphragm and significantly increasing the work of breathing. Both of these phenomena contribute to a decrease in pulmonary compliance. However, the major cause of the decrement in pulmonary compliance appears to be due to the increase in pulmonary blood volume. This restriction results in a decrease in total lung capacity and functional residual capacity (FRC), mainly from the loss of expiratory reserve volume. FRC decreases exponentially with increasing BMI, often reaching a point at which closing capacity is greater than FRC during tidal breathing, resulting in increased ventilation/perfusion mismatching in the awake state and increased shunt fraction ($\dot{Q}s/\dot{Q}t$) under general anesthesia. At rest, most morbidly obese patients experience only a modest decrease in Pao_2 and maintain $Paco_2$ via hyperventilation (low tidal volume, increased respiratory rate). On average, a 1-mm Hg drop in Pao_2 and 1-mm Hg increase in $PAO_2 - Pao_2$ occur with each additional 10-kg weight gain. These patients tolerate apnea poorly and experience up to a 50% drop in FRC on induction of general anesthesia (vs. 20% in nonobese patients). Reported $\dot{Q}s/\dot{Q}t$ for this group of patients undergoing general anesthesia can reach 10% to 25%, versus the normal 2% to 5%. The expanded pulmonary blood volume and loss of FRC also increase pulmonary vascular resistance, which then also contributes to the increased work of breathing. This loss of FRC can also accelerate the rate of uptake of inhalation anesthetic agents (shorter time constant in the lungs).

Airway anatomy becomes distorted and airway, management becomes more challenging for the anesthesia provider as the patient's level of obesity becomes more extreme. Patients may have enlarged face and cheeks, large tongue, impaired mouth opening and cervical range of motion, increasing soft tissue encroachment in the palate and pharynx, short neck, and large breasts, all of which may contribute to difficult mask ventilation, difficult direct laryngoscopy, or difficult intubation. Difficult mask ventilation has been reported to occur in up to one third of morbidly obese patients. Although older literature has suggested an incidence of difficult intubation as high as 30% in these patients, more recent prospective trials document that, in general, this is not the case and that the only two variables that appear predictive of difficulty intubating patients in this population are an increased neck circumference and a Mallampati score of 3 or more.

As BMI exceeds 30 kg/m^2, the risk of a patient having obstructive sleep apnea increases. This syndrome is due to the normal reduction in upper airway tone seen during stage 4 and rapid eye movement sleep. The excessive deposition of soft tissue in the upper airway in the obese individual accentuates this tendency and can result in periodic obstruction of the airway during sleep. Obstructive sleep apnea consists of both apneas and hypopneas and is best delineated via formal sleep evaluations with polysomnography. For more information on this topic, see Chapter 108, Obstructive Sleep Apnea.

With progressive worsening of obstructive sleep apnea, desensitization of breathing control can evolve, resulting in degrees of chronic hypoxemia and hypercarbia. Up to 50% of individuals with a BMI greater than 50 kg/m^2 have evidence of daytime hypoventilation. Eventual physiologic changes develop that consist of secondary polycythemia, pulmonary hypertension, and right ventricular failure. This apnea hypoventilation syndrome has also been referred to as the pickwickian syndrome, although the term is no longer in use.

Gastrointestinal and Hepatic Effects

Study results have suggested that the obese patient is at increased risk of aspiration due to higher residual gastric volumes and lower gastric pH. However, recent studies have questioned these conclusions, indicating no greater increased aspiration risk per se. Obese individuals have normal or accelerated rates of gastric clearance, and the incidence of gastric reflux does not differ significantly from that of the general population. However, difficult airway management by mask may predispose some to an increased aspiration risk.

Short of significant liver dysfunction due to obesity (nonalcoholic steatohepatitis with cirrhosis), there is no evidence of impaired hepatic function in individuals with morbid obesity. Neither is there any proven greater tendency to inhalation agent–induced hepatitis.

Neurologic Effects

Morbidly obese individuals have a significantly higher incidence of incurring positioning injuries involving the brachial plexus, sciatic nerve, and ulnar nerve. Special care needs to be exerted to achieve proper protection of these structures. Additionally, this population is at increased risk of developing decubiti with prolonged pressure under anesthesia.

Anesthesia for the Morbidly Obese Patient

A routine general health examination, specifically focusing on cardiac, pulmonary, airway, and metabolic issues (Table 163-2), should be performed preoperatively.

Intraoperative Anesthetic Techniques

Modification of the anesthetic technique is necessary to minimize complications related to obesity. Because of physical limitations imposed by the patient's girth, the anesthesia provider should ensure that proper "ramping" of the patient has been performed, such that the sternal notch is parallel to the angle of the mandible (Figure 163-1). This facilitates alignment of the intraoral axes for intubation. If a history of or major concerns regarding difficult intubation exist, awake fiberoptic intubation may be a reasonable option. Preoxygenation for 3 to 5 min with the patient in a mild reverse Trendelenburg position while using 10 cm H_2O of continuous positive airway pressure plus 10 cm H_2O of peak end-expiratory pressure with mask ventilation has been shown to significantly mitigate the initial drop in FRC on induction and to prolong time to desaturation. Appropriately sized oral and nasal airways should be available and used to maintain airway patency. An inability to use a mask should always be anticipated. The use of an intubating laryngeal mask airway can be highly effective in achieving successful airway maintenance when conventional mask techniques have failed.

Intraoperatively, alveolar recruitment using titrated peak end-expiratory pressure and some degree of head-up (beach-chair) positioning should be maintained. This is especially true when the operation requires introduction of a pneumoperitoneum. This technique has been proved to be more effective than the use of large tidal volume ventilation. Judicious use of colloids should be employed to maintain intravascular volume and prevent negative hemodynamic effects of excess peak end-expiratory pressure. Because of the mechanical limitations on the respiratory system and the increased sensitivity of morbidly obese patients to the effects of sedatives, opioids, and inhalation agents, spontaneous ventilation should not be used in these patients.

There is no evidence to support the use of one inhalation agent over another. Emergence times are essentially similar, especially when the agents are used in conjunction with processed electroencephalographic monitoring. The use of N_2O should be avoided, especially in the setting of pulmonary hypertension.

The dosing of intravenously administered anesthetic agents varies with lipid and solvent solubility. Lean body mass (ideal body weight + 20%) is

Table 163-2 Preoperative Assessment of the Morbidly Obese Patient

System	Assessment
Cardiovascular	Obtain baseline electrocardiogram Assess BP control Examine for symptoms or evidence of right or left ventricular dysfunction Examine for presence of CAD Obtain appropriate guided studies of heart function (echocardiography) or CAD (noninvasive or invasive evaluation of coronary circulation) Ensure appropriate preoperative drug administration for any cardiovascular comorbid conditions
Pulmonary	Assess exercise tolerance Evaluate for symptoms or history of OSA Determine compliance with CPAP or BiPAP and ensure that patient brings personal CPAP device to hospital, if on therapy* Obtain baseline ABGs on room air Obtain PFTs if appropriate
Airway	Perform a basic airway examination Look for evidence of impaired oral or cervical ROM Determine Mallampati score and neck circumference Inquire about previous difficult mask airway or intubation
Laboratory studies	Obtain electrolyte, blood glucose, and serum hemoglobin concentrations Phlebotomize patients with a hemoglobin concentration >17 g/dL
Gastrointestinal	Premedicate with metoclopramide, histamine H_2 blocker, or PPI, as appropriate
Monitoring	Consider the needs for adequate intravenous access and BP monitoring A central venous catheter may be needed to obtain reliable venous access BP cuffs should be of appropriate size (cuff bladder at least 75% of arm circumference) In some cases, the use of direct arterial monitoring may be more reliable or necessary
Miscellaneous	Ensure that plans are made for the use of an appropriately sized OR bed that can accommodate the patient's weight and size

*Refer to the American Society of Anesthesiology's Practice Guidelines for the Perioperative Management of Patients with Obstructive Sleep Apnea. An updated report by the American Society of Anesthesiologists Task Force on Perioperative Management of Patients with Obstructive Sleep Apnea. Anesthesiology. 2013 Dec 16. [Epub ahead of print].
ABGs, Arterial blood gases; BiPAP, bilevel positive airway pressure; BP, blood pressure; CAD, coronary artery disease; CPAP, continuous positive airway pressure; OR, operating room; OSA, obstructive sleep apnea; PFTs, pulmonary function tests; PPI, proton pump inhibitor; ROM, range of motion.

a good estimate for determining the dose of hydrophilic drugs, such as nondepolarizing neuromuscular blocking agents, as well as remifentanil that, although lipid soluble, behaves similarly in obese and nonobese individuals. The dose of lipid-soluble drugs and succinylcholine (increased plasma cholinesterase activity) should be based on the patient's current total body weight.

The use of multimodal analgesic agents that mitigate the use of opioids should be considered. The use of nonsteroidal anti-inflammatory agents, COX-2 inhibitors, intravenously administered lidocaine infusions, and subanesthetic doses of ketamine all help to prevent additive respiratory depression. Additionally, a marked sparing of the use of opioidergic agents without respiratory inhibition has been shown with the use of intraoperative and postoperative dexmedetomidine infusions.

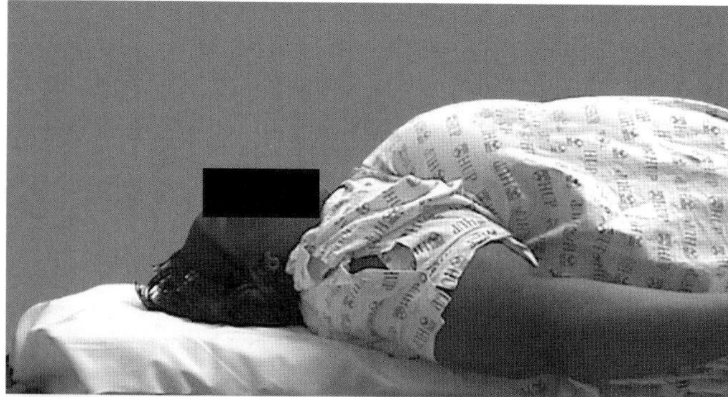

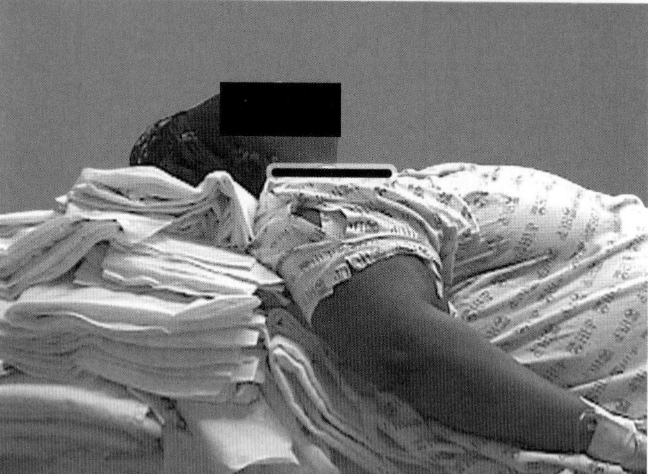

Figure 163-1 Ramping of a morbidly obese patient. (Used with permission of Richard M. Levitan, MD. Airway Cam Guide to Intubation and Practical Emergency Airway Management. Wayne, PA, Airway Cam Technologies, Inc., 2004.)

Emergence from Anesthesia

The inhalation agent should be titrated at the end of the operation to allow prompt emergence and return of airway reflexes and tone. Continuous monitoring of neuromuscular function to enable complete reversal of blockade at the conclusion of the operation is of paramount importance. The patient should be returned to the reverse Trendelenburg position if this position was not employed during the operation. Obese patients should be extubated when they are capable of maintaining a spontaneous airway with adequate tidal volume. The use of continuous positive airway pressure should be reinstituted as soon as possible.

Regional Anesthesia

Regional anesthesia is more difficult to perform in the morbidly obese patient. Landmarks are obscured, increasing the number of attempts and the potential for complications. Nonetheless, a properly performed regional blockade (peripheral or neuraxial) circumvents many of the negative respiratory and hemodynamic effects of general anesthesia. The use of ultrasound guidance for both peripheral and neuraxial blocks can markedly enhance success and accuracy.

Determining the proper doses of local anesthetic agents is more unpredictable for neuraxial blocks because morbidly obese patients have smaller cerebrospinal fluid and epidural volumes because of venous epidural engorgement and potential epidural lipomatosis. The correct dose may be decreased by as much as 20% from normal. To avoid the potentially disastrous effects of an unintended high intrathecal block, consider using a combined spinal-epidural technique, which allows more conservative intrathecal dosing with the option to augment levels via an epidural catheter.

Suggested Readings

Coetzee JF. Total intravenous anaesthesia to obese patients: largely guesswork? *Eur J Anaesthesiol*. 2009;26:359-361.

Delay JM, Sebbane M, Jung B, et al. The effectiveness of noninvasive positive pressure ventilation to enhance preoxygenation in morbidly obese patients: a randomized controlled study. *Anesth Analg*. 2008;107:1707-1713.

Fujiki M, Guta CG, Lemmens HJ, Brock-Utne JG. Is it more difficult to cannulate the right internal jugular vein in morbidly obese patients than in nonobese patients? *Obes Surg*. 2008;18:1157-1159.

Practice Guidelines for the Perioperative Management of Patients with Obstructive Sleep Apnea. An updated report by the American Society of Anesthesiologists Task Force on Perioperative Management of Patients with Obstructive Sleep Apnea. *Anesthesiology*. 2013 Dec 16. [Epub ahead of print].

Kuruba R, Koche LS, Murr MM. Preoperative assessment and perioperative care of patients undergoing bariatric surgery. *Med Clin North Am*. 2007;91: 339-351.

La Colla L, Albertin A, La Colla G, et al. No adjustment vs. adjustment formula as input weight for propofol target-controlled infusion in morbidly obese patients. *Eur J Anaesthesiol*. 2009;26:362-369.

Obesity. *Preventing and Managing the Global Epidemic*. Geneva, Switzerland: World Health Organization; 1997, Report No. 894.

Sinha AC. Some anesthetic aspects of morbid obesity. *Curr Opin Anaesthesiol*. 2009;22:442-446.

CHAPTER 164

Anesthetic Considerations for Weight Loss Surgery

Brian P. McGlinch, MD

The frequency with which weight loss surgery (WLS) is performed has increased significantly over the past 15 years, in part due to the increasing prevalence of obesity, but also because of the understanding that diet and exercise are often ineffective in producing sustained weight loss, the overwhelming evidence that WLS results in significant and sustained weight loss, that reductions occur in obesity-related comorbid conditions, and that the procedures themselves are associated with low rates of morbidity and mortality. Patients who are potential candidates for WLS typically undergo extensive medical evaluations for underlying obesity-related comorbid conditions (e.g., obstructive sleep apnea, diabetes, reactive airway disease, hyperlipidemia, gastroesophageal reflux disease), have treatment of these conditions, and improve their physical conditioning. As a result, the patient who presents for WLS is usually medically and physiologically optimized for surgery and represents a surprisingly low risk for experiencing untoward perioperative events. At the time of this writing, WLS is overwhelmingly performed laparoscopically; this chapter will focus on this surgical approach.

Obesity

Obesity is not solely a North American phenomenon. All areas of the world and all socioeconomic classes demonstrate a rapidly increasing prevalence of obesity. Obesity is defined as a body mass index (BMI, weight in kilograms divided by the square of the height in meters) greater than 30 kg/m^2. Morbid obesity is present at a BMI of 35 kg/m^2 in people who have weight-related comorbid conditions (i.e., hyperlipidemia, diabetes mellitus, obstructive sleep apnea, reactive airway disease) or a BMI of more than 40 kg/m^2 in the absence of weight-related comorbid conditions. Excessive caloric intake only partly contributes to obesity. Psychiatric, physiologic, and metabolic components are all likely factors that contribute to the obesity phenomenon. Emerging research identifying digestive hormones that influence eating behavior, metabolism, and weight gain (e.g., ghrelin, peptide YY) could potentially lead to nonsurgical therapies for obesity. However, at this time, only surgical interventions have been demonstrated to be effective in producing a significant sustained weight loss in the treatment of obesity.

Surgical Procedures for Weight Loss

Current WLS involves restrictive or restrictive-malabsorption components. Restrictive procedures (adjustable gastric banding, gastric sleeve resection) create a small stomach but do not alter how food is digested. The most common restrictive procedure at this time is the laparoscopic adjustable gastric banding procedure. The U.S. Food and Drug Administration approved the adjustable gastric band for clinical use in 2001, and its application has increased annually since its introduction. In this procedure, a limited dissection of connective tissue is performed at the top of the stomach, and an inflatable band is passed that encircles the upper stomach (Figure 164-1, *A*). The band can be adjusted via a port attached to the body wall by adding or withdrawing saline. The surgical risk is considered to be very low. In select patients, this is being performed as an outpatient procedure.

The gastric sleeve resection is typically performed laparoscopically and reduces stomach volume to approximately 100 mL by externally

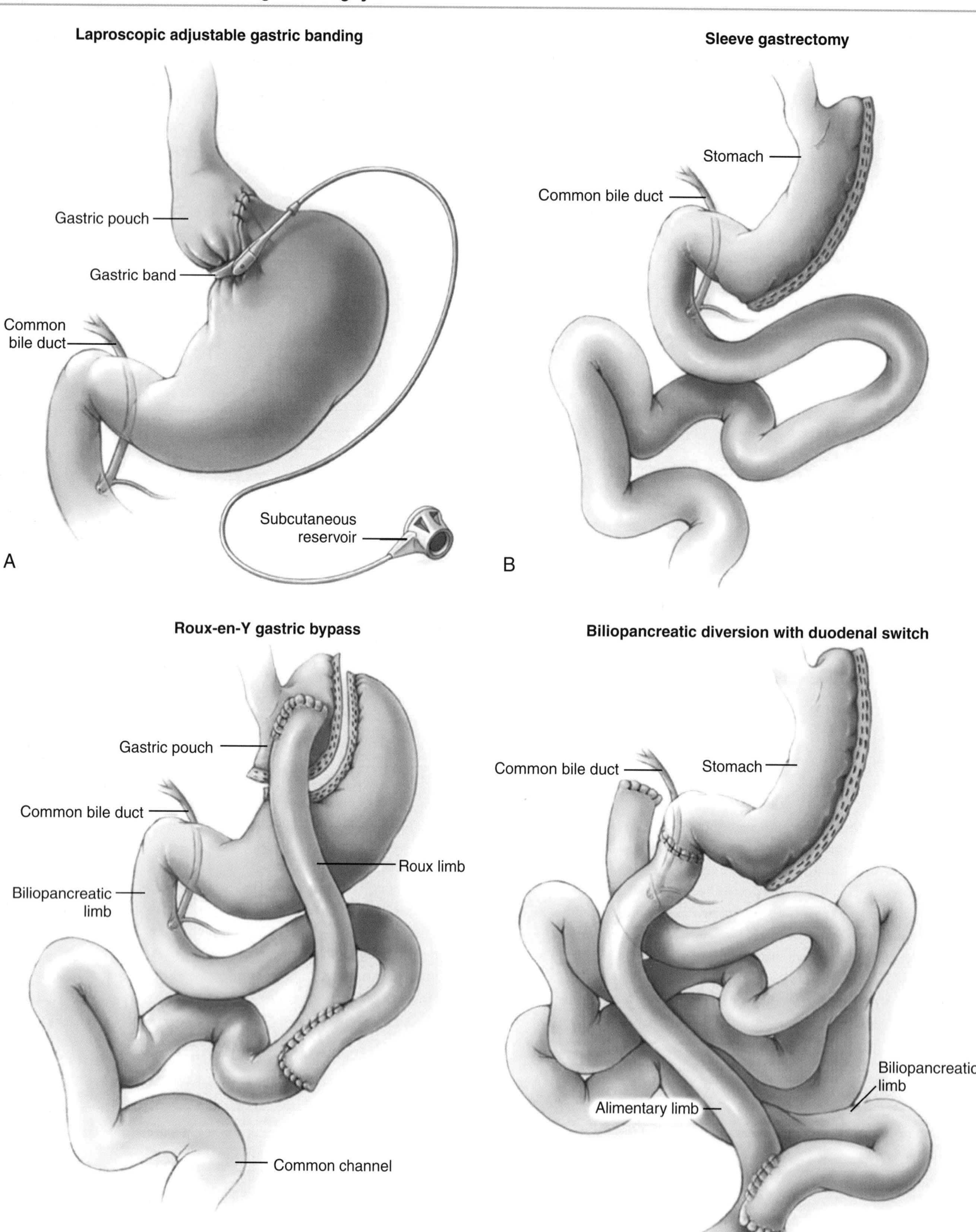

Figure 164-1 Common surgical procedures for weight loss. Restrictive operations for the treatment of morbid obesity and its coexisting conditions, popular today particularly because of laparoscopic surgical approaches, include adjustable gastric banding **(A)** and vertical (sleeve) gastrectomy **(B).** Roux-en-Y gastric bypass **(C),** a procedure that combines restriction and malabsorption, is considered by many to be the gold standard because of its high level of effectiveness and its durability. More extreme malabsorption accompanies biliopancreatic diversion procedures, commonly performed with a duodenal switch **(D),** in which a short, distal, common-channel length of small intestine severely limits caloric absorption. This procedure also includes a sleeve gastrectomy. (Reprinted, with permission, from DeMaria EJ. Bariatric surgery for morbid obesity. N Engl J Med. 2007;356:2176-2183. © 2007 Massachusetts Medical Society. All rights reserved.)

stapling the stomach to exclude the fundus and greater curvature to form a narrow tube along the lesser curvature of the stomach (Figure 164-1, *B*). Both laparoscopic adjustable gastric banding and gastric sleeve resection procedures result in significant weight loss, providing that the patients receiving these interventions comply with proper eating habits, particularly those who avoid high-caloric content (e.g., milkshakes, candy, ice cream). Blood loss is minimal. Surgical duration is relatively brief. Complications are infrequent.

The laparoscopic Roux-en-Y gastric bypass is currently the most commonly performed WLS in the United States. This procedure creates a small gastric pouch (30 mL) that empties into a limb of bowel that excludes a large portion of the small intestine (restrictive and maldigestive interventions) (Figure 164-1, *C*). As a result, satiety is achieved at relatively low volumes (restriction), and the surface area of small bowel that can absorb calories and nutrients is bypassed (maldigestion), resulting in reliable, sustained weight loss. Blood loss is minimal.

The biliopancreatic diversion/duodenal switch procedure is a more complex restrictive-malabsorptive procedure normally reserved for use in patients with a BMI in excess of 50 kg/m^2. With this procedure, a gastric sleeve resection is performed, the stomach is separated from the duodenum, and the small bowel is divided at a point proximal (approximately 100 cm) to the terminal ileum. The stomach is reanastomosed to the distal limb of small bowel, creating an "alimentary channel" where food enters but is not digested. Biliary and pancreatic fluids drain into the duodenum (now separated from the stomach) and contact food where this "biliopancreatic limb" of proximal small bowel is anastomosed to the limb of the alimentary channel (Figure 164-1, *D*). Digestive enzymes contact food late in the process, and the short segment of small bowel that is available to absorb nutrients and calories is significantly restricted. Compared with the Roux-en-Y gastric bypass, the biliopancreatic diversion/duodenal switch procedure requires considerably longer time, but blood loss and fluid shifts are not significantly different.

Anesthetic Management of Patients Undergoing Weight Loss Surgery

Fortunately, patients undergoing WLS have typically undergone a thorough preoperative evaluation based upon symptoms. Evaluations that are otherwise not indicated by symptoms and clinical findings are unnecessary. Patients without symptoms of obstructive sleep apnea do not need a polysomnographic study. Patients without cardiac symptoms do not need to have a stress test or echocardiogram unless other clinical signs (i.e., heart murmurs, pulmonary edema) warrant evaluation independent of the anticipated operation. In most circumstances, diseases typically associated with morbid obesity (e.g., obstructive sleep apnea, hyperlipidemia, diabetes, hypertension, restrictive airway disease) have been evaluated and treated, resulting in optimization of underlying conditions in advance of the operation. The anesthesia provider remains responsible for ensuring that the necessary clinical studies have been completed, that the patient is devoid of acute illness, and that other confounding issues are absent (e.g., the patient did not recently take anticoagulants) prior to inducing anesthesia.

The obese patient should not lie flat on an operating table. Obesity decreases lung compliance, reduces expiratory reserve volume, and decreases functional residual capacity well beyond that seen in nonobese patients. Dependent areas of lung collapse and close, contributing to a ventilation-perfusion mismatch. In the presence of obesity-induced increased O_2 demand and CO_2 production, these physiologic changes in pulmonary function occurring in the supine position often lead to rapid O_2 desaturations and hypercarbia during airway management and subsequent mechanical ventilation during anesthesia. Placing ramping cushions or blankets behind the patient's upper torso and neck, as well as providing 25-degree reverse Trendelenburg positioning, provides greater lung volumes, a reduced tendency for atelectasis formation and intrapulmonary shunting, and a 23% increase in O_2 saturations, compared with the supine position. Applying 10 cm H_2O of positive end-expiratory pressure (PEEP) during induction of anesthesia prolongs the duration of O_2 saturations above 92%, as compared with patients of similar size not receiving PEEP. Reestablishing these interventions (i.e., torso elevation, reverse Trendelenburg position, and application of PEEP) at the end of the surgical procedure should be considered, given the benefits demonstrated at anesthetic induction.

Compared with the nonobese patient, the obese patient will require an increased minute ventilation to maintain normocarbia. Establishing a pneumoperitoneum reduces ventilation compliance more in obese patients than it does in nonobese patients. However, oxygenation is affected by neither the presence of the pneumoperitoneum nor the Trendelenburg position commonly used in WLS. The application of PEEP is useful in improving oxygenation during these operations. However, improved oxygenation in response to PEEP is present only as long as the patient remains intubated. Regardless of the improvement in oxygenation provided by various amounts of PEEP intraoperatively (as determined by intraoperative blood gas analysis), postextubation blood gases are not significantly different from baseline nor from values from patients who do not receive PEEP intraoperatively, suggesting that there is no "best" amount of PEEP during WLS. The clinician should base ventilator-management strategies on individual patient information and the results of laboratory studies and clinical examination.

Insufflation of the peritoneum represents an important period for anesthetic management. Intraperitoneal pressure potentially obstructs venous return from the lower body and also encroaches on intrathoracic space. In most laparoscopic WLS, insufflation of the peritoneum, accompanied by maximal reverse Trendelenburg positioning (to facilitate surgical visualization of the stomach), results in significantly decreased venous return and cardiac preload. Profound hypotension and reflex bradycardia (from the abrupt reduction in cardiac preload) may occur during this period and warrant prompt recognition and treatment; the patient should be rapidly returned to the supine position, the peritoneum desufflated, and vasopressor, vagolytic, or both agents administered, as indicated. These physiologic responses to pneumoperitoneum can be attenuated by fluid loading the patient prior to insufflation. Once the pneumoperitoneum is established, tachycardia and increased mean arterial pressure are common.

Complications

Laparoscopic WLS procedures represent some of the most technically difficult procedures performed by general surgeons. The surgeon's experience performing laparoscopic procedures is likely the single most important factor that correlates with the frequency of complications. The facility in which WLS is performed also plays a significant role. Because these two aspects of WLS are, by far, the greatest contributors to complication rates, emphasis will be placed on these aspects of WLS.

Surgeon Expertise

Several studies that have evaluated outcome after WLS have concluded that surgeon experience with laparoscopic gastric bypass is inversely proportional to the incidence of postoperative complications. The most common complications (e.g., anastomotic leaks, internal hernia) occur most frequently when the surgeon has performed fewer than 75 laparoscopic WLS procedures. As surgeon experience exceeds 100 WLS procedures, major complication rates become comparable to those associated with low-risk surgical procedures.

Facility Expertise

Hospitals with high WLS volumes have overall mortality rates of 0.5%. Mortality rate is significantly lower in a high-volume facility (>100 WLS procedures per year) compared with a low-volume facility (<50 WLS procedures per year). These observed differences likely reflect familiarity with the postoperative management of patients undergoing WLS and the early recognition of the signs and symptoms suggestive of surgical complications (i.e., anastomotic leaks and internal hernia).

Summary

Laparoscopic WLS is the only therapy yielding sustained, significant weight loss and eliminating or attenuating weight-related comorbid conditions. Due to the thorough preoperative evaluations that WLS candidates undergo, anesthesia providers infrequently require additional studies or evaluations to ensure that these patients are safe for surgery. Inducing anesthesia with the patient ramped on blankets and in a modest reverse Trendelenburg position allows for improved oxygenation and ventilation. Surgeon and facility experience with WLS play significant roles in the morbidity and mortality rates associated with these procedures. Future weight-loss strategies may involve hormone therapies, but, most likely, laparoscopic WLS will remain the predominant obesity therapy offered throughout the world.

Suggested Readings

Burns EM, Naseem H, Bottle A, et al. Introduction of laparoscopic bariatric surgery in England: Observational population cohort study. *BMJ*. 2010;341:c4296.

DeMaria EJ. Bariatric surgery for morbid obesity. *N Engl J Med*. 2007;356:2176-2183.

DeMaria EJ, Sugarman HJ, Kellum JM, et al. Results of 281 consecutive total laparoscopic Roux-en-Y gastric bypasses to treat morbid obesity. *Ann Surg*. 2002;235:640-645.

Dixon BJ, Dixon JB, Carden JR, et al. Preoxygenation is more effective in the 25° head up position than the supine position in severely obese patients: A randomized controlled study. *Anesthesiology*. 2005;102:1110-1115.

Gander S, Frascarolo P, Suter M, et al. Positive end-expiratory pressure during induction of general anesthesia increases duration of nonhypoxic apnea in morbidly obese patients. *Anesth Analg*. 2005;100:580-584.

Nguyen NT, Paya M, Stevens CM, et al. The relationship between hospital volume and outcome in bariatric surgery at academic medical centers. *Ann Surg*. 2004;240:586-593.

Nguyen NT, Silver M, Robinson M, et al. Result of a national audit of bariatric surgery performed at academic centers: A 2004 University Health System Consortium Benchmarking Project. *Arch Surg*. 2006;141:445-449.

Podnos YD, Jimenez JC, Wilson SE, et al. Complications after laparoscopic gastric bypass: A review of 3464 cases. *Arch Surg*. 2003;138:957-961.

Puzziferri N, Austrheim-Smith IT, Wolfe BM, et al. Three-year follow-up of a prospective randomized trial comparing laparoscopic versus open gastric bypass. *Ann Surg*. 2006;243:181-188.

Sprung J, Whalley DG, Falcone DG, et al. The impact of morbid obesity, pneumoperitoneum, and posture on respiratory system mechanics and oxygenation during laparoscopy. *Anesth Analg*. 2002;94:1345-1350.

Whalen FX, Gajic O, Thompson GB. The effects of alveolar recruitment maneuver and positive end-expiratory pressure on arterial oxygenation during laparoscopic bariatric surgery. *Anesth Anal*. 2006;102:298-305.

CHAPTER 165
Anesthesia for Laparoscopic Surgery

Eric Werner, MD, and Michael J. Murray, MD, PhD

Compared with an open abdominal surgical procedure, a surgical procedure performed laparoscopically is less invasive, less stressful to the patient, and associated with less pain and a shorter recovery period. Over the last 2 decades, the technology for performing laparoscopic procedures, also called keyhole surgery or minimally invasive surgery, has improved significantly. With these improvements, surgeons have increased the types of procedures that they perform laparoscopically, such that laparoscopic access has become one of the most common, if not the most common, abdominal and pelvic access used by gynecologists, urologists, general surgeons, and colorectal surgeons. Patients with comorbid conditions who previously were considered to be at too high a risk to undergo an open abdominal procedure are now potentially candidates for surgery if the procedure is performed laparoscopically, resulting in an more procedures being performed in increasingly sicker patients.

Technique

For any operation other than a simple gynecologic procedure, laparoscopic surgery requires general anesthesia and controlled mechanical ventilation through a tracheal tube. After the patient is prepped and draped, the surgeon typically inserts a Veress needle or a Hasson trocar, into the patient's abdomen at the umbilicus. The insertion proceeds at an angle of approximately 45 degrees or 90 degrees, in non-obese or obese patients respectively, until a characteristic loss of resistance is felt (Figures 165-1 and 165-2). An intraperitoneal pressure of 10 mm Hg or less is usually considered to be an indicator of appropriate placement within the peritoneal cavity. CO_2 is then insufflated into the peritoneal cavity to a pressure of 20 to 30 mm Hg, lifting the anterior abdominal wall away from the abdominal viscera.

Additional trocars are inserted laterally, caudal and cephalad to the umbilicus through the abdominal wall, depending on the surgical procedure. A combined optical-access device is usually the second trocar introduced, with an endoscope inserted through it for visualizing the peritoneal space. Instruments for performing the surgical procedure are then inserted through the other trocars (Figure 165-3). The patient is then positioned—Trendelenburg for procedures performed in the pelvis; reverse Trendelenburg for procedures performed in the upper abdomen, such as laparoscopic cholecystectomies; and lateral head down for colorectal procedures, such as hemicolectomies.

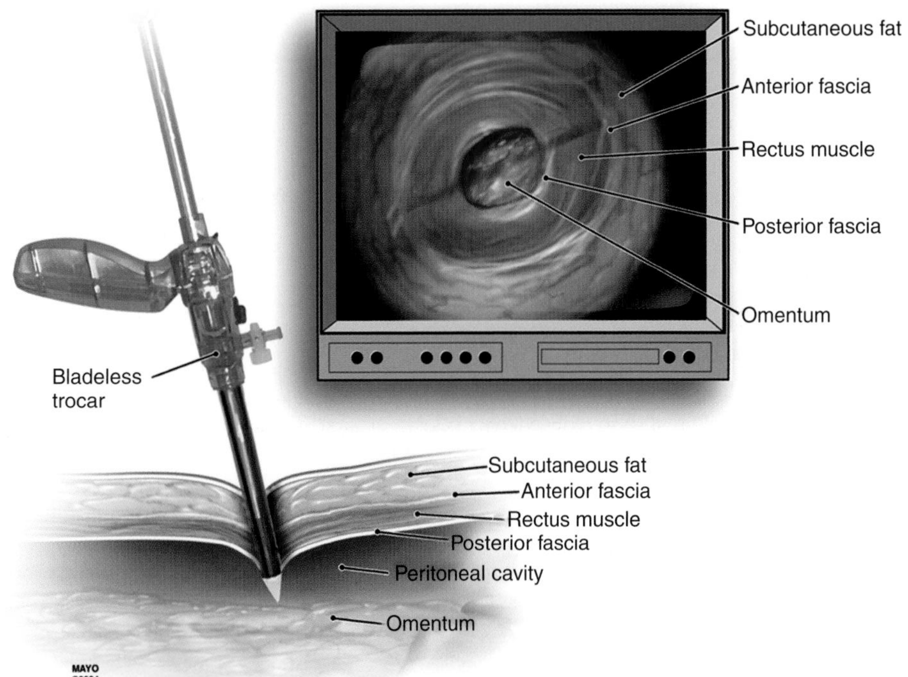

Figure 165-1 Technique for endoscopic port placement and description of anatomic layers. (Used with permission of Mayo Foundation for Medical Education and Research.)

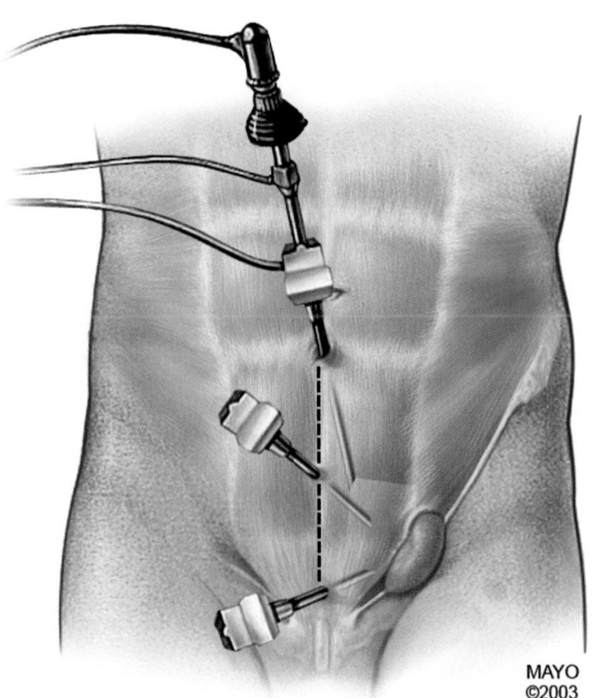

Figure 165-2 Placement of trocars and ports for laparoscopic hernia repair. (Used with permission of Mayo Foundation for Medical Education and Research.)

Physiologic Implications

During placement of trocars and insufflation of CO_2, the anesthesia provider must pay particular attention to the patient's vital signs and end-tidal CO_2 ($ETCO_2$). Patients whose cardiac output is dependent on preload may not tolerate the increased intraperitoneal pressure that occurs during CO_2 insufflation, which can compress the inferior vena cava and decrease blood return to the heart. Even patients who initially tolerate the resultant pneumoperitoneum may develop inadequate preload with decreased cardiac output and blood pressure when they are placed in the reverse Trendelenburg position.

During CO_2 insufflation, the patient's $Paco_2$ rises as CO_2 is absorbed from the peritoneal cavity until equilibrium is reached between the amount of CO_2 absorbed and the amount of CO_2 excreted through ventilation, a process that usually takes 15 to 30 minutes. However, patients with preexisting hypercarbia or with increased closing capacity may require adjustment in tidal volume prior to the establishment of equilibrium to maintain an acceptable $Paco_2$ and $ETCO_2$.

Once the patient's $Paco_2$ stabilizes, any further increase in $Paco_2$ or $ETCO_2$ warrants careful consideration of other potential causes of hypercarbia. One of the most common causes of hypercarbia is inadequate minute ventilation because of increased abdominal pressure in a patient who has been placed in a steep Trendelenburg position that impedes diaphragmatic movement. Increasing the minute ventilation by increasing the respiratory rate without increasing tidal volume may not increase alveolar ventilation enough to adequately impact $Paco_2$. However, increasing the tidal volume may require an increase in peak and plateau pressures, which may, in turn, adversely affect cardiac preload.

Challenges of Positioning

For related reasons, extremes of positioning may compromise hemodynamics (reverse Trendelenburg) or ventilation (Trendelenburg). In normal individuals placed in the Trendelenburg position, venous return, central venous pressure, and cardiac output increase, which, in turn, may activate baroreceptor reflexes, manifested by bradycardia and venodilation. Normally, though, general anesthesia suppresses the baroreceptor reflex, so it would be unusual to see hemodynamic compromise in most patients undergoing laparoscopic surgery. However, patients with cardiomyopathy may not tolerate an increase in venous return. Likewise, patients with decreased intracranial compliance

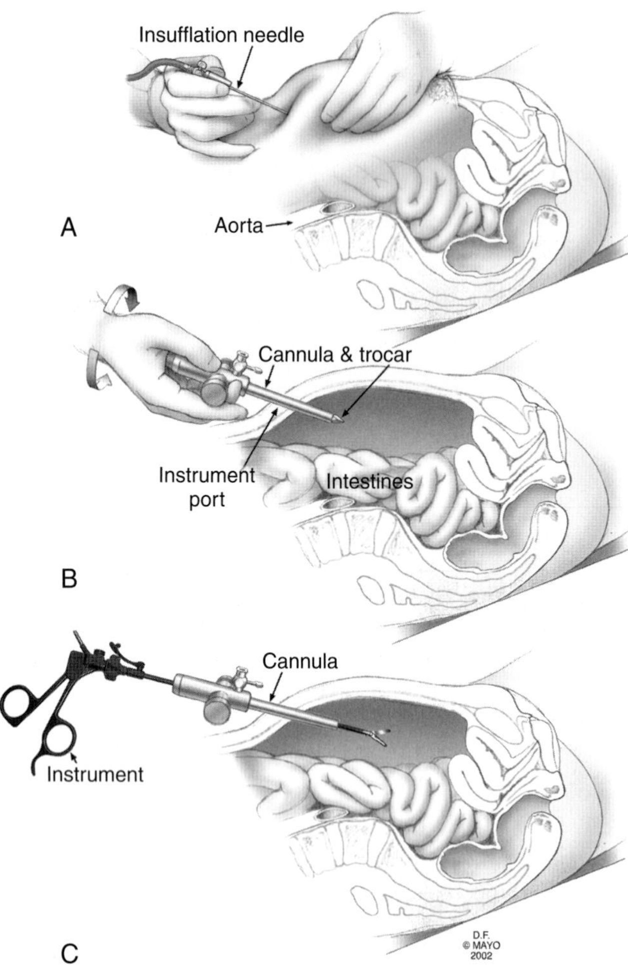

Figure 165-3 Basic laparoscopic technique. **A,** Insufflation of the abdomen. **B,** Insertion of the cannula and trocar. **C,** Trocar removed and surgical instrument inserted. (Used with permission of Mayo Foundation for Medical Education and Research.)

may experience a decrease in cerebral perfusion pressure when central venous pressure rises; similarly, the rise in intraocular pressure could adversely affect patients with poorly treated glaucoma.

The reverse Trendelenburg position has the opposite effect, compounded by the increased abdominal pressure, as mentioned earlier, further decreasing venous return and cardiac output, and, if systemic vascular resistance remains unchanged, blood pressure could also decrease.

Cases have been reported of patients sliding off the operating table if they are not adequately secured because of the extremes in the degree of head-up or head-down positioning occasionally requested by the surgeon. Most anesthesia providers pay particular attention to securing the patient to the table. In securing the patient to the table, the anesthesia provider must be careful not to restrict venous return to the extent that the patient develops a compartment syndrome in the upper extremities (when in the Trendelenburg position) or in the lower extremities (when in the reverse Trendelenburg position).

In the Trendelenburg position, central venous blood pressure increases are greater in patients with poor ventricular function because cardiac output is inadequate to handle an increase in end-diastolic volume. Similarly, patients with decreased intracranial or intraocular compliance will not tolerate the steep Trendelenburg position.

Though not ideal, laparoscopic surgery can be performed with the patient in the supine position if changes in position compromise hemodynamics, and, likewise, if the increase in $ETCO_2$ is too great, the insufflation pressure can be decreased following consultation with the surgeon.

Anesthetic Considerations

Because expertise and equipment have improved and because laparoscopic procedures are performed on an outpatient basis and in sicker patients, rendering anesthesia for laparoscopic procedures is technically difficult and challenging. A careful choice of the anesthetic technique must be tailored to the type of operation. Typically, general anesthesia with tracheal intubation and using a balanced anesthesia technique, including several intravenously administered and inhalation agents in combination with neuromuscular blocking agents, provides cardiovascular and pulmonary stability and a rapid recovery. However, peripheral nerve blocks and neuraxial anesthesia can be used for pelvic laparoscopy. Local anesthesia infiltration has been shown to be effective and safe in microlaparoscopy for limited and precise gynecologic procedures. However, intravenous sedation is sometimes required.

Adverse Effects Associated with Laparoscopic Procedures

Complications associated with the use of a Veress needle are usually less severe than those associated with introduction of the other trocars, which are associated with more significant injury to large blood vessels and the intestines. However, insertion of the Veress needle and insufflation of CO_2 has been associated with venous gas embolism, which must be treated aggressively if outcome is to be optimized. Blood vessel injury, if unrecognized, can result in significant hemorrhage—including hemorrhagic shock and death.

Suggested Readings

Aran T, Unsal MA, Guven S, et al. Carbon dioxide pneumoperitoneum induces systemic oxidative stress: A clinical study. *Eur J Obstet Gynecol Reprod Biol.* 2012;161:80-83.

Cheng Y, Lu J, Xiong X, et al. Gases for establishing pneumoperitoneum during laparoscopic abdominal surgery. *Cochrane Database Syst Rev.* 2013;1: CD009569.

De Corte W, Delrue H, Vanfleteren LJ, et al. Randomized clinical trial on the influence of anaesthesia protocol on intestinal motility during laparoscopic surgery requiring small bowel anastomosis. *Br J Surg.* 2012;99:1524-1529.

Gainsburg DM. Anesthetic concerns for robotic-assisted laparoscopic radical prostatectomy. *Minerva Anestesiol.* 2012;78:596-604.

Sharma B, Gupta R, Sehgal R, et al. ProSeal laryngeal mask airway cuff pressure changes with and without use of nitrous oxide during laparoscopic surgery. *J Anaesthesiol Clin Pharmacol.* 2013;29:47-51.

Vilos GA, Ternamian A, Dempster J, Laberge PY, The Society of Obstetricians and Gynaecologists of Canada. Laparoscopic entry: A review of techniques, technologies, and complications. *J Obstet Gynaecol Can.* 2007;29:433-465.

CHAPTER 166

Complications of Transurethral Resection of the Prostate

Marie L. De Ruyter, MD

Transurethral resection of the prostate (TURP), one of the more common surgical procedures performed in men over age 60, is the standard surgical treatment for benign prostatic hypertrophy (BPH) when symptomatic obstruction of urinary outflow occurs. A variety of factors have led to decreasing mortality and morbidity rates associated with this procedure, including increased awareness of BPH, which has led to earlier treatment, and the availability of new drugs and new surgical techniques, which are associated with lower rates of complications.

In a traditional TURP, resection of the prostate is performed during cystoscopy using a resectoscope with an electrocautery loop. The morbidity rate of 7% to 20% is associated with longer resection times (>90 min), larger gland size (>45 g), acute urinary retention, and age greater than 80 years. One of the most serious complications associated with TURP, TURP syndrome (Box 166-1) occurs in 2% to 15% of patients treated with this approach. Postoperative bleeding with the need for blood transfusion occurs in about 2% to 4.8% of patients who develop TURP syndrome.

With newer surgical techniques, however, TURP syndrome occurs in as few as 1.1% of patients, such that anesthesia providers are now unlikely to encounter patients with this complication.

Treatment

Medical Options

One of the reasons the incidence of complications of TURP is decreasing is that many men are successfully treated medically, and for those whose symptoms progress, the prostate may not be as large as it might have been without medical treatment; therefore, the operative procedure has a shorter duration and is associated with fewer complications. The medical treatment of BPH includes the oral administration of α-adrenergic antagonists (e.g., tamsulosin) or 5α-reductase inhibitors (e.g., finasteride). If medical treatment is unsuccessful or symptoms progress and the patient is a surgical candidate, a TURP may be performed to treat symptoms.

Box 166-1 Signs and Symptoms of Transurethral Resection of the Prostate Syndrome

Cardiovascular and Respiratory	Central Nervous System	Metabolic	Other
Hypertension	Agitation/confusion	Hyponatremia	Hypo-osmolality
Bradyarrhythmias/tachyarrhythmias	Seizures	Hyperglycinemia	Hemolysis
Congestive heart failure	Coma	Hyperammonemia	
Pulmonary edema and hypoxemia	Visual disturbances (blindness)		
Myocardial infarction			
Hypertension			

From Malhotra V, Sudheendra V, O'Hara J, Diwan S. Anesthesia and the renal and genitourinary systems. In: Miller RD, ed. Anesthesia. 7th ed. Vol. 2. Philadelphia: Churchill Livingstone; 2009: Chap. 65.

Surgical Options

TURP is performed under direct vision. The most common procedure in the past was performed with a modified cystoscope (resectoscope) with a monopolar electrically energized wire loop. Bleeding was controlled with a coagulating current. Continuous irrigation was used to distend the bladder and remove blood and dissected prostatic tissue. Because the prostate contains large venous sinuses, it was inevitable that irrigating solution would be absorbed into the vascular system. The volume absorbed depended on three factors: the hydrostatic pressure, duration of the resection, and number and size of the opened venous sinuses. The hydrostatic pressure is determined by the height of the irrigating fluid above the patient. Prostate venous sinuses have a pressure of approximately 10 mm Hg. The duration of the TURP was dependent upon the size of the prostate and experience of the surgeon. Approximately 10 to 30 mL of irrigating solution is absorbed per minute of resection time. The choice of irrigation solution is dependent on several factors as discussed later.

Monopolar TURP is still considered by many as the treatment of choice for very enlarged prostates (50-80 g); however, this "gold-standard" is marred by the previously mentioned significant morbidity and mortality rates.

Recently, several alternatives have been introduced that are associated with good results and fewer complications (e.g., bleeding and TURP syndrome). The use of a bipolar electrosurgical device allows the urologist to use alternative irrigation solutions, which are associated with fewer complications. "Plasma TURP" refers to a TURP in which a bipolar electrode, in the shape of a mushroom, generates a "plasma" corona on its surface. The energy simultaneously vaporizes tissue and coagulates all but the largest blood vessels; because of the type of energy used, the procedure can be performed with saline as the irrigation solution, which all but eliminates the possibility of TURP syndrome developing.

Another new technology that has been in use for about a decade is the "green-light laser"—a high-power (80-W) potassium-titanyl-phosphate laser emitting a green laser beam of light that also vaporizes and coagulates blood vessels. For some urologists, this technique has become the treatment of choice for TURP and is associated with fewer short-term (i.e., perioperative) complications.

Irrigation Solutions

The choice of which irrigating fluid to use when performing a TURP depends on many factors, including the optical properties of the fluid, its degree of ionization, and its potential for inducing hemolysis, as well as on the technology being used to resect the prostate. Distilled water was often used in the past as an irrigation solution because of its excellent optical properties and low cost, but distilled water is not often used in current practice because of its potential for inducing marked dilutional hyponatremia and intravascular red blood cell hemolysis.

Lactated Ringer's and normal saline solutions cannot be used if a monopolar electrosurgical probe is used because these solutions are highly ionized and promote current dispersion from the monopolar resectoscope. However, the newer surgical techniques mentioned above that employ a bipolar probe or a laser device can be performed with normal saline as the irrigating solution, which results in a much lower incidence of TURP syndrome. Normal saline is well tolerated when absorbed intravascularly.

Glycine (1.5%) is a low-cost, nonelectrolytic, and only slightly hypo-osmolar fluid that can be used during monopolar therapy. However, if large amounts of glycine are absorbed, transient blindness and encephalopathy can evolve, as can potential complications associated with increased fluid load.

Sorbitol (2.7%) and mannitol (0.54%) have the advantage of being nonelectrolytic, isosmolar, and rapidly cleared from the plasma but are expensive and can lead to complications resulting from increased intravascular fluid load.

Specific Complications

TURP Syndrome

TURP syndrome, a constellation of symptoms and signs caused by excessive absorption of the irrigating fluid, may occur at any time perioperatively. Patients who undergo a TURP with a neuraxial anesthetic and who remain awake will often complain of nausea, headache, and dizziness as the first manifestations of TURP syndrome, which progresses to dyspnea and confusion. Agitation often ensues, associated with elevated blood pressure and bradycardia; if no treatment is implemented, seizures and cardiac arrest may follow (see Box 166-1). Diagnosing TURP syndrome in patients who undergo TURP with general anesthesia may be difficult because the first signs are hypertension and severe refractory bradycardia, followed in short order by seizure and cardiac arrest. These signs develop most often in patients with preexisting compromised myocardial function whose compromise leaves them unable to handle the increased intravascular absorption of the irrigating solution.

The TURP syndrome develops because of circulatory overload and hyponatremia. The former is associated with the amount of irrigating solution that is absorbed, which in turn depends on cardiovascular status, amount and rapidity of absorption of irrigating solution, and amount of surgical blood loss. Dilutional hyponatremia associated with TURP is a hypervolemic hyponatremic condition representing excess total body water with normal total body sodium. If resection time is longer than 90 min or the patient has mild symptoms of TURP syndrome, such as nausea, headache, dizziness, or mild confusion, his serum sodium should be measured. If hyponatremia is present, the patient should be treated with fluid restriction and a loop diuretic (furosemide 5-20 mg administered intravenously). If serum sodium concentration is below 120 mEq/L or the patient develops severe signs and symptoms of water intoxication (twitching, visual disturbance, hypotension, dyspnea, seizures), treatment should be instituted immediately with hypertonic (3%) saline at a rate of 100 mL/h or less, allowing the most rapid correction of plasma sodium concentration. The volume of distribution of sodium equals total body water, so free water excess can be estimated from the following formula:

$$\text{Total body water} = \text{weight (in kg)} \times 0.6$$

From this, an estimation of the mEq of Na^+ necessary to normalize the plasma sodium concentration can be obtained:

$$\text{Sodium deficit} = (140 - \text{observed plasma } Na^+) \times \text{total body water}$$

Hypertonic 3% saline contains 513 mEq of Na^+ per liter and should be administered at a rate no faster than 100 mL/h. Once the symptoms have abated (or the sodium concentration rises above 120 mEq/L), the hypertonic saline should be stopped, and furosemide (40-60 mg) should be intravenously administered to aid free-water excretion by the kidneys. Frequent serum sodium measurements should be obtained. Too rapid correction of hyponatremia can cause seizures, central pontine myelinolysis, and permanent brain damage.

Glycine Toxicity

Glycine toxicity usually manifests as visual disturbances and transient blindness but may also include other signs and symptoms seen in TURP syndrome. The mechanism of action may be attributed to glycine acting as an inhibitory neurotransmitter because it has a distribution similar to that of γ-aminobutyric acid in the retina, spinal cord, and brainstem.

Ammonia Toxicity

Ammonia is a major byproduct of glycine metabolism. Hyperammonemia usually manifests with nausea and vomiting, followed by encephalopathy.

Blood Loss

Assessment of blood loss is difficult during a TURP because of dilution of blood with the absorbed irrigation fluid, which maintains intravascular volume, so that the usual hemodynamic responses to blood loss are not seen. The amount of blood loss is directly proportional to the vascularity of the prostate, length of the operation, and the weight of the prostate gland resected. Continuous postoperative bleeding may indicate a coagulopathy, since patients undergoing TURP have a higher incidence of fibrinolysis. Dilutional thrombocytopenia should also be considered in the differential diagnosis.

Hypothermia

Hypothermia, which has not been shown to be influenced by anesthetic technique, could be another cause of confusion in the elderly patient undergoing a TURP.

Bacteremia

Despite preoperative intravenous administration of antibiotics, bacteremia commonly occurs during a TURP and can lead to the development of sepsis. However, bacteremia is usually asymptomatic and is treated with antibiotics to cover gram-positive and gram-negative organisms. Sepsis has been reported to occur in as many as 6% to 7% of patients undergoing a TURP, with septic shock being the first manifestation of the condition.

Perforation of Bladder or Urethra with Extravasation

Bladder perforation most often occurs during difficult resections by the cutting loop or knife electrode. These perforations can be either extraperitoneal (most common) or intraperitoneal. In the awake patient, extraperitoneal perforation may present as pain in the periumbilical, inguinal, or suprapubic region. Intraperitoneal perforation usually occurs through the bladder wall. Pain may be generalized to the upper abdomen or referred from the diaphragm to the shoulder. Other signs and symptoms include pallor, sweating, nausea, vomiting, shortness of breath, abdominal rigidity, hypotension, and hypertension.

Prevention of Complications

In general, a TURP is an elective procedure. Therefore, optimizing the patient's preoperative state prior to surgery is always recommended and may minimize anesthetic risks. Surgical risks can be reduced by limiting the duration of the operation, using isosmotic solutions, limiting the depth of dissection, and limiting the pressure of irrigating solution (60 cm H_2O is suggested). Use of spinal anesthesia should promote earlier detection of complications.

Suggested Readings

Baazeem A, Elhilali M. Surgical management of benign prostatic hyperplasia: Current evidence. *Nat Clin Pract Urol*. 2008;5:540-549.

Gill HS, Chung B, Deem SA, Pearl RG. Transurethral resection of the prostate (TURP). In: Jaffe RA, Sammuels SI, eds. *Anesthesiologist's Manual of Surgical Procedures*. 4th ed. Philadelphia: Lippincott, Williams & Wilkins; 2009:8636.

Malhotra V. Transurethral resection of the prostate. *Anesthesiol Clin North Am*. 2000;18:883-897.

Rassweiler J, Teber D, Kuntz R, Hofmann R. Complications of transurethral resection of the prostate (TURP)—incidence, management, and prevention. *Eur Urol*. 2006;50;969-979.

CHAPTER 167

Extracorporeal Shock Wave Lithotripsy

Jonathan A. Faust, MD

Urolithiasis is a common condition with a lifetime prevalence of 12% in the United States. It is more common in men than women and most often presents in the third to fourth decade of life. Most urinary stones can be passed spontaneously; however, 10% to 30% require urologic intervention. Since the introduction of the first lithotripter in 1980, extracorporeal shock wave lithotripsy (ESWL) (Figure 167-1) has gradually replaced open and percutaneous surgical approaches as the treatment of choice for most urinary stones requiring intervention in the kidney or upper ureter.

Technical Aspects

All lithotripters consist of (1) an energy source that creates a shock wave, (2) a system to focus the energy of the shock wave, (3) a coupling medium that facilitates transfer of the shock-wave energy to the patient, and (4) an imaging system to provide localization of the stone and to guide energy delivery to the stone. First-generation lithotripters, such as the Dornier HM-3, require patients to be immersed in a water bath as the coupling medium and use a sparkplug to generate an 18-kV to 24-kV discharge. This spark causes water vaporization and a cavitation bubble that rapidly expands and then contracts, leading to the creation of a shock wave. The origin of the wave is termed the F_1 *focal point*. A semiellipsoid reflector focuses the energy wave to converge at the stone (located at the F_2 focal point) under the guidance of fluoroscopy. The shock wave travels through the water bath and the patient with little attenuation because of the similar acoustic impedance of water and body tissues. The urinary stone presents a change in impedance, resulting in the release of compressive energy and a mechanical stress on the stone. Repeated shocks (1000 or more) lead to disintegration of the stone, and stone fragments are excreted in the urine.

Some newer lithotripters use piezoelectric crystals or electromagnetic shock generators. These devices are more durable and require less frequent maintenance. Piezoelectric lithotripters have the advantage of having a wider aperture, resulting in lower energy density at the skin and, therefore, less patient discomfort. Various methods of focusing the shock wave are used. Most no longer require patient immersion in a water bath because the shock is generated within a water-filled compartment and transferred through a membrane to the patient using a coupling gel. In addition to fluoroscopy, ultrasound is used in some newer lithotripters for stone localization. Some lithotripters can synchronize shock delivery with respiration or the cardiac cycle, although this may limit the maximal rate of shock delivery.

Physiology of Water Immersion

Because first-generation lithotripters require partial immersion of the patient in a water bath, the immersion typically results in a significant redistribution of peripheral venous blood toward the central compartment, causing increased central venous and pulmonary artery pressures. The degree of these changes is related to the level of water immersion, and these effects are opposed by anesthesia (general or neuraxial) and the sitting position. Water immersion—along with the straps used to secure the patient in some devices—can contribute to a rapid, shallow breathing pattern, and functional residual capacity can be decreased by 20% to 30%. These changes, along with increased pulmonary blood flow, can lead to ventilation-perfusion mismatch and hypoxemia.

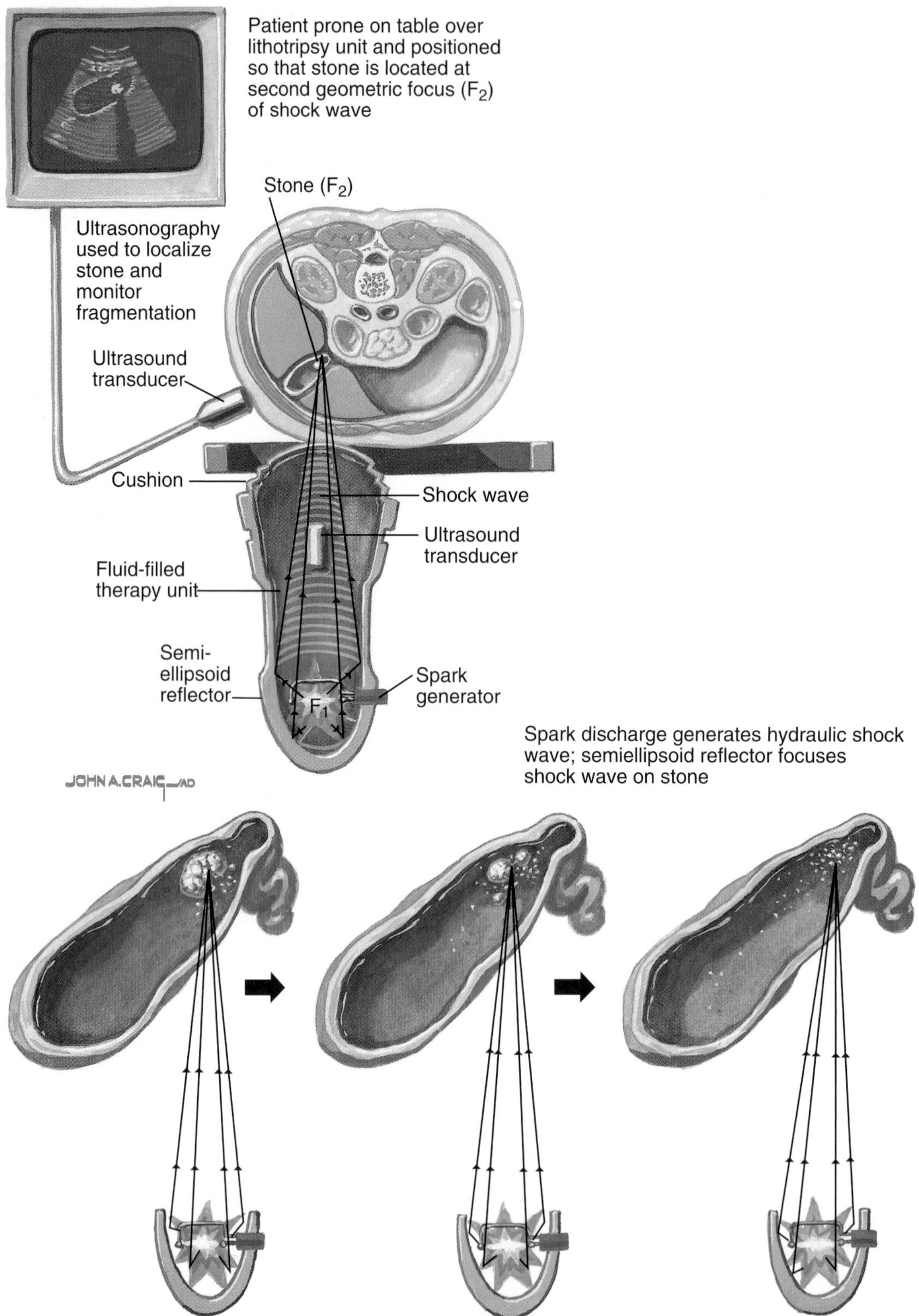

Figure 167-1 Extracorporeal shock wave lithotripsy. (Netter illustration from www.netterimages.com. © Elsevier Inc. All rights reserved.)

Patient Selection

ESWL has been used successfully to manage urinary stones in infants, children, and adults. Absolute and relative contraindications to the procedure are listed in Box 167-1. Performing ESWL on patients with untreated urinary infection and urinary obstruction distal to the location of the target stone predispose the patient to the development of urosepsis. Pregnancy is considered an absolute contraindication, because the effects of shock waves on the fetus are unknown, although ESWL has been inadvertently performed on pregnant women without apparent adverse effects on the fetus. The calcified wall of an abdominal aortic aneurysm provides an acoustic interface that can result in liberation of shock-wave energy and aneurysm rupture. Various authors have recommended minimum safe aneurysm diameters (e.g., 5 to 5.5 cm) and aneurysm-to-stone distances (e.g., at least 5 cm) along with maximum voltage settings and number of shock waves that can be safely delivered. ESWL in patients who are morbidly obese can be technically challenging and have lower success rates. ESWL can be safely performed in patients with pectorally-located implanted cardiac devices (i.e., pacemakers and automated implantable cardioverter-defibrillators), provided certain conditions are met (Box 167-2). Performing ESWL in a patient with abdominally located cardiac devices is not recommended.

Complications

Common side effects reported in the immediate postoperative period include flank pain, nausea and vomiting, and hypertension. Skin bruising at the site of shock-wave entry and flank pain lasting several days are also common. Hematuria is almost universally present due to shock wave–induced urothelial or renal parenchymal injury. Subcapsular hematoma is uncommon, with an incidence of 0.5%. Bleeding complications are more likely to occur in patients with hypertension, diabetes, or coronary artery atherosclerosis; the elderly; and patients with altered coagulation. Bleeding significant enough to require transfusion is rare. Stone fragments are generally excreted in the urine but can, occasionally, accumulate in the ureter, resulting in total obstruction (1%-5%). Air-filled alveoli within the lung present an impedance interface, and, therefore, shock waves directed toward the lungs result in liberation of shock-wave energy, alveolar rupture, and hemoptysis. In children or adults of short stature (under 48 inches), styrofoam can be used to protect the lungs from shock waves. Cardiac arrhythmias—including atrial and ventricular premature complexes, atrial fibrillation, and supraventricular and ventricular tachycardias—have been reported. Arrhythmias were extremely common in patients who had been treated with the first-generation lithotripters but are now thought to be quite rare. Some lithotripters can be programmed to deliver shock waves using "electrocardiogram gating" in an attempt to minimize the risk of an R-on-T phenomenon and subsequent ventricular arrhythmia. Pancreatitis and bowel injury resulting in rectal bleeding have been reported. There is conflicting evidence on the long-term effects of ESWL, but some studies suggest that patients who undergo ESWL may develop increased blood pressure and decreased renal function when compared with patients undergoing other treatments or observation. Elderly patients appear to be at higher risk for developing these complications.

Box 167-1 Contraindications to the Use of Extracorpeal Shock Wave Lithotripsy

Absolute Contraindications

Bleeding disorder or anticoagulation
Obstruction distal to the renal calculi
Pregnancy
Untreated urinary tract infection

Relative Contraindications

Large calcified aortic or renal artery aneurysm
Morbid obesity
Implanted cardiac devices

Adapted, with permission, from O'Hara JF, Cywinski JB, Monk TG. The renal system and anesthesia for urologic surgery. In: Barash PG, Cullen BF, Stoelting RK, eds. Clinical Anesthesia. 5th ed. Philadelphia, Lippincott, Williams & Wilkins, 2006:1030-1031.

Box 167-2 Recommendations for Management of CIEDs in Patients Undergoing ESWL

Preoperatively determine the type of device and its functional status.
Have a magnet available (and an understanding of the effect of the magnet on the device) or a programming device and a person skilled in its use.
If the patient is pacemaker dependent, ensure that an alternative method of pacing is available.
Position the patient so that the device is not in the shock-wave path.
Disable AICD functions.
Consider reprogramming the device to a nonsensing mode.

AICD, Automated implantable cardioverter-defibrillator; CIED, cardiac implantable electronic device; ESWL, extracorpeal shock wave lithotripsy.
Adapted, with permission, from O'Hara JF, Cywinski JB, Monk TG. The renal system and anesthesia for urologic surgery. In: Barash PG, Cullen BF, Stoelting RK, eds. Clinical Anesthesia. 5th ed. Philadelphia, Lippincott, Williams & Wilkins, 2006:1030-1031.

Anesthetic Considerations

Pain experienced during ESWL has cutaneous, somatic, and visceral origins. The amount of pain is directly related to the energy density of the shock wave at the skin entry site and the size of the F_2 focal zone. Modern lithotripters generally deliver shock waves of lower energy, compared with first-generation machines, and result in less patient discomfort. Additionally, piezoelectric lithotripters have a wider aperture and lower energy density at the skin entry point.

A wide variety of anesthetic techniques have been employed alone and in combination for ESWL, including general, epidural, and spinal anesthesia; flank infiltration; intercostal and paravertebral nerve blocks; topical application of EMLA (eutectic mixture of local anesthetic) cream; and intravenously and orally administered sedative and analgesic agents. Patient-controlled analgesia has been used successfully. First-generation lithotripters generally required general or neuraxial anesthesia, whereas procedures using modern lithotripters may be completed with conscious sedation and, if the patient has comorbid conditions, monitored anesthesia care. Neuraxial techniques should be performed with care to avoid the injection of air, which could provide an acoustic interface, resulting in the release of energy and tissue destruction. When neuraxial blockade is utilized, a sensory level of T6 is required.

Suggested Readings

Chow GK, Streem SB. Extracorporeal lithotripsy: Update on technology. *Urol Clin North Am.* 2000;27:315-322.

Gravenstein D. Extracorporeal shock wave lithotripsy and percutaneous nephrolithotomy. *Anesthesiol Clin North Am.* 2000;18:953-971.

Lingeman JE, Matlaga BR, Evan AP. Surgical management of upper urinary tract calculi. In: Wein AJ, Kavoussi LR, Novick AC, et al, eds. *Campbell-Walsh Urology.* 10th ed. Philadephia: Saunders Elsevier; 2012.

PART F Anesthesia for Unique Situations or for Specific Patient Populations

CHAPTER 168

Monitored Anesthesia Care

Jeffrey W. Simmons, MD, and Michael J. Murray, MD, PhD

Monitored anesthesia care (MAC) refers to a service in which an anesthesia provider monitors a patient's vital signs during a diagnostic or therapeutic intervention while administering anxiolytic and analgesic drugs for patient comfort. Occasionally during MAC, no or minimal drugs are administered to the patient—the anesthesia provider is present to closely monitor a seriously ill patient and to intervene to maintain vital functions as necessary. In these patients, who may require only minimal sedation, even the smallest doses of sedative or analgesic agents, because of the patient's comorbid conditions, could adversely affect hemodynamics or respiratory function such that immediate intervention and resuscitation are required.

At other times, the surgeon injects a local anesthetic agent or the anesthesia provider performs a peripheral nerve block for intraoperative and postoperative analgesia, and MAC is provided so that the patient has the highest level of monitoring possible and the anesthesia provider is available to intervene to maintain the patient's vital functions, with the option to convert the MAC to a general anesthetic, if necessary. This is a critical difference between MAC and moderate (conscious) sedation; the latter refers to a situation in which a physician supervises another healthcare provider, who monitors the patient and administers sedative and analgesic drugs under the supervising physician's direction while the supervising physician performs a procedure, or the physician may administer drugs himself or herself. The type and amount of medication administered to a patient are supposed to achieve a "moderate" level of sedation such that the patient's vital signs and respiratory drive are not significantly altered. Accordingly, the healthcare provider who administers moderate sedation must know how to monitor a patient's vital signs and be able to recognize the transition into deep sedation.* In this event, the provider must understand how to support the patient's vital functions and to increase the level of consciousness so that the level of sedation is again "moderate."

If a procedure being planned is likely to require a deep level of sedation or MAC, most hospitals have policies mandated by government agencies or third-party payers that specify that only a practitioner credentialed and privileged to deliver an anesthetic is permitted to perform the service. In such situations, there is a high probability that "deep" sedation will result in the patient's loss of consciousness or transition into general anesthesia. An anesthesia provider is required to monitor and manage the patient and produce the level of sedation necessary to safely complete the procedure.

*A level of consciousness induced by hypnotic, sedative, and analgesic drugs from which patients cannot be readily aroused but do respond to painful stimuli. Respiratory function may be impaired, as manifested by an inability to protect the airway; decreased respiratory rate, decreased tidal volume, or both; and hypercapnia. Patients may require assistance in maintaining a patent airway and ventilation. Blood pressure and heart rate are usually normal or decreased unless hypoxia and hypercapnia become severe.

Unfortunately, some anesthesia providers consider that MAC is less complicated and requires less vigilance than a general anesthetic. A review of the American Society of Anesthesiologists' closed-claims database has shown that claims for cases that occurred outside the operating room more often involved MAC than general anesthesia and were more likely to occur, percentage wise, than were claims that came from cases performed in operating rooms. The most common findings were insufficient oxygenation and ventilation due to inadequate monitoring, and cases with MAC outside the operating room more often resulted in death than did cases inside the operating room.

Specifics of Monitored Anesthesia Care

In essence, no difference exists between a MAC and a general anesthetic in terms of the type or level of services that the anesthesia provider delivers. The anesthesia provider evaluates the patient prior to the procedure—including reviewing the patient's history, discussing the procedure, and examining the patient (including documenting when the patient last took anything by mouth and assessing the patient's airway)—and develops an anesthetic plan. The anesthesia provider should discuss the plan with the patient, explain the options and the risks and benefits of those options (allowing the patient time to ask questions), and once those questions have been answered, obtain the patient's consent to proceed. Management of the patient in the procedure suite includes monitoring the patient's vital signs using the American Society of Anesthesiologists, standard monitors, delivering supplemental O_2 (by either a nasal cannula or a facemask), and placing an intravenous catheter with infusion of crystalloid as a carrier for any medications that may be administered during the procedure. Equipment for managing an airway and for emergency resuscitation must be readily available, as should an anesthesia workstation if conversion to a general anesthetic becomes necessary. During MAC, it would not be uncommon for a patient to lose consciousness; in reality, MAC has become a general anesthetic whether or not any airway instrumentation occurs. The anesthesia provider must be able to diagnose and treat any problems that might occur during the procedure and to provide other medical services as necessary to ensure the patient's safety during the procedure. Following the procedure, the anesthesia provider also manages the recovery of the patient, maintaining responsibility for the patient until the patient meets discharge criteria from the postanesthetic care unit or from the procedural suite in which the procedure was performed.

Medications for Monitored Anesthesia Care

For cases requiring minimal sedation, such as cataract operations, 12.5 to 25 mg of diphenhydramine or 1 to 2 mg of midazolam can be given intravenously. Along with topical application of a local anesthetic agent to the eye, this combination provides adequate sedation and operating conditions. Many procedures, such as colonoscopy or esophagoscopy, can be safely performed with a small dose of a benzodiazepine (1-2 mg of midazolam) and an opioid (25-100 μg of fentanyl). For a transesophageal echocardiogram, 30 to 50 mg of propofol given as an intravenous bolus after a local anesthetic agent is applied to the tongue allows placement of the probe, with subsequent boluses of 10 to 20 mg of propofol infused to maintain patient comfort during the acquisition of images.

For longer-lasting procedures, many providers use a bolus of a benzodiazepine at the beginning of the procedure and then a bolus followed by a continuous infusion of a hypnotic agent or a hypnotic agent and an opioid for the duration of the procedure. Propofol infused at 25 to 100 $\mu g \cdot kg^{-1} \cdot min^{-1}$ works very well for many patients undergoing many different procedures and is preferred by many anesthesia providers. Others have equal success using a combination of propofol in a lower dose (25-75 $\mu g \cdot kg^{-1} \cdot min^{-1}$), along with alfentanil, (0.3-0.4 $\mu g \cdot kg^{-1} \cdot min^{-1}$). Remifentanil has also been used by some with success, but many anesthesia providers find that the opioid-induced side effects of remifentanil limit its usefulness. As an alternative to an opioid infusion, ketamine, because of its salutary effects on the respiratory system, can be used. An infusion of a solution of 40 mL of 1% propofol, 250 μg (5 mL) of fentanyl, and 250 mg (5 mL, 50 mg/mL) of ketamine in 50 mL of saline (final concentration: 4 mg of propofol, 2.5 mg of ketamine, and 2.5 μg of fentanyl per mL) may be used because, by increasing the rate of infusion, general anesthesia can be induced with adequate analgesia and maintenance of spontaneous respiration. Adjuvants to the drugs mentioned here, to provide a more balanced approach, include the preoperative use of a nonsteroidal anti inflammatory agent, pregabalin, gabapentin, or clonidine or a bolus of a benzodiazepine and opioid (midazolam and fentanyl) followed by an infusion of the α-adrenergic receptor agonist, dexmedetomidine.

Benefits of Monitored Anesthesia Care

In patients for whom MAC is an option, studies have demonstrated that the use of MAC, as compared with general anesthesia, is associated with a shorter time to emergence and orientation, decreased time in the postanesthesia care unit, decreased time before the patient is able to leave the hospital (for those patients having an outpatient procedure), a decreased incidence of postoperative nausea and vomiting, and better patient satisfaction. Despite these benefits, it is naïve to assume that providing MAC to a patient is a straightforward easy process. For example, delivering MAC to an elderly patient in the cardiac catheterization laboratory who is undergoing an electrophysiologic procedure requires considerable skill (and patience), knowledge of pharmacology, and a very high level of vigilance. However, overall, the increase in patient satisfaction and the superior outcomes associated with MAC justify its continued use in appropriate patients.

Suggested Readings

Bhananker SM, Posner KL, Cheney FW, et al. Injury and liability associated with monitored anesthesia care: A closed claims analysis. *Anesthesiology*. 2006;104:228-234.

Metzner J, Posner KL, Domino KB. The risk and safety of anesthesia at remote locations: The US closed claims analysis. *Curr Opin Anaesthesiol*. 2009;22:502-508.

White PF, Eng M. Fast-track anesthetic techniques for ambulatory surgery. *Curr Opin Anaesthesiol*. 2007;20:545-557.

CHAPTER 169

Issues in Ambulatory Anesthesia

Brian P. McGlinch, MD

A substantial majority of surgical and invasive medical procedures in the United States are performed in ambulatory settings, from which discharge immediately following or within 24 h of the procedure is expected. Financial incentives have encouraged the performance of surgical procedures outside the inpatient or hospital setting, resulting in adoption of this practice model. Advances in surgical technology (e.g., robotic surgery) have contributed to an increasing number of procedures performed with improved patient safety, less blood loss, and minimal postoperative discomfort. Anesthetic management approaches utilizing regional anesthesia, new anesthetic agents, and multimodal therapies for treating pain and postoperative nausea and vomiting (PONV) have improved the reliability of postprocedure discharges to home. Along with the conduct of anesthesia, the anesthesia provider's role in the ambulatory setting is crucial for ensuring patient safety and practice efficiency.

Patient Screening and Evaluation

For patients to safely undergo invasive procedures in a nonhospital environment, underlying medical conditions must be identified, evaluated, and stabilized prior to the scheduled procedure. There are no contraindications for patients with significant but stable underlying disease (i.e., American Society of Anesthesiologists, [ASA] physical status categories 3 and 4) to undergo an invasive procedure or operation in an ambulatory setting if the procedure is unlikely to exacerbate the underlying condition or conditions. In 2002, the ASA issued a practice advisory indicating that preoperative testing, particularly laboratory studies, does not significantly improve the preoperative preparation nor significantly alter perioperative management decisions unless indicated by symptoms, clinical findings, or preexisting conditions that warrant evaluation. There is no evidence that perioperative adverse outcomes are influenced when preoperative evaluations are eliminated in healthy or medically stable patients.

A preoperative telephone interview with the patient can often determine the presence and stability of significant underlying diseases (e.g., angina, chronic obstructive pulmonary disease) or special anesthetic concerns (e.g., latex allergy, malignant hyperthermia, obstructive sleep apnea [OSA], a history of difficult intubations) meriting further preoperative evaluation or scheduling considerations. If the intended procedure could impact the stability of a patient's underlying condition or conditions, a more extensive evaluation can and should be performed before the day of surgery. The telephone interview also provides an opportunity for confirming with the patient the arrival time, place, and directions, as well as a review of preoperative fasting recommendations. This simple intervention reduces day-of-surgery delays and cancellations.

Preoperative fasting is a common issue that must be addressed in any setting in which sedation or anesthesia is anticipated because it influences practice efficiency. The ASA recommends the interval between ingestion and sedation or anesthesia be 2 h for clear fluids, 4 h for breast milk, and 6 h for nonhuman milk and solid food. In most circumstances, preoperative overnight fasting of both food and water has been abandoned prior to elective surgical procedures. Ingestion of clear fluids up until 2 h prior to receiving sedation or anesthesia in patients without risk for aspiration of gastric contents (e.g., no gastroesophageal reflux disease, bowel obstruction) improves patient comfort while preventing dehydration.

OSA is a common diagnosis (9% of middle-aged women, 24% of middle-aged men) of such importance to anesthesia practice that the ASA issued a practice guideline addressing this condition. At this time, there is insufficient evidence to recommend one particular anesthetic technique over another. However, OSA is negatively impacted by the use of intravenously administered sedative and hypnotic agents, as well as inhaled anesthetic agents. Postprocedure recovery and respiratory monitoring warrant significantly longer observation periods in both the inpatient and outpatient settings. The ASA guidelines recommend that, compared with patients without OSA, those with OSA be monitored for 7 h after the last episode of airway obstruction or hypoxemia while breathing room air and for 3 h longer on room air before being discharged to home. These guidelines functionally result in patients with OSA being admitted for overnight or 23-h observation in most cases of untreated OSA or for patients who are noncompliant with recommended continuous positive airway pressure therapy for OSA, as prescribed by the patient's treating physician. The presence of OSA should not automatically preclude a particular patient from being considered for an ambulatory procedure. However, consideration must be made for the potential implications for airway management and postoperative monitoring for even the most routine procedural interventions.

Anesthetic Techniques for Ambulatory Procedures

Surgical or invasive procedures performed in the ambulatory surgical setting might be prolonged but should not expose the patient to a risk for significant fluid shifts, significant postoperative discomfort, or a need for hospitalization. Similar to nearly any other surgical practice, local anesthesia, monitored anesthetic care, regional anesthesia, and general anesthesia are all reasonable approaches to patient management for ambulatory operations or other outpatient invasive procedures. Local anesthesia infrequently requires the participation of an anesthesia provider. Conscious Sedation is increasingly performed by "sedation nurses" who lack extensive anesthesia training. In circumstances in which a non–anesthesia-trained nurse (or other provider) is administering sedative agents, the potential for achieving a level of sedation that is indistinguishable from monitored anesthesia care or from a general anesthetic is quite possible. As a result, to ensure that sedation provided by individuals other than anesthesiologists, nurse anesthetists, and anesthesia assistants is conducted in a manner that affords prompt recognition and intervention of the deeply sedated or anesthetized patient, the ASA recently released a guideline for practices in which individuals other than anesthesia provider's deliver sedation. This guideline has been adopted by the Joint Commission and is followed by facilities seeking accreditation from the Joint Commission.

Regional anesthesia offers many benefits for procedures performed in ambulatory surgical centers. This anesthetic approach affords profound analgesia and anesthesia with a lower incidence of PONV, drowsiness, and pain than do general anesthetics. Peripheral nerve blocks (PNBs), however, are infrequently performed in ambulatory surgical centers. Common impediments for utilizing PNBs relate to the additional time necessary to perform the block, delayed onset time, variability of obtaining surgical anesthesia, and the lack of obvious benefit of PNB versus general anesthesia on outcomes beyond 24 h. The introduction and increasing application of ultrasound technologies to facilitate PNB placement and reliability is likely to influence PNB utilization in ambulatory settings even though patient outcomes may not be significantly influenced.

General anesthesia is the most common mode of anesthesia for ambulatory surgical procedures. However, PONV is increased after general anesthesia, compared with after regional anesthesia or PNB, occurring in nearly 30% of patients. Propofol is the anesthesia induction agent of choice because of its low incidence of associated PONV and rapid emergence. Sevoflurane and desflurane have low blood and fat solubilities, allowing more rapid patient awakening, compared with isoflurane or propofol infusions. A multimodal approach for perioperative analgesia attempts to reduce opioid-related somnolence and PONV. Fentanyl is the most commonly administered opioid in ambulatory surgery; remifentanil has a more rapid offset but is associated with a greater incidence of PONV. Nonsteroidal antiinflammatory drugs or acetaminophen, administered by mouth before the operation, or administered intravenously during the operation, demonstrate benefit in terms of patient comfort at lower opioid doses when evaluated postoperatively. The use of nonsteroidal agents is associated with increased postoperative bleeding, particularly in head and neck operations, and should be avoided in these procedures. Gabapentin (600 mg - 1200 mg) taken orally prior to the operation appears to have some benefit in reducing postoperative pain, but side effects may warrant a more selective approach for use in the perioperative period. Infiltration of surgical incision sites with local anesthetic agents has also been demonstrated to reduce opioid needs and improve postoperative comfort. There is no evidence that infiltrating the surgical site prior to incision impacts patient comfort. Installation of local anesthetic agents on surgical beds (e.g., cholecystectomy site) or intraarticular loading of opioids or local anesthetics appear to have only minimal short-lived benefit on patient comfort even though these practices are commonly performed.

Issues in the Postanesthesia Care Unit

The main source for unexpected delayed discharge or hospital admission after ambulatory surgical procedures is PONV. Without prophylactic intervention, PONV occurs in 20% to 30% of the general surgical population, with higher rates in at-risk patients (Box 169-1). At this time, antiemetic

Box 169-1 Factors Contributing to Increased Rates of Postoperative Nausea and Vomiting

- Laparoscopic abdominal operations*
- Strabismus eye operations†
- Duration of the operation and anesthetic agent
- Female sex and luteal phase‡
- History of postoperative nausea and vomiting
- History of motion sickness
- Use of opioids in any mode of administration
- Inadequate hydration and postural hypotension

*Highest incidence.
†Dependent upon the number of eye muscles corrected.
‡Premenstrual or menstrual.

medications used in anesthesia are relatively inexpensive and have minimal side effects (e.g., ondansetron), affording their routine use without significant concerns regarding overall cost or complications; the numbers required to treat to demonstrate an advantage of prophylactic antiemetic therapy is very low. Transdermal scopolamine appears to augment the effects of other antiemetics, particularly in patients with a history of motion sickness. Scopolamine should be used cautiously in men with symptoms of prostatic hypertrophy in whom urinary retention may become problematic. Although patients may initially feel well and recover from their anesthesia uneventfully, PONV may occur several hours postoperatively, suggesting a contribution from oral analgesic agents. More attention appears to be needed for improving oral analgesic-related nausea and vomiting.

The main source of patient complaint after ambulatory surgery is pain. One of the most important sources for moderate-to-severe postoperative pain is preoperative pain. Younger age is also associated with increased postoperative pain, with speculation being that younger people are more active and more likely to attempt resumption of usual activities earlier than are the elderly. Sex is not a predictor of postoperative pain but does influence the incidence of PONV.

Increasingly, prompt patient recovery from ambulatory surgical procedures, sometimes facilitated by PNB or neuraxial blockade, sometimes facilitated by new potent, ultrashort-duration medications, is allowing patients to bypass the postanesthesia care unit (PACU) immediately following the operation. Criteria addressing level of consciousness, hemodynamic stability, adequate oxygenation at low inspired O_2 concentrations, and the absence of PONV or significant pain may safely allow bypass of the PACU and improve efficiency. Reducing the number of patients in a PACU requiring treatment allows nursing resources to be better allocated and focused or to be reduced overall. The cost of newer anesthetic agents used in ambulatory settings could be offset by reduced PACU utilization.

Although the goal for patients treated at ambulatory surgical centers is to have prompt recovery and return to their preoperative state, except for those given only local anesthesia, *none* should be considered competent to drive home following the procedure. Any patient who was provided sedation in any form requires an escort who must remain present and immediately available for 24 h following discharge. The unescorted patient undergoing any procedure in which sedation is provided requires admission for observation.

Suggested Readings

Apfel CC, Philip BK, Cakamakkaya OS, et al. Who is at risk for postdischarge nausea and vomiting after ambulatory surgery? *Anesthesiology*. 2012;117:175-86.

Chung F, Yuan H, Yin L, et al. Elimination of preoperative testing in ambulatory surgery. *Anesth Analg*. 2009;108:467-475.

Gramke H, de Rijke, van Kleef M, et al. Predictive factors of postoperative pain after day-case surgery. *Clin J Pain*. 2009;25:455-460.

Practice advisory for preanesthesia evaluation. A report by the American Society of Anesthesiologists Task Force on Preanesthesia Evaluation. *Anesthesiology*. 2002;96:486-496.

Practice guidelines for the perioperative management of patients with obstructive sleep apnea. A report by the American Society of Anesthesiologists Task Force on Perioperative Management of Patients with Obstructive Sleep Apnea. *Anesthesiology*. 2006;104:1081-1093.

Practice guidelines for preoperative fasting and the use of pharmacological agents for the prevention of pulmonary aspiration. Application to healthy patients undergoing elective procedures. *Anesthesiology*. 1999;90:896-905.

Practice guidelines for sedation and analgesia by non-anesthesiologists. An updated report by the American Society of Anesthesiologists Task Force on Sedation and Analgesia by Non-Anesthesiologists. *Anesthesiology*. 2002; 96:1004-1017.

Rawal N. Postdischarge complications and rehabilitation after ambulatory surgery. *Curr Opin Anesthesiol*. 2008;21:736-742.

CHAPTER 170

Anesthesia for Patients Undergoing Magnetic Resonance Imaging Studies

Teresa M. Murray and Michael J. Murray, MD, PhD

Nuclear magnetic resonance (MR), the physical phenomenon that forms the foundation for magnetic resonance imaging (MRI), involves the absorption and emission of electromagnetic radiation by certain atomic nuclei when they are placed in the presence of a strong magnetic field. Only atomic nuclei with an odd atomic number are able to participate in this nuclear MR phenomenon. Of all such nuclei that are biologically relevant, it is the hydrogen atom that is by far the dominating species—particularly those atoms contained in water and the side chains of fatty acids. The nucleus of the hydrogen atom has a fundamental angular momentum, or spin, such that it rotates (or precesses) about an axis in the same manner as a spinning top. As it spins, the atom generates a magnetic dipole moment—a tiny magnetic field—just as the current from the power company in one of the two copper coils of an isolated power transformer generates a magnetic field as it "spins" through the coil that generates an electric current in the second copper coil. In an MRI scanner, manipulation of the magnetic dipole moments of innumerable hydrogen atoms within the human body—and the recording of their movement—is the basis for the tissue delineation provided by MRI technology.

When a hydrogen atom is placed within a static magnetic field, the dipole of the nucleus aligns to rotate about an equilibrium axis parallel to the magnetic field (Figure 170-1) at a frequency known as the Larmor frequency. Transmission of energy to the hydrogen atoms by radiofrequency (RF) pulses in the electromagnetic spectrum disrupts this equilibrium, causing the nuclei to reorient themselves away from the static field. Removal of the RF pulse allows the protons to relax to their equilibrium state. The amount of time it takes a proton to reorient in a longitudinal plane (T1, or *spin-lattice* relaxation time) and a transverse plane (T2, or *spin-spin* relaxation time) is specific to the type of tissue in which the proton is located—and whether this tissue is normal or abnormal. Images are weighted to rely on either of these two parameters, T1 or T2, for tissue contrast; scanners can also weight images by the *proton density* within a particular tissue. The actual MR signal is produced by the net movement of the magnetic dipoles within a particular volume of space (a *voxel*) in response to defined RF pulses. This net movement induces an alternating voltage in the receiver coil of the MRI machine that can be analyzed by computer software. To produce the final image, each individual voxel must be localized in three-dimensional space, which is accomplished by establishing a gradient magnetic field that varies across the patient.

Basic Magnet Safety

MRI machines produce three magnetic fields that interact with a patient to produce MR images: the static magnetic field, the RF field, and the gradient field. To work safely in an MRI suite, the anesthesia provider must be knowledgeable of the effects of each of these fields on the patient and on the environment. The RF field, the weakest of the three magnetic fields, is capable of producing localized heating and increased core temperature, although the amount of heating is limited by federal regulations. The gradient field is associated both with peripheral nerve stimulation in patients and with the characteristic noise associated with MRI scanners. The noise produced can reach in excess of 120 dB and will cause hearing damage in people who are not wearing proper protection.

The third field, the static magnetic field, is perhaps that most familiar to many people. The strength of this field must be respected at all times by anyone who works within the MRI suite. Many MRI magnets in current use create fields of up to 1.5 to 3.0 tesla (many times stronger than the earth's own magnetic field of 0.5 to 1 gauss [G]; 1000 G = 1 tesla). The static field produces forces that are capable of turning any ferromagnetic object into a high-velocity projectile—and, the larger the object, the greater the force acting upon it. Anyone who enters an MRI suite must be screened for the presence of ferromagnetic objects or implants, and all equipment must be specifically designed and designated as "MR safe." If patient care equipment is not clearly labeled as MR safe, it must not be brought into the proximity of an MRI machine.

The potential threat posed by MRI equipment to patients and care providers is related not only to the dangers of the actual static magnetic field, but also to the manner in which the field is produced. The field is created through the use of superconducting materials that are cooled to nearly absolute 0—approximately 4°K—through the use of liquid helium. In certain cases of equipment malfunction, the liquid helium can boil off in what is known as a *quench*. The volume of helium is so large and the speed at which it boils off is so rapid that specific escape valves are built into MRI suites to allow for the release of the helium to the environment. Should one of these valves fail, the oxygen within the room can be displaced, posing an asphyxiation risk to personnel and patients. For this reason, many MRI suites have detectors that warn care providers of a falling oxygen level.

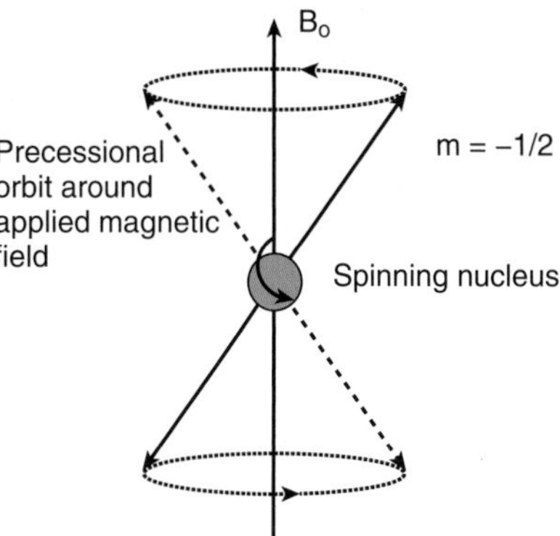

Figure 170-1 The nucleus of the hydrogen atom has a fundamental angular momentum, or spin, such that it rotates (or precesses) about an axis with a frequency known as the Larmor frequency. When placed in a magnetic field, the axis of precession is parallel to the magnetic field.

Magnetic Resonance Imaging Suite

Anesthesia providers must consider other properties of MRI scanners when providing care to a patient having an MRI scan. MRI suites are often built adjacent to, rather than within, the hospital because of the need to minimize vibration and electromagnetic interference. Some newer scanners are so sensitive that even a nearby elevator can interfere with the quality of the scans. Unlike computed tomography scanners that are placed in lead-lined rooms to protect individuals outside the room from ionizing radiation, MRI scanners are built in rooms that are 100% shielded on all sides from RF waves that can interfere with the quality of the scan. The RF shield forms a complete box around the MRI system. Everything that is to come into an MRI room must first pass through an RF filter or waveguide—the RF filter is a penetration point for data cables and electrical power, whereas the waveguide is a series of penetration points that allow a fluid (water) or gas (air conditioning, medical gas) to flow into the MRI room.

The U.S. Food and Drug Administration specifically regulates access to MRI suites; all areas in which the magnetic field is equal to or greater than 5 G must be restricted to only those individuals who have been successfully screened for potential contraindications. Any sensitive equipment, such as monitors or computed tomography scanners, should remain beyond the 5-G line. Most facilities meet these criteria by creating a series of zones that have increasing restrictions or limit people who can enter the zones (Figure 170-2 and Table 170-1).

Because of these restrictions, the MRI suite creates multiple challenges for the anesthesia provider. By being geographically at a distance from the operating rooms, MRI suites are often far from readily available additional personnel. Furthermore, because access to the suite is limited, when individuals arrive to assist in an emergency, they must first gain access to zone II.

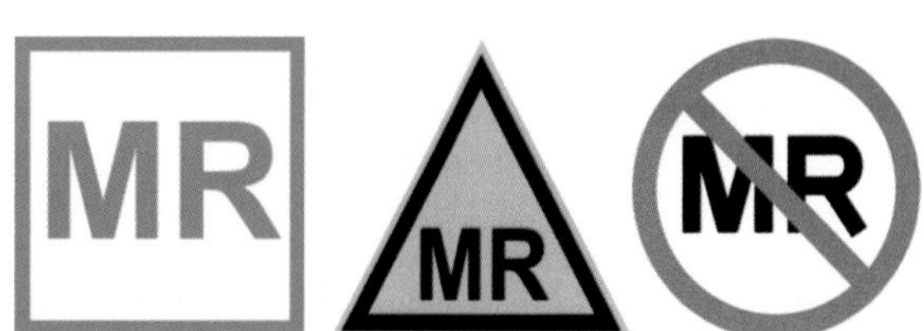

Figure 170-2 Signs and labels used to designate magnetic resonance (MR) zones. Green: safe in zone IV, nonmagnetic, nonelectrically conductive, and non–radio-frequency reactive. Yellow: may contain magnetic, electrically conductive, or radio–frequency-reactive components and is usually labeled for safe operation within fields below a certain strength (e.g., <500 gauss or <5 gauss). Red: unsafe because it contains ferromagnetic material and, therefore, has the potential to harm patients or equipment if brought into zone III or IV.

Table 170-1 Magnetic Resonance Imaging Zones, Restrictions, Locations, Hazards, and Information Pertinent to Anesthesia Providers

Zone	Restrictions on Who May Enter MRI Suite	Location	MRI-related Hazard(s)	Pertinent Information
I	None	Usually outside the MRI suite	Negligible	
II	Unscreened patients who are to undergo MRI	Interface between the publicly accessible uncontrolled zone I and the strictly controlled zone III.	Immediately outside areas of hazard	Ferromagnetic items may be left in this area. Usual site to anesthetize patients before transporting them to the MRI suite. Resuscitation equipment typically is kept here.
III	Screened patients who are to undergo MRI and approved MR personnel	Typically the control room, with access to the scanner room	Potential biostimulation interference	No ferromagnetic items may enter this zone.
IV	Screened patients undergoing MRI who are under constant direct supervision by trained MR personnel	The room with the MRI scanner	Biostimulation interference, radiofrequency heating, missile effect, cryogens	

MRI, Magnetic resonance imaging.

Monitoring a patient who is in the MRI scanner is very problematic because no ferromagnetic or unshielded electrical equipment can be used. In the event of an emergency, the patient must be immediately removed from the bore of the scanner and safely and rapidly transported to zone II. Emergency or code personnel should never be allowed in zone IV unless they have undergone appropriate screening. During cardiopulmonary arrest, the use of a defibrillator must wait until the patient is transported back to zone II.

In the rare circumstances in which shutting down the scanner becomes necessary, two options are available. The first is an emergency shutdown that will disrupt all electricity flowing into the scanner. The second is an intentional quench that will result in the collapse of the magnetic field within minutes. A quench is a significant event both in the danger it poses should the escape valves in the room fail and in the cost and effort necessary to reboot a scanner once the liquid helium has boiled off. A quench should only be used when absolutely necessary.

Patient Safety Issues

A closed-bore machine with the narrowest acceptable opening provides the best images but can be extremely confining for obese or claustrophobic patients (one of the primary reasons that anesthesia services are requested is because the patient is claustrophobic). Earplugs may protect patients and health care providers from noise, but they interfere with individuals who are attempting to communicate between zones IV and III. The strong magnetic field creates challenges for many types of patients challenges that are beyond the scope of this chapter, but about which anesthesia providers should be cognizant. The anesthesia provider who is involved in the care of a patient undergoing an MRI and the MRI personnel are jointly responsible for screening the patient for ferromagnetic implants and for being aware of conditions that may create a challenge in terms of monitoring, protecting the airway, or maintaining hemodynamic stability. Most MRI suites have guidelines for what kinds of patients, implanted devices, or materials would prohibit a scan and what changes in techniques must be made to safely image the patient. However, the anesthesia provider cannot assume anything and, therefore, has a responsibility to share any findings and concerns with the technicians and technologists in the control room. All of the standards of care that exist in the operating room apply in the MRI suite, and it is the anesthesia provider's responsibility to provide that level of care, with few exceptions. For example, diagnostic monitoring of the electrocardiogram is difficult, if not impossible, during a scan because of electrical interference created in the electrocardiogram by the magnetic field, making it difficult to monitor ST-segment changes in a patient with ischemic heart disease. Furthermore, any metal-containing cables—whether or not they contain ferromagnetic material—have the potential to generate heat in a powerful magnetic field and can burn the patient.

Health Care Worker Safety Issues

Four main issues potentially affect the health of anesthesia providers who enter zone IV. Obviously, if the provider has any implanted device or ferromagnetic material, he or she should ascertain its MRI compatibility or whether it would affect the quality of the scan. Devices to protect hearing must be used. The possibility of a quench must also be kept in mind. Finally, though there is no good evidence that magnetic fields up to 4 T have adverse effects on mammalian embryos or fetuses, guidelines suggest that elective scans should not be performed during the first trimester of a pregnancy; likewise, pregnant women who provide anesthesia care should have the option of staying out of zone IV during the first trimester of a pregnancy.

Anesthetizing a Patient for Magnetic Resonance Imaging

Monitored anesthesia care and general anesthesia have successfully been used for patients undergoing MRI scans. However, because the patient is, in essence, out of sight when in the bore of the scanner and because the patient may move and compromise the quality of the scan when only light sedation is used, many anesthesia providers use a tracheal tube or laryngeal mask airway to control the patient's airway and, therefore, prefer to use general anesthesia. Based on provider preference and the equipment available within the MRI suite, some clinicians use exclusively an inhalation agent and others use only an intravenously administered anesthetic. If monitored anesthesia care is selected, some providers use an apnea monitor to alert them if the level of sedation inhibits the patient's respiratory drive.

Independent of the anesthetic technique ultimately chosen, MRI-safe monitors should be applied in zone II. If the patient is going to have an airway placed, general anesthesia should be induced in zone II and the patient then transported through zone III and into zone IV. The patient should then be transferred to and positioned on the gantry table, and the table should then be advanced into the bore of the scanner. The ability to visualize the patient within the bore varies depending on the scanner and the construction of the room. The provider must take this into account in choosing a place to optimally visualize the patient and the monitors, either by direct vision or with video equipment. Similarly, the anesthesia monitors and workstation must be positioned to provide the level of care required but without affecting patient safety or the quality of the scan. Most anesthesia departments work with the engineering and radiology departments to select equipment that is either safe or conditionally safe provided that it remains at an adequate distance from the scanner. If such equipment is unavailable, remote monitoring is an option as long as all American Society of Anesthesiologists, Standards for Monitoring are met.

A plan should be in place to alert colleagues of the need for immediate assistance if an emergency situation develops. As part of this contingency, resuscitation equipment—including, for example, monitors, oxygen, suction, and an airway cart—should be readily available in zone II.

Some hospitals have constructed RF-shielded operating rooms in which an MRI scanner is adjacent to the operating room table. In such a situation, remote monitoring is not an option; therefore, equipment and monitors that are conditionally safe (outside the 5-G line—either tethered to a wall or placed behind a fixed barrier) must be used. Most often, an MRI scan is obtained intermittently during neurosurgical procedures to identify landmarks and the adequacy of excision of tissue. The operating room table, which is MR compatible, is turned and advanced into the bore of the scanner and withdrawn after the scan is complete, and the operation continues. Everything mentioned previously is applicable in an operating room containing an MRI scanner.

Suggested Readings

American Society of Anesthesiologists. Practice advisory on anesthetic care for magnetic resonance imaging. *Anesthesiology*. 2009;110:459-479.

Bell C. *Anesthesia in the MRI suite*. Anesthesia Patient Safety Foundation. Available at: http://www.apsf.org/resources_safety_suite.php. Accessed March 4, 2013.

Bryson EO, Frost EAM. Anesthesia in remote locations: radiology and beyond: CT and MRI. *Anesthesiol Clin*. 2009:47:11-19.

Olive D. Don't get sucked in. Anaesthesia for magnetic resonance imaging. *Australasian Anaesth*. 2005;85-96.

Reddy U, White MJ, Wilson SR. Anaesthesia for magnetic resonance imaging. *Contin Educ Anaesth Crit Care Pain*. 2012;12:140-144.

CHAPTER 171

Anesthesia for Electroconvulsive Therapy

Joseph J. Sandor, MD

Convulsive therapy for psychiatric disorders has been used since 1934. Electroconvulsive therapy (ECT), modified over the years to incorporate monitoring, intravenous administration of anesthetic drugs, neuromuscular blockade, and the use of supplemental O_2, is both safe and effective for the treatment of endogenous depression in patients whose symptoms have failed to respond to an adequate course of antidepressant drugs, who may be jeopardized by adverse events associated with the use of pharmacologic agents, who have severe melancholia, or who are suicidal.

Mechanism of Action

Seizures induced by ECT are similar to grand mal seizures. A 2-sec to 3-sec latent phase is followed by a tonic phase lasting 10 to 12 sec, then a clonic phase of 30 to 50 sec. Both the duration of individual seizures and cumulative seizure time correlate with clinical improvement of depression. The number of treatments is determined by the patient's clinical response.

Physiology

The physiologic mechanisms responsible for the therapeutic benefit of ECT are unknown; however, a variety of theories have been posited (Box 171-1).

The cardiovascular response to ECT is secondary to autonomic nervous system discharge. Parasympathetic discharge is immediate and may cause asystole, bradycardia, premature ventricular contractions, hypotension, and ventricular escape. Sympathetic discharge then follows within seconds, possibly manifesting as increased heart rate, premature ventricular contractions, bigeminy, trigeminy, sinus tachycardia, and severe hypertension. A marked increase in myocardial O_2 consumption frequently occurs.

An initial constriction of cerebral vessels is followed by increased cerebral blood flow (1.5 to 7 times baseline) from increased cerebral O_2 consumption and elevated blood pressure. Preoxygenation is used to prevent cerebral hypoxia.

The neuroendocrine response to ECT is manifest by increased levels of corticotropin, cortisol, and catecholamines. The effects on glucose levels vary; thus, patients with diabetes should have their glucose levels monitored before and after ECT.

Miscellaneous effects of ECT of importance to the anesthesia provider include increased intragastric pressure and increased intraocular pressure.

Morbidity and Mortality Rates

The mortality risk from ECT is 0.03%. Other complications include transient arrhythmias (10%-40%), gastric aspiration (2.5%), and musculoskeletal disorder (0.4%), including fractures. In addition, adverse events following ECT may include pulmonary edema, headache, memory disturbance, and agitation.

Anesthetic Management

Contraindications

A variety of contraindications to ECT, both absolute and relative, are of particular note to anesthesia providers (Box 171-2).

Box 171-1 Theories of the Physiologic Mechanism Responsible for the Therapeutic Effects of Electroconvulsive Therapy

Changes in the following
Ion transport
Permeability of the blood-brain barrier
Regional cerebral blood flow
Concentrations of
- Biogenic amines
- Electrolytes
- Neurotransmitters

Release of hormones and cytokines
Corticotropin
Hypothalamic peptides
Prolactin

Box 171-2 Relative and Absolute Contraindications to the Use of Electroconvulsive Therapy

Absolute Contraindications

Intracranial mass
Recent myocardial infarction
Recent stroke

Relative Contraindications

Angina pectoris
Chronic obstructive pulmonary disease
Congestive heart failure
Glaucoma
High-risk pregnancy
Pacemaker
Retinal detachment
Severe osteoporosis
Thrombophlebitis

Preoperative Assessment

Preoperative assessment should document cardiopulmonary, neurologic, and endocrine status; risk of gastrointestinal reflux; and history of earlier drug therapy. Ideally, monoamine oxidase inhibitors and tricyclic antidepressants should be discontinued 2 weeks before ECT. Patients receiving lithium therapy have a decreased chance of successful treatment and may experience delayed awakening, memory loss, and postictal confusion.

Anesthesia Technique

Depending on the patient's comorbid conditions, pharmacologic intervention to reduce the risks of aspiration of gastric contents may be indicated. At a minimum, the American Society of Anesthesiologists' standards for monitoring should be followed. Patients should be adequately preoxygenated after intravenous access is established. A small dose of methohexital or etomidate should be administered to produce hypnosis; 25 to 50 mg of succinylcholine is given to prevent musculoskeletal injuries; and 0.1 to 0.2 mg of glycopyrrolate is given to blunt parasympathetic response. Esmolol, in bolus doses of 2 to 3 mg/kg, can be given to diminish the sympathetic response in patients with a coronary artery disease or hypertension; a calcium channel blocker may be the preferred agent if the patient has a history, or is having an acute exacerbation, of reactive airway disease.

Suggested Readings

Anand S, Thirthalli J, Gupta A, et al. Anesthesia during electroconvulsive therapy: Importance of dosage. *J ECT.* 2010;26:145.

Bryson EO, Aloysi AS, Popeo DM, et al. Methohexital and succinylcholine dosing for electroconvulsive therapy (ECT): Actual versus ideal. *J ECT.* 2012;28: e29-30.

Bwalya GM, Srinivasan V, Wang M. Electroconvulsive therapy anesthesia practice patterns: Results of a UK postal survey. *J ECT.* 2011;27:81-85.

Gilron I, Delva N, Graf P, et al. Canadian survey of perianesthetic care for patients receiving electroconvulsive therapy. *J ECT.* 2012;28(4):219-224.

Mirzakhani H, Welch CA, Eikermann M, Nozari A. Neuromuscular blocking agents for electroconvulsive therapy: A systematic review. *Acta Anaesthesiol Scand.* 2012;56:3-16.

Reti IM, Walker M, Pulia K, et al. Safety considerations for outpatient electroconvulsive therapy. *J Psychiatr Pract.* 2012;18:130-136.

CHAPTER 172

Myasthenia Gravis and Lambert-Eaton Myasthenic Syndrome

Alaric C. LeBaron, MD

Myasthenia Gravis

The incidence of myasthenia gravis (MG), an autoimmune disease of the neuromuscular junction, is 1:20,000 in the adult population and higher in patients with other autoimmune diseases, such as thyroiditis and rheumatoid arthritis. Characterized by weakness of voluntary skeletal muscle, MG can be classified by age, etiology (Table 172-1), or the presence or absence of bulbar signs and symptoms because the muscles innervated by the cranial nerves are most frequently involved (Table 172-2).

Pathophysiology

Circulating antibodies to acetylcholine (ACh) receptors (AChRs), which are found in 70% to 90% of patients with MG, are thought to reduce the number of functional AChRs via three different mechanisms: competitive blockade of AChRs; complement-mediated lysis of the receptor and muscle end plate, resulting in blocked access to the receptor; and increased destruction and decreased production of AChRs. The net effect of these mechanisms is a motor end plate with decreased surface area and decreased functional AChRs (Figure 172-1).

Diagnosis

An electromyogram is the most specific test for the establishment of the diagnosis of MG in a patient with compatible symptoms and signs of the disease. Repetitive closely timed stimuli produce fade or progressively smaller or weaker motor responses in the muscle groups being tested. A Tensilon test (which involves administering a small dose of a short-acting acetylcholinesterase drug) is not often performed to establish the diagnosis of the disease but can be helpful in evaluating a patient with MG whose muscle weakness is worse following surgery and anesthesia to differentiate between a myasthenic crisis and a cholinergic crisis.

Treatment

The gold standard for many years for the treatment of MG was the administration of pyridostigmine, an anticholinesterase drug, which increases the amount of ACh available at the neuromuscular junction. Once the cause of the disease became known, immunosuppressive therapy with a corticosteroid, azathioprine, or cyclosporine became common. Approximately 25% of patients with thymomas have MG; because thymectomy often reduces the effect of the disease, this operation is often performed in patients with refractory MG, even if they do not have a thymoma.

A large, randomized, controlled trial should be completed in 2015 that compares thymectomy to thymectomy plus prednisone in patients with MG. In patients with acute severe exacerbations of disease, plasmapheresis and intravenous administration of immune globulin are recommended because their use is associated with rapid improvement in muscle strength.

Anesthetic Implications

Preoperative Evaluation

The duration, severity, and record of treatment of MG should be evaluated and documented. Patients with more severe disease, in whom the clinician

Table 172-1 Subgroups or Types of Myasthenia Gravis

Type	Description
Nonimmune	
Congenital myasthenic syndrome	Defects in proteins at the neuromuscular junction
Immune	
Neonatal myasthenia gravis	Transplacental passage of AChR antibodies
Juvenile myasthenia gravis	Onset before 18 years of age
Early-onset myasthenia gravis	Onset at 18 to 50 years of age
Late-onset myasthenia gravis	Onset after 50 years of age
Seronegative myasthenia gravis	No detectable AChR antibodies

AChR, Acetylcholine receptor.

Table 172-2 Signs and Symptoms Associated with the Classes of Myasthenia Gravis

Class	Signs and Symptoms
I	Any ocular muscle weakness May have weakness of eye closure All other muscle strength is normal
II	Mild weakness affecting other than ocular muscles May also have ocular muscle weakness of any severity
III	Moderate weakness affecting other than ocular muscles May also have ocular muscle weakness of any severity
IV	Severe weakness affecting other than ocular muscles May also have ocular muscle weakness of any severity
V	Defined by requirement for intubation, with or without mechanical ventilation, except when used during routine postoperative management

Etiologic and Pathophysiologic Concepts

Normal neuromuscular junction
Synaptic vesicles containing acetylcholine (ACh) form in nerve terminals. In response to a nerve impulse, vesicles discharge ACh into the synaptic cleft. ACh binds to receptor sites on muscle sarcolemma to initiate muscle contraction. Acetylcholinesterase (AChE) hydrolyzes ACh, thus limiting effect and duration of its action.

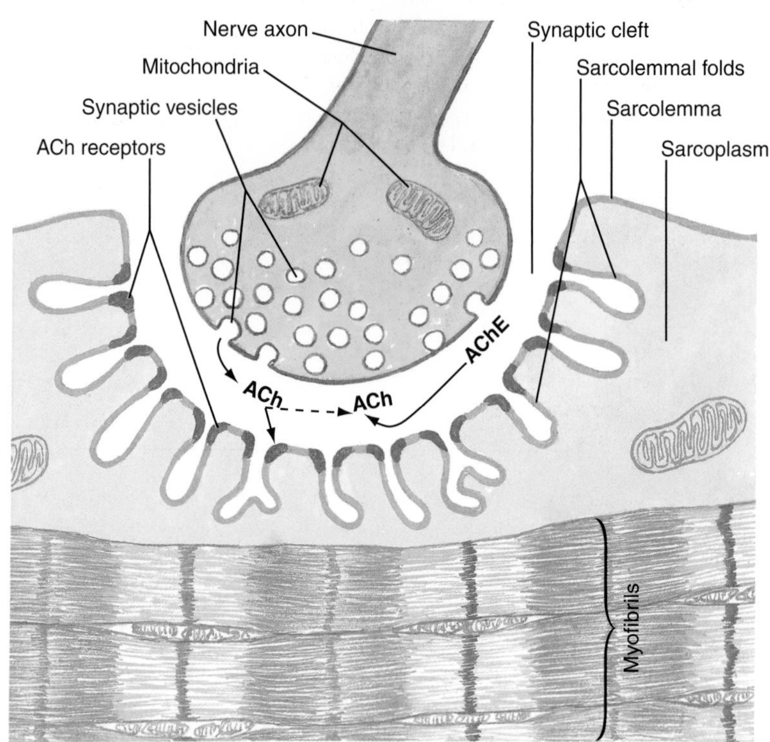

Myasthenia gravis
Marked reduction in the number and length of subneural sarcolemmal folds indicates that an underlying defect lies in the neuromuscular junction. AChE drugs increase the effectiveness and duration of ACh action by slowing its destruction by AChE.

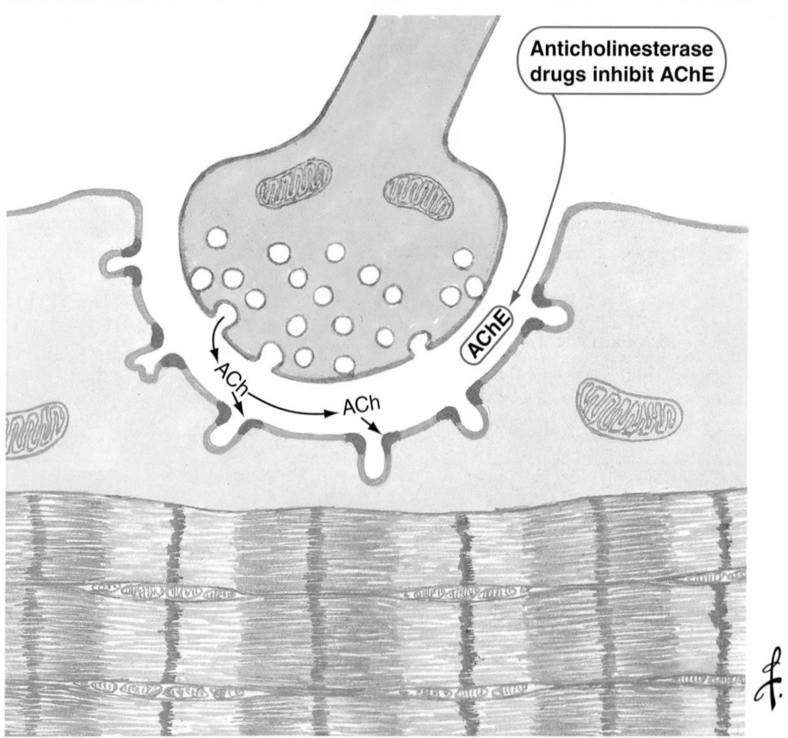

Figure 172-1 Etiologic and pathophysiologic concepts of the neuromuscular junction. (Netter illustration from www.netterimages.com. © Elsevier Inc. All rights reserved.)

is concerned about the need for postoperative mechanical ventilation, should have maximum inspiratory and expiratory ("bugle") pressures measured preoperatively to establish a baseline. Postoperative weakness and the requirement for postoperative mechanical ventilation are common, and because the trachea can be intubated without the use of neuromuscular blocking agents (NMBAs), patients should take their normal dose of pyridostigmine the morning of surgery; any alterations in this practice should be discussed with the patient's neurologist prior to surgery. Patients with MG are more sensitive to the respiratory-depressant effects of opioids and anxiolytics because these patients have reduced ventilatory reserve; therefore, these drugs should be administered with more caution than normal in patients with MG.

Intraoperative Management

Neuromuscular Blocking Agents Patients with MG have a relative resistance to the effects of depolarizing NMBAs with unpredictable responses because of decreased AChRs. Required doses of succinylcholine are usually two to three times normal, which increases the risk of a phase 2 block developing. Conversely, patients with MG are very sensitive to the effects of nondepolarizing NMBAs, often requiring as little as one tenth the normal dose, independent of the severity of the patient's symptoms and signs of disease. Most anesthesia providers, therefore, prefer to avoid the use of NMBAs in patients with MG and, if compelled to use an NMBA, use a low dose of a short-acting or intermediate-acting drug. Although sugammadex has not been approved in the United States, multiple case reports have been published of its use to reverse the effects of NMBAs in patients with MG. It is doubtful, however, that the current practice of avoiding the routine use of NMBAs in patients with MG will change.

Inhalation and Intravenously Administered Anesthetic Agents Inhalation anesthetic agents cause muscle relaxation in patients without MG but cause profound muscle relaxation in patients with MG. Intravenously administered anesthetic agents (e.g., propofol) have not been shown to have undesirable effects in patients with MG.

Regional Anesthetics To avoid the use of an NMBA, many clinicians prefer using regional anesthetic techniques, when indicated, to anesthetize patients with MG. Because patients with MG have decreased ventilatory reserve, however, the risks and benefits of neuraxial techniques (interscalene nerve blocks, phrenic nerve blockade)—essentially any technique with the potential to affect respiratory muscles—must be weighed carefully. Ester-type local anesthetic agents are degraded by pseudocholinesterase, which is also inhibited by pyridostigmine; if a regional anesthetic technique is chosen, an amide local anesthetic agent would be the preferred drug in a patient with MG who is being treated with an anticholinesterase drug.

Postoperative Management

Several factors increase the risk for patients with MG to develop postoperative ventilatory insufficiency: (1) duration of MG greater than 6 years, (2) a history of other chronic respiratory disease, (3) a pyridostigmine dose above 750 mg/day, and (4) a preoperative vital capacity of less than 2.9 L. The need for either mechanical ventilation or intensive monitoring should be anticipated. Other postoperative concerns that may arise are myasthenic crisis, cholinergic crisis (both of which can occur with perioperative changes in anticholinesterase treatment), and residual effects of anesthesia. Postoperative pain control with epidural analgesia has been shown to be of benefit in patients with MG in helping to maintain ventilatory drive.

Lambert-Eaton Myasthenic Syndrome

Lambert-Eaton myasthenic syndrome (LEMS), often confused with MG, is a rare disorder of neuromuscular transmission most often associated with carcinoma of the lung, especially oat cell carcinoma of the bronchus. Antibody-mediated destruction of presynaptic voltage-gated calcium channels leads to deficient release of ACh at the neuromuscular junction, causing muscle weakness. The skeletal muscle weakness associated with LEMS is not reliably reversed with anticholinesterase drugs or corticosteroids. Furthermore, exercise improves, rather than reduces, muscle strength in this condition. Patients with LEMS are very sensitive to the effects of both depolarizing and nondepolarizing NMBAs. The potential for LEMS should be considered in patients with known or probable carcinoma, especially of the lung (Table 172-3).

Table 172-3 Comparison of Lambert-Eaton Myasthenic Syndrome and Myasthenia Gravis

Characteristic	LEMS	Myasthenia Gravis
Manifestations		
Areas of weakness	Proximal limbs (legs more than arms)	Extraocular, bulbar, and facial muscles
Response to exercise	Improves strength	Fatigue
Muscle pain	Common	Uncommon
Reflexes	Absent or decreased	Normal
Sex	Male > female	Female > male
Coexisting pathology	Small cell carcinoma of the lung	Thymoma
Response to drugs		
Succinylcholine	Sensitive	Resistant
Nondepolarizing NMBAs	Sensitive	Sensitive
Anticholinesterase drugs	Poor	Good

LEMS, Lambert-Eaton Myasthenic syndrome; NMBAs, neuromuscular blocking agents.

Suggested Readings

Duvaldestin P, Plaud B. Sugammadex in anesthesia practice. *Expert Opin Pharmacother*. 2010;11:2759-2771.

Falkson CB, Bezjak A, Darling G, et al. The management of thymoma: A systematic review and practice guideline. *J Thorac Oncol*. 2009;4:911-919.

Farag E, Barsoum S, Spagnuolo S, et al. Anesthesia and muscle disease. *Am J Anesthesiol*. 2000;27:491-501.

Hines RL, Marschall KE, eds. Myasthenia gravis. In: *Stoelting's Anesthesia and Co-Existing Disease*. 6th ed. Philadelphia: Elsevier Saunders; 2012.

CHAPTER 173

Anesthesia for Patients with Diabetes Mellitus

Aaron M. Joffe, DO, and Douglas B. Coursin, MD

This chapter will discuss the definition and systemic complications of diabetes mellitus (DM), with particular attention given to the impact of DM on the preoperative assessment and management of anesthesia. Specific guidelines and a discussion of perioperative glycemic management are presented in Chapter 226, Perioperative Management of Blood Glucose.

The prevalence of DM has reached epidemic proportions, with roughly 13% of Americans over 20 years of age affected with type 2 DM. DM is unrecognized or undiagnosed in approximately 40% of people who have the disease. DM is defined as a metabolic disorder of varied cause characterized by chronic elevations of blood glucose and disordered carbohydrate, fat, and protein metabolism consequent to defective insulin secretion, insulin action, or both. In 1999, a World Health Organization report on the definition, diagnosis, and classification of DM and its complications suggested the application of a revised classification based upon both cause and the degree of insulin deficiency, as well as other causes of hyperglycemia. In this classification, the terms type 1 (10% of all patients with DM) and type 2 were reintroduced and reflect patients in whom the disorder is primarily a result of islet β-cell destruction typically causing an absolute insulin deficiency (type 1) or a defect in insulin secretion, almost universally accompanied by systemic insulin resistance (type 2). The terms *insulin-dependent diabetes* and *non–insulin-dependent diabetes* are to be eschewed. Type 1 DM may be autoimmune or idiopathic in origin, whereas type 2 DM is most commonly acquired secondary to obesity and inactivity but can be caused by a host of other factors, including genetic defects of β-cell function, glucose-transport abnormalities, or insulin action; exocrine pancreas malfunction; associated polyglandular endocrinopathies; pregnancy; as a side effect of medications; and infections and inflammation. A summary of the American Diabetes Association definitions for DM, prediabetes, and hyperglycemia in hospitalized patients is presented in Table 173-1.

Table 173-1 American Diabetes Association Definitions for Diabetes Mellitus, Pre-DM, and Inpatient Hyperglycemia

Diagnosis*	Results (mg/dL) or Definition
DM	
Fasting BGC	≥126
2-h BGC during 75-g OGTT	≥200
Random BGC	≥200 + symptoms of hyperglycemia
Impaired fasting glucose	
Fasting BGC	100-125
Impaired glucose tolerance	
2-h BGC during 75-g OGTT	140-199
Medical history of DM	Diagnosis of DM before hospitalization
Unrecognized DM	Symptoms of DM present, but DM not previously diagnosed
Hospital-related hyperglycemia†	
Fasting BGC	≥ 126
Random BGC	≥ 200

*Testing should be performed with the patient in an ambulatory unstressed state; the ADA recommends that any abnormal result be verified on a subsequent day to confirm the diagnosis.

†The BGC is obtained while patient is in the hospital and reverts to normal value after the patient is discharged from the hospital. Also commonly referred to as *stress hyperglycemia*.

BGC, Blood glucose concentration; DM, diabetes mellitus; OGTT, oral glucose tolerance test.

Adapted from Fahy BG, Sheehy AM, Coursin DB. Glucose control in the intensive care unit. Crit Care Med. 2009;37:1769-1776.

Complications of Diabetes

Long-term sequelae of diabetes can be categorized as either macrovascular or microvascular. Macrovascular complications include diabetic autonomic neuropathy and cardiac complications—atherosclerotic coronary artery disease, hypertension, congestive heart failure, and diastolic dysfunction—whereas microvascular complications include nephropathy, peripheral neuropathy, and retinopathy. In addition, poor glycemic control may result in diabetic ketoacidosis, nonketotic hyperosmolar syndrome, and impaired lymphocyte function and antibody formation, which may lead to an increased susceptibility to infection as well as delayed wound healing.

DM is the sixth leading cause of death in the United States, with cardiovascular disease as the leading cause of fatality in patients with DM and a strong contributor to further morbidity. A combination of hypertension, dyslipidemia, and oxidative stress with vascular inflammation leads to accelerated coronary artery disease. Inappropriate insulin signaling results in a characteristic lipid panel profile, which includes elevated triglyceride levels, decreased concentrations of high-density lipoprotein cholesterol, and an elevated low-density lipoprotein cholesterol level. These low-density lipoprotein particles in people with DM are abnormally small, dense, and more atherogenic than those in people without DM. Angina, myocardial infarction, congestive heart failure and sudden death may result. Diabetic autonomic neuropathy can affect any part of the autonomic nervous system, but cardiovascular autonomic neuropathy may be the most challenging effect for the anesthesia provider. Baroreceptor reflexes, ability to regulate vasomotor tone, and cardiovascular reactivity may be impaired, manifesting as resting tachycardia, loss of heart rate variability, orthostatic hypotension, and cardiac arrythmias. Sensitivity of central respiratory centers to hypoxia and hypercarbia may be diminished, resulting in inadequate ventilatory responses to these stimuli. This sensitivity may be of particular importance in patients with DM who receive sedative or amnestic agents or opioid analgesics prior to the induction of anesthesia, as well as during the patient's emergence and recovery from anesthesia when residual anesthesia and sedative or analgesic agents are present. Gastrointestinal manifestations include gastroparesis, which could increase the likelihood of nausea

Box 173-1 Variables and Definitions for Use of the Revised Cardiac Risk Index*

High-risk surgical procedure
- Intraperitoneal
- Intrathoracic
- Suprainguinal vascular

Ischemic heart disease
- History of myocardial infarction
- History of positive exercise test
- Current complaint of chest pain considered secondary to myocardial ischemia
- Use of nitrate therapy
- ECG with pathologic Q waves

Congestive heart failure
- History of congestive heart failure
- Pulmonary edema
- Paroxysmal nocturnal dyspnea
- Bilateral rales or S_3 gallop
- Chest radiograph showing pulmonary vascular redistribution

Cerebrovascular disease
- History of transient ischemic attack or stroke

Preoperative use of insulin therapy for DM

Preoperative serum creatinine concentration >2.0 mg/dL

*Each risk factor is assigned 1 point, and the risk level is determined based on the number of points. (See Table 173-2 for scoring of the Revised Cardiac Risk Index.)
DM, Diabetes mellitus; ECG, electrocardiogram.

Table 173-2 Scoring of the Revised Cardiac Risk Index

RCRI Category	No. of Risk Factors	Risk Level	Risk (%)
I	0	Very low	0.4
II	1	Low	0.9
III	2	Moderate	6.6
IV	≥ 3	High	11

RCRI, Revised cardiac risk index.

or vomiting occurring on induction of anesthesia. Of the microvascular complications, the most noteworthy to the an anesthesia provider is diabetic nephropathy, which, in its earliest stage, is manifested by microalbuminuria. If the patient does not have any interventions, blood urea nitrogen and serum creatinine concentrations will rise within 5 years of the patient developing microalbuminuria, with a large proportion of these patients proceeding to develop frank renal failure with a glomerular filtration rate of less than 20 mL/min. It is at this point that the kidney can no longer perform its two main functions: osmolar regulation and maintenance of normal serum electrolyte and acid-base status. Patients may ultimately become edematous with an expanded extracellular fluid volume and may become hyperkalemic and acidotic.

Preoperative Assessment

Performing a comprehensive operative risk assessment is an important initial step in the perioperative management of the patient with DM. Because the incidence of various high-risk conditions is greater among patients with DM than in the general population, particular attention should be paid to preoperative cardiac assessment. The risk for patients undergoing moderate to high-risk procedures should be stratified using the Revised Cardiac Risk Index (Box 173-1 and Table 173-2). Patients found to be at moderate risk or higher (e.g., classes III or IV) for experiencing a major cardiac event (myocardial infarction, complete heart block, pulmonary edema, and ventricular fibrillation) should potentially undergo noninvasive cardiac stress testing to rule out significant occlusive artery disease prior to the operation.

Adequacy of blood glucose control and intravascular volume and the absence of ketoacidosis should be confirmed. Elective operations should be postponed in patients who have ketoacidosis, decompensated DM with severe hyperosmolarity, or both. Information regarding antecedent glycemic control can be identified by obtaining an HbA_{1c} level, with a value of less than 7% indicating good control over the previous 2 to 3 months. A focused history and review of systems to elicit any signs and symptoms of respiratory disease, cerebral ischemia, hypertension, and renal disease should be sought. Furthermore, the musculoskeletal system should be evaluated for signs of limited joint mobility, sometimes referred to as "stiff-joint syndrome" secondary to prolonged glycosylation, with particular assessment of cervical spine mobility and mouth opening. Patients with type 1 DM may be of short stature and have limited joint mobility, whereas patients with type 2 DM are often overweight or obese. In both circumstances, difficult laryngoscopy should be anticipated.

Management of Anesthesia

The anesthesia provider must determine in advance the types of physiologic monitoring to be used during anesthesia. Selective use of arterial cannulation provides easy access for frequent sampling of blood for glucose, electrolyte, and arterial blood gas concentrations. Patients with DM who exhibit signs or symptoms of autonomic neuropathy should be assumed to have some degree of gastroparesis and impaired gastric emptying and may be at increased risk for aspirating gastric contents. However, there is little evidence to suggest that rapid sequence intubation will decrease clinically relevant aspiration upon induction of anesthesia in this patient population, because significant clinical aspiration is a rare complication in modern anesthesia: 1.4 to 6 per 100,000 patients given anesthetics for elective general surgery. Reports of delayed gastric emptying in patients with DM presenting for elective operations have not documented relevant aspiration events despite the presence of sometimes significant amounts of gastric contents. The use of metoclopramide, histamine type 2 receptor blockers, proton pump inhibitors, or nonparticulate antacids may be used before anesthesia induction to decrease gastric volume and increase pH, although the efficacy of these agents in decreasing the chances of aspiration has not been shown. Attention to the patients' intraoperative positioning is important because injuries to the limbs and nerves are more likely to occur in patients with DM because of the patients' increased vulnerability to ischemia from pressure and stretch injuries.

These patients may be more susceptible to the vasodilating and myocardial-depressant effects of intravenously administered and inhalation anesthetic agents. However, the choice of anesthetic technique may be less important than is the institution of an appropriate monitoring plan during anesthesia. If regional anesthesia is used, consideration must be given to the high incidence of peripheral neuropathies.

Summary

DM is not only a disease of abnormal metabolism but, rather, a systemic disease affecting every organ system. As more people throughout the developed world become overweight or obese, the prevalence of diabetes increases. Thus, the number of patients with DM who undergo surgical procedures, which will necessitate interaction with an anesthesiologist, is ever increasing. An understanding of the underlying pathophysiology of DM and how to assess its effects on major organ systems will allow the anesthesia provider to formulate appropriate care plans to deter perioperative complications leading to higher resource consumption and morbidity and mortality rates.

Suggested Readings

American College of Cardiology/American Heart Association Task Force on Practice Guidelines (Writing Committee to Revise the 2002 Guidelines on Perioperative Cardiovascular Evaluation for Noncardiac Surgery); American Society of Echocardiography; American Society of Nuclear Cardiology; Heart Rhythm Society; Society of Cardiovascular Anesthesiologists; Society for Cardiovascular Angiography and Interventions; Society for Vascular Medicine and Biology; Society for Vascular Surgery, Fleisher LA, Beckman JA, Brown KA, et al. ACC/AHA 2007 guidelines on perioperative cardiovascular evaluation and care for noncardiac surgery: Executive summary: A report of the American College of Cardiology/American Heart Association Task Force on Practice Guidelines (Writing Committee to Revise the 2002 Guidelines on Perioperative Cardiovascular Evaluation for Noncardiac Surgery). *Anesth Analg*. 2008;106:685-712.

Hogan K, Rusy D, Springman SR. Difficult laryngoscopy and diabetes mellitus. *Anesth Analg*. 1988;67:1162-1165.

Rodbard HW, Blonde L, Braithwaite SS, et al, AACE Diabetes Mellitus Clinical Practice Guidelines Task Force. American Association of Clinical Endocrinologists medical guidelines for clinical practice for the management of diabetes mellitus. *Endocr Pract*. 2007;13(Suppl):1-68.

Sebranek JJ, Kopp Lugli A, Coursin DB. Glycaemic control in the perioperative period. *Br J Anaesth*. 2013 in press.

CHAPTER 174

Anesthesia for Thyroid Surgery

Prith Peiris, MD

Although thyroid operations are often viewed as routine procedures, they can present a unique combination of problems for the anesthesia provider. For example, difficulties securing the airway in the presence of a large goiter and surgical trauma to the recurrent laryngeal nerves (RLN) may cause dysphonia and stridor after extubation. The presence of coexisting thyroid hyperfunction or hypofunction, particularly when poorly controlled, can impact morbidity and mortality. Anesthesia can precipitate thyroid storm in patients with hyperfunction of the thyroid; hypofunction, especially of unknown severity, can present as multisystem clinical challenges during both the intraoperative and postoperative periods. Close cooperation between the anesthesia provider and the surgeon is imperative in achieving optimal outcomes in patients undergoing thyroid operations.

General Considerations

Preoperative Assessment

Thyroid operations have been successfully completed under local, regional, and intravenous anesthesia; however, most thyroid operations require general inhalation anesthesia. For these patients, a reinforced wire spiral tracheal tube may be necessary to maintain airway patency. (Nerve integrity monitor [NIM] tracheal tubes, which will be discussed in the section Preserving and Assessing the Function of the RLN, are reinforced.)

Intubation issues and potential difficulty in securing the airway in patients with goiters should be anticipated. Positional dyspnea and hypotension may suggest that the patient's airway or great vein is compressed by a goiter. If the results of the preoperative examination and a review of the patient's medical records, including the surgeon's outpatient examination records, suggest that intubation may be difficult in any patient undergoing a thyroid operation, the results of ultrasonography or computerized tomography may assist the anesthesia provider in deciding whether a surgical airway or an awake intubation would be the safer option. In patients with goiters, a radiograph of the chest may reveal any tracheal deviation and airway collapse, but a computerized tomographic scan is better for assessing retrosternal extension, tracheal ring compression, and airway tortuosity.

Preserving and Assessing the Function of the RLN

The overall incidence of RLN damage during thyroid operations is 2% to 5%. Surgical identification and preservation of the RLNs remains the gold standard for protecting the RLN, but real-time intraoperative monitoring of RLN function may also help to reduce the incidence of damage.

To intraoperatively monitor RLN function, the anesthesia provider uses a tracheal tube with an embedded NIM to intubate the trachea under direct vision. When this tube is properly aligned, the electrodes in the NIM come into contact with both vocal cords. The anesthesia provider verifies the integrity of contact using a small stimulating current. The device provides both an audible alarm and a visual display of the action potential on a monitor whenever the RLN is stimulated. Studies have shown that such monitors detect RLN stimulation more than 70% of the time, making this technique useful in those cases in which difficulty is anticipated, such as in patients who are undergoing repeat operations or operations to excise cancer. During minimally invasive operations, monitoring of the external branch of the superior laryngeal nerve may serve as a surrogate to monitoring the RLN.

Postoperative Airway Problems

At the end of the operation, direct laryngoscopy not only will define vocal cord movement, but also may help identify factors that may cause stridor, such as glottic edema. Unilateral RLN paralysis, which occurs more often than bilateral paralysis, results in a midline ipsilateral cord on inspiration. Bilateral RLN paralysis, in which both cords are midline and is associated aphonia and stridor, requires reintubation.

Postoperative hypocalcemia secondary to parathyroid gland removal or devascularization occurs less than 2% of the time but may occur with a technically difficult operation. It may present as laryngospasm but, unlike

RLN paralysis, usually occurs 24 hours or more after the operation. Excessive bleeding is rare but should be recognized early because hemorrhage into a confined space could lead to early airway compromise.

The Patient with Undiagnosed Thyroid Disease

Up to 20% of patients with hyperthyroidism may present with atrial fibrillation as the first sign. Patients with postoperative agitation, restlessness, and tachycardia may not have anxiety or pain but, instead, impending thyroid crisis. Awareness of the possibility of thyroid dysfunction is the key to diagnosis and management.

Hypothyroidism

In patients with any thyroid dysfunction, the goal prior to elective operations is attaining a euthyroid state. In the past, surgery was usually postponed in patients with all but mild cases of hypothyroidism, but it now appears that there may not be a difference in outcome postoperatively even in patients with moderate disease. However, the anesthesia provider should always remain vigilant because the clinical expression of hypothyroidism shows much individual variation. Potential problem areas include increased aspiration risk, increased sensitivity to opioids and anesthetic agents, hypoglycemia, hypothermia, and intraoperative hypotension. Thyroxine (T_4) has a half-life of approximately 7 days, and triiodothyronine (T_3), of 1.5 days; therefore, even if both are administered preoperatively for the treatment of severe myxedema, the clinical benefit may be delayed. The cardiac effect of administered T_3/T_4 may have an onset faster than that of its other actions. Whether this is a benefit or increases the risk of the patient developing arrhythmias and acute coronary syndrome is uncertain. The risk of preoperative treatment in severe cases needs to be weighed on an individual basis and in coordination with advice from an endocrinologist and intensivist. These patients are at risk for also developing adrenal insufficiency and, therefore, should be given prophylactic steroids intraoperatively—100 mg of hydrocortisone or its equivalent every 8 h.

Hyperthyroidism

In patients with hyperthyroidism, the thyroid gland produces excess hormone, the effects of which may be subclinical or overt. In thyrotoxicosis, as the name suggests, there is excess circulating hormone, resulting in major end-organ effects. For example, patients with normal coronary vasculature may have angina pectoris. β-Blockade will relieve the tremor, palpitations, and anxiety associated with hyperthyroidism but none of the metabolic manifestations. In the presence of moderate to severe hyperthyroidism, surgery should be postponed until the patient achieves a euthyroid state, usually a period between 3 and 6 weeks. The thioamide drugs, methimazole and propylthiouracil, are the primary drugs used to treat thyrotoxicosis, but their action stops when the drug is not taken, so patient compliance should be reviewed before surgery. Pharmacologic treatment involves the use of thioamides that block the synthesis but not the release of stored hormone, stores of which may be significant in goitrous disease. In patients with Graves disease, the presence of exophthalmos requires careful eye care with lubricant and taping to avoid corneal-conjunctival desiccation and damage.

Thyroid Storm

Thyroid storm is a clinical diagnosis in which manifestations of preexisting hyperthyroidism are exacerbated into a life-threatening condition by the sudden release of T_3 and T_4. It can be induced by pregnancy, surgery, trauma, or severe illness and can take up to 24 h to develop. A chemical euthyroid state lessens the chance of a storm occurring but does not prevent it. Thyroid storm that initially manifests in the operating room may be confused with malignant hyperthermia, neuroleptic malignant syndrome, or the signs manifested by a pheochromocytoma. The signs and symptoms of a thyroid storm include confusion, high fever, tachycardia, metabolic acidosis, and congestive cardiac failure.

Once the diagnosis is made, the goal is to treat the underlying cause and to provide simultaneous supportive therapy. The patient's body should be cooled with ice packs and intravenously infused cold fluids. Propranolol has been the β-adrenergic receptor blocking agent of choice for heart rate control and inhibition of peripheral T_4 to T_3 conversion; however, intravenously administered esmolol titrated up to 300 $\mu g \cdot kg^{-1} \cdot min^{-1}$ has been shown to be effective. Vasopressors for hypotension and inotropes for heart failure may be indicated, and magnesium has been shown to be helpful in reducing catecholamine-induced arrhythmias provoked by thyroxine. Adrenal hypofunction may coexist, as in hypothyroidism; therefore, it is prudent to intravenously administer hydrocortisone. The main role of agents that inhibit hormone secretion and block their peripheral action is in their use as a part of a preoperative plan. Carbimazole, methimazole, and propylthiouracil have been used successfully in this capacity. In the operating room, their use is better postponed until after discussion with an endocrinologist. Patients with thyroid storm, which carries a significant mortality risk, should be monitored in the intensive care unit postoperatively until their condition stabilizes.

Suggested Readings

Chu KS, Tsai CJ, Lu IC, et al. Influence of nondepolarizing muscle relaxants on intraoperative neuromonitoring during thyroid surgery. *J Otolaryngol Head Neck Surg*. 2010;39:397-402.

Moitra V, Sladen RN. Monitoring endocrine function. *Anesthesiol Clin*. 2009; 27:355-364.

Schiff RL, Welsh GA. Perioperative evaluation and management of the patient with endocrine dysfunction. *Med Clin North Am*. 2003;87:175-192.

Smallridge RC. Metabolic and anatomic thyroid emergencies: A review. *Crit Care Med*. 1992;20:276-291.

Statathos N, Wartofsky L. Perioperative management of patients with hypothyroidism. *Endocrinol Metab Clin North Am*. 2003;32:503-518.

CHAPTER 175

Anesthesia for Patients with Carcinoid Tumors

Michelle A. O. Kinney, MD, John A. Dilger, MD, and Toby N. Weingarten, MD

Evaluation of Carcinoid Tumors

Carcinoid tumors are the most common gastrointestinal endocrine tumor, with an incidence of 3 per 100,000 per year in the United States. Carcinoid tumors arise from enterochromaffin cells (*entero* meaning *gut* and *chromaffin* because these cells share characteristics with chromaffin cells in the adrenal medulla) derived embryologically from epithelial stem cell precursors. Because these cells are not derived from the neural crest, they are more appropriately termed enteroendocrine than neuroendocrine. The site of origin of carcinoid tumors depends on the number of enterochromaffin cells within different organs—70% to 90% arise in the appendix, ileum, and rectum; up to 20% of tumors arise in the lungs; and less commonly, they can be found in the ovaries, thyroid, and pancreas. Enterochromaffin cells contain numerous membrane-bound neurosecretory granules composed of hormones and biogenic amines. The most prevalent compound is serotonin (80%-90% of the body's stores), produced from its precursor, 5-hydroxytryptophan, but these cells can also produce corticotropin, histamine, dopamine, substance P, neurotensin, prostaglandins, and kallikrein. Stress of any kind can stimulate tumors to release their contents of these vasoactive substances into the circulation, resulting in mild symptoms to a full-blown carcinoid crisis.

Because the vasoactive substances contained in enterochromatin cells are cleared from the circulation by the liver, carcinoid tumors that are isolated to the gastrointestinal tract usually do not result in the systemic manifestations of the carcinoid syndrome. The carcinoid syndrome occurs when these substances are secreted into the systemic venous system from a tumor that has metastasized to the liver (thus bypassing the portal circulation) or has originated in the lungs, ovaries, or thyroid. Clinical signs and symptoms of carcinoid syndrome include bronchoconstriction, episodic cutaneous flushing, abdominal pain, diarrhea, hemodynamic instability, hepatomegaly, hyperglycemia, and dysthymia.

Laboratory test results that support a diagnosis of carcinoid tumor, either primary or metastatic, include a 24-h urine test with more than 25 g of 5-hydroxyindoleacetic acid (5-HIAA), the metabolite of serotonin, or a positive serum chromogranin A (CgA) test. Serum CgA is a glycoprotein secreted with other hormones by enteroendocrine tumors and is 95% specific and almost 80% sensitive for the detection of carcinoid tumors.

In addition to performing a physical examination and history to identify associated signs and symptoms and conducting appropriate laboratory tests, a thorough heart evaluation is warranted, looking specifically for evidence of tricuspid regurgitation and pulmonary stenosis. Left-sided valvular lesions are uncommon and are usually associated with a bronchogenic tumor. Carcinoid-related valvular fibrosis has been thought to be due to longstanding exposure to elevated levels of serotonin, but other factors must be involved because serotonin inhibitors do not prevent the cardiac valvular fibrosis.

Anesthetic Management of Patients with Carcinoid Tumors

Preoperative Anesthetic Management

Most patients with carcinoid tumors who are presenting for surgery will have had a careful evaluation by an endocrinologist and cardiologist and will be taking octreotide acetate, a long-acting analog of the naturally occurring peptide somatostatin. Octreotide, which inhibits release by tumor cells of serotonin, gastrin, vasoactive intestinal peptide, secretin, motilin, and pancreatic polypeptide, can be administered intravenously or subcutaneously, depending on the desired time of onset and duration of treatment. Intravenous administration results in peak serum concentrations within approximately 3 min. Subcutaneous injections of octreotide result in peak concentrations 30 to 60 min after injection; and the plasma half-life is 113 min. The biologic duration of effect may be as long as 12 h.

The usual preoperative dose of octreotide is 50 to 300 μg. Acute administration of octreotide may be lifesaving in an acute carcinoid crisis and is generally given in 50-μg to 300-μg intravenously administered doses. Octreotide doses of 500 to 1000 μg have been reported to have been given to patients undergoing cardiac valvular operations. However, intravenously administered bolus doses of octreotide of 100 μg or greater may result in bradycardia and abnormalities in atrioventricular conduction, presumably by acting directly on the cardiac conduction system. Diluting octreotide, slowly infusing the drug, and continuously monitoring the electrocardiogram may be advisable to minimize potential adverse side effects of octreotide.

Octreotide is also now available as a once-monthly intramuscularly administered slow-release preparation. Patients who are receiving the intramuscularly administered drug who need surgery may have high sustained levels of octreotide that suppress their symptoms but that are not sufficiently high to suppress the potentially higher intraoperatively released levels of vasoactive substances. Therefore, these patients may still require subcutaneously or intravenously administered doses of octreotide in the perioperative period.

The use of preoperative sedation could be justified to minimize sympathetic stimulation, which could result in a carcinoid crisis.

Intraoperative Anesthetic Management

The presence of hypovolemia or electrolyte abnormalities and the possibility of right-sided cardiac valvular lesions should be taken into account when planning for induction and maintenance of anesthesia. Gentle surgical skin preparation to avoid tumor compression is advised (Box 175-1). The use of histamine-releasing drugs should probably be avoided in patients with carcinoid tumors, although these drugs have been used frequently in the past without complications. Phenylephrine and amrinone have been safely used in patients with carcinoid syndrome. However, even very low doses

Box 175-1 Drugs and Actions to Avoid during the Anesthetic Management of Patients with Carcinoid Syndrome

Opioids
- Meperidine and morphine

Histamine-releasing neuromuscular relaxants
- Atracurium, mivacurium, *d*-tubocurarine

Administration of exogenous catecholamines (controversial, use only in conjunction with octreotide)
- Epinephrine, norepinephrine, dopamine, isoproterenol

Release of endogenous catecholamines*

Mechanical stimulation of the tumor or tumors

Vigorous abdominal scrubbing

The use of succinylcholine†

*Anxiety, hypotension, pain, hypothermia, minimize laryngotracheal reflexes on intubation.

†The use of succinylcholine in this situation is controversial.

Adapted from Botero M, Fuchs R, Paulus DA. Carcinoid heart disease: A case report and literature review. J Clin Anesth. 2002;14:57-63.

of β-adrenergic agonists (e.g., 5 μg of intravenously administered epinephrine) have been shown to stimulate the release of vasoactive substances, but the action of these drugs can be blunted if the patient has received an adequate dose of octreotide. In a hypotensive patient, if the cause of hypotension is secondary to carcinoid crisis, additional octreotide and fluid should be administered. β-Adrenergic agonists should be used only when the cause of hypotension is thought to be secondary to decreased systemic vascular resistance or decreased cardiac output from factors unrelated to tumor activity.

Octreotide should be readily available intraoperatively for immediate treatment of carcinoid symptoms and should be administered—along with volume infusion and phenylephrine, as needed—whenever carcinoid symptoms (e.g., bronchospasm, unexpected hypotension, facial flushing) occur. The usual intravenously administered intraoperative bolus dose for the treatment of the signs of carcinoid activity is 50 to 300 μg, which may need to be repeated. The total intraoperative dose of octreotide administered in noncardiac operations may reach 4000 μg, although a dose this high is uncommon. In a study of patients with carcinoid syndrome who were undergoing cardiac operations, the median intraoperative octreotide dose was 1500 μg (mean 3666 ± 6461 μg,).

Postoperative Management

The humoral effects of metastatic carcinoid lesions are usually not eliminated by surgery. Thus, octreotide should be continued postoperatively if the patient was using it preoperatively.

Suggested Readings

Botero M, Fuchs R, Paulus DA. Carcinoid heart disease: A case report and literature review. *J Clin Anesth*. 2002;14:57-63.

Castillo JG, Filsoufi F, Adams DH, et al. Management of patients undergoing multivalvular surgery for carcinoid heart disease: The role of the anaesthetist. *Br J Anaesth*. 2008;101:618-626.

de Vries H, Verschueren RC, Willemse PH, et al. Diagnostic, surgical, and medical aspects of the midgut carcinoids. *Cancer Treat Rev*. 2002;28:11-25.

Dierdorf SF. Carcinoid tumor and carcinoid syndrome. *Curr Opin Anaesthesiol*. 2003;16:343-347.

Dilger JA, Rho EH, Que FG, Sprung J. Octreotide-induced bradycardia and heart block during surgical resection of a carcinoid tumor. *Anesth Analg*. 2004;98:318-320.

Kinney MAO, Warner ME, Nagorney DM, et al. Perianesthetic risks and outcomes of abdominal surgery for metastatic carcinoid tumours. *Br J Anaesth*. 2001;87:447-452.

Powell B, Mukhtar AA, Mills GH. Carcinoid: The disease and its implications for anaesthesia. *Contin Educ Anaesth Crit Care Pain*. 2011;11:9-13.

Weingarten TN, Abel MD, Connolly HM, et al. Intraoperative management of patients with carcinoid heart disease having valvular surgery: A review of one hundred consecutive cases. *Anesth Analg*. 2007;105:1192-1199.

CHAPTER 176

Anesthesia for the Patient Undergoing Liver Transplantation

James Y. Findlay, MB, ChB, FRCA

Liver transplantation is an established therapy for end-stage liver disease, with the more than 6000 people who receive a liver transplant every year in the United States now having a 3-year survival rate of almost 80%. Despite recent advances in the use of living donors and of split-liver grafts for pediatric and adult recipients, the number of liver transplantations remains limited by the availability of suitable donors, with approximately 16,000 people waiting to receive a transplant. Liver transplantation presents a challenge to the anesthesia provider because, in addition to the operation being complex, most patients present for transplantation with greatly altered physiology because of their end-stage liver disease.

Preoperative Evaluation

Table 176-1 lists some of the relevant physiologic consequences of liver failure and the consequences that may occur during liver transplantation. Prior to presenting for transplantation, candidates are screened for

Table 176-1 Pathophysiologic Changes Associated with Liver Failure

Organ System	Change	Consequence(s)
Cardiovascular	Hyperdynamic circulation (high cardiac output, low SVR)	Hypotension
	Portal hypertension	Varices, splenomegaly
		Bleeding (dilated vessels, thrombocytopenia)
	Ascites	Fluid shifts after drainage
	Pulmonary hypertension	High perioperative mortality rate (>80%) if severe
Respiratory	Respiratory alkalosis	
	Restrictive physiology (ascites with or without pleural effusion)	Atelectasis; reduced compliance
	Hepatopulmonary syndrome (intrapulmonary shunting)	Hypoxemia
Hematologic	Decreased factor synthesis	Bleeding potential
	Thrombocytopenia	
	Anemia	
CNS	Hepatic encephalopathy	Delayed awakening
	Cerebral edema (in fulminant failure)	Raised ICP; consider ICP monitoring
Renal	Hepatorenal syndrome	Renal failure—volume and electrolyte management concerns
	Hyponatremia	Possibility of CPM if corrected intraoperatively

CNS, Central nervous system; CPM, central pontine myelinolysis; ICP, intracranial pressure; SVR, systemic vascular resistance.

Box 176-1 Model of End-Stage Liver Disease

$$\text{Score} = 3.78[\text{Ln serum bilirubin (mg/dL)}] + 11.2[\text{Ln INR}] + 9.57[\text{Ln serum creatinine (mg/dL)}] + 6.43$$

INR, International normalized ratio for prothrombin time.

comorbid cardiopulmonary conditions: a resting echocardiogram assesses cardiac function and allows estimation of pulmonary artery pressures. A bubble test (injection of agitated saline while monitoring for echocontrast in the right side of heart chambers) can also be performed; delayed appearance of the contrast agent suggests that the patient may have hepatopulmonary syndrome. If the patient has risk factors for coronary artery disease (~40%-50% of adult patients), noninvasive testing is frequently performed, often by dobutamine stress echocardiography, because patients with significant coronary artery disease have poor peritransplant outcomes.

Renal dysfunction often accompanies end-stage liver disease from hepatorenal syndrome, acute tubular necrosis, or a combination of both. In a patient requiring renal dialysis or continuous renal replacement therapy, consideration should be given to performing continuous dialysis or ultrafiltration in the operating room if problems managing volume or electrolytes are anticipated. Washing red blood cells prior to transfusion to reduce potassium may also be helpful.

The severity of end-stage liver disease is assessed by calculating the MELD (Model of End-stage Liver Disease) score, which incorporates the patient's serum bilirubin, serum creatinine, and the international normalized ratio for prothrombin time to predict survival (Box 176-1). A higher MELD score is associated with more severe liver failure; higher MELD scores are also predictive of a greater rate of intraoperative blood product transfusion and need for vasopressors.

Intraoperative Management

Anesthesia

Induction of anesthesia may be achieved using any of the commonly used agents. Maintenance is typically achieved using a balanced technique with an inhaled agent and opioid, often fentanyl. Cisatracurium may be preferred for maintenance of neuromuscular blockade because it is not dependent on hepatic metabolism for elimination, but other neuromuscular blocking agents can be used as long as redosing is guided by train-of-four monitoring.

Invasive monitoring is the norm; direct arterial pressure is best monitored by a brachial or femoral arterial catheter rather than a radial artery catheter because these sites allow for more accurate measurement of blood pressure at reperfusion. A pulmonary artery catheter is frequently placed; additionally or alternatively, transesophageal echocardiography provides valuable cardiac and hemodynamic information. A "stat lab" in close proximity to the operating room is useful for the rapid analysis of blood gases, electrolytes, glucose, and coagulation status. Many centers use thromboelastography to provide a rapid assessment of coagulation.

Adequate large-bore venous access, which is essential because of the potential for massive hemorrhage to occur, must be obtained in the upper body because the procedure involves partial or total clamping of the inferior vena cava (IVC). A dedicated peripheral or centrally placed 8F or larger catheter connected to a rapid infusion pump is used. If venovenous bypass is planned, a second dedicated large-bore catheter is centrally placed. Red blood cell salvage is typically used. The blood bank should be able to rapidly provide large quantities of blood and blood products.

The large surgical incision, prolonged operating times, and implantation of a cold graft make hypothermia a potential problem. The use of fluid warmers and forced-air convective warming blankets can help prevent or minimize perioperative hypothermia.

Transplantation Procedure

Initial dissection and hepatectomy can result in significant blood loss from friable dilated vessels in the abdominal wall, in the abdomen, and around the liver. Excision of the liver involves mobilization and then clamping and dividing the hepatic vasculature (hepatic artery, portal vein, and IVC). Venovenous bypass is occasionally used depending on surgeons' experience and preference to overcome the loss of venous return to the heart, the lack of which can cause cardiovascular collapse. Cannulas are placed in the portal and femoral veins; blood drains by gravity to a centrifugal pump, which then returns the blood to the upper body via a large-bore cannula (Figure 176-1). An alternative surgical approach, and one more commonly used, is the "piggyback" technique, in which the surgeon separates the liver from the IVC using a side bite of the IVC (i.e., partial IVC occlusion), allowing some IVC flow to continue during surgery. With this approach, portal venous return is still lost.

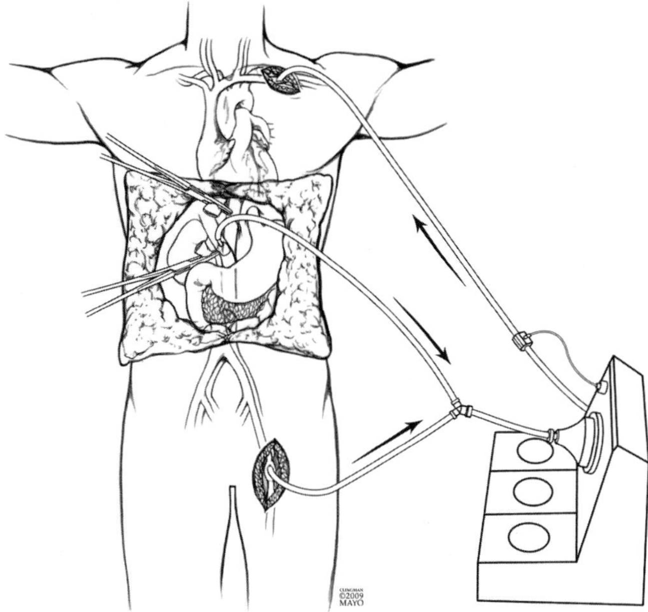

Figure 176-1 Venovenous bypass. The portal vein and inferior vena cava (via the femoral artery) are cannulated; blood drains by gravity to the pump and is then returned to a central vein in the upper body. (© Mayo Foundation for Medical Education and Research. All rights reserved.)

Once vascular anastomoses to the graft are complete, recirculation occurs. Liver inflow is restored by opening the portal vein (with or without the hepatic artery), blood is flushed through the nearly complete anastomosis, and then the IVC clamp is released. This results in the abrupt delivery of cold, potassium-containing, acidic blood to the heart, along with, occasionally, microthrombi or even air. Hypotension is common, pulmonary artery pressures elevate, and cardiac arrhythmia or even cardiac arrest may occur. Intravenously administered calcium chloride antagonizes potassium-induced changes, and low-dose epinephrine is frequently used for immediate hemodynamic support. Prolonged hypotension after recirculation, termed the postreperfusion syndrome, is most often due to systemic vasodilation; however, myocardial depression is sometimes seen. Vasopressor, inotropic, or both vasopressor and inotropic support should be used, as indicated; resolution typically occurs within 30 min. The final stage of transplantation involves hepatic artery anastomosis (if not already performed) and a biliary drainage procedure.

Intraoperative coagulation and transfusion management is often challenging; although average volumes of transfusions of blood and blood products have decreased in recent years, catastrophic bleeding still occurs. In addition to having low levels of circulating clotting factors due to decreased synthesis, most patients are thrombocytopenic as a result of sequestration and destruction of platelets in the liver and spleen. After recirculation, tissue plasminogen activator activity rises, which can result in marked fibrinolysis. Heparinoids are also released from the reperfused liver. Treatment of coagulopathy with platelets, fresh frozen plasma, and cryoprecipitate should take into account both the results of coagulation testing and the clinical situation. In the absence of significant bleeding, complete correction of coagulation abnormalities (according to the results of laboratory tests) is not undertaken because correction may increase the risk of thrombosis, particularly of the hepatic artery. Prophylactic use of antifibrinolytic agents is not usual; their use may be considered if clinically significant fibrinolysis occurs, as can be demonstrated with thromboelastography. Should catastrophic coagulopathy and bleeding occur, the use of recombinant factor VIIa is a consideration, but several deaths due to complete intravascular thrombosis following this treatment have been reported. Therefore, the use of recombinant factor VIIa should be guided by thromboelastography to ensure that the patient is not hypercoagulable. When large volumes of blood and blood products are transfused, ionized hypocalcemia secondary to citrate chelation may occur. It should also be noted that the quantity of blood and blood products transfused are both independent predictors of poor outcome in liver transplantation, so overtransfusion should be avoided. The goal of maintaining a hemoglobin concentration in the 8-g/dL to 10-g/dL range is common.

Postoperative Management

Straightforward cases can often be fast tracked, with early extubation if appropriate drug and dosing choices are planned intraoperatively. Immediate postoperative management should be in an area where adequate patient monitoring is available to detect early complications, particularly bleeding. Analgesia requirements can be surprisingly low for such a large procedure.

Suggested Readings

Kang Y, Audu P. Coagulation and liver transplantation. *Int Anesthesiol Clin.* 2006;44:17-36.

Ozier Y, Klinck JR. Anesthetic management of hepatic transplantation. *Curr Opin Anesthesiol.* 2008;21:391-400.

United Network for Organ Sharing. Available at: http://www.unos.org. Accessed August 3, 2012.

Warnaar N, Lisman T, Porte RJ. The two tales of coagulation in liver transplantation. *Curr Opin Organ Transpl.* 2008;13:298-303.

CHAPTER 177

Anesthesia for Patients with Hepatocellular Disease

Joseph J. Sandor, MD

Knowledge of the varied physiologic functions of the liver (Box 177-1) allows the anesthesia provider to anticipate potential problems when patients with hepatocellular disease present for surgery.

Patients with hepatocellular disease may have altered perioperative coagulation disorders and hypoglycemia. The pharmacokinetics and pharmacodynamics of anesthetic drugs may be altered by alcohol-induced microsomal enzyme induction, which can accelerate the metabolism of drugs and alter the amount of anesthetic drug necessary to achieve a specific anesthetic depth. Hypoalbuminemia increases the pharmacologically active fraction of several protein-bound drugs, which, combined with decreased degradation, results in an increased sensitivity to many drugs (e.g., opioids) in patients with hepatocellular disease.

Acute Hepatic Failure

Central nervous system manifestations of acute hepatic failure include encephalopathy, altered levels of consciousness, and hyperventilation from vitamin deficiency and increased serum levels of ammonia and other toxic metabolites. Hypoglycemia may result from impaired gluconeogenesis, depleted glycogen stores, and reduced insulin degradation. Cardiac output is increased from reduced systemic vascular resistance and increased arteriovenous shunting. Intrapulmonary shunting may produce hypoxemia. Patients often have coexisting renal disease and are more susceptible to developing infections. Of the proteins synthesized by the liver, factor VII has one of the shortest half-lives ($t_{1/2}$ approximately 6 h). Accordingly, the prothrombin time provides valuable information as to acute changes in hepatic function.

Surgery should be performed in patients with acute hepatic failure only in an emergency. Fresh frozen plasma and vitamin K can be given preoperatively to correct coagulation abnormalities. Because these patients have decreased rates of drug metabolism, anesthetic requirements are significantly reduced, and the effects of barbiturate and opioidergic agents are prolonged. Because plasma cholinesterase levels may be decreased but are usually adequate ($t_{1/2}$ approximately 14 days), succinylcholine does not significantly prolong apnea and, therefore, may be used. Blood glucose concentrations should be monitored.

These patients are at an increased risk of developing hypoxemia, hypotension, acidosis, hypokalemia, hypocalcemia, and hypomagnesemia. Large-bore intravenous access should be obtained preoperatively; hemodynamic measures should be invasively monitored, as appropriate; and anesthetic drugs should be carefully titrated to effect.

Box 177-1 Critical Processes Performed by the Liver

- Glucose homeostasis
  - Gluconeogenesis
  - Glycogenesis
  - Glycogenolysis
- Albumin formation
  - Maintain plasma oncotic pressure
  - Drug binding
- Protein formation
  - Albumin
  - Clotting factors
  - γ-Globulin
  - Enzymes (e.g., cholinesterase)
- Lipid metabolism
- Vitamin storage
  - Vitamin A
  - Vitamin D
  - Vitamin E
  - Vitamin K
- Vitamin synthesis
  - Vitamin A
  - Vitamin D
  - Vitamin B_{12}
- Drug and hormone degradation
- Blood storage and filtration
  - Clear degradation products of fibrinolysis
  - Prevent passage of bacteria from the gut into the blood
- Bile formation and excretion

Chronic Hepatic Disease

Anesthetic management of patients with chronic liver disease is dictated by the number and severity of cirrhosis-induced extrahepatic complications. Cardiovascular abnormalities may include increased cardiac output, increased intravascular volume, decreased blood viscosity, increased severity of arteriovenous shunting, congestive heart failure, and cardiomyopathy (e.g., ethanol-induced dilated cardiomyopathy). Arterial hypoxemia results from intrapulmonary arteriovenous shunting, ventilation/perfusion mismatch (as the result of decreased functional reserve capacity from ascites displacing the diaphragm cephalad), and recurrent pneumonia (related to decreased immunity and increased atelectasis). Hypoglycemia in the perioperative period should be anticipated. Patients with chronic hepatic disease are more likely than the general population to have cholestasis and cholelithiasis, either of which increases their susceptibility to developing cholecystitis and pancreatitis. Peptic ulcer disease occurs twice as often in people with liver disease, as compared with people without liver disease. These patients also may have gastroesophageal reflux and intestinal hypomotility.

Portal hypertension (causing varices and splenomegaly) and impaired coagulation from thrombocytopenia, factor deficiencies, disseminated intravascular coagulati[illegible]inolysis place these patients at risk for developing sudden mas[illegible]eeding. Renal disease may coexist with chronic liver disease; how[illegible], hepatorenal syndrome occurs as a manifestation of end-stage liver disease. Hepatic encephalopathy and peripheral neuropathy from nutritional deficiencies may arise.

Anesthesia Considerations

The preoperative history and physical examination of patients with hepatocellular disease should focus on identifying extrahepatic manifestations of chronic liver failure. The laboratory evaluation comprises arterial blood gas concentration, complete blood count, coagulation studies, and a chemistry panel that includes albumin and glucose concentrations. If the patient has no coagulopathy, a regional anesthetic technique may be used.

Benzodiazepine and opioidergic agents should be used cautiously. Some anesthesia providers advocate the use of H_2 antagonists, nonparticulate antacids, or proton pump inhibitors prior to induction of anesthesia to reduce these patients' risk of aspirating gastric contents.

The placement of an intraarterial catheter should be considered to facilitate perioperative monitoring of blood pressure and blood withdrawal to measure arterial blood gases; electrolyte, hemoglobin, and glucose concentrations; and coagulation status. Monitoring central venous pressure and, occasionally, pulmonary artery pressure aids in perioperative fluid management. If surgery is likely to be associated with massive blood loss, a rapid-infusion pump should be readily available. A peripheral nerve stimulator should be used to avoid administering excess amounts of neuromuscular blocking agents.

Rapid-sequence induction or awake intubation facilitates airway protection from aspiration. Doses of induction agents (etomidate, propofol) should be reduced because of the likelihood of patients having an increased sensitivity to the neurologic and cardiovascular effects of these drugs. In patients with liver disease, the hepatic arteries contribute a much greater proportion of blood to total hepatic blood flow; thus, decreases in mean arterial pressure should be avoided to prevent hepatocellular hypoxia. Avoiding light anesthesia, hypoxia, hypercarbia, and excessive positive-pressure ventilation prevents increased splanchnic vascular resistance; using halogenated inhalation agents without N_2O allows for delivery of a higher fraction of inspired O_2. Postoperative analgesic requirements are usually reduced in patients with hepatocellular disease.

Suggested Readings

Beck-Schimmer B, Breitenstein S, Urech S, et al. A randomized controlled trial on pharmacological preconditioning in liver surgery using a volatile anesthetic. *Ann Surg*. 2008;248:909-918.

Cammu G, Vermeiren K, Lecomte P, et al. Perioperative blood glucose management in patients undergoing tumor hepatectomy. *J Clin Anesth*. 2009;21: 329-335.

Craig RG, Hunter JM. Neuromuscular blocking drugs and their antagonists in patients with organ disease. *Anaesthesia*. 2009;64(Suppl 1):55-65.

Lee KH, Nam SH, Yoo SY, et al. Vecuronium requirement during liver transplantation under sevoflurane anesthesia. *J Anesth*. 2010;24(5):683-686.

Meltzer J, Brentjens TE. Renal failure in patients with cirrhosis: Hepatorenal syndrome and renal support strategies. *Curr Opin Anaesthesiol*. 2010;23: 139-144.

Shontz R, Karuparthy V, Temple R, Brennan TJ. Prevalence and risk factors predisposing to coagulopathy in patients receiving epidural analgesia for hepatic surgery. *Reg Anesth Pain Med*. 2009;34:308-311.

Stoelting RK, Dierdorf SF. Disease of the liver and biliary tract. In: Stoelting RK, Dierdorf SF, eds. *Anesthesia and Co-Existing Disease*. 5th ed. New York: Churchill Livingstone; 2008:259-278.

Tao KM, Yang LQ, Liu YT, et al. Volatile anesthetics might be more beneficial than propofol for postoperative liver function in cirrhotic patients receiving hepatectomy. *Med Hypotheses*. 2010;75(6):555-557.

Taurà P, Fuster J, Mercadal J, et al. The use of β-adrenergic drugs improves hepatic oxygen metabolism in cirrhotic patients undergoing liver resection. *J Hepatol*. 2010;52:340-347.

van Ginhoven TM, Mitchell JR, Verweij M, et al. The use of preoperative nutritional interventions to protect against hepatic ischemia-reperfusion injury. *Liver Transpl*. 2009;15:1183-1191.

Wang CH, Chen CL, Cheng KW, et al. Bispectral index monitoring in healthy, cirrhotic, and end-stage liver disease patients undergoing hepatic operation. *Transpl Proc*. 2008;40:2489-2491.

CHAPTER 178
Autonomic Dysreflexia

Michael E. Johnson, MD, PhD

Autonomic dysreflexia (AD, also referred to as autonomic hyperreflexia) is a potentially life-threatening emergency. It occurs in at least two thirds of patients with a spinal cord injury at T6 or above and is characterized by acute hypertension, usually accompanied by bradycardia, in response to a noxious stimulus below the level of the spinal cord lesion. Distention of the bladder or bowel is a frequent cause of AD.

Pathophysiology

AD results from unopposed sympathetic efferent outflow in response to noxious afferent input below the level of the spinal cord injury, with reflex activation of parasympathetic outflow above the T6 dermatomal level. The pathways involved are summarized in Figure 178-1.

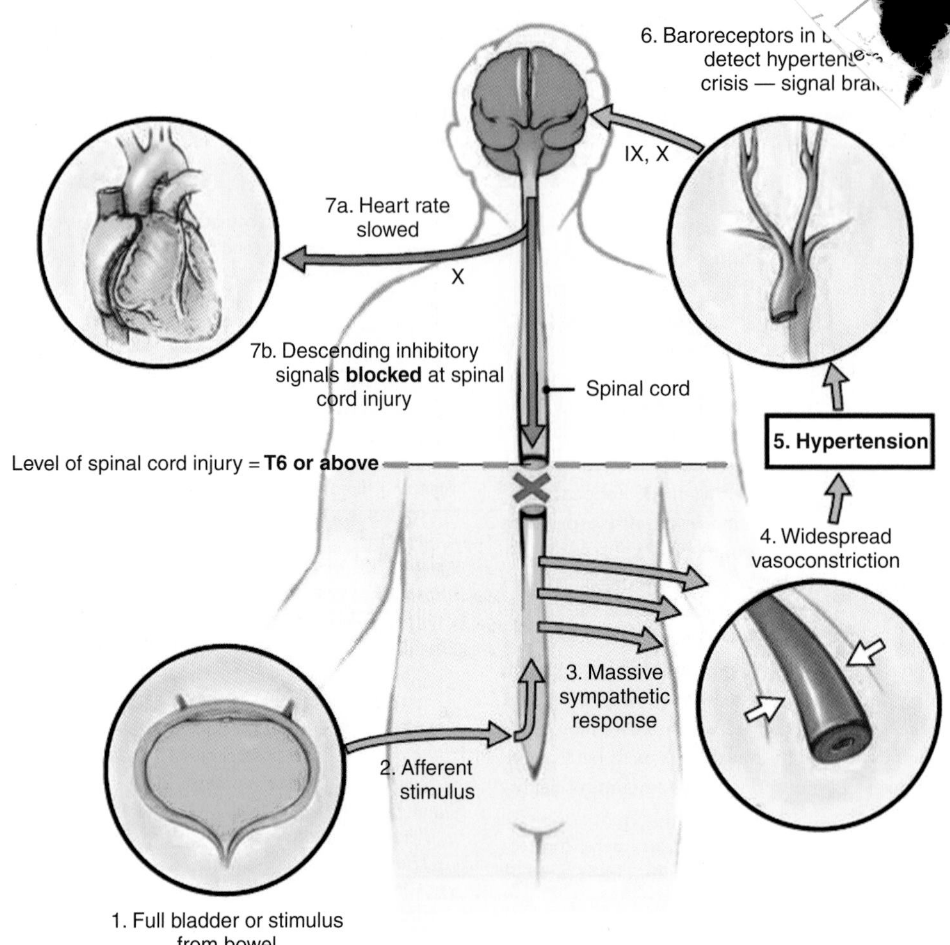

Figure 178-1 Diagram illustrating how autonomic dysreflexia occurs in a person with a spinal cord injury. The afferent stimulus—in this case, a distended bladder—triggers a peripheral sympathetic response, which results in vasoconstriction and hypertension. Descending inhibitory signals, which would normally counteract the rise in blood pressure, are blocked at the level of the spinal cord injury. The roman numerals (IX, X) refer to the cranial nerves. (Reprinted, with permission, from Blackmer J. Rehabilitation medicine: 1. Autonomic dysreflexia. Can Med Assoc J. 2003;169:931-935.)

Afferent stimuli from an insult below the level of the spinal cord injury can ascend via spinothalamic and posterior columns to activate sympathetic neurons up to the level of the cord injury, discharging these neurons as an independent reflex at the level of the cord. Ordinarily this would elicit compensatory bulbospinal sympathetic inhibition via descending spinal pathways, but these pathways are now blocked by the spinal cord injury, resulting in unopposed vasoconstriction below the injury. With a spinal cord injury at T6 or higher, noxious stimuli result in intense constriction of splanchnic vascular beds and the vasculature in the lower extremities, leading to an exaggerated hypertensive response. Cord injury below T10 does not cause AD, whereas patients with injuries at the T6 to T10 levels may have a mild blood pressure elevation without full-blown AD. AD can occur in patients with incomplete spinal cord injuries, but the AD is more severe in those with a complete injury.

Baroreceptors in the aortic arch and carotid sinus respond to hypertension by activating brainstem vasomotor reflexes, resulting in increased parasympathetic activation via the intact cranial nerve X effector pathway, which is unaffected by the spinal cord injury, usually resulting in bradycardia. Tachycardia is also possible but occurs less frequently, presumably depending on the balance between catecholamines that diffuse into the bloodstream after sympathetic neuron activation below the spinal cord lesion and vagal outflow. Parasympathetic activation also causes vasodilation above the level of the cord injury.

Although AD has been reported to occur in the acute phase of a spinal cord injury, it generally becomes evident 1 to 6 months after the initial injury. This delayed occurrence is attributed to injury-induced changes in the structure and electrophysiology of both primary afferents and spinal neurons, as well as increased sensitivity of the peripheral vasculature to α-adrenergic stimulation, which heightens the exaggerated sympathetic response to noxious stimuli.

Clinical Features

Acute hypertension is the sign of AD that is of greatest concern, causing the major morbid conditions associated with AD (e.g., myocardial ischemia, arrhythmia, congestive heart failure, cerebral ischemia, cerebral hemorrhage, and hypertensive encephalopathy). Initial blood pressure elevation may be mild and disguised by the fact that resting blood pressure in patients with high spinal cord injuries is usually low. A blood pressure of 120/80 mm Hg in a patient whose normal pressure is 90/60 mm Hg should raise concern. Blood pressures as high as 250 to 300/100 to 130 mm Hg have been reported during AD. Bradycardia and other arrhythmias often accompany the hypertension.

Other signs and symptoms can vary among patients and even among episodes of AD in the same patient and may be masked by sedative or anesthetic drugs. In an awake patient, AD often presents with the triad of severe headache, profuse sweating, and cutaneous flushing above the level of the spinal cord injury. The skin below the level of the injury may be pale and cool with piloerection. Nasal congestion, anxiety, malaise, nausea, and visual disturbances may also occur. These reactions are generally consistent with marked sympathetic activation below the cord injury, with cephalad reflex parasympathetic activity. However, the hyperhydrosis of AD is most common on the face and neck, above the level of cord injury, rather than below, where sympathetic outflow is maximal. The mechanism is not well understood, although it could involve a direct effect of catecholamines spilling over into the bloodstream, a central effect of excess catecholamines passing the blood-brain barrier, or a direct effect of intense parasympathetic stimulation on the forehead and upper lip, the only area in humans where there is parasympathetic as well as sympathetic innervation of sweat glands.

Prevention and Treatment

AD is a potential concern during any surgical procedure in which innervation of the surgical field is below the level of the spinal cord injury. Anything that would elicit pain in a patient who does not have a spinal cord injury can cause AD in an at-risk patient. A patient's history of AD should alert the anesthesia provider to the risk of the patient subsequently developing AD and to its potential magnitude in a specific patient, but any patient with a spinal cord injury at T6 or above should be considered at risk, even in the absence of previous episodes of AD. Pelvic visceral pain is a particularly potent stimulus of AD, and thus, urologic and bowel operations and childbirth are the most frequent causes of significant AD that most anesthesia providers will encounter. The magnitude of AD increases with the magnitude of the sensory stimulus and with increasing distance between the level of the cord lesion and the level of the dorsal root entry zone of the stimulus.

Prevention of AD is the ideal and can be accomplished with a dense regional block or a deep inhalation anesthetic. (This may require education of the patient and surgeon to accept the need for an anesthetic for a procedure that would not elicit any conscious sensation of pain in the patient.) Sevoflurane has been shown to prevent AD in at-risk patients undergoing transurethral litholapaxy with a half-maximal effective concentration (EC_{50}) of 3.1% and an EC_{95} of 3.8% in 50% N_2O. Although both epidurally and spinally administered local anesthetics have been used successfully to prevent AD, epidural anesthesia may not block the larger sacral nerve roots as effectively as does spinal anesthesia. It is difficult to assess the level of neuraxial block in a patient with a high cord injury, so a spinal anesthetic confirmed by cerebrospinal fluid return during placement may offer more assurance of an adequate block than would an epidural anesthetic. Anesthesia providers may encounter technical challenges in accessing the subarachnoid space in patients with spinal cord injuries and who have low resting blood pressures, but, in practice, accessing the subarachnoid space has not proved to be problematic in most patients. Topical local anesthetic agents administered alone prior to performing superficial rectal and urinary procedures has not been uniformly effective in preventing AD. Neither parenterally nor epidurally administered opioids, nor N_2O, is consistently effective in preventing AD, except for epidural meperidine, which also has some local anesthetic properties. Other intravenously administered anesthetic agents have not been extensively tested in patients with AD.

When AD does occur, it is a medical emergency and must be treated rapidly. Removal of the triggering stimulus by a temporary halt in the surgical procedure may reverse AD and allow institution of more potent prophylaxis and treatment. In mild cases, nonpharmacologic measures such as elevating the head and torso, loosening tight clothing, and relieving inadvertent bladder or bowel distention may suffice. The diagnosis of AD in the setting of an operation below the spinal cord injury in a susceptible patient is usually straightforward, but other potential causes of acute hypertension should also be considered. In a laboring parturient, preeclampsia can also cause severe hypertension, but in patients with AD, the blood pressure elevation is usually much more marked during uterine contraction, with decline during relaxation. It should also be kept in mind that obstruction of a urinary catheter and bowel impaction are frequent causes of AD in nonanesthetized patients and can occur in any susceptible patient during any surgical procedure, including those perfomed on sites above the level of the spinal cord injury.

Multiple pharmacologic agents have been used to treat AD, but for many of them, their use is supported by only anecdotal case reports. The use of sublingually administered nifedipine was widely recommended in the past but has fallen into disfavor because of reports of severe adverse reactions when nifedipine is given for acute blood pressure control in patients without AD. Case reports have shown that nitroglycerin, nitroprusside, and other nitrates have been used effectively, although the use of sildenafil or other phosphodiesterase inhibitors in the previous 24 h needs to be ruled out first. Sildenafil alone is not effective in treating AD. The oral α-adrenergic receptor blocking agents terazosin and prazosin are effective in the long-term prevention of AD outside the operating room, and intravenously administered phentolamine is acutely effective, but the effect of phenoxybenzamine is inconsistent. Intravenously administered prostaglandin E_1 and hydralazine are effective for acute treatment of AD, although hydralazine appears to be more likely to cause excessive hypotension. Labetolol and metoprolol have been used successfully in individual cases.

AD can continue into the postoperative period; therefore, patients who develop AD require careful monitoring and continued treatment. AD can also present de novo in the postanesthesia care unit, so susceptible patients should be appropriately monitored.

Suggested Readings

Blackmer J. Rehabilitation medicine: 1. Autonomic dysreflexia. *Can Med Assoc J.* 2003;169:931-935.

Hou S, Duale H, Rabchevsky AG. Intraspinal sprouting of unmyelinated pelvic afferents after complete spinal cord injury is correlated with autonomic dysreflexia induced by visceral pain. *Neuroscience.* 2009;159:369-379.

Krassioukov A, Warburton DE, Teasell R, Eng JJ, Spinal Cord Injury Rehabilitation Evidence Research Team. A systematic review of the management of autonomic dysreflexia after spinal cord injury. *Arch Phys Med Rehabil.* 2009;90:682-695.

Laird AS, Finch AM, Waite PM, Carrive P. Peripheral changes above and below injury level lead to prolonged vascular responses following high spinal cord injury. *Am J Physiol—Heart Circ Physiol.* 2008;294:H785-H792.

Murphy DB, McGuire G, Peng P. Treatment of autonomic hyperreflexia in a quadriplegic patient by epidural anesthesia in the postoperative period. *Anesth Analg.* 1999;89:148-149.

Reitz A, Schmid DM, Curt A, et al. Autonomic dysreflexia in response to pudendal nerve stimulation. *Spinal Cord.* 2003;41:539-542.

Yoo KY, Jeong CW, Kim SJ, et al. Sevoflurane concentrations required to block autonomic hyperreflexia during transurethral litholapaxy in patients with complete spinal cord injury. *Anesthesiology.* 2008;108:858-863.

CHAPTER 179

Anesthesia in Austere Environments

Craig C. McFarland, MD, and C. George Merridew, MBBS, FANCZA

For many anesthesia providers, the delivery of an anesthetic in an austere environment implies that the provider has volunteered for a humanitarian mission in a developing country or is in the military and practicing in field conditions—synonymous with an austere environment. However, any time a situation arises in which medical capability is significantly below standards that are typically available in developed countries, the provider is indeed practicing in an austere environment. Such austere environments include the following:

- Mass casualty event in which the number of cases overwhelms capacity
- Natural disaster in which the hospital is damaged or loses electricity or water
- Developing country that is disrupted by low-grade civil war
- Developing country in which health care spending is less than $5 per person per year
- Disaster (e.g., natural, industrial, terrorist) in which care is provided on site

Graduates of Western anesthesia training programs can cope well in such situations, provided that they understand the basic requisites of disaster management and the pharmacology and physiology of anesthesia. The latter allows the provider to choose among several options for delivery of a safe anesthetic—general anesthesia using a parenteral versus an inhalation technique or a regional anesthetic.

Basic Principles

The austere environment is characterized by a relative lack of medical supplies, supplemental O_2 electricity, trained health care personnel, or evacuation options. Each of these deficiencies requires proper planning to make medical care in an austere environment successful. When resupply is not a reliable option, a medical team may be forced to carry all of their supplies with them. This puts a premium on reusable items and on equipment with a low weight and a small footprint.

A lack of trained personnel or limited evacuation options make proper patient selection and selection of the appropriate surgical procedure crucial. When patients present for elective operations, care must be taken to choose the patients in whom the most benefit is likely to be obtained with the least risk. On the other hand, when patients present for emergent operations, a surgical course must be chosen that is least likely to outstrip the medical team's capability for perioperative care or to degrade the medical team's ability to care for subsequent patients. For example, an extremity mangled by a landmine explosion is better amputated if the care, equipment, and time required for limb salvage and rehabilitation are not available. The process of selecting patients for surgery, or for selecting the proper surgical treatment for patients, requires collaboration among the anesthesia provider, the surgeon, and the rest of the medical team. In an austere environment, cesarean sections and amputations would be commonly performed, whereas cardiac or neurosurgical procedures would be rare (Table 179-1).

Having a limited supply of supplemental O_2 or electricity places a premium on optimal use of anesthetic techniques that permit spontaneous ventilation, preserve hypoxic pulmonary vasoconstriction, and minimally depress consciousness. If a regional anesthesia technique is appropriate for the surgical procedure, it meets these criteria. If general anesthesia is required, one must weigh the risks and benefits of a parenteral (intramuscular versus a total intravenous anesthetic) versus an inhalation technique.

Options for Anesthesia

Regional Anesthesia

If the afferent pathways from the surgical site can be blocked with local anesthetic agents, regional anesthesia is optimal for the austere environment. Depending upon the surgical site, this may entail a field block, a peripheral nerve or nerve plexus block, a paravertebral block, or a neuraxial technique. Many of these blocks were performed historically and can still be performed in an austere environment by experienced providers using anatomic landmarks with or without the aid of a nerve stimulator. The main disadvantages of regional anesthesia are that it is not sufficient for all surgical procedures, its success is dependent upon the experience of the practitioner, and it can be time consuming to perform and resource intensive. Additionally, a spinal hematoma, although very rare, is not easily diagnosed or treated in the austere environment; on the other hand, advantages include maintenance of consciousness and of oropharyngeal reflexes and superior postoperative pain control.

General Anesthesia

Parenteral Anesthesia

Ketamine is perhaps the most useful anesthetic drug in the austere environment. It can be administered orally, intramuscularly, or intravenously and

Table 179-1 Surgical Procedures in an Austere Environment

Common Field Operations	Uncommon Field Operations
Abscess incision and drainage	Procedures requiring invasive monitoring
Fasciotomy	Procedures requiring any postoperative intensive care
Amputations	
Débridement of wounds or burns	Internal fixation of fractures
External fixation of fractures	Laparoscopy, endoscopy, arthroscopy
Emergency laparotomy	Subspecialty surgery
Emergency caesarean section	Note: Militaries from developed countries may have good ICU and evacuation capabilities
Evacuation of retained placenta	

ICU, Intensive care unit.

can be used alone or as an adjunct to other drugs. Because ketamine provides hypnosis, analgesia, and amnesia, it can be used as a total anesthetic. Ketamine maintains or even increases skeletal muscle tone, an impediment for the surgeon undertaking caesarean section with spontaneous ventilation. In comparison with other systemic anesthetic agents, at a given degree of analgesia, ketamine maintains better hemodynamics, airway control, and spontaneous ventilation. These qualities make ketamine indispensable to the anesthesia provider in an austere environment. Qualities to be aware of include the dose-dependent, although not ubiquitous, psychotomimetic effects, a tendency to promote excessive salivation, and a relative contraindication in patients with ocular and brain injuries.

Total Intravenous Anesthesia

Total intravenous anesthesia (TIVA) can be used for analgesia or sedation or as an intraoperative anesthetic. It is frequently administered as a mixture of propofol, an opioid, ketamine, and often a neuromuscular blocking drug. Such mixtures have the advantage of not requiring an anesthesia machine, an infusion pump, electricity, or batteries, resulting in a small logistical footprint. Depending upon the particular mixture of agents, TIVA may take advantage of the benefits of ketamine, conferring a decreased risk of redistribution hypothermia compared with inhalation anesthetic agents, and may not inhibit hypoxic pulmonary vasoconstriction as much as does TIVA without the addition of ketamine. An example of a TIVA recipe is found in Box 179-1. Disadvantages of TIVA include the facts that providing TIVA requires adequate intravenous access and that many anesthesia providers are unfamiliar with providing TIVA.

Inhalation Anesthesia

Inhalation anesthesia is considered by some to have the largest logistical footprint, especially if supplemental O_2 is used. Some British and Australasian anesthesia providers consider inhalation anesthesia delivered with a drawover vaporizer to be the preferred technique for use in an austere environment. Many anesthesia providers in the United States, however, may not be familiar with a drawover vaporizer, such as the Ohmeda Universal Portable Anesthesia Complete (Figure 179-1), but, given the opportunity, most providers would find it easy to set up and use, and very reliable. This device is designed to deliver inhalation agents to a spontaneously ventilating patient but can be combined with a portable ventilator, such as the Uni-Vent Eagle 754 (Impact Instrumentation, Inc.; West Caldwell, NJ). When using this technique, the anesthesia provider should select patients for whom supplemental O_2 would not be necessary unless a source of O_2 is readily available.

Other drawover vaporizers in current use include the Oxford Miniature Vaporiser (OMV), the Epstein Macintosh Oxford (EMO) both from Penlon, UK), the Diamedica Drawover Vaporiser (DDOV in the Glostavent anesthesia machine; Diamedica, UK), and the vaporizer of the Universal Anesthesia Machine (UAM; Gradian Health Systems LLC, NYNY). The latter two machines include a ventilator (basic intermittent positive pressure ventilation with or without positive end expiratory pressure), compressor and O_2 concentrator and can use partial rebreathing circuits or drawover. They are designed for missionary and other relatively fixed developing world environments with electrical generators.

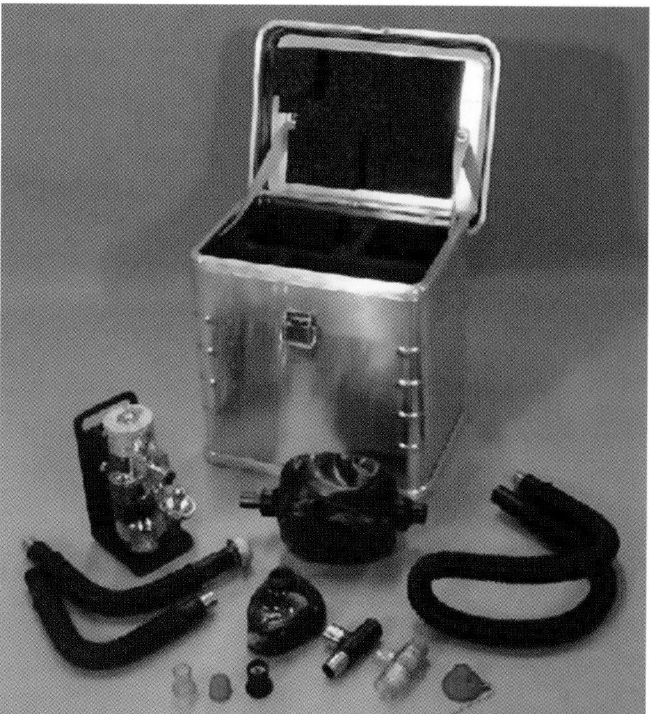

Figure 179-1 The carrying case of the universal portable anesthesia complete (PAC) contains a spill-proof, agent-specific, drawover vaporizer and an open-circuit breathing assembly. The drawover system is designed to provide anesthesia using ambient air as the main carrier of anesthetic agent. The patient's inspiratory efforts draw air through the vaporizer, in which the anesthesia provider has added an inhalation anesthetic agent. Supplementary O_2 can be added by means of an inlet. The portable anesthesia unit is suitable for use with spontaneously breathing patients or manually assisted ventilation. (Courtesy of Ohmeda, subsidiary of GE Healthcare.)

Final Thoughts

In developing countries, tragically, many children are victims of injury, burns, or surgical illness. Anesthesia providers who do not typically care for children can take comfort in knowing that their training should allow them to function well in an austere environment when treating children who require care. When new to the austere environment, the medical team should begin by treating healthier patients first while the team adjusts to its surroundings and to one another and develops experience and

Box 179-1 Recipe for Total Intravenous Anesthesia

To create the solution for infusion as a total intravenous anesthesia (TIVA), mix 40 mL of 1% propofol, 250 μg (5 mL) of fentanyl, and 250 mg (5 mL) of ketamine in 50 mL of saline (final concentration: 4 mg of propofol, 2.5 mg of ketamine, and 2.5 μg of fentanyl/mL). Using a standard 20-drops/mL drip set and assuming an 80-kg patient, 1 drop/sec equates to a propofol infusion rate of 150 $\mu g \cdot kg^{-1} \cdot min^{-1}$. One drop every 3 sec equates to a propofol infusion rate of 50 $\mu g \cdot kg^{-1} \cdot min^{-1}$. These rates provide good starting points for general anesthesia, and the infusion rates are readily titrated as needed, based on the patient's motor and cardiovascular responses to stimuli.

Box 179-2 Tips for Providing Pediatric Anesthesia in Developing Countries

Up to half the population is younger than 15 years of age in many countries.

Even in a well neonatal patient, operations may be futile if they are more complex than an inguinal hernia repair.

It may be helpful to think of a child as a frail adult with a short, narrow trachea, easily made cold and hypovolemic.

Drawover spontaneous or assisted ventilation by facemask may be used for a well 3-kg infant.

To use an Ayres T-piece with a drawover vaporizer, vapor-laden air ± added oxygen in a near-continuous stream (generated by an assistant squeezing the drawover circuit's self-inflating bag) becomes the fresh gas flow for the Ayre's T-piece circuit, applied to the patient by the anesthesia provider.

confidence with the anesthetic techniques that will be used most often. Additional tips for performing pediatric anesthesia in developing countries are listed in Box 179-2.

Obstetric anaesthesia is inevitable regardless of the main mission, and patients do not present for normal delivery. The obstetric surgery has basic indications: severe antepartum bleeding, prolonged obstructed labour, pre-eclampsia or eclampsia. Often the foetus is dead and the mother is at risk of dying. Retained placenta cases come late, with bleeding and definite septicaemia.

Suggested Readings

Buckenmaier CC 3rd, Lee EH, Shields CH, et al. Regional anesthesia in austere environments. *Reg Anesth Pain Med*. 2003;2:321-327.

Dobson MB. Anaesthesia at the district hospital. 2nd ed. World Health Organisation; 2006.

Dufour D, et al. Surgery for victims of war. 3rd ed. International Committee of the Red Cross; 1998.

Gegel BT. A field-expedient Ohmeda Universal Portable Anesthesia Complete draw-over vaporizer setup. *AANA J*. 2008;76:185-187.

Grathwohl KW, Venticinque SG. Organizational characteristics of the austere intensive care unit: The evolution of military trauma and critical care medicine; applications for civilian medical care systems. *Crit Care Med*. 2008; 36(7 Suppl):S275-283.

Hospitals for war-wounded. International Committee of the Red Cross, revised edition, 2005.

Knowlton LM, Gosney JE, Chackungal S, et al. Consensus statements regarding the multidisciplinary care of limb amputation patients in disasters or humanitarian emergencies: Report of the 2011 Humanitarian Action Summit Surgical Working Group on amputations following disasters or conflict. *Prehosp Disaster Med*. 2011;26:438-448.

Lewis S, Jagdish S. Total intravenous anaesthesia for war surgery. *J R Army Med Corps*. 2010;156(4 Suppl 1):301-307.

Mellor AJ. Anaesthesia in austere environments. *J R Army Med Corps*. 2005; 151:272-276.

Missair A, Gebhard R, Pierre E, et al. Surgery under extreme conditions in the aftermath of the 2010 Haiti earthquake: The importance of regional anesthesia. *Prehosp Disaster Med*. 2010;25:487-493.

Reynolds PC, Furukawa KT. Modern draw-over anesthetic vaporizers used to deliver anesthesia in austere and battlefield conditions. *Milit Med*. 2003;168:ii-iii.

PART G Obstetrics

CHAPTER 180

Maternal Physiologic Changes in Pregnancy

Gurinder M. S. Vasdev, MD, and Barry A. Harrison, MD

Maternal physiologic changes in pregnancy begin approximately 5 weeks after implantation and may not return to normal until 8 weeks after delivery (Table 180-1).

Respiratory System

A variety of pregnancy-related changes occur in the respiratory system and may lead to maternal airway complications, which contribute to anesthesia-related maternal mortality risk in the United States. Increased vascularity of the upper airway and nares may result in edema of the upper airway, thus necessitating the use of a smaller tracheal tube. Decreased chest wall compliance may lead to early O_2 desaturation, and decreased functional residual capacity (20%) and increased O_2 demand (60%) may result in rapid O_2 desaturation during apneic episodes.

Physiologic compensatory mechanisms in the mother yield improved fetal oxygenation. The mechanisms include a rightward shift in the maternal oxyhemoglobin dissociation curve (P_{50} = 30 mm Hg) and a 50% increase in minute ventilation. Progesterone is responsible for increasing the sensitivity of the central respiratory center to CO_2, which would cause a respiratory alkalosis; however, because renal excretion of bicarbonate is increased in pregnant women, a neutral pH is maintained. Pregnant women also have a higher Po_2 concentration, compared with the nonpregnant state.

Cardiovascular System

A myriad of cardiovascular changes occur during pregnancy. For example, maternal cardiac output increases 40% to meet the metabolic demands of both the mother and the fetus. The rise in cardiac output is initially due to an increase in stroke volume and, as pregnancy progresses, is maintained by an increase in heart rate as the stroke volume decreases. Progesterone decreases pulmonary and systemic vascular resistance, yet central venous and pulmonary artery occlusion pressures remain unchanged. Plasma volume increases up to 40% to 50% due to increased aldosterone production. Because red blood cell mass does not increase as much as does the blood volume, a dilutional anemia results.

When the pregnant woman is in the supine position, uterine compression of the inferior vena cava and aorta causes hypotension; however, this can be readily resolved by placing the parturient in a 15-degree left lateral tilt. Compression of the inferior vena cava and fluid retention also produce ankle edema and varicose veins and can enlarge portal-systemic shunts. Electrocardiographic changes (e.g., left-axis deviation, T-wave inversion in lead III) occur, with cardiac enlargement and rotation of the heart cephalad and leftward.

Gastrointestinal System

Pregnant women are more prone to developing symptomatic gastroesophageal reflux because their gastric pH is decreased, resulting from the production of gastrin by the placenta beginning at approximately 15 weeks of gestation and mechanical obstruction by the gravid uterus that delays gastric emptying and increases intragastric pressure. Lower esophageal sphincter competency is compromised when the gravid uterus causes the gastroesophageal junction to shift cephalad and posterior. Additionally, lower esophageal sphincter tone is altered by high progesterone and estrogen levels.

The risk of aspiration of gastric contents during induction of anesthesia is increased not only when the parturient undergoes emergency cesarean section (2% of deliveries in the United States) under general anesthesia, but, in reality, at any time after 18 to 20 weeks of pregnancy if the woman requires general anesthesia for a surgical procedure. Patients with larger intrauterine size (e.g., multiple gestations or polyhydramnios) are at risk even earlier during pregnancy.

Renal Function

Elevated intraabdominal pressure and changes in bladder size and shape lead to mechanical obstruction and ureteral reflux, which increases the incidence of ascending urinary tract infection. Glomerular filtration is increased by 50% above nonpregnant values and is responsible for a 40% reduction in blood urea nitrogen and creatinine levels during normal pregnancy. Glucosuria without hyperglycemia is due to a decrease in renal absorption of glucose, whereas protein excretion rises, resulting in proteinuria (up to 300 mg/day).

Hepatic Function

Minor changes in hepatic transaminase concentrations (e.g., aspartate aminotransferase [AST], lactate dehydrogenase [LDH]) may occur. Dilution of plasma proteins causes a decrease in the albumin:globulin ratio. Accordingly, the free fraction of albumin-bound medications is increased. Plasma cholinesterase levels are decreased (by dilution), but this does not result in a significant prolongation of succinylcholine-induced neuromuscular blockade.

Hematologic System

Pregnancy causes an activation of platelets, with an increased platelet turnover and shorter half-life. Levels of factors VII, VIII, X, and XII and fibrinogen are increased. The fibrinolytic system is depressed by a relative reduction of antithrombin III, resulting in a hypercoagulable state and rendering pregnant women more susceptible to developing thromboembolic disease.

Table 180-1 Maternal Physiologic Changes during Pregnancy

Parameter	Change during Pregnancy	Normal Pregnancy Value*
Cardiac		
Rate	↑	75-95 beats/min
SV	↑	
CO	↑	3-8 L/min
MAP	↓	80 mm Hg
SVR	↓	1200-1500 dyn • s^{-1} • cm^{-5}
Respiratory		
Rate	None	
V_T	↑	↑40%-45%
$\dot{V}$	↑	10.5 L/min
ERV	↓	550 mL
FRC	↓	1350 mL
Blood gas concentrations		
pH, arterial	None	7.4-7.45
P_{CO_2}	↓	25-33 mm Hg
P_{O_2}	↑	92-107 mm Hg
HCO_3^-	↓	16-22 mEq/L
Hematologic		
Blood volume	↑	4500 mL or 100 mL/kg
Plasma volume	↑	+45%
Erythrocyte volume	↑	+10%-15%
Hemoglobin	↓	11.5-15 g/dl
Hematocrit	↓	32%-36%
WBC count	↑	6000-20,000/μL
Procoagulant factors†	↑	
Anticoagulant activity‡	↓	
PAI 1 & 2	↑	
Iron	↓	30-193 μg/mL
TIBC	↑	80.1 μmol/L
Electrolytes/Renal		
Renal blood flow	↑	700 mL/min
GFR	↑	140 mL/min
Serum Cr	↓	0.53-0.9 mg/dL
Serum BUN	↓	8-10 mg/dL
HCO_3^-	None	15-20 mEq/L
Na^{2+}	↓	130-148 mEq/L
K^+	None or ↓§	3.3-5.0 mEq/L
Cl^-	↓	97-109 mEq/L
Metabolic		
Basal body temperature	↑	
O_2 consumption	↑	
Insulin resistance	↑	
Gastrointestinal		
Lower esophageal sphincter tone	↓	
Gastric emptying time	None except during labor	
Gastric acid secretion	↑	
Hepatobiliary system		
Gallbladder emptying time	↑	
Liver size	None	
ALP	↑	Up to 2-4 × normal value
Bilirubin/AST/ALT	None	
LDH	↑	650-700 U/L
Prothrombin time	None	
Albumin	↓	2.3-4.2 g/dL
Lipids		
Cholesterol	↑	141-210/219-349 mg/dL¶
Triglycerides	↑	

*Values are approximate and vary throughout pregnancy.
†Factors XII:c, VII:c, VII, and V; von Willebrand factors; and fibrinogen.
‡Activated protein C and protein S.
§Although there are total body accumulations of Na^+ and K^+, because of the retention of fluid and increase in plasma volumes, concentrations decrease.
¶First trimester/third trimester.
ALP, Alkaline phosphatase; ALT, alanine transaminase; AST, aspartate aminotransferase; BUN, blood urea nitrogen; CO, cardiac output; Cr, creatinine; ERV, expiratory reserve volume; FRC, functional residual capacity; GFR, glomerular filtration rate; LDH, lactate dehydrogenase; MAP, mean arterial pressure; PAI, plasminogen activator inhibitor; RBC, red blood cell; SV, stroke volume; SVR, systemic vascular resistance; TIBC, total iron-binding capacity; $\dot{V}$, minute ventilation; V_T, tidal volume; WBC, white blood cell.

Neurologic System

Local anesthetic requirements for neuraxial blockade are decreased during pregnancy secondary to reduced volume in the epidural space (epidural vein engorgement), decreased volume of cerebrospinal fluid, increased cerebrospinal fluid pH, and enhanced neural sensitivity to local anesthetic agents. The minimum alveolar concentration of inhalation anesthetics is also reduced 40% because of the hormone changes of pregnancy.

Uterine Physiology

Uterine blood flow and placental perfusion are affected by systemic vascular resistance, aortocaval compression, and uterine contraction. Placental blood supply is determined by spiral intervillous arteries, which are maximally dilated (Figure 180-1). They are supplied by arcuate and radial arteries, the ovarian arteries, and uterine arteries. Myometrial tension decreases the caliber of spiral arteries, reducing placental perfusion. Spiral arteries are maximally dilated and sensitive to the effects of α-adrenergic receptor agonists (e.g., phenylephrine). Vasoconstriction can cause dramatic changes in placental blood supply. The surface area and integrity of the placenta are affected by maternal and placental disorders.

Prolonged uterine contraction (hypertonia) can cause fetal asphyxia. Treatment options include fluids, bed rest, O_2 and tocolytic agents (e.g., nitroglycerin and albuterol). After delivery, uterine contraction is potentiated with massage, oxytocin, methylergonovine maleate, and carboprost tromethamine. Approximately 500 mL of blood are added to the maternal circulation with uterine contraction.

Fetal Oxygenation

Fetal oxygenation is dependent on placental blood supply, surface area integrity, and fetal cardiac output. Fetal cardiac output is rate dependent.

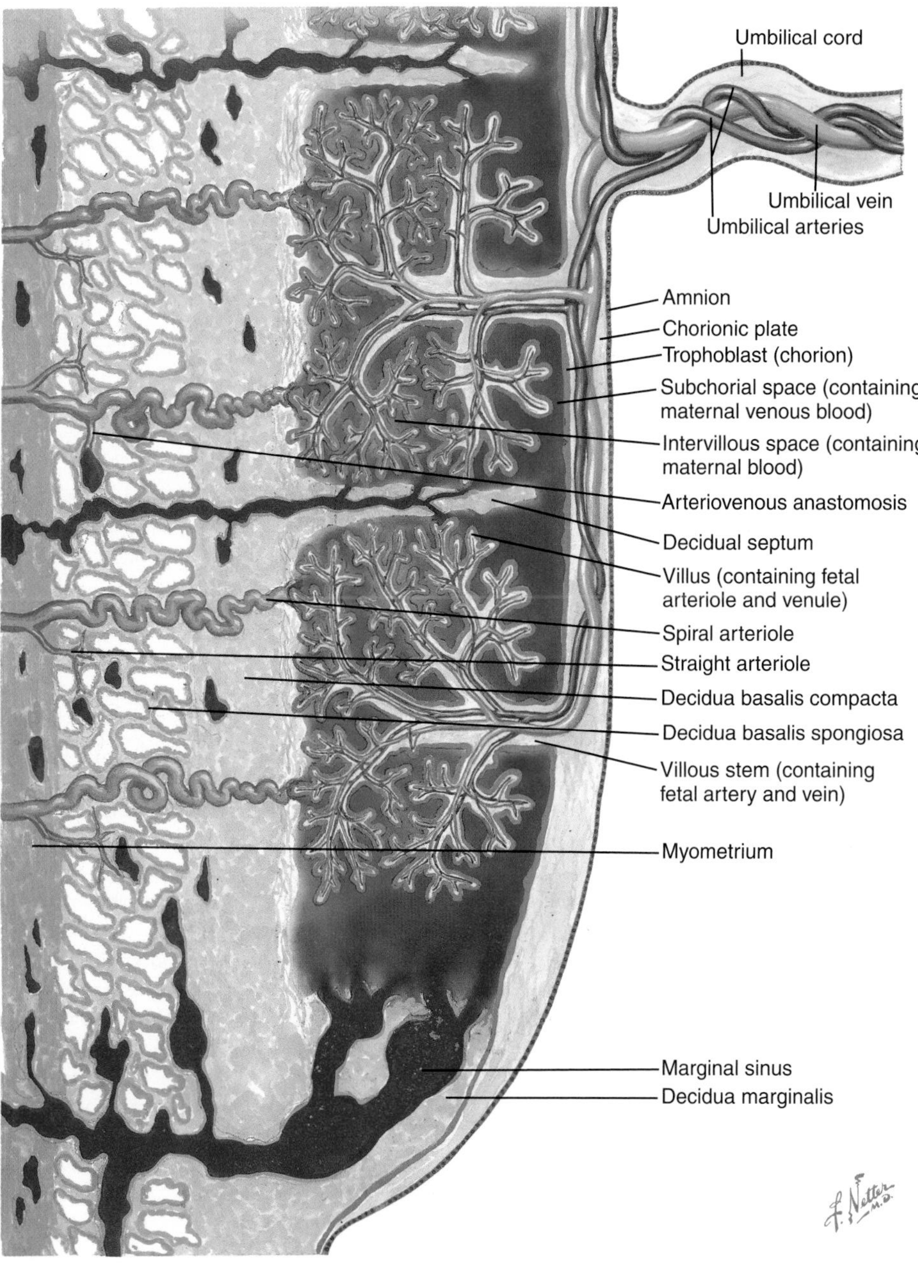

Figure 180-1 Circulation in the placenta. (Netter illustration from www.netterimages.com. © Elsevier Inc. All rights reserved.)

Mechanical compression of the umbilical cord decreases the delivery of O_2 to the fetus. Maternal-fetal O_2 transfer is facilitated by a leftward shifting of the fetal oxyhemoglobin curve. Fetal blood gas concentrations are dependent on placental perfusion and maternal ventilation. Respiratory acidosis occurs with maternal hypoventilation.

Parturition

At 40 weeks of gestation, the fetus is mature and ready for birth. Factors that control the initiation of labor are not clearly understood, but labor results from a production of prostaglandin, which increases oxytocin receptors in uterine myometria. As oxytocin levels increase, rhythmic contractions of the uterus lead to cervical dilation. The cervix is softened prior to the descent of the fetus by an ovarian hormone, relaxin.

Postpartum Period

Most of the changes that have occurred in the maternal physiology return to normal within 3 to 4 weeks after parturition but can take up to 8 weeks to return to normal.

Suggested Readings

Almeida FA, Pavan MV, Rodrigues CI. The haemodynamic, renal excretory and hormonal changes induced by resting in the left lateral position in normal pregnant women during late gestation. *Br J Obstet Gynaecol.* 2009;116:1749-1754.

Carlin A, Alfirevic Z. Physiological changes of pregnancy and monitoring. *Best Pract Res Clin Obstet Gynaecol.* 2008;22:801-823.

Cheek TG, Baird E. Anesthesia for nonobstetric surgery: Maternal and fetal considerations. *Clin Obstet Gynecol.* 2009;52:535-545.

Chestnut DH, ed. *Chestnut's Obstetric Anesthesia: Principles and Practice.* St. Louis: Mosby/Elsevier; 2009.

Gabbe SG, Niebyl JR, Simpson JL, eds. *Normal and Problem Pregnancies.* 5th ed. Philadelphia: Churchill Livingstone Elsevier; 2007.

Moertl MG, Ulrich D, Pickel KI, et al. Changes in haemodynamic and autonomous nervous system parameters measured non-invasively throughout normal pregnancy. *Eur J Obstet Gynecol Reprod Biol.* 2009;144(Suppl 1):S179-183.

Richani K, Soto E, Romero R, et al. Normal pregnancy is characterized by systemic activation of the complement system. *J Matern Fetal Neonatal Med.* 2005;17:239-245.

Varga I, Rigó J Jr, Somos P, et al. Analysis of maternal circulation and renal function in physiologic pregnancies; parallel examinations of the changes in the cardiac output and the glomerular filtration rate. *J Matern Fetal Med.* 2000;9:97-104.

CHAPTER 181
Fetal Monitoring

Jack L. Wilson, MD

Overview

Assessment of fetal well-being is conducted throughout pregnancy, labor, and delivery in an attempt to decrease the risks of fetal morbidity and mortality. Anesthetic interventions during labor and delivery can significantly alter maternal and, thus, fetal physiology. Therefore, anesthesia providers require an understanding of commonly used fetal assessment measures.

During pregnancy, fetal monitoring can aid in the diagnosis of placental dysfunction and congenital anomalies and can provide an idea of fetal maturity. Various measures are used, such as maternal urinary and plasma estrogen levels, human placental lactogen levels, and amniotic fluid analysis. The latter is particularly helpful in diagnosing fetal lung maturity by measuring the ratio of the phospholipids lecithin to sphingomyelin. A lecithin:sphingomyelin ratio of 2.0 or greater correlates with a low risk of the neonate developing respiratory distress syndrome. As pregnancy progresses, a nonstress test (no contractions stimulated) is used to assess fetal heart rate (FHR) and fetal movements, and a stress test (contractions present or induced) is used to assess FHR response to the stress of contractions.

A very useful tool during pregnancy and labor is the ultrasound scan. This noninvasive nonionizing imaging modality can aid in assessing the fetus throughout pregnancy and can provide information that guides the clinician in managing labor. Information derived from an ultrasound scan includes fetal position, placental position, causes of vaginal bleeding, quantity of amniotic fluid, and the presence or absence of significant risk factors for bleeding, including placental accreta, increta, or percreta (see Chapter 189: Peripartum Hemorrhage). Knowledge of these factors can allow the anesthesia and surgical teams to be adequately prepared at the time of delivery. Placental accreta is an abnormally adherent placenta, which can lead to devastating acute blood loss. The incidence of this problem appears to be increasing as a result of the increasing numbers of repeat cesarean deliveries. Placenta accreta vera is present when the placenta is adherent to the myometrium without invasion into the uterine muscle. Placenta increta involves myometrial adherence with invasion into the muscle, and placenta percreta involves invasion into the uterine serosa and beyond—often involving other pelvic structures.

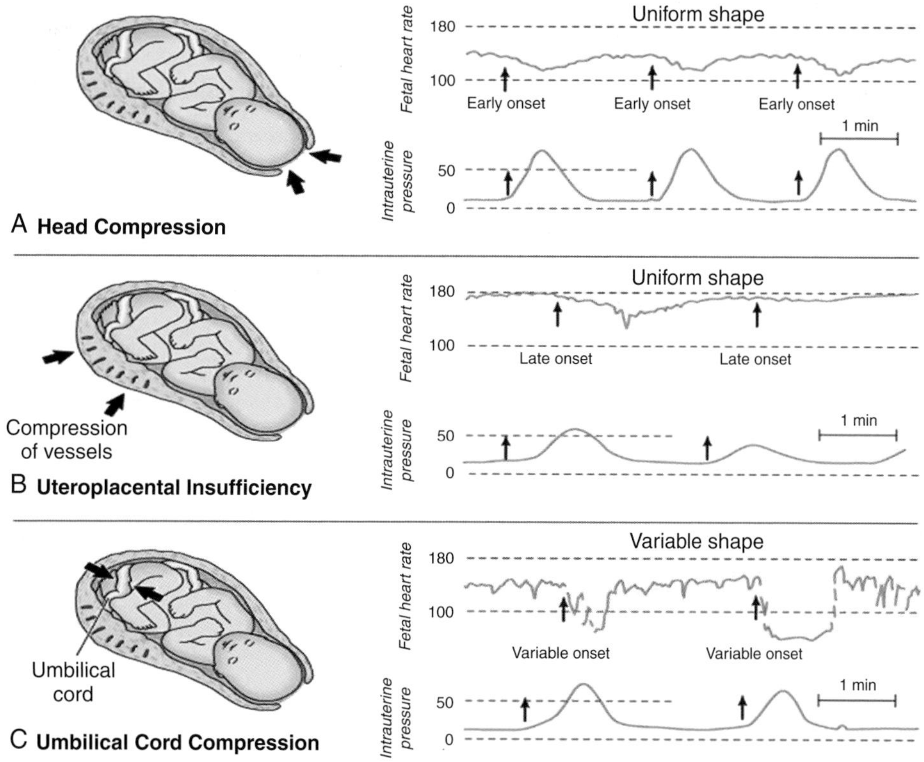

Figure 181-1 Periodic changes in fetal heart rate related to uterine contraction. **A,** Early (type I) decelerations. **B,** Late (type II) decelerations. **C,** Variable (type III) decelerations. (Modified and reproduced from Danforth DN, Scott JR. Obstetrics and Gynecology. 5th ed. Philadelphia: Lippincott; 1986.)

Electronic Intrapartum Fetal Heart Rate Monitoring

The most common form of fetal monitoring during labor is FHR monitoring (Figure 181-1). This monitoring is continuous from early labor through delivery. The FHR tracing and concurrently obtained uterine contraction tracings are displayed together so that the response of the FHR to uterine contractions can be observed. The normal FHR ranges from 110 to 160 beats/min and is controlled by fetal parasympathetic and sympathetic neural input. FHR and uterine contractions can be monitored externally (noninvasive) or internally (invasive). External monitoring consists of a Doppler ultrasound transducer for FHR monitoring and a tocodynamometer placed externally over the uterus to measure contractions. Internal, as compared with external, monitoring of the FHR provides more sensitivity in detecting FHR patterns but requires placement of an electrode into the presenting fetal part (breech or vertex). Internal monitoring is generally indicated if the external monitor tracings are of poor quality or if nonreassuring FHR patterns are evident. Internal monitoring of uterine contractions is helpful if progression of labor is slow and if inadequate force of contraction or hyperstimulation is suspected. Internal monitoring of contractions may also be useful when pharmacologic uterine stimulation is used to augment or induce labor.

Patterns of FHR are evaluated to assess fetal well-being. The baseline reading provides useful diagnostic information if the rate is too fast (>160 beats/min) or too slow (<100 beats/min). A normal baseline FHR provides the most reassurance that the fetus is not in distress when the normal rate is coupled with short-term (beat-to-beat) and long-term variability in the heart rate, as this reflects an intact higher central nervous system connection to cardiac conducting systems. Long-term variability is considered present if the amplitude range exceeds 6 beats/min. Table 181-1 lists conditions that are linked to various baseline FHRs.

Table 181-1 Conditions Related to Fetal Heart Rate

Fetal Heart Rate (beats/min)	Diagnostic Considerations
<110	Maternal hypotension; nonreassuring fetal status—hypoxemia—or congenital heart block
110-160	Normal; reassuring if variability is present
>160	Maternal fever, chorioamnionitis, thyrotoxicosis; fetal prematurity or tachyarrhythmias

Patterns of the relationship of uterine contractions to FHR are often observed continuously. Decelerations in FHR may indicate fetal distress. Early decelerations are generally not associated with fetal distress and may result from reflex vagal activity secondary to mild hypoxia or head compression. The FHR tracing usually dips fewer than 20 beats/min, and the onset and recovery mirror the uterine contraction. Variable decelerations are of more concern and may result from compression of the umbilical cord, with resulting increased vagal tone. These decelerations are also generally well tolerated, unless they become prolonged, with an FHR of less than 60 beats/min. The pattern of variable decelerations may differ in regard to onset, depth, duration, and shape. Late decelerations relate to uteroplacental insufficiency. Their onset is typically 10 to 30 sec after the onset of uterine contractions, and recovery to a normal FHR is equally delayed following the end of a contraction.

Compared with intermittent auscultation, electronic fetal monitoring has enjoyed widespread use as a real-time indicator of fetal well-being since it was introduced into clinical practice in the 1960s. Unfortunately, the use of electronic fetal monitoring has been associated with an increase in the rate of caesarean deliveries without improvement in perinatal mortality rate or fetal neurologic injury. Given the lack of predictive value for adverse outcomes, the American College of Obstetricians and Gynecologists recommends using the term *nonreassuring fetal status*, rather than the previously used descriptors *fetal distress* or *asphyxia*, when deceleration patterns or lack of variability are noted.

Suggested Readings

American Congress of Obstetricians and Gynecologists. Practice Bulletin No. 106. Intrapartum fetal heart rate monitoring: Nomenclature, interpretation, and general management principles. *Obstet Gynecol*. 2009;114:192-202.

Campbell K, Park JS, Norwitz ER. Antepartum fetal assessment and therapy. In: Chestnut DH, Polley LS, Tsen LC, Wong CA, eds. *Chestnut's Obstetric Anesthesia: Principles and Practice*. 4th ed. Philadelphia: Mosby Elsevier; 2009:89-122.

Graham EM, Petersen SM, Christo DK, Fox HE. Intrapartum electronic fetal heart rate monitoring and the prevention of perinatal brain injury. *Obstet Gynecol*. 2006;108:656-666.

Livingston EG. Intrapartum fetal assessment and therapy. In: Chestnut DH, Polley LS, Tsen LC, Wong CA, eds. *Chestnut's Obstetric Anesthesia: Principles and Practice*. 4th ed. Philadelphia: Mosby Elsevier; 2009:141-155.

Lobo AM. Fetal monitoring and resuscitation. In: Braveman FR, ed. *Obstetric and Gynecologic Anesthesia—The Requisites in Anesthesiology*. St. Louis: Mosby, Inc.; 2006:39-56.

CHAPTER 182
Analgesia for Labor

K.A. Kelly McQueen, MD, MPH

Pain relief during labor provides maternal comfort and, perhaps more importantly, prevents the maternal and fetal sequelae of maternal sympathetic activation. The drugs used for labor analgesia must be potent enough to provide relief of severe pain but must be managed effectively to limit adverse effects on the mother and the fetus. The choice of parenteral versus regional administration of drugs, as well as the medications used, should be based on several considerations, including the birthing facility and the availability of assistance in the event that complications arise.

Labor Pain

The first stage of labor begins with the onset of regular painful contractions and ends at complete dilation of the cervix. Pain in the first stage of labor is visceral and is caused by dilation of the cervix and lower uterine segment, as well as the uterine contractions themselves (Figure 182-1). Visceral afferent nerve impulses are transmitted along the sympathetic nerves, through somatic mixed spinal nerves, and then through the rami communicantes at T10, T11, T12, and L1. Referred pain can present over the cutaneous distribution of these dermatomes in the lumbar and sacral areas.

The second stage of labor begins with complete cervical dilation and ends with delivery of the baby. Pain in the second stage of labor is somatic as stretching and tearing of the pelvic ligaments and muscles occur. The stimuli for this pain are conducted along the pudendal nerves at S2, S3, and S4. In addition, uterine pain impulses continue as in the first stage of labor. Also, pain impulses during distention of the vagina and perineum just before delivery are conducted along the genitofemoral (L1, L2), ilioinguinal (L1), and posterior cutaneous nerves of the thighs (S2, S3), although they have a small role in labor pain.

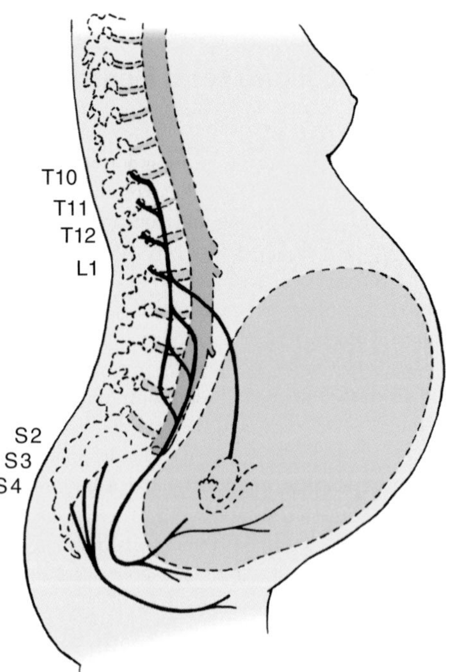

Figure 182-1 Parturition pain pathways. Afferent pain impulses from the cervix and uterus are carried by nerves that accompany sympathetic fibers and enter the neuraxis at the T10, T11, T12, and L1 spinal levels. Pain pathways from the perineum travel to S2, S3, and S4 via the pudendal nerve. (Modified from Bonica JJ, Chadwick HS. Labour pain. In: Wall PD, Melzack R, eds. Textbook of Pain. 2nd ed. New York: Churchill Livingstone; 1989:482.)

Analgesia Options for Parturients During Labor

Prior to providing any analgesic or anesthetic intervention, the anesthesia provider should obtain a maternal and perinatal history, complete a chart review, and perform an anesthesia-specific physical examination, including an airway evaluation, a heart and lung examination, and a modified neurologic examination, including evaluation of the spine. Preprocedure intravenous hydration is indicated if a regional technique is used that causes sympathectomy and subsequent hypotension. Infusing 1 L of isotonic solution is adequate, but careful evaluation and titration of fluids should be considered for parturients with preeclampsia or significant cardiac dysfunction.

Epidural Analgesia

Epidural analgesia provides excellent relief of labor pain while preserving maternal motor function and fetal circulation (Boxes 182-1 to 182-3). A continuous epidural technique is most often employed for labor, with an epidural catheter placed in a vertebral interspace between L2 and L5. Many drugs, used alone or in combination and administered via an epidural catheter, can effectively obliterate or attenuate labor pain (Table 182-1). Fentanyl used alone provides good pain relief in early labor and allows maternal ambulation ("walking epidural"). Local anesthesia, used alone or in combination with fentanyl, provides excellent pain relief throughout labor but necessitates maternal confinement because of the risk that it may cause motor weakness and hypotension. Although both bupivacaine and ropivacaine are commonly used in obstetric anesthesia practice, ropivacaine offers increased safety due to the decreased risk of hemodynamic collapse with intravascular injection. Both bupivacaine and ropivacaine are used in dilute solutions, often in combination with fentanyl (2 μg/mL) for labor pain (see Table 182-1). More concentrated bupivacaine (0.25% or lidocaine 1%) is frequently added as an epidural "top-up," when breakthrough pain is encountered, such as during the second stage of labor or episiotomy repair. In many birthing centers, after the anesthetic agent is initially administered as a bolus through the epidural catheter to achieve maternal comfort, a continuous infusion is initiated to maintain the desired level. The continuous infusion may be delivered via a standard intravenous pump or through a patient-controlled epidural analgesia pump, which allows for a continuous infusion, as well as with patient-controlled boluses, for which the time interval, volume, and lock-out interval may be set. The patient-controlled epidural analgesia pump offers the parturient excellent continuous pain control, as well as individual control of the intensity of the block without the risk of overdose. Many birthing centers report improved patient satisfaction as well as decreased need for top-ups with the use of patient-controlled epidural analgesia pumps.

Alternatively, but uncommonly, a caudal epidural block may be performed if the parturient arrives in the labor and delivery area in the latter part of stage 1 or early stage 2. A caudal block primarily affects the sacral segments and produces excellent analgesia in the second stage of labor. The block can be extended to the lumbar and lower thoracic segments by increasing the volume of drug administered. Advantages associated with the use of caudal anesthesia are few in the parturient, and sacral edema often distorts the caudal space in pregnancy, making this technique difficult to perform and infrequently used. However, the caudal technique is an option in parturients with a history of spinal surgery and in patients with dural adhesions that prevent the downward spread of local anesthesia if a lumbar technique were to be tried.

Combined Spinal/Epidural Analgesia

The need for rapid pain control combined with an unpredictable length of labor, as is the case in the young primipara, makes the option for a combined spinal-epidural analgesia technique desirable, as it provides rapid and continuous pain relief. A needle-through-needle technique is most commonly used (Figure 182-2). When using this method, the anesthesia provider intrathecally administers opioids or a local anesthetic and an opioid and then inserts an epidural catheter. Because of concern about the catheter "migrating" to an intrathecal position, two options for continued analgesia exist. One option is to test the epidural catheter using a bolus dose of medication at the upper limits of the intrathecal dose and to then start a continuous

Table 182-1 Drugs Used for Epidural and Spinal Analgesia

Drug	Concentration	Dose		
		Epidural		Spinal
		Bolus	Infusion	
Local Anesthetic Agents				
Bupivacaine	0.0625%-0.125%	12 mL	6-8 mL/h	1.25-2.5 mg
Levobupavicaine	0.0625%-0.125%	12 mL	6-8 mL/h	2.5-4.5 mg
Lidocaine	0.5%-1.0%	12 mL	6-8 mL/h	NA
Ropivacaine	0.1%-0.2%	12 mL	6-8 mL/h	2.5-4.5 mg
Opioids				
Sufentanil	NA	5-10 μg	0.2-0.33 μg/mL	1.5-5 μg
Fentanyl	NA	50-100 μg	1.5-3 μg/mL	15-25 μg
Morphine sulfate	NA	NA	NA	0.125-0.25 mg

Box 182-1 Adverse Effects of Neuraxial Analgesia

- Change in fetal heart rate tracing*
- Delayed gastric emptying
- Hypotension
- Nausea and vomiting
- Pruritus
- Recrudescence of herpes simplex virus
- Shivering
- Urinary retention

*Seen transiently with the use of sufentanil.

Box 182-2 Complications Associated with the Use of Neuraxial Analgesia

- Back pain
- Extensive motor blockade
- High neuroblockade of total spinal anesthesia
- Inadequate analgesia
- Intravascular injection of local anesthetic
- Pelvic floor injury
- Prolonged neuroblockade
- Respiratory depression
- Unintentional dural puncture

Box 182-3 Suggested Procedure for Initiation of Neuraxial Labor Analgesia

- Complete preprocedure checklist
- Position patient with the help of an assistant (lateral decubitus or sitting)
- Initiate monitoring of maternal blood pressure, maternal pulse oximetry, and fetal heart rate
- Supply supplemental O_2 via nasal cannula or face mask
- Intravenously administer a fluid bolus (500 mL lactated Ringer's solution)
- Using sterile technique, place epidural/spinal needle(s) and catheter, if used
- Administer test dose of medication if appropriate (epidural) or administer subarachnoid dose of medication
- Secure catheter if utilized, and position patient in the lateral position
- Monitor maternal blood pressure every 1 to 2.5 min for 15 to 20 min or until the parturient's blood pressure is stable
- Assess pain score and extent of sensory blockade (both cephalad and caudad)
- Initiate maintenance infusion, if indicated

Modified from Wong CA. Epidural and spinal analgesia for labor and vaginal delivery. In: Chestnut DH, Polley LS, Tsen LC, Wong CA, eds. Chestnut's Obstetric Anesthesia: Principles and Practice. 4th ed. Philadelphia: Mosby Elsevier; 2009.

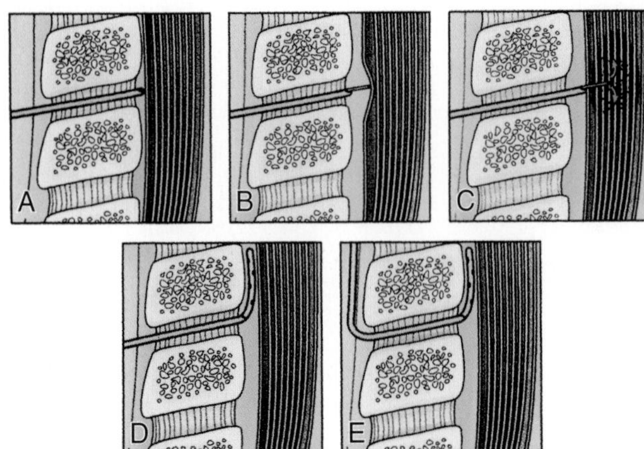

Figure 182-2 The combined spinal-epidural technique. Typically, an epidural needle is inserted in the epidural space (**A**), and a spinal needle is inserted through it (**B**). Because of the presence of air in the epidural space, the pencil-point spinal needle may considerably deform the dura before puncturing it (**C**). After the anesthetic agent is injected through the spinal needle, the needle is withdrawn, an epidural catheter is inserted (**D**), and the epidural needle is withdrawn (**E**). (Modified from Eisenach JC. Combined spinal-epidural analgesia in obstetrics. Anesthesiology. 1999;91:299-302.)

infusion. The second option is to start a continuous infusion without a bolus dose in the untested catheter following placement of the epidural catheter. Either a standard continuous infusion or a patient-controlled epidural analgesia infusion can be used safely during combined spinal/epidural anesthesia as long as the patient-controlled feature is not initiated until after the effects of the spinal anesthesia have begun to wane (approximately 1.5 h after subarachnoid dosing). Both techniques have been used effectively, and as long as the mother and fetus are adequately monitored, a clear distinction in safety is not apparent. The advantage of this technique is rapid onset and the option of continuous analgesia with an indwelling catheter. The disadvantage is a small increased risk of postdural puncture headache.

Single-Shot Spinal Analgesia

Multiparity and the rapid progression of labor may make the time required for epidural catheter placement and incremental dosing of an analgesic agent impractical. In this setting, a patient who desires pain relief can be rapidly treated with a single intrathecal dose of an opioid or an opioid combined with a local anesthetic agent. Pain relief occurs within several uterine contractions and predictably lasts 1.5 h. The disadvantages of a single-shot spinal include an increased risk of postdural puncture headache and the potential for labor outlasting the pain relief.

Continuous Spinal Analgesia

Complications associated with spinal microcatheters used for continuous spinal analgesia and anesthesia in the 1990s necessitated their removal from the market and terminated the use of continuous spinal techniques in the United States. However, experience with inadvertent dural puncture and the decision to continue a subarachnoid technique reveals that this technique may be safely utilized with the larger epidural catheter. When an inadvertent dural puncture occurs (incidence approximately 1% of the time in teaching institutions), a choice must be made as to how to proceed with the analgesic technique. Options include (1) removal of the Touhy needle and replacement of the catheter one lumbar level above the space at which the wet tap occurred or (2) placement of the epidural catheter through the dural rent and institution of a continuous drip of local anesthetic agent at approximately one-tenth the epidural infusion rate and titrated to effect. Although both a local anesthetic agent and an opioid are acceptable for continuous spinal infusion, side effects associated with opioids (pruritus) are more common when the agent is delivered into the subarachnoid space, as compared with the epidural space. When the two techniques (placement at a second lumbar epidural space versus continuous spinal infusion with an epidural catheter) are compared, a lower incidence of postdural puncture headache is noted with a continuous spinal infusion. Continuous spinal analgesia may also be the technique of choice for parturients with cardiac disease.

Other Regional Blockade

Several options exist for blockade of specific nerve plexuses during labor. These include paravertebral, lumbar sympathetic, paracervical, and pudendal blocks. Risk versus benefit profiles for these blocks during labor discourage their mainstream use when other options are available; however, in some circumstances and when performed by experienced providers, paracervical blocks offer good transient relief of the first stage of labor, and pudendal blocks offer good pain relief for the second stage of labor.

Systemically Administered Medication

Opioids are the most effective of the systemically administered medications for providing analgesia during labor. Although opioids reliably provide dose-dependent maternal analgesia, they do so at the expense of dose-dependent respiratory depression, hypoventilation, hypercarbia, and subsequent obtundation. Further, opioids are readily transported across the placenta, leading to decreased variability in the fetal heart rate and neonatal depression after birth. Therefore, systemic opioids are cautiously used in labor to reduce pain when regional analgesia is refused or cannot be used owing to maternal anatomy or coagulopathy-limiting options for regional analgesia. Other side effects common to the use of systemically administered opioids are orthostatic hypotension, nausea and vomiting, decreased gastric motility, and the possibility of decreased uterine activity in the early stages of labor.

If opioid analgesia is utilized, labor pain can be attenuated successfully with nalbuphine, fentanyl, or meperidine (with or without promethazine) in incremental doses provided by patient-controlled analgesia (Table 182-2) or at 2-h to 4-h intervals by a nurse. Fentanyl can be provided at a dose that decreases labor pain and the associated sympathetic stimulation (50-200 μg/h). Due to the rapid onset of fentanyl, it is often advised that the mother who uses patient-controlled analgesia should deliver an intravenous dose at the beginning of the contraction to attenuate the peak contraction pain and that no basal infusion rate be used to prevent oversedation and significant hypercarbia. The patient-controlled dose must be discontinued during the second stage of labor to reduce the risk of neonatal depression, necessitating intubation and ventilation of the newborn, and trained pediatric personnel must be available and present at the delivery when patient-controlled analgesia has been used during labor.

Table 182-2 Examples of Intravenously Administered Drugs Used for Patient-Controlled Analgesia for Labor Pain

Drug	Concentration	Dose		Lock-out Interval (min)
		Loading	Incremental	
Nalbuphine	1 mg/mL	5-10 mg	1 mL	6
Fentanyl	25 μg/mL	50-100 μg	0.5-1 mL	10
Meperidine	10 mg/mL	50 mg	1-1.5 mL	10

Suggested Readings

American Society of Anesthesiologists. *Practice Guidelines for Neuraxial Anesthesia in Obstetrics*. Amended by the ASA House of Delegates on October 16, 2013.

American Society of Anesthesiologists. *Practice Guidelines for Regional Anesthesia in Obstetrics*. Approved by the ASA House of Delegates on Oct 17, 2007.

Wong CA. Epidural and spinal analgesia for labor and vaginal delivery. In: Chestnut DH, Polley LS, Tsen LC, Wong CA, eds. *Chestnut's Obstetric Anesthesia: Principles and Practice*. 4th ed. Philadelphia: Mosby Elsevier; 2009.

CHAPTER 183

Preterm Labor: Tocolytics and Anesthetic Management

K.A. Kelly McQueen, MD, MPH

Preterm labor is a common occurrence associated with a diverse group of risk factors and may be precipitated by nonobstetric procedures performed during pregnancy (Box 183-1). Preterm labor necessitates the use of tocolytic therapy (Table 183-1) and fetal heart rate (FHR) monitoring, which may affect the parturient patient presenting for nonobstetric surgery or for cesarean section if the fetus demonstrates nonreassuring heart rate patterns or other indicators of non–well-being on the fetal biophysical profile. Anesthesia providers must be familiar with the pharmacokinetics and pharmacodynamics of tocolytic agents and the care of the parturient patient during preterm labor and preterm delivery.

Box 183-1 Risk Factors for Development of Preterm Labor

Demographic Characteristics/General Medical Findings

- Race: nonwhite
- Age <17 years or >35 years
- Low socioeconomic status
- Low body mass index
- Positive history of preterm labor
- Interpregnancy interval <6 months
- Abnormal uterine anatomy
- Abnormal cervical anatomy
- Abdominal surgery during pregnancy
- Acute or chronic systemic disease

Behavioral Factors

- Physical or psychological stress
- Tobacco and alcohol use
- Substance abuse

Obstetric Factors

- Vaginal bleeding
- Infection
- Multiple gestations
- Assisted reproduction (infertility intervention)
- Preterm premature rupture of membranes
- Abnormal fetal placentation
- Polyhydramnios

Fetal Factors

- Genetic abnormalities
- Fetal death

Adapted, with permission, from Muir HA, Wong CA. Preterm labor and delivery. In: Chestnut DH, Polley LS, Tsen LC, Wong CA, eds. Chestnut's Obstetric Anesthesia: Principles and Practice. 4th ed. Philadelphia: Mosby Elsevier; 2009:753.

Table 183-1 Tocolytic Pharmacologic Agents

Drug	Dose and Route	Side Effects
β-Adrenergic receptor agonists (e.g., terbutaline)	*SC*: 0.25 mg *IV infusion*: 2.5-10 μg/min	Tachycardia, anxiety
Magnesium sulfate	*Loading*: 4 g *Maintenance*: 1-4 g/h	Sedation, muscle relaxation
Cyclooxygenase inhibitors (e.g., indomethacin)	100-200 mg/d	*Maternal*: tachycardia, hypotension *Fetal*: premature closure of the ductus arteriosus, intracranial hemorrhage, necrotizing enterocolitis, oligohydramnios
Calcium channel blockers (e.g., nifedipine)	25-50 mg	Hypotension, bradycardia

IV, Intravenous; SC, subcutaneous.

Tocolytic Agents

Tocolytic agents are used to delay or stop premature labor. These agents inhibit uterine contractibility and, thus, may be used to treat preterm labor, to slow contractions if the fetus poorly tolerates labor, in the setting of breech or transverse presentation, or if the patient has an unknown type of scar from a previous cesarean section when spontaneous labor is undesired.

The β_2-adrenergic receptor agonists terbutaline and ritodrine are commonly used to treat preterm labor. Ritodrine is the only drug specifically approved by the U.S. Food and Drug Administration for tocolysis. These agents interact with β_2-receptors on the uterine myometrial cells, activating adenyl cyclase, which catalyzes the conversion of adenosine triphosphate (ATP) to cyclic adenosine monophosphate (cAMP). The increase in cAMP decreases the concentration of intracellular calcium and inhibits myosin light-chain kinase production. The combination of these effects decreases the interaction between actin and myosin and produces uterine relaxation. These agents may be administered intravenously, subcutaneously, or orally. $MgSO_4$ is often used to treat preterm labor because it has fewer cardiovascular side effects than do the β_2-receptor agonists. However, although $MgSO_4$ is known to decrease uterine activity, there is little evidence that it is effective as a tocolytic agent. $MgSO_4$ is often used to treat pregnancy-induced hypertension and to raise the seizure threshold in parturients with preeclampsia or eclampsia. The loading intravenous dose of $MgSO_4$ is 4 g over 15 min, followed by a continuous intravenous infusion of 1 to 4 g/h.

Cyclooxygenase inhibitors and the calcium channel blockers have been shown to effectively relax the uterus. By inhibiting cyclooxygenase, indomethacin prevents the synthesis of the prostaglandins that play an important role in the stimulus of uterine contractions. This drug is commonly used—either alone or with another agent—for long-term tocolysis in high-risk parturient patients with preterm labor or for refractory preterm labor. Indomethacin can be given orally or rectally, with an initial dose of 50 mg followed by 25 mg every 4 to 6 h.

Nifedipine acts by blocking cell membrane channels that are selective for calcium and by preventing the release of calcium, resulting in relaxation of smooth muscle. Nifedipine is not commonly used for tocolysis in the United States.

Contraindications to tocolytic therapy include chorioamnionitis, intrauterine demise, severe preeclampsia, and severe hemorrhage.

Anesthesia Management of Parturients on Tocolytic Therapy

Patients may present for induction of labor after preterm labor if a fetal death has occurred, in the presence of fetal anomalies incompatible with life, or when pregnancy-induced hypertension (Chapter 184) cannot be otherwise managed. Parturient patients may also present for cesarean section after a failed trial of tocolytic therapy for nonreassuring fetal status or in the presence of maternal chorioamnionitis, fever of unknown origin, or severe hemorrhage (see Chapters 181 and 189). Depending on the peripartum treatment of premature labor, the side effects of tocolytic therapy may impact or alter the anesthesia treatment plan for cesarean section.

Approximately 0.75% to 2.0% of parturient patients present for nonobstetric operations. Although few of these patients will be on tocolytic therapy preoperatively, some obstetricians advocate for the use of prophylactic perioperative tocolytic therapy for nonobstetric operations.

β_2-Adrenergic receptor agonists have little effect on the administration of either regional or general anesthesia; however, the side effects of large doses of these drugs may be of concern to the anesthesia provider. Such side effects include hypotension, tachycardia, arrhythmias, myocardial ischemia, and pulmonary edema. Fetal tachycardia commonly occurs because of the rapid placental transfer of β-adrenergic receptor agonists.

The use of $MgSO_4$ has significant side effects that may alter maternal physiology. These side effects include hypotension, maternal obtundation, muscle weakness, and prolonged effects of neuromuscular blocking agents administered during general anesthesia. $MgSO_4$ causes muscle relaxation by affecting the uptake and binding of cellular calcium. $MgSO_4$ also decreases the release of acetylcholine and alters the sensitivity of the neuromuscular junctions to acetylcholine. These effects alter the neuromuscular junction in skeletal muscle, producing prolonged muscle relaxation in the parturient patient.

The maternal side effects of indomethacin are minimal, most commonly nausea and heartburn, but fetal concerns with long-term administration of indomethacin include premature closure of the ductus arteriosus and oligohydramnios resulting from decreased fetal urine excretion. Therefore, postpartum evaluation of the newborn for these conditions is important.

Although it will be rare to encounter a patient in the United States who is receiving nifedipine for tocolysis, it is important for the anesthesia provider to be aware of the potential side effects of this drug that may affect the delivery of anesthesia. These side effects include hypotension, myocardial depression, and myocardial conduction defects. As does $MgSO_4$, nifedipine may prolong muscle relaxation.

Suggested Readings

American Society of Anesthesiologists. *Guidelines for neuraxial anesthesia in obstetrics*. Available at: https://www.asahq.org/For-Members/~/media/For%20Members/Standards%20and%20Guidelines/2014/GUIDELINES%20FOR%20NEURAXIAL%20ANESTHESIA%20IN%20OBSTETRICS.pdf. Accessed January 10, 2014.

American Society of Anesthesiologists. Optimal goals for anesthesia care in obstetrics. Available at: http://www.asahq.org/For-Members/~/media/For%20Members/documents/Standards%20Guidelines%20Stmts/Opitmal%20Goals%20Anesthesia%20Care%20Obstetrics.ashx. Accessed January 10, 2014.

American Society of Anesthesiologists Task Force on Obstetric Anesthesia. Practice guidelines for obstetric anesthesia: An updated report by the American Society of Anesthesiologists Task Force on Obstetric Anesthesia. *Anesthesiology*. 2007;106:843-863.

Blumenfeld YJ, Lyell DJ. Prematurity prevention: The role of acute tocolysis. *Curr Opin Obstet Gynecol*. 2009;21(2):136-141.

Meloni A, Melis M, Alba E, et al. Medical therapy in the management of preterm birth. *J Matern Fetal Neonatal Med*. 2009;22 Suppl 3:72-76.

Roos C, Scheepers LH, Bloemenkamp KW, et al. Assessment of perinatal outcome after sustained tocolysis in early labour (APOSTEL-II trial). *BMC Pregnancy Childbirth*. 2009;9:42.

Soraisham AS, Dalgleish S, Singhal N. Antenatal indomethacin tocolysis is associated with an increased need for surgical ligation of patent ductus arteriosus in preterm infants. *J Obstet Gynaecol Can*. 2010;32(5):435-442.

CHAPTER 184

Hypertensive Disorders During Pregnancy and Related Syndromes

K.A. Kelly McQueen, MD, MPH

A spectrum of hypertensive disorders affects 6% to 8% of pregnant women contributing to significant maternal and fetal morbidity and mortality (Box 184-1). Chronic hypertension is diagnosed if the parturient has preexisting hypertension or if she has a blood pressure reading of greater than 140/90 mm Hg before the twentieth week of the pregnancy. Preeclampsia superimposed on chronic hypertension refers to preeclampsia developing in a woman with a history of high blood pressure. Gestational hypertension typically presents in the third trimester as mild hypertension and is not associated with other organ dysfunction.

Preeclampsia, a syndrome occurring after the twentieth week of a pregnancy, is characterized by mild or severe hypertension, proteinuria, and edema. However, in 2000, the National High Blood Pressure Education Working Group on High Blood Pressure in Pregnancy emphasized that "although our current understanding of this syndrome has increased, the criteria used to identify the disorder remain subject to confusion and controversy. The confusion doubtless reflects the fact that preeclampsia is a syndrome, which means that attempts at definition use arbitrarily selected markers rather than changes of pathophysiologic importance."

In 2008, the Society of Obstetricians and Gynecologists of Canada tried to further simplify the classification of hypertension in pregnancy. Hypertension was either preexisting or gestational, with the diagnosis of *preeclampsia* added to either condition if signs or positive test results for preeclampsia were present. Preeclampsia itself can be further categorized as severe based on the criteria listed in Box 184-2 and as eclampsia if central nervous system involvement results in new-onset seizures. HELLP syndrome (a syndrome of hemolysis, elevated liver enzymes, and low platelet counts) is a severe variant of preeclampsia. Disorders of hypertension related to pregnancy usually abate within 48 h after delivery of the entire placenta.

Etiology and Pathophysiology

Preeclampsia is a multisystem disorder defined by maternal cardiovascular, respiratory, central nervous system, renal, and placental dysfunction (Box 184-3). Although associated with some well-defined risk factors (Box 184-4), the cause of preeclampsia is not well defined. The pathogenic mechanisms for preeclampsia appear to be a combination of immunologic (fetal and maternal), genetic, and endothelial factors and involve abnormalities of the clotting cascade (Figure 184-1). The final common pathway most likely involves the vascular endothelium—affected by a number of cytokines and hormones, with a decrease in the production of nitric oxide and vasodilating eicosanoids. The net result is a decrease in uterine blood flow and vasoconstriction of the spiral arteries of the myometrium. In addition to the vasoconstriction, damage caused by endothelial cell dysfunction contributes to platelet activation and a further imbalance of two eicosanoids—prostacyclin and thromboxane.

Box 184-1 Hypertensive Disorders of Pregnancy

- Chronic hypertension
- Chronic hypertension with superimposed preeclampsia
- Gestational hypertension
- Preeclampsia
  - Mild
  - Severe

Box 184-2 Criteria for Classification as Severe Preeclampsia

- Blood pressure:
  - Systolic >160 mm Hg
  - Diastolic >110 mm Hg
  - Mean arterial >120 mm Hg
- Proteinuria >5 g/24 h
- Oliguria <500 mL/24 h
- Elevated creatinine
- Cerebral or visual disturbances (headache, blurred vision, altered consciousness)
- Pulmonary edema
- Epigastric or RUQ pain
- Signs of HELLP syndrome
- Intrauterine growth restriction

HELLP, Hemolysis, elevated liver enzymes, and low platelet counts; RUQ, right upper quadrant.

Treatment

Treatment for hypertension during pregnancy includes the administration of antihypertensive agents (e.g., β-adrenergic receptor blocking agents, α-adrenergic receptor blocking agents, centrally acting α-adrenergic agonists, and methyldopa) and vasodilators (e.g., hydralazine and nitroglycerin), but once preeclampsia is diagnosed (hypertension, edema, and proteinuria), close obstetric monitoring is required. Although the definitive treatment for preeclampsia is delivery of the fetus and the placenta, if the fetus is preterm, other symptoms and signs of mild and severe preeclampsia must be specifically treated. Once the patient is hospitalized, magnesium ($MgSO_4$) can be used to lower the seizure threshold and may also lower blood pressure. Table 184-1 summarizes the effects of increasing plasma $MgSO_4$ levels. Additional blood pressure control may be obtained by either adding or increasing the dose of labetalol, hydralazine, nitroglycerin, methyldopa, clonidine, prazosin, nifedipine, or trimethaphan. Use of sodium nitroprusside is

Box 184-3 Manifestations of Preeclampsia
Central Nervous System
Cerebral edema Cerebral hemorrhage Cortical blindness Headache Hyperirritability Hyperreflexia Seizures Vertigo
Cardiovascular System
Elevated systemic vascular resistance Hemoconcentration Hypoproteinemia Hypovolemia Increased sensitivity to the effects of catecholamines, sympathomimetics, and oxytocics Left ventricular hypertrophy Myocardial dysfunction Pulmonary edema
Respiratory System
Airway edema Gastric aspiration Interstitial edema $\dot{V}/\dot{Q}$ mismatch
Renal System
Decreased glomerular filtration rate Decreased renal blood flow Elevated creatinine and blood urea nitrogen Hyperuricemia Proteinuria
Hepatic Changes
Abnormal liver function tests Decreased hepatic blood flow Decreased plasma cholinesterase levels Periportal hepatic necrosis Subcapsular hemorrhage
Hematologic Changes
Disseminated intravascular coagulation (20% of patients) Platelet dysfunction Prolonged bleeding time (25% of patients) Thrombocytopenia
Placenta
Chronic fetal hypoxia Fetal malnutrition Intrauterine growth retardation Placental abruption Premature birth Premature labor Uteroplacental insufficiency

Box 184-4 Risk Factors for Preeclampsia
Partner-Related Risk Factors
The father has fathered a preeclamptic pregnancy with another woman Mother has limited preconceptional exposure to paternal sperm Mother's first pregnancy with this partner Nulliparity
Maternal Risk Factors
Family history of preeclampsia History of placental abruption, intrauterine growth restriction, or fetal death History of preeclampsia in previous pregnancy Maternal age >35 years Non-Hispanic black
Maternal Disease Risk Factors
Behavioral Chronic hypertension Diabetes mellitus Obesity Smoking Thrombovascular disease
Pregnancy-Associated Risk Factors
Hydatidiform mole Multiple gestation

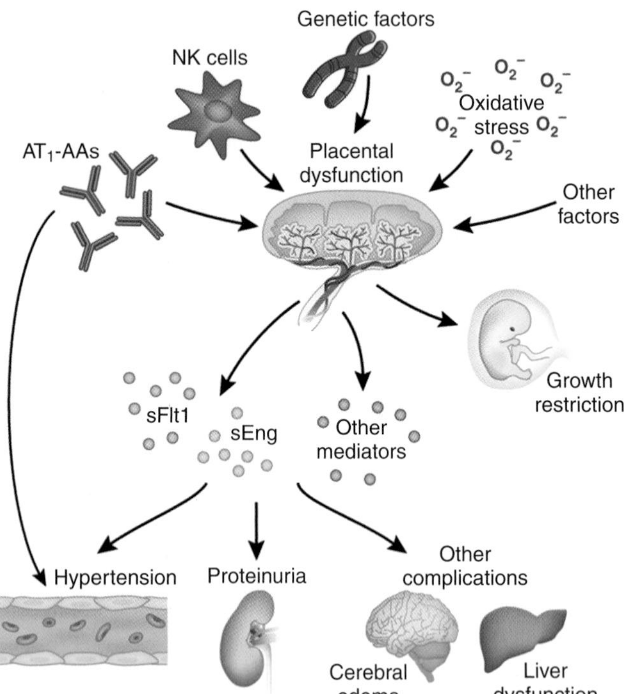

Figure 184-1 Angiotensin receptor autoantibodies (AT_1-AAs) in preeclampsia. AT_1-AAs and other factors (such as oxidative stress and genetic factors) may cause placental dysfunction, which in turn leads to the release of antiangiogenic factors (such as soluble fms-like tyrosine kinase-1 [sFlt-1] and soluble endoglin [sEng]) and other inflammatory mediators to induce preeclampsia. AT_1-AAs may also act directly on the maternal vasculature to enhance angiotensin II sensitivity and hypertension. NK, Natural killer; O_2^-, superoxide. (From Parikh SM, Karumanchi SA. Putting pressure on preeclampsia. Nat Med. 2008;14(8):810-812.)

discouraged by some clinicians because the fetus is susceptible to cyanide toxicity resulting from continuous sodium nitroprusside infusion, but it may be used for short periods of time if hypertension cannot otherwise be controlled.

Anesthetic Management

Once the fetus has reached fetal lung maturity and severe preeclampsia cannot be further managed, delivery is usually planned, and if eclampsia or HELLP syndrome develops, delivery may be urgent. The goals of the anesthesia provider include management of hypertension, intravascular volume replacement, and control of central nervous system irritability while providing analgesia for labor or anesthesia for cesarean section (see Chapter 185 for a more complete discussion of managing anesthesia for the patient with preeclampsia).

Vaginal delivery may be an option, depending on the severity of the hypertension and whether the fetus is distressed. If no contraindications to

Table 184-1 Effects of Increasing Plasma Magnesium Levels

Observed Condition	Mg^{2+} Level (mEq/L)
Normal plasma level	1.5-2.0
Therapeutic range	4.0-6.0
Electrocardiographic changes (prolonged PQ interval, widened QRS complex)	5.0-10
Loss of deep tendon reflexes	10
Sinoatrial and atrioventricular block	15
Respiratory paralysis	15
Cardiac arrest	25

placement of an epidural catheter are present, lumbar epidural analgesia provides excellent pain relief, decreases levels of circulating catecholamines, and may reduce blood pressure during labor. For the patient with preeclampsia, early placement of an epidural catheter is indicated because of the increased likelihood that the patient will need to undergo a cesarean section, potentially emergently.

Before catheter placement, it must be ascertained that the parturient does not have thrombocytopenia or another coagulopathy. Volume preloading should be carefully titrated if the patient has severe preeclampsia because, although these patients are uniformly volume contracted, they are also predisposed to developing additional capillary leakage, which can cause or exacerbate pulmonary edema. Depending on the severity of the patient's condition (e.g., the presence of pulmonary edema), central line placement for monitoring central venous pressure (and for resuscitation) should be considered prior to intravascular volume loading or dosing of the epidural catheter. In addition, anesthetic agents should be slowly and carefully infused in these patients to avoid a precipitous drop in maternal blood pressure and subsequent decelerations of the fetal heart rate.

Despite these concerns, regional anesthesia is often recommended for parturients with hypertension because the associated decrease in circulating catecholamine levels improves blood pressure and may improve blood perfusion to the uterus. Preeclamptic patients demonstrate increased sensitivity to catecholamines; therefore, the use of epinephrine is generally contraindicated in the epidural test dose and in other epidural solutions. Cesarean section is indicated for delivery when the mother's condition deteriorates or when the fetus does not tolerate labor. Nonreassuring fetal heart rate tracings include late decelerations and sustained decelerations. If an epidural catheter is in place, it may be used to provide a surgical plane of anesthesia for urgent or emergent cesarean section.

The anesthesia provider must continue to carefully monitor the patient's volume status. An initial bolus of 500 mL of crystalloid solution administered intravenously should be considered, and ephedrine or phenylephrine should be carefully used, remembering that parturients with preeclampsia may be hypersensitive to the effects of catecholamines.

Spinal anesthesia has also been shown to be a safe technique for cesarean section for severely preeclamptic patients. The more precipitous drop in systemic vascular resistance that occurs with spinal anesthesia mandates careful titration of loading fluids, with appropriate monitoring of blood pressure. In urgent circumstances, a spinal catheter should be placed only by an experienced provider, and the fetal heart rate should be monitored throughout the procedure.

General anesthesia is an acceptable way to manage preeclamptic patients, but associated risks include pulmonary aspiration, glottic edema that may compromise airway management, and acute blood pressure elevations during laryngoscopy. The brief but severe elevations in systemic and pulmonary pressures seen during laryngoscopy and tracheal intubation in preeclamptic parturients can lead to a significant risk of cerebral hemorrhage and pulmonary edema. A rapid-sequence induction technique and intubation are used, with propofol, 1.5 mg/kg, plus succinylcholine, 1.5 mg/kg, as an option. Pretreatment with intravenously administered hydralazine, lidocaine, sodium nitroprusside, nitroglycerin, or esmolol has been used with success to attenuate the hypertensive response to laryngoscopy.

Because of the possibility of glottic edema, the use of a smaller-than-usual-size cuffed tracheal tube is recommended to intubate the trachea. Anesthesia is then maintained with inhalation agents, a combination of N_2O and O_2, and neuromuscular blockade, as needed, guided by assessment of response to peripheral nerve stimulation; ergot preparations are not recommended after delivery of the placenta. Coagulopathies are managed with transfusions of platelets, fresh frozen plasma, and cryoprecipitate, as needed. After the operation is completed, the patient may be extubated once she is fully awake.

The amount of intravenously administered fluid should be guided by urine output (>1 $mL\cdot kg^{-1}\cdot h^{-1}$) and central venous pressure (4-6 cm H_2O), if such monitoring is indicated. In patients manifesting cardiopulmonary dysfunction, a pulmonary artery catheter is the preferred method of hemodynamic monitoring. Intraarterial cannulation allows continuous blood pressure monitoring and provides easy access for blood sampling (e.g., tests of coagulation, complete blood counts, arterial blood gases, electrolytes, and Mg^{2+} levels). Loop diuretics are recommended to treat pulmonary edema, and mannitol may be given to treat manifestations of cerebral edema. Because $MgSO_4$ most likely was given prior to delivery, the clinician must remember that, in addition to its therapeutic effects (i.e., antihypertensive and anticonvulsant), when administered in excess of therapeutic range, $MgSO_4$ may cause skeletal muscle weakness, respiratory depression, and cardiac arrest. Neuromuscular blockade is potentiated by $MgSO_4$, as is the sedative effect of opioids. $CaCl_2$ counteracts the adverse effects of $MgSO_4$ (see Chapter 183, Preterm Labor: Tocolytics and Anesthetic Management).

Careful postpartum monitoring should occur for parturients with preeclampsia. The risk of patients developing pulmonary edema is the highest in the postoperative period. One option for providing postoperative analgesia is patient-controlled analgesia if an epidural catheter for delivery of analgesia is not present. For the patient with HELLP syndrome, a platelet count should be obtained prior to removal of the epidural catheter; the catheter should not be removed until the platelet count is greater than 75,000 to 80,000/mm^3. Return of normal neuromuscular function should be carefully monitored, and symptoms of an epidural hematoma should be immediately evaluated with imaging studies and a neurosurgical consultation.

Suggested Readings

ACOG Practice Bulletin No. 125: Chronic hypertension in pregnancy. *Obstet Gynecol.* 2012;119:396-407.

American Society of Anesthesiologists. *Guidelines for Regional Anesthesia in Obstetrics.* Approved by the ASA HOD on Oct. 12, 1988, and last amended on Oct. 17, 2007.

Hood DD, Curry R. Spinal versus epidural anesthesia for cesarean section in severely preeclamptic patients: A retrospective survey. *Anesthesiology.* 1999;90: 1276-1282.

Magee LA, Helewa M, Moutquin JM, von Dadelszen P, Hypertension Guideline Committee, Strategic Training Initiative in Research in the Reproductive Health Sciences (STIRRHS) Scholars. Diagnosis, management, and evaluation of hypertensive disorders of pregnancy. *J Obstet Gynaecol Can.* 2008;30: S1-48.

Marik PE. Hypertensive disorders of pregnancy. *Postgrad Med.* 2009;121:69-76.

Polley LS. Hypertensive disorders. In: Chestnut DH, Polley LS, Tsen LC, Wong CA, eds. *Chestnut's Obstetrical Anesthesia: Principles and Practice.* 4th ed. Philadelphia: Mosby Elsevier; 2009:975-1007.

Practice Guidelines for Obstetric Anesthesia. An Updated Report by the American Society of Anesthesiologists Task Force on Obstetric Anesthesia. *Anesthesiology.* 2007;106:843-863.

CHAPTER 185

Anesthesia for the Patient with Preeclampsia

Joseph J. Sandor, MD

Preeclampsia—a syndrome occurring after week 20 of gestation and characterized by hypertension, proteinuria, and generalized edema—becomes eclampsia if a grand mal seizure occurs (see Chapter 184). Preeclampsia/eclampsia abates within 48 h after delivery of the entire placenta.

Etiology and Pathophysiology

The cause of preeclampsia remains unknown, although immunologic and genetic factors may play a role. Vasoconstriction of the spiral arteries of the myometrium with decreased uterine blood flow is associated with the disorder. In addition to resulting in vasoconstriction, preeclampsia causes endothelial cell damage, which contributes to platelet activation and an imbalance between vasoconstricting and vasodilating eicosanoids: thromboxane and prostacyclin, respectively.

Manifestations

Preeclampsia is a multisystem disease, affecting the central nervous system and the cardiovascular, respiratory, renal, hepatic, and hematologic systems, as well as the placenta (Table 185-1) (see Chapter 184).

Table 185-1 Manifestations of Preeclampsia

Body System	Manifestations
Central nervous system	Cerebral edema, cerebral hemorrhage, cortical blindness, headache, hyperirritability, hyperreflexia, seizures, vertigo
Cardiovascular	Hypoproteinemia; hypovolemia; hemoconcentration; left ventricular hypertrophy; myocardial dysfunction; pulmonary edema; ↑ sensitivity to catecholamines, sympathomimetics, and oxytocics; ↑ systemic vascular resistance
Hematologic	DIC,* platelet dysfunction, prolonged bleeding time,† thrombocytopenia
Hepatic	Abnormalities on liver function tests, ↓ hepatic blood flow, ↓ plasma cholinesterase levels, periportal hepatic necrosis, subcapsular hemorrhage
Placenta	Chronic fetal hypoxia, fetal malnutrition, intrauterine growth retardation, placental abruption, premature birth, premature labor, uteroplacental insufficiency
Renal	↑ Blood urea nitrogen, ↑ creatinine, ↓ glomerular filtration rate, hyperuricemia, proteinuria, ↓ renal blood flow
Respiratory	Airway edema, gastric aspiration, interstitial edema, ventilation-perfusion mismatch

*Disseminated intravascular coagulation (DIC) affects 20% of patients.
†Affects 25% of patients.

Treatment

The definitive treatment for preeclampsia is delivery of the fetus and the placenta. Goals of the anesthesia provider include treatment of hypertension, volume replacement, and control of central nervous system irritability.

Intravenous fluid administration should be guided by urine output (goal: >1 mL·kg^{-1}·h^{-1}) and central venous pressure (4-6 cm H_2O). In patients manifesting cardiopulmonary dysfunction, some clinicians advocate the use of a pulmonary artery catheter to monitor measures of cardiac function. Intraarterial cannulation allows continual blood pressure monitoring and provides easy access for blood sampling (e.g., clotting parameters, arterial blood gases, and electrolyte and Mg^{2+} concentrations). Loop diuretics are used to treat pulmonary edema, and mannitol may be given to treat cerebral edema. $MgSO_4$, with its anticonvulsant and antihypertensive properties, reduces CNS irritability, reduces irritability of the neuromuscular junction, and has direct vasodilating action on the smooth muscles of arterioles and the uterus. In excess of therapeutic range, $MgSO_4$ may cause skeletal muscle weakness, respiratory depression, and cardiac arrest. $CaCl_2$ counteracts the adverse effects of $MgSO_4$. Neuromuscular blockade is potentiated by $MgSO_4$, as is the sedative effect of opioids. Other useful antihypertensive agents include labetalol, hydralazine, nitroglycerin, methyldopa, clonidine, prazosin, nifedipine, and trimethaphan. The use of sodium nitroprusside is discouraged by some authors because the fetus is susceptible to cyanide toxicity resulting from continuous sodium nitroprusside infusion. (See Table 184-1 for a summary of the effects of increasing plasma magnesium concentrations.)

Anesthetic Management of Labor

Vaginal delivery may be performed if the fetus is not distressed. Lumbar epidural analgesia provides pain relief and a method to control blood pressure during labor. Before placing the epidural catheter, the anesthesia provider should ascertain that the parturient has no coagulopathy and that adequate volume replacement (0.5-2 L) has been achieved. When the patient has regional anesthesia, she often needs to push less (thereby attenuating elevations in blood pressure), requires lower doses of opioid analgesic agents, and has improved placental and renal blood flow. Because these patients demonstrate increased sensitivity to catecholamines, epinephrine is usually not added to the local anesthetic solution. A saddle block may be performed if the fetus is carefully monitored.

Cesarean section is indicated for delivery of a distressed fetus. If an epidural catheter has been previously placed (or if the cesarean section is elective), the catheter may be used to provide surgical anesthesia, assuming that intravascular volume has been appropriately restored (0.5-2 L).

In patients who do not have coagulopathies, neuraxial techniques have become the preferred method to provide analgesia for laboring parturients, as well as to provide anesthesia for cesarean delivery for severely preeclamptic patients.

General anesthesia is an acceptable way to manage preeclamptic patients, but there are associated risks of pulmonary aspiration, airway compromise from edema, and acute blood pressure elevations during laryngoscopy. The brief but severe elevations in systemic and pulmonary pressures seen during laryngoscopy and intubation in preeclamptic parturients can lead to a significant risk of cerebral hemorrhage and pulmonary edema. A rapid-sequence induction technique is used. Propofol (1-2 mg/kg) plus succinylcholine (1-1.5 mg/kg) is given intravenously. Earlier treatment with an intravenously administered combination of any of the following—hydralazine, lidocaine, sodium nitroprusside, nitroglycerin, labetolol, and esmolol—will attenuate the hypertensive response to laryngoscopy.

Because of the occasional severe degree of oropharyngeal edema, a smaller-than-usual cuffed tracheal tube is used to intubate the trachea. Anesthesia is then maintained with a low concentration of inhalation agents, N_2O/O_2, and neuromuscular blockade, as needed, guided by a peripheral nerve stimulator. Oxytocics may cause exaggerated blood pressure elevation, and ergot preparations should not be used after delivery of the infant. Coagulopathies are managed with transfusions of platelets, fresh frozen plasma, and cryoprecipitate, as needed. After completion of the operation, the patient may be extubated once fully awake.

Suggested Readings

Dyer RA. Maternal hemodynamic monitoring in obstetric anesthesia. *Anesthesiology*. 2008;109:765-767.

Fernando R. Gerard W. Ostheimer "What's New in Obstetric Anesthesia" lecture. *Anesthesiology*. 2007;106:615-621.

Gogarten W. Preeclampsia and anaesthesia. *Curr Opin Anaesthesiol*. 2009;22: 347-351.

Hawkins JL. Epidural analgesia for labor and delivery. *N Engl J Med*. 2010;362: 1503-1510.

Landau R. What's new in obstetric anesthesia. *Int J Obstet Anesth*. 2009;18: 368-372.

Malleeswaran S, Panda N, Mathew P, Bagga R. A randomised study of magnesium sulphate as an adjuvant to intrathecal bupivacaine in patients with mild preeclampsia undergoing caesarean section. *Int J Obstet Anesth*. 2010; 19:161-166.

Sullivan JT. What's new in obstetric anesthesia: The 2009 Gerard W. Ostheimer lecture. *Anesth Analg*. 2010;110:564-549.

Turner JA. Severe preeclampsia: Anesthetic implications of the disease and its management. *Am J Ther*. 2009;16:284-288.

CHAPTER 186

Anesthesia for Cesarean Section

K.A. Kelly McQueen, MD, MPH

Cesarean section (C/S) is the most commonly performed operation during pregnancy and the most commonly performed operation in the United States. The average annual rate of C/S is 30% in the United States, but in some high-risk birthing centers, the rate may be higher. The anesthetic implications for both mother and fetus are significant and must be carefully considered.

Preoperative Evaluation

Performing a maternal evaluation and obtaining surgical consent are essential before the anesthesia provider administers anesthesia for a C/S. Along with performing a standard preoperative maternal evaluation, including a focused history and physical examination, the anesthesia provider should also ascertain information regarding fetal gestation and pregnancy-related complications. Laboratory studies are obtained as maternal comorbid conditions and the planned procedure dictate; however, a blood sample for type and screen or crossmatch is often standard for multiparous women or for parturients with other common physiologic alterations. Preparation for elective, urgent, and emergent C/S includes aspiration prophylaxis and establishment of adequate venous access (Box 186-1).

Regional Anesthesia

Subarachnoid block and epidural anesthesia are recommended for elective C/S. When compared with general anesthesia, these techniques provide excellent anesthesia, prevent fetal depression and maternal airway management difficulties, and do not place the mother at risk for aspirating gastric contents. Local anesthetic agents, with or without the addition of an opioid, may be used for either a subarachnoid block (Table 186-1) or an epidural anesthetic (Table 186-2).

Before the anesthesia provider initiates neuraxial regional anesthesia, the patient must receive adequate hydration to prevent or attenuate maternal hypotension and uteroplacental insufficiency, regardless of whether or not an epidural anesthetic has already been instituted for labor. Intravenously administering approximately 1 L of fluid (unless preeclampsia or other maternal cardiac conditions exist) is ideal prior to infusing anesthetizing bolus doses of a local anesthetic agent. Maternal

Box 186-1 Preparing the Parturient for Cesarean Section

Obtain a focused maternal history and informed consent
Perform a physical examination
Obtain a blood sample for type and screen or crossmatch, as indicated
For elective procedures, have the patient abstain from eating solid foods for 6 to 8 h and from drinking clear liquids for 2 h before the operation
Obtain large-bore (18-gauge or 16-gauge) intravenous access in two sites
Administer nonparticulate antacid and an H_2-receptor blocking agent or metoclopramide
Administer prophylactic antibiotics

Table 186-1 Drugs Used for Subarachnoid Block for Cesarean Section

Drug	Dose
Bupivacaine	7.5-15 mg
Lidocaine*	60-80 mg
Levobupivacaine	7.5-15 mg
Ropivacaine	15-25 mg
Fentanyl	10-25 μg
Morphine	0.1-0.2 mg
Sufentanil	2.5-5 μg
Meperidine	60-70 mg
	Clonidine 20 μg

*Epinephrine, 0.1-0.2 mg, may be used as an adjuvant.

Table 186-2 Drugs Used for Epidural Anesthesia

Drug	Strength	Dose
Chloroprocaine	3%	450-750 mg
Bupivacaine*	0.5%	75-125 mg
Lidocaine*	2%	300-500 mg
Fentanyl		50-100 μg
Morphine		3-4 mg
Sufentanil		10-20 μg
Meperidine		50-75 mg

*Epinephrine, 5 μg/mL, and bicarbonate may be added to lidocaine.

hypotensive episodes are ideally treated with intravenous hydration, and if these episodes are persistent or involve changes in fetal heart rate, an indirect-acting sympathomimetic agent (e.g., ephedrine, titrated to effect) or direct-acting sympathomimetic agent (e.g., phenylephrine) should be administered intravenously. Regardless of anesthetic technique used, patients should be positioned to provide left uterine displacement to prevent aortocaval syndrome.

Emergent or Urgent Cesarean Section

The need for an emergency C/S is a constant threat during labor. An operating room set up for a "crash" induction must always be available. Time is critical to ensure delivery of a healthy fetus. Although general anesthesia is usually the most expedient option for use in a true emergency situation, regional anesthesia may be a viable option provided that (1) the fetal heart rate returns to normal after obstetric management of nonreassuring fetal status (e.g., optimize maternal position, provide supplemental O_2, improve maternal circulation, discontinue oxytocin, administer a tocolytic agent for uterine hypertonus) and (2) an experienced anesthesia provider can place a subarachnoid block in a timely fashion, with ongoing monitoring of the fetal heart rate. Communication between the anesthesia and obstetric teams is essential.

Box 186-2 Rapid-Sequence Induction of General Anesthesia

Maintain continuous cricoid pressure
Administer propofol, 1-2 mg/kg
Administer succinylcholine, 1.5 mg/kg
Consider using a smaller tracheal tube (6.5) and stylet

If general anesthesia is required, rapid-sequence induction (Box 186-2) with cricoid pressure should be initiated *after* the abdomen is prepped and draped. The surgical team is notified that they can safely proceed as soon as proper tracheal tube placement is confirmed. Maintenance with low-concentration inhalation anesthetic agents (e.g., isoflurane or sevoflurane), 50% O_2, and N_2O is used until the umbilical cord has been clamped and the neonate is delivered. Nondepolarizing neuromuscular blocking agents may be given once motor end plate function has recovered from the effects of succinylcholine. After the umbilical cord is clamped, opioids may be administered, given that there is no longer any concern about neonatal respiratory depression. In addition, midazolam may be administered at this time to prevent the patient from experiencing recall while simultaneously allowing for the use of a lower dose of inhalation anesthetic agents (i.e., drugs known to relax uterine smooth muscle), thereby decreasing the risk of uterine hypotonia and persistent uterine bleeding. Following delivery of the placenta, oxytocin (Pitocin, 20 to 40 IU in 1 L of crystalloid solution) may be given to facilitate uterine contractions. If hypotonia persists, oxytocin (as a slow intravenous push) or methylergonovine mesylate (Methergine, 0.2 mg intramuscularly) may be given. Both oxytocin and methylergonovine produce hemodynamic sequelae (see Chapter 189).

The prophylactic use of antibiotics has been shown to decrease the incidence and severity of infections after C/S, and, therefore, antibiotics should be administered either before the abdominal incision is made or immediately after the umbilical cord is clamped. The time of delivery and Apgar scores should be noted on the anesthetic record. Following the operation, the patient should not be extubated until she is awake to minimize the ongoing risk of aspiration.

Suggested Readings

American Society of Anesthesiologists. Guidelines for regional anesthesia in obstetrics. Available at: http://www.asahq.org/publicationsAndServices/standards/45.pdf. Accessed September 15, 2009.

American Society of Anesthesiologists. Practice guidelines for obstetric anesthesia. Available at: http://www.asahq.org/publications/pc-119-4-practiceguidelines-for-obstetrical-anesthesia.aspx. Accessed September 15, 2009.

American Society of Anesthesiologists Task Force on Obstetric Anesthesia. Practice guidelines for obstetric anesthesia: An updated report by the American Society of Anesthesiologists Task Force on Obstetric Anesthesia. *Anesthesiology*. 2007;106:843-863.

Dahl JB, Jeppesen IS, Jorgensen H, et al. Intraoperative and postoperative analgesic efficacy and adverse effects of intrathecal opioids in patients undergoing cesarean section with spinal anesthesia. *Anesthesiology*. 1999;91:1919-1927.

Tsen LC. Anesthesia for cesarean delivery. In: Chestnut D, ed. *Chestnut's Obstetric Anesthesia: Principles and Practice*. 4th ed. Philadelphia: Mosby Elsevier; 2009:521-574.

CHAPTER 187

Effects of High Maternal Oxygen Concentrations on the Fetus

Inge Falk van Rooyen, MD

When necessary, 100% O_2 may be given to a parturient to improve fetal oxygenation; however, maternal hyperoxygenation may have a harmful effect on the developing fetal vascular beds. For more than a century, research has shown that, as a result of the harmful effects of free O_2 radicals and oxidative stress, O_2 can be toxic, particularly to the vascular beds of the central nervous system, the eye, and pulmonary circulation. It is also now clear that preterm infants are more susceptible to O_2 toxicity than are full-term infants. Several factors are known to affect severity of injury related to O_2 toxicity (Box 187-1).

Within the fetomaternal circulation, the highest possible partial pressure gradient of O_2 that can be delivered to the fetus in utero is limited by the fetomaternal gas-exchange mechanisms (Figure 187-1). The placenta is 15 times less efficient at gas exchange than is the lung; however, the unloading of O_2 to the fetus is enhanced by several biochemical mechanisms.

Placental Transfer of O_2

Increasing maternal oxygenation will increase the partial pressure of O_2 (Po_2) in the fetal umbilical artery and umbilical vein. Because of limited flow exchange (placental), an increase in maternal Pao_2 does not produce an increase of equal magnitude in the fetus. Even with a maternal inspired O_2 concentration of 100%, fetal Po_2 in the umbilical vein will be less than 50 mm Hg. It has been shown in an animal model that, by increasing the maternal inspired O_2 concentration from 0.21 to 1.0, the Po_2 in the umbilical vein increases by only 10 mm Hg at 1 atm pressure.

Hyperbaric O_2 delivery to the mother will significantly increase fetal Po_2. It has been shown that hyperbaric O_2 delivery to a pregnant ewe to achieve an arterial Po_2 of 1300 mm Hg will raise umbilical vein Po_2 to nearly 600 mm Hg. No fall in uteroplacental or umbilical blood flow occurs.

Toxic Effects of High Maternal O_2 Concentration

Three anatomic sites are considered to be most at risk for the toxic effects of hyperoxia: the lung, eye, and brain. Sequelae include bronchopulmonary dysplasia, retinopathy, and periventricular leukomalacia.

Box 187-1 Factors Affecting the Severity of Fetal Injury Resulting from Exposure to High Maternal O_2 Concentrations

- Duration of O_2 exposure
- Steep gradient between maternal Fio_2 and fetal Pao_2
- Extent of prematurity of the fetus
- Preexisting fetal and maternal pathology

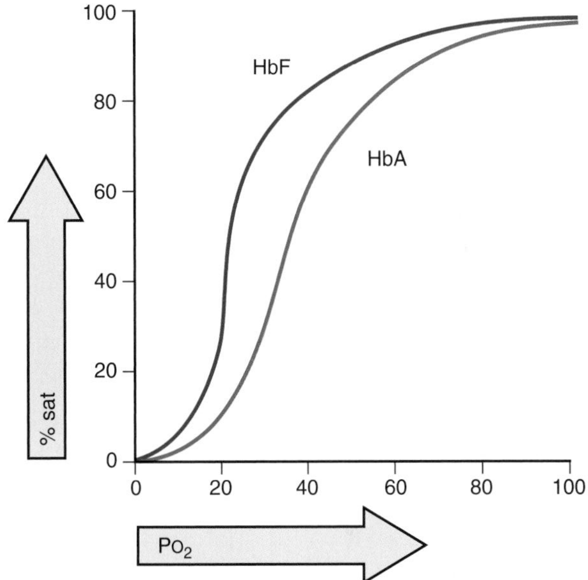

Figure 187-1 Dissociation curves of fetal hemoglobin (HbF) and adult hemoglobin (HbA). In the placenta, the HbA frees up its O_2 in favor of the HbF, which possesses a higher affinity for O_2.

Bronchopulmonary Dysplasia and O_2 Toxicity

Chronic lung disease or bronchopulmonary dysplasia is a severe complication of prematurity. Pathologic mechanisms of tissue injury are complex. However, injury may be caused by direct reactive O_2 species production in response to hyperoxia or indirectly by reactive O_2 species due to phagocyte activation and inflammation. Recent studies in newborn mice exposed to 100% O_2 at normal atmospheric pressure for up to 6 weeks resulted in pulmonary changes comprising deposition of dense fibrous tissue, chronic bronchitis, bronchiolitis, and emphysema. Survival of the experimental animals also decreased with the duration of O_2 exposure.

Retinopathy of Prematurity

Treatment with supplemental O_2 in premature infants who have incompletely vascularized retinas (a process that is usually completed at 36 weeks of gestation) may cause hyperoxia and vasoconstriction. This leads to local hypoxia, deposition of fibrous tissue, excessive tissue vascularization, and the further mechanisms of visual loss from retinopathy of prematurity.

O_2 and Brain Injury

Oxidative stress and damage to premyelinating oligodendrocytes in cerebral white matter has been proposed as a mechanism of periventricular leukomalacia, increasing the risk of cerebral palsy and cognitive deficit in preterm infants.

Fetal Abnormalities

No fetal abnormalities have been found in human or animal models with administration to the parturient of up to 100% O_2 at 1 atm pressure. However, hyperbaric O_2 delivery has been shown to be teratogenic in animals. In one study, hamsters that received 100% O_2 delivered at 2 atm for 3 h or 3 atm for 2 h gave birth to offspring with a number of congenital anomalies, including spina bifida, exencephaly, and limb defects. In another experiment, hyperbaric O_2 administered to rabbits late in pregnancy resulted in retrolental fibroplasia, retinal detachment, microphthalmia, and stillbirth.

Optimal Maternal O_2 Concentration

To date, there is insufficient evidence available to suggest what the optimal O_2 saturation or PaO_2 values are in preterm infants (who receive supplemental O_2) to prevent O_2 toxicity while providing adequate O_2 delivery to tissues.

Suggested Readings

Heidary G, Vanderveen D, Smith LE. Retinopathy of prematurity: Current concepts in molecular pathogenesis. *Semin Ophthalmol.* 2009;24:77-81.

Jobe AH, Bancalari E. Bronchopulmonary dysplasia. *Am J Respir Crit Care Med.* 2001;163:1723-1729.

Maternal physiology. In: Cunningham FG, Leveno KJ, Bloom SL, et al, eds. *Williams Obstetrics.* 23rd ed. New York: McGraw-Hill; 2009:79-107.

Rasanen J, Wood DC, Debbs RH, et al. Reactivity of the human fetal pulmonary circulation to maternal hyperoxygenation increases during the second half of pregnancy: A randomized study. *Circulation.* 1998;97:257-262.

Shaul PW, Farrer MA, Zellers TM. Oxygen modulates endothelium-derived relaxing factor production in fetal pulmonary arteries. *Am J Physiol.* 1992; 262:H355-364.

Simchen MJ, Tesler J, Azami T, et al. Effects of maternal hyperoxia with and without normocapnia in uteroplacental and fetal Doppler studies. *Ultrasound Obstet Gynecol.* 2005;26:495-499.

CHAPTER 188

Maternal Diabetes: Neonatal Effects

Jack L. Wilson, MD

As the obesity epidemic becomes even greater in the United States, the incidence of diabetes mellitus is also increasing. The disease prevalence in the United States is 2.6% to 4.5% of the general adult population, and 3% to 7% of pregnancies result in a new diagnosis of gestational diabetes mellitus (GDM). Diabetes may complicate pregnancy, delivery, and fetal outcomes. The majority of parturients experiencing diabetes have GDM resulting from insulin resistance that occurs during pregnancy secondary to hormonal factors. This type of diabetes often resolves following pregnancy and delivery, but many of these patients are susceptible to developing type 2 diabetes later in life. However, approximately 10% of diabetic parturients have preexisting diabetes. Table 188-1 lists the classification scheme for diabetes complicating pregnancies.

Traditionally, GDM has been linked to increased fetal risks (Box 188-1), particularly associations with fetal macrosomia, birth trauma, and a higher incidence of cesarean delivery. Although no clear evidence of increased perinatal mortality rate in the offspring of women with GDM exists, a more confounding question is whether the association of fetal macrosomia results from the diabetes, or from obesity, and if treatment of maternal hyperglycemia improves outcomes—including a decreased rate of cesarean section. There is some evidence that identifying and treating gestational diabetes can decrease the incidence of macrosomia.

Table 188-1 White's Classification System of Diabetes During Pregnancy

Class	Definition
A1	Gestational diabetes that is diet controlled
A2	Gestational diabetes that requires insulin
B	Preexisting diabetes with onset before age 20 and duration <10 years without complications
C	Preexisting diabetes with onset between ages 10 and 19 or duration <10 years (ages 10 to 19) without complications
D	Preexisting diabetes with onset before age 10 or duration >20 years without complications
F	Preexisting diabetes complicated by nephropathy
R	Preexisting diabetes complicated by proliferative retinopathy
T	Preexisting diabetes and status post kidney transplantation
H	Preexisting diabetes complicated by ischemic heart disease

From Braveman FR: The Requisites in Anesthesiology. St. Louis: Mosby; 2006:96, Table 8-2.

Box 188-1 Neonatal and Maternal Morbidity Associated with Maternal Diabetes Mellitus

Fetal macrosomia (>4-4.5 kg)
- Shoulder dystocia
- Birth trauma

Fetal pulmonary hypoplasia
Increased propensity for cesarean delivery
Increased risk of congenital anomalies*
Increased risk of intrauterine fetal death
Intrauterine infections
Maternal diabetic ketoacidosis†
Maternal hypoglycemia†
Neonatal hypoglycemia
Nonreassuring fetal status
Preeclampsia or eclampsia
Polyhydramnios
Reduction in uteroplacental perfusion‡

*Especially cardiovascular and central nervous system anomalies.
†In parturients with type 1 diabetes.
‡Compared with parturients without diabetes, 35% to 40% lower.

Many obstetricians increase the frequency of fetal assessments during the third trimester in parturients with GDM to more closely monitor the progress of the pregnancy and to make decisions regarding timing of delivery. Even if the results of fetal assessments are reassuring, many obstetricians will induce labor in diabetic patients at 38 to 40 weeks of gestation to avoid the possibility of a late stillbirth and also to reduce the risks of delivering a macrosomic infant—with potential shoulder dystocia, birth trauma, and increased incidence of cesarean delivery.

Following delivery, the most common problem neonates of mothers with GDM may face is hypoglycemia, occurring in 5% to 12% of cases. The proposed cause relates to increased secretion of insulin by the fetus in response to maternal hyperglycemia. In terms of fetal anomalies, there is a difference between infants born to women with pregestational diabetes and those born to women with GDM. The former group is associated with a 6% to 18% incidence of major anomalies (most commonly cardiovascular and central nervous system), whereas the latter group is associated with a lower 3% to 8% incidence—still higher than in nondiabetic parturients. Clinical data, although inconclusive, point to a benefit of strict glycemic control in diabetic parturients—in terms of preventing neonatal adverse outcomes and anomalies.

Suggested Readings

Crowther CA, Hiller JE, Moss JR, et al, for the Australian Carbohydrate Intolerance Study in Pregnant Women (ACHOIS) Trial Group. Effect of treatment of gestational diabetes mellitus on pregnancy outcomes. *N Engl J Med.* 2005;352:2477-2486.

Fragneto RY. The high-risk obstetric patient. In: Braveman FR, ed. *Obstetric and Gynecologic Anesthesia—The Requisites in Anesthesiology.* Philadelphia: Mosby; 2006, Chap. 8.

Greene MF, Solomon CG. Gestational diabetes mellitus—Time to treat. *N Engl J Med.* 2005;352:2544-2546.

Wissler RN. Endocrine disorders. In: Chestnut DH, ed. *Obstetric Anesthesia Principles and Practice.* 3rd ed. Philadelphia: Elsevier Mosby; 2004, Chap. 41.

CHAPTER 189

Peripartum Hemorrhage

K.A. Kelly McQueen, MD, MPH

Despite advances in obstetric care and improved diagnostic testing, peripartum hemorrhage remains a leading cause of maternal morbidity and death. Severe bleeding is most common in the third trimester of pregnancy and near the time of delivery.

Antepartum Hemorrhage

Causes of Antepartum Hemorrhage

Severe antepartum hemorrhage is most commonly associated with placenta previa, abruptio placentae, and uterine rupture.

Placenta Previa

Placenta previa is defined as abnormal implantation of the placenta on the lower uterine segment with partial to complete occlusion of the internal cervical os. It occurs in 1 in 200 to 1 in 250 deliveries and is associated with maternal mortality rate of up to 0.9%. The multiparous patient and the older patient are at increased risk for developing placenta previa, as are patients undergoing repeat cesarean section (C/S). The chance of recurrence in a subsequent pregnancy is approximately 5%.

Abruptio Placentae

Abruptio placentae results from separation of a normally implanted placenta after 20 weeks of gestation and before birth. It occurs in 1 in 75 to 1 in 226 deliveries. Maternal mortality rate is 1.8% to 2.8%, and fetal mortality rate may be as high as 50%. Risk factors include hypertensive disorders, high parity, uterine abnormalities, trauma, intravenous drug use, and history of previous abruption. Bleeding may be apparent (external) or concealed (internal) and varies in severity from mild (<100 mL) to severe (>500 mL).

The type of delivery and the timing will depend on the severity of hemorrhage. With limited blood loss, vaginal delivery is often possible. If the mother or fetus is in distress, then rapid delivery by C/S is required. In mild or moderate abruptions with fetal death, maternal coagulation must be evaluated before regional anesthetic is administered because disseminated intravascular coagulation may occur within 8 h of fetal demise.

Uterine Rupture

Uterine rupture is a rare but serious cause of hemorrhage occurring in 0.1% to 0.3% of pregnancies. Risk factors include previous uterine surgery, past history of uterine rupture, abnormal fetal presentation, operative vaginal delivery, use of uterotonic agents, and uterine distention. Maternal mortality rate approaches 5%, and fetal mortality rate is as high as 50%. Presenting signs and symptoms include atypical abdominal pain, shoulder pain, vaginal bleeding, uterine tenderness, hypotension, tachycardia, and shock.

Anesthetic Management of Antepartum Hemorrhage

Anesthetic management includes ensuring the availability of blood and blood products and securing adequate venous access through placement of large-bore central cannulas, peripheral cannulas, or both. If an emergency C/S is required, general anesthesia is usually recommended because of maternal intravascular hypovolemia, coagulopathy, positioning problems during regional anesthetic administration, and surgical urgency.

When possible, before a C/S is undertaken, all efforts should be made to stabilize the mother while maintaining uterine perfusion pressure (uterine arterial pressure minus uterine venous pressure) and maximizing oxygenation. If time permits, maternal laboratory evaluation, including platelet concentration, prothrombin time, activated partial thromboplastin time, fibrinogen level, and hemoglobin concentration, should be ordered. If maternal hemodynamic status is stable and coagulation status is normal, then regional anesthesia can be used for the urgent C/S.

Postpartum Hemorrhage

The vast majority of cases of severe postpartum hemorrhage occur within a few minutes after delivery. Postpartum hemorrhage is the most common hemorrhagic condition in obstetrics and is typically defined as a blood loss of 500 mL or more within 24 h of delivery. Postpartum hemorrhage can be massive and sudden and may require aggressive therapy. The three most common causes of postpartum hemorrhage are retained placenta and membranes, uterine atony, and genital tract disruption (Box 189-1).

Causes of Postpartum Hemorrhage

Placenta Accreta

Placental accreta is an abnormally adherent placenta, which can lead to devastating acute blood loss. The incidence of this problem appears to be increasing as a result of the increasing numbers of repeat cesarean deliveries. Placenta accreta vera is present when the placenta is adherent to the myometrium without invasion into the uterine muscle. Placenta increta involves myometrial adherence with invasion into the muscle, and placenta percreta involves invasion into the uterine serosa and beyond—often involving other pelvic structures.

Table 189-1 Pharmacologic Treatment of Uterine Atony and Postpartum Hemorrhage

Medication	Dose	Side Effect(s)
Oxytocin (Pitocin)	10-40 units/L of IV fluid	Hypotension
Methylergonovine maleate (Methergine)*	0.2 mg IM	N/V
15-Methylprostaglandin $F_{2\alpha}$ (Hemabate)	250 μg IM or IV	Bronchospasm
Misoprostol (Cytotec)	600 μg PO or sublingual	Shivering, ↑ temperature, N/V, diarrhea

*Contraindicated in patients with preeclampsia.
IM, Intramuscular(ly); IV, intravenous(ly); N/V, nausea and vomiting; PO, per os (by mouth).

Retained Placenta and Membranes

The placenta and membranes are retained in about 1% of vaginal deliveries. Treatment usually includes manual exploration of the uterus, which may require treatment to provide uterine relaxation. Commonly used agents to facilitate exploration include intravenously administered nitroglycerin, sedation with ketamine or opioids, low doses of inhalation anesthetic agents, and induction of general anesthesia.

Uterine Atony

Uterine atony of varying severity commonly occurs after vaginal delivery. Blood loss can be massive and sudden and is sometimes delayed for several hours. Risk factors include multiparity, multiple births, polyhydramnios, intrauterine manipulation, and retained placenta. Initial treatments include uterine massage and pharmacologic therapy (Table 189-1). Persistent uterine atony and maternal hemorrhage may necessitate massive blood transfusions and, in extreme cases, hysterectomy.

Genital Tract Disruption

Genital tract disruption may result in severe postpartum hemorrhage. Lacerations may occur in the vagina, cervix, or body of the uterus. An episiotomy incision is another possible source of bleeding. Vigilance must be maintained after delivery, as blood loss may be delayed.

Treatment of Postpartum Hemorrhage

Treatment is similar to that for antepartum hemorrhage. Early diagnosis and aggressive treatment are important to decrease maternal morbidity and mortality risks. After the diagnosis is established, large-bore intravenous access should be secured as soon as possible. Preparations should be made for

Box 189-1 Etiology of Antepartum and Postpartum Hemorrhage

Antepartum Hemorrhage

Abruptio placentae
Placenta previa
Uterine rupture
Vasa previa

Postpartum Hemorrhage

Genital trauma
Placenta accreta
Retained placenta
Uterine atony
Uterine inversion

Box 189-2 General Anesthesia for Emergency Cesarean Section for Maternal Hemorrhage

Administer nonparticulate oral antacid
Insert two large-bore IV catheters
Replace blood loss with crystalloids or colloids
Type and crossmatch 2 units of blood
Have access to a rapid-infusion blood-warming device
Preoxygenate
Maintain ongoing fluid resuscitation
Use a rapid-sequence induction while providing cricoid pressure
Induction agent
    Etomidate, 0.3 mg/kg
    Ketamine, 0.5-1 mg/kg

massive transfusion; adequate supplies of crystalloids, colloids, blood, and blood products should be available. Blood warmers should be used to prevent hypothermia. The use of invasive hemodynamic monitoring—including arterial catheterization and central venous pressure monitoring—should be considered (Box 189-2), as should the use of a rapid-infusion device.

The treatment for uterine atony and retained products of conception (once extracted) include oxytocic and other vasoconstriction pharmacologic therapy. Oxytocic agents stimulate the smooth muscle of the uterus, thereby producing or augmenting uterine contractions. Oxytocin is a posterior pituitary hormone that stimulates uterine smooth muscle. The synthetic derivative of oxytocin, Pitocin, is the drug of choice to treat uterine atony because it has less antidiuretic and cardiovascular activity than does vasopressin. Pitocin is primarily given as an intravenous bolus, a continuous infusion, or both a bolus and an infusion titrated to effect; the use of Pitocin requires monitoring uterine contractions during labor and in the postoperative period. Pitocin generally affects the uterus by causing slow generalized contractions with periods of relaxation between contractions. The side effects of Pitocin include hypotension, especially when given as a bolus, and secondary tachycardia; these effects usually occur immediately after administration of the drug and are typically transient. Transient electrocardiographic changes, including T-wave flattening and inversion and a prolonged QT interval, may occur. When given in large doses or over extended periods, Pitocin may produce water intoxication and hyponatremia.

Methylergonovine Maleate

A purified semisynthetic ergot alkaloid, methylergonovine maleate (Methergine) is typically given as a 0.2-mg intramuscular injection to augment uterine contractions if Pitocin does not produce the desired effect. Methergine is used exclusively in the postpartum period because it produces tonic contractions more quickly, as compared with Pitocin, that significantly limit blood flow. The major side effects include nausea, vomiting, and significant hypertension due to direct peripheral vasoconstriction. For this reason, intravenous administration of Methergine is controversial, and the drug must be carefully administered to parturients with essential hypertension or pregnancy-induced hypertension.

Prostaglandin $F_{2\alpha}$

Severe uterine atony and postpartum hemorrhage may necessitate the use of prostaglandin $F_{2\alpha}$ ($PGF_{2\alpha}$), a biochemical produced by the pregnant uterus that induces uterine contractions. $PGF_{2\alpha}$ can also cause bronchospasm. The 15-methyl analog of $PGF_{2\alpha}$ (Hemabate) acts similarly to $PGF_{2\alpha}$ but promotes stronger sustained uterine contractions, limiting blood flow to the uterus. 15-Methyl $PGF_{2\alpha}$ (250 μg) is administered intramuscularly or intramyometrially only after Pitocin and Methergine have been used and have failed to achieve the desired results because of the nausea, vomiting, and diarrhea associated with the use of 15-methyl $PGF_{2\alpha}$.

For some patients with persistent postpartum hemorrhage whose bleeding fails to respond to pharmacologic interventions, angiographic uterine artery embolization may be an option. This procedure can be performed in the presence of coagulopathy and under local anesthesia. During angiography, the radiologist can identify the vessels responsible for bleeding and embolize these vessels effectively with Gelfoam, a technique that allows for return of flow over time, thereby preserving fecundity.

If pharmacologic and radiologic interventions fail, or if the cause of postpartum hemorrhage is only amenable to surgery (repair of genital tract disruption), a surgical approach may be necessary to control bleeding. Surgical approaches include bilateral hypogastric artery ligation, bilateral ovarian artery ligation, and uterine artery ligation. In rare cases, emergency hysterectomy is required to treat postpartum hemorrhage. Postpartum hysterectomy is the definitive treatment for postpartum hemorrhage.

Suggested Readings

Mayer DC, Smith KA. Antepartum and postpartum hemorrhage. In: Chestnut DH, ed. *Obstetric Anesthesia: Principles and Practice*. 4th ed. Philadelphia: Mosby Elsevier; 2009:811-852.

Practice guidelines for obstetric anesthesia. An updated report by the American Society of Anesthesiologists Task Force on Obstetric Anesthesia. *Anesthesiology*. 2007;106:843-863.

CHAPTER 190

Anesthesia for Tubal Ligation

Scott A. Gammel, MD

Tubal ligations are performed either as an interval (not postpartum) procedure or as an immediate postpartum procedure using local, regional, or general anesthesia.

Interval Tubal Ligations

Laparoscopy is the most common surgical approach for interval tubal ligations. Anesthetic considerations include those related to pneumoperitoneum, head-down positioning (with related cardiovascular and pulmonary changes), and other potential complications.

Pneumoperitoneum is performed via a needle inserted at the lower margin of the umbilicus (a relatively avascular and thin portion of the abdominal wall). An incorrectly placed needle can lead to insufflation of the abdominal wall, retroperitoneum, mesentery, omentum, or bowel. CO_2 is the gas of choice to perform pneumoperitoneum because it is highly soluble, is rapidly absorbed postoperatively, and provides a margin of safety if injected intravascularly. N_2O is less soluble and is not eliminated as quickly, but its use is associated with less peritoneal and diaphragmatic irritation and less postoperative shoulder pain.

Head-down (Trendelenburg) positioning is associated with brachial plexus injury if shoulder rests are used (as a result of clavicular compression of nerve roots); however, current guidelines recommend that shoulder rests *not* be used for patients in the Trendelenburg position. Because the Trendelenburg position results in decreased functional residual capacity, decreased pulmonary compliance, and altered stomach position, tracheal intubation will reduce the risk of pulmonary aspiration and atelectasis. Mainstem intubation may result from cephalad shift of the mediastinum and carina.

Cardiovascular changes result from increased intraabdominal pressure, patient position, anesthesia, and hypercarbia. Decreases in cardiac output, increased peripheral and pulmonary vascular resistance, increased arterial pressure, and arrhythmias may result.

Respiratory changes include decreased vital capacity, decreased functional residual capacity, increased blood volume, and decreased pulmonary compliance, which can lead to atelectasis. Peak inspiratory pressures increase. A significant increase in arterial CO_2 (15% to 25%) and decrease in pH occur during general anesthesia when CO_2 is used for insufflation because of absorption of CO_2 from the pneumoperitoneum. Spontaneous ventilation can also lead to significant hypercarbia.

Other complications include hemorrhage, (accounting for almost half of complications), cardiac arrhythmias (some of which may result from reflex increases in vagal tone from peritoneal stretching or electrocautery of fallopian tubes), gas embolism, pneumothorax, pneumomediastinum, pneumopericardium, and mesenteric ischemia. Complications from creation of pneumoperitoneum and placement of trocars are more common with laparoscopy performed for tubal ligation than with laparoscopy for gastrointestinal surgery.

Anesthetic Techniques

General Anesthesia

After intravenous induction takes place, O_2, N_2O, and an inhaled anesthetic agent are used to maintain anesthesia. This is supplemented with short-acting opioids and neuromuscular blocking agents.

Common postoperative complications of general anesthesia are abdominal and shoulder pain and postoperative nausea and vomiting (PONV). Increasing the volume of infused preoperative and intraoperative fluids reduces the incidence of PONV and improves hemodynamic response to pneumoperitoneum and postoperative recovery.

Metoclopramide (10-20 mg, administered intravenously 15-30 min before induction) and droperidol (0.5-1.0 mg, administered 3-6 min before induction) are synergistic in decreasing nausea, vomiting, and recovery time. Droperidol alone (0.625-2.15 mg) administered after intubation is an effective antiemetic for outpatient tubal ligation, and its use shortens time in the postanesthesia care unit. Ondansetron (4-8 mg, administered intravenously) before induction also significantly reduces the incidence of PONV.

Neuraxial Anesthesia

Regional anesthesia is not often used for interval tubal sterilization because the block may take too long to develop and spinal headache is more likely to occur in this patient group. The ability to maintain spontaneous ventilation may be difficult for the patient, especially when she is in the steep head-down position, but neuraxial anesthesia does not have a major detrimental effect on ventilation. The incidence of PONV and the metabolic response is lower in patients who receive neuraxial anesthesia, compared with general anesthesia.

Local Anesthesia

Although local anesthesia is not commonly used for laparoscopy in the United States, it is the number one technique used throughout the world—for either intermittent or postpartum tubal ligation. The use of local anesthesia for tubal ligation produces fewer hemodynamic changes (less likelihood of hypertension, hypotension, or tachycardia), less PONV, quicker recovery, and earlier diagnosis of complications. It is also reported to produce shorter surgical time and be significantly less expensive. Success of local anesthesia demands gentle and precise surgical technique. Sedation improves management of patient anxiety and pain from organ and tissue manipulation.

Postpartum Tubal Ligation

The American Society of Anesthesiologists provides published guidelines concerning postpartum tubal ligations in section VI of their "Practice Guidelines for Obstetric Anesthesia" (Box 190-1). In addition to following these guidelines, it is prudent to also check the patient's preoperative hemoglobin level because determining blood loss at delivery may be difficult.

Anesthetic Techniques

General Anesthesia

The increased risk of aspiration occurring in the postpartum period probably warrants the prophylactic use of an H_2-receptor antagonist, nonparticulate antacid, and metoclopramide with rapid sequence induction and application of cricoid pressure for the postpartum woman undergoing tubal ligation.

Halogenated inhaled anesthetic agents cause dose-related uterine relaxation and, therefore, increase the risk of hemorrhage, especially in multiparous women. The reduced minimum alveolar concentration of an inhaled anesthetic agent that occurs in the postpartum period returns to normal 12 to 36 h after delivery. Propofol anesthesia (induction and maintenance) provides a lower incidence of PONV and rapid awakening, with low concentrations in breast milk 4 and 8 h postoperatively.

Plasma cholinesterase activity is significantly lower in postpartum women than in women who are not postpartum, even compared with pregnant women; therefore, blockade with succinylcholine, rocuronium, mivacurium, or vecuronium is prolonged in the postpartum period; however, when the dose of rocuronium is based on lean body mass, blockade is

Box 190-1 Summary of Postpartum Tubal Anesthesia Guidelines from American Society of Anesthesiologists Practice Guidelines for Obstetric Anesthesia

Statements

There is insufficient literature to evaluate the benefits of neuraxial, compared with general, anesthesia.
There is insufficient literature to evaluate the impact of timing of procedure on maternal outcome.
Neuraxial, compared with general, anesthesia reduces complications.
The consultants agree that performing postpartum tubal ligation within 8 h of delivery does not increase maternal complications.

Recommendations

No oral intake of solid foods for 6-8 h prior to surgery.
Aspiration prophylaxis should be considered.
The timing of the procedure and the anesthetic technique should be individualized and based on anesthetic risk factors, obstetric risk factors (e.g., blood loss), and patient preference. However, neuraxial techniques are preferred to general anesthesia for most postpartum tubal ligations.
The anesthesiologist should be aware that gastric emptying will be delayed if the patient received opioids during labor.
The anesthesiologist should be aware that an epidural catheter used for labor will be more likely to fail the longer the postdelivery-to-surgery time interval.

not prolonged. Neuromuscular blockade is unchanged with atracurium and is shortened with cisatracurium. Metoclopramide inhibits plasma cholinesterase and prolongs succinylcholine neuromuscular blockade by 100% to 200%.

Neuraxial Anesthesia

Neuraxial anesthesia for postpartum tubal sterilizations provides excellent operating conditions and is the most common anesthetic technique used for this indication in the United States. Airway risk (obstruction, hypoventilation, and aspiration) is significantly reduced, as compared with general anesthesia. A T4 block provides excellent operating conditions and pain relief. A T10 block may be inadequate, especially if it is difficult to mobilize the uterus during surgery. Sedation that prolongs postoperative amnesia should be avoided to improve early maternal-neonate interaction and bonding.

Although epidural catheters used for labor are more likely to fail when used for tubal ligation if surgery is delayed for more than 10 h after delivery, success rates are still high for up to 24 h after delivery. Postpartum use of an epidural catheter is more likely to be successful when a multiorifice catheter is placed 4 to 6 cm into the epidural space and secured to the patient's skin while her back is not flexed.

Starting 18 h postpartum, there is a progressive decrease in dermatomal spread of epidural anesthesia, compared with the spread in patients given epidurals for cesarean section. At 36 h postpartum, there is no significant difference in spread between women who have recently delivered and nonpregnant patients.

Spinal anesthesia has a very positive risk-benefit profile. The risk of local anesthetic toxicity is almost nil compared with epidural anesthesia. Rapidity of onset (and offset) and density of block are very favorable. The risk of postdural puncture headache when using small-gauge or pencil-point-design spinal needles is low and may be no different than with epidural anesthesia.

Local anesthetic requirements (which are lessened by 30% in pregnant women) return to nonpregnant levels within 12 to 36 h after delivery and appear to be associated with rapid decline in progesterone levels. There is a faster onset, higher level, and longer duration of spinal anesthesia in term patients than in young gynecologic patients. There is also a progressive decline in duration of block during the first 3 days postpartum.

Cardiovascular effects are markedly decreased in postpartum patients (no aortocaval compression and maternal autotransfusion at delivery), as compared with pregnant women. The need for treatment of hypotension after spinal anesthesia is lower (<10%), compared with patients undergoing cesarean section (>80%).

To avoid the transient neurologic symptoms associated with the use of hyperbaric lidocaine and hyperbaric bupivacaine, preservative-free meperidine (intrathecal formulation) at a dose of 1 mg/kg based on the patient's prepregnant weight (usual range 50-80 mg) may be used. The onset time of intrathecal meperidine is 3 to 5 min, with a duration of 30 to 60 min. The use of 60 mg of meperidine or 70 mg of 5% lidocaine have similar rates of PONV and patient satisfaction, but meperidine provides a notably longer postoperative analgesia. Pruritus occurs more often with meperidine.

Local Anesthesia

Local anesthesia is the most commonly used technique worldwide to provide anesthesia for a tubal ligation. See earlier discussions on Anesthetic Techniques in Interval Tubal Ligation for a discussion of the use of local anesthesia in tubal ligation.

Suggested Readings

American Society of Anesthesiologists Task Force on Obstetric Anesthesia. Practice guidelines for obstetric anesthesia: An updated report by the American Society of Anesthesiologists Task Force on Obstetric Anesthesia. *Anesthesiology*. 2007;106:843-863.

Balestrieri PJ. Epidural chloroprocaine-standard of care for postpartum bilateral tubal ligation. *Anesth Analg*. 2005;101:1241.

Bucklin BA. Postpartum tubal ligation: Timing and other anesthetic considerations. *Clin Obstet Gynecol*. 2003;46:657-666.

Gupta L, Sinha SK, Pande M, Vajifdar H. Ambulatory laparoscopic tubal ligation: A comparison of general anaesthesia with local anaesthesia and sedation. *J Anaesthesiol Clin Pharmacol*. 2011;27:97-100.

Hawkins JL. Postpartum tubal ligation. In: Chestnut DH, Polley LS, Tsen LC, Wong CA, eds. *Obstetric Anesthesia*. 4th ed. Philadelphia: Mosby Elsevier; 2009: 505-517.

Lawrie TA, Nardin JM, Kulier R, Boulvain M. Techniques for the interruption of tubal patency for female sterilisation. *Cochrane Database Syst Rev*. 2011; 16:CD003034.

McKenzie R, Kovac A, O'Conner T, et al. Comparison of ondansetron versus placebo to prevent postoperative nausea vomiting in women undergoing ambulatory gynecologic surgery. *Anesthesiology*. 1993;78:21-28.

Panni MK, George RB, Allen TK, et al. Minimum effective dose of spinal ropivacaine with and without fentanyl for postpartum tubal ligation. *Int J Obstet Anesth*. 2010;19:390-394.

PART H Pediatrics

CHAPTER 191

Neonatal Cardiovascular Physiology

William C. Oliver Jr., MD

To better understand neonatal cardiac physiology, it is necessary to have knowledge of the fetal circulation, knowledge of the neonatal circulation, and knowledge of the transition between the two.

Fetal Circulation

Compared with the postnatal circulation (in which the right ventricle and left ventricle are in series), in the fetal circulation, the two ventricles are in parallel. The parallel circulation is created by several shunts and preferential flow patterns that deliver relatively well-oxygenated blood from the placenta to those fetal organs that have increased metabolic demand. The most important structures that shunt blood in the fetal circulation are the ductus venosus (DV), the foramen ovale (FO), and the ductus arteriosus (DA).

From the placenta, blood with a partial pressure of oxygen (Po_2) of 30 to 35 mm Hg flows to the fetus via the umbilical vein (UV) (Figure 191-1), which, in the liver of the fetus, separates into two branches, with one branch joining the portal vein and the other becoming the DV, which joins the inferior vena cava (IVC). Approximately 30% to 50% of the oxygenated blood flowing through the UV will bypass the liver and flow directly through the DV into the IVC, flowing along its posterior wall. As this oxygenated blood enters the right atrium, it is directed across the FO into the left atrium by the eustachian valve, flowing through the left ventricle (~35% of fetal circulation) into the aorta to supply the head and upper torso.

The deoxygenated blood returning from the superior vena cava, from the myocardium via the coronary sinus, and from the IVC flows through the right ventricle into the pulmonary artery. Most of this deoxygenated blood returns to the descending aorta via the DA; however, approximately 5% to 10% passes through the high-resistance pulmonary circulation. Blood in the descending aorta either flows through the umbilical arteries to be reoxygenated in the placenta or continues to supply the lower limbs. The fetal circulation therefore runs in parallel, with the left ventricle providing 35% and the right 65% of cardiac output. Fetal cardiac output is therefore measured as a combined ventricular output (CVO).

The three major shunts are under autonomic, neural, and hormonal control. The DV, for example, is not a passive shunt; the vessel is trumpet-shaped, with a sphincter at its distal end that regulates flow by β-adrenergic dilation or α-adrenergic constriction. Hypoxemia, presumably via release of endothelial nitric oxide, results in significant vasodilation. Prostaglandins ostensibly have an important role, as they do in the DA, in maintaining patency and in closure following birth.

The second major shunt, the FO, provides a communication between the right and left atria, directing flow from the inferior venous inlet. As the stream of oxygenated blood ascends along the posterior wall of the IVC into the right atrium, it encounters the interatrial ridge, which separates into two arms. The left arm fills like a windsock formed by the FO valve and the atrial septum to direct the oxygenated blood through the FO into the left atrium. The right arm of the interatrial ridge directs deoxygenated blood toward the right atrium to join with the flow from the superior vena cava and coronary sinus to the tricuspid valve. Channeling of this blood flow is sensitive to a number of factors and is easily influenced by differences in systemic and pulmonary pressures.

The last shunt, the DA, is a wide muscular vessel that connects the pulmonary artery to the descending aorta. The majority of blood ejected from the right ventricle into the pulmonary artery crosses the DA and flows to the lower torso and umbilical arteries. A small fraction, anywhere between 5% and 10%, of the right ventricular output flows beyond the DA into the pulmonary circulation because, prior to birth and inflation of the lungs, the pulmonary vascular resistance (PVR) is quite high because the alveoli are collapsed, compressing the interstitium of the lung. However small the fraction is, it is sufficient to meet the metabolic needs for development and growth of the lungs.

Fetal cardiac output increases from 210 mL/min at 20 weeks of gestation to 1900 mL/min at term. Two thirds of the total aortic flow goes to the placenta because the systemic vascular resistance (SVR) within the placental blood vessels is relatively low, compared with the resistance in the blood vessels within the fetal organs and tissues. Placental blood flow is relatively stable, unaffected by autonomic or neural inputs, correlating best with maternal arterial blood pressure.

The fetal ventricles are poorly compliant, with the right less so than the left, in part from the constraint of the pericardium, collapsed lungs, and constrained chest wall. They are therefore limited in their ability to increase stroke volume, so that an increase in cardiac output is achieved by an increase in heart rate. Conversely, if heart rate decreases, so too does cardiac output. Unlike during the postnatal state, in the prenatal state, there is very little difference between fetal right and left ventricular pressures.

Transition to Neonatal Circulation

Transition to the postnatal circulation is initiated by two abrupt changes: (1) a dramatic increase in SVR caused by removal of the placenta (low SVR) from the fetal circulation and (2) following inflation of the lungs, an equally dramatic decrease in PVR mediated by increased production of endogenous nitric oxide. Normally, smaller vessels in the lungs continue to dilate for 24 h after birth. However, the pulmonary vasculature of the neonate is very sensitive to hypoxia and hypercarbia, which may trigger pulmonary vasoconstriction and dilation, respectively, rather than closure of the DA. If the precipitating factors are left untreated, a life-threatening condition known as persistent fetal circulation (PFC) may develop.

The changes in oxygenation, SVR, and PVR that occur at birth functionally close the fetal shunts, and the ventricles begin working in series.

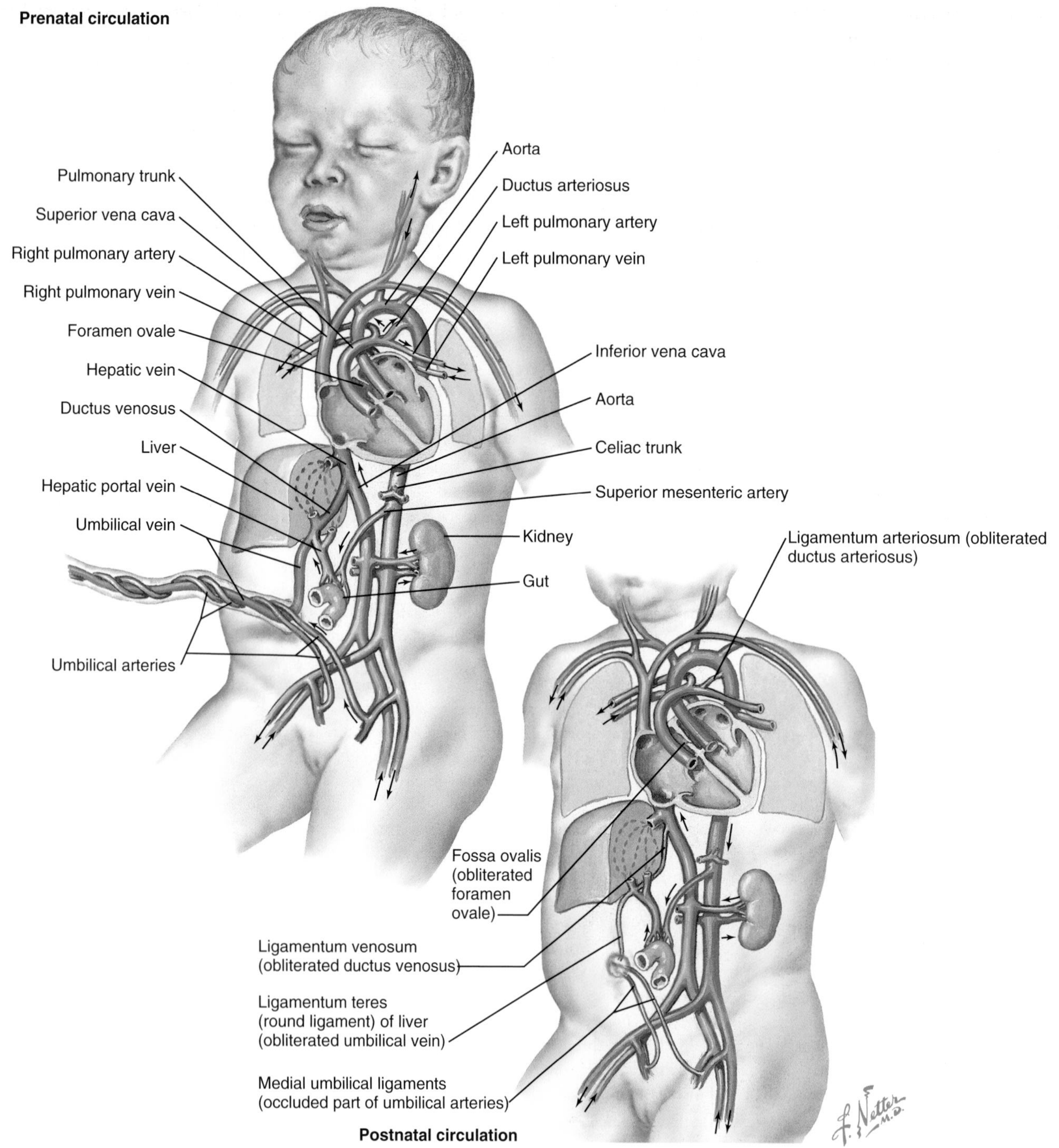

Figure 191-1 Prenatal and postnatal circulation. Prenatally, inferior vena caval blood is largely diverted across the foramen ovale to the left atrium, while the superior vena caval blood enters the right ventricle. Blood from the right ventricle is shunted away from the pulmonary circulation through the ductus arteriosus. (Netter illustration from www.netterimages.com. © Elsevier Inc. All rights reserved.)

The DV starts to wither once the UV flow disappears following placental separation. Its demise is a passive event that occurs functionally between 3 and 7 days after birth and is obliterated by 1 to 3 weeks. Unlike the DA, there is no identifiable trigger for its closure.

Flow through the DA changes from a right-to-left shunt to a left-to-right shunt until functional closure occurs, usually within 24 h. Anatomic closure normally occurs within 4 to 8 weeks of life; however, the DA will remain patent in the presence of hypoxemia.

The closure of the FO is based on pressure differences between the right and left atria. Following birth, pulmonary venous return increases, significantly raising left atrial pressure, which forces the flap of the FO to press against the septum, functionally closing the opening between the right and left atria. Anatomic closure may occur as early as 3 months of age but often is delayed until 5 years of age.

Neonatal Cardiovascular Physiology

Fetal myocytes are morphologically different from those of adults in that they are smaller, have fewer myofibrils, and display greater myofibril disorganization. Growth of the fetal heart occurs by hyperplasia of the myocytes, accounting for the increased size of the heart temporarily after birth. The right ventricle is larger than the left at birth because of the nature of the fetal circulation, but within a few months after birth, the left ventricle increases in size by a factor of 3 secondary to its increased afterload.

Immediately after birth, the neonate's stroke volume nearly doubles because of an increased preload (removal of the placenta) and because of increased thoracic compliance (decreased mechanical encroachment on the mediastinum).

Diastolic function of the heart depends on myocardial relaxation and compliance. Initially, the neonatal heart is much less compliant than the adult heart due to immaturity of the sarcoplasmic reticulum and its inability to sequester calcium during diastole. The decreased compliance limits the ventricular response to preload; excessive preload places the ventricle on the downslope to the right of the Starling curve. Although diastolic function improves with age, neonatal cardiac output is as dependent on heart rate as it was *in utero*. The typical neonatal heart rate is above 140 beats/min to achieve a cardiac output (150 $mL \cdot kg^{-1} \cdot min^{-1}$) twice the adult value based on weight because of the need to meet high neonatal O_2 requirements.

Because of the decreased compliance of the ventricles and immaturity of the autonomic nervous system, cardiac output in neonates is more affected by changes in SVR than it is in infants, and much more so than in the adult heart. Beat-to-beat variability improves over time as the autonomic nervous system matures.

Neonatal blood pressure is typically 75/50 mm Hg. Mean arterial pressure is more dependent on vascular tone than myocardial function. Baroreflexes are impaired after birth, manifested by hypotension with relatively small decreases in preload. Because of the immature autonomic nervous system, direct agonists, as compared with indirect agonists, are more effective for increasing heart rate and blood pressure in neonates.

Neonatal PVR remains relatively high after birth because the pulmonary arterioles have a thicker layer of muscle relative to their diameter, as compared with infants or adults, that results in greater sensitivity to hypoxemia and hypercarbia, sometimes causing PFC. When diagnosing PFC, the clinician must exclude parenchymal lung disease or congenital heart disease as causes of the patient's symptoms and signs. There are many causes of PFC, but, once PFC is diagnosed, the administration of nitric oxide or a vasodilating prostaglandin decreases PVR; attenuates, if not abolishes, the PFC; and eliminates the right-to-left shunt.

Suggested Readings

Abdulla R, Blew GA, Holterman MJ. Cardiovascular embryology. *Pediatr Cardiol.* 2004;25:191-200.

Benson DW. Advances in cardiovascular genetics and embryology: Role of transcription factors in congenital heart disease. *Curr Opin Pediatr.* 2000;12: 497-500.

Kiserud T. Physiology of the fetal circulation. *Semin Fetal Neonatal Med.* 2005;10:493-503.

Lake CL, Booker PD, eds. *Pediatric Cardiac Anesthesia.* 4th ed. Philadelphia: Lippincott, Williams & Wilkins; 2005; 21-22.

Rudolph AM. Myocardial growth before and after birth: Clinical implications. *Acta Paediatr.* 2000;89:129-133.

Soufan AT, van den Berg G, Moerland PD, et al. Three-dimensional measurement and visualization of morphogenesis applied to cardiac embryology. *J Microsc.* 2007;225:269-274.

CHAPTER 192

Differences Between the Infant and Adult Airway

Nicole W. Pelly, MD

The infant airway differs from the adult airway in structure and in functionality (Figure 192-1). Understanding these differences is important for airway management and, when necessary, for successful tracheal intubation of neonatal, infant, and pediatric airways.

Anatomy

Head Size

The head of an infant is proportionally larger than that of an adult because of the infant's large occiput. Elevation of the head to produce an anatomic sniffing position in an infant or child is not needed. An infant or child with a large occiput can sometimes benefit from placing a small folded towel under the shoulders and neck, which slightly elevates the thorax. In addition, the head can be stabilized to prevent side-to-side movement.

Laryngeal Position

The infant larynx is more cephalad than the adult larynx. At birth, the larynx is located opposite the first and second cervical vertebrae (C1 and C2), and the cricoid cartilage is opposite C3. This relationship provides a functional separation between breathing and swallowing so that the infant can suck, swallow, and breathe at the same time without aspirating. By the time a child is 2 years old, the larynx and cricoid have descended to C3-C4. The infant and pediatric larynx is in a more anterior position, and distances between the tongue, hyoid bone, epiglottis, and other oral structures are smaller than in an adult. In adults, the laryngeal opening is opposite the C5-C6 interspace, and the lower cricoid cartilage is located opposite the top of C7. The laryngeal position changes throughout childhood and, by age 8, is in the adult position.

Figure 192-1 Differences between the pediatric and adult airway. (By permission of Mayo Foundation for Medical Research and Education. All rights reserved.)

Tongue

The infant tongue is proportionally larger than the adult tongue and is a common cause of airway obstruction. When infants or children are being mask ventilated, their airways are often enhanced by using an oral airway to relieve this obstruction.

Epiglottis

The infant epiglottis is proportionally longer, compared with the adult epiglottis. It is often omega-shaped, whereas the adult epiglottis is flatter and more flexible. The hyoid bone in the infant overlaps the superior aspect of the thyroid cartilage, which causes the base of the tongue to depress the epiglottis and leads to its protrusion into the pharyngeal cavity. With age, the hyoid and thyroid cartilage separate, and the epiglottis becomes more flexible.

Vocal Folds

The vocal folds are composed of the vocal ligament anteriorly and the cartilaginous vocal process of the arytenoid posteriorly. The anterior vocal ligament in an infant is attached in a more caudal position, which causes the vocal folds to be angled. In an adult, the vocal folds are perpendicular to the trachea. Infantile vocal folds are concave, whereas concavity is minimal in the adult. Forward movement of the thyroid cartilage with growth straightens the folds. The angle of the vocal folds in an infant can sometimes cause difficulty in passage of the tracheal tube because the tip of the tube can be caught by the anterior commissure of the vocal folds. This difficulty can sometimes be relieved by gentle rotation of the tracheal tube.

Subglottis

The subglottic region in an infant is funnel-shaped as a result of the structure of the cricoid cartilage. The cricoid ring is the only complete cartilage in the larynx and is nonexpandable, whereas the trachea has a membranous muscle in its posterior aspect that allows for increased compliance with respiration. Classic teaching is that the narrowest point in an infant airway is at the level of the cricoid cartilage, whereas the vocal folds are the narrowest point in an adult. It is now understood that the funnel shape of the larynx is present in adults as well. Because the diameter of an adult trachea is usually still larger than the diameters of most commonly used adult tracheal tubes, a tracheal tube that passes the vocal folds in an adult usually also passes the cricoid ring. In infants and children, a tube that cannot pass beyond the vocal folds is usually too large to pass through the cricoid ring and should be replaced with a smaller tracheal tube. Failure to do so may result in trauma, airway edema, and postextubation stridor and can lead to the development of subglottic stenosis.

Table 192-1 Sizes of Tracheal Tubes

Age	Size
Premature (<2.5 kg)	2.5
Term neonate	3.0
2-8 months	3.5
8-12 months	4.0
18-24 months	4.5
Older than 24 months	(Age in years/4) + 4

Tracheal Tube

Size and Type

Choosing the correct size of tracheal tube in infants and children is dependent upon the size of the child. Table 192-1 gives some approximate tracheal tube sizes used in infants and children. The presence of an air leak around the tracheal tube is critically important in preventing postintubation edema of the trachea. An air leak should be present at less than 30 cm H_2O peak inflation pressure (the approximate capillary pressure of the tracheal mucosa). If it is not, then the tube should be replaced with the next half-size smaller. Airway resistance is inversely proportional to the radius of the lumen to the fourth power for laminar flow. Therefore, in an infant airway, 1 mm of edema will obstruct the airway by more than 40%, according to the law of Poiseuille.

A cuffed tracheal tube is acceptable for pediatric use as long as a leak is present at less than 30 cm H_2O. However, it is important to remember that the presence of a cuff contributes a half size to the tracheal tube (4.0 cuffed tracheal tube is equivalent to a 4.5 uncuffed tracheal tube). A cuffed tracheal tube should not be automatically inflated with air because the presence of the cuff itself is sometimes enough to decrease the leak. An air leak should occur between 12 and 25 cm H_2O. If a leak is present at less than 12 cm H_2O and interferes with the ability to ventilate the child, then air can be carefully added to the cuff. However, this air should be titrated to an ideal leak between 15 and 20 cm H_2O to prevent airway edema.

Length

The position of the tracheal tube in the trachea is critically important in infants because a small movement can cause mainstem bronchus intubation or an accidental extubation. Preterm infants have an insertion distance of between 6 and 9 cm, depending on their weight. Term newborns have an insertion distance of approximately 10 cm; a 1-year-old child, 11 cm; and a 2-year-old child, 12 cm. An approximate formula for tube insertion distance is three times the size of the tracheal tube. After the tracheal tube is inserted, it is important to auscultate bilaterally in the axillae and to watch for equal anterior chest wall movement. A small but persistent change in O_2 saturation in an infant should cause a reassessment of the position of the tracheal tube. Although there are many formulas for estimating tube insertion distance, it is important to clinically assess and confirm the position in each individual child.

Suggested Readings

Finucane BT, Santora AH. *Principles of Airway Management*. 3rd ed. New York: Springer; 2003.

Wheeler M, Cote C, Todres ID. The pediatric airway. In: Cote C, Lerman J, Todres ID, eds. *A Practice of Anesthesia for Infants and Children*. 4th ed. Philadelphia: Saunders Elsevier; 2009:237-254.

CHAPTER 193

Pediatric Breathing Circuits

Dawit T. Haile, MD

Anesthetic breathing circuits function to deliver O_2 and anesthetic gases to patients and to eliminate CO_2 from patients. They are classified according to (1) the presence or absence of unidirectional valves, (2) the presence and the position of a reservoir bag, (3) the means by which CO_2 is eliminated, (4) the ability of the circuit to permit or prevent rebreathing, and (5) the efficiency of the circuit at preventing rebreathing.

Mapleson Circuits

The first anesthesia breathing systems delivered NO_2-O_2 mixtures for dental anesthesia via a reservoir bag directly connected to an expiratory valve and a facemask. Sir Ivan Magill improved this circuit by distancing the reservoir bag from the expiratory valve and facemask with a reservoir tube to improve surgical access for facial operations. The Magill attachment, also referred to as Mapleson A, was popular for more than 50 years.

By the 1950s, several types of semiclosed circuits were used to deliver anesthetic gases. Semiclosed circuits under optimal conditions prevent rebreathing of alveolar gases. In 1954, the physicist William W. Mapleson analyzed five of these circuits and proposed optimal conditions that would prevent rebreathing. The efficiency of a nonrebreather is determined by the amount of fresh-gas flow, as well as by the positions of the inflow of fresh gas, the expiratory valve, and the reservoir bag. Mapleson labeled these circuits A, B, C, D, and E (Figure 193-1); subsequently, these circuits have been referred to as the Mapleson circuits, and Mapleson's theoretical analyses have been verified empirically by others.

The Mapleson (A, B, C, D, and E) circuits lack unidirectional valves and a CO_2 absorber. They have the advantage of reduced airflow resistance, which is ideal for use in pediatric patients. The Mapleson circuit removes CO_2 by venting exhausted gas to the atmosphere, in contrast with circle systems, in which CO_2 is removed by a CO_2 absorber. Because Mapleson circuits lack a unidirectional valve, the fresh gas and alveolar gases mix, and significant rebreathing occurs if the fresh-gas flow is not adequate. The Mapleson A and D circuits have been analyzed most extensively, the B and the C circuits are rarely used, and the E circuit is basically a T-piece system. The D circuit is the most commonly used Mapleson circuit, and the A circuit is infrequently used but has a historical and a functional significance.

Mapleson A Circuit

The Mapleson A circuit, as described earlier, comprises a reservoir tubing (corrugated tubing) separating, at one end, the fresh-gas flow passing through a reservoir bag and, at the opposite end, an adjustable pressure-limiting valve (APL valve) near the facemask. The system is the most efficient and, with spontaneous ventilation, requires less fresh-gas flow than with controlled ventilation. To explain these differences, the breathing cycle can be artificially divided into three phases: the inspiratory, the expiratory, and the expiratory-pause phase.

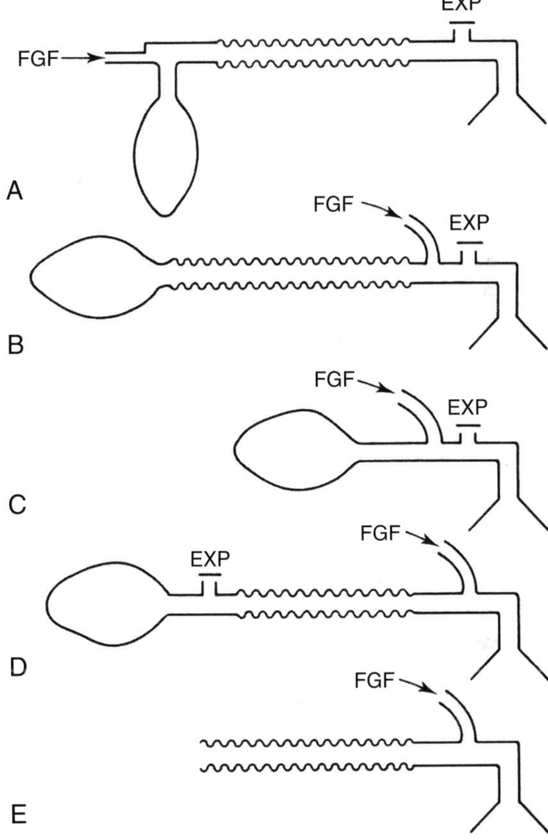

Figure 193-1 Mapleson breathing circuits A through E. Note that E is a T-piece system. EXP, Expiratory valve; FGF, fresh-gas flow. (Redrawn from Ward CS. Anaesthetic Equipment: Physical Principles and Maintenance. 2nd ed. London: Bailliere Tindall (WB Saunders); 1985:122-126.)

Immediately before the inspiratory phase of spontaneous ventilation occurs, continuous fresh gas flows into the reservoir bag and the circuit (Figure 193-2). As the patient inhales, the reservoir bag begins to empty. The lower the fresh-gas flow, or the higher the tidal volume, the emptier the reservoir bag becomes. During the expiratory phase, the reservoir bag completely fills with fresh gas, and, when the fresh-gas flow exceeds 70% of minute ventilation, enough pressure develops to vent alveolar and fresh gas through the APL valve. At the last stage of the expiratory phase, a pause occurs before the initiation of the next cycle. During the expiratory pause, fresh-gas flow further drives alveolar gas through the APL valve and virtually eliminates rebreathing.

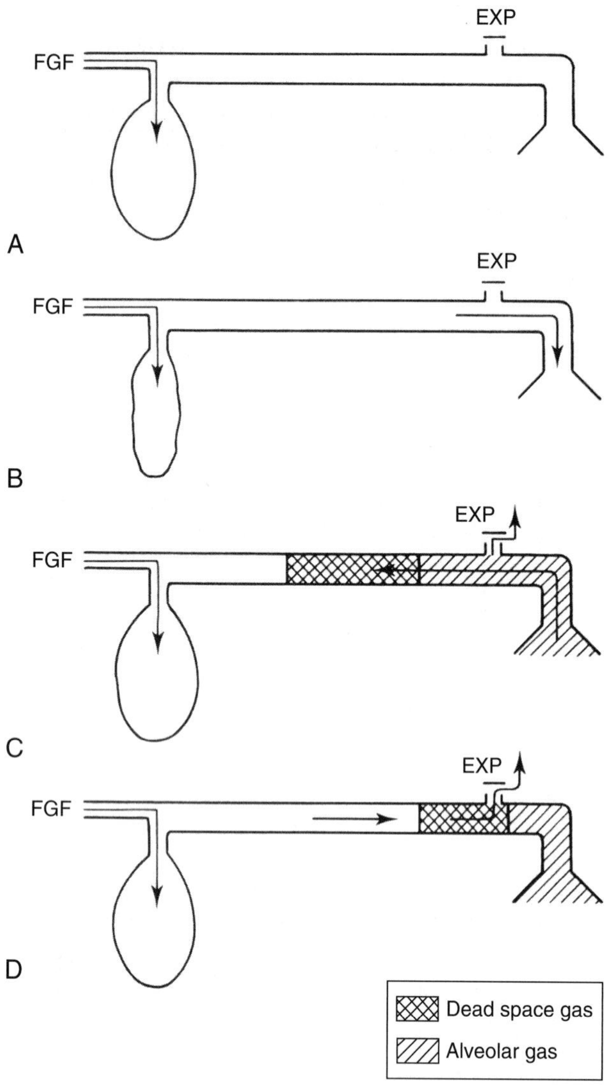

Figure 193-2 Mapleson A circuit: Spontaneous ventilation. **A,** Prior to the inspiratory phase, continuous fresh gas flows into the reservoir bag and the circuit. **B,** The reservoir bag empties during inspiration. **C,** During expiratory phase, the reservoir bag fills with fresh gas, and when it exceeds 70% of minute ventilation, alveolar gas is pushed through APL valve. **D,** During the last phase of expiration, fresh gas further pushes alveolar gas through the APL and virtually eliminates rebreathing. EXP, Expiratory valve; FGF, fresh-gas flow. (Redrawn from Ward CS. Anaesthetic Equipment: Physical Principles and Maintenance. 2nd ed. London: Bailliere Tindall (WB Saunders); 1985:122-126.)

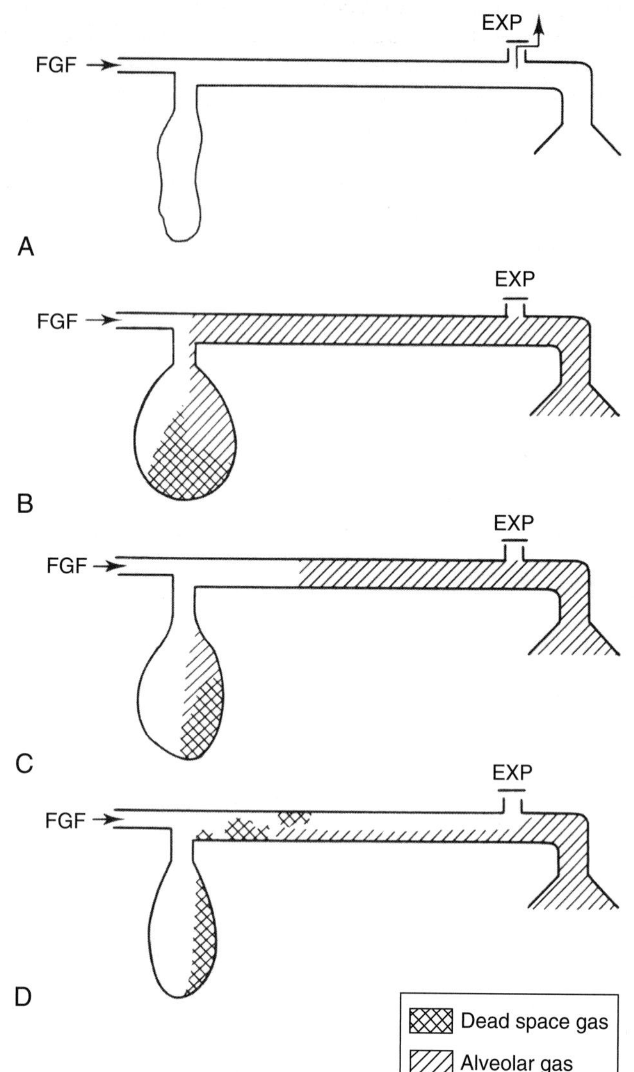

Figure 193-3 Mapleson A circuit: Controlled ventilation. **A,** At the end of the inspiratory phase, the reservoir bag is empty. **B,** During expiration, the reservoir bag refills with alveolar gas, fresh gas, and dead-space gas. **C,** The expiratory pause is minimal, and **(D)** the alveolar gas retention in the circuit is quite high. EXP, Expiratory valve; FGF, fresh-gas flow. (Redrawn from Ward CS. Anaesthetic Equipment: Physical Principles and Maintenance. 2nd ed. London: Bailliere Tindall (WB Saunders); 1985:122-126.)

How can a fresh gas flow that is only 70% of minute ventilation prevent rebreathing? The answer is "dead-space gas." The gas in the reservoir tubing immediately before exhalation is dead-space gas because it is has not been exchanged within the patient's lung and, therefore, does not contain alveolar gases. During the expiratory pause, all of the alveolar gases in the reservoir tubing and some of the dead-space gases are pushed by the fresh-gas flow and expelled through the APL valve. However, not all of the dead-space gas is expired before the next cycle. Because of this residual dead-space gas, the amount of fresh gas required to eliminate rebreathing in the Mapleson A circuit during spontaneous ventilation is less than the minute ventilation.

In contrast with spontaneous ventilation, controlled ventilation (hand ventilation) of the Mapleson A circuit empties the reservoir bag at the end of the inspiratory phase (Figure 193-3). The reservoir bag refills with a mixture of alveolar gases, fresh gas, and dead-space gases during the expiratory phase. During controlled ventilation, the expiratory pause is minimal, which increases the likelihood of alveolar gas retention in the reservoir tubing and increases the amount of alveolar gases present with the initiation of the next inspiratory phase. Among the Mapleson circuits, the Mapleson A circuit under controlled ventilation is considered to be the least efficient at preventing rebreathing; rebreathing is overcome by increasing fresh-gas flow far exceeding minute ventilation.

Mapleson D Circuit

In the Mapleson D circuit, compared with the Mapleson A circuit, the positions of the APL valve and the fresh-gas-flow nipple are reversed; the fresh-gas-flow nipple is located at the patient's end of the circuit, and the APL valve is next to the reservoir bag at the opposite end. The Mapleson D circuit is considered to be a modification of a T-piece circuit; the T-piece circuit is modified into a Mapleson D circuit by adding a reservoir bag and APL valve to the distal end of the reservoir tubing. This circuit requires slightly more fresh-gas flow to eliminate rebreathing than does the Mapleson A circuit. However, for controlled mechanical ventilation, circuit D is the most efficient of the Mapleson circuits.

During spontaneous ventilation with the Mapleson D circuit (Figure 193-4), the alveolar gases are immediately mixed with fresh-gas flow as the gases pass down the reservoir tubing and fill the reservoir bag. When the reservoir bag is filled with a mixture of alveolar and fresh gases, the mixed gas is vented out the APL valve. The first gas to exit through the APL is the dead-space gas, followed by the mixture of alveolar and fresh gases. During the expiratory pause, fresh-gas flow expels most of the alveolar mixed gas if the minute ventilation is adequate. Therefore, to prevent rebreathing, the fresh-gas flow has to be twice the minute ventilation, and the expiratory pause has to be sufficiently long to allow all of the alveolar mixed gases to be expelled.

During the expiratory phase of controlled ventilation with the Mapleson D circuit (Figure 193-5), the fresh-gas flow drives the mixed alveolar gases

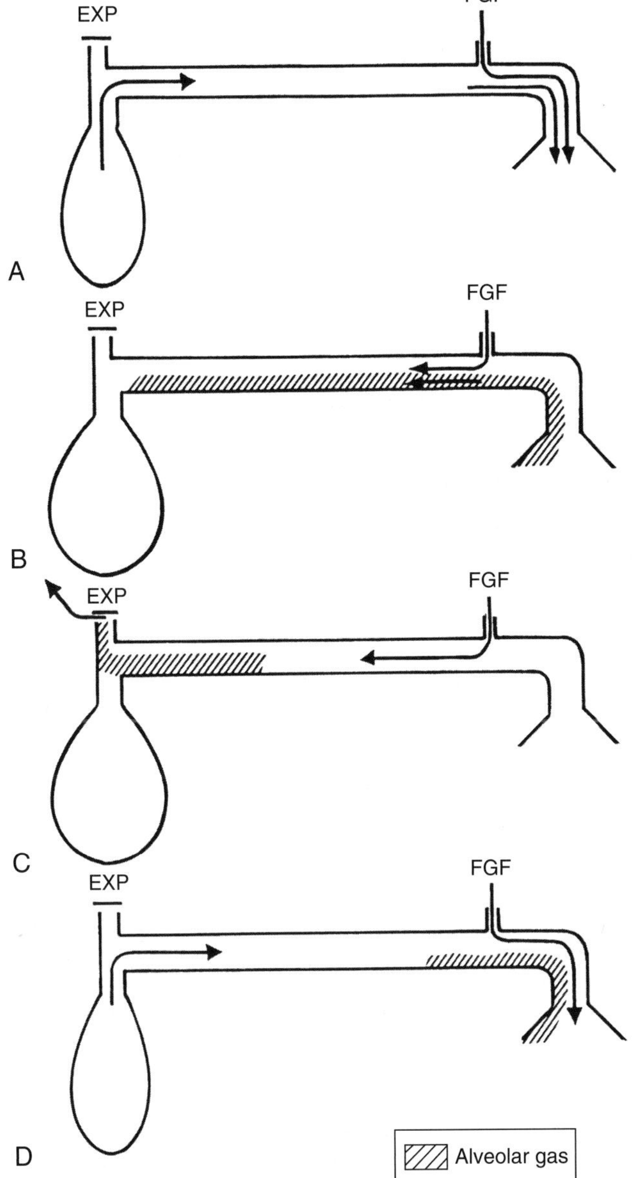

Figure 193-4 Mapleson D circuit: Spontaneous ventilation. **A,** The fresh gas flow nipple is at the patient's end of the circuit, and the APL is at the opposite end with the reservoir bag, and therefore **(B)** alveolar and fresh gas mix in the circuit during expiration and **(C)** the alveolar gas is not completely evacuated before **(D)** the next inspiratory phase of spontaneous respiration. EXP, Expiratory valve; FGF, fresh-gas flow. (Redrawn from Ward CS. Anaesthetic Equipment: Physical Principles and Maintenance. 2nd ed. London: Bailliere Tindall (WB Saunders); 1985:122-126.)

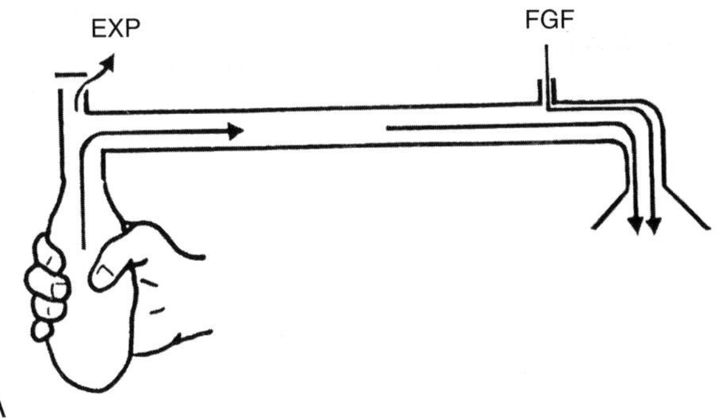

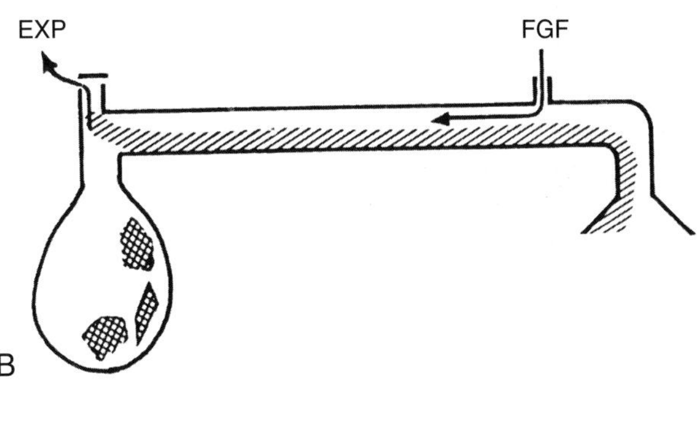

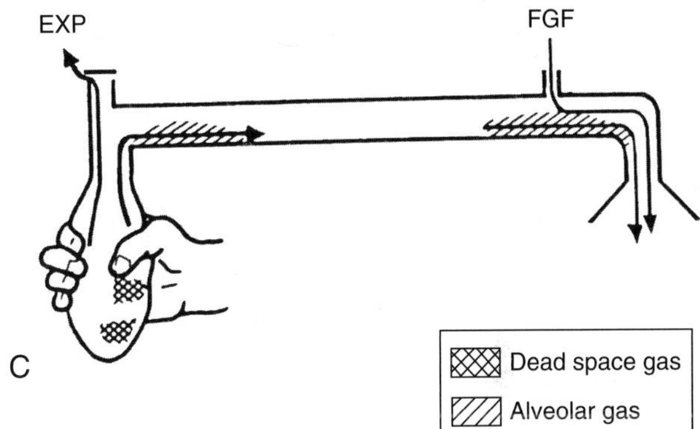

Figure 193-5 Mapleson D circuit: Controlled ventilation. **A,** During inspiratory phase, the positive pressure (with hand bag-squeeze) will build pressure to expel alveolar mixed gases through APL and the fresh gas flow will also push through APL **(B)** and provide fresh gas to the patient **(C).** EXP, Expiratory valve; FGF, fresh-gas flow. (Redrawn from Ward CS. Anaesthetic Equipment: Physical Principles and Maintenance. 2nd ed. London: Bailliere Tindall (WB Saunders); 1985:122-126.)

and dead-space gases out of the APL valve. Furthermore, during the inhalation phase, the mixed alveolar gases are pushed and expelled not only by the continuous fresh-gas flow, but also by the positive pressure of controlled ventilation. The amount of fresh-gas flow necessary to minimize rebreathing is greater than the patient's minute ventilation.

The Bain circuit is a modification of the Mapleson D; the two circuits have the same efficiency, but the Bain circuit provides improved humidification of the inspired air and is the most compact of the Mapleson circuits. The position of the reservoir bag, APL valve, and the fresh-gas inflow in these two devices is the same except that the tube carrying fresh gas is an inner coaxial tube within the corrugated tube in the Bain circuit. The inner tube enters the circuit at the reservoir-bag end, and the fresh gas empties at the patient's end of the circuit. The advantages of the Bain circuit over the Mapleson D include the following: (1) less equipment to interfere with the surgical field, (2) less likelihood of kinking the tracheal tube or extubating the patient because the system is lightweight, and (3) the ability to mount the Bain circuit on the anesthesia machine, allowing for expired gases to be scavenged. Gas flows and minute ventilation requirements are similar to those for the Mapleson D circuit.

Circle System

The circle system is the standard anesthetic circuit on most modern anesthesia machines. Defined by unidirectional valves and a CO_2 absorber, the system requires low fresh-gas flow, enabling conservation of heat, humidity, and anesthetic gases. Pediatric circle breathing systems have been developed but are not often used. They are modified to minimize resistance by incorporating narrow-caliber hoses and a smaller CO_2 absorber. These pediatric circuits have not been marketed with disposable material, and the adaptation to modern anesthesia is suboptimal.

Summary

The relevance of the Mapleson circuits, other than the Mapleson D and Bain circuits, is purely academic. However, the relative efficiency of rebreathing prevention and the requirement of fresh-gas flow of these circuits have been described as follows. For spontaneous ventilation, the most efficient to the least efficient is A > DE > CB. During controlled ventilation, the most efficient to the least efficient is DE > BC > A.

Most children are anesthetized with an adult circle breathing system. Infants and neonates who are too small or have sensitive mechanical ventilation requirements need a different class of modern ventilator (e.g., Siemens 300, Dräger Evita, and others). The discussion of the technology behind this class of ventilators is beyond the scope of this chapter. However, these ventilators utilize technology that can meet the oxygenation and ventilation needs of low-weight infants and neonates and that minimize lung injury more effectively than do the adult anesthesia machines.

Suggested Readings

Coté CJ. Pediatric breathing circuits and anesthesia machines. *Int Anesth Clin*. 1992;30:51-52.

Bain JA, Spoerel WE. Flow requirements for a modified Mapleson D system during controlled ventilation. *Can Anaesth Soc J*. 1973;20:629.

Mapleson WW. Fifty years after—Reflections on "The elimination of rebreathing in various semi-closed anaesthetic systems." *Br J Anaesth*. 2004;93(3): 319-321.

Fisher DM. Anesthesia equipment for pediatrics. In: Gregory GA, ed. *Pediatric Anesthesia*. 4th ed. New York: Churchill Livingstone; 2001:214-216.

CHAPTER 194

Fluid Management in Infants

William Shakespeare, MD, and Randall P. Flick, MD, MPH

The normal newborn is particularly prone to developing derangements in fluids and electrolyte concentrations. In the face of significant illness or injury or in the setting of an invasive surgical procedure, fluid balance becomes even more precarious. This propensity arises from several factors that are unique to the neonate and infant. Total body water in neonates and infants makes up a substantially larger proportion of body mass than in the older child or adult (80% vs. 60%). Body surface area, when compared with body mass, is also much larger in neonates and infants, leading to greater insensible fluid losses, especially when a major body cavity is opened. Finally, limited ability to communicate hunger and thirst makes the young child dependent on thoughtful fluid and electrolyte management by a vigilant clinician throughout the perioperative period.

Maintenance Fluids

Reliance on the method of Holliday and Segar continues despite concern regarding its relevance to the perioperative care of young children. In their seminal 1957 paper, the authors provided a simplified method for estimating maintenance fluids and electrolytes based on energy requirements: 1-kg to 10-kg infants need about 100 $cal \cdot kg^{-1} \cdot 24\ h^{-1}$; each kilogram over 10 kg and up to 20 kg requires an additional 50 $cal \cdot kg^{-1} \cdot 24\ h^{-1}$; after 20 kg, each additional kilogram requires 20 $cal \cdot kg^{-1} \cdot 24\ h^{-1}$. Approximately 1 mL of water is needed for each calorie expended. This method can be simplified (Table 194-1). These recommendations were intended to guide maintainence fluid therapy for hospitalized children, however, and *not* for intraoperative care.

Table 194-1 Maintenance Fluid Therapy for Hospitalized Neonates and Infants*

Weight (kg)	Fluid Needed ($mL \cdot kg^{-1} \cdot h^{-1}$)
< 10	4
10-20	2
> 20	1

*Based on the method of Holliday and Segar.
Note: These recommendations are NOT intended to be used intraoperatively.

Table 194-2 Guidelines for Third-Space Fluid Replacement

Probability of Fluid Translocation	Example Procedure	Additional Fluid Replacement ($mL \cdot kg^{-1} \cdot h^{-1}$)
Little or no	Craniotomy	0
Mild	Inguinal hernia	2
Moderate	Thoracotomy	4
Severe	Bowel obstruction	6

Table 194-3 Mechanisms of Complications of Massive Transfusion

Complication	Mechanism
Acidosis	Poor O_2 delivery, lactate accumulation
Alkalosis	Citrate metabolism to bicarbonate by the liver
Hypocalcemia	Citrate binding of calcium
Hyperglycemia	Dextrose preservative in packed red blood cells
Hypothermia	Transfusion of cold blood products
Hyperkalemia	Multifactorial

Fluid Replacement

The fluid deficit in a patient receiving nothing by mouth can be calculated by multiplying the number of hours that the patient is not receiving anything by mouth by the maintenance fluid requirement. Although a scientific basis for the following recommendation is lacking, common practice is to not only provide maintenance requirements, but also replace half of the fluid deficit in 1 h, one fourth of the deficit in the second hour, and the final one fourth of the deficit in the third hour. Likewise, limited data exist to support the practice of replacing third-space losses, as has been described in most standard texts of pediatric anesthesia (Table 194-2). Many factors may influence fluid requirements in the very young, making the use of simplified formulas problematic and potentially dangerous. In the neonate, insensible water loss is increased by fever, crying, sweating, hyperventilation, bilirubin lights, and radiant heaters. Adequacy of fluid therapy is best monitored by clinical signs (heart rate, blood pressure, urine output, capillary refill, central venous pressure) rather than by blind adherence to a poorly validated formula. A few simple rules that will help to avoid problems occasionaly encountered in fluid management:

- Intravenously administered hypotonic fluids should, in general, not be used in the operating room. Hyponatremia in the perioperative setting is a concern and has been associated with many deaths. However, replacement of sodium should rarely be undertaken in the operating room. Alterations in serum sodium are more often a reflection of abnormalities in total body water than in sodium, and, more importantly, rapid replacement of sodium can result in devastating neurologic injury.
- Metabolic acidosis is most often a reflection of poor tissue perfusion and should first prompt the anesthesia provider to evaluate the patient's volume status. If a decision has been made to treat metabolic acidosis, give one half of the HCO_3^- calculated requirement, and then reassess the acid-base status: calculated HCO_3^- (mEq) = base deficit × weight (kg) × 0.3 (0.4 for infants).
- Potassium replacement is rarely indicated in young children and carries significant risk. If undertaken, replacement should be accomplished slowly, with frequent monitoring of serum potassium concentration. Replace at a maximum of 3 $mEq \cdot kg^{-1} \cdot 24\ h^{-1}$ at a rate not to exceed 0.5 $mEq \cdot kg^{-1} \cdot h^{-1}$. Ideally, urine output should be maintained at 0.5 to 1.0 $mL \cdot kg^{-1} \cdot h^{-1}$.
- Hypocalcemia is a frequent complication of massive transfusion (Table 194-3). Tissue loss from extravasation of calcium chloride given through a peripheral intravenous line is an unfortunate occurrence that can be avoided by employing central venous access or through the use of calcium gluconate. The typical dose of calcium chloride is up to 10 mg/kg and, for calcium gluconate, 30 mg/kg.

Blood Replacement

In the first 3 months of life, infants experience a physiologic anemia, decreasing their mean hemoglobin of 16.8 g/dL at term to a nadir of 10.5 to 11.5 g/dL at age 8 to 12 weeks. In premature infants, this decrease may be even more profound and may occur around week 6 post partum. Infants undergoing surgical interventions during this time do not require transfusion therapy unless they have clinical indications to do so. There are only two accepted indications for the transfusion of red blood cells: (1) to increase O_2-carrying capacity (O_2 delivery = cardiac output × hemoglobin × O_2 saturation) or to avoid an impending inadequate O_2-carrying state and (2) to suppress production, or dilute the amount, of endogenous hemoglobin in selected patients with thalassemia or sickle cell disease.

In 1996, the American Society of Anesthesiologists Task Force on Blood Component Therapy published transfusion practice guidelines that are probably applicable to pediatric patients *without* cardiopulmonary disease. The points regarding red blood cell transfusions are summarized here. Guidelines specific to pediatric patients older than 4 months of age have been published (Box 194-1).

- Transfusion is rarely indicated when hemoglobin concentration is above 10 g/L and is almost always indicated when the hemoglobin concentration is less than 6 g/L, especially if the anemia is acute.
- The determination of whether intermediate hemoglobin concentrations (6-10 g/L) justify transfusion should be based on the patient's risk for developing complications related to inadequate oxygenation.
- The use of a single hemoglobin trigger for all patients is not recommended.

Box 194-1 Indications for Transfusion of Red Blood Cells in Patients Older Than 4 Months of Age

Acute blood loss with hypovolemia not responsive to other therapy
Chronic transfusion programs for disorders of red blood cell production*
Emergency surgical procedure in a patient with clinically significant preoperative anemia
To preoperatively increase hemoglobin to 10 g/dL when general anesthesia is planned and no other therapy is available
Hematocrit < 24%
- During the perioperative period in a patient with signs and symptoms of anemia
- While receiving chemotherapy or radiation
- With chronic congenital or acquired symptomatic anemia

Hematocrit < 40%
- With severe pulmonary disease
- Extracorporeal membrane oxygenation

Intraoperative blood loss ≥ 15% of total blood volume
Sickle cell disease and any of the following
- Cerebrovascular accident
- Acute chest syndrome
- Splenic sequestration
- Recurrent priapism

*Such as thalassemia major or Diamond-Blackfan syndrome unresponsive to therapy.
Adapted from Roseff SD, Luban NL, Manno CS. Guidelines for assessing appropriateness of pediatric transfusion. Transfusion. 2002;42:1398-1413.

A number of calculations have been presented for the evaluation of transfusion thresholds. One such formula proposes that the maximum allowable blood loss should equal the estimated blood volume multiplied by the hematocrit minus the target hematocrit divided by the hematocrit. In clinical practice, these calculations have limited utility as they are dependent on estimates of blood loss that have been repeatedly shown to be inaccurate. In children, transfusion is best guided by close monitoring of hemodynamic parameters and frequent determination of hemoglobin concentration. Estimated blood volume for various ages is shown in Table 194-4.

Table 194-4 Estimated Blood Volume in Infants and Children

Age Group	Estimated Blood Volume (mL/kg)
Premature infants	90-100
Term newborns	80-90
Infants younger than 1 year	75-80
Older children	70-75

Red Blood Cell Products

The transfusion of fresh whole blood (≤5 days old) would appear to be the obvious choice for resuscitation of a bleeding child because it replaces all of the components being lost. If fresh whole blood is not obtainable but its use is required, stored red blood cells can be reconstituted with fresh frozen plasma. It may be appropriate to ask the blood bank to split units to limit donor exposure and waste. For neonates, it is recommended that red blood cells be cytomegalovirus negative and leukocyte reduced via filtration or irradiated to prevent infection and graft-versus-host disease.

Glucose Management

Much controversy exists over the need for the administration of supplemental glucose in infants and children. Some recommend the use of glucose-containing fluids for all children under anesthesia, whereas others suggest that only infants and younger children need intraoperative glucose supplementation. A third option is to measure the patient's glucose concentration during the operation and to supplement only when needed. Any of these options is acceptable as long as care is taken to prevent hyperglycemia and, more importantly, hypoglycemia. The simplest means of preventing either is to use a solution of 2.5% dextrose in lactated Ringer's solution infused at a maintenance rate. This solution should be used in all infants and young children and may be sufficient for those at risk for developing hypoglycemia (those with metabolic or liver disease). Premature infants and neonates, however, may require a solution containing 5% dextrose, as their glucose consumption may be as high as 8 $mg \cdot kg^{-1} \cdot min^{-1}$. Infants receiving concentrated glucose solutions preoperatively should continue to receive at least half the rate intraoperatively. When in doubt, the serum glucose concentration should be measured at regular intervals. No data exist to support tight intraoperative glucose control in children, as has been advocated for adults. The risk of profound neurologic injury resulting from hypoglycemia must be weighed against the uncertain benefit of tight glucose control.

Suggested Readings

Holliday MA, Segar WE. Maintenance need for water in parenteral fluid therapy. *Pediatrics*. 1957;19:823.

Neville KA, Sandeman DJ, Rubinstein A, et al. Prevention of hyponatremia during maintenance intravenous fluid administration: A prospective randomized study of fluid type versus fluid rate. *J Pediatr*. 2010;156:313-319.

Ramez Salem M. Blood conservation in infants and children. In: Motoyoma E, Davis P, eds. *Smith's Anesthesia for Infants and Children*. 7th ed. Philadelphia: Mosby; 2005:396-343.

Roseff SD, Luban NL, Manno CS. Guidelines for assessing appropriateness of pediatric transfusion. *Transfusion*. 2002;42:1398-1413.

Smith HM, Farrow SJ, Ackerman JD, et al. Cardiac arrests associated with hyperkalemia during red blood cell transfusion: A case series. *Anesth Analg*. 2008; 106:1062-1069.

CHAPTER 195

Neuromuscular Blocking Agents in Infants

Wayne H. Wallender, DO

The neuromuscular system is incompletely developed at birth and does not mature until after the first year of life. The motor nerve end plates of neonates release greatly reduced amounts of acetylcholine, likely resulting in the increased sensitivity of the neonatal neuromuscular junction to the effects of nondepolarizing neuromuscular blocking agents (NMBAs). In addition to differences between the neuromuscular systems in neonates and adults, the higher cardiac output and increases in extracellular fluid volumes in infants, as compared with adults, also affect dosing requirements. During the first months of life, the infant diaphragm and intercostal muscles show a progressive increase in the percentage of slow-twitch muscle fibers, which support prolonged repetitive efforts. In neonates, the use of NMBAs paralyzes the diaphragm simultaneously with peripheral muscles, in contrast with the resistance to diaphragmatic paralysis seen in adults. Infants have a greater extracellular fluid and blood volume in proportion to skeletal muscle weight, as compared with older children and adults, resulting in increased drug requirements for some agents in infants. The reduced glomerular filtration rate in neonates is responsible for slower elimination of agents or metabolites excreted by the kidneys.

Specific Agents and Unique Characteristics in Neonates

Depolarizing Neuromuscular Blocking Agents

Succinylcholine is the only depolarizing NMBA used today, but its use can be problematic in children. Neonates have a decreased sensitivity to its effects (50% less response than an adult to an equivalent dose). There is evidence that this resistance to succinylcholine persists even when the larger relative volume of distribution in the infant is taken into consideration, suggesting that the nicotinic receptors are immature at birth. Succinylcholine is hydrolyzed rapidly in plasma (90%) by pseudocholinesterase. Even though term neonates have only about 50% of the plasma pseudocholinesterase of an adult, no prolongation of effect is seen. Newborns have adult levels of plasma pseudocholinesterase by 2 weeks of age. The duration of muscle paralysis from succinylcholine is shorter in neonates, probably because of dilution factors and more rapid redistribution away from effector sites resulting from their high cardiac output. Neonates develop tachyphylaxis after about 3 mg/kg of succinylcholine.

It is uncommon for neonatal muscles to fasciculate following an intravenously administered dose of succinylcholine of 1 to 2 mg/kg. An increase in plasma myoglobin occurs in 60% of prepubescent children. Elevated plasma creatine phosphokinase (CK), an indicator of muscle injury, occurs in 75% of patients and is not age related. An increase in serum potassium of about 0.5 mEq/L occurs after intravenous administration of succinylcholine and is not prevented by pretreatment.

Isolated masseter muscle spasm can occur after succinylcholine administration. Controversy exists as to the actual incidence of malignant hyperthermia associated with masseter spasm. Approximately 50% of such patients have positive halothane-caffeine contracture testing on muscle biopsy. Some have suggested that anesthesia be continued in cases of isolated masseter muscle spasm if the patient has no other evidence of malignant hyperthermia and careful monitoring is performed.

Bradycardia, which can occur with an intravenously administered bolus of succinylcholine, is vagally mediated and can be prevented by pretreatment with atropine or glycopyrrolate. The incidence of bradycardia increases with repeated doses and is higher with the use of halothane than with isoflurane.

Instances of hyperkalemic cardiac arrest in young males with undiagnosed muscular dystrophy have been reported, although they are rare. In 1994, the U.S. Food and Drug Administration recommended that succinylcholine use should be reserved for emergency intubation and instances in which immediate securing of the airway is necessary (boxed warning against the elective use). Because of these concerns, many pediatric anesthesia providers completely avoid the use of succinylcholine.

Depolarizing Neuromuscular Blocking Agents

Pancuronium

Children of all ages are reported to be more resistant to the effects of pancuronium than are adults. Recovery may be prolonged in sick premature infants because of renal disease or increased volume of distribution from anasarca. There is also an increased incidence of intracranial hemorrhage in premature infants who are given pancuronium and who are not anesthetized, possibly because of a combination of increased blood pressure and increased levels of circulating catecholamines.

Atracurium

Atracurium is an intermediate agent that is metabolized by nonspecific esterases and spontaneously decomposes by Hofmann degradation. The effective dose (ED_{95}) of atracurium varies with patient age and is lowest in neonates (i.e., neonates are most sensitive to its effects). Effects are further influenced by age and temperature. Neonates younger than 48 h require less atracurium to induce nearly complete paralysis than do those who are 48 h old or older (300 μg/kg vs. 500 μg/kg). Recovery also takes longer in neonates younger than 48 h, and neonates with body temperatures below 36°C have a longer duration of paralysis. Adverse effects are mainly related to histamine release.

Cisatracurium

Cisatracurium is 1 of 10 stereoisomers that make up atracurium. It is more potent than atracurium and has greater specificity of action, fewer side effects, and a slower onset of action than atracurium.

Vecuronium

Vecuronium induces paralysis more rapidly in infants than in adults, has a longer duration of block in neonates (probably because of the larger volume of distribution), and has a longer recovery time. It is considered to be a long-acting drug in neonates and infants.

Mivacurium

Mivacurium is a short-acting agent metabolized by plasma cholinesterase that can stimulate histamine release at larger doses. In infants, the time required to produce complete blockade is similar to that of succinylcholine, although coughing and diaphragmatic movements may be more common with intubation. Clearance in infants is more rapid than in children, presumably because of a larger volume of distribution.

Rocuronium

Rocuronium is a nondepolarizing steroid NMBA similar to vecuronium but with one tenth the potency. The onset is more rapid than that of vecuronium. Time to recovery is twice as long in infants as it is in children aged 1 to 5 years.

Reversal of Neuromuscular Blockade

In the past, children were believed to need more neostigmine than adults to reverse neuromuscular blockade. However, it has been demonstrated that neostigmine dose requirements are actually lower in pediatric patients.

The dose-response relationship for edrophonium does not differ between children and adults, although the elimination half-life is shorter in neonates, resulting in more rapid clearance. A larger dose of edrophonium is usually recommended for children (1 mg/kg) compared with adults (0.5 mg/kg). To minimize cardiovascular effects, atropine, 0.01 mg/kg, should be given 30 sec before neostigmine or edrophonium. After adequate doses of reversal agents are administered, failure of reversal or the recurrence of blockade indicates the presence of other factors that can prolong neuromuscular blockade (Box 195-1).

Box 195-1 Factors Prolonging Neuromuscular Blockade in Infants

Abnormal variant or deficient pseudocholinesterase	Hypermagnesemia
Antibiotics	Hypokalemia
Aminoglycosides	Hypothermia
Tetracyclines	Lithium
Lincomycins	Local anesthetic agents (e.g., lidocaine)
Polymyxins	Phase II block, if succinylcholine used
Chemotherapy agents	Residual inhalation agents
Dantrolene	Respiratory acidosis
Hepatic dysfunction	

Suggested Readings

Davis PJ, Bosenberg A, Davidson A, et al. Pharmacology of pediatric anesthesia. In: Davis PJ, Cladis FP, Motoyama EK, eds. *Smith's Anesthesia for Infants and Children*. 8th ed. St. Louis: Elsevier Mosby; 2011:239-257.

Johnson PN, Miller J, Gormley AK. Continuous-infusion neuromuscular blocking agents in critically ill neonates and children. *Pharmacotherapy*. 2011;31: 609-620.

Littleford JA, Patel LR, Bose D, et al. Masseter muscle spasm in children: implications of continuing the triggering anesthetic. *Anesth Analg*. 1991;72: 151-160.

Meretoja OA. Neuromuscular blocking agents in paediatric patients: influence of age on the response. *Anaesth Intensive Care*. 1990;18:440.

CHAPTER 196

Regional Anesthesia and Pain Relief in Children

Robert J. Friedhoff, MD

Regional anesthesia in the pediatric patient has been undergoing a revival since the early 1990s. These advances have been particularly advantageous for the pediatric patient undergoing outpatient surgery. Regional anesthesia is usually provided along with general anesthesia in the pediatric patient because a regional anesthetic technique can provide prolonged and predictable intraoperative anesthesia and postoperative analgesia. Performance of the nerve block after the induction of anesthesia but prior to the beginning of the operation allows the concentration of general anesthetic agents to be reduced once the block is established. The clinician should be familiar with the anatomic, physiologic, and pharmacologic differences between adult and pediatric patients.

Anatomy

In pediatric patients, target nerves are smaller, closer to other anatomic structures (vessels), and closer to the skin. The caudal extent of the dura and spinal cord extends approximately two interspaces lower in an infant than in an older child or adult, down to S3 to S4 and L3, respectively, but by the time the child is 12 months of age, the anatomy is similar to that of an adult. The epidural fat is more gelatinous and less fibrous in an infant, favoring the spread of local anesthetic agents and the passage of epidural catheters, but by 8 years of age, the child's epidural space is similar to an adult's.

Physiology

Clinically significant decreases in blood pressure secondary to sympathectomy from central neuraxis blockade are rare in children younger than 8 years of age.

Pharmacology

The potential for local anesthetic toxicity is increased in infants due to their reduced binding proteins (α_1-acid glycoprotein), resulting in an increased concentration of free local anesthetic drug. Maximum recommended doses for commonly used local anesthetic agents are found in Table 196-1.

Table 196-1 Maximum Recommended Doses for Commonly Used Local Anesthetic Agents

Drug	Dose (mg/kg)
Lidocaine*	3.0
Bupivacaine	2.6
Ropivacaine	3.0

*With epinephrine 6 mg/kg.

Cooperation

Essentially all regional techniques, with the exception of spinal anesthesia for the high-risk premature infant, are performed in a heavily sedated or anesthetized patient. The use of a peripheral nerve stimulator can be very helpful in performing some of the nerve blocks. The use of ultrasound in identifying nerves can be of benefit in certain circumstances (see later).

Test Doses

Use of epinephrine to detect unanticipated intravascular injection in patients under inhalation anesthetics is unreliable and controversial. If used, it is recommended that the local anesthetic agent be injected slowly and with frequent aspiration. Observing the electrocardiographic tracing for changes during injection is recommended.

Topical Blocks

EMLA cream is a combination of prilocaine and lidocaine that can be placed on the skin and covered with a transparent film dressing at least 1 h before an invasive procedure (e.g., needlestick, circumcision, separation of preputial adhesions).

Lidocaine iontophoresis requires approximately 10 min but also entails an apparatus that provides a tingly sensation, which can be troublesome to the pediatric patient.

Specific Techniques

Ilioinguinal/Iliohypogastric Nerve Block

Indication

Ilioinguinal or iliohypogastric nerve blocks are used during hernia repairs and orchidopexy.

Technique

The key to performing an ilioinguinal or iliohypogastric nerve block is to identify the anterior superior iliac spine and place a 23-gauge needle 1 to 2 cm (1 fingerbreadth) medial and inferior to it, feeling the "pop" as the needle passes through the fascia, and then fanning the local anesthetic from lateral to medial. The wound edge is infiltrated prior to surgical closure, or alternatively, the local anesthetic agent can be instilled prior to closure (enough to fill the wound after dissection). Use of ultrasound can confirm the proper needle placement and deposition of drug.

Drug

The most commonly used local anesthetic agent in an ilioinguinal or iliohypogastric nerve block is bupivacaine, 0.25% to 0.5%, at a dose of 2 to 10 mL, depending on the size of the patient.

Rectus Sheath Block

Indication

The rectus sheath is a potential space located between the rectus abdominis muscle and the posterior rectus sheath, where thoracic intercostal nerves pass through to provide sensation to the anterior abdominal wall. A rectus sheath block is used most often for repair of an umbilical hernia.

Technique

Using ultrasound guidance, the lateral edge of the rectus sheath is identified bilaterally at the level of the umbilicus, and a 22-gauge B (blunt) or 23-gauge needle is inserted into the rectus sheath while simultaneously feeling and seeing the needle pop through.

Drug

The local anesthetic agent most commonly used in the rectal sheath block is bupivacaine, 0.25% to 0.5%, at a dose of 0.1 mL/kg on each side of the abdomen.

Penile Block

Indication

Penile blocks are used during circumcision and hypospadias repairs.

Technique

When performing a penile block, the base of the penis is ringed with a superficial wheal of local anesthetic agent, or, while pulling the penis toward the patient's feet, a needle is inserted at 90 degrees, just below the symphysis pubis into the dorsum of the penis. A "pop" will be felt as the needle passes through the Buck fascia—this needs to be repeated twice, with half of the drug injected at 11 o'clock and half at 1 o'clock.

Drug

The local anesthetic agent most commonly used in the penile block is bupivacaine, 0.25%, at a dose of 2 to 10 mL, depending on the patient; epinephrine should not be used.

Femoral Nerve Block

Indication

The femoral nerve block is most commonly used for biopsy of the quadriceps muscle, when the femoral shaft is fractured, or during knee operations.

Technique

The key to performing the femoral nerve block is to remember NAVEL (nerve, artery, vein, empty space, ligament)—the nerve is lateral to the artery. When performing the femoral nerve block, a line is drawn from the anterior superior iliac spine to the pubic tubercle, demarcating the inguinal ligament. Just below (0.5-1.0 cm) the inguinal ligament, an insulated needle attached to a nerve stimulator is placed lateral to the femoral artery pulsations. (The patient must not be paralyzed with a neuromuscular blocking agent.) The twitch monitor is set at 1 per second, and the nerve is stimulated at the lowest possible setting until a twitch is noted in the patella. Ultrasound can be helpful in visualizing the anatomic structures as well.

Drug

The drugs most commonly used in a femoral nerve block are bupivacaine, 0.25% to 0.5%, or ropivacaine, 0.2%, at a dose of 5 to 20 mL, depending on the patient's size.

Lateral Femoral Cutaneous Nerve Block

Indication

The lateral femoral cutaneous nerve is often blocked in conjunction with the femoral nerve.

Technique

A needle is advanced 1 cm below and medial to the inguinal ligament and the anterior superior iliac spine. The drug is injected after "popping" through the fascia lata.

Drug

The local anesthetic agent most commonly used in the lateral femoral cutaneous nerve block is bupivacaine, 0.5%, at a dose of 0.1 to 0.2 mL/kg.

Popliteal Fossa Block

Indication

The popliteal fossa block is most commonly used for blocks below the knee.

Technique

Correct positioning of most children undergoing a popliteal fossa block involves simply lifting the supine child's leg with the knee and thigh flexed. The apex of the popliteal fossa triangle (formed by the biceps femoris tendon laterally and semimembranous and semitendinous tendons medially) is identified, and this triangle is divided into medial and lateral halves. The point of needle insertion is 1 cm lateral to this line, 1 to 2 cm proximal to the popliteal crease, and lateral to the popliteal artery. A blunt insulated needle, directed perpendicular to the skin, is advanced until a distinct pop is felt and muscle stimulation resulting in plantar flexion or dorsiflexion of the foot occurs. Ultrasound can provide visualization of the sciatic nerve bifurcating into the common peroneal and tibial nerves.

Drug

The local anesthetic agent most commonly used in the popliteal fossa block is bupivacaine, 0.25%, at a dose of 0.5 to 1.0 mL/kg.

Axillary Block

Indication

An axillary block is used when operations involve the upper extremity.

Technique
As in adults, axillary blocks in children are performed with a nerve stimulator (in patients who have not received a neuromuscular blocking agent). Alternatively, the axillary artery in the axilla can be palpated, and the skin can be punctured with a 20-gauge needle. A 22-gauge B (blunt) needle is then inserted through the puncture site, aiming toward the artery, until a "pop" is felt as the needle goes through the fascia or "septa" of the axillary sheath. Upon demonstration of a negative aspiration, the local anesthetic agent can be injected. Ultrasound can also provide assistance in performing this block.

Drug
The local anesthetic agents most commonly used in the axillary block are bupivacaine, 0.25%, or ropivacaine, 0.2%, with epinephrine, 1/200,000, at a dose of 0.5 mL/kg.

Caudal Block

Single-Shot Caudal Block
Indication The single-shot caudal block is used most often in operations with an operative field below the diaphragm.

Technique With the patient in the lateral decubitus position (left lateral for a right-handed clinician, right lateral for a left-handed clinician) and the knees flexed up into the abdomen, the thumbnail is used to palpate and identify the two sacral cornua above the gluteal fold. Using aseptic technique, a 22-gauge Jelco, 22-gauge B-bevel needle, or a 23-gauge needle is placed at 45 degrees to the skin and advanced until a "pop" is felt through the sacrococcygeal ligament. The needle is then lowered, parallel to the skin, and advanced 1 cm. After ascertaining that aspiration for blood and cerebrospinal fluid is negative, the local anesthetic agent is slowly injected while observing the electrocardiogram for T-wave changes. Injection of the local anesthetic agent should be easy; any resistance indicates incorrect needle placement.

Drug The local anesthetic agents most commonly used in the single-shot caudal block are bupivacaine, 0.125% to 0.25%, or ropivacaine, 0.2%, with the dose dependent upon the patient's age and the location of the incision: penile operation, 0.5 to 0.8 mL/kg; inguinal operations, 1.0 mL/kg up to 20 mL. Other analgesic agents such as the α-adrenergic agonist clonidine (dose of 2 μg/kg) or preservative-free ketamine (dose of 0.5 mg/kg) can be added to the bupivacaine solution to prolong the duration of the block for an additional 3 to 12 h. Adverse effects include sedation and minor hypotension.

Continuous Caudal Block
Indication The continuous caudal block is used most often for prolonged pain relief after operations. The catheter tip is placed at the level of the incision.

Caution The dressing for a continuous caudal block, which is in the sacral area, must be kept clean, and access must be maintained to the site; therefore, the patient cannot have a spica cast.

Technique The technique for a continuous caudal block is similar to that of a single-shot caudal block. The caudal space is identified under sterile technique, and then either an 18-gauge angiocatheter or a Crawford needle is advanced. The epidural catheter is then threaded through the needle for 3 cm or to the level of the incision. A sterile transparent film dressing is applied.

Drug The choice of drug for a continuous caudal block is dependent upon catheter position and the operation.

Lumbar Epidural Block

Indications
Indications and contraindications for lumbar epidural blocks are similar to those in adults.

Technique
Techniques for performing a lumbar epidural block in children are similar to those used in adults. For patients weighing less than 30 kg, a 2-inch, 18-gauge Weiss or Crawford needle can be used.

Drug
The drugs most commonly used in a lumbar epidural block are lidocaine, bupivacaine, fentanyl, morphine (Duramorph), or hydromorphone, depending on the patient and the operation.

Spinal Block

Indication
A spinal block is used most often in high-risk neonates who were born prematurely and are having lower abdominal operations.

Technique
The spinal block should be placed, if possible, with the patient in the sitting position, upright, with special attention to the head so as not to flex it and obstruct the airway. The depth of the subarachnoid space is about 0.7 cm in premature infants and 1.0 cm in full-term infants. It is best to avoid sedation, if possible, including ketamine, to prevent postoperative apnea. Placing the blood pressure cuff on a lower extremity will avoid stimulating the restless infant.

Drugs
The drug most commonly used in a spinal block is tetracaine, 1 mg/kg, plus dextrose.

Newer Techniques
The use of ultrasound-guided blocks in pediatric patients has some advantages (e.g., shorter block performance time, faster onset time, higher success rates, longer block duration, and less volume of anesthetic used) over the traditional nerve stimulation techniques, but improved safety has been shown to be beneficial only while performing an ilioinguinal nerve block.

Suggested Readings
Bosenberg A. Benefits of regional anesthesia in children. *Paediatr Anaesth.* 2012;22:10-18.

Bosenberg A, Flick RP. Regional anesthesia in neonates and infants. *Clin Perinatol.* 2013;40:525-538.

Chandrakantan A, Glass PS. Multimodal therapies for postoperative nausea and vomiting, and pain. *Br J Anaesth.* 2011;107:i27-40.

Ecoffey C. Safety in pediatric regional anesthesia. *Paediatr Anaesth.* 2012;22:25-30.

Kokki H. Spinal blocks. *Paediatr Anaesth.* 2012;22:56-64.

Mai CL, Young MJ, Quraishi SA. Clinical implications of the transversus abdominis plane block in pediatric anesthesia. *Paediatr Anaesth.* 2012;22:831-840.

Marhofer P, Willschke H, Kettner SC. Ultrasound-guided upper extremity blocks—Tips and tricks to improve the clinical practice. *Paediatr Anaesth.* 2012;22:65-71.

Mossetti V, Vicchio N, Ivani G. Local anesthesia and adjuvants in pediatric regional anesthesia. *Curr Drug Targets.* 2012;13:952-960.

O'Sullivan MJ, Mislovic B, Alexander E. Dorsal penile nerve block for male pediatric circumcision—Randomized comparison of ultrasound-guided vs. anatomical landmark technique. *Paediatr Anaesth.* 2011;21:1214-1218.

Polaner DM, Taenzer AH, Walker BJ, et al. Pediatric Regional Anesthesia Network (PRAN): A multi-institutional study of the use and incidence of complications of pediatric regional anesthesia. *Anesth Analg.* 2012;115(6):1353-1364.

Rubin K, Sullivan D, Sadhasivam S. Are peripheral nerve blocks with ultrasound guidance more effective and safe in children? *Paediatric Anesth.* 2009;19:92-96.

Suresh S, Birmingham PK, Kozlowski RJ. Pediatric pain management. *Anesthesiol Clin.* 2012;30(1):101-117.

Willschke H, Kettner S. Pediatric regional anesthesia: Abdominal wall blocks. *Paediatr Anaesth.* 2012;22:88-92.

CHAPTER 197

Anesthetic Risks Associated with Prematurity

Wayne H. Wallender, DO

Approximately 12% of infants (one of every eight) born in the United States are born prematurely. Prematurity was previously defined as infants born before 38 weeks of gestation or with a weight of less than 2500 g at birth, but current definitions take into account that morbidity and mortality risks are more closely related to gestational age than to birth weight. The World Health Organization currently defines prematurity as a gestational age of less than 37 completed weeks regardless of birth weight. More than 90% of premature infants who weigh at least 800 g survive. Preterm birth is often due to a combination of fetal, placental, uterine, and maternal factors (Box 197-1).

Premature infants rarely present for surgery unless they are severely ill, and most will have multiorgan disorders. The underlying medical conditions are usually life-threatening respiratory, cardiovascular, or bowel crises (Box 197-2). Premature infants have a higher-than-normal perioperative complication rate following even minor operations. Anesthetic morbidity rate increases directly with the degree of prematurity.

Anesthetic Considerations in Premature Infants

Temperature Instability

Impaired temperature regulation in premature infants can be due to a variety of factors, including increased surface-to-volume ratio; lack of adipose tissue, which insulates neonates from their environment; fewer brown fat cells (cells stimulated by norepinephrine to increase heat production)

Box 197-1 Factors That Increase the Risk of Preterm Birth

Fetal

Fetal distress
Multiple gestation

Placental

Abruptio placentae
Placenta previa

Uterine

Incompetent cervix

Maternal

Preeclampsia
Heart disease
Drug abuse (cocaine, nicotine)
African-American
Lower socioeconomic status
Younger or older age

Other

Premature rupture of membranes
Polyhydramnios

Box 197-2 Organ System Pathology in Premature Neonates

Neurologic

Intraventricular hemorrhage*
Delayed development
Seizures
Hydrocephalus
Cerebral Palsy

Cardiovascular

Congenital malformation
Persistent patent ductus arteriosus

Respiratory

Apnea
Respiratory distress syndrome*
Bronchopulmonary dysplasia*
Pneumothorax
Pneumonia

Gastrointestinal

Necrotizing enterocolitis*
Hyperbilirubinemia
Disordered swallowing/sucking
Gastroesophageal reflux
Bowel obstruction

Hepatic

Hepatic failure
Hyperalimentation hepatitis

Hematologic

Anemia
Vitamin K deficiency

Endocrinologic

Hypoglycemia
Hypocalcemia

Renal

Chronic renal failure
Renal tubular acidosis
Electrolyte abnormalities
- Hyponatremia
- Hypernatremia
- Hyperkalemia

Visual

Retinopathy of prematurity

Other

Malnutrition
Sepsis*

*Major causes of morbidity.

than in full-term infants; and thin skin, resulting in heat and water loss. (The epidermis is not mature until after 32 weeks of gestation.)

Hypothermia is associated with hypoglycemia, respiratory distress, jaundice, and sepsis. Outcome is improved if premature (and sick) infants are cared for in a neutral thermal environment. Therefore, when anesthetizing such patients, the anesthesia provider must maintain patient temperature at or about 37° C through the use of radiant warmers, maintenance of warmer-than-normal room temperature, etc.

Respiratory Distress Syndrome

Many premature infants have respiratory distress syndrome (RDS), also known as hyaline membrane disease. RDS is rare after 34 weeks of gestation in otherwise normal neonates and occurs three times more often in infants born via cesarean section than in those born vaginally. Immediate treatment with artificial surfactant has reduced mortality risk associated with RDS. A pneumothorax should be considered in any neonate whose oxygenation deteriorates suddenly.

Bronchopulmonary Dysplasia

Bronchopulmonary dysplasia (BPD), defined as O_2 dependence at 36 weeks postconception age (>28 days of total O_2 therapy), is a chronic disorder, usually occurring in infants with a history of RDS. The more severe the RDS, the greater the degree of BPD. The incidence of BPD has not decreased in recent times despite improved neonatal care.

Although the cause of BPD is unknown, risk factors associated with BPD include increased inspired fraction of O_2, the use of positive-pressure ventilation, infection, patent ductus arteriosus (PDA), and fluid overload in the first 5 to 6 days of life. BPD is characterized by increased airway resistance, decreased pulmonary compliance, ventilation/perfusion mismatch, decreased Po_2, tachypnea, increased O_2 consumption, and an increased number of pulmonary infections.

Apnea

All premature infants have some degree of periodic breathing. Apnea, defined as cessation of breathing that lasts for 15 sec or longer or a shorter respiratory pause associated with pallor or bradycardia (heart rate <100), is more common in premature infants than in full-term infants. The more premature the infant, the greater the likelihood that he or she will develop apnea spells. The risk of apnea spells is increased postoperatively, especially in preterm infants less than 44 weeks postconception age (the risk decreases after 44 to 60 weeks postconception age). In-hospital respiratory monitoring is recommended for at least 12 h after a preterm infant has undergone any surgical procedure, and some authorities recommend monitoring overnight in the hospital.

Patent Ductus Arteriosus

PDA results in a left-to-right shunt, left ventricular hypertrophy, and increased pulmonary blood flow and can lead to congestive heart failure, which manifests as respiratory failure. The first line of treatment is usually an attempt to close the PDA medically with indomethacin, fluid restriction, and diuresis before surgical ligation.

Infection

Infection is a constant threat to premature infants because these infants have reduced cellular and tissue immunity; pneumonia, sepsis, and meningitis are common. Sepsis can develop in the absence of a positive blood culture, elevated white blood cell count, or fever. The first signs of infection may be apnea, bradycardia, or acidosis. Strict compliance with handwashing and maintenance of universal precautions is mandatory when providing care to these infants.

Necrotizing Enterocolitis

Primarily a disease of small preterm infants, necrotizing enterocolitis has a multifactorial cause, but hypoperfusion of the gastrointestinal tract, resulting in ischemia, seems to be a primary factor. Small preterm infants (<32 weeks of gestation and 1500 g) are at greatest risk for developing necrotizing enterocolitis. Initial signs are abdominal distention and bloody feces; shock may develop from multiple bowel perforations. Patients are often hypovolemic and require fluid resuscitation before anesthesia is induced. Rapid fluid administration to preterm neonates may cause intracranial hemorrhage or reopening of the ductus arteriosus. Necrotizing enterocolitis is often associated with disseminated intravascular coagulopathy and thrombocytopenia. The use of N_2O should be avoided, and perioperative blood pressure should be maintained.

Retinopathy of Prematurity

Premature infants are at increased risk of developing retinopathy of prematurity (ROP). The risk of ROP is inversely related to birth weight, with the risk highest in infants weighing less than 1000 g. The cause of ROP is multifactorial. Although the role of O_2 as a risk factor is controversial, minimizing O_2 exposure is prudent in premature infants less than 44 weeks postconception age. There is little convincing evidence that brief exposure to 100% O_2 is a risk factor for the development of ROP in infants of any age. Nonetheless, it is recommended that the Po_2 be maintained between 60 and 80 mm Hg whenever possible to reduce the risk of ROP in susceptible infants. Fortunately, most retinal changes regress spontaneously.

Intracranial Hemorrhage

The four types of intracranial hemorrhage that may occur in premature neonates are subdural, primary subarachnoid, periventricular-intraventricular (the most common), and intracerebral. Newborn immaturity is the single most important risk factor for the development of intracranial hemorrhage, which rarely occurs after 10 days after birth, with the vast majority of bleeds occurring in the first 3 days.

A variety of mechanisms are involved in intracranial hemorrhage. Impaired autoregulation of cerebral blood flow (CBF) occurs in stressed neonates. An elevation in blood pressure causes increased CBF, which may, in turn, result in hemorrhage. Arterial hypoxemia and hypercapnia that occur during asphyxia can also precipitate hemorrhage. The effects of anesthesia on CBF in neonates are not known, but it is prudent to prevent hypoxemia and hypercapnia and to avoid cerebral hyperperfusion by maintaining blood pressure in the normal range. Hyperosmolarity is also a contributing factor. Therefore, the use of hyperosmolar fluids should be avoided (e.g., dilute bicarbonate and give slowly).

An inverse correlation between IQ and the frequency of general anesthesia in infants has been shown. However, many clinicians maintain that the association between IQ and exposure to general anesthesia is secondary to the fact that many premature infants also have multiple organ problems and are, therefore, frequently anesthetized for operations and that chronic disease is the real cause of the decrease in IQ. Independent of concerns about general anesthesia on the developing brain, other issues also have an impact on the effects of drugs on preterm infants. Hepatic metabolism is decreased and renal clearance of almost all drugs secreted in the urine is also decreased in premature infants. Many drugs and drug doses safe for adults may be harmful in premature infants.

Suggested Readings

Coté CH, Lerman J, Todres ID. *A Practice of Anesthesia for Infants and Children*. 4th ed. Philadelphia: Elsevier Health Sciences; 2009.

Montoyama E, Davis P, eds. *Smith's Anesthesia for Infants and Children*. 7th ed. Philadelphia: Elsevier Health Sciences; 2005.

Stoll BJ, Adams-Chapman I. The high-risk infant: Prematurity and intrauterine growth retardation. In: Kleigman RM, Behrman RE, Jenson HB, Stanton MD, eds. *Nelson Textbook of Pediatrics*. 18th ed. Philadelphia: WB Saunders; 2007:701-709.

CHAPTER 198

Neonatal Resuscitation

Brian Emerson, MD, and Heather L. Naumann, MD

Two maternal uterine arteries supply the placenta—oxygenated blood travels from the mother through the placenta; O_2 diffuses across the placenta, binds with neonatal hemoglobin, and is then carried by a single umbilical vein to the body of the fetus. Deoxygenated blood is returned from the fetus to the placenta by two umbilical arteries. As one would expect, at birth, umbilical arterial blood is lower in pH and O_2 and higher in CO_2 compared with umbilical venous blood (Table 198-1). Umbilical cord blood gas measurements can serve to assess the fetal condition immediately after delivery. Umbilical arterial measurements represent the fetal condition, whereas umbilical vein measurements would represent the maternal condition if the blood were withdrawn prior to cross-clamping the umbilical cord, as well as uterine placental gas exchange.

The majority of births do not require active intervention to establish adequate cardiorespiratory function in the newborn because most newborns undergo a relatively smooth physiologic transition at birth. However, it is of utmost importance to have skilled practitioners available at the time of birth to provide dedicated assessment and resuscitation of the newborn as needed. Such individuals should be capable of managing the airway and have a working knowledge of neonatal physiology and pathology, including vital sign parameters, laboratory values, common congenital anomalies, and their immediate implications. Adequate equipment and resources should be available and checked prior to delivery and should include, at the very minimum, airway supplies (e.g., appropriately sized laryngoscopes, tracheal tubes, and masks), a warming device, suction catheters connected to a suction system, O_2, and the ability to provide positive-pressure ventilation, in addition to emergency medications.

When the infant is born, initial maneuvers—such as suctioning of the nose, mouth, and pharynx, as well as stimulation (flicking the feet or rubbing the back)—may be necessary to facilitate regular spontaneous breathing. Infants not responding to such measures may require a range of therapies, including administration of O_2, bag-mask ventilation, tracheal intubation and suctioning, chest compressions, and pharmaceutical intervention. Simultaneously, the infant's color, heart rate, and respiratory effort should be assessed. The goals of such resuscitative efforts are to prevent hypoxic or ischemic injury and to restore adequate spontaneous respiration and cardiac output.

Table 198-1 Newborn Blood Gas Values

Variable	Umbilical Vein at Birth	Umbilical Artery at Birth	60 Minutes	24 Hours	Adult and Child
pH	7.35 (7.3-7.4)	7.28 (7.23-7.33)	7.3-7.35		7.4
PCO_2 (mm Hg)	40 (33-43)	50 (42-58)	30	30	40
PO_2 (mm Hg)	30 (25-35)	20 (12-25)	60	70	100

The Apgar scoring system, a rapid assessment tool based on physiologic responses to birth, is used to evaluate the need for resuscitation of a newborn. Created and first utilized in 1953 by an anesthesiologist, Dr. Virginia Apgar, the absolute utility of the system remains in debate today. At intervals of 1 min and 5 min after birth, an experienced and qualified examiner evaluates five physiologic parameters (Table 198-2). Although this assessment may be helpful in evaluating newborns in need of attention, patients may require immediate resuscitation prior to the 1-min scoring.

Guidelines for neonatal resuscitation require simultaneous and continuous assessment and treatment (Figure 198-1), which generally consists of a simplified ABCD approach that requires some qualification and clarification. The fundamental principles include evaluating the **a**irway, establishing effective respiration (**b**reathing), determining adequate **c**irculation, and administering medications (**d**rugs).

A review of maternal and prenatal history conducted prior to the neonate's birth may guide resuscitation efforts. Initially, an infant should be placed in a warmer with his or her head down and the head slightly extended. The neonate's oropharynx should then be suctioned, while she or he is stimulated and assessed (color, heart rate, respiration).

Meconium staining of amniotic fluid necessitates immediate suctioning of the hypopharynx, nose, and mouth. The decision to perform tracheal suctioning was previously based upon the quality of the meconium present; however, that decision is now based upon the infant's appearance. If the infant is vigorous, has adequate respiratory effort, and has a heart rate of more than 100 beats/min, tracheal intubation to attempt to aspirate possible meconium should not be attempted. However, if the infant's respiratory rate

Table 198-2 Apgar Scoring System

Score Component	Points Assigned: 0	1	2
Heart rate (beats/min)	None	<100	>100
Respiration	None	Slow, irregular	Good, crying
Muscle tone	None	Some extremity flexion	Arms and legs well flexed
Reflex irritability	None	Grimace	Cry, withdraw from stimulus
Color	Blue body	Pink body, blue extremities	Pink all over

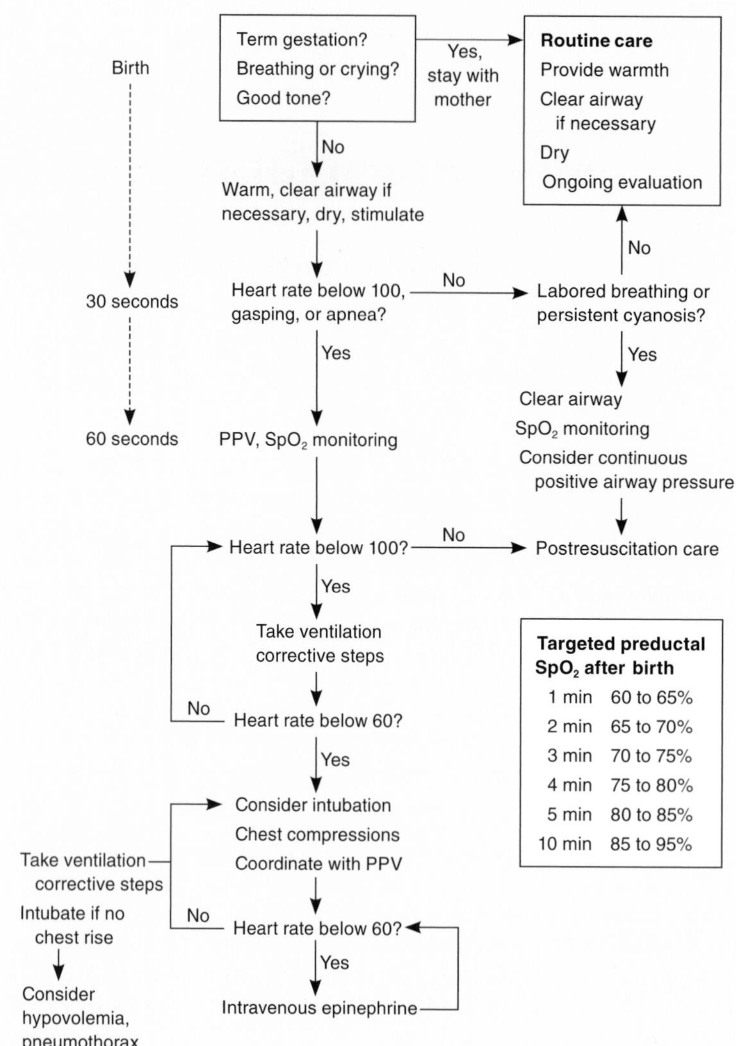

Figure 198-1 Algorithm outlining neonatal resuscitation. (PPV, Positive pressure ventilation; SpO2, oxygen saturation as measured by pulse oximetry.) Reprinted with permission from Kattwinkel J, Perlman JM, Aziz K, et al. Part 15: Neonatal resuscitation: 2010 American Heart Association guidelines for cardiopulmonary resuscitation and emergency cardiovascular care. Circulation. 2010;122(18 suppl 3):S910.

and heart rate are depressed and the infant has poor tone, intubation should be undertaken and further tracheal suctioning performed.

The infant's breathing should be closely monitored and, if necessary, a patent airway should be established by suctioning or intubation. Adequate breathing should be ensured by use of tactile stimulation or positive-pressure ventilation by bag-mask or tracheal tube. Sufficient circulation should be maintained with chest compressions and medications, if required. For further details, refer to the steps outlined in Figure 198-1.

If the infant's condition deteriorates or does not improve over 30 sec, efforts should be escalated. Currently, room air is recommended for resuscitation and if there is no increase in heart rate or in oxygenation as measured by a pulse oximeter, then supplemental O_2 should be considered. Pressures as high as 30 to 40 cm of H_2O may be required to ensure adequate ventilation at a rate of 40 to 60 breaths/min. Beware of forcing excessive air into the stomach if performing bag-mask ventilation. Adequate chest rise, symmetrical breath sounds, and presence of end-tidal CO_2 should be established.

Chest compression and medications are not needed for most neonates who have mild to moderate cardiac or respiratory depression at birth. Typically, most bradycardia is secondary to hypoxia and responds to effective ventilation. If the heart rate remains lower than 60 beats/min despite adequate ventilation and chest compressions, administration of epinephrine, volume expansion (10 mL/kg of an isotonic crystalloid), or both may be considered. The recommended dose of intravenously administered epinephrine is 0.01 to 0.03 mg/kg per dose. Doses of up to 0.1 mg/kg by tracheal tube may be used if necessary. In rare instances, an opioid antagonist or vasopressors may prove useful. Following resuscitation, the infant may require admission to a neonatal intensive care unit, based on the reasons for and circumstances of the resuscitation.

Suggested Readings

American Society of Anesthesiologists Committee on Obstetric Anesthesiology. ACOG Committee Opinion No. 256, May 2001.

Chestnut DH. *Obstetric Anesthesia*. 3rd ed. Philadelphia: Mosby; 2004, Chap 9.

Kattwinkel J, Bloom RS, eds. *Neonatal Resuscitation Textbook*. 5th ed. Elk Grove, IL: American Academy of Pediatrics, American Heart Association; 2006.

Kattwinkel J, Perlman JM, Aziz K, et al. Part 15: neonatal resuscitation: 2010 American Heart Association Guidelines for Cardiopulmonary Resuscitation and Emergency Cardiovascular Care. *Circulation*. 2010;122:S909-S919.

Kliegman RM, Stanton B, St. Geme J, et al. *Nelson Textbook of Pediatrics*. 19th ed. Philadelphia: Saunders Elsevier; 2011, Part XI, Chap. 100.

CHAPTER 199

Meconium Aspiration and Meconium Aspiration Syndrome

Inge Falk van Rooyen, MD

The leading cause of respiratory death in the full-term newborn is meconium aspiration—defined as the presence of meconium below the vocal cords—and ensuing aspiration pneumonitis. Meconium aspiration syndrome (MAS) is defined as respiratory distress developing shortly after birth in an infant born through meconium-stained amniotic fluid whose symptoms cannot otherwise be explained.

Intratracheal meconium aspiration occurs in 55% to 60% of total aspirations, and death occurs in up to 20% of infants with MAS (Figure 199-1). A number of fetal and maternal conditions are associated with an increased incidence of meconium aspiration (Box 199-1). The severity of physiologic symptoms and extent of respiratory, cardiac, and neurologic sequelae vary significantly in individual patients.

Box 199-1 Conditions Associated with an Increased Prevalence of Meconium Staining

- Postmaturity (>42 weeks of gestation)
- Uteroplacental insufficiency
  - Cord prolapse
  - Cord compression
- Intrauterine growth retardation (fetal weight <10th percentile for gestational age)
- Maternal conditions
  - Hypertension
  - Placenta previa
  - Pulmonary hypertension
  - Placentae abruptio

Pathophysiology of Meconium Passage in Utero

Meconium is seen in late pregnancy, rarely before 36 weeks of gestation. Meconium passage in utero can occur with fetal hypoxia, which stimulates gastric peristalsis and relaxation of the rectal sphincter with passage of meconium. In many circumstances however, passage of meconium is a manifestation of a mature gastrointestinal tract; as many as 25% of postterm deliveries, of infants older than 40 weeks, will have evidence of meconium in the amniotic fluid.

Consequences of Meconium Passage or Aspiration

Meconium aspiration can occur before, during, or after birth. Under normal conditions, the fetus will inhale approximately 1 mL of amniotic fluid. When "gasping," as often occurs during fetal hypoxic distress, the fetus will inhale up to 60 mL of amniotic fluid, resulting in meconium aspiration.

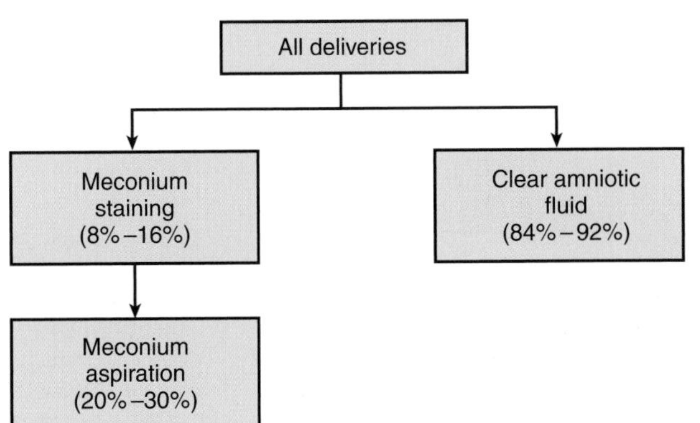

Figure 199-1 Of all full-term neonates in the United States, between 8% and 16% will have meconium staining. Of these, 20% to 30% will develop meconium aspiration syndrome.

Meconium directly alters amniotic fluid by reducing the antibacterial activity of the fluid and thereby increasing the risk of perinatal bacterial infection. It also irritates fetal skin, which, in turn, increases the incidence of erythema toxicum. However, of greatest consequence to the fetus are the effects on the respiratory (Figure 199-2) and cardiac systems. The outcomes related to partial mechanical obstruction of the airway from meconium aspiration include ball-and-valve effects, pneumothorax, pneumomediastinum, or pneumopericardium. Complete tracheal obstruction may result in fetal death.

Treatment

Prevention is a key component of treatment and remains a primary aspect of care. Because meconium aspiration can occur prior to the time of delivery because of chronic asphyxia and infection, perhaps the most critical preventive strategy is good prenatal care, including the detection and prevention of fetal hypoxemia and the avoidance of postdate deliveries. During labor, it is critical that the fetus be monitored for signs of fetal distress, with intervention begun immediately upon determining that the fetus is distressed. Approaches to the prevention and treatment of MAS have changed over the past half century and are somewhat controversial.

Treatment Before Delivery

In a multinational, multicenter, randomized controlled trial involving 1998 women with thick meconium-stained amniotic fluid, amnioinfusion—the transvaginal instillation of warm sterile saline into the amniotic cavity—failed to show an effect on the incidence of MAS or death. Thus, current consensus is that a large number of infants born through meconium-stained

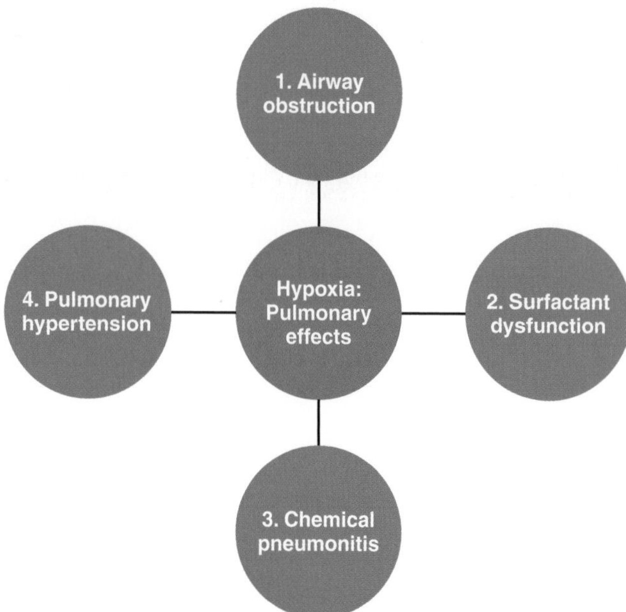

Figure 199-2 The potential pulmonary effects associated with meconium aspiration syndrome.

amniotic fluid will have aspirated meconium before an amnioinfusion can be performed, therefore prompting the issuance of an American College of Obstetricians and Gynecologists' opinion stating that "routine prophylactic amnioinfusion for the dilution of meconium-stained amniotic fluid should be done only in the setting of additional clinical trials."

Treatment During and After Delivery

Once the infant has been delivered, treatment focuses on immediate transfer of the newborn to the neonatal team members, who initiate management of the airway, as indicated, depending on the infant's signs and symptoms.

No randomized controlled trials have been conducted to provide clear recommendations on the use of tracheal suctioning during delivery before the shoulders are delivered or immediately after delivery. However, the American Heart Association and the American College of Obstetricians and Gynecologists recommend against the use of tracheal suctioning in vigorous neonates with meconium-stained amniotic fluid. Tracheal suctioning is recommended in nonvigorous neonates. If intubation is deemed necessary and attempts to intubate the trachea are not successful or are prolonged, the infant, particularly if bradycardic, may need to be ventilated with a bag and mask prior to placement of the tracheal tube (Figure 199-3).

The goals of continued care in the neonatal intensive care unit include limiting O_2 consumption and optimizing $Pa{O_2}$ with minimal airway pressures and preventing air trapping. Rescue therapies include high-frequency oscillation or jet ventilation, as an alternative to mechanical ventilation, and surfactant therapy. Nitric oxide may be used to prevent persistent pulmonary hypertension of the newborn, a not uncommon occurrence with neonates who have MAS. Because its use is associated with a high incidence of poor neurologic outcome, extracorporeal membrane oxygenation should be used as a last resort.

Avoiding hypocapnia and alkalosis will help to optimize cerebral perfusion pressures. Cardiac complications, which are the result of chronic in utero hypoxia, include persistent fetal circulation and persistent pulmonary hypertension of the newborn. Minimizing right-to-left pulmonary shunting—by keeping systemic pressures greater than pulmonary pressures—will decrease the incidence of patent ductus arteriosus. Persistent pulmonary hypertension of the newborn is associated with the greatest risk of death in neonates with MAS.

Suggested Readings

ACOG Committee on Obstetric Practice. ACOG Committee Opinion No. 346, October 2006: Amnioinfusion does not prevent meconium aspiration syndrome. *Obstet Gynecol*. 2006;108:1053.

ACOG Committee on Obstetric Practice. ACOG Committee Opinion No. 379, September 2007: Management of delivery of a newborn with meconium-stained amniotic fluid. *Obstet Gynecol*. 2007;110:739.

Fanaroff AA. Meconium aspiration syndrome: Historical aspects. *J Perinatal*. 2008;28(Suppl 3):S3-7.

Hofmeyr GJ, Xu H. Amnioinfusion for meconium-stained liquor in labour. *Cochrane Database Syst Rev*. 2010:CD000014.

Kattwinkle J. *Textbook of Neonatal Resuscitation*. 5th ed. Chicago: American Academy of Pediatrics; 2005.

Kattwinkel J, Perlman JM, Aziz K, et al. Part 15: Neonatal resuscitation: 2010 American Heart Association Guidelines for Cardiopulmonary Resuscitation and Emergency Cardiovascular Care. *Circulation*. 2010;122(18 Suppl 3): S909-919.

Roggensack A, Jefferies AL, Farine D. Management of meconium at birth. *J Obstet Gynaecol Can*. 2009;31:353-354.

Vain NE, Szyld EG, Prudent LM, et al. Oropharyngeal and nasopharyngeal suctioning of meconium-stained neonates before delivery of their shoulders: Multicentre, randomized controlled trial. *Lancet*. 2004;364:597-602.

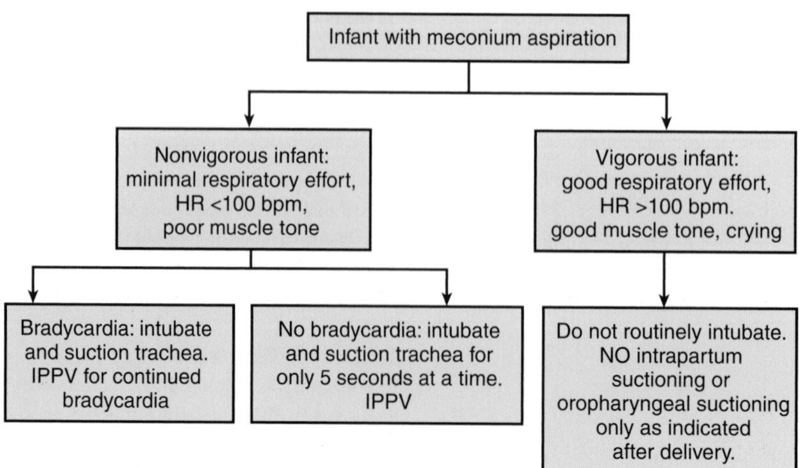

Figure 199-3 Management of neonate if amniotic fluid is stained with meconium. bpm, Beats per minute; HR, heart rate; IPPV, intermittent positive-pressure ventilation.

CHAPTER 200

Congenital Pediatric Airway Problems

Wayne H. Wallender, DO

The upper airway is more easily compromised in infants and children than in adults. Anatomically, compared with an adult, the tongue of an infant or child is relatively larger within the mouth, the larynx is more cephalad, the glottic opening and airways are narrower, the arytenoid cartilages are more prominent, and the occiput is larger, resulting in greater resistance to airflow. Infants' and children's respiratory physiology further complicates the management of the airway. Because infants have higher weight-adjusted basal metabolic rates, O_2 consumption and CO_2 production rates are higher. In addition, the functional residual reserve of infants, per kilogram, is less than that of adults. Congenital abnormalities associated with airway problems can cause further difficulties with airway management.

Management of the difficult pediatric airway should include spontaneous ventilation with the consideration that direct laryngoscopy has a significant failure rate. As a general approach, these patients can be divided into those who will be difficult to intubate but can be ventilated by mask and those who are difficult or impossible to ventilate by mask. The latter group poses a more difficult anesthetic challenge and may require emergency tracheostomy. If a child can be ventilated by mask, then a number of options can be safely employed until the trachea is successfully intubated. The anesthetic goals are always a safe induction and intubation as well as a safe extubation.

Congenital Abnormalities of the Airway

Mucopolysaccharidoses

Hurler syndrome is associated with severe mental retardation, gargoyle facies, deafness, stiff joints, dwarfism, pectus excavatum, kyphoscoliosis, abnormal tracheobronchial cartilage, hepatosplenomegaly, severe cardiac valvular disease, and early coronary artery disease. Children with Hunter syndrome often have course facial features, deafness, hypertrichosis, stiff joints, macrocephaly, and carpal tunnel syndrome. Children with Morquio syndrome often appear healthy at birth; however, as the child ages, manifestations may include coarse facial features, prognathism, odontoid hypoplasia, atlantoaxial instability resulting from thoracic or lumbar kyphosis, aortic valve incompetence, hepatomegaly, inguinal hernias, mixed hearing loss, ocular complications, and limb abnormalities.

Upper airway obstruction and difficult intubation are common in children with mucopolysaccharidosis because of infiltration of lymphoid tissue, enlarged tongue, small mouth, and profuse thick secretions. A difficult airway should be expected and, as the infant ages, the airway may become even more difficult to manage.

Pierre Robin Syndrome

Children with Pierre Robin syndrome may have cleft palate, micrognathia, glossoptosis (posterior displacement of the tongue), and congenital heart disease. Affected infants can present with significant airway problems almost immediately after birth. Intubation may be very difficult and should initially be attempted with the infant awake. Tracheostomy should be considered early. Airway obstruction may be relieved by positioning the patient prone, pulling the tongue forward, or using a nasopharyngeal airway. A suture may be placed to maintain the tongue position.

Treacher Collins Syndrome

This syndrome is the most common of the mandibulofacial synostoses. Clinical features include micrognathia, aplastic zygomatic arches, microstomia (small mouth), choanal atresia, and congenital heart disease. These children usually present with less severe airway and intubation difficulties than are seen in children with Pierre Robin deformities.

Goldenhar Syndrome

Patients with Goldenhar syndrome are characterized by unilateral facial hypoplasia associated with mandibular hypoplasia (60%), congenital heart disease (20%), and eye, ear, and vertebral abnormalities on the affected side. The difficulty of tracheal intubation is highly variable in these patients.

Crouzon Syndrome

This form of congenital craniofacial synostosis combines a wide towering skull with proptosis, maxillary hypoplasia, and a beaked nose. Premature closure of the cranial sutures does not begin until after birth; thus, cranial shape can vary. Life span and intelligence are usually normal. A high-arched palate and malocclusion can occur. Maxillary hypoplasia can make mask ventilation difficult, but intubation is usually not a challenge. Long-duration open surgical repairs often have significant blood loss and postoperative swelling of the airway, thus mandating perioperative intubation.

Cleft Lip and Palate

Considered together, cleft lip and palate represent some of the most common congenital anomalies and are associated with more than 300 syndromes. The incidence of cleft lip (with or without cleft palate) varies by sex (higher rate in males, with isolated cleft palate higher in females) and ethnicity, with Asian Americans and Native Americans having the highest incidence and African Americans, the lowest. In European Americans, the incidence of cleft lip with or without cleft palate is 1 in 750 births; that of cleft palate alone is approximately 1 in 2500.

These patients may have other associated anomalies. Middle ear infections are quite common in this population. Infants with cleft lip or palate have difficulty swallowing and are at risk for developing pulmonary aspiration.

Anesthetic management depends on the degree of airway abnormality and can be relatively straightforward in uncomplicated cases. Large defects of the palate are usually not associated with airway obstruction, unless the defect is so extensive that the tongue prolapses into the nasopharynx. However, large defects can cause difficulty with intubation if the laryngoscope blade wedges into the cleft, or, if the patient is already intubated, the oral tracheal tube can migrate into the cleft, resulting in extubation. Postoperative airway problems are also common after a palatoplasty. Surgical edema in children with small oral cavities can result in airway obstruction requiring reintubation.

Anesthetic Management of the Difficult Pediatric Airway

Regardless of the congenital anomaly that causes an airway that may be difficult to manage, problems should be anticipated and managed expectantly. In most cases, preservation of spontaneous ventilation is strongly recommended, and fiberoptic intubation should be employed only when difficulty is suspected and difficult direct laryngoscopy is anticipated. Suggestions for management include the following:

- The preoperative use of H_2-receptor blocking agents may be considered in infants at risk for aspirating.
- Intravenous access should be established either before or as soon as possible after induction.
- The use of intravenously administered sedatives, opioids, or neuromuscular blocking agents should be avoided.
- Atropine should be administered before laryngoscopy is attempted.
- The intravenous administration of lidocaine, 1 mg/kg, before intubation may decrease the risk of laryngeal spasm. Alternatively, topical translaryngeal lidocaine can be given, remembering that transmucosal absorption of lidocaine is close to that of intravenously administered lidocaine.
- Preoxygenation is strongly recommended.
- A variety of laryngoscopy blades, tracheal tubes, and stylets should be readily available.
- Laryngoscopy should be performed under deep anesthesia.
- The use of either mask ventilation or a laryngeal mask airway may be warranted (Box 200-1).
- Several intubation approaches should be considered (e.g., awake, blind nasal, fiberoptic), but alternative methods must be immediately available, including facilities for cricothyrotomy or tracheostomy.
- Induction with sevoflurane via spontaneous ventilation is preferred if awake intubation is not possible. Sevoflurane has a rapid onset of action, provides a smooth induction, and will not sensitize the heart to endogenous catecholamines, such as halothane does (halothane is no longer used in the United States but it may still be used in developing countries by anesthesia providers who provide humanitarian care there to pediatric patients." Desflurane should not be used for induction because of its pungency and propensity to irritate the airway.
- Spontaneous ventilation should be maintained.
- Fiberoptic intubation is becoming more desirable in pediatric patients as smaller bronchoscopes become available. Currently, pediatric bronchoscopes are available that will fit through a 3.0-mm tracheal tube, although they do not have suction ports.

Box 200-1 Advantages and Disadvantages with Use of Laryngeal Mask Airway

Advantages	Disadvantages
Can be used as main airway device	Does not protect against aspiration
Can be used to ventilate and as conduit for fiberoptic intubation	May be difficult to ventilate patients with acute lung injury
Is available in multiple sizes:	Can be easily dislodged

LMA Size	*Patient Weight (kg)*
1	<1
1.5	5-10
2	10-20
2.5	20-30
3	>30

LMA, Laryngeal Mask Airway.

Because children are very prone to developing laryngospasm at the time of extubation, all equipment for ventilation and reintubation must be available before extubation is attempted. These children should usually not be extubated until awake. Mild laryngospasm can be treated with positive-pressure ventilation with O_2 by mask. Severe laryngospasm usually responds to a small dose of succinylcholine (0.3 mg/kg).

Suggested Readings

Hardcastle T. Anaesthesia for repair of cleft lip and palate. *J Perioper Pract.* 2009;19:20-23.

Nargozian C. The airway in patients with craniofacial abnormalities. *Paediatr Anaesth.* 2004;14:53-59.

Semjen F, Bordes M, Cros AM. Intubation of infants with Pierre Robin syndrome: The use of the paraglossal approach combined with a gum-elastic bougie in six consecutive cases. *Anaesthesia.* 2008;63:147-150.

Ward CF. Pediatric head and neck syndromes. In: Katz J, Steward DJ, eds. *Anesthesia and Uncommon Pediatric Diseases.* 2nd ed. Philadelphia: WB Saunders; 1993:319-363.

CHAPTER 201

Congenital Diaphragmatic Hernia

Wayne H. Wallender, DO

Congenital diaphragmatic hernia (CDH) most commonly presents as respiratory distress and cyanosis in a baby shortly after birth and is a true surgical emergency. Because the diaphragmatic malformation originates early in fetal development, the presence of intestines in the thorax inhibits lung development, resulting in the primary problem in CDH—hypoplasia of the lung parenchyma and pulmonary vasculature. CDH is often associated with other congenital problems that may affect the management of anesthesia (Table 201-1).

Incidence and Classification

CDH occurs in about 1 in every 2500 live births. Classification is based on location of the defect, with the most common and significant being the posterior lateral aspect of the diaphragm, through the foramen of Bochdalek (80%). Left-sided hernias occur five times more often than right-sided ones. Hernias through the esophageal hiatus are generally small, with no compromise of pulmonary function, and do not usually present in the neonatal period. Figure 201-1 illustrates other sites in which hernias may be evidenced. Incomplete muscularization of the diaphragm (eventration) may occur, resulting in the development of a hernia sac. Many cases are asymptomatic, but severe cases may present identically to CDH.

Embryology

In the fetus, the pleuroperitoneal cavity begins as a single compartment. The development and closure of the diaphragm are usually complete by the ninth fetal week, with return of the gut to the peritoneal cavity in the tenth week. Gut return from the yolk stalk occurring early or diaphragmatic formation occurring late produces the potential for a diaphragmatic hernia. Anatomic defects of the lung occur because bronchial development can be impeded by the herniated abdominal contents.

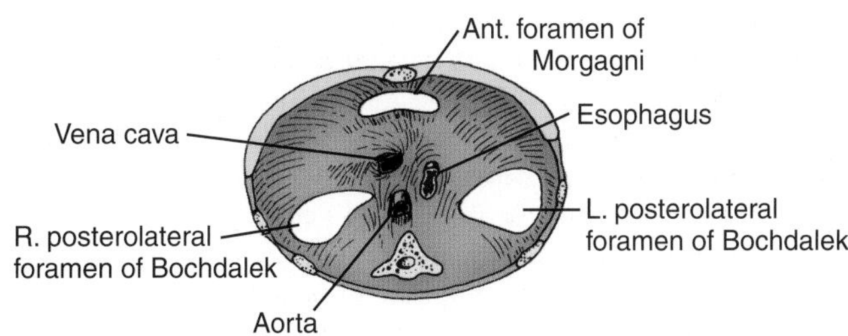

Figure 201-1 Potential sites of herniation of abdominal contents with congenital diaphragmatic hernia. Ant, Anterior; L, left; R, right. (From Morray JP, Krane EJ. Anesthesia for Thoracic Surgery. In: Gregory GA, ed. Pediatric Anesthesia. 2nd ed. New York: Churchill Livingstone; 1989:893.)

Table 201-1 Congenital Problems Associated with Congenital Diaphragmatic Hernia

System	Frequency (% of Affected Neonates)	Associated Problem(s)
Central nervous system	28	Encephalopathy, hydrocephalus, spina bifida
Polyhydramnios, without gastrointestinal anomalies	30	
Gastrointestinal	20	Intestinal atresia, malrotation
Genitourinary	15	Hypospadias
Cardiac	13-23	Atrial septal defect, coarctation, tetralogy of Fallot, ventricular septal defect

Clinical Presentation

CDH may be suspected in utero because about 30% of cases are associated with polyhydramnios. Severe CDH is usually discovered by ultrasound prenatally, immediately after birth, or within the first 6 h of life. Some visceral herniations can act as an evolving lesion and may present at birth, even though the diaphragmatic defect occurs in gestation. The infant presents with cyanosis and respiratory distress. Physical findings include shifted cardiac sounds, scaphoid abdomen, and diminished breath sounds on the affected side. The primary cause of death is progressive hypoxemia and acidosis. Radiographs are usually confirmatory. The immediate therapy is tracheal intubation and mechanical ventilation along with placement of a nasogastric tube to decompress the gut. Significant degrees of postsurgical hypoxemia and acidosis may result in persistent fetal circulation, with right-to-left shunting of desaturated blood. Progressive deterioration and death can result from the subsequent high pulmonary pressures. Ligation of a patent ductus arteriosus in infants with severe persistent fetal circulation is controversial because acute right ventricular failure and death can occur. Prior to delivery, parturients who are anticipated to deliver an infant with CDH should be transferred to a facility that is equipped to provide specialized therapies (e.g., extracorporeal membrane oxygenation [ECMO]) and drugs (e.g., inhaled nitric oxide).

Anesthetic Management

Most infants with CDH are urgently intubated in the delivery room. If the infant is not intubated before coming to the operating room, the tracheal tube can be placed while the infant is awake, or a rapid sequence intravenous induction can be planned. The neonate is preoxygenated, cricoid pressure is applied, and precautions are taken to prevent aspiration of stomach contents. Positive-pressure ventilation with bag and mask prior to intubation should be avoided because it may cause further distention of the gut. The use of standard monitors, along with arterial and central venous pressure catheters, is recommended. Because heat loss is rapid, the operating room should be warmed, and a source of radiant heat provided.

Selection of anesthetic agent and technique depends on the infant's condition. The usual technique is O_2/opioid/neuromuscular blocking agent. The use of N_2O is contraindicated. Any sudden deterioration in heart rate, blood pressure, Spo_2, or lung compliance suggests a contralateral pneumothorax, which should be promptly treated by inserting a chest tube. Some practitioners advocate the prophylactic insertion of a contralateral chest tube. A peak inspiratory pressure of less than 30 cm H_2O is recommended.

Two factors that affect pulmonary vascular resistance are Po_2 and Pco_2. The Pao_2 should be maintained in the 90- to 100-mm Hg range. The lungs should be hyperventilated to achieve a $Paco_2$ of 25 to 30 mm Hg (to decrease pulmonary vascular resistance). After repair of the diaphragmatic defect, the infant's abdomen may be primarily closed, or a staged closure may be performed with a Silastic pouch. After surgery, the infant should be transferred to an intensive care unit and remain intubated, mechanically ventilated, and paralyzed in a warmed incubator unit. Attempts to expand the ipsilateral lung may lead to excessive airway pressure and pneumothorax.

Postoperative Care

The postoperative care of infants with CDH is critical. ECMO may be required. Infants with relatively normal lungs usually do well, but those with varying degrees of pulmonary hypoplasia have difficulty maintaining adequate oxygenation because of persistent fetal circulation. The postoperative use of positive-pressure ventilation usually will be necessary. Bilateral chest tubes are also frequently needed. Gastric suction should be continued. Pain management is important and may include epidural or caudal analgesia.

The Use of Extracorporeal Membrane Oxygenation

Criteria have been established to identify infants with CHD who do not respond to pharmacologic and ventilatory therapy, a group that might benefit from a period of ECMO to provide time for pulmonary growth and remodeling. Selection criteria for ECMO include hemodynamic instability, persistent acidosis, and pneumothoraces, as well as severe pulmonary hypertension unresponsive to pharmacologic intervention. However, the use of ECMO is associated with significant risks, and contraindications do exist (Box 201-1). ECMO is discontinued if irreversible brain damage or lethal organ failure occurs or when lung function improves. The overall survival rate of infants with CDH treated with ECMO is reported to be between 50% and 87%.

Box 201-1 Contraindications to the Use of Extracorporeal Membrane Oxygenation

Gestational age < 35 weeks
Weight < 2000 g
Preexisting intracranial hemorrhage
Congenital or neurologic anomalies incompatible with good outcome
Aggressive ventilatory therapy > 1 week
Congenital heart disease

The prenatal diagnosis of CDH is important, but unfortunately, ultrasound diagnosis of CDH is, in most cases, an incidental finding. The possible association with chromosomal anomalies or syndromes is an important prognostic factor. Fetal liver herniation into the chest can also be prognostic. The lung-to-head circumference ratio is a measurement of the contralateral lung taken by ultrasound at the four-chamber heart view and compared with the head circumference. A value less than 1.0 is associated with increased morbidity and an increased need for ECMO.

Mortality Rate

Overall mortality rate in patients with CDH remains high (20% to 80%, average 50%). The survivors lead fairly normal lives, despite having some residual hypoplastic lung disease. Long-term sequelae include bronchopulmonary dysplasia, pulmonary hypoperfusion, and abnormal findings on pulmonary function tests (i.e., decreased forced expiratory volume in 1 sec and decreased maximum voluntary ventilation) but normal functional residual capacity.

Suggested Readings

Chou HC, Hsu WM. New evolutions in congenital diaphragmatic hernia. *Pediatr Neonatol*. 2010;51:80-82.

Hendrick HL, Danzer E, Merchant A, et al. Liver position and lung to head ratio for prediction of extracorporeal membrane oxygenation and survival in isolated left congenital diaphragmatic hernia. *Am J Obstet Gynecol*. 2007:197:422.e1-4.

Holzman RS, Mancuso TJ, Polaner DM. *A Practical Approach to Pediatric Anesthesia*. Philadelphia: Lippincott, Williams & Wilkins; 2008.

Schaible T, Hermle D, Loersch F, et al. A 20-year experience on neonatal extracorporeal membrane oxygenation in a referral center. *Intensive Care Med*. 2010;36:1229-1234.

Tsao K, Allison ND, Harting MT, et al. Congenital diaphragmatic hernia in the preterm infant. *Surgery*. 2010;148:404-410.

CHAPTER 202

Congenital Heart Disease: Congestive Heart Failure

William C. Oliver Jr., MD

Anesthetic management of a patient with congenital heart disease (CHD) and congestive heart failure (CHF) requires a thorough understanding of human anatomy and physiology. Anesthesia is more frequently employed in the setting of cardiac surgery; however, as life expectancy increases in this patient population, anesthesia is increasingly necessary for the performance of noncardiac procedures.

The fetal circulation is perfectly designed to adapt to the intrauterine environment; the anatomic and physiologic characteristics of the fetal circulation also allow the fetus to tolerate CHD. It is with the transition from fetal to postnatal circulation that characteristic physiologic changes usually appear that point to the presence of a cardiac anomaly. The degree of "fetal" circulation that persists after birth determines the impact of extrauterine life; consequently, the diagnosis of CHD may be made immediately after birth or may be delayed for days to months. Certain CHDs typically result in poor ventricular function and hemodynamics with progression to CHF. Unfortunately, the cause of CHF is not always readily apparent in neonates and infants. In addition to CHF, patients with CHD may have secondary effects, such as pulmonary hypertension.

CHD has been classified using numerous systems that represent the biases and interests of their authors, but none have been universally accepted. For this discussion, CHD will be classified according to the presence or absence of cyanosis. Cyanotic lesions are caused by shunting of blood from the pulmonary circulation to the systemic circulation, which results in poor pulmonary blood flow and progressive arterial desaturation. In contrast, lesions without cyanosis (acyanotic) are characterized by pulmonary overcirculation because of shunt from the systemic to pulmonary circulation that eventually causes CHF. Excessive blood to the lung reduces lung compliance and increases the work of breathing by two mechanisms: (1) increased left atrial pressure resulting in pulmonary venous congestion and pulmonary edema, which decreases the compliance of the lung itself, and (2) increased size of pulmonary vessels, causing greater obstruction to airflow in both large and small airways. A typical example of acyanotic CHD with CHF is the preterm infant with a ductus arteriosus that does not close postnatally (patent ductus arteriosus, or PDA). A large left-to-right (L-to-R) shunt causes systemic circulatory steal, pulmonary overcirculation, and diastolic hypotension. Pharmacologic or surgical closure of the PDA is required to resolve the CHF.

The orifice of the shunt in a PDA may be described as restrictive or nonrestrictive. If the orifice is restrictive, the primary determinant of shunt fraction is the radius of the orifice and pressure gradient. If the orifice is nonrestrictive, the shunt direction and magnitude depend on the relative resistances of the pulmonary and systemic vascular circulations, which can be manipulated as part of the care of individuals until closure of the PDA.

CHF can also occur from obstructive cardiac defects more quickly than from L-to-R shunts and may progress to circulatory collapse without immediate intervention. Obstructive defects are characterized as subvalvular, primary valvular, or supravalvular obstructions causing reduced left ventricular reserve, hypotension, and ventricular hypertrophy. Furthermore, myocardial ischemia is especially common in obstructive lesions of both ventricles, which show signs of failure. Patients with obstructive defects are at increased risk for developing arrhythmias, such as ventricular fibrillation, in part because of the tenuous myocardial O_2 supply-to-demand ratio. Isolated obstructive lesions can be seen in the right ventricle and are exacerbated by increased pulmonary vascular resistance (PVR), resulting in right-sided heart failure.

Anesthetic Management

The presence of CHF in a patient with CHD should raise concern, especially if the patient has pulmonary hypertension or an obstructive outflow lesion, because these patients are at increased risk for experiencing serious perioperative morbidity and death. In some patients, the stress of surgery may be enough to lead to acute cardiac decompensation, typically reflected by a respiratory, as well as metabolic, acidosis. There is no single anesthetic technique that has been identified as "ideal" for these patients. Anesthetic management must include knowledge of the individual physiologic aspects of the cardiac anatomy (shunt flow) and a plan to minimize myocardial depression and maintain baseline hemodynamic parameters.

Central to the anesthetic management of patients with CHF secondary to L-to-R shunting is to avoid increasing the shunt and pulmonary overcirculation. Repeated cardiopulmonary evaluations are important to identify influences on the patient that would increase systemic vascular resistance or decrease PVR (Table 202-1). One of the foremost responsibilities of the anesthesia team is to consider factors that may adversely affect shunt flow. However, the team must be cautious about the degree to which the L-to R-shunt is manipulated to reduce pulmonary overcirculation. Efforts to aggressively reduce systemic vascular resistance or increase PVR to reduce

Table 202-1 Manipulations That Alter Pulmonary Vascular Resistance (PVR)

↑ PVR	↓ PVR
Hypoxia	O_2
Hypercarbia	Hypocarbia
Acidosis	Alkalosis
Hyperinflation	Normal functional residual capacity (FRC)
Atelectasis	Low hematocrit
Sympathetic stimulation	Blocking sympathetic stimulation
High hematocrit	Nitric oxide
Surgical constriction	

pulmonary overcirculation and, hence, improve CHF will lessen the L-to-R shunt; however, the ensuing hypotension or pulmonary hypertension, respectively, reduces coronary perfusion and stresses a poorly functioning right ventricle, leading to hemodynamic deterioration. In contrast, cyanotic CHD with R-to-L shunts can be improved dramatically with aggressive measures to increase systemic vascular resistance or decrease PVR, often in association with immediate hemodynamic improvement.

Altering ventilation or oxygenation or both are important ways to influence either L-to-R or R-to-L shunts. The pulmonary vasculature is very sensitive to changes in $Paco_2$. Values of $Paco_2$ between 28 and 32 mm Hg are associated with pulmonary vasodilation that will worsen CHF in patients with L-to-R shunts. A $Paco_2$ above 55 mm Hg raises PVR and lessens pulmonary overcirculation in these patients. However, the patient will tolerate hypercarbia only until the associated respiratory acidosis results in worsening myocardial function and compromised hemodynamics, overcoming any benefit from reduced L-to-R shunt. The effect of O_2 as a potent pulmonary vasodilator often goes unnoticed in patients with shunts. The patient's inspired O_2 concentration (Fio_2) should be lowered incrementally after induction of anesthesia to avoid hyperoxia, which decreases PVR and could worsen pulmonary overcirculation.

Patients with CHF secondary to L-to-R shunts or obstructive lesions will benefit from anesthetic medications that do not change or only minimally decrease myocardial contractility. Administering appropriate doses of synthetic opioids, ketamine, or both (which have minimal to no negative inotropic effects) provides excellent hemodynamic stability for these patients. Ketamine is widely used for neonates and infants with CHF because it maintains cardiac output and perfusion pressures by enhanced sympathetic stimulation. Propofol has been used infrequently in this patient population, but even with careful dose adjustments, the use of these drugs poses risks to hemodynamic stability. The use of propofol has been associated with significant vasodilation and hypotension in adults. Preservation of baseline heart rate is essential in the neonate or infant because neonates and infants, unlike adults, are unable to augment cardiac output with increases in stroke volume. Ketamine preserves the heart rate better than does any other anesthetic agent and prevents the bradycardia often associated with the administration of fentanyl alone. A benefit to the use of synthetic opioids in patients with CHD and CHF is the ability of these drugs to attenuate increases in PVR. Though these patients with CHD and CHF may have hypertrophied pulmonary vasculature, the vasculature can be very reactive. Any insult that increases PVR may cause severe systemic hypotension by decreasing left ventricular preload and hypoxemia by decreasing perfusion of the lungs.

If the intravenous route is not an option for induction of anesthesia, intramuscular or inhalation techniques may be used. For intramuscular induction, ketamine is the drug of choice for use when obtaining venous access by causing dissociative anesthesia. A major advantage of ketamine over other medications for intramuscular induction is the limited respiratory depression and maintenance of airway reflexes caused by ketamine, which increases safety until venous access is obtained. Halogenated inhalation agents have been used for induction for years in pediatric patients with CHD and CHF. In the past, the nonirritating airway effects of halothane made it a popular choice for induction, but the associated significant myocardial depression, bradyarrhythmia, and prolonged time to induction were particularly disadvantageous for neonates and infants with CHD, who responded with a greater degree of hypotension to the use of inhalation agents than do older children and adults. Hypotension occurs with the use of inhalation agents (see Chapter 66) as a result of a combination of reduced myocardial contractility, increased vasodilation, lower heart rate, and inhibition of compensatory reflex mechanisms.

The development of inhalation agents with low solubility and less myocardial depression (desflurane and sevoflurane) since the 1990s has been very beneficial, creating an opportunity to use these inhalation agents in managing the care of neonates and infants with CHF. The lower solubility of these inhalation agents results in more rapid induction and emergence. Unlike desflurane, sevoflurane has been evaluated repeatedly in neonates and infants with either cyanotic or acyanotic CHD and has been found to be acceptable in terms of cardiopulmonary side effects when used appropriately for induction and maintenance of anesthesia. It has replaced halothane as the agent of choice for inhalation induction because it results in more rapid inductions, reasonably well maintained hemodynamics, fewer arrhythmias, better contractility, and more rapid emergence and possesses the nonirritating airway effects of halothane. Furthermore, the use of sevoflurane has been shown to be associated with less breath holding, coughing, and laryngospasm, as compared with halothane.

Anesthesia can be induced by sevoflurane in patients with obstructive lesions, but at the concentration often used for an inhalation induction, the negative inotropic effect and risk of hypotension present a risk of hemodynamic collapse, a phenomenon not seen when ketamine is used to induce anesthesia. However, compared with the hypotension associated with the use of other inhalation agents, hypotension from sevoflurane can be quickly corrected by decreasing the concentration of inhaled drug. When inhalation induction with sevoflurane is used, an intravenously administered induction agent should be substituted to complete induction as soon as intravenous access is obtained because, irrespective of the inhalation agent used, a ketamine-based or an opioid-based anesthetic induction is more likely to provide greater hemodynamic stability in this population of patients.

Suggested Readings

Gregory GA, ed. *Pediatric Anesthesia*. 4th ed. New York: Churchill Livingstone; 2002; 477-480.

Hillier SC, Krishna G, Brasoveanu E. Neonatal anesthesia. *Semin Pediatr Surg*. 2004;13:142-151.

Ulke ZS, Kartal U, Sunger MO, et al. Comparison of sevoflurane and ketamine for anesthetic induction in children with congenital heart disease. *Paediatr Anesth*. 2008;18:715-721.

Walker A, Stokes M, Moriarty A. Anesthesia for major general surgery in neonates with complex cardiac defects. *Paediatr Anesth*. 2009;19:119-125.

CHAPTER 203

Other Neonatal Emergencies: Tracheoesophageal Fistula and Omphalocele

Robert J. Friedhoff, MD

Tracheoesophageal Fistula

Tracheoesophageal fistula (TEF) occurs as the result of failure of the tracheal bud to develop normally from the primitive foregut. TEF occurs in several forms (Figure 203-1); type C—esophageal atresia (more correctly agenesis because the proximal part of the primitive foregut develops primarily into a trachea rather than an esophagus) with a distal TEF—is the most common form (accounts for 90% of all TEFs). Maternal polyhydramnios may indicate the presence of the lesion before birth. Diagnosis is suspected at birth when the neonate has excessive drooling, cyanotic episodes, or coughing relieved by suctioning or the clinician is unable to pass a soft catheter into the infant's stomach. TEF can be confirmed by radiography by showing a curled catheter in the upper esophageal pouch with an air bubble in the stomach. Contrast medium is unnecessary and contraindicated because the neonate may aspirate the medium. Associated conditions include prematurity (20%-25%), congenital heart disease (20%-25%), and other midline defects.

Preoperative Management

Preoperative assessment is directed at detecting associated congenital lesions and assessing the patient's pulmonary status. The infant should be fed in the semiupright position, and continuous suction should be applied to the upper esophageal pouch to prevent aspiration. Respiratory support with humidified O_2 should be provided. Routine newborn preoperative laboratory studies (i.e., hemoglobin, electrolytes, glucose, and calcium concentration with or without arterial blood gases) and echocardiography to detect cardiac anomalies, including a right aortic arch (5% of neonates with TEF), should be performed. Pulmonary complications of TEF will not resolve until the fistula is ligated. A preliminary gastrostomy is often performed under local anesthesia.

Intraoperative Management

Induction techniques for repair of a TEF include the use of inhalation agents with a rapid sequence or awake intubation. The use of N_2O, which will add to gastric distention, should be avoided. Care must be taken to avoid intubating the fistula. A tracheal tube with the Murphy eye facing anteriorly should be inserted into the right main bronchus while listening for unilateral breath sounds; the tracheal tube is then pulled back until bilateral breath sounds are heard. Some clinicians prefer to cut the distal end of the tracheal tube, eliminating the Murphy eye. Use of a cuffed tracheal tube to both ventilate and occlude the fistula has been reported. Placement of a Fogarty catheter to identify and occlude the fistula using a pediatric bronchoscope can be attempted. Spontaneous ventilation, to avoid gastric distention until the fistula has been ligated, should be performed, and then controlled ventilation can be used.

Thoracoscopic repair of the fistula will avoid a thoracotomy and its sequelae. Use of a Fogarty catheter placed in the right main bronchus with the aid of a bronchoscope will facilitate one-lung ventilation. An alternative technique is to manipulate the tracheal tube to the left main bronchus with a bronchoscope. Surgical insufflation of CO_2 (5-6 mm Hg) into the right hemithorax will cause right lung collapse and possible hypercapnia and

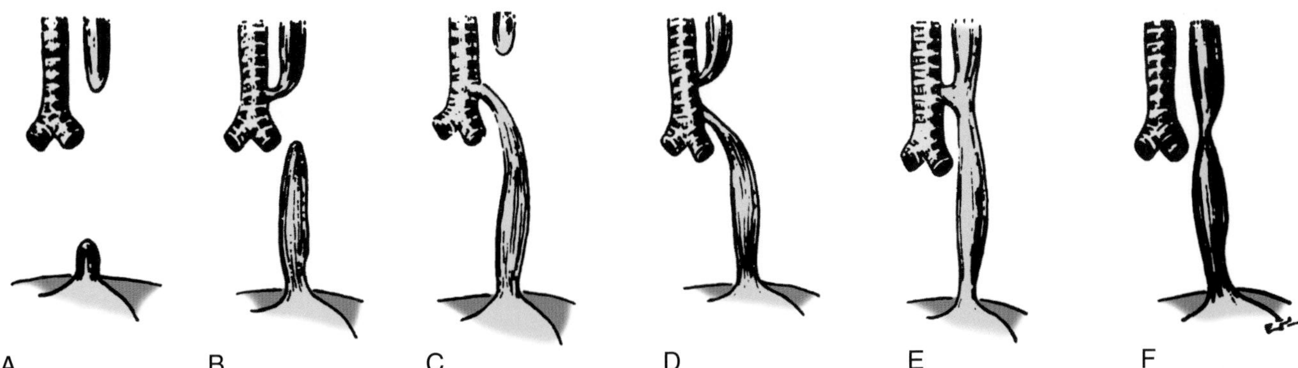

Figure 203-1 Types of congenital abnormalities of the esophagus. **A,** Esophageal atresia, no esophageal communication with the trachea. **B,** Esophageal atresia, the upper segment communicating with the trachea. **C,** Esophageal atresia, the lower segment communicating with the back of the trachea. More than 90% of all esophageal malformations fall into this group. **D,** Esophageal atresia, both segments communicating with trachea. **E,** Esophagus has no disruption of its continuity but has a tracheoesophageal fistula. **F,** Esophageal stenosis. (Modified from Gross RE. The Surgery of Infancy and Childhood. Philadelphia: WB Saunders; 1953.)

hypoxemia. Time to extubation and discharge from the neonatal intensive care unit are decreased with thoracoscopic repair.

A precordial stethoscope should be placed under the dependent lung. Routine intraoperative monitors and an arterial catheter are typically used. Regional anesthesia can be added as an adjuvant.

Postoperative Care

Respiratory status in the intensive care unit can be optimized with the use of tracheal intubation and mechanical ventilation. Damage to the esophageal anastomosis can be avoided by marking a suction catheter so that it is not inadvertently extended past the anastomosis during nasopharyngeal suctioning.

Postoperative Complications

Tracheal compression secondary to tracheomalacia may occur. Infants with TEF typically have abnormal swallowing; 68% have gastroesophageal reflux, leading to possible aspiration. Esophageal stricture is common. A tracheal diverticulum may persist, causing problems with subsequent intubations.

Omphalocele

Anesthetic management for omphalocele and gastroschisis are essentially the same, but knowledge of the associated anomalies will influence anesthetic decisions. Omphalocele and gastroschisis are congenital defects of the anterior abdominal wall, permitting external herniation of abdominal viscera. Gastroschisis is not midline (usually occurs on the right), has a normally situated umbilical cord (not covered with a hernia sac), and is rarely associated with other congenital anomalies but is associated with an increased incidence of prematurity.

Omphalocele has a 75% incidence of other congenital defects, including cardiac anomalies (ventricular septal defects most common), trisomy 21, and Beckwith-Wiedemann syndrome (omphalocele, organomegaly, macroglossia, and hypoglycemia). Epigastric omphaloceles are associated with cardiac and lung anomalies. Hypogastric omphaloceles are associated with exstrophy of the bladder and other genitourinary anomalies.

Preoperative Care

The exposed viscera must be covered with a sterile plastic bag or film to limit evaporative heat loss from exposed bowel. Deficits of fluid and electrolytes (often excessive) need to be replaced prior to operative repair. Hypoglycemia should be corrected slowly with a glucose infusion (6-8 $mg{\cdot}kg^{-1}{\cdot}min^{-1}$). Severe rebound hypoglycemia may occur after bolus doses of glucose. The stomach should be decompressed using a nasogastric tube.

Intraoperative Management

General tracheal anesthesia, using a combination of an inhaled anesthetic agent (N_2O should be avoided) and a parenteral opioid, along with controlled ventilation is required. Preoxygenation followed by awake or rapid sequence intubation is preferred.

Routine monitors, along with an arterial catheter and central venous line for measurement of intravascular pressures, are recommended. Elevated intra abdominal pressures, high ventilatory pressures, and inferior vena cava compression, which can result in circulatory stasis in the lower limbs, should be avoided.

Postoperative Management

Problems seen intraoperatively with ventilation, elevated intra abdominal pressure causing compression of the inferior vena cava and impaired visceral blood flow, prolonged ileus, and decreased hepatic clearance of drugs can continue postoperatively. Urine output should be monitored closely.

Suggested Readings

Alabbad SI, Shaw K, Puligandla PS, et al. The pitfalls of endotracheal intubation beyond the fistula in babies with type C esophageal atresia. *Semin Pediatr Surg*. 2009;18:116-118.

Broemling N, Campbell F. Anesthetic management of congenital tracheoesophageal fistula. *Paediatr Anaesth*. 2011;21:1092-1099.

Deanovic D, Gerber AC, Dodge-Khatami A, et al. Tracheoscopy assisted repair of tracheo-esophageal fistula (TARTEF): A 10-year experience. *Paediatr Anaesth*. 2007;17:557-562.

Gayle JA, Gómez SL, Baluch A, et al. Anesthetic considerations for the neonate with tracheoesophageal fistula. *Middle East J Anesthesiol*. 2008;19: 1241-1254.

Ho AM, Wong JC, Chui PT, Karmakar MK. Case report: Use of two balloon tipped catheters during thoracoscopic repair of type C tracheoesophageal fistula in a neonate. *Can J Anesth*. 2007;54:223-226.

Kinottenbelt G, Skinner A, Seefelder C. Tracheo-oesophageal fistula (TOF) and oesophageal atresia (OA). *Best Pract Res Clin Anaesthesiol*. 2010;24:387-401.

Knottenbelt G, Costi D, Stephens P, et al. An audit of anesthetic management and complications of tracheo-esophageal fistula and esophageal atresia repair. *Paediatr Anaesth*. 2012;22:268-274.

CHAPTER 204

Pyloric Stenosis

Robert J. Friedhoff, MD

Pyloric stenosis is one of the most common gastrointestinal abnormalities occurring during the first 6 months of life. The incidence is 1 in 500 live births in whites and 1 in 2000 in blacks, with males having a two to four times increased incidence, compared with females. It is especially common in first-born sons of parents who had pyloric stenosis.

Pyloric stenosis usually presents at 3 to 5 weeks of age in the preterm or term infant. Although the cause is unknown, proposed mechanisms include an imbalance in the autonomic nervous system, humoral imbalances, infection, or edema with muscular hypertrophy. Hirschsprung first described pyloric stenosis in 1888, although he could offer no effective treatment. Ramstedt described the optimal surgical therapy in 1912. Since then, improvements in fluid therapy and anesthetic technique have decreased the mortality rate from 25% to 0.01% to 0.1%.

Presentation

In pyloric stenosis, a thickening of the circular muscular fibers in the lesser curvature of the stomach and pylorus (from both hypertrophy and an increased number of fibers) causes obstruction of the pyloric lumen. The typical presentation is an infant with persistent bile-free vomiting who is dehydrated and lethargic. The skin is cool to touch, capillary refill is usually greater than 15 sec, and the eyes are sunken. The infant may present at less than its birth weight. Vomiting can be projectile (2 to 3 feet), occurring after every feeding, thus resulting in loss of hydrogen, chloride, sodium, and potassium ions from the stomach.

A metabolic alkalosis develops for several reasons. First and foremost is the loss of hydrogen ions from the stomach. The vomitus does not contain any of the alkaline secretions of the small intestine because the obstruction is proximal (at the gastric outlet). Bicarbonate is one of the ions contained in pancreatic secretions, but because little food reaches the duodenum, pancreatic output is decreased, and bicarbonate remains in plasma (instead of being secreted by the pancreas).

Volume depletion stimulates aldosterone secretion, the distal tubules and collecting ducts retain fluid and sodium and, initially, chloride. As chloride concentration in the plasma and glomerular filtrate decreases, the kidneys begin to retain bicarbonate over chloride, the net result of which is a profound hypokalemic hypochloremic metabolic alkalosis. Eventually, acidic urine is produced because, as the volume and electrolyte concentrations worsen, potassium, rather than hydrogen, is retained preferentially. At this stage, maximal chloride ion conservation in the kidney results in a urinary chloride concentration less than 20 mEq/L.

When examining the infant, the clinician can palpate an olive-sized mass in the midepigastrium. This finding, along with the history, is diagnostic in 99% of cases of pyloric stenosis. Noninvasive diagnostic tests include ultrasound, which can confirm the diagnosis. The "string sign" on barium swallow shows elongation and narrowing of the pyloric canal. Elevated levels of unconjugated bilirubin are seen in 20% of patients with pyloric stenosis.

Pyloric stenosis is a medical emergency, not a surgical emergency. The degree of dehydration may be determined by weighing the infant and measuring bicarbonate and chloride levels. Treatment is instituted with intravenously administered normal saline with 5% dextrose at a rate of 3 $L \cdot m^{-2} \cdot day$. After urine output is established, 40 mmol of potassium can be added to each liter of fluid. Therapy is aimed at repleting intravascular volume and correcting electrolyte and acid-base abnormalities. A urine chloride concentration greater than 20 mEq/L implies that the volume status has been corrected. The plasma chloride concentration should then be greater than 105 mEq/L.

Management of Anesthesia

Anesthetic considerations for pyloric stenosis include the usual neonatal anesthetic concerns; fluid, electrolyte, and glucose balance; anesthesia for a patient with a full stomach who is prone to vomit; and postoperative complications. Patients with pyloric stenosis are at increased risk of vomiting and aspirating gastric contents. After intravenously administering atropine (20 μg/kg) but immediately before inducing anesthesia, the anesthesia provider should empty the patient's stomach as completely as possible by passing a large-bore (14F multiorifice) orogastric tube two to three times because gastric volume prior to induction averages 96 mL ± 7 mL independent of the fasting interval, prior use of a nasogastric tube, or barium studies. Routine monitors should be applied. The preferred method of induction is either through a rapid sequence or modified rapid sequence intravenous induction using cricoid pressure. Awake oral tracheal intubation, or even intubation after an inhalation induction, has also been described, although these techniques are rarely used.

After general anesthesia is induced, a nasogastric tube should be inserted and left in place during the operation to allow testing of the integrity of the pyloric wall after the surgeon performs the pyloromyotomy. Laparoscopic surgical repair has the advantage of shorter times to full feeding and shorter hospital stays, compared with the traditional open approach. Anesthesia is maintained with inhalation agents without N_2O. Skeletal muscle relaxation may not be needed after induction. Additional opioid analgesia may not be necessary in this age group, which has increased respiratory sensitivity. Rectal acetaminophen can be given in the postanesthesia recovery room.

Postoperatively, the infant may be lethargic. Respiratory depression and apnea may occur and are related to cerebrospinal fluid pH and hyperventilation. For these reasons, the infant should be fully awake and able to sustain a regular respiratory pattern before being extubated. Hypoglycemia, which may occur 2 or 3 h after surgical correction of the stenosis, is probably caused by cessation of intravenously administered glucose infusions and the depletion of glycogen stores from the liver. Small frequent feedings are usually begun 4 to 6 h postoperatively. An uneventful recovery should result in discharge from the hospital in 24 to 48 h.

Suggested Readings

Bissonnette B, Sullivan P. Continuing medical education: Pyloric stenosis. *Can J Anaesth*. 1991;38:668.

Cook-Sather SD, Tulloch HV, Cnaan A, et al. A comparison of awake versus paralyzed tracheal intubation for infants with pyloric stenosis. *Anesth Analg*. 1998;86:945-951.

Cook-Sather SD, Tulloch HV, Liacouras CA, Schreiner MS. Gastric fluid volume in infants for pyloromyotomy. *Can J Anaesth*. 1997;44:278-283.

Hal NJ, Pacilli M, Eaton S, et al. Recovery after open versus laparoscopic pyloromyotomy for pyloric stenosis: A double-blind multicentre randomized controlled trial. *Lancet*. 2009;373:358-360.

Hammer G, Hall S, Davis PJ. Anesthesia for general, urologic, and plastic surgery. In: Davis PJ, Cladis FP, Motoyama EK, eds. *Smith's Anesthesia for Infants and Children*. 8th ed. Philadelphia: Elsevier Mosby; 2010: 745-785.

Stoelting RK, Dierdorf SF. Diseases common to pediatric patients. In: Stoelting RK, Dierdorf SF, eds. *Anesthesia and Co-Existing Disease*. 3rd ed. New York: Churchill Livingstone; 1993:579.

Yemen TA. Gastrointestinal diseases. In: Berry FA, Steward DJ, eds. *Pediatrics for the Anesthesiologist*. New York: Churchill Livingstone; 1993:101.

CHAPTER 205

Croup Versus Epiglottitis

Peter Radell, MD, PhD, and **Sten Lindahl**, MD, PhD, FRAC

Respiratory distress is one of the most common presenting symptoms among pediatric patients emergency departments and one of the most common reasons for admission to general pediatric intensive care units. Both acute epiglottitis (supraglottic inflammation) and croup (laryngotracheobronchitis or spasmodic croup, subglottic inflammation) present with evidence of airway obstruction. In 80% of all pediatric patients with acquired stridor, infection is the cause. Of these, 90% are due to laryngotracheobronchitis, and a minority are cases of epiglottitis. Other causes of respiratory distress, such as a foreign body, subglottic stenosis, bacterial tracheitis, and retropharyngeal abscess, also must be considered in the differential diagnosis.

Vaccination against *Haemophilus influenzae* has resulted in a dramatic reduction in the incidence of epiglottitis in children since the late 1980s. The incidence in adults has been less affected, and the prevalence of other bacterial infections—e.g. *Staphylococcus*, *Streptococcus*, *Klebsiella*, *Pseudomonas*—has increased relatively.

Because of the possibility of rapid clinical progression to complete obstruction, acute epiglottitis requires early and prompt intervention. To provide the appropriate therapeutic interventions, one must be able to differentiate between acute epiglottitis and laryngotracheobronchitis. Table 205-1 compares these two causes of severe stridor.

Management

Croup

The treatment of croup varies according to the severity of the illness. In mild cases, conservative measures—such as humidification of air, fever control, and hydration—are usually effective. The cause is usually viral—most commonly parainfluenza viruses, influenza A and B viruses, and respiratory syncytial virus. Radiography can be performed to exclude other diagnoses, such as a foreign body, and may show the classic "steeple sign" characteristic of croup. In patients who are nontoxic and and whose condition is stable, it is increasingly common that flexible endoscopy of supraglottic structures is carried out to eliminate other diagnoses in the differential diagnosis of croup. In more severe cases, racemic epinephrine inhalations delivered by intermittent positive-pressure breathing or a simple nebulizer mask produce improvement and decrease the rate of hospital admission. L-Isomer epinephrine can be used with equal efficacy. Racemic epinephrine, 0.2 to 0.5 mL mixed in 2 to 3 mL of normal saline, can be administered over 15 to 20 min. The use of epinephrine requires subsequent observation to exclude rebound worsening when positive effects abate after 2 to 3 h, although mandatory admission does not seem necessary if observation for 3 to 6 h is carried out and reliable supervision is ensured.

If no improvement is seen after inhalation treatment, reconsider the diagnosis (e.g., bacterial tracheitis). Some patients require more than a single treatment, however. The use of steroid therapy has been controversial, but increasing evidence indicates benefit in terms of hospital admission and need for intubation. Dexamethasone, 0.6 mg/kg, can be administered orally, intramuscularly, or parenterally with equal efficacy. The use of He_2/O_2 (Heliox) has increased because the low density of He_2 attenuates the effects of turbulent flow in the airways. Mixtures of 70:30 or possibly 60:40 $He_2{:}O_2$ are needed to achieve an effect, making Heliox inappropriate for use in patients with significant O_2 requirements. In rare cases (less than 3%) of laryngotracheobronchitis, humidification, epinephrine, steroids, and Heliox are insufficient, and intubation or tracheostomy becomes necessary. Antibiotics are needed only if a secondary bacterial infection develops.

Acute Epiglottitis

In cases with a more toxic presentation (see Table 205-1) or imminent respiratory collapse, a diagnosis of epiglottitis (supraglottitis) must be

Table 205-1 Acute Epiglottitis Versus Croup

Clinical Feature	Acute Epiglottitis	Croup
Age (years)	3-7	0.5-5
Family history	No	Yes
Prodrome	Usually none ± dysphagia	Usually URI
Onset	Abrupt (6-24 h)	Gradual (days)
Clinical course	Rapid, may progress to cardiorespiratory arrest	Usually self-limited
Signs and symptoms		
Temperature (° C)	38-40	38
Hoarseness	No	Yes
Dysphagia	Yes	No
Dyspnea	Severe	No
Inspiratory stridor	Yes	Yes
Appearance	Toxic, anxious, sitting upright, leaning forward, mouth open, exaggerated sniffing position	Nontoxic
Oral cavity	Pharyngitis with excessive salivation	Minimal pharyngitis
Epiglottis	Cherry red, edematous	Normal
Radiographic studies		
Neck	Enlarged epiglottis (thumb sign)	Narrow epiglottis
Anteroposterior	Tracheal narrowing	Subglottic narrowing (steeple sign)
Laboratory studies		
WBC count	Marked elevation with left shift	Variable
Bacteriology	*Haemophilus influenzae* type b, *Staphylococcus, Streptococcus*	Viral etiology, parainfluenza usually

URI, Upper respiratory infection; WBC, white blood cell.

suspected. Consider the four "Ds" of epiglottitis—drooling, dysphagia, dysphonia, and dyspnea. The child with acute epiglottitis should be disturbed as little as possible (e.g. by radiography examinations or phlebotomy). Transport the child to the operating room in the sitting position with airway equipment readily available for possible ventilatory support. Do not attempt to visualize the pharynx, which may cause acute obstruction. The operating room should be set up for direct laryngoscopy, emergency bronchoscopy, and possible tracheostomy. Monitoring should include blood pressure, electrocardiography, precordial stethoscope, and pulse oximetry. Induction of anesthesia with O_2 and an inhalation anesthetic agent (sevoflurane or halothane, if it is available), with the child seated, should be performed. Because of the unpredictable variation in the amount of edema, and the potential anatomic distortion and difficulty with ventilation, the use of neuromuscular blocking agents and barbiturates should be avoided.

When anesthesia is induced, the child should be gently laid down. Assisted ventilation may be needed. Intravenous access should be obtained, and atropine, 0.02 mg/kg, should be intravenously administered to attenuate reflex bradycardia, and lidocaine, 1 mg/kg, is given to minimize the risk of coughing and laryngospasm. The use of racemic epinephrine, which may precipitate complete airway obstruction, should be avoided. Laryngoscopy should be performed and the trachea intubated orally with a tube that is 0.5 to 1.0 mm smaller than predicted for age. Once the child is anesthetized and well oxygenated, the oral tracheal tube can be replaced with a nasotracheal tube (again, 0.5 to 1.0 mm smaller than predicted for age). A chest radiograph should be obtained to confirm tube placement and to identify any infiltrate or atelectasis. After the airway is secured in the operating room, admission to an intensive care unit is essential. Intravenous sedation and restraints help prevent accidental extubation. Inspired gases should be humidified and the nasotracheal tube regularly suctioned. Extubation should be considered when pyrexia has resolved (usually within 12 to 36 h) and an air leak has developed around the tracheal tube.

Because the cause of epiglottitis is often uncertain, a broad-spectrum cephalosporin, such as cefotaxime (200 $\mu g \cdot kg^{-1} \cdot day^{-1}$), is initiated after blood and epiglottic cultures have been obtained. The use of corticosteroids has not been shown to be beneficial.

Suggested Readings

Cherry JD. Croup. *N Engl J Med*. 2008;358:384-391.

Fleisher GR, Ludwig S, eds. *Textbook of Pediatric Emergency Medicine*. 6th ed. Philadelphia: Lippincott, Williams & Wilkins; 2010.

Gregory GA, ed. *Pediatric Anesthesia*, 4th ed. New York: Churchill Livingstone; 2002.

Rotta AT, Wiryawan B. Respiratory emergencies in children. *Respir Care*. 2003;48:248-258.

Steward DJ. *Manual of Pediatric Anesthesia*. 5th ed. New York: Churchill Livingstone; 2001.

Stroud RH, Friedman NR. An update on inflammatory disorders of the pediatric airway: Epiglottitis, croup and tracheitis. *Am J Otolaryngol*. 2001;22:268-275.

CHAPTER 206

Sickle Cell Anemia: Anesthetic Implications

Barbara E. Switzer, MD, and Michael J. Murray, MD, PhD

Sickle cell disease (SCD)—an inherited hemoglobinopathy characterized by erythrocytes that assume a rigid sickle shape under relatively hypoxic conditions—is more prevalent in people who themselves or whose forebearers came from tropical or subtropical sub-Saharan regions with current or previously endemic malaria.

In utero, at the end of the first trimester, erythrocytes contain hemoglobin (Hb)F ($\alpha_2\gamma_2$), which, like HbA ($\alpha_2\beta_2$) and HbA_2 ($\alpha_2\delta_2$), is composed of four protein (globin) molecules, each binding one of four hematoporphyrin rings. The P_{50} of HbF is 19 mm Hg (compared with the P_{50} of HbA of 26.8 mm Hg), that is, HbF has a higher affinity for O_2, which is necessary for the fetus to extract O_2 from the placenta and the maternal erythrocytes. Within 6 months of birth, HbF is replaced by adult Hb (HbA), except in individuals with hemoglobinopathies, of which there are close to 300 variants. In people with SCD, the amino acid valine is substituted for glutamic acid in the β-globulin chain. In the United States, approximately 1 in 500 African American children and 2 in 36,000 Hispanic American children have SCD. These children may initially have normal Hb values but, over time, develop anemia (sickle cell anemia [SCA]).

People with SCA, also referred to as HbSS because they have homozygosity for the gene encoding the β chain of hemoglobin (mutant S), develop sickling of erythrocytes in small arterioles at O_2 tensions of 40 to 45 mm Hg (the P_{50} of HbS is approximately 49 mm Hg). However, although hypoxia may cause these cells to "sickle," the process is far more complex, involving erythrocyte-endothelial cell interactions, viscosity of the blood, and probably cytokines released locally as part of a systemic inflammatory response. Patients with sickle cell trait, also called HbAS because of the heterozygosity for the mutation, can develop sickling of erythrocytes at O_2 tensions of 20 to 25 mm Hg. Other, rarer forms of SCD—such as sickle cell–hemoglobin C disease (HbSC), sickle cell–hemoglobin D disease (HbSD), sickle cell β-plus-thalassemia (HbS/β^+), and sickle cell β-zero-thalassemia (HbS/β^0)—are compound heterozygous states in which the affected individual has only one copy of the mutation that causes HbS and one copy of another abnormal hemoglobin allele. These cells can also "sickle," but people with these heterozygous conditions tend to have higher Hb levels (approximately 10 g/dL) than do people with HbSS.

Although the term *sickle cell crisis* is commonly used, in reality, a variety of crises are subsumed under this term, including vaso-occlusive, splenic sequestration, aplastic, and hemolytic crises. Patients with SCA have increased perioperative morbidity and mortality rates, as compared with the general population, likely due to vaso-occlusion from sickled erythrocytes, resulting in acute tissue injury and chronic organ damage (Table 206-1). People with SCA also undergo more operations and at an earlier age; the most commonly performed surgical procedures are cholecystectomy (due to an increased rate of formation of pigmented gallstones and cholelithiasis in this population), splenectomy (because of splenic sequestration and splenic pooling), and hip arthroplasty (related to the 50% rate of osteonecrosis in the femoral head among individuals with SCA who are 35 years of age and older). In addition, postoperative hospital length of stay is typically longer in this population.

Women with SCA are more likely to experience complications during pregnancy. Fifty-four percent of pregnancies in women with SCD result in a live birth, with the average gestational age at delivery being 34 weeks.

Anesthetic Implications

Because hypoxia, hypercarbia, hypothermia, acidosis, dehydration, and low-flow conditions promote erythrocyte sickling, anesthesia providers should be particularly cognizant of these issues and take steps to avoid them during the perioperative period.

Preoperative Considerations

The preoperative assessment of patients who are at risk for having SCD should include Hb phenotype, past medical history, and risk status. For those patients who have an established diagnosis of SCD, the frequency, pattern, and severity of recent exacerbations, as well as the extent of any organ damage, should be ascertained. For those patients who have severe organ damage, pulmonary function tests, chest radiographs, arterial blood gas assessment, an electrocardiogram, and neurologic imaging may be indicated.

Although many anesthesia providers advocate the use of preoperative transfusions to reduce perioperative complications in patients with SCD, few controlled trials document this benefit, and transfusion is associated with significant risks. A 2012 Cochrane Review found that conservative preoperative transfusion protocols appear to be as effective as aggressive therapy in preparing people with SCD for surgery. A small, prospective, randomized trial, with results published in 2013 (Howard and associates), compared preoperative transfusion and no transfusion in patients with SCD who were scheduled to undergo low-risk or medium-risk operations. This study was terminated early because of an elevated rate of adverse events in the no-transfusion group; the investigators concluded that patients with HbSS who have baseline hemoglobin concentrations lower than 9 g/dL and are scheduled to undergo low-risk or medium-risk operations should receive a preoperative transfusion to reduce the risk of developing perioperative acute chest syndrome.

Intraoperative Considerations

Microcirculatory abnormalities, chronic anemia, and progressive renal insufficiency may alter the pharmacologic response of patients with SCD to anesthetic agents. For example, in patients with SCD, the onset of the neuromuscular blocking effect of atracurium is prolonged, but the duration of action is unchanged. The use of premedication with agents that cause respiratory depressions should be avoided. Upon arrival in the operating room—and throughout the procedure—the patient should be carefully

Table 206-1 Effects of Vaso-occlusive Insults from Sickled Erythrocytes on Organ Systems in Patients with Sickle Cell Disease

System	Effect	Cause	Finding(s)
Cardiac	Cardiomegaly Hyperdynamic circulation	Long-term increased cardiac output and gradual occlusion of pulmonary vascular bed	Full pulses Murmurs
Pulmonary	↓ Total lung capacity ↓ Vital capacity ↑ Risk of contracting pneumococcal pneumonia	In patients with SCD, $\dot{V}/\dot{Q}$ mismatch and pulmonary sickling add to their likelihood of developing pulmonary infarction and infection perioperatively. When compared with the general population, these patients have a 10-fold higher risk of serious perioperative pulmonary complications.	Resting Sao_2 70-90 mm Hg
Renal	Papillary necrosis and nephrotic syndrome	The relatively hypoxic, hypertonic, and acidotic environment in the medulla leads to sickling of RBCs with consequent vaso-occlusion, resulting in decreased renal medullary blood flow. Hematuria, which often occurs in patients with sickle cell nephropathy, increases venous pressure, further worsening the ischemia of the renal medulla and predisposing the patient to further RBC sickling.	Large dilute urine volume
Hepatic	Cirrhosis, hepatitis, hepatic sequestration, hepatosplenomegaly, and cholelithiasis Hemosiderosis Hemochromatosis	Both the vascular complications from the sickling process itself and the fact that patients with SCD have often received multiple transfusions increase their risk for developing viral hepatitis, iron overload, and (combined with the effects of chronic hemolysis) pigmented gallstones.	A combination of the following findings, depending on the hepatic cause: fever, pain, jaundice, elevated AST/ALT, cutaneous leukocytoclastic vasculitis, essential mixed cryoglobulinemia with purpura, arthralgias, glomerulonephritis, and peripheral neuropathy, positive PCR assay for viral RNA, elevated serum ferritin, Kupffer cell hyperplasia with erythrophagocytosis, sinusoidal distention with aggregates of sickled erythrocytes, and fine fibrosis in the space of Disse

AST/ALT, Aspartate transaminase/alanine transaminase; PCR, polymerase chain reaction; RBCs, red blood cells; SCD, sickle cell disease; $\dot{V}/\dot{Q}$, ventilation-perfusion.

positioned to avoid venous stasis. The use of a tourniquet on an extremity is relatively contraindicated.

Throughout the procedure and in the postanesthesia care unit or intensive care unit, intravenously administered fluids should be provided, and blood loss should be replaced as indicated. Acid-base status, renal function, and cardiopulmonary status should be carefully monitored both intraoperatively as well as postoperatively. An Sao_2 of 100% and a Pao_2 of 90 mm Hg should be maintained, again throughout the procedure and in the immediate postoperative period (with a close-fitting, nonrebreathing facemask, at 100% O_2, if necessary).

Postoperative Considerations

Common postoperative morbidities associated with SCD include painful sickle cell crisis and acute chest syndrome, a phenomenon due to pulmonary sequestration of sickled cells, with symptoms that range from fever and respiratory distress to abdominal discomfort. Acute chest syndrome typically manifests on approximately postoperative day 3 and lasts for 8 days, on average. When acute chest syndrome is severe, the associated mortality rate in postoperative patients is 25% to 50%. Ventilation-perfusion mismatch and pulmonary sickling increase the risk that patients with SCD will develop pulmonary infarction and infection perioperatively. When compared with the general population, patients with SCD have a 10-fold higher risk of developing serious perioperative pulmonary complications. Therefore, atelectasis and pulmonary complications should be aggressively treated.

Suggested Readings

Adam S, Jonassaint J, Kruger H, et al. Surgical and obstetric outcomes in adults with sickle cell disease. *Am J Med.* 2008;121:916-921.

Dulvadestin P, Gilton A, Hernigou P, Marty J. The onset time of atracurium is prolonged in patients with sickle cell disease. *Anesth Analg.* 2008;107:113-116.

Firth PG. Anesthesia and hemoglobinopathies. *Anesthesiol Clin.* 2009;27:321-336.

Firth PG, McMillan KN, Haberkern CM, et al. A survey of perioperative management of sickle cell disease in North America. *Paediatr Anaesth.* 2011;21:43-49.

Hirst C, Williamson L. Preoperative blood transfusions for sickle cell disease. *Cochrane Database Syst Rev.* 2012;1:CD003149.

Howard J, Malfroy M, Llewelyn C, et al. The Transfusion Alternatives Preoperatively in Sickle Cell Disease (TAPS) study: A randomised, controlled, multicentre clinical trial. *Lancet.* 2013;381:930-938.

Koshy M, Weiner SJ, Miller ST, et al. Surgery and anesthesia in sickle cell disease. Cooperative Study of Sickle Cell Diseases. *Blood.* 1995;86:3676-3684.

CHAPTER 207

Anesthetic Considerations in the Patient with Down Syndrome

Michael J. Murray, MD, PhD, Jennifer A. Rabbitts, MB, ChB

Trisomy 21 (three copies of chromosome 21) accounts for 95% of the cases of Down syndrome (DS), the most common chromosomal abnormality (1:691 live births, according to the Centers for Disease Prevention and Control) and also the most common genetic cause of intellectual disability. The other 5% of patients have DS due to mosaicism (two populations of cells in the same individual, some with two copies of chromosome 21, the rest with three copies of chromosome 21) or due to translocation of part of chromosome 21 onto another chromosome such that there are triplicate copies of a sufficient number of genes to produce the syndrome.

How trisomy 21 causes the multiple genetic deficits associated with DS is not known, but progress is being made. Chromosome 21 is the smallest of the human chromosomes, but it is a very small part of the chromosome that is most likely involved in the genesis of DS. Because of areas of synteny (the correspondence of genes located on the same chromosome in several species) between the human and mouse genomes, researchers have been able to use mouse models to pinpoint the specific genes on human chromosome 21 that are most likely involved in producing symptoms of DS. The Ts65Dn mouse, which carries 132 genes that are syntenic with human chromosome 21, has facial characteristics, memory and learning problems, and age-related changes in the forebrain similar to what is seen in human DS. Studies in other animal models suggest that more than 400 genes are triplicated in DS. Scientists are of the opinion that the deficits seen in DS are not due to a single triplicate copy of one gene but, rather, to several genes or the interaction of several genes. Most recently, investigators have developed a pluripotent stem cell line that contains triplicate copies of genes of interest; the investigators have been able to transform some of these cells into neurons that display reduced synaptic activity, affecting excitatory and inhibitory synapses equally, deficits that are consistent with the cognitive deficits seen in individuals with DS.

The most significant risk factor for trisomy 21—maternal age—was thought more than a century ago to be due to "uterine exhaustion." However, we now know that older mothers have more babies with DS because the frequency of meiotic nondisjunction increases with increasing maternal age. The American College of Obstetricians and Gynecologists recommends that all pregnant women undergo nuchal translucency ultrasound, amniocentesis, or chorionic villus sampling during the first few months of pregnancy to check for DS.

Clinical Manifestations

Abnormalities associated with DS, including abnormalities of the nasal structures and decreased blood flow into the right atrium, are apparent in utero via ultrasound by about 12 weeks. At birth, infants with DS have hypotonia, characteristic oblique palpebral fissures, flat faces, inner canthal folds, hyperflexible joints, a single palmar crease, and dysplastic middle phalanx of the fifth digit. More than half will have congenital cardiac malformations (about half have endocardial cushion defects and another 25% have ventricular septal defects). Although DS is universally associated with mental impairment, the degree of impairment varies.

Neurologic Manifestations

In addition to the delayed mental development, social development is also delayed, resulting in common problems such as impulsive behavior, poor judgment, short attention span, and slow learning. As the child ages and becomes aware of his or her limitations, behavior may become increasingly unmanageable, with frequent outbursts noted. Independent of the degree of mental impairment early in life, those individuals with DS who survive into later adulthood are at increased risk for developing dementia, compared with individuals who do not have DS.

Head and Neck Abnormalities

Because patients with DS often have abnormalities of the head and neck, the anesthesia provider should assess any patient with DS seen in the preoperative clinic for these abnormalities (Box 207-1). Despite the many airway abnormalities described, patients with DS are typically not difficult to intubate, though they may be difficult to ventilate by mask. Cervical spinal malformations have been reported in association with trisomy 21,

Box 207-1 Anesthetic Concerns in Patients with Trisomy 21

- General
  - Difficult intravenous access
  - Limited cognitive abilities
  - Obesity
  - Generalized hypotonia
  - Increased prevalence of obstructive sleep apnea
- Airway
  - Abnormal dentition
  - Large tongue
  - Large tonsils and adenoids
  - Small subglottic area
- Spine
  - Cervical spinal stenosis
  - Atlantoaxial subluxation
- Cardiac
  - Ventricular septal defect
  - Other endocardial cushion defects
  - Atrial septal defect
  - Tetralogy of Fallot
  - Patent ductus arteriosis
- Pulmonary hypertension

with 10% of patients having cervical spinal stenosis and 30% having atlantoaxial instability, although only 1% to 2% of these patients will become symptomatic.

Cardiac Abnormalities

As previously mentioned, patients with DS have a high incidence of congenital cardiac abnormalities, the most prevalent of which are atrial septal defects and ventricular septal defects. If the child has not had a previous echocardiogram, depending on the nature of the procedure for which the anesthesia provider is seeing the child, obtaining a cardiac consultation or performing an echocardiogram should be considered. Any child with uncorrected or corrected cardiac abnormalities should be considered a candidate for endocarditis prophylaxis, again depending on the nature of the surgery, and in keeping with American Heart Association guidelines.

Respiratory Manifestations

Because of the prevalence of cardiac abnormalities in patients with DS, insufficient attention is typically given to the pulmonary problems that children and adolescents with DS can have. Common pulmonary problems include recurrent bronchitis or pneumonia, sleep-disordered breathing, laryngomalacia, tracheobronchomalacia, tracheal bronchus (a bronchus that originates above the carina, more commonly on the right), pulmonary hypertension, subpleural cysts, and subglottic stenosis. Less common abnormalities include complete tracheal rings and interstitial lung disease.

Gastrointestinal Manifestations

Anesthesia providers involved in the resuscitation of a neonate with DS should be aware that early and massive vomiting may be a sign of gastrointestinal obstruction due to esophageal atresia or duodenal atresia. Adolescents and adults with DS may have problems with constipation.

Endocrinologic Considerations

Older children, adolescents, and adults with DS are frequently obese (which may increase their likelihood of developing obstructive sleep apnea) and may have metabolic syndrome (obesity, hypertension, diabetes). Patients with DS also are at increased risk of developing hypothyroidism.

Musculoskeletal Abnormalities

As mentioned previously, patients with DS are at increased risk of having spinal abnormalities, including atlanto-occipatal subluxation and spinal stenosis. Other musculoskeletal abnormalities include separated joints between the bones of the skull (sutures), a single crease in the palm of the hand, wide short hands with short fingers, and a dysplastic middle phalanx of the fifth digit. Physical development is often slower than normal. Most children with DS never reach average adult height.

Perioperative Management

Preoperative Evaluation

Because of the many problems these children have, they frequently undergo surgical procedures. Educating and preparing them for surgery, ensuring that they have not eaten for the requisite period of time prior to surgery, and assessing their pain postoperatively can be a challenge.

As with any other patient, a complete history and physical examination should be performed in compliance with the American Society of Anesthesiologists guidelines and third-party requirements. The primary reason for doing so, however, is and always should be for the effect on patient outcome. The five most important items in the preoperative assessment of a patient with DS are evaluation of the airway, of the cardiac system, and of the pulmonary system; assessment of the cervical spine; and discussion of postoperative pain management.

The preoperative assessment should focus on a number of factors related to atlantoaxial instability. The anesthesia provider should conduct a thorough history and physical examination looking for symptoms or signs suggestive of cord compression and should particularly focus on identifying abnormal range of motion or tenderness in the neck, gait abnormalities, and weakness, spasticity, increased deep tendon reflexes, or clonus of the lower extremities. All patients with trisomy 21 who are to undergo a surgical procedure that includes an anesthetic should have their cervical spines radiographically evaluated if this evaluation has not previously taken place. Examining the patient's joints for laxity will help to identify those patients who are at risk for developing atlanto-occipital dislocation. Any patient who is identified during the preoperative assessment as having evidence of atlantoaxial instability should be referred for further evaluation of neck stabilization. Elective procedures should be postponed until this determination is made.

Finally, depending on how independent the patient is, postoperative pain management should be discussed with the patient and the patient's care provider. If the patient's intellectual functioning is insufficient, plans for managing the patient's pain postoperatively should be discussed, with the patient's assent and the care provider's consent.

Operative Management

Anesthetic management in patients with DS is dictated by the patient's cognitive abilities and associated abnormalities, especially congenital cardiac anomalies and atlantoaxial instability. Patients with DS have an increased incidence of hip problems, the most significant of which is subluxation due to laxity of ligaments and tendons. This needs to be borne in mind when positioning the patient for any procedure, but especially for procedures performed with the patient in the lithotomy position or on the lower extremities.

Atropine premedication, the use of which was previously thought to be inadvisable in patients with DS, is now considered safe but would be dependent on the surgical procedure, the evaluation of the patient, and the degree of preoperative salivation and in keeping with the anesthesia department's practice. Response to preoperative sedation varies in patients with DS because of their different levels of cognitive functioning.

Induction of anesthesia may be accomplished using either inhalation or intravenous techniques, although difficulty in obtaining intravenous access should be anticipated, especially in patients who are obese and who are uncooperative. The minimum alveolar concentration of inhalation anesthetic agents is not reported to differ in patients with DS, as compared with the general population, and maintenance of anesthesia may be achieved with either inhalation or intravenous agents. Care must be taken in choosing an appropriately sized tracheal tube, with awareness of the possibility of subglottic narrowing. Intubation should be performed with care taken to not hyperextend the cervical spine and to avoid undue pressure with the laryngoscope blade on malpositioned teeth. Though these patients have small mouths and large tongues, most should be considered to be candidates for direct laryngoscopy or videolaryngoscopy to secure the airway. If a fiberoptic bronchoscope must be used, it would probably best be performed with the patient receiving monitored anesthesia care, obtaining a view of the airway with a videolaryngoscope, and then passing the bronchoscope into the glottic opening and sliding a tracheal tube of appropriate size off the bronchoscope and into the trachea.

Due caution should be exercised on extubation, and the possibility of upper airway obstruction and postextubation stridor should be anticipated.

Postanesthesia Care

At this juncture, if a plan has not already been developed for addressing the issue of obstructive sleep apnea, the patient's preoperative status, hospital policy, and how the patient does in the postanesthesia care unit will dictate whether intervention is necessary. Per the American Society of Anesthesiologists guidelines, there are no firm recommendations whether or not the patient should be admitted to the hospital overnight or should be discharged, but one must consider the patient's history, appropriately evaluate the patient, and proceed accordingly.

Suggested Readings

Bhattarai B, Kulkarni AH, Rao ST, Mairpadi A. Anesthetic consideration in Down's syndrome—A review. *Nepal Med Coll J*. 2008;10:199-203.

Graham RJ, Wachendorf MT, Burns JP, Mancuso TJ. Successful and safe delivery of anesthesia and perioperative care for children with complex special health care needs. *J Clin Anesth*. 2009;21:165-172.

McDowell KM, Craven DI. Pulmonary complications of Down syndrome during childhood. *J Pediatr*. 2011;158:319-325.

Meitzner MC, Skurnowicz JA. Anesthetic considerations for patients with Down syndrome. *AANA J*. 2005;73:103-107.

Walker SM. Perioperative care of neonates with Down's syndrome: should it be different? *Br J Anaesth*. 2012;108:177-179.

Weick JP, Held DL, Bonadurer GF 3rd, et al. Deficits in human trisomy 21 iPSCs and neurons. *Proc Natl Acad Sci U S A*. 2013;110(24):9962-9967.

CHAPTER 208 Pediatric Neuromuscular Disorders

Andrea P. Dutoit, MD, and Randall P. Flick, MD, MPH

Neuromuscular disorders (NMDs) affect a diverse group of pediatric patients with muscular and neurologic disease of varying complexity and origin. Perioperative concerns and management differ greatly depending on the specific cause of the disorder and the patient's signs and symptoms, making it very important to be familiar with the precise underlying pathophysiology of the NMDs. This information is not always known, making anesthetic management of patients with NMDs challenging.

NMDs are often associated with other congenital disorders; pediatric patients with NMDs often present for elective surgical procedures to correct various deformities or for diagnostic purposes. The major and most common anesthetic concerns when caring for pediatric patients with NMDs are listed in Box 208-1. Several types of NMDs are briefly considered here, along with their major perioperative concerns.

Box 208-1 Anesthetic Considerations for Children with Neuromuscular Disorders

- Aspiration risk is increased due to decreased airway reflexes and increased oral secretions.
- The use of succinylcholine should be avoided, except in emergency situations, due to the increased risk of hyperkalemia developing.
- The risk of MH or rhabdomyolysis with MH-triggering anesthetic agents is unclear.
- Patients may have an increased resistance to the effects of nondepolarizing neuromuscular blocking agents.
- The MAC may be decreased.
- Patients with NMDs may have an increased sensitivity to the effects of opioids.
- Patients with NMDs may have an increased risk of experiencing perioperative blood loss, factor deficiency, or thrombocytopenia.
- Patients with NMDs may be more prone to developing hypothermia.

MAC, Minimum alveolar concentration; MH, malignant hyperthermia; NMD, neuromuscular disorders.

Cerebral Palsy

Cerebral palsy (CP) and static encephalopathy are terms used for a collective group of nonprogressive disorders of movement involving abnormal development or prenatal injury to the brain. Although genetic abnormalities, perinatal anoxia, infection, and trauma have been proposed as etiologic factors in CP, no single cause has been identified. CP has a prevalence of 2 to 4 in 1000 live births, and patients with CP will have a variety of presentations, from near normal functional status to complete incapacitation. Clinical manifestations include disorders of posture due to spasticity or hypotonia of lower extremity or upper extremity muscle groups and abnormal speech or vision. Gastroesophageal reflux, behavior problems, mental retardation, and epilepsy can occur in some children with CP.

Muscular Dystrophy

The muscular dystrophies (MDs) are characterized by progressive degeneration of skeletal muscles without signs of denervation. Duchenne MD (DMD) is an X-linked recessive disorder present in about 1 in 3500 male births. Symptoms of DMD are more severe than those that are part of Becker MD, although both disorders result from abnormalities of the dystrophin protein. In patients with DMD, affected muscles increase in size (pseudohypertrophy) as as result of muscle replacement with fat and connective tissue. Muscle weakness may not become evident until the patient is 2 to 5 years of age, but the weakness is rapidly progressive such that children are often wheelchair bound by 8 to 10 years of age and die by age 25. When succinylcholine is used in patients with MD, hyperkalemia may occur, whether or not the MD is clinically apparent. Because the manifestations of MD do not necessarily occur until children are older, many anesthesia providers avoid the use of succinylcholine in all males under the age of 10 years unless its use is indicated in emergency situations.

The preanesthetic evaluation of patients with MD should include an assessment of preexisting associated problems, such as kyphoscoliosis, as well as a thorough review of the cardiac system, given the increased prevalence of cardiomyopathy and the risk during anesthesia of cardiac complications occurring, such as heart failure or arrhythmias due to fibrosis of the electrical conduction system of the heart. The anesthesia provider should consider the potential for the patient to have respiratory muscle weakness and need postoperative mechanical ventilation and to be at increased risk for experiencing aspiration due to decreased laryngeal reflexes and gastric atony. The use of an inhalation agent for either induction or maintenance of anesthesia is controversial because of the perceived increased risk of children with MD developing malignant hyperthermia (MH), although studies have shown no clear association (see discussion later).

Mitochondrial Myopathies

Mitochondrial myopathies are a very rare complex group of disorders characterized by defects in the electron transport chain or oxidative phosphorylation of skeletal muscle. The manifestations include generalized muscle fatiguability, progressive weakness, hypoglycemia, metabolic and respiratory acidosis, and stroke. Affected organ systems include not only those with high O_2 demands, such as the brain and heart, but also the liver and kidneys.

Surgical stress can decrease the O_2 supply-demand ratio because of an increase in O_2 demand, leading to hypoxia in the patient who is under anesthesia. Mitochondrial disorders have no direct link to MH but it has been suggested that the use of propofol in these patients may lead to a progressive metabolic acidosis similar to that seen in the propofol infusion syndrome.

Malignant Hyperthermia and Neuromuscular Disorders

Despite continuing controversy, it is widely assumed that children with known or suspected myopathies are at increased risk for developing MH. Previous reports have suggested a relationship between MH risk and a variety of NMDs, including DMD, osteogenesis imperfecta, myotonia congenita, Schwartz-Jampel syndrome, Kearns-Sayre syndrome, and others. A clear link to MH has been established for only two disorders: central core disease and King syndrome. Both are quite rare, well-defined clinically, autosomal dominant, and frequently diagnosed without muscle biopsy.

Much of the difficulty associated with defining the relationship between MH and MD is related to the phenomenon of acute rhabdomyolysis. Acute rhabdomyolysis leading to hyperkalemic cardiac arrest has been reported to occur in association with MDs and with myopathies and has been understandably confused with MH. Presenting symptoms and signs of acute rhabdomyolysis are very similar to those of MH and include fever, hypercarbia, tachycardia, acidosis, hyperkalemia, arrhythmias, and elevated creatine kinase levels. If untreated, both rhabdomyolysis and MH may result in death. Similar to MH, most reported cases of rhabdomyolysis have been associated with the use of succinylcholine, although several cases have occurred in its absence. Inhalation anesthetic agents have subsequently been implicated as well, although the mechanism by which this occurs remains, to a large extent, unexplained. For these reasons, it is common to avoid the use of triggering anesthetic agents (succinylcholine and inhalation agents) in patients with MD.

The most commonly mentioned alternative to the use of inhalation anesthetics agent in this population is total intravenous anesthesia (e.g., propofol). Theoretically, the use of propofol in patients with MD is also controversial given the reports of rhabdomyolysis, unrelenting acidosis, and death that have occurred when propofol was used at high doses in children. It has been recommended that anesthesia providers who administer anesthesia to children who have or may have mitochondrial disorders consider avoiding the use of propofol due to concerns that this group may be at particular risk for developing the propofol infusion syndrome.

Because of the rarity of both MH and rhabdomyolysis, most studies are underpowered to be able to demonstrate the safety of using inhalation anesthetic agents in the setting of suspected myopathy. Studies that include small groups of patients have shown that, in a diverse population of children undergoing muscle biopsy for known or suspected myopathy, the incidence of MH or rhabdomyolysis is extremely uncommon even when succinylcholine or inhalation anesthetic agents have been used. The estimated risk of MH or rhabdomyolysis attributed to the use of these agents is probably less than 1.0%. Each anesthesia provider must decide, based on these results, whether the risk is sufficient to justify the use of an alternative anesthetic agent, such as propofol, or some other approach, such as the use of etomidate (adrenal suppression), dexmedetomidine (bradycardia and hypotension), ketamine (hallucinations), or a regional technique (acceptance/cooperation).

Suggested Readings

Baum VC, O'Flaherty JE, eds. *Anesthesia for Genetic Metabolic and Dysmorphic Syndromes of Childhood*. 2nd ed. Philadelphia: Lippincott, Williams & Wilkins; 2007.

Flick RP, Gleich SJ, Herr MM, Wedel DJ. The risk of malignant hyperthermia in children undergoing muscle biopsy for suspected neuromuscular disorder. *Pediatr Anesth*. 2007;17:22-27.

CHAPTER 209

Anesthesia for Myotonic Dystrophy

Joseph J. Sandor, MD

Myotonia—the repetitive firing of muscle action potentials causing prolonged muscle contractions even after mechanical stimulations to the muscles have ceased—is a hallmark of myotonic dystrophy. The grip test is a quick and easy way to determine the presence of active myotonia. Patients with myotonic dystrophy are unable to relax the muscles of the hand after forming a fist.

Myotonic dystrophies are autosomal dominantly transmitted disorders and classified as DM1 (Steinert disease) or DM2 (proximal myotonic myopathy), with DM1 further subdivided by age of onset. Prominent features of classic DM1, the most common myotonic dystrophy, include slowly progressive muscle weakness (dystrophy), cataracts, endocrine disturbances, and functional abnormalities of the cardiorespiratory system and gastrointestinal tract (Table 209-1).

An abnormality in the intracellular adenosine triphosphate (ATP) system that fails to return calcium to the sarcoplasmic reticulum is the theoretical pathologic mechanism of the myotonia. Contractions are not relieved by nondepolarizing neuromuscular blocking agents (NMBAs), regional anesthesia, or deep anesthesia; however, infiltration of local anesthetic agents into involved muscle may produce relaxation. Depression of rapid sodium flux into muscle cells by the use of phenytoin, procainamide, quinine, tocainide, or mexiletine may alleviate contractions by delaying membrane excitability.

Coexisting Organ System Dysfunction

Cardiac involvement is characterized by conduction system abnormalities, supraventricular and ventricular arrhythmias, and, less commonly, myocardial dysfunction and ischemic heart disease. Mitral valve prolapse occurs in 20% of affected individuals. Sudden death is usually related to abrupt onset of atrioventricular block. Cardiomyopathy is rare.

Pulmonary pathophysiology may be both structural and functional. Pulmonary function testing reveals a restrictive lung disease pattern due to contractures of intercostal muscles. Ventilatory responses to hypoxia and hypercarbia are impaired. Patients are predisposed to developing pneumonia as a result of reduced lung volume and ineffective cough mechanisms.

Table 209-1 Genetics of Myotonic Dystrophy

	Type	
Feature	**DM1**	**DM2**
Alternative name	Steinert disease	Proximal myotonic myopathy
Chromosome	19q13.3	3q21
Defect		
Gene	*DMPK*	*ZNF9*
Repeat	CTG	CCTG

Gastrointestinal abnormalities that predispose patients with myotonic dystrophy to aspirating gastric content include dysphagia because of pharyngeal muscle weakness with impaired airway protection, gastric atony, and intestinal hypomotility. Additional gastrointestinal abnormalities include dysphagia, constipation, gallbladder stones, and pseudoobstruction.

Central nervous system manifestations include attention disorders, cognitive impairment, and mental retardation. Endocrine abnormalities include diabetes mellitus, thyroid dysfunction, adrenal dysfunction, and hypogonadism. Because insulin resistance is common in patients with myotonic dystrophy—likely related to reduced relative capacity of the myocyte insulin receptor in these patients—maintaining optimal glycemic control is often difficult.

Pregnancy exacerbates myotonic dystrophy, probably secondary to elevated progesterone levels. Women with myotonic dystrophy have a high incidence of obstetric complications, including polyhydramnios, premature onset of labor, breech presentation, impaired cervical dilation, uterine atony, retained placenta, and postpartum hemorrhage.

Anesthetic Management

Patients with DM1 have an increased risk of developing complications related to anesthesia, with reported complication rates ranging from 10% to 42.9%; comparatively, the risk of serious complications occurring in patients with DM2 is low (0.6%), likely related to the general lack of impairment of respiratory muscles in DM2. Risk factors that appear to be related to a higher incidence of perioperative adverse events, at least in children, appear to be a high score on the muscular impairment rating scale, prolonged operative time (>1 h), perioperative morphine use, and lack of reversal of NMBAs.

The preoperative evaluation of a patient with myotonic dystrophy should focus on pulmonary function, the patient's ability to protect the airway, cardiac conduction abnormalities, and cardiac reserve. Preoperative medications might include orally administered nonparticulate antacids and metoclopramide. Patients with DM1 have an increased sensitivity to preoperative sedative medications, and these agents should be avoided, if possible. These patients also have an increased sensitivity to intravenously administered induction agents; thus, these drugs should be used cautiously and titrated to effect. Etomidate may cause myoclonus and may precipitate fasciculations.

Depolarizing neuromuscular blockade is to be avoided because it may exacerbate fasciculations and contractures. Succinylcholine-induced fasciculation can lead to contractions severe enough to impair ventilation. Because patients with myotonic dystrophy often have impaired airway-protective mechanisms, placement of a cuffed tracheal tube is recommended.

Tracheal intubation can be performed while the patient is awake or as a rapid-sequence induction with cricoid pressure along with a reduced dose of an intravenously administered induction agent. Neuromuscular blockade might not be needed to facilitate intubation. Maintenance of anesthesia is best achieved with a balance of inhalation agent, opioids, and NMBA, all titrated to effect. Total intravenous anesthesia with propofol may also be a valuable and effective anesthetic technique for patients with myotonic dystrophy.

Myocardial depression may result with the use of any induction agents, but cautious use may minimize these effects and obviate the need for intravenously administered NMBAs. Exaggerated respiratory depressant effects from opioidergic agents used for anesthetic maintenance should be anticipated. The use of short-acting opioids (fentanyl, alfentanil, or remifentanil) for supplemental analgesia is recommended.

If neuromuscular blockade is needed, careful titration of shorter-acting agents (cisatracurium or mivacurium) is guided by the use of a peripheral nerve stimulator, the use of which is recommended throughout the procedure. Use of an anticholinesterase agent for reversal of neuromuscular blockade could theoretically precipitate myoclonus because of acetylcholine-facilitated depolarization at the neuromuscular junction. Use of short-acting NMBAs may eliminate the need for pharmacologic reversal.

Postoperative shivering should be avoided because shivering may precipitate fasciculation, myoclonus, or both. Patients' core temperature should be maintained at 36.5° C or higher through the use of a body warmer and whatever other measures are appropriate.

Extubation should be performed when the patient can protect his or her airway.

Suggested Readings

Kirzinger L, Schmidt A, Kornblum C, et al. Side effects of anesthesia in DM2 as compared to DM1: A comparative retrospective study. *Eur J Neurol.* 2010;17(6):842-845.

Morimoto Y, Mii M, Hirata T, et al. Target-controlled infusion of propofol in a patient with myotonic dystrophy. *J Anesth.* 2005;19:336-338.

Sinclair JL, Reed PW. Risk factors for perioperative adverse events in children with myotonic dystrophy. *Paediatr Anaesth.* 2009;19:740-747.

Turner C, Hilton-Jones D. The myotonic dystrophies: Diagnosis and management. *J Neurol Neurosurg Psychiatry.* 2010;81:358-367.

Weingarten TN, Hofer RE, Milone M, Sprung J. Anesthesia and myotonic dystrophy type 2: A case series. *Can J Anaesth.* 2010;57:248-255.

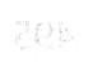

CHAPTER 210

Preemptive Analgesia and Postoperative Pain: The Transition from an Acute to a Chronic State

Tony L. Yaksh, PhD, and Qinghao Xu, PhD

Acute high-threshold stimuli activate small afferents and dorsal horn circuits and evoke a pain report that mirrors the time course and intensity of the stimuli. Blocking small (high-threshold), but not large (low-threshold mechanoreceptor), afferent traffic prevents or diminishes the pain report.

Persistent Pain States

There is now evidence suggesting that, in the face of local tissue trauma, reactive changes lead to an enhanced response to subsequent aversive (e.g., hyperalgesia) or innocuous (low-threshold mechanoreceptors: allodynia) requiring additional analgesic management. This enhanced pain response may reflect events that occur perioperatively over intervals of hours to days. Other events that reflect fundamental changes in pain processing occur over intervals of weeks to months or longer and rise to meet the criterion of a "chronic" pain state (e.g., total knee arthroplasty, thoracotomy, or inguinal herniorrhaphy) (Figure 210-1).

Underlying Mechanisms

Let us consider potential events that may underlie these two postoperative events. In the face of local tissue trauma, after the initial activation of the chemosensitive Aδ and C afferents, there appears persistent, ongoing, afferent traffic in these same nerve fibers and an enhanced response in these nerve fibers to subsequent stimuli. This condition is accompanied by a pain experience wherein, *after* removal of the stimulus (e.g., the incision, burn, or needlestick), there is an ongoing pain sensation and an enhanced behavioral response to not only subsequent stimuli applied to the site of injury (e.g., primary hyperalgesia), but also to otherwise innocuous stimuli applied to dermatomes adjacent to the injury site (e.g., secondary hyperalgesia/allodynia). The primary hyperalgesia is believed to reflect first a sensitization of the terminals of the sensory afferent fibers innervating the injured tissue (somatic or visceral) by the chemical milieu at the injury site. Thus, injury evokes the appearance of (1) extracellular K^+, H^+, a myriad of mediators derived from fatty acids (e.g., prostaglandins and thromboxanes), or clotting factors (e.g., the kininogen cascade); (2) circulating blood products (e.g., extravasated monocytes, platelets) that release a multitude of factors (amines, superoxides, growth factors, cytokines); and (3) an innate immune response (evidenced by the migration of inflammatory cells, degranulation of mast cells). All of these products act through eponymous receptors known to be present on the afferent nerve terminal to depolarize the terminal (increasing afferent traffic) and increase the concentrations of intracellular calcium. The increased calcium leads to activation of intraterminal protein kinases that phosphorylate local membrane ion channels (sodium) and receptors (e.g., TRPV1, TRPA1, bradykinin) that enhance their response to subsequent stimuli. At the level of the dorsal horn, the ongoing afferent traffic initiated by the injury leads to a change in spinal dorsal horn sensory processing. The biology underlying this enhanced response will be considered further later in this chapter. However, since the mid-1960s, it has been appreciated that persistent small afferent input (as generated by tissue injury and ectopic activity in injured nerves) leads to an enhanced excitability of dorsal horn projection neurons, and this facilitated state in animal models parallels the behaviorally enhanced response to otherwise innocuous stimuli applied to the injured dermatome, as well as to areas adjacent to the injury site. Importantly, these changes in the dorsal horn of the spinal cord provide insight as to why local injuries can yield an enhanced response to stimuli applied outside of the area of injury that manifest as a persistent pain state (e.g., secondary tactile allodynia).

The electrophysiologic expression of this facilitated state outlined above has been referred to as "wind-up." This nomenclature specifically refers to the enhanced responsivity of dorsal horn–wide dynamic-range neurons caused by repetitive C fiber stimulation. The underlying biology of this small afferent evoked sensitization is complex but includes (1) events mediated at the level of the first-order primary afferent synapse when repetitive input leads to increased intracellular calcium and activation of intracellular phosphorylation cascades that enhance membrane neuronal excitability (by phosphorylating voltage-gated channels for sodium and calcium and various receptors, such as the glutamatergic NMDA receptor); (2) reduced activation of local inhibitory interneurons that otherwise attenuate the excitability of the projection neuron in response to large low-threshold afferent stimulation; (3) activation of nonneuronal cells (astrocytes and microglia), which release proexcitatory products (glutamate, lipids, growth factors, adenosine triphosphate [ATP], free radicals, cytokines); and (4) bulbospinal input (typically serotonergic), which can enhance the excitability of dorsal horn projection neurons. Finally, the signaling outlined earlier, particularly that which leads to increased intracellular calcium, leads to activation of a variety of kinases that lead to enhanced transcription (e.g., such as P38 mitogen-activated protein kinase). Such enhanced transcription leads to increased synthesis of enzymes, such as cyclooxygenase-2 and nitric oxide synthase. In short, persistent small afferent activity can initiate ongoing enhancement of pronociceptive processing that leads to changes in function that outlast the initiating stimulus by intervals of hours to days or longer.

Aside from the previously mentioned cascades, traumatic stimuli may injure the peripheral nerve itself. Such injuries lead independently to

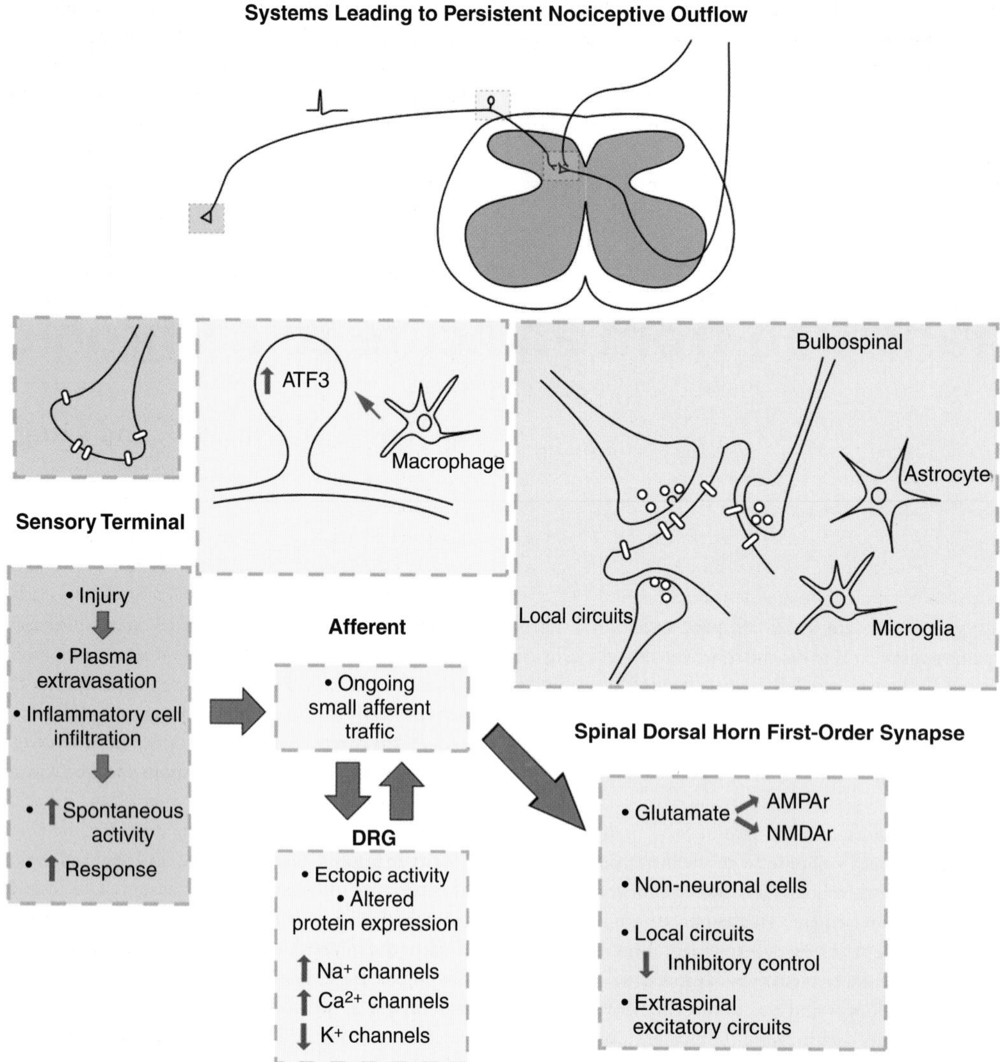

Figure 210-1 Summary of events leading to persistent pain states after local tissue injury. As indicated, injury leads to the altered local milieu that initiates sensitization of the peripheral terminal and initiates the ongoing activity. Such afferent traffic leads to activation of central sensitization that results in altered expression and excitability of local projection neurons. In the face of ongoing input, there are changes in the phenotype of the primary afferent, resulting in changes resembling those associated with nerve injury. These changes lead to a net increase in dorsal horn reactivity and ongoing afferent activation. Block of the afferent traffic prior to the initiation of the sensitizing process can, in a variety of models, reduce the sensitization process. Not shown are the events that arise secondary to the nerve injury phenotype that is reviewed in the text. AMPAr, α-Amino-3-hydroxyl-5-methyl-4-isoxazole propionate receptor; ATF_3, activating transcription factor 3; DRG, dorsal root ganglia; NMDAr, *N*-methyl-D-aspartate receptor.

pronounced change in function: (1) the evolution of ectopic sensory activity from the injured nerve after the formation of a neuroma and the dorsal root ganglia, a response that occurs over time in all classes of injured axons (small and large) and (2) reactive change in dorsal horn processing wherein large, low-threshold afferent nerves acquire the ability to initiate a pain state. Numerous mechanisms are thought to underlie these post–nerve-injury events, including (1) change in the expression of ion channels in nerve membranes that lead to an enhanced excitability (increased Na^+ channels, decreased K^+ channels), (2) loss of dorsal horn inhibitory interneurons, (3) change in inhibitory phenotype wherein inhibitory systems such as the γ-aminobutyric acid (GABA) or glycine receptors become excitatory, (4) release of excitatory products from nonneuronal cells, and (5) potential sprouting of local terminals altering patterns of afferent connectivity. These events are believed to result, over an interval of days to weeks, in ongoing pain (dysesthesia) and pain initiated by low-threshold afferents.

The presence of nerve injury indeed provides a model for an enduring pain phenotype, though, in many cases, the presence of evident nerve injury is not obvious. Of particular interest, however, is current work that suggests that, in the face of a chronic inflammatory condition, changes occur that resemble a nerve injury. Thus, after nerve injury, markers, such as ATF_3 (activating transcription factor 3), appear in the dorsal root ganglion, and macrophages invade this ganglion. More recently, it has become evident that, in the face of chronic peripheral inflammation, these changes may be similarly observed. These events suggest that phenotypic changes initiated by nerve injury and chronic afferent input may converge over time. These events have led to the concept of preempting the facilitated state by instituting antinociceptive therapies before the nociceptive stimulus occurs, a concept that has captured the attention of many investigators and clinicians alike.

Prevention of the Facilitated State

Preemptive analgesia is an antinociceptive modality that prevents the establishment of central hyperexcitability that follows a nociceptive stimulus. This is not as easy to determine or measure as many studies presume. Reduction of postoperative pain medication requirements and lower scores on visual analog scales for pain will perhaps indicate the possibility of a preemptive effect, but, by themselves, they do not reliably confirm a preemptive effect from any given intervention.

The phenomenon of wind-up is routinely studied in animals that are in a surgical plane of anesthesia induced by intravenously administered anesthetic agents (e.g., thiopental) or inhaled anesthetic drugs (e.g., halothane) that produces a state of no reactivity but does *not* wind up. In contrast, agents such as opiates and α_2-receptor agonists, as well as inhibitors of ionotropic glutamate receptors (NMDA [*N*-methyl-D-aspartate] and AMPA [α-amino-3-hydroxyl-5-methyl-4-isoxazole propionate], are able to prevent the wind-up. The actions of these several families of "analgesic agents" in the first-order synapse stand in contrast to the *failure* of centrally acting anesthetic agents (barbiturates and inhaled anesthetic agents) to do so. Importantly, such anesthetics do not block release of small afferent transmitters, indicating that the membrane of the second-order neurons will still manifest the effects of activating the local dorsal horn receptors (e.g., AMPA/ NMDA/ NK1), leading to persistent changes in protein expression, the effects of which are apparent when the anesthetic state is reversed. The phenomenon of preemptive analgesia then reflects the events that lead to downstream augmentation of sensory processing at the spinal level that leads to a persistent facilitated state. For example, in the formalin animal model, it can be shown that application of opiates during the initial injury when there is increased afferent nerve traffic will reduce the magnitude of the secondary phase, the facilitated pain state. In contrast, a short-lasting general anesthetic agent administered during the first phase has no effect upon the activity observed during the second phase.

One of the problems with direct application of these findings to the clinical situation is that, unlike many experimental models that use a short-lived nociceptive stimulus, continued afferent stimulation from a surgical wound persists during the period of wound healing, allowing central sensitization even in the postoperative period. A single "preemptive" intervention may well reduce the amount of pain experienced postoperatively but, due to its short duration, is usually ineffective in preventing the secondary hypersensitivity phase of the pain response. Animal studies using a sustained nociceptive stimulus (carrageenan injection) fail to show any effects from preemption. Unless the treatment or intervention is effective for the entire duration of the noxious stimuli, spinal sensitization can still occur.

The results of many clinical studies evaluating the value of preemptive analgesic modalities have been inconclusive, in part because of the difficulty in providing an effective antinociceptive intervention that covers the entire postoperative period. A compounding factor is the inability to establish a control group of patients because we have a responsibility to our patients to provide humane care, adequate pain relief, and anxiolysis throughout the perioperative period. The net result is minimal differences between experimental and control groups.

Role of Regional Anesthesia

Local anesthetic infiltration of surgical wounds has some potential in providing preemptive analgesia. In addition to blocking neuronal transmission from the surgical site, local anesthetic agents may reduce neurogenic inflammation by blocking the axon reflex and sympathetic efferent pathways to the site of injury. Local anesthetic agents have also been shown to have effects on nonneuronal aspects of the inflammatory response. Antimicrobial activity of local anesthetics, inhibition of leukocyte migration to the surgical site, and inhibition of inflammatory activity at the surgical site may have implications in terms of outcome and wound healing that are well beyond the scope of investigations regarding effects on analgesia.

Preoperative local anesthetic administration, by either local tissue infiltration or nerve block, has proved to be effective in reducing postoperative pain in patients undergoing surgery under general anesthesia. This result has been demonstrated in a variety of surgical settings, including tonsillectomy, inguinal herniorrhaphy, cholecystectomy, and dental extractions. There is some evidence to suggest that continuous infusion of local anesthetic agents may be of greater benefit than single-dose administration. Local infiltration and peripheral nerve blocks seem to be more efficacious than central neuraxial anesthetic techniques in reducing postoperative pain. In one study, patients undergoing inguinal herniorrhaphy under spinal anesthesia had less postoperative pain than did those who received general anesthesia alone, but the effect was less pronounced than that seen with general anesthesia plus local infiltration. Yet another study evaluated the efficacy of ilioinguinal/iliohypogastric nerve block with 10 mL of 0.5% bupivacaine as an adjunct to spinal anesthesia for inguinal herniorrhaphy. The study found significant differences in pain at 3, 6, 24, and 48 h after surgery. Similar results have been found in patients undergoing total knee arthroplasty under spinal anesthesia either with or without femoral nerve block.

The differences found in these studies should not surprise practitioners who routinely use regional anesthetic techniques in their clinical practice. The profundity of conduction blockade would be expected to be greatest when the local anesthetic agent is placed on or near peripheral nerves. Epidural and spinal blockade may not provide complete conduction blockade, thereby potentially allowing some degree of central sensitization to occur. This is not to diminish the effectiveness of epidural or spinal anesthesia in reducing postoperative pain. There are many clinical situations in which local infiltration or nerve block is not technically feasible. In these circumstances, neuraxial anesthesia can be quite effective in reducing postoperative pain.

A recent study of patients undergoing radical retropubic prostatectomy found significant reductions in long-term pain and increased activity levels in patients whose epidurals were injected with local anesthetic agents and opioids before incision versus at the time of closure. The combination of local anesthetic agents and opioids for perioperative epidural infusions may be superior to opioids alone. Another study looking at patients having partial colectomy found significantly better pain relief and return of bowel function 1.5 days earlier in those patients whose epidural infusion included both opioids and local anesthetic agents rather than only opioids. Current investigations are focusing on other receptor populations within the spinal cord in which the roles of α_2-receptor agonists, NMDA antagonists, and GABA agonists have yet to be clearly defined.

Although the goal of providing a true preemptive analgesic intervention may be elusive or even impractical in many clinical circumstances, as clinicians, we should have a goal of providing a relatively pain-free perioperative experience for our patients. Modification of the pain response can occur at several different levels—the site of the injury itself with infiltration of local anesthetic agents or administration of systemic nonsteroidal antiinflammatory drugs, peripheral neural blockade, and central neuraxial administration of local anesthetic agents and opioids. There remain many questions regarding the timing and duration of antinociceptive interventions, optimal combinations and doses of agents, patient selection, and cost effectiveness.

Acknowledgment

The author and editors would like to thank Beth A. Elliott, MD, for her work on this chapter in previous editions.

Suggested Readings

Chiang CY, Sessle BJ, Dostrovsky JO. Role of astrocytes in pain. *Neurochem Res.* 2012;37(11):2419-31.

Christianson CA, Corr M, Firestein GS, et al. Characterization of the acute and persistent pain state present in K/BxN serum transfer arthritis. *Pain.* 2010;151(2):394-403.

Jacob AK, Walsh MT, Dilger JA. Role of regional anesthesia in the ambulatory environment. *Anesthesiol Clin.* 2010;28:251-266.

Katz J, Seltzer Z. Transition from acute to chronic postsurgical pain: Risk factors and protective factors. *Expert Rev Neurother.* 2009;9:723-744.

Kehlet H, Jensen TS, Woolf CJ. Persistent postsurgical pain: Risk factors and prevention. *Lancet.* 2006;367:1618-1625.

Latremoliere A, Woolf CJ. Central sensitization: a generator of pain hypersensitivity by central neural plasticity. *J Pain.* 2009 Sep;10(9):895-926. doi: 10.1016/j.jpain.2009.06.012.

Pogatzki-Zahn EM, Zahn PK. From preemptive to preventive analgesia. *Curr Opin Anaesthesiol.* 2006;19:551-555.

Reichling DB, Levine JD. Critical role of nociceptor plasticity in chronic pain. *Trends Neurosci.* 2009;32:611-618.

Schaible HG, von Banchet GS, Boettger MK, et al. The role of proinflammatory cytokines in the generation and maintenance of joint pain. *Ann N Y Acad Sci.* 2010;1193:60-69.

Takasusuki T, Yamaguchi S, Hamaguchi S, Yaksh TL. Effects of general anesthetics on substance P release and c-Fos expression in the spinal dorsal horn. *Anesthesiology.* 2013 Aug;119(2):433-42.

Tsuda M, Beggs S, Salter MW, Inoue K. Microglia and intractable chronic pain. *Glia.* 2013 Jan;61(1):55-61.

Van de Ven TJ, John Hsia HL. Causes and prevention of chronic postsurgical pain. *Curr Opin Crit Care.* 2012 Aug;18(4):366-71.

Xu Q, Yaksh TL. A brief comparison of the pathophysiology of inflammatory versus neuropathic pain. *Curr Opin Anaesthesiol.* 2011 Aug;24(4):400-7.

Yaksh TL, Sorkin LS. Mechanisms of neuropathic pain. *Curr Med Chem.* 2005;5:129-140.

CHAPTER 211

Patient-Controlled Analgesia

Martin L. De Ruyter, MD

As many as 50% of patients who receive conventional therapy for their postoperative pain do *not* have adequate analgesia. In a report by Sommer et al, 41% of 1490 surgical patients under the care of an acute pain protocol reported having moderate to severe pain on the day of surgery, 30% on their first postoperative day, and 19% on postoperative day 2.

Development and Application of Patient-Controlled Analgesia

In 1968, Sechzer first described patient-controlled analgesia (PCA) with intermittent intravenous (IV) doses of opioids delivered "on-demand" by the patient, which gave patients the ability to better control their level of analgesia, balanced against their level of sedation and, therefore, the risks of side effects such as respiratory depression. In current practice, an infusion pump is programmed to provide a preset dose of an analgesic agent when the patient presses a button on a handheld controller; the "lockout" time—the interval before the next dose can be delivered—is also preset. Although IV PCA with opioids is the most widely used modality to treat postoperative pain, cancer-related pain, and pain associated with nonmalignant conditions (e.g., acute nephrolithiasis and pancreatitis), other PCA modes have been developed. These other PCA modes include patient-controlled epidural analgesia and patient-controlled peripheral nerve catheter analgesia. Unlike IV PCA, patient-controlled epidural analgesia is not limited to infusion of opioids and often includes the coadministration of a local anesthetic agent, whereas patient-controlled peripheral nerve catheter analgesia primarily involves delivery of only local anesthetic agents. A complete discussion of the various types of PCA is beyond the scope of this section; therefore this chapter will be limited to IV PCA with opioids.

Intravenous Patient-Controlled Analgesia

Advantages

The main advantage of IV PCA with opioids is that it is "patient-controlled." Traditional intermittent nurse-administered parenteral analgesia is inherently labor intensive and fraught with problems. Patients receive a "scheduled" or an "as-needed" dose of an analgesic drug, one that is targeted for a broad patient population, with little thought given to the pharmacokinetics and pharmacodynamics of a drug in an individual patient. Doses of analgesic drugs are relatively large, sometimes exceeding the minimal effective dose, to achieve a more sustained effect. The time to redosing is often prolonged, resulting in low serum drug concentrations and the recurrence of pain. The "as-needed" administration of analgesic drugs is an even less favorable regimen because patients often wait until their pain is significant before calling the nursing staff, nurses must be able to respond to the call, the analgesic drug must be obtained from the pharmacy or the medication-dispensing device, and then, after the elapse of some time, patients receive their pain medication. With both regimens, patients can experience "peaks" of supratherapeutic analgesia, which can increase the risk of complications such as respiratory depression, nausea, and emesis, followed by "valleys" of low serum opioid levels, during which patients experience "breakthrough" pain. These subtherapeutic levels, with their associated inadequate analgesia, may limit patients' progress, as evidenced by inadequate pulmonary hygiene, an unwillingness to get out of bed, and refusal to participate in postoperative rehabilitation. In a study of patients administered opioid analgesic agents intramuscularly every 3 to 4 h, the subsequent serum drug concentration met (or exceeded) the minimal analgesic concentration only 35% of the time (Figure 211-1). The other 65% of the time, the dose was inadequate for the patient to achieve adequate analgesia, which, in turn, was associated with adverse perioperative outcomes and patient dissatisfaction.

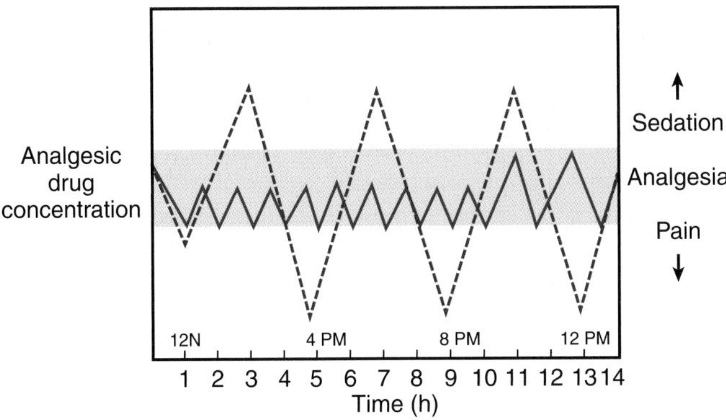

Figure 211-1 Serum levels of analgesic drugs comparing intravenously administered patient-controlled analgesia *(solid lines)* versus intramuscular administration *(dashed lines)*. (Adapted from White PF. Use of patient-controlled analgesia for management of acute pain. JAMA. 1988;259:243.)

Box 211-1 Advantages of Intravenously Administered Opioids via Patient-Controlled Analgesia

- Compared with other forms of analgesia, IV PCA provides superior pain relief with less medication.
- The use of IV PCA decreases the potential delay between patients' requests for analgesics and the administration of the drug.
- Postoperative pulmonary function is improved in patients receiving IV PCA.
- IV PCA allows for accommodation for diurnal changes in drug requirements and variable range of analgesic needs.
- Less daytime sedation occurs with the use of IV PCA.
- Patients who receive IV PCA are able to mobilize sooner after surgery.
- Patients report high levels of acceptance and satisfaction with IV PCA.
- Less inappropriate "screening" by nursing staff occurs with the use of IV PCA.
- Patients receiving IV PCA experience fewer postoperative pulmonary complications.
- The potential for overdose is low when small doses per activation are prescribed.
- Patients' sleep patterns improve when IV PCA is used.
- The use of IV PCA is cost effective.

IV PCA; Intravenously administered patient-controlled analgesia.

Because the dose of analgesic agent and lockout interval are better individualized, and because it eliminates a second person as a decision maker (i.e., the nurse), IV PCA maintains more effective serum analgesic drug concentrations, minimizes adverse effects, and improves patient satisfaction. Other reported advantages of IV PCA are listed in Box 211-1.

Choice of Opioids

Morphine, hydromorphone, and fentanyl are the opioids commonly administered via IV PCA. Meperidine, in the past an often used agent, is less frequently used because of the potential adverse effects (i.e., seizures) associated with its active metabolite, normeperidine, and the recognition of better alternative agents. (Table 211-1).

Initial Setup

When prescribing IV PCA with opioids, the anesthesia provider must determine the loading dose, the demand dose, the lockout interval, and the maximum dose limit. The loading dose administered at the initiation of IV PCA is intended to quickly establish an effective serum concentration of drug. The loading dose of the opioid is typically administered over five minutes until satisfactory analgesia is achieved. Satisfactory analgesia is maintained with subsequent demand doses delivered in a predetermined window or frequency. The demand dose of the drug should be adjusted for the patient's age, comorbid conditions, and concomitant medications. Smaller loading and demand doses of opioids should be prescribed for patients who are elderly, have pulmonary disease (i.e., chronic obstructive pulmonary disease or obstructive sleep apnea), whose hemodynamic status is tenuous, or who are receiving drugs that may act synergistically with opioids, whereas patients with chronic pain and opioid tolerance will likely need higher or more frequent doses. The maximum dose allowed is usually the cumulative dose allowed at 1 or 4 h as a safety measure to ensure that patients do not exceed a total cumulative dose of opioids. Bolus doses are similar to loading doses that can be administered to a patient by a health care provider if the patient does not have adequate analgesia achieved with the initial settings.

Most clinicians do not routinely prescribe a continuous or basal infusion of an opioid that is delivered independent of patient demand unless the patient is opioid tolerant and now has acute pain superimposed on chronic pain. By monitoring the number of patient demands relative to the number of doses delivered, clinicians can tailor and adjust the demand dose and lockout interval to better meet the analgesic needs of the patient. For example, 15 attempts per hour by a patient with a PCA setting of 1 delivery every 10 min implies that the patient's analgesic needs are not being met. Appropriate responses include decreasing the lockout interval, increasing the demand dose, adding a basal infusion, or using a combination of these strategies.

Adverse Effects and Outcomes

IV PCA with opioids is not without side effects and adverse outcomes (Box 211-2). Nausea, vomiting, and pruritus are not uncommon, and excessive somnolence has been observed. In a group of patients who underwent total hip arthroplasty and received an IV PCA for postoperative analgesia, investigators observed that, on postoperative day 2, more than 50% of patients experienced episodes of desaturation ($Spo_2 < 90\%$) and one patient experienced a respiratory arrest. To improve the safety of IV PCA, many hospitals have guidelines that recommend staff members have regular interaction with patients and measure and document the patient's pain scores (using a metric such as numeric or visual analog scores), respiratory rate, O_2 saturation via pulse oximetry, state of arousal, and level of sedation. In opioid-related respiratory depression, O_2 desaturation is a delayed observation. With the advancement of technology and recent more widespread availability, end-tidal CO_2 monitors are used more often. As these devices become more accepted in clinical practice, it is hoped that IV PCA will become a safer modality for analgesic administration.

Table 211-1 Suggested Dosing Regimens for Opioid-Naïve Patients* Receiving Opioids via Intravenous Patient-Controlled Analgesia

Drug	Concentration, mg/mL	Loading Dose†, mg maximum	Demand Dose, mg	Lockout Interval, min	Basal Infusion‡, mg/h	1-h Limit, mg	4-h Limit, mg
Morphine	1	2-4	1-2	6-10	0-1.0	7.5	30
Hydromorphone	0.2	0.4	0.2-0.4	6-10	0-0.2	1.5	6
Fentanyl	0.01	0.02-0.04	0.01-0.03	6-10	0-0.02	0.1-0.2	0.4-0.8

*Elderly patients (>65 y) and patients on chronic opioids may need adjustment of these guidelines.
†The loading dose is given as a bolus every 5 min until the patient is comfortable and then the patient-controlled analgesia is started.
‡Most practitioners do not recommend a continuous infusion for most patients.

Box 211-2 Disadvantages of Intravenously Administered Opioids via Patient-Controlled Analgesia

- Patients using patient-controlled analgesia must be mentally alert, physically able to push the button, and able to understand the concept of IV PCA and follow instructions.
- IV PCA should be used with caution in patients with significant liver, renal, or pulmonary disease.
- Patients with obstructive sleep apnea are at increased risk of experiencing opioid-induced respiratory depression.
- Pruritus is more common with IV PCA than with intramuscular administration but less common than with epidural administration.
- Surrogate (nonpatient, i.e., family members or nursing staff) "pushers" of the button may subject patients to overdosing levels of opioids.
- Some anesthesia providers consider opioid addiction to be relatively contraindicated.
- Hypovolemia is associated with excessive rates of opioid-induced respiratory depression.
- Direct costs are increased because of the need for special equipment, setup, and staff training.

IV-PCA; Intravenously administered patient-controlled analgesia.

Conclusion

In summary, IV PCA is a significant improvement over opioids administered intermittently by another person, particularly for acute postoperative pain. Although IV PCA is associated with relatively high startup costs, provided there is adequate monitoring for, and treatment of, adverse events, IV PCA is very cost effective because its use is associated with improved outcomes and patient satisfaction.

Suggested Readings

Elliott JA. Patient-controlled analgesia. In: Smith HS, ed. *Current Therapy in Pain*. Philadelphia: Saunders Elsevier; 2009:73-77.

Sechzer PH. Objective measurement of pain. *Anesthesiology*. 1968;29:209-210.

Sommer M, de Rijke JM, van Kleef M, et al. The prevalence of postoperative pain in a sample of 1490 surgical inpatients. *Eur J Anaesthesiol*. 2008;25: 267-274.

Stone JG, Cozine KA, Wald A. Nocturnal oxygenation during patient-controlled analgesia. *Anesth Analg*. 1999;89:104-110.

CHAPTER 212 Neuraxial Opioids

Paul E. Carns, MD

Opioids were first introduced into the central neuraxis in 1979. Since that time, epidurally and intrathecally administered opioids have been used for both acute and chronic pain control and are commonly administered in combination with other neuraxial adjuvant compounds, such as local anesthetics and α_2-adrenoreceptor agonists. The clinical benefits of epidural and intrathecal opioids include excellent analgesia in the absence of motor, sensory, and autonomic blockade. Downstream benefits then occur, which include earlier ambulation and improved pulmonary function.

The sites of action are the opioid receptors found mainly within layers 4 and 5 of the substantia gelatinosa in the dorsolateral horn of the spinal cord. When activated, these receptors inhibit the release of excitatory nociceptive neurotransmitters within the spinal cord. In addition to producing direct spinal effects, neuraxially administered opioids may also activate cerebral opioid receptors when cephalad spread of the drug occurs via cerebrospinal fluid (CSF). Systemic effects may also be seen because some drug is absorbed into the vasculature.

The lipid solubility of each opioid, determined by the octanol/water partition coefficient, is the most critical pharmacokinetic property to consider when administering opioid doses near the neuraxis. Molecular weight, dose, and volume of injectate may also play a role in dural transfer (Table 212-1).

Hydrophilic opioids (those with low octanol/water partition coefficients, e.g. morphine) have a high degree of solubility within the CSF, permitting significant cephalad spread. Therefore, thoracic analgesia may be accomplished when either epidural or intrathecal doses are administered at the lumbar level. The epidural or intrathecal dose of morphine is significantly less than that required to achieve an equianalgesic effect through intravenous administration.

Hydrophilic opioids, used epidurally (Table 212-2), have a slow onset and prolonged duration of action. An initial epidural bolus dose is required, which may be followed by a continuous infusion through an epidural catheter. Because of their slow onset of action, hydrophilic opioids are less suitable for patient-controlled epidural analgesia than are lipophilic opioids. When hydrophilic opioids are used intrathecally, onset of action is more rapid and very low doses are required, resulting in less systemic toxicity. Effective analgesia may be provided for up to 24 h. This method is less expensive because no catheter is used.

Lipophilic opioids (those with a high octanol/water partition coefficient, e.g., fentanyl) have a rapid onset and a much shorter duration of action. When used epidurally (see Table 212-2), these drugs are rapidly taken up by epidural fat and redistributed into the systemic circulation, resulting in poor bioavailability to the spinal cord. Neuraxial doses of lipophilic opioids needed to achieve equianalgesic effect are nearly equal to intravenous doses. Plasma levels attained with equal doses of epidural and intravenous infusions of fentanyl are nearly identical, suggesting a significant systemic mode

Table 212-1 Octanol/Water Partition Coefficients and Molecular Weights of Common Opioids

Drug	Octanol/Water Partition Coefficient	Molecular Weight (g/mol)
Morphine	1.4	285
Hydromorphone	2	285
Meperidine	39	247
Alfentanil	145	452
Fentanyl citrate	813	528
Sufentanil citrate	1778	578

of action. Low CSF solubility permits only a limited amount of cephalad spread. Doses should be placed near the dermatome or dermatomes at which analgesia is desired. Therefore, lumbar administration of a lipophilic opioid would be a poor choice for thoracic analgesia. Side effects are generally fewer, with a lower incidence of delayed respiratory depression. These drugs are ideal for continuous infusions and patient-controlled epidural analgesia.

Epidural doses of hydrophilic opioids produce a biphasic pattern of respiratory depression. A portion of the initial bolus dose is absorbed systemically, accounting for the initial phase, and usually occurs within 2 h of the bolus dose being administered. Remaining drug within the CSF slowly spreads rostrally, producing a second phase as the drug reaches the brainstem 6 to 18 h later, resulting in direct depression of the respiratory nuclei and chemoreceptors. Intrathecal doses of hydrophilic opioids produce only a uniphasic pattern of respiratory depression. Effective doses of intrathecally administered hydrophilic opioid are very low compared with the larger epidural doses, and early respiratory depression is typically not seen. The slow rostral spread of drug deposited directly within the CSF is responsible for the pattern of delayed respiratory depression. Mechanical ventilation and Valsalva maneuvers (coughing/vomiting) that raise intrathoracic pressure may promote rostral spread. Somnolence usually precedes the onset of significant respiratory depression. Patients should be closely monitored; monitoring should include continuous pulse oximetry for the 24-h period following a neuraxial dose of morphine. If an infusion is planned, monitoring is necessary throughout its duration.

Side effects after neuraxial administration of opioids are dose dependent and are generally similar when used either epidurally or intrathecally. They include respiratory depression, somnolence, pruritus, nausea and vomiting, and urinary retention. Generalized pruritus is the most common and least dangerous side effect seen with the use of neuraxial opioids. The mechanism is unclear, but it is not thought to be secondary to histamine release—rather, it is more likely to be brainstem mediated. Treatment includes dilute naloxone infusions and low-dose mixed agonist/antagonist opioids (nalbuphine). Antihistamines may also be beneficial for the sedation they may provide.

Nausea and vomiting are common complications of neuraxial opioid administration. They also often occur with parenteral opioid use. Reversible causes, such as hypotension, must be initially ruled out and corrected. Rostral spread of opioids directly stimulates the medullary vomiting center. Treatment options include the administration of butyrophenones (droperidol), phenothiazines (prochlorperazine), 5-HT_3 antagonists (ondansetron or granisetron), and antihistamines. Phenothiazines may cause significant drowsiness, however, which may hinder evaluation of somnolence secondary to the opioid effects.

Opioids may reduce the sacral parasympathetic outflow, resulting in urinary retention. Although this may be reversed by direct antagonism with naloxone, the doses of naloxone required are often high and may also result in reversal of analgesia. Placement of an indwelling urinary catheter should be considered.

Suggested Readings

Bonnet MP, Marret E, Josserand J, Mercier FJ. Effect of prophylactic 5-HT_3 receptor antagonists on pruritus induced by neuraxial opioids: A quantitative systematic review. *Br J Anaesth*. 2008;101:311-319.

Carvalho B. Respiratory depression after neuraxial opioids in the obstetric setting. *Anesth Analg*. 2008;107:956-961.

Cook TM, Counsell D, Wildsmith JA, Royal College of Anaesthetists Third National Audit Project. Major complications of central neuraxial block: Report on the Third National Audit Project of the Royal College of Anaesthetists. *Br J Anaesth*. 2009;102:179-190.

D'Angelo R. All parturients receiving neuraxial morphine should be monitored with continuous pulse oximetry. *Int J Obstet Anesth*. 2010;19:202-204.

Horlocker TT, Burton AW, Connis RT, et al, American Society of Anesthesiologists Task Force on Neuraxial Opioids. Practice guidelines for the prevention, detection, and management of respiratory depression associated with neuraxial opioid administration. *Anesthesiology*. 2009;110:218-230.

Schug SA, Saunders D, Kurowski I, Paech MJ. Neuraxial drug administration: A review of treatment options for anaesthesia and analgesia. *CNS Drugs*. 2006;20:917-933.

Yaksh TL. Spinal opiate analgesia: Characteristics and principles of action. *Pain*. 1981;11:293-346.

Table 212-2 Clinical Pharmacology of Epidural Opioids*

Property	Advantages	Disadvantages
Hydrophilic Opioids		
Slow onset		Delayed onset of analgesia
Long duration	Prolonged single-dose analgesia	Unpredictable duration
High CSF solubility	Minimal dose compared with intravenous administration	Higher incidence of side effects
Extensive CSF spread	Thoracic analgesia with lumbar administration	Delayed respiratory depression
Lipophilic Opioids		
Rapid onset	Rapid analgesia	
Short duration	Decreased side effects	Brief single-dose analgesia
Low CSF solubility	Ideal for continuous infusion or PCEA	Systemic absorption
Minimal CSF spread		Limited thoracic analgesia with lumbar administration

CSF, Cerebrospinal fluid; PCEA, patient-controlled epidural analgesia.
*Modified from Grass JA. Epidural analgesia. Probl Anesth. 1998;10:45-70.

CHAPTER 213

Complex Regional Pain Syndrome

Nicole M. Dawson, MD

Terminology

Complex regional pain syndrome (CRPS) types I and II—formerly known as reflex sympathetic dystrophy and causalgia, respectively—are chronic pain disorders characterized by varying degrees of hyperalgesia, allodynia, edema, vasomotor and sudomotor instability, trophic changes, and bone rarefaction.

In CRPS type I, the initial event, whether spontaneous or a major insult, does not affect any particular nerve. The hallmark of CRPS type I is continuing pain disproportionately more severe than expected given the injury. The pain, dystrophy, and features of autonomic instability progress and affect regions of the extremity not involved in the initial injury. Severe cases may involve the entire limb or the contralateral extremity. CRPS type I can result from ischemia of the viscera, cardiac myocytes, or cerebrovascular bed.

Conversely, CRPS type II results from injury to an identifiable nerve. It is distinct from a peripheral mononeuropathy in that the afflicted region extends beyond the predicted nerve distribution.

Etiology

The pathophysiology underlying both types of CRPS remains incompletely understood. Emerging research points to an element of peripheral sensitization in disease development. Upregulation and hypersensitivity of adrenergic receptors and functional coupling between sympathetic efferent and sensory afferent fibers may provide the basis for the sympathetic nervous system abnormalities characteristic of CRPS. Central sensitization or "wind-up" of the dorsal horn neurons, brainstem, or thalamus, along with remodeling of the primary somatosensory cortex and disinhibition of the motor cortex, appear to play key roles in more severe forms of CRPS.

Sympathetically mediated pain responding to central or peripheral sympathetic blockade variably contributes to the overall pain experienced by patients. Additional sympathetically independent mediators have been identified. Elevated levels of circulating free radicals, inflammatory cytokines (e.g., interleukin 6 and tumor necrosis factor-α), neuropeptides (substance P, bradykinin, neuropeptide Y, and calcitonin G-related protein), and cerebrospinal fluid levels of glutamate have been measured in patients with CRPS. Associations have been demonstrated between disease onset, responsiveness to treatment, features of dystonia, and the presence of HLA class I and II polymorphisms among patients with CRPS, suggesting a possible genetic component to the disease.

Diagnosis

Diagnosis is made by clinical observation, because currently no objective diagnostic criteria exist. In an effort to improve diagnostic predictability, it has been suggested that patients report at least one symptom in each category and demonstrate at minimum one sign in two or more categories (Table 213-1). Using these clinical criteria based on the International Association for the Study of Pain (IASP) guidelines improves diagnostic specificity (94%) at the expense of sensitivity (70%). The differential diagnosis includes small-fiber and diabetic neuropathies, entrapment, degenerative disc disease, thoracic outlet syndrome, cellulitis, vascular insufficiency, thrombophlebitis, lymphedema, angioedema, erythromelalgia, and deep venous thrombosis.

Laboratory studies may provide objective results to assist in the diagnosis of CRPS. Thermometry, quantitative sudomotor axon reflex test (QSART), thermoregulatory sweat testing, laser Doppler flowmetry, three-phase bone scintigraphy, plain radiographs, and magnetic resonance imaging studies have been shown to be useful in the diagnosis of CRPS. In the past, CRPS types I and II were thought to progress through several stages, which vary significantly in temporal duration (Table 213-2).

Treatment

Several multimodal treatments are in clinical use. Because of the lack of diagnostic criteria and inherent heterogeneity of CRPS, high-quality studies evidencing therapeutic efficacy remain scarce.

Occupational Therapy

Prompt initiation of functional restoration has been considered a therapeutic mainstay. Gentle range-of-motion exercises, bandaging for control of

Table 213-1 International Association for the Study of Pain Criteria for the Diagnosis of Complex Regional Pain Syndrome*

Category	Signs and Symptoms
Sensory	Allodynia Hyperalgesia Hyperesthesia Hypoalgesia
Vasomotor	Livedo reticularis Skin color changes Temperature variability
Sudomotor	Edema Hyperhidrosis Hypohidrosis
Motor	Decreased range of motion Neglect Tremor Weakness

*Diagnostic predictability improves when patients report at least one symptom in each category and one sign in two or more categories.

Table 213-2 Stages of Complex Regional Pain Syndrome

Stage	Presentation
Acute/warm	Burning or aching pain increasing with physical contact or emotional stress Edema Unstable temperature and color of limb Increased periarticular uptake on scintigraphy Accelerated hair and nail growth Joint stiffness Muscle spasm
Dystrophic	Indurated, cool, hyperhidrotic, cyanotic, mottled skin Joint space narrowing Muscle weakness Osteoporotic changes on radiography
Atrophic/cold	Ankylosis Hair loss Muscle atrophy Tendon contractures Thickening of fascia Thin shiny skin

edema, and a progressive increase in weight-bearing activities aid in recovery, although controversy exists regarding the long-term benefit of these interventions. Gradual desensitization can be accomplished through exposure of the limb to warm and cool contrast baths and to fabrics of varying textures.

Psychiatric Therapy

Depression, anxiety, posttraumatic stress disorder, and kinesophobia often accompany CRPS and, if present, should be addressed promptly through cognitive behavioral therapy and pharmacologic adjuncts if necessary.

Pharmacologic Therapy

Randomized controlled trials conducted on patients with CRPS support the use of alendronate, corticosteroids, parenteral and topical ketamine, antiepileptics (gabapentin), N-acetylcysteine for the treatment of "cold" CRPS, dimethylsulfoxide (DMSO) for the treatment of "warm" CRPS, epidural clonidine, vitamin C for prevention, and intrathecal administration of γ-aminobutyric acid (GABA)-agonists (baclofen) for symptomatic relief of dystonia.

Additional treatments in practice but with less conclusive or conflicting evidence supporting their use in this patient population include nonsteroidal antiinflammatory agents; opioids; tricyclic antidepressants, selective norepinephrine reuptake inhibitors, or other antidepressants; sarpogrelate; topical capsaicin; calcitonin; intravenously administered lidocaine; and topically applied local anesthetic agents.

Procedural Techniques

Intravenously administered regional blockade using guanethidine and reserpine is not supported by evidence based on randomized controlled trials. However, one small (n = 12) published, randomized, controlled trial of intravenously administered regional blockade using bretylium and lidocaine, compared with lidocaine alone, demonstrated a statistically significant improvement in analgesia.

Traditionally, sympathetic blockade techniques such as stellate ganglion and lumbar plexus blocks have been viewed as a gold standard for CRPS treatment, yet there is a remarkable paucity of data supporting their therapeutic use. Permanent chemical, thermal, and surgical neurolysis are also used in clinical practice, but controlled studies regarding their long-term utility are lacking. Sympathetic blockade is at times employed to facilitate functional restoration exercises and has been shown to aid in the prediction of successful treatment with spinal cord stimulation (SCS).

Literature supporting SCS is similarly limited to studies comprising small numbers of patients. A nonrandomized prospective trial of SCS in patients with CRPS responsive to sympathetic blockade demonstrated significant improvement in pain relief and strength over a mean of 35 months. In a different randomized study comparing patients with CRPS treated with physical therapy to patients undergoing physical therapy and SCS, SCS plus physical therapy resulted in decreased pain intensity and improved global perceived effect for a duration of up to 2 years; these significant findings were not apparent at 5-year follow-up.

Limited evidence supports the use of permanent peripheral nerve stimulators in the treatment of CRPS type II. Mirror and motor imagery therapies have been shown in preliminary, randomized, crossover studies to significantly decrease pain and improve functionality.

CRPS may resolve spontaneously, but significant disability can persist for years with periods of remission and relapse despite treatment. Cold CRPS appears to prognosticate a worse outcome. Estimated rates of return to original functional status vary from 20% to 40%.

Suggested Readings

de Mos M, Sturkenboom CJM, Hugyen FJ. Current understandings on complex regional pain syndrome. *Pain Practice*. 2009;9:86-99.

Harden RN. Complex regional pain syndrome. *Br J Anesth*. 2001;87:99-106.

Tran DQ, Duong S, Bertini P, Finlayson RJ. Treatment of complex regional pain syndrome: A review of the evidence. *Can J Anesth*. 2010;57:149-166.

Williams KA, Hurley RW, Lin EE, Wu CL. Neuropathic pain syndromes. In: Benzon HP, Rathmell JP, Wu CL, et al, eds. *Raj's Practical Management of Pain*. 4th ed. Philadelphia: Mosby; 2008:427-431.

CHAPTER 214

Postoperative Headache

Terrence L. Trentman, MD

Postoperative symptoms—including pain, nausea and vomiting, fatigue, drowsiness, backache, sore throat, muscle aches, and headache—are common, can delay discharge, and can contribute to patients' suffering and dissatisfaction with their care. Postoperative headache may result from an intentional (e.g., to administer a local anesthetic agent for a spinal anesthetic) or inadvertent (e.g., during placement or maintenance of an epidural catheter) dural puncture, from an inhaled anesthetic agent, or from certain other procedures.

Postdural Puncture Headache

A cerebrospinal fluid (CSF) leak that results in headache may be spontaneous or iatrogenic (from a diagnostic lumbar puncture or during a procedure to administer neuraxial analgesia or anesthesia). The International Headache Society defines a postdural puncture headache (PDPHA) as "a bilateral headache that develops within 7 days after a lumbar puncture and disappears within 14 days. The headache increases in intensity within 15 minutes of assuming the upright position and disappears or improves within 30 minutes of resuming the recumbent position." These criteria help to distinguish PDPHA from a migraine headache. A PDPHA typically presents within 48 h after the patient has undergone a dural puncture, although much longer delays have been reported.

Traditional teaching held that PDPHA was secondary to traction on pain-sensitive meninges, but it is more likely that headache results from compensatory venous hypervolemia and dilation of pain-sensitive dural venous sinuses in response to low intracranial CSF volume. Intrathecal air from dural puncture during an air-based epidural loss-of-resistance technique can also cause a headache. Classic symptoms of PDPHA include a dull or throbbing postural headache and stiff neck. Patients may complain of hearing impairment, photophobia, nausea, vertigo, and occasionally diplopia (usually due to an abducens nerve palsy). Complications of CSF leak, such as subdural hematoma and Chiari malformation, may also amplify the underlying headache, result in persistent headache (even in the supine position), or both. Women are at higher risk than men for developing PDPHAs. Risk is inversely related to age and may correlate with low body mass index. A previous PDPHA increases the risk of a subsequent PDPHA occurring.

Prevention

The incidence of PDPHA can be reduced with several techniques. First, the smallest-gauge pencil-point (vs. cutting or Quincke) needle should be used. The bevel of the cutting needle should be parallel to the dural fibers (i.e., parallel to the spinal longitudinal axis), although not all studies confirm that this technique reduces the prevalence or volume of CSF leak. If the dura is unintentionally punctured during epidural placement, an intrathecal catheter left in place for 24 h may lessen the PDPHA risk by inducing an inflammatory response (to the catheter) that promotes sealing of the breach. For the parturient, avoidance of pushing during the second stage of labor has been shown to decrease the incidence of PDPHA. Bed rest will not lessen the risk, although symptomatic patients typically do not want to be ambulatory.

Treatment

In addition to bed rest, hydration, analgesics, abdominal binders, and various medications (including sumatriptan, caffeine, methylergonovine maleate, hydrocortisone, and gabapentin) have been used to treat PDPHA. Most of the supporting evidence for these therapies is weak, as is the use of caffeine for preventing and treating PDPHA.

Epidural saline infusions may provide short-term benefit. An epidural blood patch (EBP) is used to treat persistent and severe symptoms, although EBPs performed less than 24 h after dural puncture are associated with a lower success rate. Risks of EBP are low but not negligible; back pain is most common, with rare reports of arachnoiditis occurring after inadvertent intrathecal injection of autologous blood. The mechanism of action of the EBP may be twofold: immediate headache relief results from compression of the intrathecal space by the iatrogenic epidural hematoma, resulting in increased CSF pressure and headache resolution; long-term relief is due to sealing of the dural tear.

Other Postoperative Headaches

Headaches are common in postpartum women, even in the absence of a dural puncture. Myalgias, tension-type headache, and migraine are common; cerebral imaging in refractory cases has revealed intracranial hemorrhage, vasculopathy (e.g., reversible cerebral vasoconstriction syndrome), and cerebrovenous sinus thrombosis.

Preoperative headache is considered a risk factor for postoperative headache. Caffeine withdrawal has been cited as a common cause of postoperative headache in surgical patients. Intravenous or oral caffeine has been used successfully in some cases. Inhalation anesthetic agents are associated with postoperative headaches. Treatment is symptomatic.

Certain neurosurgical procedures have been associated with postoperative headache. Headache has been reported in up to 75% of patients undergoing a craniotomy for acoustic neuroma or other cerebellopontine angle tumors, though headache can occur after any craniotomy. The clinical characteristics of the headache following craniotomy suggest a combination of tension-type and "site-of-injury" headache overlying the surgical site and are similar to the headaches described following head trauma. Although the pathogenesis of postcraniotomy headache remains unclear, recent evidence demonstrates that meningeal nerves infiltrate the periosteum through the calvarial sutures and may mediate headache caused by head trauma, including surgical trauma. In view of the concentration of sensory fibers in the sutures, it may be useful to avoid drilling the sutures in patients undergoing craniotomies for a variety of neurosurgical procedures.

A pneumocephalus with associated headache can occur after spine operations. Otolaryngologic (e.g., sinus) and ophthalmologic operations have also been complicated by postoperative headache.

The hyperperfusion syndrome and associated headache has been described after carotid endarterectomy. Carotid endarterectomy can be associated with headache even in the absence of hyperperfusion, perhaps due to damage to the sympathetic plexus and altered sympathetic tone.

Suggested Readings

Gaiser R. Postdural puncture headache. *Curr Opin Anaesthesiol*. 2006;19:249-253.

Gee JR, Ishaq Y, Vijayan N. Postcraniotomy headache. *Headache*. 2003;43:276-278.

Halker RB, Demaerschalk BM, Wellick KE, et al. Caffeine for the prevention and treatment of postdural puncture headache: Debunking the myth. *Neurologist*. 2007;13:323-327.

Kosaras B, Jakubowski M, Kainz V, Burstein R. Sensory innervation of the calvarial bones of the mouse. *J Comp Neurol*. 2009;515:331-348.

Olesen J, Bousser M-G, Diener H-C, et al. The International Classification of Headache Disorders. 2nd ed. *Cephalalgia*. 2004;24:9-160.

Stella CL, Jodicke CD, How HY, et al. Postpartum headache: Is your work-up complete? *Am J Obstet Gynecol*. 2007;196:318e1-327.

Thew M, Paech M. Management of postdural puncture headache in the obstetric patient. *Curr Opin Anesth*. 2008;21:288-292.

Vandam LD, Dripps RD. Long-term follow-up of patients who received 10,098 spinal anesthetics. *JAMA*. 1954;156:1486-1491.

Wagner W, Cossman DV, Farber A, et al. Hyperperfusion syndrome after carotid endarterectomy. *Ann Vasc Surg*. 2005;19:479-486.

Wu CL, Berenholtz SM, Pronovost PJ, Fleisher LA. Systematic review and analysis of postdischarge symptoms after outpatient surgery. *Anesthesiology*. 2002;96:994-1003.

Wu CL, Rowlingson AJ, Cohen SR, et al. Gender and post-dural puncture headache. *Anesthesiology*. 2006;105:613-618.

Zeidan A, Farhat O, Maaliki H, Baraka A. Does postdural puncture headache left untreated lead to subdural hematoma? Case report and review of the literature. *Int J Obstet Anesth*. 2006;15:50-58.

CHAPTER 215

Treatment of Cancer-Related Pain

Tim J. Lamer, MD, and Stephanie A. Neuman, MD

Pain is exceedingly prevalent among patients with malignancies and is often suboptimally managed. It is estimated that approximately two thirds of patients with metastatic cancer have pain. One third of patients have pain while undergoing active therapy for disease, and more than three quarters have pain during the last stages of illness. With the use of pharmacologic agents, interventional therapies, and other modalities, effective analgesia can be attained for 70% to 90% of people with cancer.

Mechanisms of Cancer Pain

Two major pain categories exist: nociceptive pain and neuropathic pain. Nociceptive pain results from tissue damage and can be further subdivided into somatic and visceral pain. Somatic pain may originate from multiple sites—including skin, muscle, joints, connective tissue, or bone—and is mediated by somatic afferent fibers (Aδ and C fibers). Somatic pain is most often described as sharp, throbbing, and well localized if it is superficial, or it is described as dull, aching, and less well localized if it is deep. Visceral pain originates from solid or hollow visceral organs and is mediated by visceral nociceptive afferent fibers that travel along with visceral sympathetic efferent fibers. Visceral pain is often described as a dull diffuse pain that is frequently referred in a dermatomal fashion.

Neuropathic pain occurs when there is damage to or dysfunction of nerves in the peripheral or central nervous system. The pain frequently has dysesthetic (e.g., burning, pricking) or paroxysmal (e.g., stabbing, shooting, electric shock-like) qualities and may be associated with sensory, motor, or autonomic dysfunction. Neuropathic pain may be centrally or peripherally generated. When the pain is coupled with loss of sensory input, it is referred to as deafferentation pain (e.g., phantom limb pain). When dysregulation of the autonomic nervous system plays a major role, the pain is referred to as sympathetically mediated pain (e.g., complex regional pain syndrome). Sympathetically mediated pain may occur after a nerve or limb injury; the patient often has diffuse burning pain of the affected extremity associated with allodynia, hyperpathia, sudomotor dysfunction, and signs of impaired blood flow regulation to the extremity. This pain is believed to be mediated, at least in part, by sympathetic efferent fibers. Deafferentation pain and sympathetically mediated pain are examples of centrally generated neuropathic pain. Examples of peripherally generated pain include polyneuropathies and mononeuropathies. Compared with nociceptive pain, neuropathic pain is often less responsive to conventional pharmacologic therapy.

One or more of these mechanisms may contribute to a patient's pain and may occur as a result of the primary cancerous lesion, metastatic disease, neural compression, or treatments, such as radiation therapy, chemotherapy, or surgery. Pain may also originate from secondary nonmalignant sources (e.g., herniated nucleus pulposus, spinal stenosis, myofascial pain syndrome).

Medical Therapy

The World Health Organization's three-step analgesic ladder is a validated, clinical pain treatment algorithm that is very helpful in outlining a therapeutic pain management strategy for patients with cancer. The analgesic ladder progresses in a stepwise approach as pain increases and is utilized to meet individual needs. The approach begins with nonopioids; then, as necessary, it progresses to intermediate-potency opioids for moderate pain and then to more potent opioids for severe pain. Nonopioid medications and adjuvant medications may be used at each step depending on the type or types of pain being treated.

Adjuvant analgesic agents play a major role in treating patients with malignancies (Table 215-1). Most of these medications have a primary indication other than pain but have analgesic properties. The choice of adjuvant is made based on several assessments, including the type of pain, pharmacologic characteristics and adverse effects of the drug, interactions with other medications, and patient comorbid conditions (e.g., depression). Adjuvant agents comprise a diverse group of medications and can be broadly classified into multipurpose adjuvant analgesic agents and adjuvants specific for neuropathic pain, bone pain, musculoskeletal pain, and bowel obstruction.

Tricyclic antidepressants are the most common antidepressant used in the treatment of chronic pain conditions; however, their use may be limited by the frequent occurrence of associated adverse effects, such as orthostatic hypotension, sedation, cardiotoxicity, and drug-induced confusion. Corticosteroids are useful for bone pain, neuropathic pain, headaches secondary to increased intracranial pressure, spinal cord compression, and pain due to obstruction of a hollow viscus or organ-capsule distention. Corticosteroids may have other benefits, including improvement in appetite, nausea, malaise, and overall quality of life. The α_2-adrenergic agonists clonidine and tizanidine are also useful. Intraspinally administered clonidine has been shown to be beneficial in severe, intractable cancer pain. Neuroleptic agents, such as olanzapine, have been found to decrease pain and opioid consumption and to improve cognitive function and anxiety.

Cancer-related neuropathic pain is widely treated with anticonvulsants. Gabapentin is considered a first-line agent. Pregabalin is a similar anticonvulsant with evidence of analgesic efficacy in certain neuropathic pain states. Orally and parenterally administered local anesthetic agents have analgesic properties in patients with neuropathic pain. The NMDA (*N*-methyl-D-aspartic acid) receptor antagonists have been shown to have analgesic effects, with ketamine, specifically, being found to reduce opioid requirements and relieve cancer pain.

Bone pain and pathologic fractures are common in patients with cancer. Radiation therapy is administered when possible. Adjuvants that have been found to be valuable in treating bone pain include calcitonin, bisphosphonates, and certain radiopharmaceuticals (radionuclides that are absorbed at areas of high bone turnover).

If surgical decompression is not feasible in patients with a malignant bowel obstruction, the use of the somatostatin analog octreotide, anticholinergic drugs (hyoscine, glycopyrrolate), and corticosteroids may be beneficial.

Other systemically administered drugs such as baclofen, cannabinoids, benzodiazepines, and psychostimulants have also been used as adjuvant analgesics. The 5% lidocaine patch, EMLA cream (a eutectic mixture of the local anesthetic agents prilocaine and lidocaine), and capsaicin (an ingredient in chili pepper that causes release of substance P) may be useful in patients with localized pain syndromes, such as chest pain after mastectomy, radiation-induced dermatitis, post-thoracotomy pain, and others.

Not all cancer-related pain can be managed with orally or parenterally administered medications alone. Pain may be inadequately controlled, or doses may be limited by intolerable systemic adverse effects of the analgesic agent. In these situations, interventional therapy is often undertaken.

Table 215-1 Adjuvant Analgesic Agents for the Treatment of Cancer-Related Pain: Major Classes

Drug Class	Example(s)
Multipurpose Analgesic Agents	
Antidepressants	
Tricyclic antidepressants	Amitriptyline, desipramine, nortriptyline
SSRIs	Citalopram, paroxetine
NSRIs	Duloxetine, venlafaxine
Other agents	Bupropion
Corticosteroids	Dexamethasone, prednisone
α_2-Adrenergic agonists	Clonidine, tizanidine
Neuroleptic agents	Olanzapine
Adjuvants for Neuropathic Pain	
Anticonvulsants	Carbamazepine, gabapentin, phenytoin, pregabalin, topiramate
Local anesthetic agents	Lidocaine, mexiletine
NMDA receptor antagonists	Dextromethorphan, ketamine
Other agents	Baclofen, cannabinoids, capsaicin, lidocaine, lidocaine/prilocaine, psychostimulants (methylphenidate, modafinil)
Topical drugs	Capsaicin, EMLA cream, lidocaine patch 5%
Adjuvants for Bone Pain	
Corticosteroids	Dexamethasone, prednisone
Calcitonin	
Bisphosphonates	Clodronate, pamidronate, zoledronic acid
Radiopharmaceuticals	Samarium-153, strontium-89
Adjuvants for Musculoskeletal Pain	
Muscle relaxants	Carisoprodol, cyclobenzaprine, metaxalone, methocarbamol, orphenadrine
Baclofen	
Benzodiazepines	Clonazepam, diazepam, lorazepam
Tizanidine	
Adjuvants for Pain from Bowel Obstruction	
Anticholinergics	Glycopyrrolate, scopolamine
Corticosteroids	Dexamethasone, prednisone
Octreotide	

EMLA, Eutectic mixture of local anesthetics [prilocaine and lidocaine]; NMDA, *N*-methyl-D-aspartate; NSRIs, norepinephrine-serotonin reuptake inhibitors; SSRIs, selective serotonin reuptake inhibitors.

Interventional Therapy

Given that the use of the World Health Organization's analgesic ladder does not provide adequate analgesia for all patients with cancer, a revised stepwise approach has been developed that includes the use of interventional techniques (Figure 215-1).

For those patients with pain that is refractory to treatment with medications, multiple interventional therapies exist to provide relief. Options include

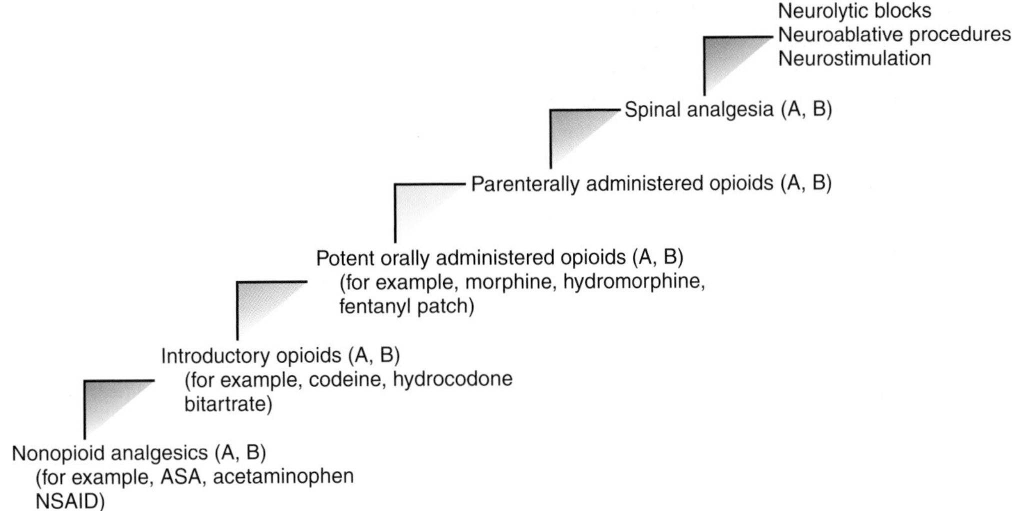

Figure 215-1 Revised stepladder approach to the management of cancer pain. ASA, Acetylsalicylic acid; NSAID, nonsteroidal antiinflammatory drug. (Modified, with permission, from Lamer TJ. Treatment of cancer-related pain: When orally administered medications fail. Mayo Clinic Proc. 1994;69:473-480.)

nerve blocks and other injection therapies (e.g., joint and trigger-point injections), neurolytic blocks, epidurally and intrathecally administered analgesia, neuromodulation (e.g., spinal cord stimulator), and advanced neurosurgical techniques (e.g., cordotomy, midline myelotomy, rhizotomy, neurostimulation).

Neuraxially Administered Analgesia

Drug toxicity secondary to high-dose opioids and adjuvant medications is a leading cause of failure in the management of cancer-related pain. By changing the route of drug administration to an epidural or intrathecal route, toxicities are reduced. In addition to reducing systemic adverse effects, implantable intrathecal drug-delivery systems have been found to provide better pain relief and to extend survival in patients with cancer. Little consensus exists on when to use intrathecal versus epidural routes of administration and when to use an implantable versus an external pump. Epidurally administered analgesia is often chosen if there is a need for more focal analgesia and if a large amount of local anesthetic agent is required because the patient has extreme opioid intolerance. Intrathecally administered analgesia is favored if the pain is more diffuse or if there is abnormal pathology in the epidural space. In general, an external system is used if the patient has a short life expectancy (<3 months), needs frequent self-administered doses of analgesic agents, or needs an epidural infusion (generally requires infusion volumes too great for an implanted pump) or if reprogramming or refilling capabilities are not near the patient's home. Factors that lead to the decision to place an implantable pump include a longer life expectancy (>3 months), access to pump refill or reprograming capabilities, diffuse pain (e.g., widespread metastasis), and a favorable response to an intrathecal trial. Numerous medications are available for neuraxially administered analgesia, including opioids, α_2-adrenergic agonists, calcium channel blockers, and local anesthetic agents. Single agents or a combination of agents may be used, depending upon the pain mechanism involved.

Nerve Blocks and Ablative Procedures

Neurolytic nerve blocks and ablative procedures can be effective for treating refractory pain. Neurolytic blocks with phenol, ethanol, radiofrequency ablation, or cryoablation are most appropriate for patients with advanced disease and decreased life expectancy when other, less invasive, options have failed to provide adequate relief. Celiac plexus block is very effective for intra abdominal malignancies, particularly pancreatic cancer. For tumors of the pelvis, lumbar sympathetic, superior hypogastric plexus, or ganglion impar neurolytic blocks are useful. Intercostal and paravertebral blocks are valuable for treating chest pain (e.g., rib metastasis). For perineal pain, sacral nerve neurolytic blocks are beneficial, and trigeminal nerve blocks are often effective for facial pain.

Surgical Procedures

Anterolateral cordotomy was the first effective surgical procedure on the spinal cord that was introduced for pain relief. However, significant complications can occur (e.g., incontinence, respiratory problems) with this operation. Bilateral anterocordotomy and commissural myelotomy are additional surgical techniques that can be used to relieve midline pain in a very small subset of carefully selected patients. Punctate midline myelotomy (a neuroablative operation that interrupts the midline of the dorsal column) is a newer surgical technique that was developed to treat otherwise intractable abdominal and pelvic cancer-related pain.

As with all interventional techniques, these interventions are not without potential complications; therefore, the provider must carefully weigh the risks and benefits for each patient individually (Table 215-2).

Other Approaches

Therapies other than medications and procedures have been effective for treating cancer-related pain. Relaxation techniques, massage, therapeutic exercise, heat, ice, electrical stimulation, counseling, and other modalities may be valuable. A multidisciplinary or team approach to the management of cancer-related pain, with the participation of oncologists, nurses, psychologists, palliative care specialists, and pain management specialists, will likely produce the most beneficial treatment program.

Table 215-2 Potential Complications of Invasive Procedures for the Treatment of Cancer-Related Pain

Treatment	Potential Adverse Effects
Neurolytic blocks	Sensorimotor impairment Sympathetic or parasympathetic impairment Postural hypotension Bowel or bladder dysfunction Pain recurrence Deafferentation pain Pneumothorax*
Spinally administered opioids	Respiratory depression Pruritus Urinary retention Nausea and vomiting
Spinally administered clonidine	Hypotension Sedation
Spinally administered local anesthetic agent	Sympathetic blockade[†] Exaggerated spread[‡] Motor block
Neurosurgical procedures	Bladder dysfunction Motor weakness Deafferentation pain Respiratory dysfunction[§]
Neuraxial catheters	Catheter break or leak Catheter obstruction Infection[¶] CSF leak
Spinally administered ziconotide	Psychiatric symptoms[#] Motor deficits Meningitis Seizures

CSF, Cerebrospinal fluid.
*Celiac plexus.
†Hypotension, urinary retention.
‡High block.
§Cervical cordotomy.
¶Cellulitis, epidural abscess, meningitis.
#Hallucinations, new or worsening depression, suicidal ideation.

Suggested Readings

Burton AW, Rajagopal A, Shah HN, et al. Epidural and intrathecal analgesia is effective in treating refractory cancer pain. *Pain Med.* 2004;5:239-247.

Gralow J, Tripathy D. Managing metastatic bone pain: The role of bisphosphonates. *J Pain Symptom Manage.* 2007;33:462-472.

Green E, Zwaal C, Beals C, et al. Cancer-related pain management: A report of evidence-based recommendations to guide practice. *Clin J Pain.* 2010;26:449-462.

Lussier D, Huskey AG, Portenoy RK. Adjuvant analgesics in cancer pain management. *Oncologist.* 2004;9:571-591.

Smith TJ, Staats PS, Deer T, et al. Randomized clinical trial of an implantable drug delivery system compared with comprehensive medical management for refractory cancer pain: Impact on pain, drug-related toxicity, and survival. *J Clin Oncol.* 2002;20:4040-4049.

Wong GY, Schroeder DR, Carns PE, et al. Effect of neurolytic celiac plexus block on pain relief, quality of life, and survival in patients with unresectable pancreatic cancer. *JAMA.* 2004;291:1092-1099.

CHAPTER 216

Postherpetic Neuralgia

Salim Michel Ghazi, MD

The syndrome of postherpetic neuralgia (PHN) is defined as the onset of persistent chronic pain following an attack of acute herpes zoster (AHZ). AHZ is itself a reactivation of the varicella virus that had been dormant following an episode of chickenpox, which usually occurred during childhood.

The pain of AHZ typically subsides within 3 weeks. Whenever the pain of AHZ lasts for more than 4 to 6 weeks, a diagnosis of PHN is suspected. Although PHN has been defined in different ways, recent data support making a distinction among acute herpetic neuralgia (within 30 days of rash onset), subacute herpetic neuralgia (30-120 days after rash onset), and PHN (defined as pain lasting at least 120 days from rash onset).

Overall, pain persists in a chronic form in 10% to 15% of patients following AHZ infection. This incidence is higher if the following well-established risk factors are present: older age, greater severity of acute pain during AHZ infection, more severe rash, a prodrome of dermatomal pain before onset of the rash, cancer, diabetes, immunosuppression, and lymphoproliferative disorders. Patients with these risk factors may have as much as a 50% to 75% risk of having pain that persists for at least 6 months after rash onset. PHN is more common after ophthalmic herpes than after the spinal segment type.

Description of the Syndrome

The persistence of pain—described as continuous, burning, and lancinating—that spreads along a single dermatome from the central dorsal line in a ventral direction following the initial rash of AHZ is the most typical manifestation of the syndrome of PHN. The pain is unilateral, most commonly affecting a thoracic dermatome or the ophthalmic division V_1 of the trigeminal nerve (cranial nerve V). Lumbar, cervical, and sacral involvement is less common. Occasionally, but rarely, the pain of PHN can occur without a preceding rash.

In PHN, the affected area typically shows changes in the form of pigmentation and scarring where the vesicles of AHZ have healed. Hyperesthesia, hyperpathia, and allodynia may be present. The pain can often be excruciating and intractable, impairing quality of life to the point that the patient may contemplate suicide. The pain of PHN is purely neuropathic.

Pathophysiology

After the initial infection of herpes zoster, usually many years previously, the virus remains dormant in the dorsal root ganglion of the peripheral nerve. The cause of its reactivation is not fully understood but could be related to a perturbation in the immune system, an increase in stress, or both. The reactivation causes the findings seen in AHZ. The dermatomal distribution of the vesicular rash seen in AHZ is related to the transport of the reactivated virus along the sensory nerve fiber to the skin.

Pathologic changes in AHZ and PHN are characterized by inflammatory changes, followed by necrosis and then scarring of the dorsal root ganglion, leading to degeneration and destruction of the emerging sensory and motor fibers. The inflammatory processes can also involve the anterior and posterior horns of the spinal cord.

Despite the descriptive pathologic changes noted in AHZ and PHN, the exact mechanism of how pain is generated is unclear. Both peripheral and central mechanisms may be involved.

The peripheral mechanism can be explained by the preferential loss of large-caliber neurons found in PHN. According to the gate control theory of pain, decreased activity of large-fiber neurons may allow increased rates of pain impulses to reach the dorsal horn of the spinal cord.

The central mechanism involves a very complex, anatomic, synaptic reorganization in the dorsal horn caused by increased chronic afferent painful input to the cord and ending in a hyperexcitable state in which nonpainful stimuli are now perceived as pain (wind-up phenomenon).

Treatment

Because of the complex nature of the pathology of PHN, no definitive treatment is available. For this reason, prevention of the PHN is vital and consists of recommendations that individuals older than 60 years of age be vaccinated and, when recurrence is diagnosed, that the AHZ episode be treated early with appropriate antiviral medication and steroids.

Since the pain is purely neuropathic, multiple modalities of therapy have been recommended. They are divided into pharmacotherapy, nerve blocks, and surgical intervention. A balanced combination of modalities has the best potential to achieve the goal of decreasing pain to a level that allows patients a better functional status and improves their quality of life (Table 216-1). Referral to a pain rehabilitation center is recommended when the disease is debilitating to the patient and when the patient's functional status, emotional status, and quality of life are severely impaired.

Because transcutaneous electrical nerve stimulation has minimal side effects and typically provides at least moderate results, these units should also be tried along with pharmacotherapy.

Pharmacotherapy

Pharmacotherapy should include an initial trial of the antiepileptic agent gabapentin, starting at a low dose and gradually increasing the dose to reach 1800 to 2400 mg/day, unless improvement or major adverse effects occur. If the patient does not tolerate gabapentin, pregabalin can be tried to a maximum dose of 300 to 600 mg/day. Tricyclic antidepressant medications can also be used if no results were obtained with gabapentin or pregabalin or adverse effects were not tolerated. Amitriptyline (25-50 mg initial dose at night), nortriptyline, trazodone, and doxepin have been used with variable success. Other medications used with variable success include nonsteroidal antiinflammatory drugs; tramadol; various topical creams, including capsaicin and EMLA cream (eutectic mixture of local anesthetics); and a lidocaine patch. Recently, a patch containing high concentration of capsaicin (8%) was made available in the United States.

Table 216-1 Treatment Options for Postherpetic Neuralgia

Pharmacotherapy	Nerve Blocks	Surgical Interventions
Gabapentin Pregabalin Amitriptyline NSAIDs Tramadol EMLA cream Lidoderm cream and patch Opioids Capsaicin cream and patch	Epidural local anesthetic injection Intrathecal steroid injection Lumbar sympathetic block Pulsed radiofrequency denervation of DRG Radiofrequency denervation of intercostal nerves SCS Subcutaneous nerve stimulation	DREZ Motor cortex stimulation Nucleotractotomy

EMLA, Eutectic mixture of local anesthetics; DREZ, dorsal root entry zone lesioning; DRG, dorsal root ganglion; NSAIDs, nonsteroidal antiinflammatory drugs; SCS, spinal cord stimulation.

Opioid medications can be used and have been found to be helpful in well-selected patients. The use of opioid medications for patients with chronic long-term nonmalignant pain should follow strict rules, with the patient being well informed on the proper use of the medication and establishing treatment goals in association with the health care provider, understanding the risks and consequences of nonadherence to well-detailed instructions. Methadone, long-acting morphine, and long-acting oxycodone have been used for the treatment of PHN, with short-acting medications provided for breakthrough pain. The medication dose should be titrated to effectiveness. If or when patients develop tolerance, they should be switched to another opioid medication. Patients who are receiving opioid medications for the treatment of PHN should be informed that, if they show any sign of abuse, they will be switched to a different treatment.

Nerve Blocks

Central, spinal, and sympathetic nerve blocks have shown good but variable results in the treatment of PHN. One study indicated that lumbar sympathetic blocks provided up to 90% improvement in pain score up to 29 months. Intrathecal injection of steroids may be effective, but this treatment is still controversial. Another technique that has been used with some success is the epidural injection of a local anesthetic agent with steroids during the first 2 months of an AHZ infection. More randomized controlled trials are needed to reach a better understanding of the true efficacy of these procedures.

Emerging interventions for the treatment of PHN have been numerous in the last few years and include pulsed or routine radiofrequency denervation of the intercostal nerve roots/dorsal root ganglion, implanted spinal cord stimulators, and implanted subcutaneous peripheral nerve stimulation (not to be confused with transcutaneous nerve stimulation). Of all of these interventions, spinal cord stimulation looks most promising in controlling the pain of PHN over the long term and in improving quality of life.

Surgical Procedures

Surgical interventions for the treatment of PHN include dorsal root entry zone lesioning, spinal trigeminal nucleotractotomy, and stereotactic radiosurgery of the trigeminal root. These procedures should be used only when all other modalities have failed.

Nicolas Chamfort, an eighteenth century French writer, said, "Philosophy, like medicine, has plenty of drugs, few good remedies, and hardly any specific cure."

Suggested Readings

Kuman V, Krone K, Mathieu A. Neuraxial and sympathetic blocks in herpes zoster and postherpetic neuralgia: An appraisal of current evidence. *Reg Anesth Pain Med.* 2004;*29*:454-461.

Niv D, Maltsman-Tseikhin A, Lang E. Postherpetic neuralgia: What do we know and where are we heading? *Pain Physician*. 2004;*7*:239-247.

Raja SN, Haythornwaite JA, Pappagallo M, et al. Opioids versus antidepressants in postherpetic neuralgia. *Neurology*. 2002;*59*:1015-1021.

CHAPTER 217

Epidural Steroid Injection for Low Back Pain

Caridad Bravo-Fernandez, MD

Low back pain (LBP) is common among those seeking medical care; the lifetime prevalence of LBP varies between 60% and 80%. Recurrent episodes of LBP are also common, especially within 12 months of the first occurrence. For manual laborers, LBP may cause absence from work from 30 weeks to 140 weeks over an entire 40-year career.

Multiple therapeutic measures and techniques have been used to treat acute episodes of LBP, and almost all are equally effective—whatever the intervention, the LBP usually resolves within 2 weeks. However, an alternate treatment path may be appropriate for those patients whose pain persists longer than 2 weeks and who, on evaluation, are found to have evidence of radicular pain or of a radiculopathy and whose imaging studies are indicative of spinal stenosis, spondylolysis, or a protruding nucleus pulposus of an intervertebral disk. Many believe that a herniated disk causes radicular pain only if it initiates an inflammatory process mediated through interleukins and tumor necrosis factor-α. In these patients, a course of 1 to 3 epidural steroid injections (ESIs) with or without a local anesthetic (occasionally also with an opioid or clonidine) may be indicated to inhibit the release of these cytokines and to diminish inflammation, subsequently diminishing pain.

Site of Injection

The translaminar approach has been the traditional approach to the epidural space—using anatomic landmarks and a loss-of-resistance technique to place a Tuohy needle in the epidural space—and is still commonly used in many academic pain departments. The practice is changing, however, and many anesthesia providers especially those in private practice, are more likely to use fluoroscopy and the transforaminal approach to deposit solution at the site of the nerve root that is involved in the radiculopathy or radiculitis. When administering epidural injections under fluoroscopic guidance, nonionic radiographic dyes, such as iopamidol (Isovue) and iohexol (Omnipaque), are used to confirm location but may precipitate an allergic response. The use of fluoroscopy and contrast dye provides evidence of delivery of medication to the appropriate nerve root. When the transforaminal approach is used, the volume of injectate is smaller than that used for the translaminar approach; with the latter, saline is usually used to increase the injectate volume, increasing the likelihood that the active medications—steroids, local anesthetic agents, or a combination of both—will reach the affected site.

The caudal approach from the sacral canal was used frequently in the past, but it is not commonly used in current practice. However, good results have been demonstrated with the lumbar approach.

Technique

Few studies have evaluated the use of sedation in performing ESIs, but the existing evidence suggests that many practitioners provide some sedation, with appropriate monitoring, using either small amounts of midazolam or fentanyl. Translaminar needle placement is usually performed with the patient in the sitting, lateral, or prone position. The patient is usually prone for transforaminal injections, using the fluoroscope to take lateral images of the spine. As with any invasive procedure, documentation of the appropriate patient, site, and intervention are mandatory, as is the use of sterile technique.

Medications Used

Steroids commonly used in ESI include triamcinolone, methylprednisolone, betamethasone, and dexamethasone (Table 217-1) and are often combined with a local anesthetic agent, such as lidocaine, bupivacaine, or ropivacaine.

Table 217-1 Steroids Commonly Used for Epidural Injection

Drug	Dose (mg)
Betamethasone	4-12
Dexamethasone	4
Methylprednisolone acetate	40-80
Triamcinolone diacetate	50-80

Contraindications and Adverse Effects

The use of ESI is contraindicated in patients with coagulopathy or who use anticoagulant therapy and in patients who have an active systemic infection or a history of adverse reactions to steroids or any other drug being used. ESI should be used with caution in patients with diabetes.

The use of ESI is associated with a variety of adverse effects (Box 217-1) and is not without risks that must be weighed when assessing the potential benefits. The risks can be divided among those related to placement of the needle and to the adverse effects associated with the drugs. As with the placement of any epidural needle, dural puncture (spinal headache), intrathecal (or intravascular) injection of drug, bleeding and hematoma, infection (e.g., meningitis, abscess), and direct trauma to the cord, nerve roots, or nerves can occur. There are isolated case reports of pneumothorax and quadriplegia or paraplegia occurring.

Box 217-1 Adverse Effects Associated with the Use of Epidural Steroid Injections

Adverse Effects	Severe Adverse Effects
Accidental dural puncture	Arachnoiditis
Adrenal suppression	Aseptic necrosis of major joints
Cushingoid symptoms	Cauda equina
Dizziness	Diskitis
Headache	Epidural abscess
Hyperglycemia	Meningitis—septic and aseptic
Immune suppression	Paraplegia
Nausea/vomiting	Paraspinal abscess
Sodium and fluid retention	
Transient local pain	

Conclusion

Limited evidence indicates that ESIs may be effective in treating LBP in some patients, with a long-term success rate of approximately 20%. The best results seem to be obtained in patients with acute radicular symptoms; conversely, the poorest results are in patients with chronic symptoms of axial back pain who have had surgery and those who smoke. In addition, ESIs are being used to provide pain relief from diskogenic pain. Even with all the recent controversies about the lack of randomized controlled studies, ESIs continue to be used and these procedures can be done safely and effectively, providing pain relief to many patients.

Suggested Readings

Abram SE. Treatment of lumbosacral radiculopathy with epidural steroids. *Anesthesiology*. 1999;91:1937-1941.

Benyamin RM, Manchikanti L, Parr AT, et al. The effectiveness of lumbar interlaminar epidural injections in managing chronic low back and lower extremity pain. *Pain Physician*. 2012;15:E363-404.

Buenaventura RM, Datta S, Abdi S, Smith HS. Systematic review of therapeutic lumbar transforaminal epidural steroid injections. *Pain Physician*. 2009;12:233-251.

Cluff R, Mehio AK, Cohen SP, et al. The technical aspects of epidural steroid injections: A national survey. *Anesth Analg*. 2002;95:403-408.

DePalma MJ, Slipman CW. Evidence-informed management of chronic low back pain with epidural steroid injections. *Spine J*. 2008;8:45-55.

Huntoon MA, Burgher AH. Back to the future: The end of the steroid century? *Pain Physician*. 2008;11:713-716.

Manchikanti L, Buenaventura RM, Manchikanti KN, et al. Effectiveness of therapeutic lumbar transforaminal epidural steroid injections in managing lumbar spinal pain. *Pain Physician*. 2012;15:E199-245.

Manchikanti L, Singh V, Cash KA, et al. Effect of fluoroscopically guided caudal epidural steroid or local anesthetic injections in the treatment of lumbar disc herniation and radiculitis: A randomized, controlled, double blind trial with a two-year follow-up. *Pain Physician*. 2012;15:273-286.

Parr AT, Manchikanti L, Hameed H, et al. Caudal epidural injections in the management of chronic low back pain: A systematic appraisal of the literature. *Pain Physician*. 2012;15:E159-198.

Radcliff K, Hilibrand A, Lurie JD, et al. The impact of epidural steroid injections on the outcomes of patients treated for lumbar disc herniation: A subgroup analysis of the SPORT Trial. *J Bone Joint Surg Am*. 2012;94(15):1353-1358.

Smith HS, Chopra P, Patel VB, et al. Systematic review of the role of sedation in diagnostic spinal interventional techniques. *Pain Physician*. 2009;12:195-206.

Staal JB, de Bie RA, de Vet HC, et al. Injection therapy for subacute and chronic low back pain: An updated Cochrane review. *Spine*. 2009;34:49-59.

CHAPTER 218

Stellate Ganglion Block

Glenn E. Woodworth, MD

Indications

Indications for stellate ganglion block include circulatory insufficiency in the arm resulting from traumatic or embolic occlusion of the arterial supply of the arm, postembolectomy vasospasm, postreimplantation of a traumatic amputation, or arteriopathy from whatever cause; pain caused by complex regional pain syndrome, herpes zoster, neoplasm, phantom limb pain, Paget disease, or lesions in the central nervous system; and other problems, such as hyperhidrosis, Sudeck atrophy, tinnitus, and sympathetically maintained pain in the upper extremity, head, or neck. It has even been suggested as a treatment for cerebral vasospasm due to embolus or thrombosis and for upper extremity tourniquet-induced hypertension.

Anatomy

The peripheral sympathetic nervous system arises from the intermediolateral column of the spinal cord. The efferent preganglionic fibers pass out of the spinal cord via the ventral roots from T1 to L2. The fibers then enter the sympathetic chain through the white rami communicantes. The preganglionic fibers may travel for a variable distance within the sympathetic chain before synapsing in ganglia or exiting the chain to synapse in peripheral ganglia.

The sympathetic chain lies along the anterolateral aspect of the vertebral bodies in a fascial space bounded posteriorly by the prevertebral muscles and in the cervical region anteriorly by the carotid sheath. The nerve fibers in the cervicothoracic chain originate from preganglionic sympathetic fibers from T1 to T6 and visceral afferent fibers from the head, neck, and upper extremity (see Chapter 40). These fibers are distributed to the brain, meninges, eye, ear, glands, skin, and vessels of the head, neck, upper extremity, and some thoracic viscera. The efferent and afferent fibers form several ganglia; the first thoracic and inferior cervical ganglia lie in close proximity and are often fused to form the stellate ganglion, which is oval and about 1 inch long by 0.5 inch wide. It lies within the fascial space described earlier. It is bounded posteriorly by the neck of the first rib and the transverse process of C7 and anteriorly by the dome of the pleura, the carotid sheath, and the vertebral artery. The medial boundary is the vertebral column. It is important to note that some thoracic preganglionic sympathetic fibers may bypass the stellate ganglion.

Technique

Although posterior and anterior approaches have been described, a paratracheal route is used most frequently. The patient is instructed to lie supine with the head supported by a pillow. The head is kept in the midline in slight extension. The patient's mouth should be slightly open to relax the neck muscles. The stellate ganglion can be blocked at the level of C6 or C7, but, because of the risk of pleural puncture, the approach to the fascial space is often made slightly superior to the ganglion at the level of C6 (Chassaignac tubercle) (Figure 218-1). Two fingerbreadths (1.5-2 cm) above the clavicular head, the trachea, sternocleidomastoid muscle, and carotid sheath are palpated (approximately at the level of the cricoid cartilage). The anesthesia provider presses two fingers gently down onto the lateral edge of the transverse process of C6 (the most readily palpable cervical anterior tubercle) while simultaneously drawing the contents of the carotid sheath laterally (Figure 218-2). A 1.5-in to 3-in, 23-gauge or 25-gauge B (blunt) bevel needle is inserted just lateral to the trachea after skin infiltration with a local anesthetic agent. The transverse process of C6 should be encountered between the two palpating fingers at a depth of 1.5 to 2 cm. The needle is withdrawn 2 mm to place it in the correct fascial plane, and 8 to 10 mL of local anesthetic agent is injected incrementally after careful aspiration. A 0.5-mL test dose is recommended to rule out a vertebral artery injection. A generalized seizure can occur with as little as 0.5 mL of local anesthetic agent injected into the vertebral artery. If blockage of the sympathetic supply to the upper extremity is desired, the patient is placed in a 30-degree head-up position to encourage caudal diffusion of the local anesthetic agent to the upper thoracic ganglia. In addition, a larger volume of local anesthetic agent may be necessary. Position of the needle and spread of solution may be confirmed by fluoroscopy.

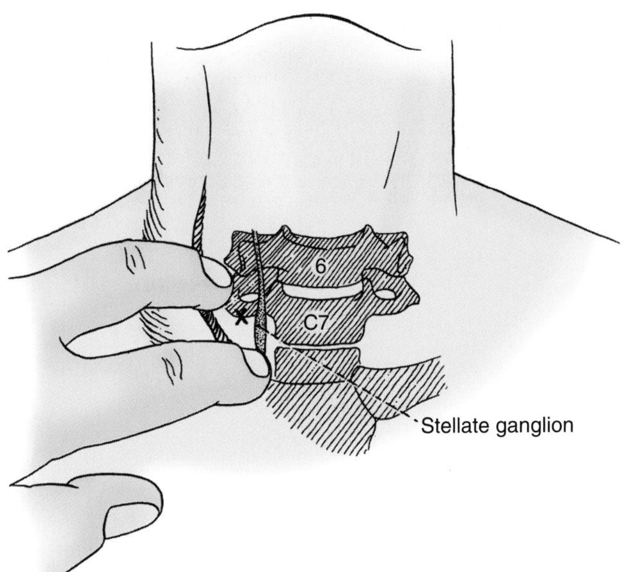

Figure 218-1 Landmarks for injection of the stellate ganglion at the level of C7. (Modified from Adriani J. Labat's Regional Anesthesia: Techniques and Clinical Applications. Philadelphia, WB Saunders, 1967.)

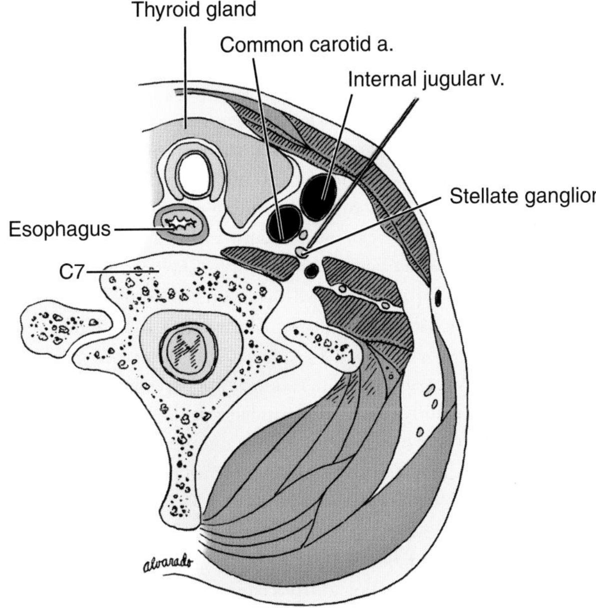

Figure 218-2 Cross-section of the neck at the level of the body of the seventh cervical vertebra. The carotid bundle is retracted laterally for the stellate ganglion block. Note the proximity of the vertebral artery (immediately posterior to the stellate ganglion). (Modified from Adriani J. Labat's Regional Anesthesia: Techniques and Clinical Applications. Philadelphia, WB Saunders, 1967.)

Box 218-1 Signs of a Successful Stellate Ganglion Block

Flushing of the conjunctiva and skin
Horner syndrome (ptosis, miosis, enophthalmos)
Ipsilateral nasal congestion
Temperature increase in the ipsilateral arm and hand

Box 218-2 Side Effects and Complications of a Stellate Ganglion Block

Common Side Effects and Complications

Hematoma
Sensation of "a lump in the throat"
Temporary hoarseness and dysphagia because of recurrent laryngeal block (a 60% prevalence rate)
Unpleasant effects of Horner syndrome

Uncommon Complications

Brachial plexus block (rare)
Cardioaccelerator nerve block with hypotension or bradycardia
Epidural or subarachnoid block
Osteitis of the transverse process or vertebral body
Phrenic nerve block
Pneumothorax (1% prevalence rate)
Puncture of esophagus
Puncture of intervertebral disk

Potentially Severe Complications

Intradural injection causing total spinal block
Osteomyelitis of the vertebral body or diskitis
Vertebral artery injection causing loss of consciousness and seizure

A large number of different types of nerve blocks, including stellate ganglion blocks, are being performed under ultrasound guidance to improve success of the block and to decrease complications. Real-time ultrasound of the neck can delineate the carotid artery, internal jugular vein, esophagus, thyroid, longus colli muscle, root of C6, and the transverse process of C6. The needle tip is directed to penetrate the prevertebral fascia covering the longus colli, and the injection is performed under direct ultrasound visualization. Signs of a successful stellate ganglion block and complications and side effects of a stellate ganglion block are outlined in Boxes 218-1 and 218-2, respectively.

Suggested Readings

Brown DA. *Atlas of Regional Anesthesia*. 4th ed. Philadelphia: Saunders Elsevier; 2010:183-191.

Fujiwara S, Komatsu T. A new approach of ultrasound-guided stellate ganglion block. *Anesth Analg*. 2007;105:550-551.

Katz J. *Atlas of Regional Anesthesia*. Norwalk, CT: Appleton-Century-Crofts; 1985.

Lofstrom J, Cousins M. Sympathetic neural blockade of upper and lower extremity. In: Cousins M, Bridenbaugh P, eds. *Neural Blockade in Clinical Anesthesia and Management of Pain*. 2nd ed. Philadelphia: Lippincott; 1988.

CHAPTER 219
Lumbar Sympathetic Blockade

David M. Rosenfeld, MD

Lumbar sympathetic blockade was first fully described by Mandl in 1926. Currently, the modality is widely used as a diagnostic and therapeutic procedure in the treatment of a wide variety of medical conditions.

Relevant Anatomy

The lumbar sympathetic ganglia are known to control the sympathetic impulses to the lower extremities. These structures may represent either a single fused elongated mass or up to six separate ganglia spanning the L1 to L5 vertebra. As the sympathetic trunk passes into the abdomen, it begins a migration from a position that is more anterior to the vertebral bodies to a true anterolateral position by the midlumbar levels. On the right side, the sympathetic trunk is positioned posterior to the inferior vena cava, and, on the left, it is lateral and slightly posterior to the aorta. Injection techniques that position needles from L2 through L4 have been described. When approaching the ganglia, the best starting point is the area just cephalad to the middle of the body of the L3 vertebral body. This level has the highest probability of encountering the ganglia, variation is less, as compared with at L2 or L4, and the psoas muscle may terminate at the lower part of the L3 vertebra. The psoas muscle is well positioned posterior to the sympathetic chain, thus separating it from the somatic lumbar plexus and leading to fewer complications after injection, compared with other levels of the sympathetic chain.

Indications

The indications for lumbar sympathetic blockade fall into three main categories and serve both diagnostic and therapeutic purposes. First are conditions that result in circulatory insufficiency of the lower extremity, including atherosclerotic disease, arterial embolism, thromboangiitis, Raynaud phenomenon, frostbite, and following reconstructive vascular operations. Many of these conditions, such as claudication, rest pain, ischemic ulcers, and gangrene, are painful. The institution of continuous sympathetic blockade can transiently improve regional blood flow and predict the success of surgical sympathectomy or neurolytic therapy.

The second category involves pain from nonvascular causes and includes phantom or stump pain after amputation, varicella zoster or postherpetic neuralgia, renal colic, interstitial cystitis, complex regional pain syndrome, and labor analgesia. For complex regional pain syndrome, blocks are often performed in succession or continuously via a catheter and can improve analgesia and function in conjunction with pharmacologic and physical therapy. Lumbar sympathetic blockade is known to provide relief from the pain associated with the first stage of labor. Lack of effectiveness of lumbar sympathetic blockade for pain relief during the second stage of labor, concerns over potential intrathecal injection, technical difficulty, and the relative efficiency and ease of epidural analgesia have rendered lumbar sympathetic blockade rare in labor and delivery.

A third miscellaneous category includes nonpainful conditions such as lower extremity hyperhidrosis. The block is primarily used for diagnostic and predictive purposes prior to neurolysis or surgical sympathectomy. It has also been attempted on a limited basis to transiently improve renal function in patients with hepatorenal syndrome.

Technique

Patients are generally positioned prone, with pillow support provided beneath the lower abdomen to decrease lumbar lordosis and improve exposure of the L2 through L4 vertebrae. Establishment of intravenous access is recommended. Local infiltration of an anesthetic agent is mandatory along the needle track, and some clinicians use varying levels of conscious sedation in patients for whom specific diagnostic interaction is not necessary. The procedure routinely can be accomplished in 30 min and should be performed by clinicians who are experienced in performing percutaneous procedures and have knowledge of the relevant anatomy. Historically, the procedure was performed without radiographic assistance; however, currently, many clinicians use fluoroscopic guidance with anteroposterior, oblique, and lateral views to improve safety and precision. A myelographic iodinated contrast agent should be used if possible to help avoid intravascular injection and to enhance needle position and injection spread within the distribution of the ganglion. Currently, ultrasound-guided needle placement is being investigated, and some clinicians even employ computed tomography to guide needle placement. Transcutaneous temperature monitoring should be utilized to verify blockade; increases between 1°C and 8°C can be seen.

Brown Single-Needle Technique

With this technique, the patient is placed in the prone position, and pillow support is provided. The needle is inserted 12.5 cm lateral to the spine at the level of the L4 vertebra, 1 cm cephalad to the ileum. A 22-gauge 14-cm needle is inserted at an angle of 35 to 40 degrees to the skin. The needle is directed medially until bone is contacted, and the needle lies at the anterolateral surface of the vertebra. The patient is then placed in a 5- to 140-degree Trendelenburg position, and 20 mL of local anesthetic agent is injected; the anesthetic agent should spread as high as L2. This oblique approach with insertion of the needle at the level of L4, versus a more cephalad position, is mandatory to avoid kidney injury. The Brown single-needle technique is infrequently used.

Lateral Approach First Described by Reid

With this technique, the patient is again placed in the prone position with pillow support of the lower abdomen. Fluoroscopy is used for assistance in properly placing the needle. The spinous processes of L2, L3, and L4 are marked, and a site that is 7 to 8 cm lateral to midline at approximately the L2 to L3 transition is located. A spot that is perpendicular to the caudal aspect of the L2 vertebra, which corresponds to the interspace between the transverse process of L2 and L3, is marked. Reid described 7 cm as the optimal position to gain the proper trajectory to the ganglion of the vertebral body and to avoid injury to the renal parenchyma. This technique can be employed with a single needle at L3 or with as many as three needles positioned at L2, L3, and L4.

A 22-gauge 12-cm to 18-cm needle is advanced until it contacts the vertebral body at the cephalad portion of L3. The typical angle of insertion is 45 degrees, but this angle may be modified depending upon the patient's body habitus. If bone is encountered soon after inserting the needle, the clinician has likely come into contact with a transverse process, and the needle trajectory should be modified cephalad or caudad to avoid contact with bone. If this occurs, the needle depth is noted, and the needle is retracted to skin level and redirected at a steeper angle under fluoroscopy to clear the lateral margin of the vertebra and position the tip at the anterolateral border of the vertebral body (Figure 219-1). The needle should be anterior to the psoas fascia. The needle is aspirated to verify extravascular position, taking into account the proximity of the aorta and vena cava. A small volume of iodinated contrast agent is injected, and spread should ideally be seen from L2 to L4. If spread is limited, additional needles can be placed at L2 and L4. Obtaining anteroposterior and lateral radiographic views helps to assess contrast spread, and, if striations (psoas stripe) are seen on fluoroscopy, the needle position may be too posterior.

It is helpful to initially inject 10 to 15 mL of lidocaine to document distal temperature rise and then follow with an additional 10 to 15 mL of bupivacaine. If temperature rise is not seen with initial injection, the needle should be repositioned and the local anesthetic agent reinjected, taking care to not exceed the maximum recommended dose of local anesthetic agent. The patient should be carefully monitored for the presence of lower extremity weakness and toxicity from the local anesthetic agent.

Mandl Technique

With the Mandl technique, the spinous processes of L2 to L4 are marked, and a skin wheal is placed approximately 10 cm off midline with a local anesthetic agent injected at the L2 level and infiltrated to the transverse process. A 20-gauge, 12-cm needle is inserted to the level of the transverse process and then redirected medially toward the vertebral body 45 degrees to the coronal plane between the transverse processes. The needle is

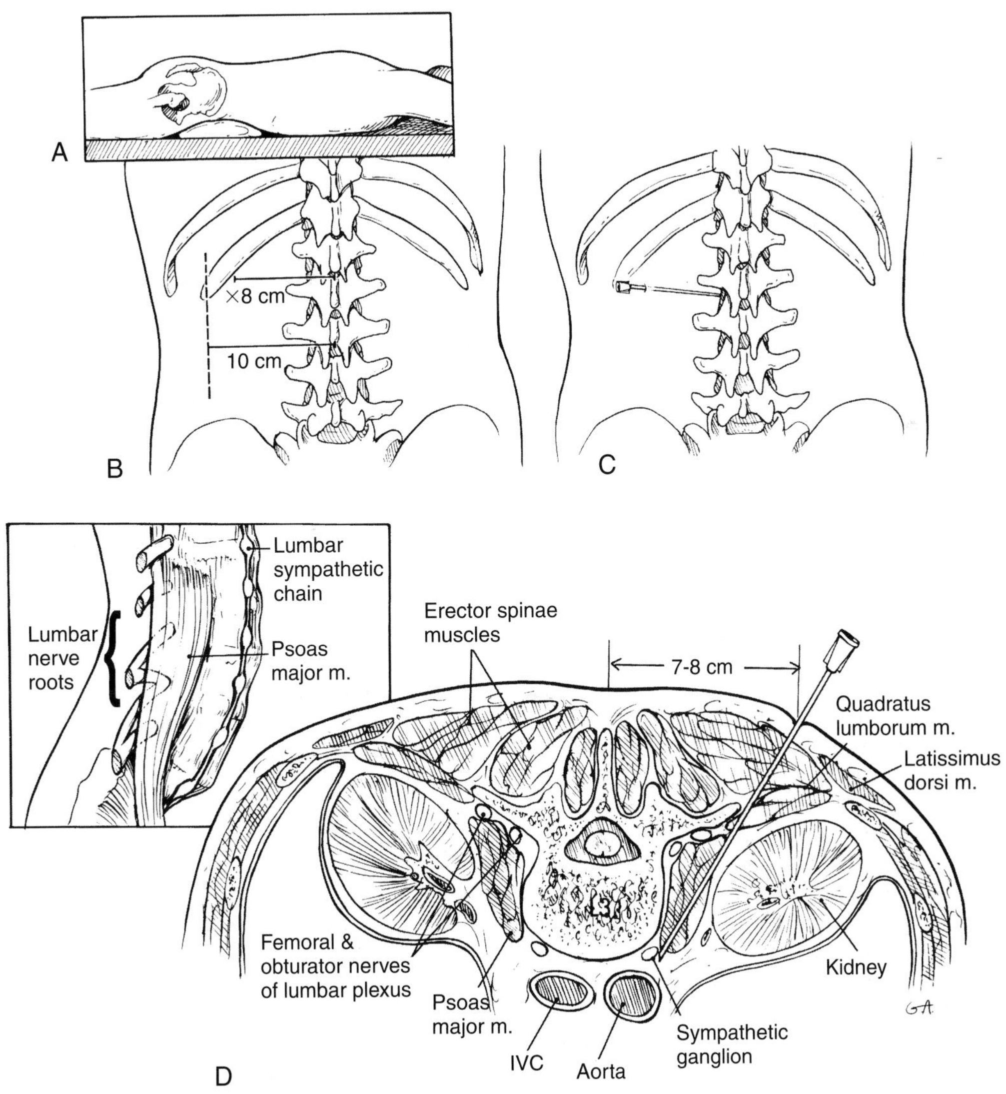

Figure 219-1 Lateral approach described by Reid. **A,** The patient should be positioned prone, with a pillow beneath the anterior iliac spines. **B,** Skin landmarks include the twelfth rib, the posterior iliac crest, and the cephalad tip of the L2 spinous process. **C,** Insertion of the needle is 7 to 8 cm from the midline, perpendicular to the spinal canal at L2. **D,** Cross-sectional view of the final needle placement. IVC, Inferior vena cava. (From Rauck R. Sympathetic nerve blocks: Head, neck, and trunk. In: Raj P, ed. Practical Management of Pain. 3rd ed. Philadelphia: Elsevier; 2000:674.)

advanced, with the bevel toward the vertebral body, until contact is made; the needle is then adjusted to a position that allows it to slide 1 cm off the vertebral body. The position can be verified by loss of resistance and negative aspiration for cerebrospinal fluid, blood, or urine. Movement of the needle with normal respiration indicates lateral positioning in the diaphragmatic crus. Radiographic screening with contrast injection is recommended to ensure proper needle positioning, especially for neurolytic blocks. Alternatively, ultrasonography may be used, sparing the patient and physician radiation exposure. The procedure is repeated at the L4 level. Catheters may be placed if an 18-gauge needle is used.

Adverse Events

Back pain from needle trauma is common after the procedure and usually resolves in a few days; it may be treated with heat, ice, and rest. Blockade of the genitofemoral nerve or lumbar plexus within the psoas muscle may occur and may result in numbness in the groin, thigh, or quadriceps and may cause prolonged neuralgia and burning pain, especially in the groin, if a neurolytic agent is injected. Other adverse effects include renal or urethral trauma, hematoma, infection, abscess, intravascular injection, perforation of a disk, diskitis, ejaculatory failure, somatic nerve injury, and chronic back pain.

Suggested Readings

Breivik H, Cousins MJ. Sympathetic neural blockade of upper and lower extremity. In: Cousins M, Bridenbaugh P, eds. *Neural Blockade in Clinical Anesthesia and Management of Pain*. 4th ed. Philadelphia: Lippincott, Williams & Wilkins; 2008:872-879.

Brown EM, Kunjappan V. Single needle lateral approach for lumbar sympathetic block. *Anesth Analg*. 1975;54:725-729.

Rauck R. Sympathetic nerve blocks: Head, neck, and trunk. In: Raj PP, ed. *Practical Management of Pain*. 3rd ed. St. Louis: Mosby; 2000:673-678.

Reid W, Watt JK, Gray TG. Phenol injection of the sympathetic chain. *Br J Surg*. 1970;57:45-50.

Rocco AG, Palombi D, Racke D. Anatomy of the lumbar sympathetic chain. *Reg Anesth*. 1995;20:13-19.

Sayson SC, Ramamurthy S. Sympathetic blocks. In: Warfield C, Bajwa Z, eds. *Principles and Practice of Pain Medicine*. 2nd ed. New York: McGraw-Hill; 2004:705-708.

CHAPTER 220
Celiac Plexus Block

David P. Martin, MD, PhD

Indications

The celiac plexus provides sensory innervation and sympathetic outflow to most of the upper abdominal viscera (see Chapter 40). Neurolytic blockade of the celiac plexus is most commonly used to control pain caused by pancreatic cancer, although it can be useful for managing pain related to malignancies of the gastrointestinal tract from the lower esophageal sphincter to the splenic flexure, as well as the liver, spleen, and kidneys. Although potentially long-lasting, neurolytic celiac plexus block is not "permanent" because the nerves in the plexus regenerate in 3 to 6 months. The block can be repeated in such circumstances, but many patients with pancreatic cancer do not outlive the effective duration of neurolytic celiac plexus block. The median survival after diagnosis with pancreatic cancer is 3 to 6 months. Most patients with pancreatic cancer still require some oral analgesics even after neurolytic celiac plexus block.

Temporary diagnostic blockade of the celiac plexus can be used to differentiate visceral pain from somatic pain. Visceral pain is poorly localized and can be referred to somatic areas. For example, pancreatic pain often presents as epigastric tenderness radiating to the back. Relief of pain after celiac plexus block suggests a visceral origin of the pain. If pain persists after celiac plexus block, it is more likely to be somatic in origin. In addition to its neurolytic and diagnostic uses, celiac plexus injection with a local anesthetic agent and a corticosteroid is sometimes used to treat the pain associated with chronic pancreatitis.

Anatomy

The celiac plexus is primarily a sympathetic nervous system structure that lies anterior to the aorta near the celiac arterial trunk (Figure 220-1). Preganglionic sympathetic fibers originate from the nerve roots of T5-T12 and combine to form the splanchnic nerves. The splanchnic nerves cross the crura of the diaphragm before joining the vagus nerve to form the celiac plexus anterior to the aorta. The location of the plexus varies from T12 to L2 vertebral levels; approaches to the block are directed at the T12-L1 level.

Effective visceral pain relief can be achieved by either blocking the splanchnic nerves before they pierce the diaphragm or blocking the nerves and ganglia anterior to the diaphragmatic crura. The splanchnic nerve block (retrocrural) is also termed the *classic* celiac plexus block, as opposed to *true* blockade of the plexus and ganglia (intercrural).

Procedure

Several approaches to the celiac plexus have been described, including endoscopic, ventral, and dorsal. The endoscopic route is convenient when

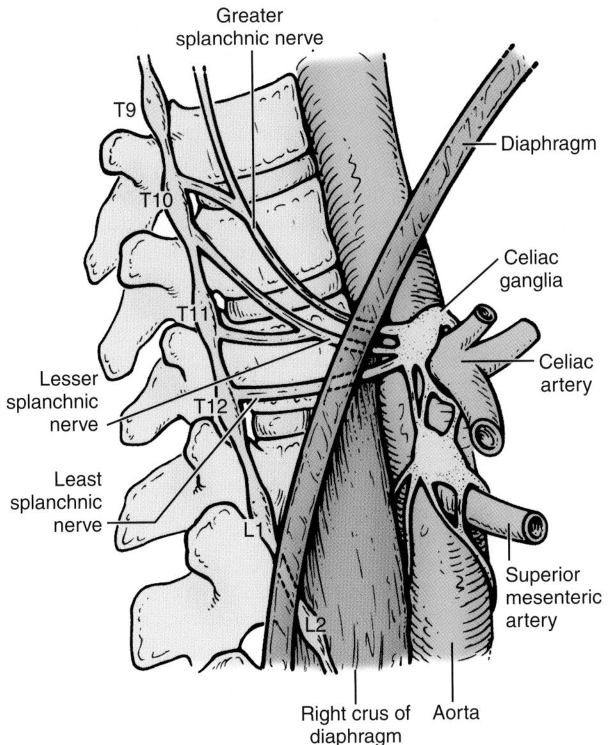

Figure 220-1 Anatomy. The celiac ganglion lies anterior to the aorta just superior to the celiac artery. It receives preganglionic fibers from the splanchnic nerves. Visceral analgesia can be achieved by blocking the splanchnic nerves before they pierce the diaphragm or by blocking the plexus and ganglion anterior to the diaphragmatic crura. (Modified from Stanton-Hicks MB. Lumbar sympathetic nerve block and neurolysis. In: Waldman SD, Winnie AP, eds. Interventional Pain Management. Philadelphia: WB Saunders; 1996:353-359.)

combined with endoscopic retrograde cholangiopancreatography (ERCP). The ventral approach can be advantageous if tumor blocks the dorsal route, but it has a higher risk of bowel injury and infection. The most common route used by anesthesia providers is via the dorsal approach and is performed with the patient in the prone position with a pillow under the hips. Landmarks are identified and marked on the skin surface, indicating the twelfth rib and the thoracolumbar spinous processes. Needles are inserted bilaterally at a site approximately 7.5 cm lateral to midline at a point 2 cm inferior to the twelfth rib. The initial pass is directed to contact the L1 vertebral body at an angle approximately 45 degrees from the sagittal plane (Figure 220-2). The path of the needle is approximately parallel to the inferior border of the twelfth rib, directed toward the middle of the L1 vertebral body. After noting the depth at which bone is contacted, the needle is withdrawn to skin level and redirected more steeply, so that it passes just lateral to the L1 body, and is then advanced an additional 1 to 2 cm. Ideal positioning is anterolateral to the body of the L1 vertebral body.

Once the needle is placed, careful aspiration is performed to exclude a vascular or intrathecal position. Proper drug distribution can be confirmed with the injection of radiocontrast dye under fluoroscopy. It is important to ensure that the injectant is not within the psoas muscle, which could result in blockade of the lumbar plexus. Bupivacaine, 0.25% to 0.5%, is a reasonable choice for the diagnostic nerve block. Typically, 10 to 15 mL is injected on each side.

For diagnostic blocks, the procedure ends at this point. At least 15 to 20 min must elapse until the effects of blockade can be assessed. In addition to pain relief, motor function should also be tested. If a neurolytic block is planned, the needles can be left in place during this assessment.

If pain is relieved and no motor deficits are observed after injecting a local anesthetic, it is reasonable to proceed with neurolysis. For neurolytic procedures, 50% to 100% alcohol is the most commonly used agent. Typically, 10 mL is injected on each side. A small volume of local anesthetic agent

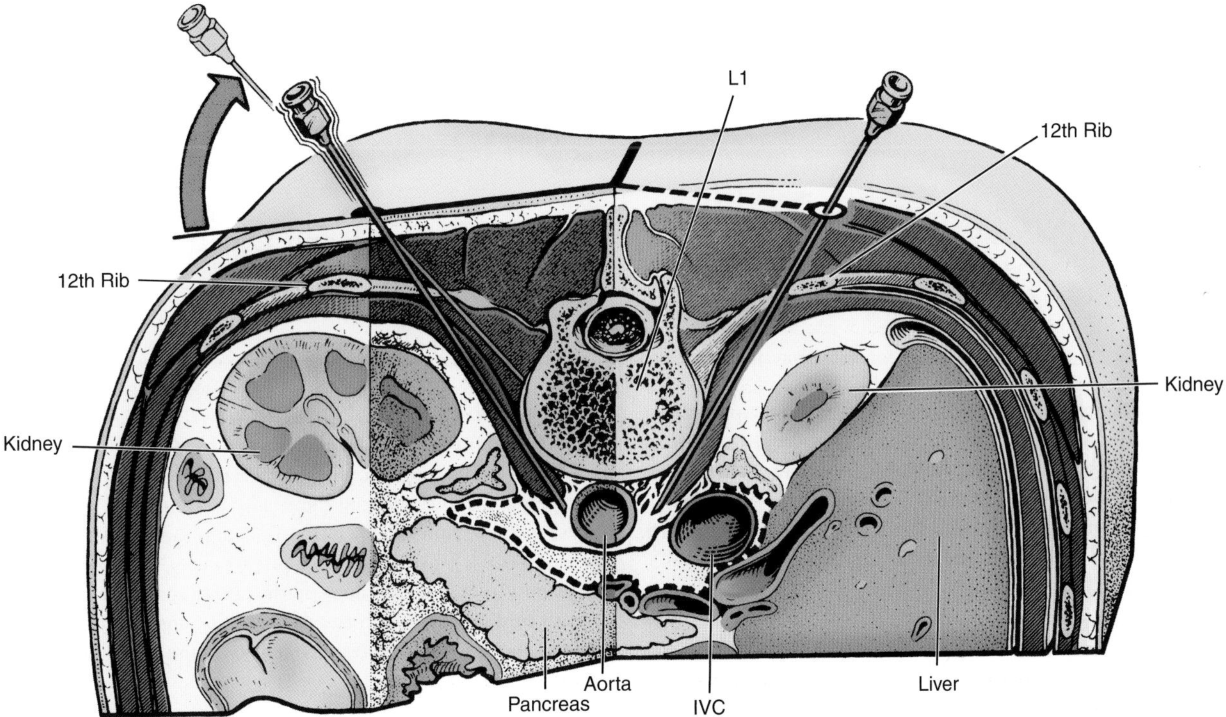

Figure 220-2 Performing the celiac plexus block. The needle is inserted approximately 7.5 cm lateral to the midline along a path inferior to the twelfth rib. The initial needle path is at a 45 degree angle from the sagittal plane to contact the vertebral body of L1. The needle is then withdrawn and redirected to pass anterolateral to L1. IVC, Inferior vena cava. (Modified from Kopacz DJ, Thompson GE. Celiac and hypogastric plexus, intercostal, interpleural, and peripheral neural blockade of the thorax and abdomen. In Cousins MJ, Bridenbaugh PO, eds. Neural Blockade in Clinical Anesthesia and Management of Pain. 3rd ed. Philadelphia: Lippincott; 1998:451-485.)

can be injected while withdrawing the needles to prevent alcohol from tracking to more superficial tissue.

Expected Side Effects

The procedure itself can cause local soreness and bruising. These symptoms are usually transient and can be treated with ice. Psoas spasm is not uncommon after neurolytic celiac plexus block and can be minimized by preventing the escape of neurolytic agent through the needle tract. Psoas spasm often responds well to intravenously or intramuscularly injected ketorolac.

Interruption of sympathetic innervation to the viscera can blunt normal postural hemodynamic reflexes, resulting in orthostatic hypotension. Patients should be cautioned that they may feel lightheaded upon standing. The sympathectomy can also cause increased gastrointestinal motility and possibly diarrhea. However, the effect of sympatholysis on intestinal motility can be beneficial in counteracting the constipation caused by orally administered opioids. Finally, celiac plexus block may mask early presenting symptoms of other intra abdominal diseases, such as cholecystitis and gastric ulceration.

Adverse Effects

As with any injection, sterile technique should be observed with the performance of a celiac plexus block to minimize the risk of infection. Because of the close proximity of the celiac plexus to the aorta, vascular injury is possible; hematoma formation, aortic dissection, and distal (lower extremity) ischemia have been reported. Intravascular injection of a local anesthetic agent can cause mental status changes, seizures, and possible hemodynamic collapse.

Unintentional intrathecal or epidural spread can cause spinal nerve block. The spread of neurolytic agent to unintended nerve or vascular structures introduces the risk of permanent neurologic injury, including paralysis. Therefore, careful neurologic evaluation after injection of a local anesthetic is essential before injecting the neurolytic agent. The most common nerve injury after celiac plexus block is genitofemoral neuralgia. Despite these risks, celiac plexus block is relatively safe when performed by experienced physicians.

Suggested Readings

Brown DL, ed. Celiac plexus block. In: *Atlas of Regional Anesthesia*. 2nd ed. Philadelphia: WB Saunders; 1999:283-291.

Burton AW, Phan PC, Cousins MJ. Treatment of cancer pain: Role of neural blockade and neuromodulation. In: Cousins MJ, Carr DB, Horlocker TT, Bridenbaugh PO, eds. *Neural Blockade in Clinical Anesthesia and Pain Medicine*. 4th ed. Philadelphia: Lippincott; 2009:1124-1133.

Lamer TJ. Sympathetic nerve blocks. In: Brown DL, ed. *Regional Anesthesia and Analgesia*. Philadelphia: WB Saunders; 1996:357-384.

Stanton-Hicks MB. Lumbar sympathetic nerve block and neurolysis. In: Waldman SD, Winnie AP, eds. *Interventional Pain Management*. Philadelphia: WB Saunders; 1996:353-359.

Wong GY, Brown DL. Celiac plexus block for cancer pain. *Tech Reg Anesth Pain Manage*. 1997;1:18-26.

Wong GY, Schroeder DR, Carns PE, et al. Effect of neurolytic celiac plexus block on pain relief, quality of life, and survival in patients with unresectable pancreatic cancer. *JAMA*. 2004;291:1092-1099.

CHAPTER 221

Spinal Cord Stimulation

Deepesh M. Shah, MD, and David P. Seamans, MD

Spinal cord stimulation (SCS) was first used in 1967 and approved by the U.S. Food and Drug Administration for the management of chronic pain in 1989; since then, SCS has become an important interventional adjuvant. In the United States, common indications for SCS include failed back surgery syndrome (postlaminectomy pain syndrome), complex regional pain syndrome (CRPS), and lumbar radiculopathy.

Mechanism of Action

Several theories have been postulated regarding the potential mechanism of action behind SCS. To date, the most accepted is the gate control theory, which was introduced by Melzack and Wall in 1965. This theory proposes that pulsed energy from neurostimulator electrodes (placed in the epidural space so that, if possible, the points of stimulation are cephalad and caudal to the dermatomes from which the noxious stimuli arise) activates large myelinated Aβ fibers that inhibit or "close the gate" to painful peripheral stimuli carried by Aδ and C fibers. Ideally, an electrical field is created that stimulates the appropriate spinal cord structures without affecting the nearby nerve roots. Another potential mechanism of pain relief is release of neuromodulators (γ-aminobutyric acid [GABA], 5-hydroxytryptamine [5-HT], glycine, and adenosine) in proximity to the dorsal horn of the spinal cord that inhibits afferent spinal cord impulses. SCS has also been demonstrated to activate supraspinal nuclei, with an increase in activity of inhibitory descending pathways in the spinal cord.

Placement of a Spinal Cord Stimulator

The process of SCS involves two phases. The first phase, or trial phase, involves implantation of a percutaneous lead into the epidural space under fluoroscopic guidance. Trial stimulation is performed to elicit paresthesia over the painful area. The patient then "test drives" the device for 3 to 10 days. The trial is considered successful if the patient experiences pain relief of more than 50%, regains functionality, or is able to decrease the use of pain medication.

If the first phase is successful, the second phase is implemented, entailing placement of a permanent lead (cylindrical or flat; Figures 221-1 and 221-2) in the same location. Leads are surgically placed (via a midline laminotomy or a minimally invasive technique); paddle-lead electrodes are spaced wider than those on cylindrical leads. The lead is then connected to an implanted pulse generator (Figure 221-3).

Criteria for implantation require that the patient have primary neuropathic pain, have failed conservative therapy (e.g., injections, medications, physical therapy), be devoid of major psychiatric conditions, and have had a successful trial phase. Because of the high overlap of psychiatric illnesses in patients with chronic pain, a psychiatric evaluation must be obtained prior to implantation.

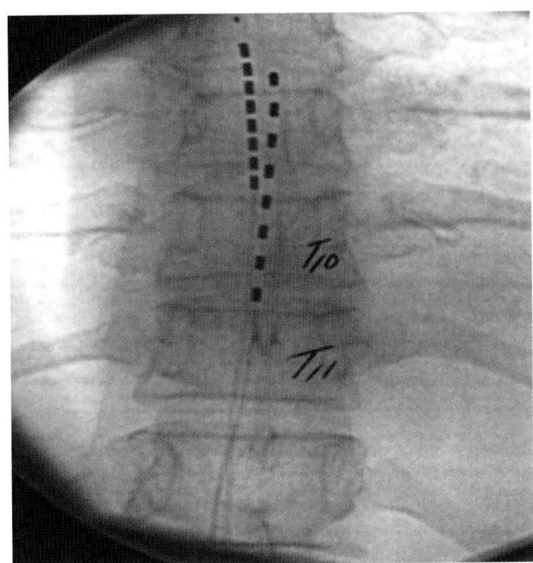

Figure 221-3 Fluoroscopic view of cylindrical lead in the epidural space.

Outcome Studies

Several studies have reported favorable responses to SCS in patients with either postlaminectomy pain syndrome or CRPS. In 2005, North and associates randomly assigned 50 patients—who had previously undergone back operations and were candidates for repeat operations—to SCS (n = 24) or repeat laminectomy (n = 26). Patients were excluded if they had major neurologic deficits, gross spinal instability, large disk fragments, severe spinal stenosis, or major psychiatric comorbidity, including opioid dependency. After 6 months, patients were allowed to cross over from one treatment group to the other. By the 3-year follow-up, 54% elected to cross over from reoperation to SCS, whereas only 21% crossed over from SCS to reoperation; 47% in the primary SCS group continued to have a significant reduction in pain, compared with only 12% in the primary reoperation group. No patients who crossed over from SCS to reoperation had a significant reduction in pain. Opioid use was also significantly higher in the reoperation group; however, activities of daily living and work status did not differ. North and associates concluded that SCS was more effective than repeat surgery.

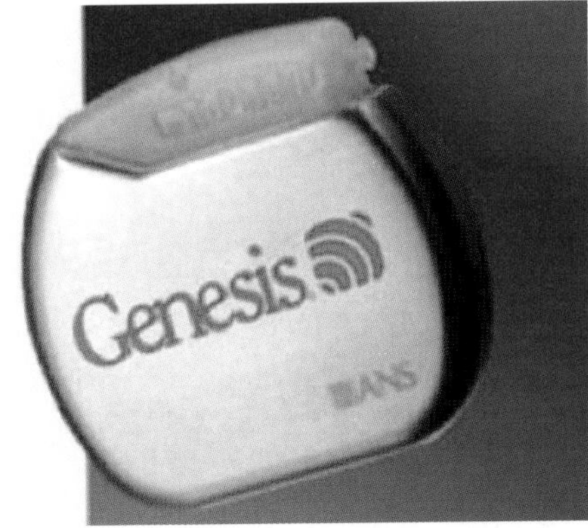

Figure 221-1 Internal pulse generator. (Courtesy of Advanced Neuromodulation Systems, Inc./St. Jude Medical, St. Paul, MN.)

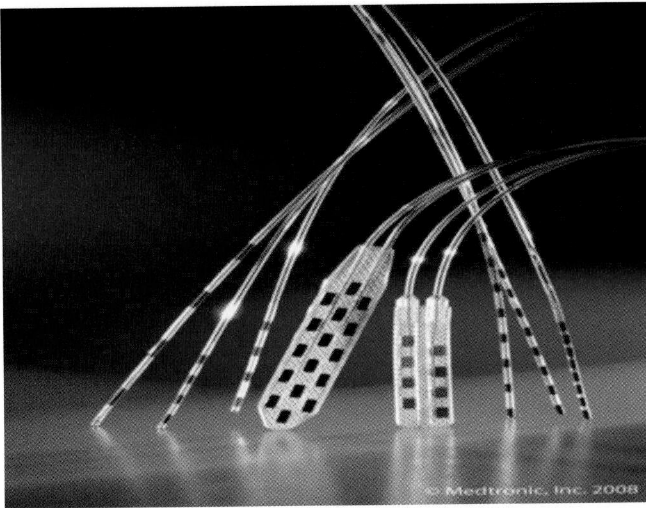

Figure 221-2 Variety of leads—cylindrical and paddle. (Courtesy of Medtronic, Inc., Minneapolis, MN.)

In 2006, Kumar and colleagues undertook a prospective multicenter study that included 100 patients with postlaminectomy pain syndrome. Patients were randomly assigned to receive either conventional medical management alone or conventional medical management in combination with SCS. Conventional medical management included any therapy advised by the physician except reoperation, implantation of an intrathecal drug-delivery system, or SCS. At 6 months, the SCS group had a statistically significant reduction in pain, as compared with the conventional medical management group (48% versus 9%, respectively). The SCS group also had improved functionality and improved patient satisfaction. These results were consistent up to the 24-month follow-up visit.

Several studies have analyzed the medical costs of SCS therapy in the setting of postlaminectomy pain syndrome. The consensus remains that, by reducing the demand for medical care, SCS therapy (if effective) pays for itself within 2.1 years.

In 2000, Kemler and coworkers published a prospective clinical trial comparing SCS to conservative therapy in patients with CRPS. Patients with a 6-month or longer history of CRPS were randomly assigned to SCS plus physical therapy (n = 36) or to physical therapy alone (n = 18). The SCS was implanted only if test stimulation was successful. Outcomes measures included intensity of pain, the global perceived effect of SCS, functional status, and quality of life. The trial stimulation was successful in 24 patients with SCS; the 12 who did not have a successful stimulation trial did not receive implanted stimulators. Investigators reported a mean 2.4-point reduction in the visual analog pain score at 6 months in patients who received SCS, compared with a 0.2-point increase in the physical therapy group ($p < 0.001$). Global perceived effect was "much improved" in

39% of patients who had an SCS implanted, versus 6% of patients who received only physical therapy ($p = 0.01$). Quality of life also improved; however, functional status did not. Overall, SCS was more effective in reducing pain and improving quality of life and led to a greater patient satisfaction than did physical therapy at 6 months.

Complications

Complications from the use of SCS may occur. Fortunately, severe complications are extremely rare. In 2004, Cameron published a 20-year literature review looking at the complication rates in 2700 patients who had undergone SCS. The overall complication rate was 34%. The most common complications were lead migration (13%) and lead fracture (9%). Complications that occurred less frequently included infection, undesired stimulation, cerebrospinal fluid leak, allergic reaction, and hematoma.

Future Directions

The role of neurostimulation has expanded, and SCS is now being used for various peripheral neuropathies, peripheral vascular diseases, and angina. The use of direct nerve stimulation versus peripheral field stimulation has been considered for use in various conditions, including supraorbital/infraorbital neuralgia, intercostal neuralgia, occipital neuralgia, intractable migraines, and ilioinguinal neuralgia. Stimulation is achieved either via direct placement of the lead on the affected nerve or with lead placement within the field covering the affected nerve. Peripheral vascular disease and angina in patients who are not candidates for surgery are common indications for neurostimulation in Europe, based on the theories that SCS decreases sympathetic outflow, increases regional blood flow, and decreases myocardial O_2 consumption.

Suggested Readings

Bala MM, Riemsma RP, Nixon J, Kleijnen J. Systematic review of the (cost-) effectiveness of spinal cord stimulation for people with failed back surgery syndrome. *Clin J Pain*. 2008;24:741-756.

Benzon HT, Raja SN, Mallou RE, et al, eds. *Essentials of Pain Medicine and Regional Anesthesia*. 2nd ed. Philadelphia: Churchill Livingstone; 2005:454-463.

Cameron T. Safety and efficacy of spinal cord stimulation for the treatment of chronic pain: A 20-year literature review. *J Neurosurg*. 2004;100:254-267.

Kemler M, Barendse GA, van Kleef M, et al. Spinal cord stimulation in patients with chronic reflex sympathetic dystrophy. *N Engl J Med*. 2000;343:618-624.

Kumar K, Taylor RS, Jacques L, et al. Spinal cord stimulation versus conventional medical management for neuropathic pain: A multicenter randomized control trial in patients with failed back surgery syndrome. *Pain*. 2007;132: 179-188.

North RB, Kidd DH, Farrokhi F, Piantadosi SA. Spinal cord stimulation versus repeated lumbosacral spine surgery for chronic pain: A randomized, controlled trial. *Neurosurgery*. 2005;56:98-107.

Shealy CN, Mortimer JT, Resnick J. Electrical inhibition of pain by stimulation of the dorsal column. *J Int Anesth Res Soc*. 1967;46:489-491.

Winfree C. Neurostimulation techniques for painful peripheral nerve disorders. *Neurosurg Clin North Am*. 2009;20:111-120.

CHAPTER 222

Advanced Cardiac Life Support

Kjetil Sunde, MD, PhD, and Petter A. Steen, MD, PhD

The annual incidence of out-of-hospital sudden cardiac arrest in the United States is estimated to be 350,000 to 400,000, with approximately 200,000 individuals being treated for in-hospital cardiac arrest. The incidence of ventricular fibrillation (VF) as initial rhythm has declined to less than 30% of the sudden cardiac arrests, both in and out of the hospital, possibly because, as the care of cardiac disease has improved, people who arrest have more severe disease.

Survival to hospital discharge varies greatly among communities in the United States: from 1% to 2% to greater than 20% for patients who receive cardiopulmonary resuscitation (CPR) for any abnormal rhythm out of hospital, and 24% for in-hospital adult cardiac arrests from Get With the Guidelines-Resuscitation 2012 data. The key to successful resuscitation is a well-organized community program, consisting of early recognition and activation, early institution of effective CPR, early defibrillation, and postresuscitation care. Survival has been discouragingly unchanged over decades despite factors such as the number of education programs, the increased availability of defibrillators in public places, and the number of first responders. However, over the last several years, there have been reports of improvements due to changes in CPR, most of which have been compiled in the American Heart Association's 2010 CPR guidelines, which focus on the most important components of resuscitation—the delivery and effectiveness of those components—and postresuscitation care.

The 2010 guidelines place more emphasis on chest compressions of sufficient depth and rate with minimal interruptions because studies have demonstrated that, in the past, approximately one third of compressions were performed at less than the recommended depth, and pauses in compressions frequently accounted for half of the CPR time. Inadequate compression depth and compression pauses decrease the chance of successful defibrillation occurring, whereas periods of continuous chest compressions before shocks are delivered have been reported to increase the defibrillation success rate for ambulance response times of more than 4 to 5 min. Compressions should be at least 2 inches deep at a rate of 100/min, allowing full chest recoil after each compression.

Other changes during the past decade have been in the type of defibrillator used and in the recommendations for defibrillation. Termination of VF is higher with biphasic defibrillators. Delivering only one shock is recommended, not stacks of three, and the shock should be immediately followed by 2 min of CPR before rhythm or pulse checks are performed (Figure 222-1). In patients with continuous electrocardiographic and hemodynamic monitoring (as might occur in the hospital setting), performance of defibrillation may be modified by the physician in charge, especially for arrests of very short duration, such as in the operating room or intensive care unit. If the patient does not have a secured airway, chest compressions and ventilations are given in a 30:2 ratio, but the importance of ventilation is being questioned, particularly for patients with cardiac arrest of cardiac origin. If the patient has an advanced airway device in place (supraglottic airways are increasingly being recommended, particularly for paramedics and emergency medical technicians), compressions are given without pausing for ventilations, which can be interposed at a rate of 8 to 10/min while 100% O_2 is delivered. No consensus has been reached on whether the use of mechanical chest compressions or other adjuncts increase survival, as compared with performance of standard manual CPR. To avoid deterioration in the quality of CPR when performing manual CPR, the person performing compressions should change every 2 min (see Figure 222-1).

Both amiodarone, 300 mg, given in shock-refractory VF and epinephrine, 1 mg, given every 3 to 5 min, increase the rate of return of spontaneous circulation (ROSC), but no drug (including these, other vasopressors, fibrinolytic agents, or buffers) administered during CPR has been shown to improve final outcome.

The high rate of noncompliance with CPR guidelines has triggered a search for technologies that provide real-time feedback on CPR effectiveness. During CPR, end-tidal CO_2 ($ETCO_2$) correlates more with chest compressions than with adequacy of effective ventilation and is therefore an indicator of cardiac output. In addition, return to normal levels of $ETCO_2$ during CPR is a good indicator of ROSC. As an indicator of correct tracheal tube placement, $ETCO_2$ is not a good measure of CO_2 returned to the lungs during CPR. For example, ventilation through a tracheal tube placed in the esophagus can result in relatively high $ETCO_2$ with the initial breaths because it is actually measuring exhaled breath forced into the stomach during mouth-to-mouth resuscitation before the tracheal tube was placed, providing an erroneous measurement, which may be interpreted as correct tube placement. Carotid or femoral pulses cannot be used to indicate adequate coronary perfusion pressure (aortic–right atrial decompression or "diastolic" pressure). With invasive monitoring in place, coronary perfusion pressure can guide therapy and should be kept at a minimum of 15 mm Hg, which has been shown to increase ROSC rate. Most modern defibrillators used for CPR collect data on chest compressions, ventilations, and changes in VF frequency spectra, which are very useful for evaluating CPR quality in debriefing sessions. Some defibrillators use the same data to provide automated real-time auditory and visual feedback during the actual CPR event. Both uses have been shown to improve quality of CPR.

The importance of the postresuscitation phase is increasingly recognized. Therapeutic hypothermia improved neurologic outcome in randomized studies of patients with initial VF who remained unconscious after ROSC. The optimal target temperature or duration is not known, but the present recommendation is to cool to 32° C to 34° C for 12 to 24 h. However, the recommendation may change when new guidelines are developed that include the results of two recent studies that call into question the benefit of

ACLS Cardiac Arrest Algorithm

Adult Cardiac Arrest

Shout for Help/Activate Emergency Response

1 **Start CPR**
- Give oxygen
- Attach monitor/defibrillator

Rhythm shockable?

Yes → 2 VF/VT

No → 9 Asystole/PEA

3 Shock

4 **CPR 2 min**
- IV/IO access

Rhythm shockable? (No → 12)

Yes

5 Shock

6 **CPR 2 min**
- **Epinephrine** every 3-5 min
- Consider advanced airway, capnography

Rhythm shockable? (No → 12)

Yes

7 Shock

8 **CPR 2 min**
- **Amiodarone**
- Treat reversible causes

10 **CPR 2 min**
- IV/IO access
- **Epinephrine** every 3-5 min
- Consider advanced airway, capnography

Rhythm shockable? (Yes → Go to 5 or 7)

No

11 **CPR 2 min**
- Treat reversible causes

Rhythm shockable?

No → 12

Yes → Go to 5 or 7

12
- If no signs of return of spontaneous circulation (ROSC), go to **10** or **11**
- If ROSC, go to Post–Cardiac Arrest Care

Go to 5 or 7

CPR Quality
- Push hard (≥2 inches [5 cm]) and fast (≥100/min) and allow complete chest recoil
- Minimize interruptions in compressions
- Avoid excessive ventilation
- Rotate compressor every 2 minutes
- If no advanced airway, 30:2 compression-ventilation ratio
- Quantitative waveform capnography
  - If P_{ETCO_2} <10 mm Hg, attempt to improve CPR quality
- Intra-arterial pressure
  - If relaxation phase (diastolic) pressure <20 mm Hg, attempt to improve CPR quality

Return of Spontaneous Circulation (ROSC)
- Pulse and blood pressure
- Abrupt sustained increase in P_{ETCO_2} (typically ≥40 mm Hg)
- Spontaneous arterial pressure waves with intra-arterial monitoring

Shock Energy
- **Biphasic:** Manufacturer recommendation (eg, initial dose of 120-200 J); if unknown, use maximum available. Second and subsequent doses should be equivalent, and higher doses may be considered.
- **Monophasic:** 360 J

Drug Therapy
- **Epinephrine IV/IO Dose:** 1 mg every 3-5 minutes
- **Vasopressin IV/IO Dose:** 40 units can replace first or second dose of epinephrine
- **Amiodarone IV/IO Dose:** First dose: 300 mg bolus. Second dose: 150 mg.

Advanced Airway
- Supraglottic advanced airway or endotracheal intubation
- Waveform capnography to confirm and monitor ET tube placement
- 8-10 breaths per minute with continuous chest compressions

Reversible Causes
- Hypovolemia
- Hypoxia
- Hydrogen ion (acidosis)
- Hypo-/hyperkalemia
- Hypothermia
- Tension pneumothorax
- Tamponade, cardiac
- Toxins
- Thrombosis, pulmonary
- Thrombosis, coronary

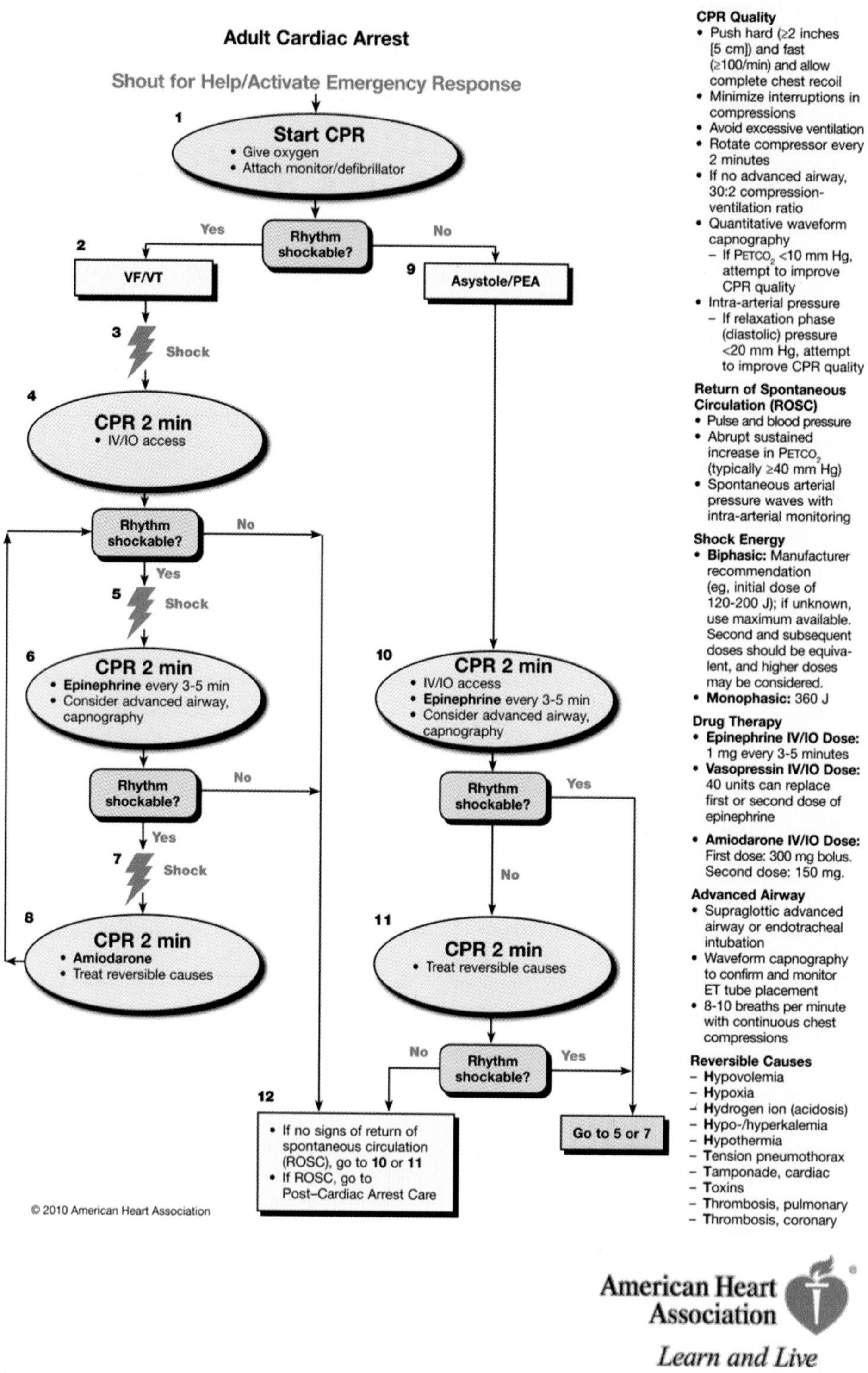

Figure 222-1 Advanced Cardiac Life Support (ACLS) cardiac arrest algorithm. CPR, Cardiopulmonary resuscitation; ET, endotracheal; IO, intraosseous; IV, intravenous; PEA, pulseless electrical activity; VF, ventricular fibrillation; VT, ventricular tachycardia. (Reprinted with permission from 2010 American Heart Association Guidelines for Cardiopulmonary Resuscitation and Emergency Cardiovascular Care, Part 8: Adult Advanced Cardiovascular Life Support. Circulation. 2010;122[Suppl 3]:S729-S767, © 2010 American Heart Association, Inc.)

hypothermia following cardiac arrest. Few well-controlled studies have evaluated other factors after ROSC, but some hospital systems report doubling of survival to hospital discharge with good neurologic outcome after introduction of well-defined standardized post-ROSC protocols. Such protocols usually recommend (1) using therapeutic hypothermia in all unconscious patients regardless of initial pulseless rhythm if active treatment is required; (2) undertaking coronary angiography with coronary revascularization, as indicated, as soon as possible after ROSC; (3) avoiding high levels of glucose (>180-200 mg/dL); (4) treating seizures recognized clinically or on electroencephalography; and (5) optimizing vital organ perfusion. Reversible postresuscitation myocardial dysfunction (myocardial stunning) is normally present in the early phase after ROSC, requiring several efforts to optimize organ perfusion, such as a positive fluid balance and the use of vasopressor agents, inotropes, an intraaortic balloon pump, or a combination thereof. Echocardiography should initially be undertaken daily. Unless the patient is conscious after ROSC, ventilation should be controlled, but hyperventilation ($Paco_2$ < 35 mm Hg) might worsen cerebral perfusion, and, thus, neurologic outcome, and should be avoided. The optimal level of oxygenation has not been established, but with recognized increased production of reactive O_2 species in the reperfusion phase, it is reasonable to monitor arterial O_2 saturation and avoid hyperoxygenation.

Because unconscious patients after ROSC require high levels of care, prognostication with high predictive accuracy is desirable as early as possible so that futile efforts can be discontinued. Before the introduction of therapeutic hypothermia, absence of corneal or pupillary light reflexes, motor response to pain no better than extension, bilateral absence of somatosensory evoked potentials, or high levels of neuron-specific enolase and protein S-100B 48 to 72 h after cardiac arrest have been used as prognosticators for poor outcome (severe brain damage, permanent coma, or death) with 100% specificity and tight confidence intervals. Studies from the hypothermia era are sparse, but data so far indicate that futility decisions are more difficult and should probably not be undertaken until 72 h after rewarming in still-comatose patients. Self-fulfilling prophecies might lead to early treatment withdrawal in potentially successful survivors.

Suggested Readings

Abella BS, Alvarado JP, Myklebust H, et al. Quality of cardiopulmonary resuscitation during in-hospital cardiac arrest. *JAMA*. 2005;293:305-310.

El-Menyar AA. The resuscitation outcome: Revisit the story of the stony heart. *Chest*. 2005;128:2835-2846.

Go AS, Mozaffarian D, Roger VL, et al. Heart disease and stroke statistics – 2013 Update. A report from the American Heart Association. *Circulation*. 2013; 127:e6-e245.

Kim F, Nichol G, Maynard C, et al. Effect of prehospital induction of mild hypothermia on survival and neurological status among adults with cardiac arrest: A randomized clinical trial. *JAMA*. 2014;311:45-52.

Nielsen N, Wetterslev J, Cronberg T, et al. Targeted temperature management at 33°C versus 36°C after cardiac arrest. *N Engl J Med*. 2013;369:2197-2206.

Rea TD, Eisenberg MS, Sinibaldi G, White RD. Incidence of EMS-treated out-of-hospital cardiac arrest in the United States. *Resuscitation*. 2004;63:17-24.

Sunde K, Pytte M, Jacobsen D, et al. Implementation of a standardised treatment protocol for post resuscitation care after out-of-hospital cardiac arrest. *Resuscitation*. 2007;73:29-39.

Travers AH, Rea TD, Bobrow BJ, et al. Part 4: CPR overview: 2010 American Heart Association Guidelines for Cardiopulmonary Resuscitation and Emergency Cardiovascular Care. *Circulation*. 2010;122(18 Suppl 3):S676-684.

CHAPTER 223

Positive-Pressure Mechanical Ventilation

Edmund Carton, MD

Many advances have occurred in intraoperative mechanical ventilation (MV) in the past 5 decades. Multiple modes of ventilatory support can now be delivered by microprocessor-driven mechanical ventilators. Closed-loop technology can provide protective ventilatory strategies with low total gas flows. N_2O, He, or air may be added to O_2, and the inspired gas and inhaled anesthetic agents are delivered by electronic flowmeters. Contemporary airway circuit technology allows efficient CO_2 absorption and improved scavenging. There are also alarm systems for multiple parameters including end-tidal carbon dioxide ($ETCO_2$), tidal volume (V_T), respiratory rate, minute ventilation, fraction of inspired O_2 (FIO_2), and airway pressure to ensure adequate O_2 delivery and ventilation.

In addition to these industry-derived improvements, our understanding of intraoperative changes in respiratory mechanics has also improved so that appropriate MV settings can be used in patients with airflow obstruction or lung or chest wall abnormalities. Recent concern about the risk of developing acute lung injury in previously healthy patients after intraoperative MV is also discussed in this chapter. A list of the abbreviations for terms commonly used in respiratory physiology is provided in Box 223-1.

Respiratory Mechanics

Two independent patient-related forces have to be overcome to achieve lung inflation by positive-pressure MV (Figure 223-1): (1) resistance to the flow of gases within the airway and (2) compliance and elastance of the lung and chest wall, respectively. The latter concept can be difficult for the anesthesia provider to understand. In an inflated lung, the elastin within the lung is stretched. If you then remove a lung from the thoracic cavity and if the airway is open, the lung will collapse. This does not happen within the thoracic cavity because the parietal pleura is adherent to the thoracic cavity. In an intubated paralyzed patient at end expiration, or when the lungs are at their functional residual capacity, positive pressure must be applied to expand the lungs to deliver a breath. The amount of pressure (plateau pressure [Pplat]) applied to expand the lungs to a known volume is a measure of the compliance of the lung (Compliance = $\Delta V/\Delta P$). For example, 5 cm of H_2O pressure in a patient with a V_T of 500 would equal a compliance of 100. In a patient with a diseased lung (e.g., with severe acute respiratory distress syndrome), the compliance would typically be less than 20.

Box 223-1 List of Abbreviations Used in Respiratory Physiology

$ETCO_2$: end-tidal CO_2
f: frequency, or respiratory rate (number of breaths per minute)
FIO_2: fractional inspired O_2 concentration (100% O_2: FIO_2 = 1.0)
I:E ratio: ratio of inspiratory time to expiratory time
MV: mechanical ventilation
PBW: predicted body weight based on sex and height:
 Female patients: 45.5 + 0.89 (height in cm – 152.4)
 Male patients: 48.2 + 1.07 (height in cm – 152.4)
PEEP: positive end-expiratory pressure
Ppeak: peak airway pressure
Pplat: plateau airway pressure (end-inspiratory hold or pause pressure)
SaO_2: O_2 saturation of arterial blood
TE: expiratory time
TI: inspiratory time
Ttot: total cycle time
VT: tidal volume

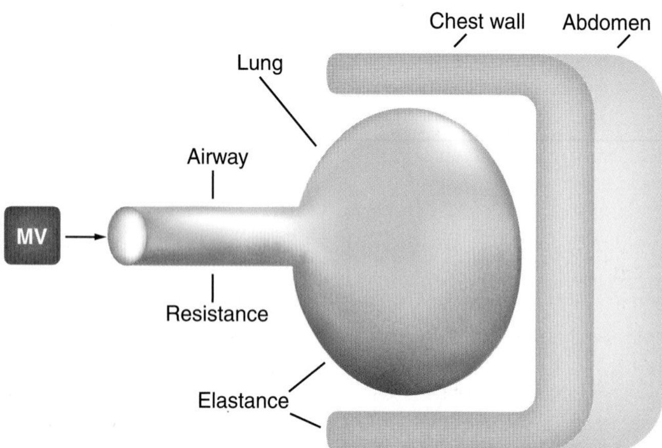

Figure 223-1 Schematic of respiratory system showing the components of respiratory system impedance (resistance plus-elastance or compliance). MV, Mechanical ventilation.

The reciprocal of compliance, elastance, is defined as the ΔP/ΔV and is more commonly used to describe the pressure-volume relationships within the thoracic cavity. Unlike the lung, which collapses if opened, the chest wall or cavity would expand if opened.

Taken together the resistive and elastic properties (also referred to as compliance) of the lung and chest wall make up the patient-related *impedance* during any mode of positive-pressure inspiration. During each MV inflation, a dynamic interaction occurs between these patient-related variables (airway, lung, and chest wall) and MV settings (VT, airway pressure, and inspiratory flow). Airway pressure is equal to the sum of the pressure required to overcome the resistive component of the respiratory system (influenced by airway resistance and inspiratory flow) plus the pressure required to overcome the elastic component of the respiratory system (influenced by lung compliance, chest wall elastance, and VT):

$$\text{Airway pressure} = (\text{Resistance} \times \text{Flow}) + (\text{Compliance} \times V_T)$$

Mode of Mechanical Ventilation

In contemporary mechanical ventilators, microprocessor-controlled valves rapidly adjust airflow and pressure during inspiration to achieve the desired lung inflation. Conventional intraoperative MV usually provides complete ventilatory support (control ventilation) when the patient is expected to have no spontaneous ventilatory effort. The common modes of intraoperative ventilatory support include *volume* control or *vv* control at respiratory rates less than 60 breaths/min.

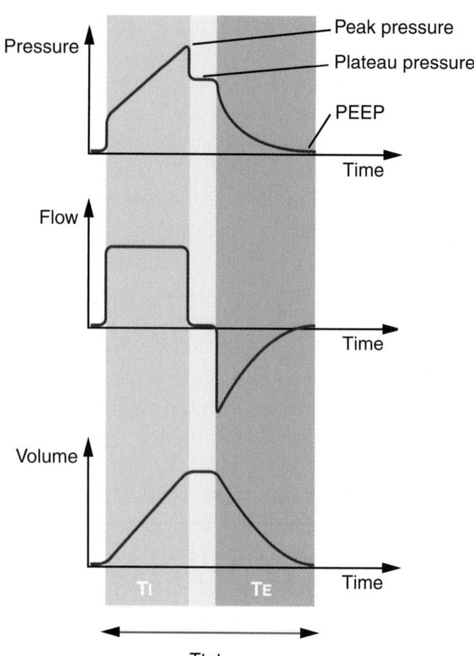

Figure 223-2 Volume-control mechanical ventilation: pressure, flow, and volume are plotted against time. Peak pressure, plateau pressure, positive end-expiratory pressure (PEEP), inspiratory time (TI), expiratory time (TE) and total cycle time (Ttot) are shown.

Volume Control Mechanical Ventilation

During volume control mode, VT and TI (or respiratory rate and inspiratory: expiratory [I:E] ratio) are set by the clinician and inspiratory flow remains constant (Figure 223-2). In volume control MV, the resistive impedance (transmission of the VT through the airway) and the elastic impedance (compliance of the lung or chest wall) both contribute to the peak airway pressure (Ppeak).

A short end-inspiratory pause may be included in the respiratory cycle in volume control MV so that, after the VT has been fully delivered and just prior to exhalation, airflow is reduced to zero for a fixed proportion of TI. The airway pressure recorded during this end-inspiratory interval is called the plateau (Pplat), pause, or end-inspiratory hold pressure (see Figure 223-2). In many anesthesia ventilators, the default setting in volume control mode may include no end-inspiratory pause so that only Ppeak is recorded. However, it is always possible (and desirable) to include an end-inspiratory pause when using volume control MV so that both Ppeak and Pplat are recorded.

In contrast to Ppeak, which is influenced by both resistive and elastic components, Pplat is influenced only by compliance factors, as there is no resistive contribution during zero-flow conditions. When we use volume control MV and include an end-inspiratory pause, Pplat provides a more accurate estimate of the maximal distending pressure inside the alveolar sac than does Ppeak.

Pressure Control Mechanical Ventilation

In pressure control MV, inspiratory pressure and TI (or respiratory rate and I:E ratio) are set by the clinician and remain constant, but the delivered VT and inspiratory flow will vary during inspiration (Figure 223-3). In pressure control MV, in which inspiratory pressure remains constant for the duration of TI, no Ppeak or end-inspiratory Pplat is registered (as occurs in volume control mode when an end-inspiratory pause is added into the respiratory cycle). Therefore, the relationship between Ppeak and Pplat that is informative in volume control MV cannot be used in pressure control MV.

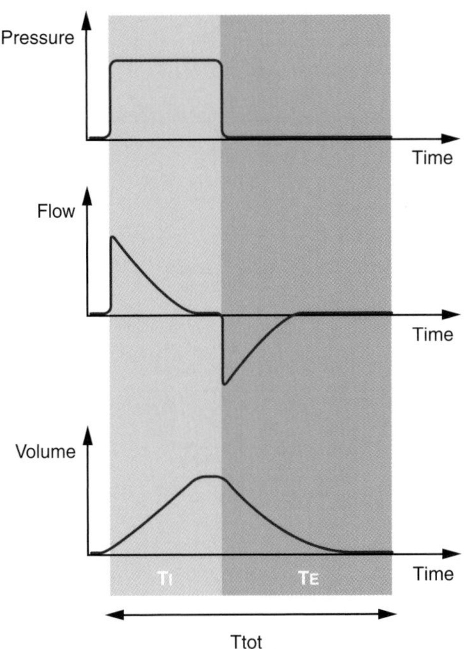

Figure 223-3 Pressure control mechanical ventilation: pressure, flow, and volume versus time. TE, Expiratory time; TI, inspiratory time; Ttot, total cycle time.

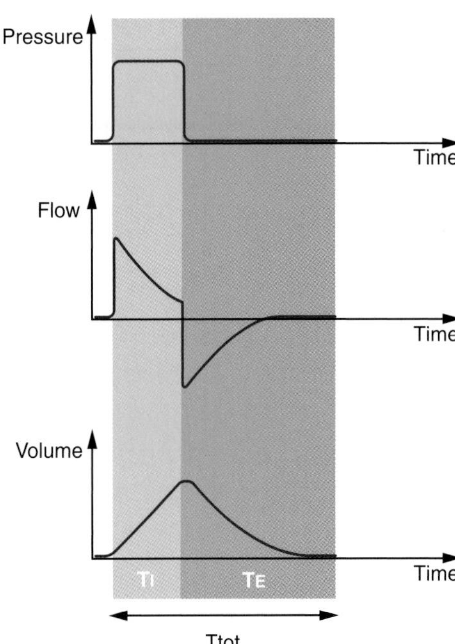

Figure 223-4 Pressure support mechanical ventilation: pressure, flow, and volume versus time. TE, Expiratory time; TI, inspiratory time; Ttot, total cycle time.

Intraoperative Mechanical Ventilation: Which Mode Should We Use?

No particular mode of ventilation (e.g., volume or pressure control mode) has been shown to be superior for any adult patient subgroup during intraoperative MV. It is more important to appreciate the limitations and the appropriate application of both volume and pressure control mode during intraoperative MV. Traditionally, volume control MV has been used intraoperatively in adult patients to maintain a secure minimum level of alveolar ventilation regardless of temporary changes in airway resistance or respiratory system compliance or elastance. When using volume control MV, an end-inspiratory pause should be routinely included in the respiratory cycle so that the distinction between increased airway resistance and decreased compliance can be observed. Pressure control MV could equally be used in adult patients as long as appropriate adjustments are made to MV settings with intraoperative changes in respiratory system mechanics.

Contemporary anesthetic machines now provide modes of ventilatory support similar to those used in critical care ventilators. Use of assisted (rather than control) modes of ventilatory support during a surgical procedure depends on the intraoperative conditions, patient-related factors (there is no difference between control mode and assisted mode if the patient has received a neuromuscular blocking agent and has a train-of-four of zero and therefore cannot initiate any respiratory effort), the airway device used, and the preference of the individual clinician involved. In pressure support mode, the ventilator delivers a constant inspiratory pressure until the ventilator cycles into expiration. The trigger to change from inspiration to expiration is when the inspiratory flow declines to a set proportion of peak inspiratory flow (Figure 223-4).

The VT and inspiratory flow will vary with each breath, depending on the patient effort and the prevailing respiratory system impedance. The patient must initiate all pressure support breaths and a mode of mandatory minute ventilation should always be used if the triggering of the pressure support breaths is unreliable for any reason.

Transpulmonary Pressure in Volume or Pressure Control Mechanical Ventilation

The transpulmonary pressure (also called transmural pressure), the maximal distending pressure for the alveolar sac, is the difference between maximal intraalveolar and extraalveolar pressure. In either volume or pressure control MV, transpulmonary pressures greater than 30 cm H_2O are associated with alveolar overdistention. The extraalveolar pressure is not usually measured in clinical practice but can be clinically estimated by the pleural pressure or by measuring esophageal balloon pressure.

During volume control MV, the maximal intraalveolar pressure is indicated by Pplat and the extraalveolar pressure in normal patients is considered close to atmospheric pressure so that transpulmonary pressure is reflected by Pplat alone. When extraalveolar pressure is thought to be elevated (e.g., pneumoperitoneum) a higher Ppeak and Pplat will be recorded, but the transpulmonary pressure (Pplat – pleural pressure) and the delivered VT will remain unchanged.

In pressure control MV, the maximal intraalveolar pressure is indicated by the inspiratory pressure set by the clinician. When extraalveolar pressure is close to atmospheric pressure, as in patients with normal respiratory dynamics, the transpulmonary pressure is reflected by the set inspiratory pressure alone. If pleural pressure is elevated (e.g., pneumoperitoneum), the transpulmonary pressure (constant set inspiratory pressure – pleural pressure) will be decreased, leading to a reduction in inspiratory flow and VT.

Inspiratory Time, Respiratory Rate, and I:E Ratio

On many anesthesia machine ventilators, respiratory rate and I:E ratio are adjusted directly by the clinician, and TI must be calculated. When the respiratory rate (f) is chosen, the total cycle time (Ttot) is easily calculated: Ttot = 60/f. Once Ttot is known, TI can be calculated from the I:E ratio.

Exhalation

The MV settings discussed thus far define only the inspiratory phase of ventilation. With anesthesia and neuromuscular blockade (no expiratory muscle activity), exhalation after a mechanical ventilator-delivered VT occurs passively and varies exponentially with time. Exhalation is dependent on the time constant of the patient's respiratory system (resistance and elastance or compliance) and the VT/TE settings on the ventilator. During one time constant, approximately two thirds of the expired

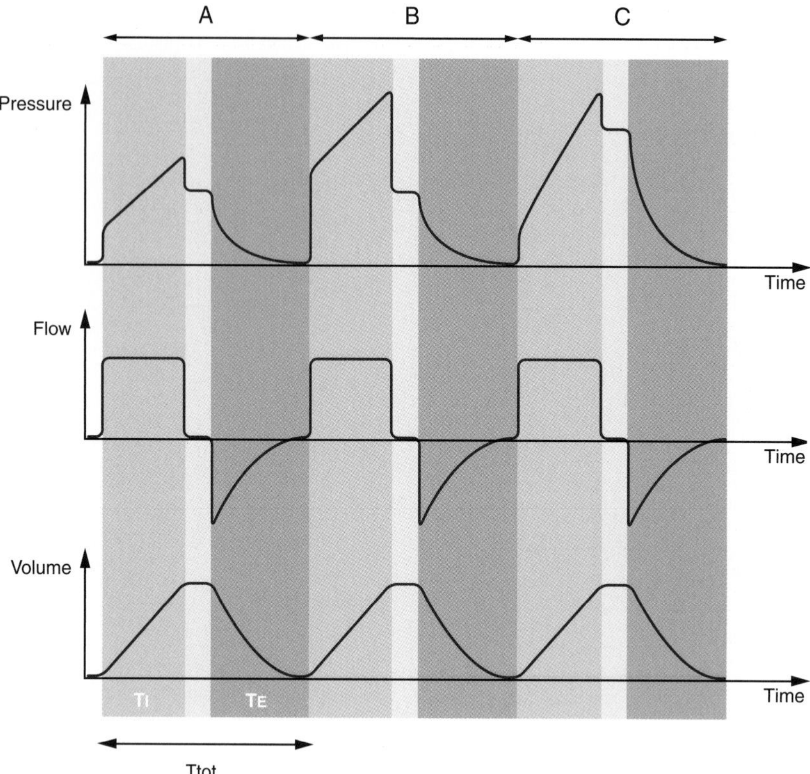

Figure 223-5 Volume control mechanical ventilation: pressure, flow, and volume versus time. **A,** Normal airway resistance, normal lung/chest wall/abdominal stiffness. **B,** Increased airway resistance, normal lung/chest wall/abdominal stiffness. **C,** Normal airway resistance, increased lung/chest wall/abdominal stiffness. TE, expiratory time; TI, inspiratory time; Ttot, total cycle time.

volume is exhaled. In patients with increased airway resistance and decreased elastance (e.g., emphysema) the time constant for exhalation will be prolonged.

Dynamic hyperinflation (also referred to as intrinsic or auto-positive end-expiratory pressure) occurs during MV, particularly in patients with airflow obstruction, when complete exhalation has not been achieved prior to delivery of the next mechanical inflation. The high intrathoracic pressure generated by dynamic hyperinflation has physiologic consequences (decreased venous return and cardiac output, increased risk of barotrauma, displacement of the diaphragm and inspiratory muscles from their optimal functional position) similar to those of high levels of externally applied positive end-expiratory pressure (PEEP).

At the end of expiration, airway pressure returns to atmospheric pressure or to a defined PEEP set by the clinician. In patients with hypoxic respiratory failure, PEEP helps to recruit collapsed or flooded lung units and improve oxygenation. In mechanically ventilated patients with chronic obstructive lung disease, PEEP reduces small-airway collapse during expiration in mechanically ventilated patients with emphysema, allowing more complete exhalation, and reduces the work of breathing in spontaneously breathing patients.

Clinical Application of Intraoperative Mechanical Ventilation

Even in previously healthy patients, anesthesia, neuromuscular blocking agents, and MV may lead to atelectasis with an increased venous admixture and dead space ventilation. The normal homogeneous pattern of ventilation/perfusion matching is disrupted, because of the regional differences in lung compliance due to atelectasis. In addition, tidal ventilation delivered by the MV as a uniform wave of positive airway pressure will be distributed primarily to the higher-compliance nonatelectic lung units.

In volume control MV, an increase in respiratory system impedance (either increased resistance or decreased compliance) will lead to the set VT being delivered during the set TI but at the expense of higher airway pressures. Importantly, an increase in airway resistance or decrease in lung compliance can be differentiated by observing the associated changes in Ppeak and Pplat. An increase in airway resistance is reflected by an increase in Ppeak with a relatively unchanged Pplat (Figure 223-5, *B*) so that the difference between Ppeak and Pplat is increased. In volume control MV, a decrease in lung compliance will increase both Ppeak and Pplat so that the difference between Ppeak and Pplat remains unchanged (Figure 223-5, C).

In pressure control MV (constant inspiratory pressure and TI), any increase in airway resistance or decrease in lung compliance will lead to a decrease in inspiratory flow and delivered VT (Figure 223-6). In contrast to volume control MV, in pressure control MV, there is no way of identifying which factor (airway resistance or lung compliance) is responsible for the decrease in alveolar ventilation.

Mechanical Ventilation in Patients with Airway Obstruction

During volume control MV in patients with airflow obstruction, Ppeak and the difference between Ppeak and Pplat can be increased, but the delivered VT remains constant, and there is no change in the transpulmonary pressure. During pressure control MV in patients with airflow obstruction, the achieved VT can be reduced, and, if so, an increase in the set inspiratory pressure or TI should be considered.

During any mode of MV, if an increase in airway resistance is suspected (increase Ppeak but relatively unchanged Pplat during volume control MV or a decrease in achieved VT during pressure control MV), an immediate examination (including passage of a suction catheter) of the patency and position of the tracheal tube or for the presence of bronchospasm should be performed.

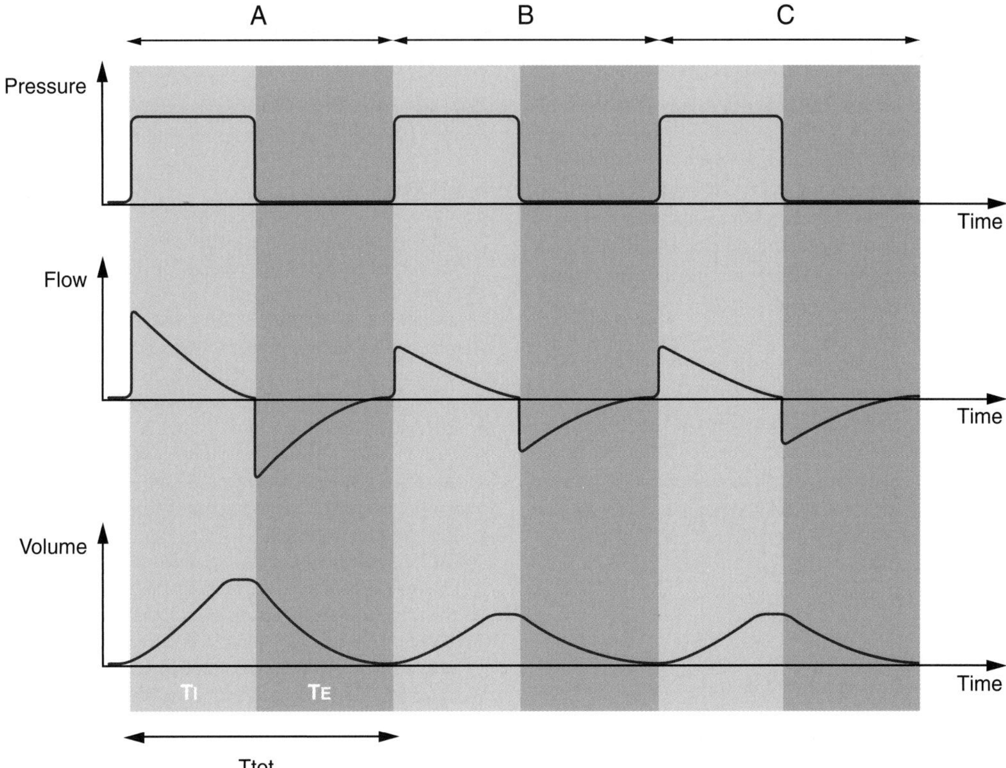

Figure 223-6 Pressure control mechanical ventilation: pressure, flow, and volume versus time. **A,** Normal airway resistance, normal chest wall/abdominal stiffness. **B,** Increased airway resistance, normal chest wall/abdominal stiffness. **C,** Normal airway resistance, increased chest wall/abdominal stiffness. TE, Expiratory time; TI, inspiratory time; Ttot, total cycle time.

Regardless of the mode of MV in patients with airflow obstruction, the expiratory time constant will be prolonged because of the increased airway resistance. The incomplete exhalation prior to delivery of the next scheduled MV breath leads to breathstacking or dynamic hyperinflation. An important MV goal in patients with airflow obstruction is to maintain the lowest end-expiratory volume.

Ventilator adjustments designed to minimize dynamic hyperinflation include reducing VT and extending TE. Extending TE is primarily achieved by decreasing the respiratory rate. Additional measures include increasing inspiratory flow or decreasing the I:E ratio, which will inevitably increase inspiratory pressures and achieve only a modest prolongation of TE. These changes in MV settings will lead to a reduction in minute ventilation, but the resultant respiratory acidosis is generally well tolerated.

Mechanical Ventilation in Patients with Decreased Respiratory Compliance

During volume control MV in patients with decreased compliance of the lung, both Ppeak and Pplat are elevated, and the difference between them remains unaltered. The set VT is delivered unchanged at the expense of higher airway pressures. During pressure control MV, the achieved VT and inspiratory flow are reduced despite the constant inspiratory pressure during the set TI.

An unusual feature of intraoperative MV is that there may be transient but significant changes in chest wall or abdominal elastance during the course of the operation (e.g., head-down position, insufflation of CO_2 into the peritoneum or hemithorax for laparoscopic procedures). These intraoperative events are associated with significant changes in pleural (and extraalveolar) pressure.

During volume control MV, the increased Ppeak and Pplat (and unchanged gap between them) associated with an abrupt increase in pleural pressure is not associated with an increased risk of barotrauma because the transpulmonary pressure (Pplat – pleural pressure) is unchanged and the set VT is not reduced. When the pleural pressure is decreased to normal (e.g., deflation of pneumoperitoneum), the Pplat and pleural pressure will return to their original settings with no change in the delivered VT.

During pressure control MV, an abrupt increase in pleural pressure (e.g., pneumoperitoneum) will lead to a reduction in the achieved VT but an unchanged airway pressure tracing on the monitor. The decrease in VT will be indicated by an increase in $ETCO_2$, and a decrease in VT and minute ventilation. Under these circumstances, it is appropriate to increase the inspiratory pressure or TI to restore minute ventilation to its prior level. Again, this increase in inspired pressure will not be associated with barotrauma because the transpulmonary pressure (inspired pressure – pleural pressure) remains unchanged. When the pleural pressure is returned to normal, the inspired pressure should also be reduced to achieve an appropriate VT.

Intraoperative Mechanical Ventilation and Acute Lung Injury

MV has been used to ensure satisfactory gas exchange during general anesthesia for decades. In 1963, Bendixen and associates advocated using a high VT (>10 mL/kg predicted body weight [PBW]) during intraoperative MV to reduce atelectasis, and this practice has continued almost unchanged until recently. Over the same time period, robust evidence has been accumulated for the existence of ventilator-induced lung injury. In the critical care setting, it has now become widely accepted to use protective lung ventilation settings in patients with acute respiratory distress syndrome.

In the past 10 years, the risk of intraoperative MV settings inducing or predisposing previously healthy patients to similar lung injury has been hotly debated. Multiple studies in previously healthy surgical patients have demonstrated that, compared with high V_T (12-15 mL/kg PBW) MV, low V_T (6-8 mL/kg PBW) MV is associated with the generation of lower levels of proinflammatory biomarkers. Perioperative patients at increased risk of developing acute lung injury (sepsis, shock states, multiple trauma and blood transfusion, patients undergoing high-risk operations) should be identified, and recent reviews support using protective ventilation settings in these patients during intraoperative MV. Measures commonly employed include low V_T (6-8 mL/kg PBW), maintaining Pplat less than 30 cm H_2O if pleural pressure is normal, use of PEEP and recruitment maneuvers, reduced F_{IO_2}, and permissive hypercapnia.

In previously healthy patients at low risk of developing acute lung injury and having elective surgical procedures with a short period (<5 h) of MV, there is little evidence to guide optimal intraoperative MV settings. Some authors suggest that it is reasonable to apply protective MV settings in all patients to avoid sensitizing the lung to any further potential injury. In the face of the very many patients having uneventful intraoperative MV, other authors have questioned whether protective MV settings are necessary or indeed feasible for all patients.

Summary

The improvements in intraoperative ventilatory equipment and a better understanding of the important changes in respiratory mechanics during anesthesia and surgery have led to a more focused clinical application of intraoperative MV. In each mode of MV, it is important to recognize which MV parameters will remain constant and which parameters will change when alterations in airway resistance or lung compliance occur intraoperatively. In patients at risk of developing acute lung injury, protective MV settings should be used intraoperatively. Several ongoing studies may give us more clarity about the place of protective MV settings in healthy patients undergoing elective procedures.

Suggested Readings

Bendixen HH, Hedley-Whyte J, Laver MB. Impaired oxygenation in surgical patients during general anesthesia with controlled ventilation. A concept of atelectasis. *N Engl J Med.* 1963;269:991-996.

Hubmayr RD. Point: Is low tidal volume mechanical ventilation preferred for all patients on ventilation? Yes. *Chest.* 2011;140:9-11.

Hubmayr RD, Abel MD, Rehder K. Physiologic approach to mechanical ventilation. *Crit Care Med.* 1990;18:103-113.

Kilpatrick B, Slinger P. Lung protective strategies in anaesthesia. *Br J Anaesth.* 2010;105:108-116.

Lellouche F, Lipes J. Prophylactic protective ventilation: Lower tidal volumes for all critically ill patients? *Intensive Care Med.* 2013;39:6-15.

Marini JJ. Lower tidal volumes for everyone: Principle or prescription? *Intensive Care Med.* 2013;39:3-5.

The Acute Respiratory Distress Syndrome Network. Ventilation with lower tidal volumes as compared to traditional tidal volumes for acute lung injury and the acute respiratory distress syndrome. *N Engl J Med.* 2000;342:1301-1308.

Tremblay LN, Slutsky AS. Ventilator-induced lung injury: From the bench to the bedside. *Intensive Care Med.* 2006;321:24-33.

Wolthuis EK, Choi G, Dessing MC, et al. Mechanical ventilation with lower tidal volumes and positive end-expiratory pressure prevents pulmonary inflammation in patients without preexisting lung injury. *Anesthesiology.* 2008; 108:46-54.

CHAPTER 224

Hyperbaric Oxygen Therapy

Klaus D. Torp, MD, Neil G. Feinglass, MD, FASE, FCCP, and Timothy S.J. Shine, MD

Hyperbaric O_2 therapy (HBOT) refers to the inhalation of 100% O_2 in an environment in which the barometric pressure is greater than 1 atmosphere. Note that 1 atmosphere absolute (ATA) is the pressure at sea level. For every increase in ambient pressure of 760 mm Hg, or 14.7 psi or 33 feet of seawater, the pressure increases by 1 ATA. Exposure to increased gas pressures can occur in other situations, such as breathing compressed gas mixtures while diving (scuba) or working in underground tunnels (caisson workers). For HBOT, the pressure in a hyperbaric chamber is typically at least 1.4 ATA.

All gases follow fundamental gas laws:

Boyle's law: A volume of gas is inversely proportional to pressure at a constant temperature:

$$PV = k$$

where P is absolute pressure, V is volume, and k is a constant representative of the pressure and volume of the system.

Dalton's law: The total pressure of a mixture of gases is equal to the sum of the partial pressures of the component gases.

Henry's law: At constant temperature, the amount of gas dissolved in a liquid is directly proportional to the partial pressure of that gas in equilibrium with the liquid.

In clinical medicine, the liquid of interest is blood and the dissolved gas is O_2. The driving pressure of O_2 into blood is the partial pressure of O_2 in alveoli (P_{AO_2}). Note that it is the partial pressure of O_2 and not the percentage of O_2 that is responsible for its effects (Table 224-1). As the Pa_{O_2} increases in arterial blood, the saturation of hemoglobin approaches 100% (at Pa_{O_2} ~100 mm Hg). Above this level, all additional

Table 224-1 Expected Gas Tensions and Arterial Blood O_2 Content at Various Ambient Pressures in a Normal Individual*

Atm	FIO_2	Inspired PO_2 (mm Hg)	PAO_2 (mm Hg)	PaO_2 (mm Hg)	CaO_2 (mL/dL)		$PaCO_2$ (mm Hg)
					Total	Dissolved	
1	0.21	150	102	87	18.7	0.3	40
1	1.0	713	673	572	21.2	1.7	40
2	1.0	1473	1433	1218	23.1	3.7	40
3	1.0	2233	2193	1864	25.1	5.6	40
6	0.21	898	848	>750	21.8	2.3	40

*Hemoglobin = 14 g/dL.
Modified, with permission, from Moon RE, Camporesi EM. Clinical care in altered environments: At high and low pressure and in space. In: Miller RD, ed. Anesthesia. 6th ed. Philadelphia: Churchill Livingstone; 2005:2665-2701.

O_2-carrying capacity of blood comes from the oxygen dissolved in the plasma. HBOT can therefore increase O_2 content in the face of severe anemia and increase O_2 delivery in areas of partial obstruction to blood flow. In addition, the increased barometric pressure can reduce intravascular air bubbles in patients with decompression sickness or air embolism, improving perfusion and increasing the removal of N from the blood (Figure 224-1).

The effectiveness of HBOT has been established for several indications, and the basic mechanisms for its effect on the body have been demonstrated. Table 224-2 lists conditions that are recommended for HBOT by the Undersea and Hyperbaric Medical Society, as well as those that are reimbursed by the Centers for Medicare and Medicaid Services. For any other indications, one should first examine how the basic mechanisms of HBOT (Box 224-1) will affect the underlying pathophysiology of the disease.

Effects of Hyperbaric Oxygen

Pulmonary Effects

A high PO_2 is thought to overcome the body's scavenging system for free radicals, resulting in the formation of reactive O_2 species, such as superoxides, hydrogen peroxide, and hydroxyl radicals. Reactive O_2 species can cause pulmonary O_2 toxicity symptoms, such as retrosternal burning, coughing, and fibrosis and can lead to a measurable decrease in vital capacity. The pulmonary toxicity is dependent upon duration and PO_2, and its effect is cumulative. Most HBOT protocols reduce toxicity by introducing room air breaks between O_2 treatment periods.

Central Nervous System Effects

HBOT decreases cerebral blood flow that, in turn, decreases intracranial pressure and central nervous system (CNS) edema formation by up to 20%. CNS toxicity manifests when breathing 100% O_2 at approximately 3 ATA at rest (or less at exercise). Common signs and symptoms of toxicity include nausea, facial numbness, facial twitching, and unpleasant taste or smell. Unrecognized CNS toxicity can progress to full tonic/clonic seizures.

Cardiovascular Effects

A PaO_2 above 1500 mm Hg can increase systemic vascular resistance and peripheral blood pressure, with a resultant reflex bradycardia. Flow to the periphery is reduced; however, total O_2 delivery to tissues is markedly increased. Diffusion of O_2 away from the vascular bed into the tissues is greatly enhanced, which is the basis for most of the indications for HBOT. Pulmonary vascular resistance is decreased under hyperbaric conditions.

Effects on Air-Containing Cavities

Nasal sinuses, the middle ear, and noncommunicating pulmonary bullae may be affected by the pressure changes in a HBOT chamber.

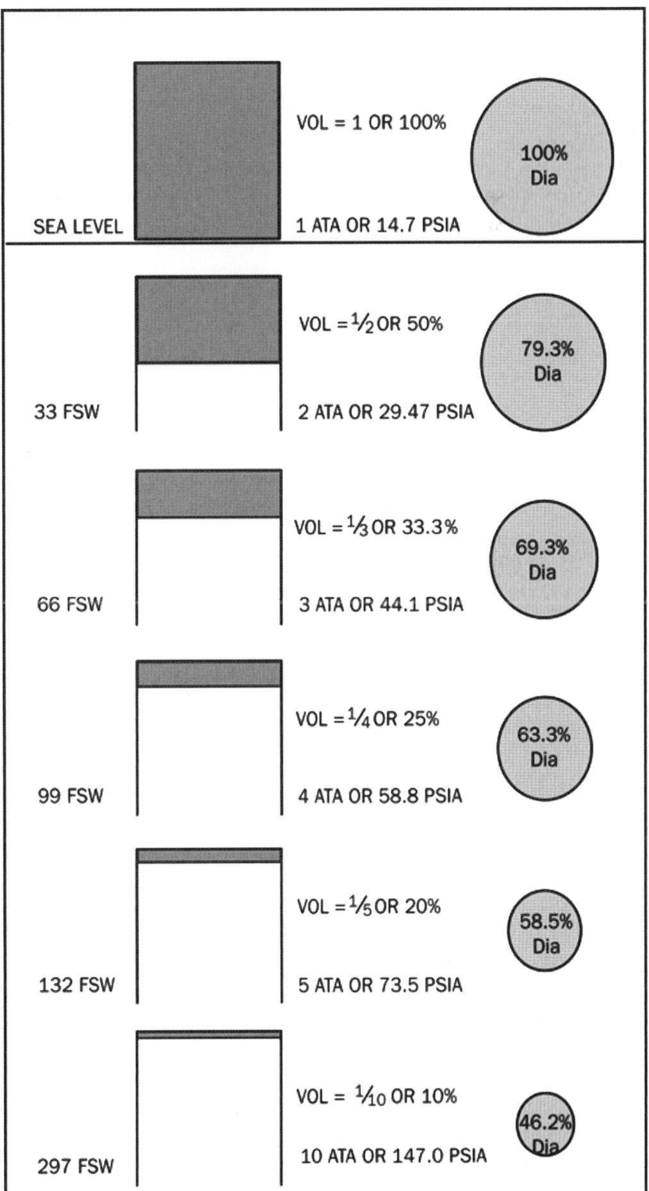

Figure 224-1 Gas volume (Vol) and bubble size as a function of depth: Boyle's law. ATA, Atmosphere(s) absolute pressure; Dia, diameter; FSW, feet of sea water; PSIA, pounds per square inch absolute.

Table 224-2 Recommended (UHMS) and Reimbursed (CMS) Indications for Hyperbaric O_2 Therapy

Indication	UHMS	CMS
Air or gas embolism	X	X
Carbon monoxide poisoning	X	X
Carbon monoxide poisoning complicated by cyanide poisoning	X	X
Clostridial myositis and myonecrosis (gas gangrene)	X	X
Crush injury, compartment syndrome, and other acute traumatic ischemias	X	X
Decompression sickness	X	X
Enhancement of healing in selected problem wounds	X	
Exceptional blood loss (anemia)	X	
Intracranial abscess	X	
Necrotizing soft tissue infections	X	X
Osteomyelitis (refractory)	X	X
Delayed radiation injury (soft tissue and bony necrosis)	X	X
Skin grafts and flaps (compromised)	X	X
Thermal burns	X	
Acute peripheral arterial insufficiency	X	X
Refractory actinomycosis		X
Diabetic wounds of the lower extremities in patients who meet certain criteria		X
Idiopathic Sudden Sensorineural Hearing Loss	X	
Central Retinal Artery Occlusion	X	

CMS, Centers for Medicare and Medicaid Services; UHMS, Undersea and Hyperbaric Medical Society.

Box 224-1 Basic Mechanisms of Hyperbaric O_2 Therapy

Hyperoxygenation
Vasoconstriction
Neovascularization
Increasing pressure and gas gradients (to decrease bubble size and increase off-gassing of bubble content)
Altering cellular functions, such as inhibiting β_2-integrin molecules on white blood cells or increasing killing power of neutrophils by increasing O_2 radicals

Middle ear barotrauma is the most common problem but highly variable with 2% to 45%. Nonsurgical therapies are usually effective, but myringotomy tubes may be needed. Pulmonary barotrauma is a rare complication, that may need needle or chest tube decompression.

Effects on Blood Sugar

In patients with diabetes, HBOT may lead to a drop in blood sugar, which should be monitored before and after each hyperbaric treatment.

Anesthetic Management in an HBOT Chamber

Provision of general anesthesia in a hyperbaric chamber is rare. Potential indications include double-lung lavage and emergent surgical procedures in patients who cannot be brought out of the chamber in a timely manner. The anesthesia provider may, however, be called for airway management or to sedate and provide support for critically ill patients. All personnel have to be pressure tested and properly trained before entering an HBOT chamber. The induction of anesthesia by inhalation agents depends on the partial pressure of those agents in the brain, not on the concentration that is inhaled. If 1.1 minimum alveolar concentration (MAC) of isoflurane (about 8 mm Hg) produces anesthesia at sea level (1 ATA), then the same effect will be produced by 0.33 MAC of isoflurane at 3 ATA because partial pressure of the drug in the alveoli and brain will still be 8 mm Hg.

Increasing pressure on variable bypass vaporizers leads to a decrease in the concentration of anesthetic agent leaving the vaporizer, but, because nearly the same partial pressure of agent in the CNS is produced, the clinical changes are imperceptible. A vaporizer with a heating element should not be taken into an HBOT chamber. Nitrous oxide has been used successfully in a hyperbaric chamber before, but should be avoided, because of it's increased solubility and the complex changes in pressure and breathing gases in a hyperbaric chamber. Total intravenous anesthesia is preferred over the use of inhalation anesthetic agents in an HBOT chamber because total intravenous anesthesia requires less equipment and eliminates pollution of the HBOT chamber with anesthetic gases. Regional anesthesia is also a very good choice, but the local anesthetic agent should be devoid of any air bubbles when injected.

Increased gas density caused by the increase in atmospheric pressure decreases flow through rotameter flowmeters, leading to falsely high readings under hyperbaric conditions. Gas cylinders should function normally but are usually not found inside an HBOT chamber.

Anesthesia equipment needs to be rated for use in an HBOT chamber because it may not function normally. Cuffs on tracheal tubes and intravenous and bladder catheters should be filled with fluid. Air-filled cuffs will undergo large volume changes with changes in pressure, as will drip chambers on intravenous lines, which require frequent observation during pressure changes to rapidly identify air and avoid an intravenous air embolus. Mechanical ventilators should be rated for use in an HBOT chamber or, at the least, tested for accuracy and safety under pressure. Petroleum-based lubricants and alcohol must be avoided because they are a fire hazard in an O_2-enriched environment.

Suggested Readings

Moon RE, Camporesi EM. Clinical care in altered environments: At high and low pressure and in space. In: Miller RD, ed. *Miller's Anesthesia*, 7 ed. Philadelphia: Churchill Livingstone; 2010:2485-2502.

Neuman TS, Thom SR, eds. *Physiology and Medicine of Hyperbaric Oxygen Therapy*. Philadelphia: Saunders Elsevier; 2008.

Weaver LK, ed. *Hyperbaric Oxygen Therapy Indications*. 13th ed. North Palm Beach, FL: Best Publishing Co.; 2014.

CHAPTER 225

Nutrition Support in the Hospitalized Patient

Nichole T. Townsend, RN, MD, and Michael J. Murray, MD, PhD

Most patients, and certainly critically ill patients, almost by definition, are catabolic and often hypermetabolic. Although the medical team often orders early nutrition support, it has recently been found that only approximately 50% of the calories prescribed are being delivered to patients during their first 2 weeks of care in the intensive care unit (ICU). However, a number of relatively new recommendations based on recent clinical trials have been made to provide specific nutrients at a particular time and dose during a patient's hospital course to reduce their risk of infection, improve their physiologic function, and, above all, save lives. These recent trials also emphasize that clinicians should view some of these nutrients not as "food," but as drugs—nutraceuticals—and administer them accordingly.

Feeding the Critically Ill: the When and How

Malnutrition that occurs among hospitalized patients is associated with an increased risk of complications and hospital costs, with as many as 40% to 50% of hospitalized patients being malnourished. This is often confounded by the old adage of nil per os (NPO) following surgery until the patient's bowel sounds and function return. An overwhelming amount of data now indicate that this practice likely worsens patient outcomes, including survival.

Based on expert opinion, current guidelines recommend that feedings should start early when patients are admitted to the ICU—as soon as the patient has been initially resuscitated and stabilized. There are no prospective randomized controlled studies to support early feedings, although several studies have shown a blunted catabolic response and a correlation with early feedings and patient outcomes; however, correlation does not prove cause and effect.

Shock, severe illness, starvation, trauma, and the use of total parenteral nutrition (TPN) are associated with changes in the small intestine, resulting in villous and mucosal atrophy and concomitant changes in permeability, potentially allowing for translocation of bacteria. There is no doubt that, if the gastrointestinal (GI) tract is patent, enteral nutrition is the route of choice for providing nutrients.

If the GI tract is not patent, TPN should be started at some point in time. A recent large study demonstrated that patients for whom enteral feedings were inadequate to meet caloric goals had better outcomes if TPN was started 8 days after, as opposed to within 48 h of, admission to the ICU. The late-initiation group had fewer infections and fewer days on mechanical ventilatory support and on renal replacement therapy, if they required either of those therapies. At least in this patient group, supplying more calories parenterally early in the ICU stay did not correlate with better outcomes.

Other sequelae are associated with the route with which nutrition is delivered. Because it is relatively easier to overfeed with TPN than with enteral nutrition, the use of TPN is associated with cholestasis and fatty infiltration of the liver. Enteral feedings, on the other hand, release cholecystokinin, stimulating bile flow and decreasing the incidence of cholehepatic complications. Early enteral feeding has also been shown to attenuate the hormone response to inflammation. Despite early aggressive nutrition, as mentioned earlier, patients remain catabolic, and acute phase reactants (proteins) are synthesized at the expense of visceral protein; no currently available therapy has been demonstrated to completely reverse the decrease in lean mass (protein wasting) that occurs in catabolic patients.

Early enteral feeding may also have a protective effect on the gut by restoring GI blood flow, which is often compromised in critical illness. Trace elements are regulated via the GI tract, but it is not known if regulation continues when trace elements are given parenterally. TPN requires central venous access, which has its own mechanical and infectious hazards. The intravenous infusion of lipid emulsions has been associated with immunosuppression. The use of TPN is also associated with frequent severe metabolic changes, such as hyperglycemia, acid-base disturbances (hyperchloremic metabolic acidosis), and electrolyte abnormalities (hypophosphatemia due to the refeeding syndrome).

Most clinical evidence supports improved outcomes in patients fed enterally as opposed to parenterally. Though the benefit to enteral nutrition is thought by many to relate to its physiologic effect on the GI tract, it makes little difference whether it is the avoidance of problems associated with TPN, as opposed to any physiologic benefit of enteral nutrition. The adage "if the gut works, use it" still holds.

Enteral nutrition should ideally be administered through a feeding tube passed through the pylorus beginning within the first 24 to 36 h of critically ill patients' admission. When being fed enterally, the patient should have the head of the bed elevated to at least 30 degrees, and residual feeding volumes in the stomach should be assessed on a regular basis—every 4 h initially and then changing to every 8 h when the patient's condition is stable. Depending on where the patient is hospitalized and the institution's practices, residual volumes of 200 to 500 mL result in holding the feeding for 1 to 4 h and restarting the feedings at a lower rate.

Nutrition Goals

Protein

Although numerous studies have been conducted comparing intravenously administered amino acid supplementation with intravenously administered saline, no statistically significant difference in the rate of protein synthesis between the groups has been found. In critically ill patients, even patients in renal failure—if critically ill—should receive 1.0 to 1.4 g of protein per kilogram per day.

Branched-Chain Amino Acids

Some patients with hepatic encephalopathy have an improvement in mental status with the administration of products containing an increased concentration of branched-chain amino acids (valine, leucine, isoleucine) as their protein source.

Arginine

If augmented in patients who have had traumatic injury, arginine, another essential amino acid, is associated with a reduction in infection rates and shortened length of stay.

Glutamine

Glutamine is an amino acid that serves as a precursor for a number of biochemicals that serve important physiologic functions, most notably as a precursor for glutathione (antioxidant) and as fuel for the endothelium in the GI tract. A recent meta-analysis demonstrated a reduction in mortality rates in ICU patients who received glutamine, regardless of admission diagnosis. The optimal dose of glutamine has been found to be 0.3 to 0.5 g/kg per day to improve patient survival.

Box 225-1 Recommendations for Nutrition Support in Patients in the Intensive Care Unit

Critically ill patients have increased nutrient requirements and are hypermetabolic.
Improved clinical outcomes as a result of nutrition support have been inadequately studied.
Nutrition should be instituted in patients not expected to resume oral feeding for 7 to 10 days.
Trauma patients who are enterally fed have fewer complications than do those who are parenterally fed.
No conclusions can be reached regarding the efficiency of specialized substances and formulas.

Carbohydrate

Glucose remains the most physiologic and most widely used carbohydrate. There is no difference in oxidative rate between patients receiving 4 g/kg per day of 20% D-glucose and patients receiving fewer grams of glucose per day. Although fructose is not used in the United States, the administration of fructose as a parenteral carbohydrate source remains a clinical option in Europe because of an associated reduction in adverse effects with its use.

Lipids

Whole-body lipolysis rates are decreased with the administration of a mixture of medium-chain and long-chain triglycerides, compared with only long-chain triglycerides. Patients who receive no lipids develop a deficiency in the level of essential (ω-3 and ω-6) fatty acids, manifested by an exfoliative dermatitis.

The ω-3 fatty acids are precursors to eicosanoids that have anti-inflammatory properties, and their use is advocated for cardiac and neurologic benefits. The administration of a combination of ω-3 and ω-6 fatty acids is thought to be beneficial in patients with acute lung injury, though a recent prospective study by the ARDS Network failed to confirm this belief.

Specific Critical Illness

Participants at an intersociety (National Institutes of Health, American Society for Parenteral and Enteral Nutrition, and American Society for Clinical Nutrition) conference held in Bethesda, MD, in 1996 reviewed the available published data in reference to critical illness (trauma, sepsis, systemic inflammatory response syndrome, multiple organ dysfunction syndrome, burns, acute lung injury, acute renal failure). Despite the large volume of material reviewed, the nature of the majority of nutrition data led to remarkably scant conclusions (Box 225-1).

Guidelines recently released from the Society of Critical Care Medicine are more optimistic, and, fortunately, there are a few recently conducted, prospective, randomized, controlled studies to prove the efficacy of a more aggressive approach to nutrition support in hospitalized patients and, in particular, to patients who are critically ill.

Conclusions

Investigators continue to find improved outcomes by providing nutrition support to critically ill patients, especially to those patients who are malnourished at the time they are injured or develop an acute illness. Consensus has been reached that critically ill patients should be fed enterally rather than parenterally, that the makeup of the components of the nutrition-support formula plays a role, and that subgroups of patients would benefit from targeted nutrition-support therapies. Currently, more definitive recommendations for ICU patients await the completion of prospective, randomized, controlled studies of how best to feed critically ill patients.

Suggested Readings

Kerrie JP, Bagshaw SM, Brindley PG. Early versus late parenteral nutrition in the adult ICU: Feeding the patient or our conscience? *Can J Anaesth*. 2012; 59(5):494-498.

Klein S, Kinney J, Jeejeebhoy K, et al. Nutrition support in clinical practice: Review of published data and recommendations for future research directions. National Institutes of Health, American Society for Parenteral and Enteral Nutrition, and American Society for Clinical Nutrition. *JPEN*. 1997;21:133-156.

Martindale RG, McClave SA, Vanek VW, et al. Guidelines for the provision and assessment of nutrition support therapy in the adult critically ill patient: Society of Critical Care Medicine and American Society for Parenteral and Enteral Nutrition: Executive summary. *Crit Care Med*. 2009;37:1757-1761.

Ukleja A, Freeman KL, Gilbert K, et al. The Task Force on Standards for Nutrition Support: Adult Hospitalized Patients, and the American Society for Parenteral and Enteral Nutrition Board of Directors. Standards for nutrition support: Adult hospitalized patients. *Nutr Clin Pract*. 2010;25:403-414.

Wischmeyer P. Nutritional pharmacology in surgery and critical care: "You must unlearn what you have learned." *Curr Opin Anesth*. 2011;24:381-388.

CHAPTER 226

Perioperative Management of Blood Glucose

Aaron M. Joffe, DO, and Douglas B. Coursin, MD

Critical illness, anesthesia, and the metabolic stress of surgery result in neurohormone and metabolic dysregulation, leading to elevated rates of perioperative hyperglycemia. Although perioperative hyperglycemia was once believed to be a normal adaptive response supplying more substrate to stressed organs, it is now clear that outcomes are worse in patients who have hyperglycemia. Unfortunately, a dearth of direct evidence is available to guide anesthesia providers within the operating room as to what is an acceptable blood glucose level and how to achieve that level; most of the current recommendations are based on data extrapolated from studies of patients admitted to general medical or surgical wards or the intensive care unit.

The avoidance of hyperglycemia, hypoglycemia, loss of electrolytes, and loss of free water and the prevention of ketogenesis are the main goals of perioperative glycemic control. To accomplish these goals, consideration should be paid to the type of diabetes mellitus (DM) the patient has, the antecedent pharmacologic therapy of the DM, the degree of metabolic control prior to surgery, and the type and duration of the operation the patient is to undergo. A summary of this approach is presented in Table 226-1.

Preoperative Management of Glycemic Control

All oral agents should be held the day of surgery, and a preoperative blood glucose level obtained. In a stable nonhypotensive patient undergoing an elective procedure, a fingerstick point-of-care (POC) measurement will suffice (see later discussion under "Blood Glucose Measurement"). Patients whose DM is well controlled with diet and exercise alone do not require any special preoperative glucose intervention. Patients with type 2 DM not routinely treated with insulin, who exhibit fair chronic glycemic control (preoperative fasting glucose concentration 130-180 mg/dL) and who are undergoing minor operations, may not require insulin or can be given a small dose of rapid-acting insulin in the holding area. In patients with poorer glycemic control (preoperative fasting glucose concentration > 180 mg/dL), consideration should be given to providing a larger dose of rapid-acting insulin, particularly if the operation is expected to be short in duration. However, for longer operations and for those patients who will be admitted to the hospital for postoperative care, a continuous insulin infusion is recommended. Patients with type 1 and type 2 DM treated chronically with insulin who undergo minor operations and exhibit fair glycemic control may be given half of their intermediate-acting insulin the morning of surgery and may be supplemented with short-acting insulin if, for whatever reason, the preoperative holding time is extended and, thus, the patient is receiving nothing by mouth for longer than 4 to 6 h and a repeat glucose determination continues to indicate only fair glycemic control. Patients receiving insulin glargine should be given their usual basal dose, and those with a continuous insulin pump should be continued on their usual basal rate. Continuous insulin infusion is recommended when glycemic control is poor. All insulin-requiring patients with DM

Table 226-1 Perioperative Management of Patients with Diabetes Mellitus

Surgical Scenario	Fasting BGC	Treatment
Minor operation, patient has type 2 DM, NOT treated with insulin	All patients	Hold oral agents day of operation.
	<180 mg/dL*	Cover with regular or rapid-acting insulin (lispro, aspart, glulisine) as needed.
	>180 mg/dL†	Plan to initiate a continuous insulin infusion.
	All patients	Target BGC 80-180 mg/dL.
Minor operation, patient has type 1 or type 2 DM, treated with insulin	<180 mg/dL*	Give ½ of intermediate-acting insulin dose morning of operation.
		Consider adding 5% dextrose-containing solution to IV infusion with or without potassium, depending on starting lab values and time of NPO.
		Check serial BGC q4-6 h while patient is NPO and supplement with short-acting insulin.
		Those taking basal insulin, by injection or continuous pump, should receive their usual basal dose or infusion rate.
		Restart preadmission insulin therapy once oral intake tolerated.
	180 mg/dL†	Start continuous insulin infusion and check BGC q1-2 h.
Major operation, patient has type 1 or type 2 DM treated with insulin	All patients	Hold oral agents day of surgery.
		Start continuous insulin infusion in OR and continue postoperatively.
		Target BGC of 150 mg/dL; avoid hypoglycemia (<80 mg/dL).

*Fair control.
†Poor control.
BGC, Blood glucose concentration; DM, diabetes mellitus; NPO, nothing by mouth (*nil per os*); OR, operating room.
Adapted with permission from Smiley DD, Umpierrez GE. Perioperative glucose control in the diabetic or nondiabetic patient. South Med J. 2006;99:580-589.

undergoing major operations should be started on a continuous insulin infusion, as needed, after induction of anesthesia. Serial blood glucose levels should be monitored along with serum potassium, which may require supplementation.

Intraoperative Management of Glycemic Control

Current recommendations are based largely upon the understanding of physiologic derangements related to hyperglycemia and outcome studies in cardiac surgical and critically ill patients. The issue of what to do for many surgical patients undergoing noncardiac operations is further confounded by the wide range of targeted blood glucose concentrations among available studies (125-200 mg/dL, 100-150 mg/dL, 125-175 mg/dL, 150-200 mg/dL, <180 mg/dL, and 80-110 mg/dL), their control ranges (<250 mg/dL, ≤180 mg/dL, or <200 mg/dL), the population studied, and the constituents of the infusion itself. Some studies have employed a glucose-potassium-insulin mixture rather than insulin alone. To date, the results of only two prospective randomized trials of intraoperative glycemic control, both in patients undergoing cardiac operations, are available. One showed a decrease in the length of stay and the rate of postoperative arrhythmia, wound infections, and mortality rate at 2 years, whereas the other found no difference in a composite endpoint of death, sternal infections, prolonged mechanical ventilation, arrhythmia, stroke, and renal failure at 30 days. Data on intraoperative glucose control in noncardiac surgical patients are lacking. The result of this discordant information is a general recommendation to initiate insulin therapy when the plasma glucose concentration exceeds 180 mg/dL and to target a goal of approximately 150 mg/dL. Consensus is that such a target should minimize the potential for hypoglycemic episodes, which would be otherwise silent and potentially catastrophic in anesthetized patients. The reader should note that variation exists among guidelines from various organizations and such guidance may change in the future.

Postoperative Management of Glycemic Control

A recent consensus statement of the American Association of Clinical Endocrinologists and the American Diabetes Association recommends a premeal blood glucose concentration of less than 140 mg/dL and a random blood glucose concentration of less than 180 mg/dL for non–critically ill hospitalized patients. They further recommend that these targets be achieved and maintained with the use of scheduled subcutaneously administered insulin with basal, nutrition, and correction components. The use of "sliding-scale" insulin dosing as the sole insulin preparation or the administration of oral hypoglycemic agents is strongly discouraged. Although not identical, these recommendations are comparable with those published in 2007 by the American College of Endocrinology and in 2008 by the Canadian Diabetes Association and seem to be a justifiable goal in the postoperative period. Currently, there is no single universally accepted target for blood glucose control for all critically ill patients. Investigators who studied the morbidity and mortality benefits derived from intensive glucose control (80-110 mg/dL) in a predominantly postcardiac surgical population were unable to reproduce the results in an exclusively medical population. Subsequently, the Efficacy of Volume Substitution and Insulin Therapy in Severe Sepsis (VISEP) trial was suspended after the first safety analysis because of an increased number of severe hypoglycemic episodes (<40 mg/dL) in the intensive glucose-control group versus conventional insulin therapy. Most recently, the Normoglycemia in Intensive Care Evaluation and Survival Using Glucose Algorithm Regulation (NICE-SUGAR) Trial reported a significantly increased mortality rate in adult patients in the intensive care unit who were treated with intensive glucose control (81-108 mg/dL), compared with a control group treated to maintain blood glucose concentration less than 180 mg/dL. Based upon these data and others not specifically discussed here, maintenance of blood glucose concentration in critically ill adults at less than 150 mg/dL, as advocated by the Surviving Sepsis Campaign guidelines, is a reasonable target. The mechanism of hyperglycemia should also be taken into account when considering treatment and goals of therapy. Patients without known DM who exhibit stress-induced hyperglycemia appear to benefit more from stricter glucose targets than do those patients with preexisting DM. Although no prospective studies have specifically examined the impact of intensive insulin therapy (IIT) on patients with DM versus hyperglycemic patients without known DM, subgroup analyses of critical care data suggest it may be reasonable to initiate insulin therapy earlier, say, at a level of 150 mg/dL, rather than at 180 mg/dL, and to target a level between 110 and 140 mg/dL in these acutely ill hospitalized patients.

Blood Glucose Measurement

It is not commonly appreciated that blood glucose measurements are not direct determinations of blood glucose concentrations. Rather, all glucose measurement devices in current clinical use, whether a central laboratory or POC device, utilize an indirect enzyme technique. Glucose oxidase, glucose 1-dehydrogenase, and hexokinase are the three enzyme systems most commonly employed. Of these, the hexokinase reaction is used most commonly in central laboratories and is considered to be the gold standard. Further, POC devices measure whole blood, not plasma, and are calibrated to then report plasma values, in contrast with central laboratory devices, which directly report plasma glucose concentrations. This is important because the glucose concentration in plasma is approximately 11% higher than in whole blood and the physiologic activity of glucose corresponds more closely with plasma concentration. Therefore, it is not surprising that a variety of factors—including sampling site, peripheral vasoconstriction, anemia, high or low Pao_2, interference from other sugars or medications, electrolyte abnormalities, hyperbilirubinemia, and hyperuricemia—can all affect POC glucose determinations. Underscoring this fact, POC measurements utilizing glucose testing strips, whether from capillary blood or arterial blood, disagree 15% of the time. It is important to note that discordance is defined by a deviation of greater than 20%. Furthermore, agreement between methods becomes worse in the presence of hypoglycemia, with the tendency for overestimation to occur. Despite their widespread clinical use among hospital wards, the intensive care unit, and the operating room, POC devices have never received U.S. Food and Drug Administration approval for such use. In these settings, the use of venous blood samples is recommended.

Treatment Protocols

A variety of IIT protocols have been used to achieve glycemic control with varying degrees of success. Whether automated, based upon a computer-generated algorithm, or paper-based utilizing simple bedside calculations, the goal is to obtain blood glucose values within the specified target range for the most time possible without causing significant hypoglycemia. The majority of these IIT protocols were developed for and tested in acutely ill hospitalized patients and were nurse driven; staffing was plentiful. An implementation study performed at the University of California at San Francisco reported that each glucose determination required an average of 7 min of nursing time and that, considering the usual nursing-to-patient ratio of 1:2, if both patients had been on an IIT protocol, nearly 17% of a 12-h shift would have been spent solely on obtaining samples, performing tests, and following the IIT protocol. Inasmuch as the anesthesia provider is often caring for a patient in the operating room alone, with many tasks to perform, it is not surprising that a study of intraoperative IIT in patients without diabetes who were undergoing cardiac operations was terminated early due to "unobtainable" glucose goals. The reader should be aware that the Surgical Care Improvement Project, a joint effort between the Joint Commission and Centers for Medicare and Medicaid Services, which ultimately determines the perceived quality of care of a particular institution, requires that patients who have had cardiac operations have a morning blood glucose concentration less than 200 mg/dL on postoperative days 1 and 2—regardless of the impact of achieving that goal on patient care. Although, the benchmark of 200 mg/dL is entirely arbitrary and not based on current evidence, it is being used to define, along with other predetermined quality benchmarks, "top-performing" hospitals and reimbursement levels.

Summary

The stress of surgery, anesthesia, and critical illness often results in patients developing hyperglycemia in the perioperative period. Anesthesia providers should consider patient factors (type, duration, and control of diabetes) as well as surgical factors (duration, degree of insult, and pathophysiologic derangement) when choosing perioperative glycemic control management strategies. Despite the acknowledgment that hyperglycemia is deleterious, there is no universally agreed upon blood glucose level for which insulin therapy should be initiated, nor is a single glucose concentration target suitable for all patients. Further, hypoglycemia is a real possibility in perioperative patients even when some higher-risk patients (sepsis, renal failure, those on continuous venovenous hemofiltration or receiving inotropic agents) are not receiving insulin. Individuals may have limited signs or symptoms of significant hypoglycemia, which may be unrecognized if POC devices are routinely used to measure blood glucose, and may have increased morbidity and mortality risks.

Suggested Readings

Akhtar S, Barash PG, Inzucchi SE. Scientific principles and clinical implications of perioperative glucose regulation and control. *Anesth Analg*. 2010;110:478-497.

Lipshutz AK, Gropper MA. Perioperative glycemic control: An evidence-based review. *Anesthesiology*. 2009;110:408-421.

Moghissi ES, Korytkowski MT, DiNardo M, et al. American Association of Clinical Endocrinologists, American Diabetes Association. American Association of Clinical Endocrinologists and American Diabetes Association consensus statement on inpatient glycemic control. *Endocr Pract*. 2009;15:353-369.

Smiley DD, Umpierrez GE. Perioperative glucose control in the diabetic or non-diabetic patient. *South Med J*. 2006;99:580-589.

Sebranek JJ, Koop Lugli A, Coursin DB. Glycemic control in the perioperative period. *Br J Anaesth*. 2013;111:i18-i34.

CHAPTER 227

The Acute Respiratory Distress Syndrome

Mark T. Keegan, MB, MRCPI, MSc

Background and Definitions

The acute respiratory distress syndrome (ARDS) is an inflammatory lung condition with associated noncardiogenic pulmonary edema and impairment of gas exchange. ARDS is a major cause of respiratory failure in patients in the intensive care unit (ICU). In the perioperative period, patients who are undergoing major surgical procedures, who are seriously ill, or who aspirate are susceptible to developing ARDS. In 2012, ARDS was redefined according to the Berlin definition (Table 227-1) in an effort to overcome some of the inadequacies of the previously used American-European Consensus definition, which dated from 1994 (Table 227-2). Compared with the prior definition, the Berlin definition defines "acute," clarifies the methods to exclude hydrostatic edema, adds minimal ventilator-setting requirements, drops the term "acute lung injury," and classifies ARDS into three categories of severity.

ARDS may result from a direct insult to the lung, such as from pneumonia or from aspiration of gastric contents. Direct injury may also be related to pulmonary contusion, fat embolus, inhalation or drowning injury, or transfusion of blood products. Secondary ARDS occurs as part of a systemic illness or may be related to trauma and may be thought of as the lung manifestation of the systemic inflammatory response, just as oliguria, mental status changes, and hypotension are manifestations of sepsis in the kidney, brain, and cardiovascular systems, respectively.

ARDS manifests as noncardiogenic pulmonary edema with hypoxemia. An alteration in the relationship between the alveolar epithelium and the capillary endothelium allows influx of protein-rich edema fluid into the alveoli. Injury to type II alveolar cells results in disruption of epithelial fluid transport, impairs removal of alveolar fluid, and alters surfactant production. These changes lead to abnormalities in gas exchange. Pulmonary neutrophils play a key role in the generation of an inflammatory response, and this inflammatory process may be augmented by inappropriate mechanical ventilation (see later discussion).

A prospective study in 1999 to 2000 estimated an incidence of ARDS in the United States of almost 200,000 adult patients per year. The incidence appears to have decreased over the subsequent decade, probably because of the use of lung-protective ventilation, more conservative use of blood products, and a reduction in nosocomial infections. ARDS remains, however, a major ICU disease entity. Approximately 10% to 15% of patients admitted to the ICU and up to 20% of those requiring mechanical ventilation have ARDS.

ARDS has been divided into a number of pathologic stages. Diffuse alveolar damage seen in the initial "exudative" stage gives way over the first week to a "proliferative" stage, during which type II alveolar cells predominate and interstitial inflammation develops. A later "fibrotic" stage occurs in some patients, during which normal lung architecture is disrupted by deposition of collagen.

Table 227-1 Berlin Definition of Acute Respiratory Distress Syndrome

Feature	Description
Timing	Onset within 1 week of a known clinical insult or new or worsening respiratory symptoms
Chest imaging*	Bilateral opacities—not fully explained by effusions, lobar/lung collapse, or nodules
Origin of edema	Respiratory failure not fully explained by cardiac failure or fluid overload; need objective assessment (e.g., echocardiography) to exclude hydrostatic edema if no risk factor is present
Oxygenation†	
Mild	200 mm Hg < PaO_2/FIO_2 ≤ 300 mm Hg with PEEP or CPAP ≥ 5 cm H_2O‡
Moderate	100 mm Hg < PaO_2/FIO_2 ≤ 200 mm Hg with PEEP ≥ 5 cm H_2O
Severe	PaO_2/FIO_2 ≤ 100 mm Hg with PEEP ≥ 5 cm H_2O

*Chest radiograph or computed tomography scan.
†If altitude is greater than 1000 m, the correction factor should be calculated as follows: (PaO_2/FIO_2) × (Barometric pressure/760).
‡This may be delivered noninvasively in the mild ARDS group.
ARDS, Acute respiratory distress syndrome; CPAP, continuous positive airway pressure; FIO_2, fraction of inspired O_2; PaO_2, partial pressure of arterial O_2; PEEP, positive end-expiratory pressure.
Modified from ARDS Definition Task Force. Acute respiratory distress syndrome: The Berlin definition. JAMA. 2012;307:2526-2533.

Table 227-2 American-European Consensus Conference Definitions for Acute Lung Injury and Acute Respiratory Distress Syndrome*

Feature	ALI	ARDS
Timing	Acute	Acute
Findings on chest radiograph	Bilateral diffuse infiltrates	Bilateral diffuse infiltrates
PCOP (mm Hg)	≤18	≤18
PaO_2/FIO_2	≤300	≤200

*The original intent with these definitions was to designate acute respiratory distress syndrome (ARDS) as a subset of acute lung injury (ALI). In practice, however, many clinicians used the term ALI exclusively to indicate those patients with ALI but without ARDS (i.e., a PaO_2/FIO_2 ratio of 201-300). The Berlin definition dropped the "ALI" category. (Although superseded by the Berlin definition, these criteria were used as a basis for interventional and epidemiologic studies between 1994 and 2012.)
FIO_2, Fraction of inspired oxygen; PaO_2, partial pressure of arterial oxygen; PCOP, pulmonary capillary occlusion pressure.

Clinical manifestations of ARDS include rapidly worsening dyspnea, tachypnea, and hypoxemia with diffuse rales on lung auscultation. Arterial blood gas analysis shows an elevated alveolar-arterial O_2 gradient with severe hypoxemia, consistent with right-to-left shunt physiology. Pulmonary hypertension may develop. Although a respiratory alkalosis may be present in early ARDS, respiratory acidosis usually develops later in the course of the condition. Diffuse "fluffy" bilateral infiltrates are apparent on chest radiography. A computed tomography scan will show areas of alveolar filling, consolidation, and atelectasis, especially in the dependent lung zones. Despite the heterogeneity of the computed tomographic findings, the whole lung is involved in the inflammatory process, and bronchoalveolar lavage of even the relatively spared areas will show inflammatory changes.

Patients with ARDS almost invariably need mechanical ventilation, which is the mainstay of supportive therapy. Noninvasive ventilation, such as continuous positive airway pressure or biphasic positive airway pressure, may be sufficient in some patients, but most patients with moderate or severe ARDS require tracheal intubation. Although oxygenation tends to improve over the course of the first few days as pulmonary edema resolves, the presence of continued hypoxemia, high minute ventilation requirements, and poor lung compliance necessitate prolonged ventilation in a significant number of patients. Large doses of sedative agents and, on occasion, the use of infusions of neuromuscular blocking agents may be required to enable appropriate ventilation of the patient with ARDS. Current guidelines (2012) from the Society of Critical Care Medicine, based on the results of one prospective study, advocate a short course (≤48 h) of a neuromuscular blocking agent for septic patients with ARDS.

Ventilator-associated lung injury is a major concern (Figure 227-1). Inspired gas flows preferentially to relatively uninvolved alveoli, potentially causing overdistention and lung injury due to volutrauma and barotrauma. Constant opening and closing of derecruited lung units can lead to shear stress (atelectrauma). These physical forces can lead to an increase in the injurious inflammatory response (biotrauma). Laboratory investigations have suggested that a "safe zone" exists on the pulmonary pressure-volume curve defined by lower and upper "inflection points" in which ventilation should occur. At the lower end of the pressure-volume curve, lung units are susceptible to derecruitment and atelectasis, and, at the upper end of the pressure-volume curve, overdistention leads to lung injury (Figure 227-2).

The National Heart Lung and Blood Institute ARDSNet investigators have conducted a number of randomized, multicenter, clinical trials evaluating the role of therapies in ARDS. The ARDSNet lower tidal volume trial (ARMA) proved that use of lower tidal volumes (6 mL/kg predicted body weight) decreases fatality caused by lung overdistention and ventilator-associated lung injury. Predicted body weight is based on patient height and sex. Low tidal volume ventilation has become a standard of care in the management of patients with ARDS in the ICU. Although volume-control ventilation was used in the ARDSNet low tidal volume study, pressure-control ventilation—which may provide superior oxygenation because of its flow pattern—can be used instead, providing tidal volumes are limited.

Application of positive end-expiratory pressure (PEEP) has been advocated as a method of improving oxygenation and preventing atelectasis, thus allowing ventilation above the lower inflection point. PEEP levels of up to 22 to 24 cm H_2O have been used. The optimal level of PEEP in ARDS has not been determined, despite a number of prospective studies having been conducted.

Treatment

A variety of techniques have been used in patients with ARDS to allow adequate oxygenation and ventilation while attempting to minimize ventilator-induced lung injury. Selected major clinical trials of therapeutic interventions for ARDS are listed in Table 227-3.

Diuresis

Studies have demonstrated improved oxygenation and a decreased duration of mechanical ventilation with the use of a conservative fluid strategy. When any period of active volume resuscitation has ended, diuretics should be administered, as tolerated, in an effort to decrease extravascular lung water. The desire to keep the lungs "dry" must be balanced by the need to preserve perfusion to other organs.

Recruitment Maneuvers

Application of high levels (e.g., 40 cm H_2O) of continuous positive airway pressure for 30 to 40 sec may open alveoli that have collapsed, thus improving oxygenation. Such recruitment maneuvers may be especially beneficial after the patient has been temporarily disconnected from the ventilator (e.g., transport, suctioning), but the effect of routine use of such recruitment maneuvers on outcome is controversial.

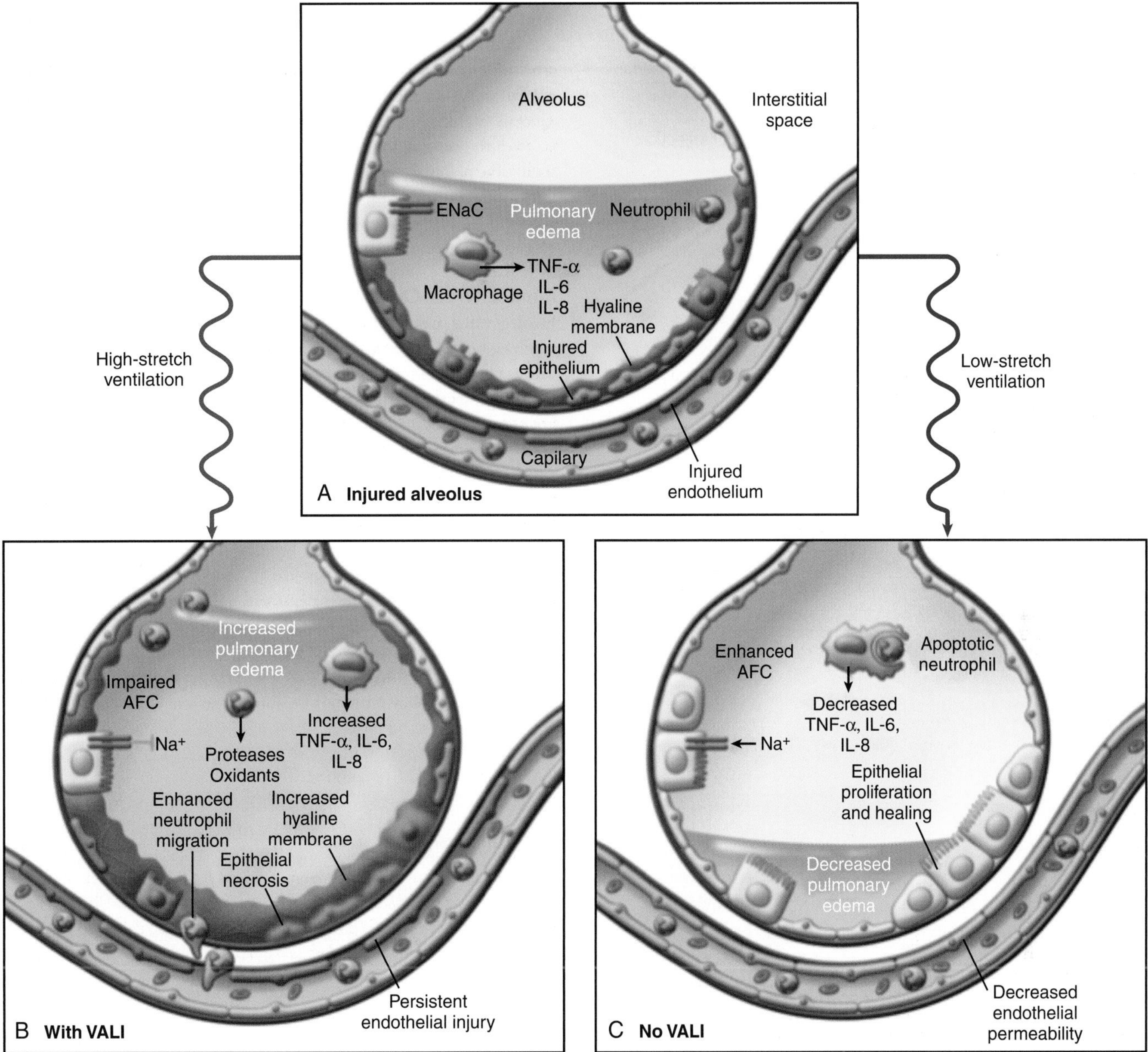

Figure 227-1 Mechanisms of ventilator-associated lung injury (VALI). **A,** Acute respiratory distress syndrome (ARDS) leads to lung endothelial and epithelial injury, increased permeability of the alveolar-capillary barrier, flooding of the airspace with protein-rich pulmonary edema fluid, activation of alveolar macrophages with release of proinflammatory chemokines and cytokines, enhanced neutrophil migration and activation, and fibrin deposition (hyaline membranes). **B,** If the injured lung is ventilated with high tidal volumes and high inflation pressures (high-stretch ventilation), then lung injury is exacerbated, with increased lung endothelial and epithelial injury and necrosis, enhanced neutrophil margination, release of injurious neutrophil products such as proteases and oxidants, increased release of proinflammatory cytokines from alveolar macrophages and the lung epithelium, increased fibrin deposition, and increased hyaline membrane formation. Injurious mechanical ventilation can also impair alveolar fluid clearance (AFC) mechanisms. **C,** In contrast, a protective ventilatory strategy (low-stretch ventilation) can limit further lung endothelial and epithelial injury, reduce the release of proinflammatory cytokines, and enhance alveolar fluid clearance through the active transport of sodium and chloride across the alveolar epithelium, thereby reducing the quantity of pulmonary edema and allowing endothelial and epithelial repair to occur. Epithelial repair occurs through migration, proliferation, and differentiation of alveolar epithelial type II cells to repopulate the denuded basement membrane. Acute inflammation resolves through apoptosis of neutrophils, which are phagocytosed by alveolar macrophages. ENaC, Epithelial sodium channels; IL, interleukin; TNF, tumor necrosis factor. (Modified from Matthay MA, Ware LB, Zimmerman GA. The acute respiratory distress syndrome. J Clin Invest. 2012;122:2731-2740.)

Permissive Hypercapnia

Maintenance of minute ventilation when a low tidal volume strategy is used requires an increase in respiratory rate. At high respiratory rates (usually in the mid- to high-30s range), dynamic hyperinflation—also known as intrinsic PEEP or auto-PEEP—develops. This leads to a potentially deleterious reduction in cardiac output. Permissive hypercapnia is a technique in which the $Paco_2$ is allowed to increase, even to the point of acidemia. Over time, the respiratory acidosis will be compensated for by renal retention of bicarbonate to bring the pH back toward normal. Some practitioners administer buffer solutions to maintain a neutral pH when using permissive hypercapnia.

Tracheal Gas Insufflation

In some patients with ARDS, the presence of a large physiologic dead space may require the use of a very high minute ventilation (e.g., 20 L/min). Even

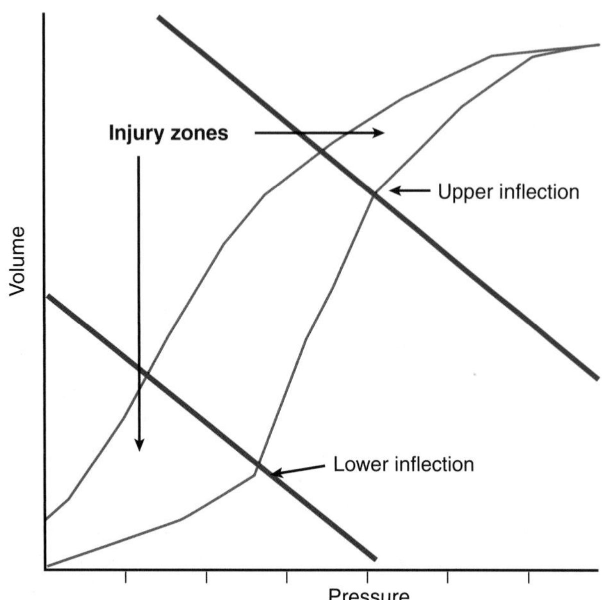

Figure 227-2 Pressure-volume curve in acute respiratory distress syndrome (ARDS) showing the "injury zones." The zones at the bottom and top represent the zones of derecruitment and atelectasis and the zone of overdistention, respectively. Between the upper and lower "inflection points" on the pressure-volume curve is a "safe zone" in which ventilation should occur. (Modified from Frank JA, Matthay MA. Science review: Mechanisms of ventilator-induced injury. Crit Care. 2003;7(3):233-241.)

such minute ventilation may not maintain normocapnia because increasing respiratory rate to increase minute ventilation without increasing tidal volume does not change the ratio of dead space ventilation to alveolar ventilation. Although the patient may tolerate hypercapnia, the development of cardiac arrhythmias or the presence of intracranial disease may require additional efforts to increase the clearance of CO_2. Tracheal gas insufflation involves the continuous flow of fresh O_2 (usually ~6 L/min) through a small tube placed through or alongside the tracheal tube and exiting above the carina. The gas washes out CO_2 as an adjunct to the CO_2 removal provided by the regular ventilatory circuit. Care must be taken to avoid damaging the carina by means of high pressures or "catheter whip."

Inhaled Nitric Oxide and Prostaglandin E_1

Inhaled nitric oxide (INO), a selective pulmonary vasodilator, may be administered through the breathing circuit by a dedicated delivery system. The gas is delivered to those lung units that are ventilated, and it dilates the local pulmonary arterioles. The pulmonary vasculature of nonventilated lung units is not affected. INO thus improves ventilation and perfusion matching and increases Pao_2. INO is rapidly metabolized and has no systemic effects. In addition to improving oxygenation (at doses of 3-20 ppm), when used at higher doses (up to 80 ppm), INO decreases pulmonary arterial pressure and pulmonary vascular resistance, increases right ventricular ejection fraction, and causes mild bronchodilation. Despite improvements in physiologic parameters, the use of INO has not been associated with improvement in outcomes in patients with ARDS.

Inhaled prostaglandin E_1 works in a manner similar to INO. The drug is delivered by nebulizer into the breathing circuit and is used at a dose of 10 to 40 $ng{\cdot}kg^{-1}{\cdot}h^{-1}$. As with INO, prostaglandin E_1 improves oxygenation but has not been shown to improve outcome in a randomized trial.

Table 227-3 Selected Major Clinical Trials in Acute Respiratory Distress Syndrome

Intervention	Study	No. of Patients	Result
Lung-protective strategy	ARDSNet Investigators, 2000 (ARDSNet ARMA trial)	861	Ventilation with 6 mL/kg IBW decreased mortality rate (versus 12 mL/kg)
High PEEP	Brower RG, et al, 2004 (ARDSNet ALVEOLI trial)	549	No difference in mortality rate with high (versus low) PEEP strategy
Fluid strategy	Wiedemann HP, et al, 2006 (ARDSNet FACTT)	1000	More ventilator-free days with fluid-conservative strategy
PAC versus CVC	Wheeler AP, et al, 2006 (ARDSNet FACTT)	1000	No improvement in survival or organ function but more complications with PAC-guided therapy
Neuromuscular blockade	Papazian L, et al, 2010 (ACURASYS study)	340	Decrease in mortality rate with 48 hours of neuromuscular blockade in severe ARDS
Methylprednisolone	Steinberg KP, et al, 2006 (ARDSNet LASRS study)	180	No difference in mortality rate with steroid administration in late-phase ARDS
Prone position	Taccone P, et al, 2009 (PRONE-SUPINE II Study Group)	342	No difference in mortality rate
Extracorporeal membrane oxygenation	Peek GJ, et al, 2009 (CESAR study)	180	Decrease in mortality rate but results not conclusive
Inhaled nitric oxide	Taylor RW, et al, 2004	385	No difference in mortality rate
β_2-Agonist	Gao Smith F, et al, 2012 (BALTI-2 trial)	324	Increase in mortality with intravenous β_2-agonist
ω-3 fatty acid, γ-linoleic acid, and antioxidant supplementation	Rice TW, et al, 2011 (OMEGA study)	272	No difference in ventilator-free days or mortality rate
HFOV	Ferguson ND, et al, 2013 (OSCILLATE trial)	548	HFOV does not reduce, and may increase, in-hospital mortality rate

ARDSNet, Acute Respiratory Distress Syndrome Network (of the National Heart, Lung, and Blood Institute); CVC, central venous catheter; HFOV, high-frequency oscillatory ventilation; IBW, ideal body weight; PAC, pulmonary artery catheter; PEEP, positive end-expiratory pressure.

Prone Positioning

Placement of a patient in the prone position increases end-expiratory lung volume, improves ventilation-perfusion matching, and causes regional changes in ventilation associated with alterations in chest wall mechanics. Oxygenation is thus improved, and this improvement may or may not be sustained when the patient is turned back supine. The introduction of specialized rotating beds may lead to an increase in the use of the prone position. However, use of the prone position has not been demonstrated in randomized trials to improve outcome in ARDS.

High-Frequency Oscillatory Ventilation

The recognition that conventional mechanical ventilation can lead to a worsening of lung injury makes the use of high-frequency oscillatory ventilation (HFOV) attractive. An oscillator is used to deliver very low tidal volume breaths at rates of 3 to 15 Hz. HFOV can provide excellent lung recruitment without causing overdistention while maintaining near-normal arterial blood gases. It permits higher *mean* airway pressures without exposing the lungs to high pressures during tidal excursions. The technique decouples oxygenation and ventilation: oxygenation is proportional to mean airway pressure, and the pressure amplitude controls ventilation. CO_2 removal is *decreased* by increases in frequency. Gas exchange relies on less obvious mechanisms of gas transport, such as bulk convection, pendelluft, cardiogenic oscillations, augmented dispersion, and molecular diffusion. Although this technique is theoretically attractive, large studies of HFOV in ARDS have failed to show a benefit and have even suggested harm.

Extracorporeal Membrane Oxygenation

Extracorporeal membrane oxygenation (ECMO) has been used extensively in neonatal respiratory failure and after repair of congenital heart defects. Only one study—the multicenter CESAR trial—provided supportive evidence for the use of ECMO in adults with ARDS, but, unfortunately, it was not truly a prospective randomized trial. ECMO may be especially beneficial in young patients with influenza who have a higher mortality risk due to hypoxia—as opposed to other groups in whom mortality risk is primarily due to multiple organ dysfunction syndrome.

Other Therapeutic Interventions

The use of corticosteroids has not been demonstrated to be advantageous in either early-phase or late-phase ARDS. Despite initial enthusiasm for the use of corticosteroids in the fibroproliferative stage of ARDS, the ARDSNet Late Steroid Rescue Study failed to show an outcome benefit. Steroids are indicated, however, in certain circumstances (e.g., ARDS associated with "peri-engraft syndrome" in patients after hematopoietic stem cell transplantation). Immunomodulatory nutrition formulations, β-adrenergic receptor agonists, and novel surfactant preparations have also been investigated as adjunctive therapies for ARDS, but, so far, the results have been disappointing (see Table 227-3).

Mortality and Morbidity

The mortality rate associated with ARDS has decreased over the past decade. Recent clinical trials in ARDS have demonstrated mortality rates of approximately 25% to 45%, with lower mortality rates reported in young patients who developed ARDS following polytrauma and higher mortality rates in older patients admitted to medical ICUs (Figure 227-3). As alluded to previously, although some patients die as a result of hypoxemia, most deaths are due to sepsis, multiple organ failure, and the underlying disease rather than to ARDS itself. Initial indices of oxygenation and ventilation do not predict outcome, although failure to improve after 1 week of therapy and persistently high minute ventilation requirements are signs of poor prognosis. Advanced age and the presence of comorbid conditions also increase the chance of death.

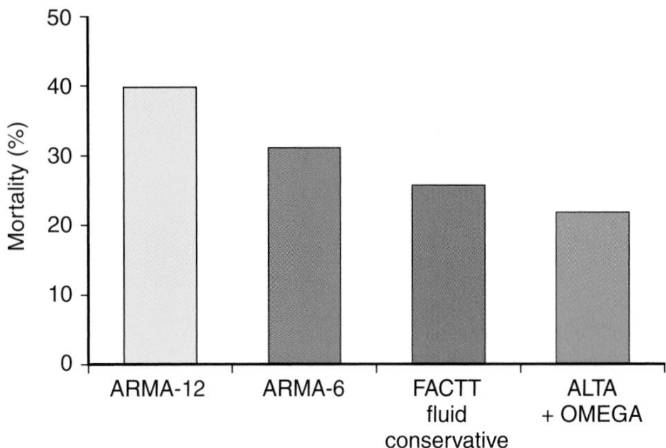

Figure 227-3 Mortality rates in acute respiratory distress syndrome (ARDS). Shown is the 60-day mortality rate reported in randomized clinical trials from the ARDS Network published between 2000 and 2011. *ARMA-12* refers to the mortality rate of 431 patients enrolled into the higher tidal volume arm (12 mL tidal volume/kg predicted body weight), and *ARMA-6* refers to the mortality rate of 430 patients enrolled in the lower tidal volume arm (6 mL tidal volume/kg predicted body weight) of the ARDSNet low tidal volume study (2000). *FACTT* fluid conservative refers to the mortality rate of the 500 patients enrolled into the fluid-conservative arm of the Fluid and Catheter Treatment Trial (2006). *ALTA + OMEGA* refers to the combined mortality rates of studies of albuterol and nutritional/antioxidant (2011). (N = 517 in both trials combined.) (Modified from Matthay MA, Ware LB, Zimmerman GA. The acute respiratory distress syndrome. J Clin Invest. 2012;122:2731-2740.)

Survivors of ARDS may have significant short-term to medium-term disability. Many patients will require a tracheostomy and a significant period of ventilator weaning. Prolonged immobility may lead to the development of critical illness polymyoneuropathy requiring lengthy periods of rehabilitation. Dysfunction of other organs (e.g., renal failure) may be due to the initiating illness or secondary to nosocomial infection. In the long term, lung function usually returns to near normal, but mild abnormalities on pulmonary function tests may persist.

Suggested Readings

ARDS Definition Task Force. Acute respiratory distress syndrome: The Berlin Definition. *JAMA*. 2012;307:2526-2533.

ARDSNet Investigators. Ventilation with lower tidal volumes as compared with traditional tidal volumes for acute lung injury and the acute respiratory distress syndrome. *N Engl J Med*. 2000;342:1301-1308.

Bernard GR, Artigas A, Brigham KL, et al. The American-European Consensus Conference on ARDS. Definitions, mechanisms, relevant outcomes, and clinical trial coordination. *Am J Respir Crit Care Med*. 1994;149:818-824.

Brower RG, Lanken PN, MacIntyre N, et al. Higher versus lower positive end-expiratory pressures in patients with the acute respiratory distress syndrome. *N Engl J Med*. 2004;351:327-336.

Fan E, Needham DM, Stewart TE. Ventilatory management of acute lung injury and acute respiratory distress syndrome. *JAMA*. 2005;294:2889-2896.

Ferguson ND, Cook DJ, Guyatt GH, et al. High frequency oscillation in early acute respiratory distress syndrome. *N Engl J Med*. 2013;368:795-805.

Gao Smith F, Perkins GD, Gates S, et al. Effect of intravenous β-2 agonist treatment on clinical outcomes in acute respiratory distress syndrome (BALTI-2): A multicentre, randomized controlled trial. *Lancet*. 2012;379:229-235.

Herridge MS, Cheung AM, Tansey CM, et al. One-year outcomes in survivors of the acute respiratory distress syndrome. *N Engl J Med*. 2003;348:683-693.

Matthay MA, Ware LB, Zimmerman GA. The acute respiratory distress syndrome. *J Clin Invest*. 2012;122:2731-2740.

Papazian L, Forel JM, Gacouin A, et al. Neuromuscular blockers in early acute respiratory distress syndrome. *N Engl J Med*. 2010;363:1107-1116.

Peek GJ, Mugford M, Tiruvoipati R, et al. Efficacy and economic assessment of conventional ventilatory support versus extracorporeal membrane oxygenation for severe adult respiratory failure (CESAR): A multicentre randomized controlled trial. *Lancet*. 2009;374:1351-1363.

Rice TW, Wheeler AP, Thompson BT, et al. Enteral omega-3 fatty acid, gamma-linolenic acid, and antioxidant supplementation in acute lung injury. *JAMA*. 2011;306:1574-1581.

Steinberg KP, Hudson LD, Goodman RB, et al. Efficacy and safety of corticosteroids for persistent acute respiratory distress syndrome. *N Engl J Med*. 2006;354:1671-1684.

Taccone P, Pesenti A, Latini R, et al. Prone positioning in patients with moderate and severe acute respiratory distress syndrome: A randomized controlled trial. *JAMA*. 2009;302:1977-1984.

Taylor RW, Zimmerman JL, Dellinger RP, et al. Low-dose inhaled nitric oxide in patients with acute lung injury: A randomized controlled trial. *JAMA*. 2004;291:1603-1609.

Wheeler AP, Bernard GR, Thompson BT, et al. Pulmonary-artery versus central venous catheter to guide treatment of acute lung injury. *N Engl J Med*. 2006;354:2213-2224.

Wiedemann HP, Wheeler AP, Bernard GR, et al. Comparison of two fluid-management strategies in acute lung injury. *N Engl J Med*. 2006;354:2564-2575.

CHAPTER 228

Pulmonary Arterial Hypertension

Barry A. Harrison, MD

Pulmonary arterial hypertension (PAH) is an uncommon disease entity manifested by vasoconstriction of the arterioles within the lung, thickening of the vessel wall, and thrombosis in situ that leads to an increase in pulmonary vascular resistance (PVR). The right ventricle is not capable of handling a large pressure load, so, over time, the right ventricle fails, and if PAH is untreated, patients usually die within approximately 3 years after diagnosis. Men and women of all ages can develop the disease, but it is more common in women between the ages of 20 and 40. The initial symptoms of the disease are easy fatigability, dyspnea on exertion, and dizziness. As the disease progresses, the patient experiences shortness of breath at rest, palpitations, and chest pain. As the right ventricle begins to fail, the patient may develop syncope and signs of right ventricular failure, which are evidence of severe disease.

Diagnosis

In a patient suspected of having PAH, a right-sided heart catheterization is performed to measure pulmonary arterial pressures, allowing the calculation of the PVR, which is equal to the decrease in pressure across the pulmonary vascular system (mean pulmonary arterial pressure [mPAP] minus the pulmonary arterial occlusion pressure [PAOP]—an indirect measure of left atrial pressure) divided by the cardiac output (CO):

$$PVR = \frac{(mPAP - PAOP)}{CO}$$

The normal resting mPAP value is 14 ± 3.3 mm Hg; the World Health Organization defines PAH as a sustained elevation of mPAP to more than 25 mm Hg at rest or to more than 30 mm Hg with exercise, with a mean PAOP or left ventricular end-diastolic pressure of less than 15 mm Hg. The World Health Organization classifies PAH as primary or secondary, with recognition that considerable overlap exists between groups, and further divides secondary PAH into left-sided heart disease, PAH from hypoxemia, PAH from pulmonary thrombotic disease, and PAH from miscellaneous causes (Box 228-1). The distinguishing feature between PAH caused by left-sided heart disease and other causes of PAH is that the latter diagnoses require a PVR greater than 3 Wood units (1 Wood unit = 80 dyn·sec^{-1}·cm^{-5}). If left atrial (PAOP) pressure is high (e.g., in patients with mitral valve insufficiency), then PVR is unlikely to be greater than 3 Wood units, and the PAH is secondary to left-sided heart disease.

Box 228-1 Clinical Classification of Pulmonary Arterial Hypertension

Primary

- Idiopathic*
- Familial†
- Caused by drugs or toxins
- Associated with other diseases
  - Connective tissue disease
  - Portopulmonary hypertension
  - Schistosomiasis
  - Human immunodeficiency virus (HIV) infection

Secondary

- Heart disease
  - Systolic
  - Diastolic
  - Valvular
- Hypoxia and lung disease
- Chronic thromboembolic pulmonary hypertension
- Miscellaneous‡

*Previously known as primary pulmonary artery hypertension.
†Genetic
‡Pulmonary hypertension with associated multiple ill-defined mechanisms.

Treatment

Once a diagnosis of PAH is made, treatment first focuses on correcting any secondary causes of the disease; these treatments include, for example, supplemental O_2 to treat hypoxemia, surgery to correct mitral insufficiency, and pulmonary thromboendarterectomy to treat chronic thromboembolic disease. Ultimately, however, most patients with PAH will require pharmacologic therapy to treat the vasoconstriction, smooth muscle cell and endothelial cell proliferation, and prothrombotic state.

Pharmacologic Treatment

Currently, four classes of drugs are used to treat patients with primary PAH, and these drugs are often used in combination. Calcium channel blockers are relatively inexpensive and, with the exception of verapamil (the use of which is associated with too much negative inotropy), can be used if the patient responds with at least a 10% decrease in mPAP.

Studies have demonstrated an association between PAH and decreased endogenous prostacyclin synthase; prostacyclin is a potent endogenous pulmonary vasodilator. Several prostacyclin analogs are therefore used to treat PAH. Epoprostenol (prostacyclin) is given by continuous intravenous infusion, whereas iloprost (a prostacyclin analogue) is delivered by an aerosol route.

Phosphodiesterase inhibitors, especially sildenafil, have a role in the treatment of PAH by inhibiting the breakdown of cyclic guanosine monophosphate, which, in turn, leads to relaxation in smooth muscle cells within the vascular intima, resulting in vasodilation.

Endothelin receptor antagonists are a newer class of drugs that block endothelin receptors, decreasing the vasoconstrictive and vascular remodeling effects of endothelin-1. Bosentan, an oral preparation, increases exercise capacity and delays disease progression but, unfortunately, is hepatotoxic, is teratogenic, and causes anemia.

Anesthetic Management of the Patient with Pulmonary Arterial Hypertension

As mentioned earlier, without treatment, an early death is not uncommon; however, with better awareness, improved diagnosis, and therapy, patients with PAH are surviving much longer and are more likely to present for surgery for unrelated reasons. Because of their underlying condition, these patients have significant perioperative morbidity and mortality rates; one study found a perioperative mortality rate of 7%.

Preoperative Evaluation

When evaluating a patient with PAH, an easy maxim to remember is that the worse the patient's dyspnea at rest, the more severe the PAH. A history of syncope is a harbinger of a poor outcome. The patient likewise should be evaluated for symptoms and signs of right-sided heart failure. A right atrial pressure of more than 20 mm Hg, pericardial effusion, and a cardiac output of less than 2 $L \cdot min^{-1} \cdot m^{-2}$ have each been associated with adverse perioperative outcomes. Patients with significant dyspnea and evidence of right-sided heart failure who present for elective operations but who have not undergone any other diagnostic testing should probably be seen by a cardiologist prior to anesthesia and surgery.

All medications that the patient is taking to treat PAH should be continued throughout the perioperative period, especially any of the prostacyclin analogs, because abrupt discontinuation can result in severe rebound pulmonary hypertension.

Intraoperative Management

Pulse oximetry and end-tidal CO_2 monitoring are considered essential monitors by the American Society of Anesthesiologists and are particularly important for patients with PAH. Consideration should be given to placing an arterial cannula and a pulmonary artery catheter and even to using transesophageal echocardiography in patients with PAH who are undergoing complex operations in which the risk of hemorrhage is high, large fluid shifts are anticipated, or the patient is positioned other than supine.

Both regional and general anesthetic techniques have been used successfully to anesthetize patients with PAH. More important than the technique used is the avoidance or prompt treatment of hypoxia, hypercapnia, acidosis, hypothermia, and pain because all increase PVR and right ventricular afterload. A decreased right ventricular stroke volume leads to decreased left ventricular preload, which is further compromised by the septal displacement from the enlarged right ventricle into the left ventricle. If left ventricular stroke volume decreases (and along with it, aortic root perfusion pressure), coronary blood flow to the right ventricle is decreased, further compromising the performance of the right ventricle. Goals for these patients then include maintaining normal sinus rhythm, with a heart rate of approximately 80 to 90 beats/min, to optimize cardiac output. Right ventricular function is sensitive to both intravascular volume depletion and excess; therefore, fluids should be administered slowly and in small volumes, with a goal of maintaining a central venous pressure of 12 mm Hg or less (Box 228-2).

Intravenously administered anesthesia agents (e.g., propofol) should be carefully titrated to avoid precipitous decreases in systemic arterial pressure. Etomidate may be a better choice for the induction of anesthesia in patients with PAH. Nitrous oxide should be avoided because of its pulmonary vasoconstrictive properties. α-Adrenergic agents, which also increase mPAP, should be used with caution, if at all, in these patients. If allowed to breathe spontaneously, patients who have a laryngeal mask airway in place, and who have received any of a number of drugs that shift the CO_2 response curve to the right, have a significant risk of developing hypercapnia and hypoxia, which will worsen the PAH. The use of mechanical ventilation is neither indicated nor contraindicated. High tidal volumes and peak airway pressures increase mean airway pressure, thereby increasing PVR; however, extremely low tidal volumes will also increase PVR. High peak end-expiratory pressures (>10 cm H_2O) will also increase PVR.

Neuraxial anesthesia may be indicated, especially for procedures below the level of the umbilicus, but it must be borne in mind that prostacyclin

Box 228-2 Suggested Management Strategies for Acute Decompensation of Pulmonary Artery Hypertension and Right-Sided Heart Failure

Administer O_2 to correct hypoxemia and decrease PVR.
- Decrease PVR by correcting hypercapnia, acidosis, and hypothermia.
- Manage systemic hemodynamics.

If hypovolemia, CVP <8-10 mm Hg, use cautious fluid administration.
- Avoid CVP >12 mm Hg.

Maintain normal sinus rhythm, aim for heart rate 80-90 beats/min.

Maintain adequate systemic arterial pressure, use α_1-agonists, vasopressin cautiously.

Manage pulmonary hemodynamics.

Pharmacologic management
- Intravascular inodilators—milrinone (load 50 μg/kg, infuse 0.25-0.75 μg/kg/min) and dobutamine (2-5 $\mu g \cdot kg^{-1} \cdot min^{-1}$)*—will increase right ventricular contractility and decrease mPAP. Systemic hypotension may result, requiring the use of vasopressors.

Inhaled pulmonary artery vasodilators
- Nitric oxide (gas) up to 30 ppm—continuous administration usually via a ventilator.
- Inhaled prostacyclin (liquid) — continuous or intermittent administration via a nebulizer.

Mechanical devices
- An intraaortic balloon pump may be of benefit by augmenting myocardium perfusion, improving function of both ventricles.
- A right ventricular assist device may be of benefit, especially if the patient's right ventricular failure has been exacerbated by left ventricular failure, or vice versa.

*Levosimendan is an inodilator that is not currently approved by the Food and Drug Administration in the United States.

CVP, Central venous pressure; mPAP, mean pulmonary arterial pressure; PVR, pulmonary vascular resistance.

analogs have an inhibitory effect on platelet aggregation. Neuraxial anesthesia and analgesia can result in significant systemic vasodilation, which can result in decreased coronary artery perfusion pressure to the right ventricle and in decreased preload to the right ventricle.

Postoperative Management

Supplemental O_2 should be administered to all patients with PAH in the postoperative period; O_2 saturation and intravascular volume should be monitored. Opioids must be carefully titrated, if used at all, to minimize the potential for hypercapnia. Treatment of pain with multimodal analgesia with nonopioid medications and techniques is preferred.

Conclusion

Patients with PAH have much better prognoses today than they did even 20 years ago. When these patients present for elective operations, it is incumbent on the anesthesia provider to be cognizant of the complex pathophysiology of the disease, be familiar with the multiple drugs the patient may be taking, develop an anesthetic plan that minimizes the chances of increasing PVR, and be prepared to intervene if the patient develops acute right-sided heart failure.

Suggested Readings

Prittis C, Pearl RG. Anesthesia for patients with pulmonary hypertension. *Curr Opin Anesth*. 2010;23:411-416.

Ramakrishna G, Sprung J, Ravi BS, et al. Impact of pulmonary hypertension on the outcomes of non cardiac surgery: Predictors of perioperative morbidity and mortality. *J Am Coll Cardiol*. 2005;45:1691-1699.

Strumpher J, Jacobsohn E. Pulmonary hypertension and right ventricular dysfunction: Physiology and perioperative management. *J Cardiothorac Vasc Anesth*. 2011;25:687-704.

Teo YW, Greenhalgh DL. Update on anaesthetic approach to pulmonary hypertension. *Eur J Anesth*. 2010;27:317-323.

CHAPTER 229

Management of Stroke

William David Freeman, MD

Pathophysiology

Ischemic strokes, which make up 85% of all strokes, occur when a large intracranial artery (e.g., middle cerebral artery, 3-4 mm in diameter) or small perforating intracranial artery (50-200 μm in diameter) is occluded, causing ischemia to downstream brain tissue. The cause of ischemic stroke is multifactorial (Box 229-1).

Brain tissue has high aerobic metabolic demand and receives a large proportion of cardiac output (15%) relative to the organ's mass (average, 1500 g). Compromised cerebral blood flow (CBF) results in inadequate O_2 delivery to the brain, metabolic failure (i.e., conversion of aerobic to anaerobic metabolism), loss of CBF autoregulation (regionally or globally), depletion of high-energy phosphates (e.g., adenosine triphosphate [ATP]), and subsequent accumulation of neurotoxic substances (e.g., lactate, aspartate, and glutamate). The magnitude of ischemia is both time and CBF-threshold dependent. On average, normal global CBF is approximately 50 $mL \cdot 100\ g^{-1} \cdot min^{-1}$, whereas the ischemic threshold is 12 $mL \cdot 100\ g^{-1} \cdot min^{-1}$. The area of complete cellular death is termed the *infarct core* and is not salvageable after a few minutes. In contrast, brain tissue that is potentially salvageable is termed the *penumbra*. Brain tissue in the penumbra will infarct, similar to core regions, in a time-dependent fashion unless reperfusion of the occluded vessel occurs.

Box 229-1 Causes of Ischemic Stroke

- Cardioembolic
- Large artery atherosclerosis to distal artery
- Small vessel occlusion
- Other mechanism (e.g., vasculitis, vasculopathy, dissection)
- Cryptogenic (stroke of undetermined cause)

Hemorrhagic strokes, which account for 15% of all strokes, result from a ruptured intracranial vessel. Spontaneous (nontraumatic) intraparenchymal hemorrhage (IPH) occurs in about two thirds of hemorrhagic strokes, with two thirds of them occurring in deep locations (basal ganglia, pons, or cerebellum) from a ruptured Charcot-Bouchard microaneurysm (submillimeter) caused by chronic hypertension, and the remaining one third of IPH occurring in corticosubcortical locations, typically from cerebral amyloid angiopathy. IPH volume is a powerful predictor of mortality risk, with increasing IPH volumes associated with increased risk of mortality. Subarachnoid hemorrhage, which accounts for about 5% of strokes, occurs typically from a ruptured cerebral aneurysm around the circle of Willis. Other causes of intracranial bleeding include spontaneous or traumatic epidural hematoma, subdural hematoma, and intraventricular hematomas, which may occur from a vascular anomaly such as an aneurysm or arteriovenous malformation. When compared with ischemic strokes (except massive ischemic stroke with cerebral edema), hemorrhagic stroke is more commonly associated with increased intracranial pressure (ICP). Increased ICP is proportionate to the volume of blood introduced into the closed intracranial vault (i.e., Monro-Kellie doctrine). The presence of intracranial blood may further increase ICP by obstructing cerebrospinal fluid pathways (obstructive hydrocephalus) or diffusely obstructing the arachnoid granulations, preventing absorption of cerebrospinal fluid (communicating hydrocephalus). Regardless of the mechanism, increased ICP can compromise global cerebral perfusion pressure (which equals the mean arterial pressure [MAP] minus the ICP) and induce brain ischemia.

Anesthetic Management

Preoperative Evaluation

In patients who have had a stroke, it is important to perform a baseline neurologic examination and to document the results thereof. If feasible, patients with an acute stroke should have elective operations postponed to enable the care team to elucidate the cause of the stroke and to initiate therapy, as well as to allow the patient's recovery of CBF autoregulation. It is important for the anesthesia provider to know the patient's preoperative baseline systemic blood pressure, given that chronic hypertension shifts the autoregulation curve to the right, thereby necessitating higher MAP to maintain CBF. Overall, a 20% acute reduction in MAP is generally well tolerated. Intra operative and postoperative stroke risk is higher in patients with high-grade carotid artery stenosis (>70%-99% by ultrasound) or high-grade extracranial/intracranial vascular stenosis or vessel occlusion.

Intraoperative Monitoring

When a patient is undergoing general anesthesia, new-onset neurologic deficits are impossible to recognize until the patient emerges from anesthesia. Therefore, to detect ischemia as early as possible, intraoperative neuromonitoring techniques (e.g., somatosensory evoked potentials, motor evoked potentials, electromyography, electroencephalography, jugular venous O_2 saturation, frontal near-infrared spectroscopy, and transcranial Doppler) may be used. Discovery of intraoperative ischemia by neuromonitoring should lead to immediate action to reverse the deficit (e.g., correcting surgical clamping of a carotid artery, increasing MAP, and optimizing O_2-carrying capacity). The use of inhalation anesthetic agents impairs cerebrovascular resistance to react to changes in cerebral perfusion pressure (CPP), which can can make CBF linearly dependent on CPP (i.e., CBF = CPP divided by cerebrovascular resistance [CVR]). This in turn can lead to reduced brain perfusion (CBF) in cerebrovascular disease patients with existing large vessel extracranial or intracranial artery stenosis or occlusions, impaired vascular reserve or collaterals or lack of a complete Circle of Willis, impaired vascular autoregulation either from ischemia or drugs that impair CVR, chronic hypertensive patients with rightward shifted autoregulation, or a combination of these cerebrovascular diseases.

Postoperative Management

The differential diagnosis of postoperative stroke-like symptoms includes cerebrovascular accident, hypoglycemia, hypotension, seizure, complicated migraine, hypertensive encephalopathy, and conversion disorder. Acute stroke management comprises obtaining an emergency neurology consultation, assessing the patient's O_2-carrying capacity (e.g., serum hemoglobin concentration, arterial blood gas analysis), performing other serologic tests (e.g., glucose concentration, coagulation studies, troponin I or troponin T tests), and acquiring noncontrast cerebral computed tomography scans to distinguish ischemic from hemorrhagic stroke. Intensive care unit management and thrombolytic therapy (in the setting of ischemic stroke) are appropriate considerations.

If the patient has a seizure after experiencing a stroke, benzodiazepines (e.g., lorazepam) are considered first-line agents. If the patient has more than one seizure, benzodiazepines followed by fosphenytoin, 15 mg/kg, should be administered intravenously for subsequent seizure prophylaxis (rate not to exceed 150 mg/min because of the risk of the patient developing hypotension and AV junctional rhythms). The routine use of antiepileptic drug (AED) for seizure prophylaxis in patients who have a stroke is generally not recommended. Patients with lobar IPH however have a relatively higher risk of early seizures (<1 week) and in which short-term use of prophylactic AED is considered optional.

In patients given tissue plasminogen activator intravenously, heparin and aspirin should be avoided for the first 24 h. Patients who have intracranial hemorrhage who were therapeutically anticoagulated (international normalized ratio [INR] > 2.0, or heparin activated partial thromboplastin time > 36 sec) prior to surgery should have rapid anticoagulation reversal to prevent hematoma expansion. For patients taking warfarin, the INR should be normalized with intravenous administration of vitamin K (10 mg, slow infusion over 30 min) or fresh frozen plasma (15 mL/kg). Some centers give prothrombin complex concentrate or recombinant factor VIIa instead of fresh frozen plasma, depending on the availability of these products, which normalize the INR more quickly than do vitamin K and fresh frozen plasma but are associated with significantly higher cost (prothrombin complex concentrate ~ $900, recombinant factor VIIa ~ $7500) with little comparative efficacy data and at least a 6% to 7% risk of the patient developing thromboembolic complications.

"Permissive hypertension" is allowed in acute ischemic stroke. If the computed tomographic examination reveals intracranial hemorrhage, blood pressure is more tightly regulated than it is in ischemic stroke because of concerns that hypertension may cause more bleeding in patients with intracranial hemorrhage. Given that ICP is a key determinant of cerebral perfusion pressure, patients with an increased ICP require a different blood pressure management scheme. The cerebral perfusion pressure should be maintained at a minimum of 70 mm Hg. The use of continuous cardiac monitoring or telemetry is advised because of the high rate of cardiac arrhythmias and electrocardiographic abnormalities that occur in patients after stroke. The use of hypotonic fluids should be avoided because of a "leaky" blood-brain barrier and the attendant risks of worsening cerebral edema.

Obtunded patients who have had a stroke (e.g., Glasgow Coma Scale < 8, loss of central respiratory drive, or loss of protective respiratory reflexes) should have their airway secured to control ventilation and mitigate aspiration risk. Coughing, performing the Valsalva maneuver, and excessive straining should be avoided in patients with increased ICP during tracheal intubation. In patients with increased ICP, inducing mild hyperventilation and hypocapnia ($Paco_2$ 30-35 mm Hg) may be used temporarily until definitive neurosurgical intervention (e.g., surgical decompression or placement of an external ventricular drain) can take place.

Stress ulcer prophylaxis with an H_2-receptor blocking agent or a proton pump inhibitor is recommended. A core body temperature of 38.5° C or higher should be treated with antipyretic medications to avoid temperature-mediated exacerbations of neurologic injury.

Suggested Readings

Blacker DJ, Flemming KD, Link MJ, Brown RD. The preoperative cerebrovascular consultation: Common cerebrovascular questions before general or cardiac surgery. *Mayo Clin Proc*. 2004;79:223-229.

Jauch EC, Saver JL, Adams HP Jr, et al Guidelines for the early management of patients with acute ischemic stroke: A guideline for healthcare professionals from the American Heart Association/American Stroke Association. *Stroke*. 2013;44:870-947.

Morgenstern LB, Hemphill JC 3rd, Anderson C, et al. Guidelines for the management of spontaneous intracerebral hemorrhage: A guideline for healthcare professionals from the American Heart Association/American Stroke Association. *Stroke*. 2010;41:2108-2129.

Qureshi AI. Antihypertensive treatment of acute cerebral hemorrhage (ATACH): Rationale and design. *Neurocrit Care*. 2007;6:56-66.

Selim M. Perioperative stroke. *N Engl J Med*. 2007;356:706-713.

CHAPTER 230

Carbon Monoxide Poisoning

John M. VanErdewyk, MD

Carbon monoxide (CO) is a colorless, odorless, tasteless, and nonirritating gas produced by the incomplete combustion of materials containing carbon. Its effects on the O_2-carrying capacity of blood are profound: CO is responsible for approximately 3500 accidental and suicide deaths each year in the United States and is the major cause of death in patients exposed to smoke inhalation from fires. Many additional people are exposed to concentrations of CO that produce major morbidity.

Pathophysiology

CO is emitted from almost any flame or combustion device. A 3% to 7% concentration is present in the exhaust of internal combustion engines. Much higher concentrations can be generated during the burning of most illuminating and heating gases. Both CO and O_2 compete for binding with hemoglobin; however, the affinity of hemoglobin for CO is 200 times greater than that for O_2. CO binding results in carboxyhemoglobin (HbCO), which is incapable of off loading significant quantities of O_2 in tissues. A HbCO level of approximately 25% is a critical level at which the central nervous system is profoundly affected. The HbCO level depends on the CO concentration in the air and on the duration of exposure. Besides decreasing O_2-carrying capacity, HbCO also interferes with the release of O_2 from oxyhemoglobin (i.e., a leftward shift in the oxyhemoglobin dissociation curve), further reducing the amount of O_2 available to the tissues, which is the cause of tissue anoxia in CO-poisoned patients.

Small amounts of CO are present in all individuals because CO is a byproduct of erythrocyte destruction, resulting in an HbCO concentration of approximately 1%. Cigarette smokers often have HbCO levels exceeding 5%.

Signs and Symptoms

Signs and symptoms of HbCO poisoning vary, depending on the concentration of HbCO present, the tissue O_2 demands, and the hemoglobin concentration. Small amounts of HbCO in the blood may manifest as irritability, headache, nausea or vomiting, confusion, dizziness, visual disturbances, and dyspnea. Increasing concentrations of HbCO may produce respiratory failure, agitation, seizures, coma, or death (when HbCO concentrations reach 50%).The classic cherry-red color of the skin is usually a sign of high CO concentrations in the blood; however, cyanosis may be seen in patients with severe CO poisoning.

Significant hypoxemia can be present despite apparently normal oximeter readings. Conventional pulse oximetry (most oximeters emit only two wavelengths of light—660 nm and 940 nm) overestimates the true Spo_2 because HbCO competes with oxyhemoglobin in the absorption spectrum. Independent of the true oxyhemoglobin concentration, the pulse oximeter will display a reading of no less than 84% to 86% even with a HbCO of 50% and an oxyhemoglobin of 50%. The concentration of HbCO can be accurately measured with a co-oximeter that is based on fractional oximetry (in which the oximeter emits five wavelengths of light to detect all hemoglobin species).

Treatment

The first step in treatment is to remove the patient from the environment containing CO to prevent further exposure. The next is to administer 100% O_2. Because the binding of CO to hemoglobin is competitive with O_2, increasing the inspired concentration of O_2 to 100% will cause more O_2 to displace CO from the hemoglobin molecule, shortening the elimination half-life. Thus, the half-life of CO elimination can be shortened from 4 h to 40 min by ventilation of the lungs with 100% O_2. The administration of 100% O_2 will also partially relieve tissue hypoxia by increasing the amount of O_2 dissolved in the plasma. Tracheal intubation and mechanical ventilation may be necessary. Hyperbaric O_2 therapy is indicated for the treatment of severe CO poisoning; the use of hyperbaric O_2 therapy can decrease the HbCO elimination half-life to 15 to 30 min. Transfusion of red blood cells (thereby increasing O_2-carrying capacity) may also be helpful. The use of diuretics, steroids, or both may be indicated if the patient develops cerebral edema.

Carbon Monoxide Production from CO_2 Absorbers

CO may be produced when any currently used inhalation anesthetic (desflurane > isoflurane >>> sevoflurane) reacts with a desiccated CO_2 absorber containing strong bases (KOH > NaOH). For further details, see Chapter 8, Carbon Dioxide Absorption.

Suggested Readings

Coppens MJ, Versichelen LF, Rolly G, et al. The mechanisms of carbon monoxide production by inhalational agents. *Anaesthesia*. 2006;61:462-468.

Weaver LK. Clinical practice. Carbon monoxide poisoning. *N Engl J Med*. 2009;360:1217-1225.

Wissing H, Kuhn I, Warnken U, Dudziak R. Carbon monoxide production from desflurane, enflurane, halothane, isoflurane, and sevoflurane with dry soda lime. *Anesthesiology*. 2001;95:1205-1212.

CHAPTER 231

Acute Renal Failure

Patrick O. McConville, MD, and Robert M. Craft, MD

Varying degrees of renal dysfunction are frequently present in patients presenting for surgery; the hemodynamic sequelae of anesthesia and of surgical intervention, along with the renal toxicity of some of the drugs that anesthesia providers use, may further compromise the ability of the kidneys to maintain fluid and electrolyte homeostasis. Maintaining fluid and electrolyte balance while preventing injury to the kidneys during the perioperative period is the goal of all anesthesia providers and is especially important in patients with preexisting renal disease.

Incidence and Signs and Symptoms

Some degree of acute renal failure (ARF), a decline in the ability of the kidneys to maintain electrolyte and fluid homeostasis and excrete waste products, affects 5% to 7% of hospitalized patients. Clinical symptoms are typically absent until the glomerular filtration rate (GFR) is 25% to 40% below normal values. Function within this range is often categorized as renal insufficiency, at which point the only symptom may be nocturia. The uremic syndrome is associated with a GFR of 10% of baseline or less and is manifested by symptoms of volume overload (e.g., pulmonary and lower extremity edema). Electrolyte abnormalities—including metabolic acidosis, hyperphosphatemia, hypocalcemia or hypercalcemia, hyponatremia, hypermagnesemia, and hyperkalemia—may manifest as any combination of cardiac arrhythmias, neuropathy, myocardial dysfunction and ischemia, lethargy, nausea, diarrhea, encephalopathy, tremors, or seizures.

Risk Factors

The most important risk factor for perioperative renal failure is preoperative renal dysfunction. The administration of radiocontrast dyes or other nephrotoxic drugs is responsible for additional iatrogenic sources of perioperative renal failure. Patients with advanced age, coronary artery disease, or congestive heart failure and those undergoing major operative procedures associated with large fluid shifts and that involve cross-clamping of the aorta are also at increased risk for developing ARF during the perioperative period. Multiple organ system failure, systemic inflammatory response syndrome, sepsis, and traumatic injury with myoglobinemia and inadequate resuscitation and restoration of normal hemodynamics present additional risks for the development of renal failure.

Laboratory Analysis

ARF can be categorized as prerenal ARF, intrinsic renal failure, or postrenal ARF. Diagnosing the type of renal failure is important because treatment for each is different. Although laboratory tests (such as urine flow rate, urine specific gravity, urine osmolality, urine/plasma creatinine and blood urea nitrogen, serum creatinine and blood urea nitrogen, and urine sodium) may indicate ARF, creatinine clearance is the best available test to differentiate prerenal from early acute tubular necrosis. Differentiation may allow earlier treatment before progression of renal failure. The measurement of creatinine clearance traditionally requires a 24-h urine collection, but a creatinine clearance measurement based on a 2-h urine collection correlates reasonably well with the test performed on a 24-h urine sample and can be used to screen at-risk patients.

Causes and Treatment

Prerenal Acute Renal Failure

Timely treatment of prerenal causes of ARF can reverse kidney dysfunction. Administering fluids, packed red blood cells, or fluids and packed red blood cells; providing blood pressure support; and maintaining oxygenation may be effective in increasing renal perfusion and O_2 delivery, thus limiting further renal damage. Monitoring central venous pressure may assist in estimating blood volume status and response to fluid administration. Serial hematocrit levels may be useful in guiding transfusion in situations involving ongoing blood loss. When hypotension is present, invasive measurement of arterial pressure may be useful in guiding vasopressor therapy. The use of a pulmonary artery catheter or a transesophageal echocardiographic probe to monitor cardiac function may be advantageous when decreased cardiac contractility is suspected as a cause for decreased renal blood flow. Oxygen saturation in this situation should be maintained at 94% or greater.

Intrinsic Renal Failure

Intrinsic renal failure is most often caused by acute tubular necrosis, which, in turn, is most often due to ischemia. In addition to ischemia, nephrotoxic drugs (antibiotics, nonsteroidal antiinflammatory agents, intravenous contrast material used for imaging studies, chemotherapeutic drugs), solvents (ethylene glycol), and myoglobinemia are sources of intrinsic renal failure.

Other sources of intrinsic renal failure include interstitial nephritis, sepsis, drug administration, and acute glomerulonephritis. Glomerulonephritis occurs due to antigen-antibody deposition from streptococcal infections and collagen disorders. Withdrawal of the offending drugs and providing supportive therapy and corticosteroid therapy may be indicated, depending on the suspected source of intrinsic renal failure.

Postrenal Azotemia

Postrenal azotemia is caused by obstruction of urine flow in the ureter, bladder, or urethra. Investigation for nephrolithiasis, tumors, prostatic hypertrophy, and kinked catheters may yield a reversible cause.

Management

If, prior to surgery, a patient undergoes imaging studies in which radiocontrast agents will be injected intravenously, adequate intravascular volume must be assured and sufficient fluid should be administered to induce a brisk diuresis. Some anesthesia providers administer N-acetylcysteine and others may administer sodium bicarbonate, but there is little evidence to support the use of continuous renal replacement therapy to reduce the incidence of radiocontrast agent–induced ARF. Once patients develop ARF, their medications should be reviewed and consideration should be given to discontinuing those that are associated with nephrotoxicity. Treatment is mostly supportive, including fluid or blood products to maintain cardiac output, mean arterial pressure, and O_2 delivery—and correcting electrolyte abnormalities. Hemofiltration and hemodialysis, when indicated, should probably be instituted sooner, rather than later. Although isolated ARF carries a mortality rate of less than 10%, ARF in the setting of multiple organ failure has a mortality rate of up to 90%.

Complications

Complications of ARF include platelet dysfunction secondary to uremia, pulmonary edema (resulting in respiratory failure), myocardial infarction from arrhythmias or increased myocardial demand, and sepsis due to impaired immunity associated uremia or the presence of indwelling catheters. Gastrointestinal complications (due to the failure of the kidneys to excrete toxins) can cause ileus, nausea, anorexia, and weight loss. Somnolence, confusion, and seizures may result from the accumulation of neural toxins.

Suggested Readings

Kheterpal S, Tremper K, Englesbe MJ, et al. Predictors of postoperative acute renal failure after noncardiac surgery in patients with previously normal renal function. *Anesthesiology*. 2007;107:892-902.

Uchino S, Kellum JA, Bellomo R, et al. Acute renal failure in critically ill patients. A multinational, multicenter study free. *JAMA*. 2005;294:813-818.

Ympa YP, Sakr Y, Reinhart K, Vincent J-L. Has mortality from acute renal failure decreased? A systematic review of the literature. *Am J Med*. 2005;118: 827-832.

CHAPTER 232

Systemic Inflammatory Response Syndrome and Sepsis

Mark T. Keegan, MB, MRCPI, MSc

The systemic inflammatory response syndrome (SIRS) and sepsis are complex syndromes resulting from an inciting insult that causes systemic inflammation, leading to widespread tissue injury. In the case of sepsis, the initial insult is an infection. Sepsis is the leading cause of death in critically ill patients. In the Unites States, sepsis occurs in 750,000 people every year, and more than 200,000 of them die. The incidence of sepsis is increasing, and it is especially common in the elderly. Both SIRS and sepsis may be seen in the perioperative period and are common causes of admission to the surgical intensive care unit.

The American College of Chest Physicians and the Society of Critical Care Medicine published consensus-derived definitions of SIRS, sepsis, and organ failure in 1992 (Table 232-1). In 2001, a list of signs and laboratory findings that should prompt a clinician to consider sepsis in the differential diagnosis was proposed. In addition to tachypnea, tachycardia, and alterations in temperature and white blood cell count, these findings include chills, poor capillary refill, decreased skin perfusion, thrombocytopenia, hypoglycemia, oliguria, alteration in mental status, and skin mottling.

SIRS occurs in the absence of infection and may be secondary to surgical insult, trauma, or inflammatory conditions, such as pancreatitis. Sepsis is the result of a complex interaction among the patient's immune, inflammatory, and coagulation systems and an infecting organism. In both SIRS and sepsis, at the site of injury or infection, a local inflammatory response is antagonized by a local antiinflammatory response (Figure 232-1). Such proinflammatory and antiinflammatory responses often become systemic. Both excessive and inadequate host-immune responses can lead to progression of disease and organ dysfunction. Further, a large inciting stimulus or a virulent infectious agent may cause organ dysfunction even in the presence of a competent immune system. Neutrophils play a key role in the development of sepsis. An initial toxic stimulus (e.g., bacterial endotoxin) leads to production of proinflammatory cytokines, such as interleukin 1 and tumor necrosis factor. Migration of neutrophils to vascular endothelium subsequently occurs, with concomitant activation of clotting and generation of secondary inflammatory mediators.

Multiple organ dysfunction syndrome (MODS) may result from SIRS or sepsis. Organ dysfunction tends to follow a predictable course—independent of the inciting insult—unless the process is halted by therapeutic interventions. Intravascular volume depletion and vasodilation initially lead to hypotension. The acute respiratory distress syndrome (ARDS) may also occur relatively early. Subsequently, acute kidney injury, ileus, mental status changes, and hepatic dysfunction may occur. As the process continues, direct myocardial depression and bone marrow suppression may develop.

Common sites of infection, in descending order of frequency, include the lung, the abdominopelvic region, urinary tract, and soft tissue. In 20% to 30% of patients, a definite site of infection is not identified, and blood cultures may be positive only 30% of the time.

Table 232-1 Consensus Definitions for Sepsis and Organ Failure

Term	Definition
SIRS	Two or more of the following • Temperature >38° C or <36° C • Heart rate >90 beats/min • Respiratory rate >20 breaths/min or $Paco_2$ <32 mm Hg • WBC count >12 × 10^9/L or <4 × 10^9/L or >10% immature band forms
Sepsis	The presence of SIRS and either of the following • An infection suspected or documented by the presence of pathogenic microorganisms on culture or Gram stain of blood, sputum, urine, or normally sterile body fluids • The focus of infection identified by visual inspection (e.g., wound with purulent discharge)
Severe sepsis*	Sepsis associated with organ dysfunction, hypoperfusion, or hypotension. Hypoperfusion and perfusion abnormalities include, but are not limited to, lactic acidosis, oliguria, or mental status changes
Sepsis-induced hypotension*	Systolic blood pressure <90 mm Hg, or reduction of >40 mm Hg, in the absence of other causes for hypotension
Septic shock*	Sepsis-induced hypotension despite adequate fluid resuscitation plus perfusion abnormalities including, but not limited to, lactic acidosis, oliguria, and mental status changes; patients who receive vasopressor or inotropic agents to maintain blood pressure are considered to be in shock even if they are not hypotensive

*Or systemic inflammatory response syndrome (SIRS), depending on whether or not infection is present.
WBC, white blood cell.

Sepsis and SIRS are associated with a vasodilated state; intravascular volume depletion results from "third spacing." The classic picture shows a hyperdynamic, high cardiac output state with a low systemic vascular resistance. However, this hemodynamic pattern may be absent in the early stages before adequate volume resuscitation has taken place or when sepsis-associated myocardial depression leads to a decrease in stroke volume.

Severe sepsis and septic shock are medical emergencies requiring prompt intervention. Guidelines for management have been developed by a multinational multidisciplinary collaboration of experts as part of an education initiative known as the Surviving Sepsis Campaign, the latest iteration being the 2012 version. Many institutions have incorporated these therapies into "sepsis bundles" to promote best practice. Suggested algorithms for investigating potential sepsis and managing patients with sepsis are provided in Figures 232-2 and 232-3. Elements of sepsis management include initial resuscitation, diagnosis, antibiotic therapy, source control, and supportive therapy.

Initial Resuscitation

Fluid resuscitation and identification of the infection with surgical site control, if possible, are hallmarks of treatment. Intravenously administered large-volume fluid resuscitation is required to reverse organ hypoperfusion. In adults, the deficit is often more than 6 L, and both crystalloids and colloids may be administered, preferably according to a protocol. The multicenter SAFE (Saline versus Albumin Fluid Evaluation) study failed to show a benefit of colloid (albumin) over crystalloid (saline) in most patient populations; in patients with traumatic brain injury, albumin was found in a posthoc analysis to be harmful. Arterial and central venous catheters for measuring central venous pressure and venous oximetry are often placed to guide resuscitation. "Early goal-directed" resuscitation has

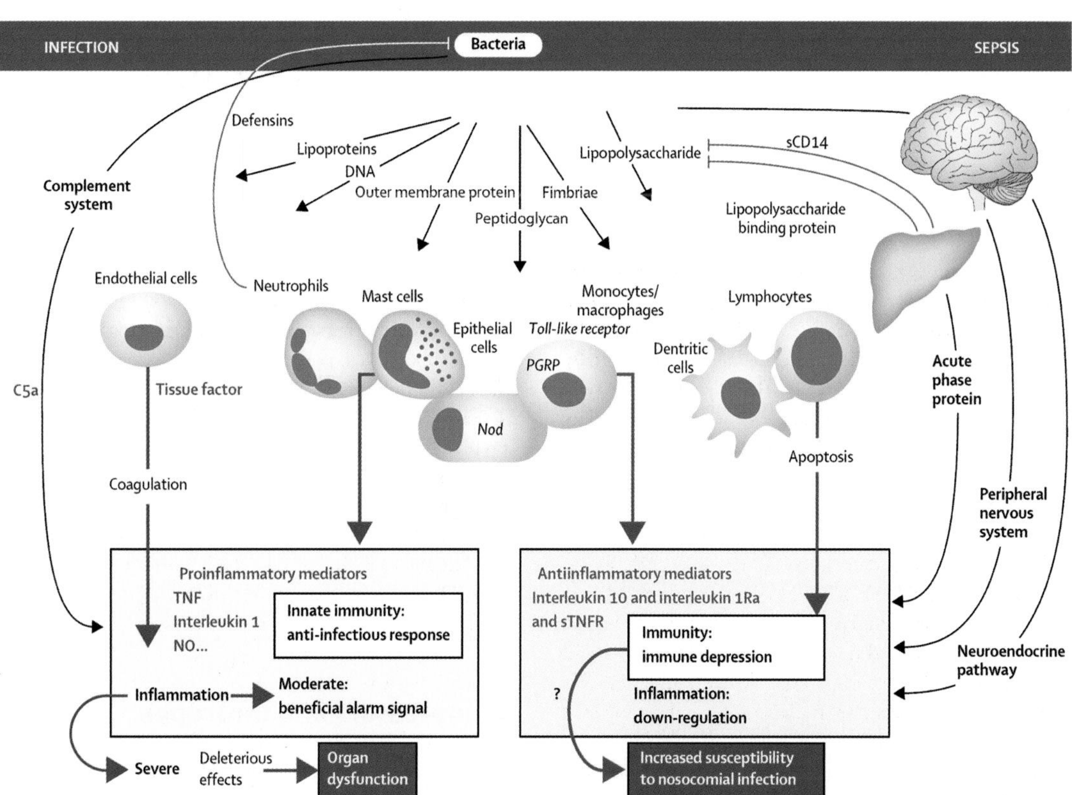

Figure 232-1 Mechanisms of disease after bacterial infection. Barred lines indicate inhibition; lines with arrows, activation or consequences. C5a., Complement component 5a; NO, nitric oxide; Nod, nucleotide-binding oligomerization domain; PGRP, peptidoglycan recognition proteins; sCD14, soluble CD14; sTNFR, soluble tumor necrosis factor (TNF) receptor. (From Annane D, Bellissant E, Cavaillon JM. Septic shock. Lancet. 2005;365:63-78.)

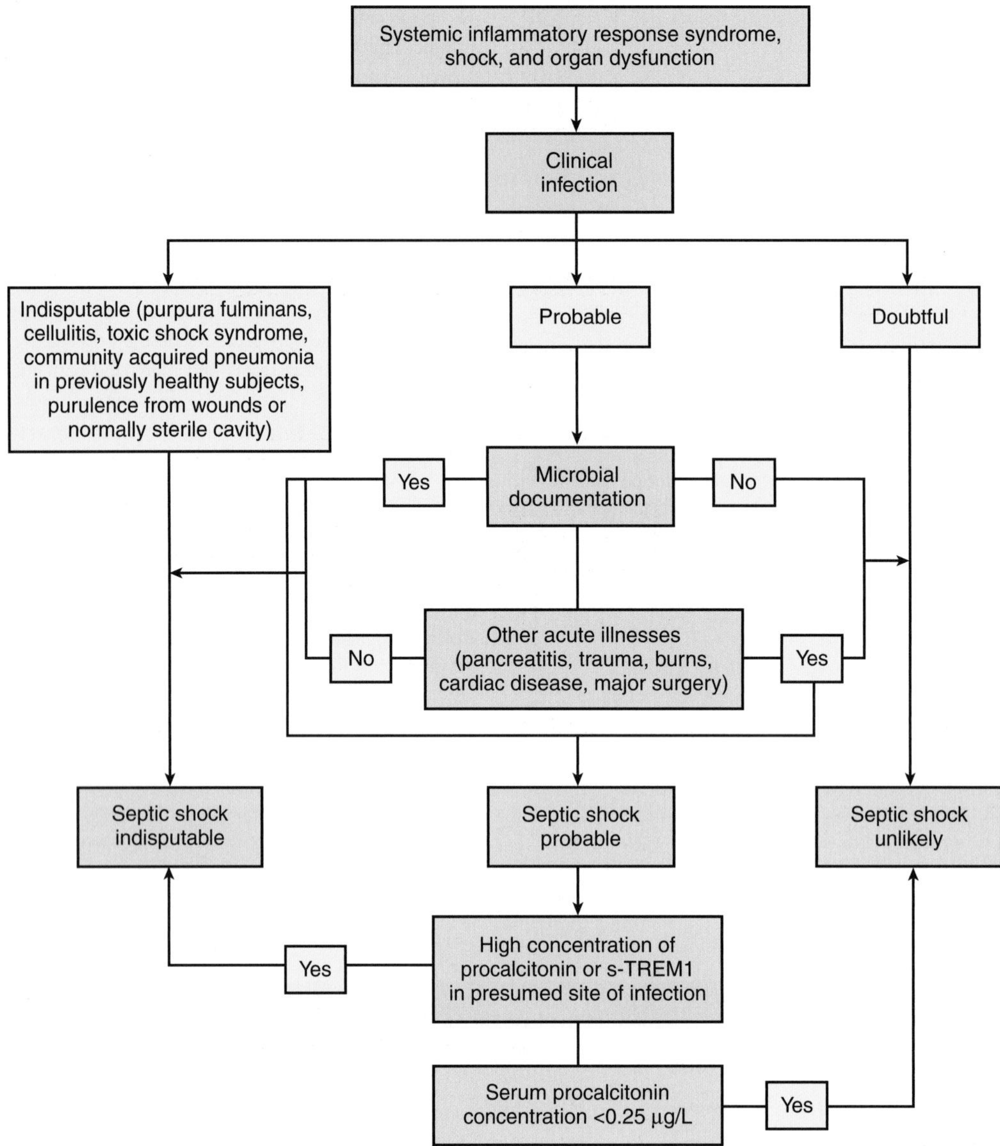

Figure 232-2 Decision tree for the diagnosis of septic shock. sTREM1, Soluble triggering receptor expressed on myeloid cells. (From Annane D, Bellissant E, Cavaillon JM. Septic shock. Lancet. 2005;365:63-78.)

been demonstrated to improve outcomes in septic shock, although the details are debated. Reasonable targets for fluid resuscitation include a central venous pressure of 8 to 12 mm Hg, a mean arterial pressure of at least 65 mm Hg, and a central venous O_2 saturation of at least 70% or mixed venous O_2 saturation of at least 65%.

Evidence supports, during the first 6 h of resuscitation, transfusion of packed red blood cells to a hematocrit of at least 30%, administration of dobutamine (up to 20 $\mu g \cdot kg^{-1} \cdot min^{-1}$), or both to achieve hemodynamic goals if they are not met by fluid administration alone. Although nonspecific, measurement of serum lactate, C-reactive protein, and procalcitonin concentrations may be useful markers.

Diagnosis

Appropriate cultures should be obtained before antimicrobial therapy is initiated, assuming that performance of such cultures does not significantly delay antibiotic administration. Two sets of blood cultures should be drawn in addition to appropriate cultures of other potential sites of infection. Imaging studies should be performed expeditiously, weighing the risk of transport, if required, against the potential benefit of the study.

Antibiotic Therapy and Source Control

Antibiotic therapy, directed against likely pathogens, should be intravenously administered as soon as possible and within the first hour after severe sepsis or septic shock is recognized. Antimicrobial agents that effectively penetrate into the presumed site of infection should be chosen. The initial therapy should cover a wide spectrum of pathogens, with subsequent daily reassessment based on culture data and clinical response. Antimicrobial options are presented in Table 232-2. Identification of an anatomic site of infection should prompt consideration of intervention to control the source (e.g., drainage of empyema or intraabdominal abscess, débridement of infected necrotic tissue, removal of an infected device.)

Vasopressors and Inotropes

Mean arterial pressure should be maintained at a minimum of 65 mm Hg, though preexisting comorbid conditions (e.g., longstanding hypertension) may alter this pressure goal. Surviving Sepsis Campaign recommendations for hemodynamic support are provided in Box 232-1. Norepinephrine is recommended as the first-choice vasopressure in septic shock,

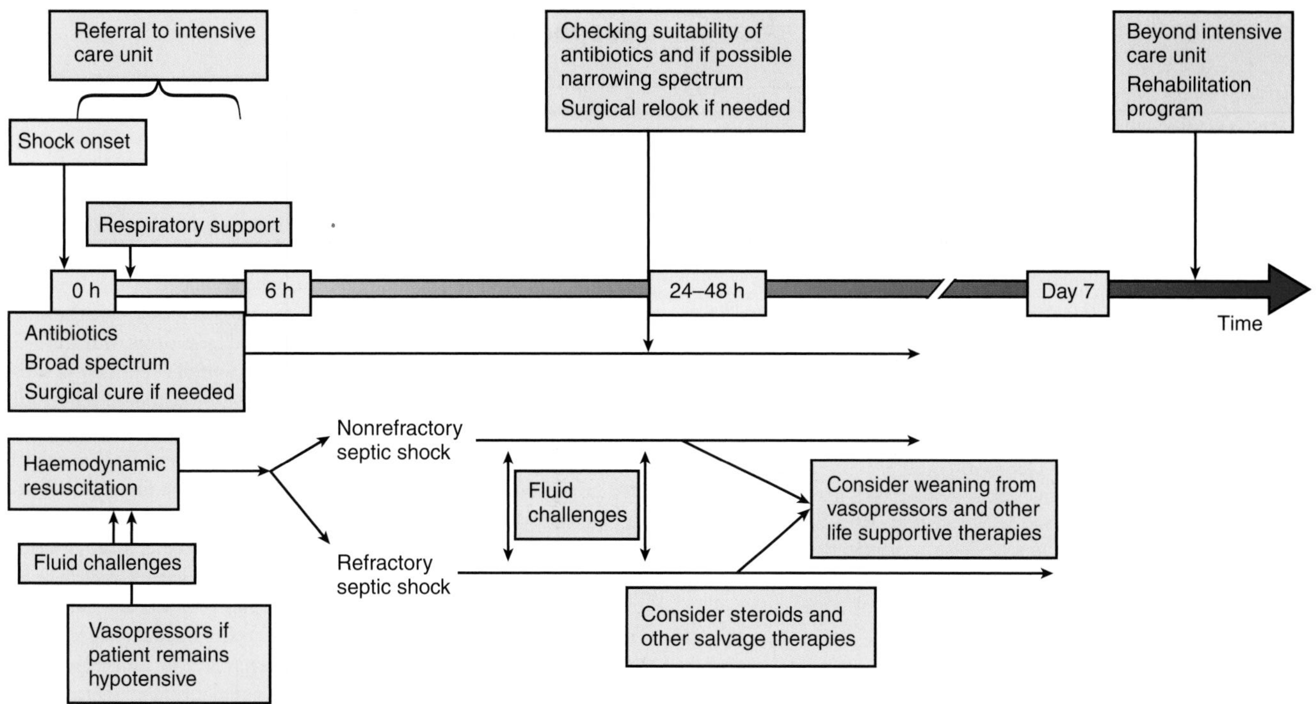

Figure 232-3 Principles of the treatment of septic shock. Pink boxes refer to interventions; brackets, timing of interventions. (Modified from Annane D, Bellissant E, Cavaillon JM. Septic shock. Lancet. 2005;365:63-78.)

Table 232-2 Antimicrobial Choices in Sepsis

Patient Population/ Site of Infection	Likely Pathogen	Recommended Antimicrobial Agent or Agents
Immunocompetent	Gram-positive Gram-negative	Give ureidopenicillins + one of the following β-Lactamase inhibitors Carbapenems Third- and fourth-generation cephalosporins Add antipseudomonal fluoroquinolone if *Pseudomonas aeruginosa* is a likely pathogen. Add vancomycin or linezolid if there is concern for MRSA. Add linezolid if there is concern for VRE.
Immunocompromised	Gram-positive Gram-negative Fungal	Treat as for an immunocompetent patient, with inclusion of vancomycin or linezolid and antipseudomonal agent. Add antifungal (amphotericin B, caspofungin, or voriconazole) if patient is at high risk for fungal infection.
Intravascular catheter–related infections	Gram-positive Gram-negative Fungal	Provide broad-spectrum antimicrobial coverage In settings with a significant MRSA prevalence, vancomycin should be administered. Add antipseudomonal agent in immunocompromised patients. Add intravenously administered amphotericin B or fluconazole if fungemia is suspected.
VAP, HCAP, HAP*	*Streptococcus pneumoniae, Haemophilus influenzae*, MSSA, enteric gram-negative bacilli	In the absence of risk factors that necessitate use of broad-spectrum antibiotics, fluoroquinolone, ampicillin/sulbactam, or ceftriaxone can be given. With recognized risk factors, use antipseudomonal cephalosporin (cefipime, ceftazidime), antipseudomonal carbapenem (imipenem, meropenem), or piperacillin/tazobactam AND antipseudomonal fluoroquinolone (ciprofloxacin, levofloxacin) or aminoglycoside. Add vancomycin or linezolid if there is concern for MRSA. Add macrolide or fluoroquinolone if there is concern for *Legionella pneumophila*.
Severe community-acquired pneumonia	Typical organisms (*S. pneumoniae, H. influenzae, S. aureus*) and atypical organisms (*Mycoplasma pneumoniae, Chlamydia pneumoniae, L. pneumophila*)	Give third-generation cephalosporin and intravenously administered macrolide or non-pseudomonal fluoroquinolone. Give antipseudomonal fluoroquinolone if *Pseudomonas aeruginosa* is a likely pathogen.
Fungal infections	*Candida* spp., *Aspergillus*	Caspofungin, amphotericin B, voriconazole, itraconazole, or fluconazole may be chosen depending on individual patient and organism factors.

*Certain patients (e.g., those with recent antibiotic therapy, prolonged hospitalization, or immunosuppression or on dialysis) require broad-spectrum antibiotics targeting gram-positive, gram-negative, and atypical organisms, such as *Legionella pneumophila* and MRSA. (methicillin-resistant *Staphylococcus aureus*)

HAP, Hospital-acquired pneumonia; HCAP, health care–associated pneumonia; MSSA, methicillin-sensitive *Staphylococcus aureus*; VAP, ventilator-associated pneumonia; VRE, vancomycin-resistant *Enterococcus*.

Box 232-1 Surviving Sepsis Campaign 2012 Recommendations for Hemodynamic Therapy

Crystalloids should be the initial resuscitation fluid in severe sepsis and septic shock. Albumin should be added when substantial amounts of crystalloids are required. Hydroxyethyl starches are not recommended.
A fluid bolus of 30 mL/kg should be administered in hypoperfusion states with presumed hypovolemia. Fluid challenges should be repeated based on response (change in pulse pressure, stroke volume variation, arterial pressure, heart rate).
Vasopressor therapy should target a MAP of 65 mm Hg.
Norepinephrine is the first-choice vasopressor. Epinephrine should be added or substituted when an additional agent is needed to maintain MAP. Vasopressin may be added to increase MAP or decrease norepinephrine dose. Vasopressin should not be used as a single agent, and its use in doses of >0.03-0.04 unit/min should be reserved for refractory cases.
Dopamine and phenylephrine should be used only in highly selected cases. Dopamine should not be used for renal protection.
Dobutamine should be added if myocardial dysfunction is present or if there are signs of hypoperfusion despite adequate intravascular volume and MAP. There is no benefit to achieving a "supranormal" cardiac index.

MAP, Mean arterial pressure.

though epinephrine may be used as an alternative when the patient is poorly responsive to the initial choice. Patients with sepsis may have a relative vasopressin deficiency that contributes to vasodilatation, and intravenously administered vasopressin is increasingly used by many as a vasoconstrictor. Phenylephrine is devoid of β-adrenergic effects and is not recommended as a first-line agent because it is likely to decrease stroke volume. Vasopressor agents should be administered through a central venous catheter as soon as a catheter is available. When myocardial dysfunction is suggested by elevated cardiac filling pressures and low cardiac output, dobutamine should be administered to attain a normal (though not *supra*normal) cardiac index.

Corticosteroids

Relative adrenal insufficiency may be a feature of the "endocrinopathy of critical illness." Although the results of some studies have suggested that supplementation with corticosteroids in patients with septic shock might be beneficial, recent multicenter trials (e.g., CORTICUS [Corticosteroid Therapy of Septic Shock]) have failed to demonstrate a survival benefit in patients with septic shock who received steroids. If hemodynamic stability is not achieved by the use of fluids, vasopressors, and inotropes alone, the administration of hydrocortisone at 200 mg/day may be considered. Patients who have documented adrenal insufficiency or who are likely to have suppression of the hypothalamic-pituitary-adrenal axis because of long-term steroid use should receive supplemental intravenously administered hydrocortisone during episodes of critical illness.

Recombinant Human Activated Protein C

A randomized controlled trial in adult patients with severe sepsis and septic shock demonstrated a survival advantage with the use of the antiinflammatory, antithrombotic, profibrinolytic agent recombinant human activated protein C (rhAPC). This was the first drug targeting the mechanism of sepsis that appeared to offer a survival benefit. Further studies clarified the indications for rhAPC and the contraindications for its use—patients with severe sepsis and a low risk of death or children because of the risk of hemorrhagic complications. Careful consideration was given to the use and timing of administration of rhAPC in surgical patients because anticoagulation was a predictable side effect of the drug. As more studies were conducted, however, other concerns were demonstrated, and the manufacturer withdrew the product from the market in October 2011.

Supportive Therapy

Multiple supportive therapies are often required for patients with sepsis. Noninvasive or invasive mechanical ventilation may be needed for patients with acute respiratory distress syndrome. Mechanical ventilatory support should be based on the principles discussed in Chapter 227. When required, sedation should be guided by protocols that target predetermined end points (e.g., sedation scales), with daily interruption or lightening of sedation with awakening and retitration of sedative agents. Neuromuscular blocking agents should be avoided, if possible, to decrease the likelihood of the development of critical illness polyneuromyopathy, although a short (≤ 48 h) course of neuromuscular blocking agents is recommended for patients with acute respiratory distress syndrome and sepsis. Glycemic control in critically ill patients has been the subject of considerable debate, with evolution of target values over the past decade. The NICE-SUGAR (Normoglycaemia in Intensive Care Evaluation and Survival Using Glucose Algorithm Regulation) study has greatly influenced the Surviving Sepsis Guidelines in this regard. A use of a protocol-based approach is recommended, commencing with intravenously administered insulin when two consecutive blood glucose levels are greater than 180 mg/dL, and targeting an upper blood glucose level of 180 mg/dL or less.

Renal failure is common in patients with septic shock, and renal replacement therapy should be initiated as appropriate. Continuous renal replacement therapy and intermittent hemodialysis are equivalent in patients with severe sepsis and acute renal failure, but continuous techniques may facilitate management of fluid balance in hemodynamically unstable patients.

In addition to the aforementioned therapies, other proven practices (e.g., deep venous thrombosis and stress ulcer prophylaxis, optimal nutrition support) should be used in patients with sepsis.

Unfortunately, septic shock has a mortality rate between 25% and 50%, which is directly related to the number of organ failures. An important aspect of management is communication of likely outcomes to family members or health care surrogates and, when appropriate, consideration for limitation of support.

Suggested Readings

American Thoracic Society and the Infectious Disease Society of America. Guidelines for the management of adults with hospital-acquired, ventilator-associated, and healthcare-associated pneumonia. *Am J Respir Crit Care Med.* 2005;171:388-416.
Angus DC, Linde-Zwirble WT, Lidicker MA, et al. Epidemiology of severe sepsis in the United States: Analysis of incidence, outcome, and associated costs of care. *Crit Care Med.* 2001;29:1303-1310.
Annane D, Bellissant E, Cavaillon JM. Septic shock. *Lancet.* 2005;365:63-78.
Bone RC, Balk RA, Cerra FB, et al. Definitions for sepsis and organ failure and guidelines for the use of innovative therapies in sepsis. The ACCP/SCCM Consensus Conference Committee. American College of Chest Physicians/Society of Critical Care Medicine. *Chest.* 1992;101:1644-1655.
Dellinger RP, Levy MM, Rhodes A, et al. Surviving Sepsis Campaign: International Guidelines for management of severe sepsis and septic shock: 2012. *Crit Care Med.* 2013;41:580-637.
Finfer S, Bellomo R, Boyce N, et al. SAFE Study Investigators. A comparison of albumin and saline for fluid resuscitation in the intensive care unit. *N Engl J Med.* 2004;350:2247-2256.
Finfer S, Chittock DR, Su SY, et al. NICE-SUGAR Study Investigators. Intensive versus conventional glucose control in critically ill patients. *N Engl J Med.* 2009;360:1283-1297.
Hotchkiss RS, Karl IE. The pathophysiology and treatment of sepsis. *N Engl J Med.* 2003;348:138-150.
Levy MM, Fink MP, Marshall JC, et al. 2001 SCCM/ESICM/ACCP/ATS/SIS International Sepsis Definitions Conference. *Crit Care Med.* 2003;31:1250-1256.
Rivers E, Nguyen B, Havstad S, et al. Early goal-directed therapy in the treatment of severe sepsis and septic shock. *N Engl J Med.* 2001;8:1368-1377.
Russell JA. Management of sepsis. *N Engl J Med.* 2006;355:1699-1713.
Sprung CL, Annane D, Keh D, et al. The CORTICUS Study Group. Hydrocortisone therapy for patients with septic shock. *N Engl J Med.* 2008;358(2):111-124.
Wheeler AP, Bernard GR. Treating patients with severe sepsis. *N Engl J Med.* 1999;340:207-214.

CHAPTER 233

Anesthesia for Burn-Injured Patients

Christopher V. Maani, MD, Peter A. DeSocio, DO, and Kenneth C. Harris, MD

Patients with thermal injuries may have problems in the perioperative period that are distinct from those of other surgical populations. These issues require consideration and planning by the anesthesia provider and surgical team to obtain optimal outcomes.

Acute Injury

The first 24 to 48 h after a major burn occurs is considered the resuscitation phase. Depending on the extent of injury, the patient will often require massive amounts of intravascular fluids to maintain intravascular volume, cardiac output, and urine output. Several different formulas can be used to guide therapy, but the primary goal is to administer sufficient fluid to maintain urine output between 0.5 and 1.0 mL·kg^{-1}·h^{-1}, not to restore intravascular euvolemia. During this phase, the patient may require escharotomy or fasciotomy to preserve blood flow to extremities or to allow for chest expansion. Less commonly, a laparotomy may be required to treat abdominal hypertension (abdominal compartment syndrome). Blood transfusion is typically not required during these initial procedures.

For patients with burns that cover less than 40% of total body surface area (TBSA), tracheal intubation is rarely required; however, almost all patients with burns that cover more than 60% of TBSA require intubation. Patients with inhalation injury may require intubation to protect their airways regardless of the size of their burn. The decision to intubate a given patient often requires considerable judgment, but, once the decision has been made, the procedure does not require any unusual considerations beyond those for any other patient with a traumatic injury. If the decision to intubate is delayed until the patient is in respiratory distress, the time remaining before complete arrest occurs may indeed be short. In this situation, because of the increased risk that these patients may develop glottis edema, an "awake" intubation may be indicated. Larger-than-normal tracheal tubes are preferred due to the likely need for bronchoscopy and suctioning of clots or mucous plugs.

General Burn Care

Full-thickness burns, unless very small, must be treated with excision and grafting. Partial-thickness burns may require excision and grafting depending on their depth, size, and location. Antibiotic creams and solutions—silver sulfadiazine or mafenide acetate, a carbonic anhydrase inhibitor—are the drugs most commonly used on some partial-thickness and full-thickness burns. Silver sulfadiazine is considered less painful to apply but does not penetrate intact burn eschar. Silver sulfadiazine may also cause significant leukopenia, typically in the first few days of use. Mafenide acetate cream penetrates burn eschar but can be painful to apply. In patients with large burns or renal failure, a hyperchloremic metabolic acidosis is occasionally seen that may be attributable to the application of mafenide acetate cream and may not resolve until the drug use is discontinued.

Excision and Grafting

Excision of burned skin and placement of skin grafts are the primary reason that patients with burns make frequent trips to the operating room (OR). Some controversy exists over the exact timing of surgery but this approach has changed from delayed intervention to the current practice in which many burn surgeons will operate within 24 to 48 h of the patient's admission; other surgeons will wait 48 h to ensure that the patient has been adequately resuscitated.

Excision may be either tangential, in which the burn is shaved off until unburned tissue is reached, or fascial, in which all skin and underlying fat is removed down to fascia, usually by using an electrocautery device. Tangential excisions generally produce a better functional and cosmetic result. Fascial excisions may be faster to perform and usually result in less blood loss, as compared with tangential excisions. Whichever method is chosen, these procedures can be quite bloody, with blood loss varying from 123 to 387 mL for each 1% of TBSA of burned tissue excised. Several factors affect the volume of blood loss (Table 233-1).

The use of tourniquets and fibrin glue may substantially reduce blood loss. Harvesting of the skin graft may produce considerable blood loss itself, especially if scalp is harvested, but bleeding can be decreased with the infiltration of epinephrine solution into the area to be harvested. Pitkin solution, lactated Ringer's solutions with 1 to 2 mg/L of epinephrine, or other combinations of vasoconstrictors in crystalloid solutions are often used to try to decrease blood loss.

Preoperative Evaluation of the Patient with Burns

In addition to the standard preoperative evaluation, several aspects of the preoperative evaluation in patients with burns deserve special attention and will be covered in the following sections.

Airway

Patients should be examined for scarring that may limit mouth opening or neck extension. The anesthesia provider should anticipate a difficult mask ventilation if the patient has antibiotic cream or bandages on the face. Additional personnel should be present in the OR to assist in managing the airway. A small towel or washcloth that can be placed over cream

Table 233-1 Factors Related to Blood Loss in Patients with Burns

	Blood Loss	
Factor	**Decreases**	**Increases**
Excision technique	Fascial	Tangential
Age of burns	Fresh	Older
Location of burns	Torso	Hands, feet, or shoulders

on the skin should be available should the need arise to provide a tight interface between the mask and skin when managing the airway.

Pulmonary Care

The fraction of inspired O_2, arterial blood gas results, and ventilator settings if the patient is intubated and mechanically ventilated should be noted; burn patients typically have a minute ventilation that is higher than normal.

Patients with inhalation injuries frequently produce plugs or clots that can obstruct a tracheal tube; if this occurs when the patient is in the prone position, the results can be fatal. The anesthesia team should have a plan for dealing with such an emergency should it occur, and that plan should be discussed in advance with other personnel in the OR.

Circulation

Patients who survive their initial burn injury have essentially passed a cardiac stress test, so most of these patients do not require further cardiac evaluations. A burn that involves a large TBSA frequently results in a rise in troponin levels independent of any cardiac injury. Patients with burns are typically hyperdynamic; heart rates in adults of 110 to 120 beats/min are typical. Hypotension that occurs preoperatively should be treated with volume resuscitation; decreased systemic vascular resistance as the cause of hypotension is not typically an issue until later in the patient's hospital course.

Neurologic Care

The primary neurologic issues related to burns are pain and anxiety. Patients may receive large doses of opioids or benzodiazepines and remain surprisingly awake. Assessing a patient's level of consciousness and current drug doses helps the anesthesia provider in developing the anesthetic plan.

Vascular Access

In addition to having an 18-gauge or larger peripheral intravenous line, patients with burns should also have central access established if copious bleeding is anticipated. In such a patient, an arterial cannula should also be placed to monitor blood pressure and for drawing blood for laboratory tests. Plasma-Lyte is the crystalloid most often administered at most burn centers.

Nutrition

Because patients with burns are so catabolic, interruption of alimentation should be minimized as much as possible. Though it is common practice to stop enteral feedings prior to the patient coming to the OR, there are few data to support the practice.

Parenteral Infusions

Patients who are in an intensive care unit may be on many different infusions of drugs, most of which should be stopped prior to the patient coming to the OR unless the infusions are essential.

Care in the Operating Room

Setup

The OR should be heated to 90° F or as close to that temperature as possible. The patient's entire body must often be exposed, thus limiting the usefulness of warming blankets. A rapid blood infusion system should be available. Two to six units of crossmatched packed red blood cells (pRBCs) should be immediately available, with the understanding that, for patients who will require excisions of large amounts of TBSA, 10 to 20 units may be needed, as will fresh frozen plasma and platelets. For patients with facial burns who will be intubated in the OR, the anesthesia provider should plan to secure the tracheal tube with cloth ties; suturing the tracheal tube to a tooth is another viable option, as is intubation with ties around the nasal septum.

Patient Care

Consideration should be given to induction of anesthesia on the patient's bed if movement is especially painful for the patient. Standard placement of monitors is usually routine but may be limited by injuries and dressings. Because standard electrocardiographic lead placement is rarely essential, leads are placed where space permits; in unusual situations, leads may be stapled in place after induction of anesthesia. Noninvasive blood pressure cuffs work surprisingly well over most dressings. Creativity may be needed in placing the probe for a pulse oximeter; the ears, nose, lips, forehead, and hard palate have all been used successfully. Monitoring of body temperature is always required; patients' inability to maintain a temperature of 36°C warrants maximum effort to warm the patient. A Foley catheter should be used for most patients.

Several people, all with clearly defined roles, should be involved in transferring the patient to, or from, the operating table to minimize the risk of inadvertent removal of vascular cannulas or tubes.

Following induction of anesthesia, neuromuscular blocking agents are usually administered, either to facilitate tracheal intubation or as part of a balanced anesthetic. The use of succinylcholine is safe for the first 24 h after a burn, but, beyond that period and for up to a year afterward, can result in dramatic and fatal hyperkalemia. Nondepolarizing neuromuscular blocking agents are regularly used in patients with burns but at larger and more frequent doses than in patients without burns. The exception is mivacurium, which lasts as long or longer in patients with burns, as compared with patients without burns.

With the exception of opioids and catecholamines (e.g., phenylephrine), to which they may be relatively resistant, patients with burns typically respond normally to the usual induction agents. Following induction and intubation, the use of inhalation agents supplemented with opioids works well for most patients. Propofol may be used if the anesthesia provider wishes to administer a total intravenous anesthetic. Ketamine, a traditional agent used for many patients with burns, is also acceptable either as the primary agent or as part of a balanced anesthetic. Emergence delirium is seldom an issue with the use of ketamine because most of these patients receive a benzodiazepine.

Blood loss during the excision portion of the operation may be dramatic, with 1 to 2 L of blood not uncommonly lost in a short period of time. Young healthy adults can easily tolerate hematocrit concentrations of 20%, but once the hematocrit level drops below 18%, patients typically become hypotensive. Older patients with comorbid conditions are less tolerant of hematocrit concentrations of 24% or less. Serum ionized calcium levels should be monitored in patients receiving a large number of pRBCs over a short period of time. At many centers, the patient who has traumatic injury in addition to the thermal injury will receive a ratio of fresh frozen plasma to pRBCs of 1:1. However, the need for non-RBC products varies considerably from case to case and is usually driven by laboratory values, clinically observed bleeding, and judgment. Recombinant activated factor VIIa has been used occasionally in patients who develop coagulopathy, but, at present, there are no outcome data to support its use.

Hypotension secondary to a decrease in systemic vascular resistance from bacteremia or other factors released during excision of the wound is not uncommon but, assuming that the patient's intravascular volume is adequate, responds well to vasopressin, norepinephrine, or phenylephrine.

After skin grafts are placed, they may be covered with a negative pressure dressing or conventional gauze dressings. For those patients who are to be extubated at the end of the operation, care should be taken to provide a smooth emergence from anesthesia to decrease the chance that patient movement (i.e., thrashing about on the bed) may damage the grafts.

Postoperative Care

Appropriate patients are transported to the intensive care unit and returned to the care of the surgical or intensive care unit team. Patients who are not in the intensive care unit should recover in the postanesthesia care unit, where the personnel should ensure that the negative pressure dressings are connected to suction upon arrival to the unit, and are discharged from the unit when they meet discharge criteria.

Care Outside of the Operating Room

Anesthesia providers often assist in caring for patients who require bedside wound care and whose pain cannot be controlled with standard doses of benzodiazepines and opioids. Propofol, at rates of 50 to 200 $\mu g \cdot kg^{-1} \cdot min^{-1}$, is usually well tolerated. Patients frequently require jaw lift to maintain spontaneous ventilation, especially after they receive a bolus dose of propofol, but apnea is uncommon unless opioids have also been given. If propofol alone is inadequate, small doses of ketamine can be added, typically 10 to 20 mg at a time, up to 1 mg/kg. These cases are routinely performed without need for positive-pressure ventilation or supplemental O_2. Pulse oximetry is sufficient monitoring for most patients in this situation.

Electrical Injuries

Electrical injuries are similar to thermal injuries, with a few distinctions. When people have contact with high-voltage sources, they may have extensive underlying tissue destruction beyond the obvious contact point, resulting in extensive muscle necrosis. In such situations, potassium, creatine phosphokinase, blood urea, and creatinine levels must be monitored. Patients with electrical injuries, no matter how small the injuries, are usually monitored for cardiac arrhythmias for 24 h, even though significant arrhythmias are rare.

Nonthermal Skin Diseases

Patients with toxic epidermal necrolysis are frequently provided care in a burn unit. These patients do not require skin grafting, but the anesthesia provider may be involved for management of the airway, which can be challenging because mucous membranes may slough and cause bleeding when manipulated. Direct laryngoscopy in a patient with toxic epidermal necrolysis may result in bleeding sufficient to obscure the view of the airway. The first attempt at laryngoscopy may provide the only good view, and fiberoptic bronchoscopy may be difficult or impossible to perform once bleeding begins.

Conclusion

Providing anesthesia service to patients with thermal injuries requires knowledge of, and preparation for, specific issues. With proper planning and close coordination with the surgical and burn care team, anesthesia providers can safely manage the care of these patients with many of these patients having excellent outcomes with good functional recovery. Because many patients with burns return to the OR multiple times over the course of days to weeks, the anesthesia provider has the opportunity to provide continuity of care that they seldom have with other patients, as well as the satisfaction of seeing patients recover, some quite dramatically.

Suggested Readings

Barret JP, Herndon DN. Effects of burn wound excision on bacterial colonization and invasion. *Plast Reconstr Surg*. 2003;111:744-750.

Cartotto R, Musgrave MA, Beveridge M, et al. Minimizing blood loss in burn surgery. *J Trauma*. 2000;49:1034-1039.

Ducic I, Shalom A, Rising W, et al. Outcome of patients with toxic epidermal necrolysis syndrome revisited. *Plast Reconstr Surg*. 2002;110:768-773.

Han T, Kim H, Bae J, et al. Neuromuscular pharmacodynamics of rocuronium in patients with major burns. *Anesth Analg*. 2004;99:386-392.

Hart DW, Wolf SE, Beauford RB, et al. Determinants of blood loss during primary burn excision. *Surgery*. 2001;130:396-402.

Hettiaratchy S, Dziewulski P. ABC of burns: Pathophysiology and types of burns. *BMJ*. 2004;328:1427-1429.

Ivy ME, Atweh NA, Palmer J, et al. Intra-abdominal hypertension and abdominal compartment syndrome in burn patients. *J Trauma*. 2000;49:387-391.

Johnson KB, Egan TD, Kern SE, et al. Influence of hemorrhagic shock followed by crystalloid resuscitation on propofol: A pharmacokinetic and pharmacodynamic analysis. *Anesthesiology*. 2004;101:647-659.

Martyn JA, Chang Y, Goudsouzian NG, Patel SS. Pharmacodynamics of mivacurium chloride in 13- to 18-yr-old adolescents with thermal injury. *Br J Anaesth*. 2002;89:580-585.

Wolf SE, Kauvar DS, Wade CE, et al. Comparison between civilian burns and combat burns from Operation Iraqi Freedom and Operation Enduring Freedom. *Ann Surg*. 2006;243:786-792.

CHAPTER 234

Perioperative Corticosteroids

Michael J. Murray, MD, PhD

Within a very short period of time after their discovery, corticosteroids were being used for a variety of medical conditions with outstanding results. Unfortunately, within an equally short period of time—just a few years—the adverse effects associated with the use of exogenous corticosteroid administration were recognized, attenuating the initial enthusiasm for these drugs. In the early 1950s, reports began to appear in the medical literature of patients who had been chronically receiving corticosteroids who developed refractory circulatory shock when undergoing major surgical procedures. Clinicians quickly recognized that exogenous corticosteroids suppressed the hypothalamic-pituitary-adrenal (HPA) axis. During any major insult to homeostasis, individuals with a suppressed HPA axis do not release adrenocorticotropic hormone (ACTH, or corticotropin) in sufficient quantities, and, therefore, the adrenal glands do not release an adequate amount of endogenous corticosteroids to handle the stress.

In the past, the solution to suppression of the HPA axis was to administer corticosteroids in sufficient quantities to match what the adrenal glands would have released when maximally stimulated. Because even 2 weeks of corticosteroid use within the previous 3 months has been found to inhibit the HPA axis, recommendations were developed that such patients should receive exogenous corticosteroids when they were undergoing major operations. For these criteria to have been met, the dose of corticosteroids that the patient should have taken would have had to have been high enough to suppress the HPA axis—20 mg of prednisone or its equivalent (Table 234-1). However, because the dose and duration of the use of corticosteroids varied so much, it was not always clear which patients should receive perioperative corticosteroids. Some patients using topical, ophthalmic, or inhaled corticosteroids were found to have suppressed HPA axes.

An ACTH stimulation test in which cosyntropin is administered can test the viability of the HPA axis. In the low-dose version of this test, serum cortisol levels are measured immediately before and 30 min after intravenous injection of a 1-μg/1.73 m^2 or 0.5-μg/1.73 m^2 dose of cosyntropin. In the high-dose version, serum cortisol levels are measured immediately before and 30 and 60 min after intravenous injection of 250 μg of cosyntropin. A serum cortisol concentration of less than 18 μg/dL at 30 min denotes impaired adrenocortical reserve, and the patient may not release sufficient ACTH from the adrenal gland to mount an adequate response to a major stressor. However, cosyntropin stimulation tests are expensive and time consuming to perform. An easier, less expensive alternative has been advocated and adopted for perioperative steroid replacement therapy. Typically, a 100-mg dose of hydrocortisone or its equivalent is administered the day of surgery, with the first dose of steroids administered the morning of surgery.

Table 234-1 Glucocorticosteroid Equivalencies

Agent	Glucocorticoid Activity	Mineralocorticoid Activity	Equivalent Oral or Intravenous Dose (mg)
Cortisol	1	1	20
Cortisone	0.8	0.8	25
Prednisone	4	0.8	5
Prednisolone	4	0.8	5
Methylprednisolone	5	0.5	4
Triamcinolone	5	0	4
Betamethasone	25	0	0.75
Dexamethasone	25	0	0.75

The Role of Corticosteroids in Attenuating Stress Response

In response to major stress (e.g., hemorrhage or sepsis) or if the stress is severe enough to cause a decrease in blood pressure (in the former, from a decrease in preload, stroke volume, and cardiac output; in the latter, from a decrease in systemic vascular resistance), the sympathetic nervous system is activated, and the parasympathetic system is inhibited. Efferent activity in the sympathetic nervous system increases. Postganglionic efferent nerves release norepinephrine in close proximity to smooth muscle cells in the peripheral vasculature. Norepinephrine binds to α-adrenergic receptors, thereby increasing cytoplasmic concentrations of Ca^{2+}. (Think of a "wave" of Ca^{2+} sweeping across the cell—both the height [concentration] and periodicity [rate] have an effect.) The increased Ca^{2+} concentration stimulates binding of actin to myosin, causing the cell to contract. The lumens of the peripheral arterioles narrow, and systemic vascular resistance and blood pressure increase. The sympathetic efferent nerve cells simultaneously stimulate the adrenal medulla to release epinephrine into the adrenal vein, which empties into the renal vein or directly into the inferior vena cava. From the entry site into the inferior vena cava, it is but a short distance to the right atrium. Within the right atrium and subsequent cardiac chambers, epinephrine increases chronotropy (heart rate), inotropy (cardiac contractility), dromotropy (conduction velocity), and lusitropy (myocardial relaxation), all of which increase cardiac output. The α-adrenergic receptors are downregulated within minutes of activation, certainly within 30 min. If nothing intervenes to restore the sensitivity of the α-receptors, blood pressure will fall progressively (especially if hemorrhage or sepsis continues unabated).

When the sympathetic nervous system is activated, a simultaneous activation occurs in the HPA axis. The pituitary gland releases ACTH, which, when it reaches the adrenal gland, stimulates the adrenal cortex to release corticosteroids. These corticosteroids bind to receptors on the smooth muscles in the peripheral vasculature, but they do not stimulate release of Ca^{2+} in the cytoplasm; instead, a complex interaction between the Ca^{2+} and the α-receptors restores the sensitivity to catecholamines.

Treatment of Adrenal Suppression

As described earlier, rather than performing the cosyntropin stimulation test, current practice is to administer hydrocortisone the day of surgery to all patients who are currently taking at least a 10-mg dose of hydrocortisone or its equivalent (enough to suppress the HPA axis) or who have taken that amount of corticosteroids for 14 days at any time in the preceding 3 months. (Previous recommendations were to administer perioperative steroids to any patients who had received this amount of corticosteroid in the previous year, but such recommendations have been found to be too liberal. Three months is sufficient for most patients to regain functionality of the HPA axis.)

Patients currently taking corticosteroids should take their regular dose of corticosteroids the morning of surgery and should then receive 100 mg of hydrocortisone or its equivalent over the next 24 h (Table 234-2). If dexamethasone is chosen, 10 mg before surgery may be adequate to protect the patient because of its potency and duration. These recommendations are the same if the patient is not currently taking corticosteroids but has taken an HPA axis–suppressive dose for 14 days in the previous 3 months.

The recommendation is to space the hydrocortisone dose over 24 h, but, obviously, a patient who was receiving a replacement dose of corticosteroids and develops hypotension intraoperatively that is refractory to treatment should be given a dose of corticosteroids intraoperatively. In fact, because some patients in the intensive care unit who are sufficiently stressed have been demonstrated to have suppression of the HPA axis, corticosteroids are used to treat hypotension in these patients. Similarly, some anesthesia providers who treat trauma patients routinely administer corticosteroids in the operating room to patients who have sustained traumatic injury.

Treatment of Airway Edema

Because of their antiinflammatory properties, corticosteroids have long been used to treat patients with or at risk of developing airway edema. Otorhinolaryngologists performing surgery often administer 4 to 10 mg of dexamethasone to reduce the risk of edema in the nose, pharynx, or larynx. Similarly, anesthesia providers will administer a comparable dose of dexamethasone when anesthetizing children with a small airway, in whom even a minimal amount of edema would compromise the airway, such as those who require a tracheal tube smaller than 4.5 mm or adults who require a wire spiral tracheal tube (usually used because the patient's neck will be flexed or turned so much that a standard tracheal tube might collapse). A similar strategy is often used for patients who have been intubated for several days in the intensive care unit and who are anticipated to be imminently extubated. This is done because even a small amount of edema in a child's airway will decrease the diameter of the airway, will significantly decrease the cross-sectional area of the airway, and will decrease the flow of air by an even greater amount. Similarly, if the anesthesia provider is apprehensive enough to intubate the trachea with a wire spiral tube because of concerns about positioning of the head, there is a high probability that venous drainage of the head will be compromised, which would increase the likelihood of edema developing in the airway or glottic opening. Finally, traction associated with a tracheal tube that has been in place for some time, especially in patients who are able to move their heads, will cause a small amount of repeated movement of the tube, which, in turn, will create friction between the tube and the tracheal mucosa, leading to inflammation. When the tube is in place, the tube stents the airway open, but once the tube is removed, edema will begin to form, narrowing the airway over time.

Table 234-2 Recommended Perioperative Steroid Coverage for Patients Currently Taking Steroids or Who Have Taken Steroids in the Previous 3 Months

Current Daily Dose of Steroid (mg)	Type of Operation	Perioperative Hydrocortisone Coverage
<10	Any	No additional coverage needed*
≥10	Minor	25 mg at induction
≥10	Moderate	Usual preoperative dose + 25 mg at induction + 100 mg over the 24 h after surgery
≥10	Major	Usual preoperative dose + 25 mg at induction + 100 mg/24 h for 48-72 h after surgery

*Assume normal hypothalamic-pituitary-adrenal axis response.

Timing of Administration of the Dose of Corticosteroids

If time is sufficient in patients who have prolonged intubation, the patient should receive a dose of dexamethasone 6 to 8 h before extubation (onset of dexamethasone is 6-8 h), with a second dose administered when the patient is extubated. If only one dose of dexamethasone is planned, it should be given when the patient is extubated. For pediatric patients and for adults undergoing surgery on the head or neck, the dexamethasone, if it is to be given, should be administered at the beginning of the procedure—usually after induction and intubation of the airway. These guidelines are only suggestions, given that no large prospective, randomized, controlled study has shown a benefit with this use of dexamethasone. The results of smaller studies are mixed. Because of their belief that one to two doses of dexamethasone have minimal side effects, many anesthesia providers continue to administer dexamethasone to decrease the chance that patients will develop airway edema.

Treatment of Postoperative Nausea and Vomiting

Postoperative nausea and vomiting (PONV) can occur in up to 33% of patients undergoing anesthesia and surgery (see Chapter 109), depending on the patient's sex, age, and history (smoking, motion sickness, previous PONV) and type of operation the patient has undergone. As in many other situations, an ounce of prevention is worth a pound of cure. Typically, 5-HT_3-receptor blocking agents—because of onset and duration of action—are administered to patients at the end of a surgical procedure, with prochlorperazine and other related compounds used for rescue therapy. In years past, droperidol was administered prophylactically at the beginning of surgical procedures because of its efficacy and duration of action. However, when the U.S. Food and Drug Administration required a boxed warning on the label of droperidol in 2001 regarding the development of *torsades de pointes* in patients with long QT syndrome who received an intravenously administered bolus of more than 1.25 mg of droperidol, the use of droperidol fell out of favor. Some clinicians and departments of anesthesia continue to use droperidol, albeit in smaller doses (0.625-1.2 mg) for prophylaxis of PONV, but others have changed to the use of corticosteroids. Dexamethasone has been found to have the most efficacy—usually at a dose of 4 to 10 mg administered intravenously while the patient is still in the preoperative holding area prior to the patient's transport to the operating room.

The Use of Corticosteroids for Antiinflammatory Properties

Because of their antiinflammatory properties, corticosteroids have been used in the past, and are still used by some, to treat systemic and localized inflammatory responses. In the past, some clinicians used corticosteroids to treat the generalized inflammatory response associated with cardiopulmonary bypass, transfusion reactions, allergic reactions, and anaphylaxis. As techniques for cardiopulmonary bypass have improved, there is less need for the administration of antiinflammatory drugs. With respect to allergic reactions, whether they are caused by transfusion of blood products or drugs, there are better medications that specifically block the degranulation of mast cells and that inhibit H_1 and H_2 receptors. Special note should be made of transfusion-related acute lung injury caused by a reaction between antibodies in transfused fresh frozen plasma (especially if the plasma is obtained from multiparous women) and antigens on the recipient's white blood cells. Corticosteroids have no role in the treatment of transfusion-related acute lung injury, nor in the treatment of acute respiratory distress syndrome.

Anesthesia providers often administer corticosteroids during organ transplantation, but, in this circumstance, the corticosteroids are administered as part of the immunosuppression regimen and will be continued postoperatively, often indefinitely. Such use is beyond the scope of this chapter and will not be discussed further.

Adverse Effects Associated with the Use of Corticosteroids

Corticosteroids have multiple actions (Table 234-3) that highlight their role in maintaining homeostasis during a stress of sufficient magnitude to activate the fight-or-flight response (Figure 234-1). The sequelae of corticosteroid use are not so much adverse effects as they are the primary effects associated with the corticosteroids in general. However, for the purpose of this discussion, we consider these effects to be "adverse effects" when one or two doses of corticosteroids are administered for the treatment or prevention of PONV or edema.

Table 234-3 Effects of Glucocorticoids

System	Effect(s)
Immune	Up-regulate the expression of antiinflammatory proteins Down-regulate the expression of proinflammatory proteins
Metabolic	Stimulate gluconeogenesis Metabolize amino acids from extrahepatic tissue Inhibit glucose uptake in muscle and adipose tissue Stimulate fat breakdown in adipose tissue
Fetal development	Stimulate lung maturation
Arousal and cognition	Enhance memory, vigilance, and cognition
Fluid homeostasis	Normalize extracellular fluid volume: Inhibit dehydration-induced water intake Induce diuresis

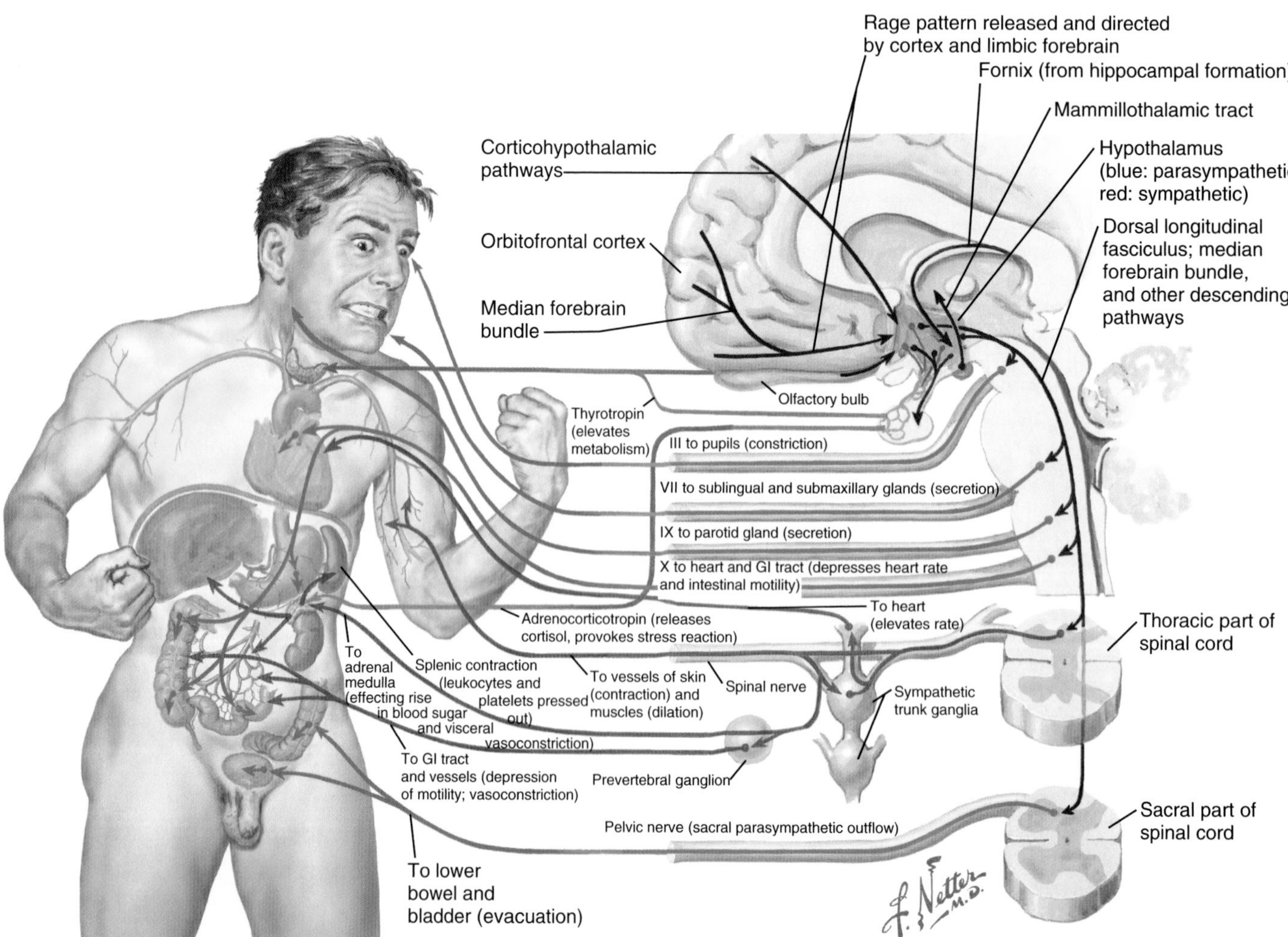

Figure 234-1 Neural, neuroendocrine, and systemic components of rage reaction. (Netter illustration from www.netterimages.com. © Elsevier Inc. All rights reserved.)

The most recognized adverse effect of corticosteroids is hyperglycemia, which can be seen following one or two doses, usually in obese (but not in overweight) patients. Because of the emphasis on maintaining patients' blood glucose levels at less than 180 to 200 mg/dL (depending upon which guidelines are used), obese patients (body mass index $\geq$ 30 kg/m^2) who have received a corticosteroid intraoperatively should have a blood glucose level checked either intraoperatively or in the postanesthesia care unit.

Anesthesia providers should at least be aware of the potential negative effects of corticosteroid use on wound healing and surgical site infection, although no studies have confirmed these associations when only one or two doses of corticosteroids are administered perioperatively. However, these adverse effects should give anesthesia providers cause for concern if they plan to administer more than one or two doses of corticosteroids.

Suggested Readings

Augoustides JG. Integrating outcome benefit into anesthetic design: The promise of steroids and statins. *J Cardiothorac Vasc Anesth*. 2011;25:880-884.

De Oliveira GS Jr, Almeida MD, Benzon HT, McCarthy RJ. Perioperative single dose systemic dexamethasone for postoperative pain: A meta-analysis of randomized controlled trials. *Anesthesiology*. 2011;115:575-588.

Hammond K, Margolin DA, Beck DE, et al. Variations in perioperative steroid management among surgical subspecialists. *Am Surg*. 2010;76:1363-1367.

Mechanick JI, Youdim A, Jones DB, et al. Clinical practice guidelines for the perioperative nutritional, metabolic, and nonsurgical support of the bariatric surgery patient—2013 update: Cosponsored by American Association of Clinical Endocrinologists, The Obesity Society, and American Society for Metabolic and Bariatric Surgery. *Obesity (Silver Spring)*. 2013;21(Suppl 1):S1-27.

Shaw M. When is perioperative "steroid coverage" necessary? *Cleve Clin J Med*. 2002;69:9-11.

Waldron NH, Jones CA, Gan TJ, et al. Impact of perioperative dexamethasone on postoperative analgesia and side effects: Systematic review and meta-analysis. *Br J Anaesth*. 2013;110:191-200.

Yong SL, Coulthard P, Wrzosek A. Supplemental perioperative steroids for surgical patients with adrenal insufficiency. *Cochrane Database Syst Rev*. 2012; 12:CD005367.

CHAPTER 235

Medical Ethics

Keith H. Berge, MD

Medical practice is a complex undertaking, fraught with ambiguity and uncertainty. A clinician is often forced to choose between alternate courses of action when there is little in the way of guidance for his or her actions. How, then, is a decision to be reached in the face of such ambiguity, especially if the decision creates a moral conflict for the physician? Although medical ethics focus on the "oughts" and "shoulds" of patient care, the study of medical ethics will usually fail to reveal a single "right" course of action. However, clarification of the relevant issues of the case at hand will often allow a decision to be reached in a manner that is not capricious or based on a visceral reaction to the clinical facts.

Medical ethics have been an integral part of the practice of medicine for ages. Perhaps the most famous code of ethics is the Oath of Hippocrates, which states many of the principles that still guide the modern-day physician. As modern medical practice has evolved, many ethical dilemmas have become manifest as a result of advances in technology. This has forced a rapid evolution in medical ethics from the relatively simplistic codes that have guided the "virtuous" physician for centuries. Hand in hand with this evolution has been an evolution in the laws regarding a vast array of complex biomedical issues, such as assisted suicide and euthanasia, abortion, surrogate motherhood, genetic testing of minors, withdrawal of artificial nutrition and hydration, and allocation of scarce resources. No broad consensus exists on most of these topics, reflecting the wide range of values within our pluralistic society.

Principles of Medical Ethics

The principles of autonomy, beneficence, nonmaleficence, and justice, expounded on at length by Beauchamp and Childress, are cornerstones of current ethical writings.

Autonomy

Autonomy is derived from the Greek root words *autos* (self) and *nomos* (rule, governance, or law). The autonomous person retains personal rule of the self while remaining free from both controlling interferences by others and personal limitations, such as coercion or inadequate understanding, that prevent meaningful choice. For example, courts and medical ethicists have long agreed that any patient with the capacity to understand the consequences of her or his actions has the right to reject any medical care, even "lifesaving" care, for herself or himself.

Beneficence

Beneficence is an obligation to help others further their important and legitimate interests. This requires the removal of harm as well as the provision of benefit and an effort to balance the benefits and harms of alternate plans of action so as to maximize the benefit. An example of this is the obligation for a physician to render emergency assistance when necessary.

Nonmaleficence

Nonmaleficence is an obligation not to inflict evil or harm on others. It is clearly associated with the maxim *primum non nocere*, "above all, do no harm." The Hippocratic Oath addresses the duty to both nonmaleficence and beneficence with the statement, "I will use treatment to help the sick according to my ability and judgment, but I will never use it to injure or wrong them."

Justice

Justice is giving to each his or her due. This principle has been focused in medical ethics to address just distribution of medical resources. In other words, what characteristics, if any, give one person or group of persons an entitlement to more health care opportunities than others? The principle of justice lies at the very heart of the debate regarding health care reform. That is, if it is now necessary to do less than everything for some people, on what basis do we choose who gets less and how much does each of us "deserve"?

There is no societal consensus on the hierarchical ordering of these principles, but altering the priority of the principles can lead to dramatically different, and yet equally "ethical," solutions to an ethical dilemma. As such, only a naïve person will look to these principles for absolute answers to an ethical dilemma. How, then, is one to bring any order from such seeming chaos? Common sense and an orderly approach are required.

A Method of Resolving an Ethical Dilemma

As proposed by Jonsen and associates and outlined only briefly here, an ethical dilemma can be approached in much the same way as a routine patient history. The familiar chief complaint, history of the present illness, past medical history, and review of systems are replaced with analogous historical features. Ethical features in a clinical case include (1) medical indications (risk:benefit), (2) patient preferences, (3) quality of life, and (4) the contextual features surrounding the case, such as social, economic, legal, and administrative features. Most difficult and ambiguous patient care situations become easier to manage once these issues have been clarified.

Ethical Dilemmas Encountered in Anesthesia Practice

Most of the common ethical dilemmas encountered by the anesthesiologist in the operating room or intensive care unit are primarily questions about the limits of patient autonomy. An example of such a dilemma is the patient who is a Jehovah's Witness and who refuses a potentially lifesaving blood transfusion despite full disclosure of the risks and benefits of this decision. Another example would be the patient who demands to retain a do-not-resuscitate status throughout the perioperative period. Excellent reviews of these two topics can be found in the recent literature. In both of these circumstances, and, indeed, in any circumstance in which a competent adult rejects medical intervention for herself or himself, the courts have been consistent in requiring that the patient's wishes be honored.

Further complexity is introduced into these already difficult situations when these decisions are being either made or related by a surrogate decision maker (e.g., a spouse or family member) on behalf of an incompetent patient. Reflecting growing societal interest and concern brought about by court decisions in so-called "right-to-die" cases, such as that of Nancy Cruzan, Congress enacted the Patient Self-Determination Act in 1991 in an effort to increase the use of advance directives. "Living wills" and "durable powers of attorney for health care" are mechanisms for a patient to give advance directives for care in the event that he or she becomes incompetent. A living will can be difficult to use because its terms can be hard to define and interpret and the conditions can change at various stages of an illness. What do "extraordinary measures" mean for this patient? The patient may have requested no mechanical ventilation, but wouldn't the patient want to be mechanically ventilated until she or he regains consciousness after this anesthetic?

Durable powers of attorney for health care can be more workable in that decisions can be made by an appointed relative, spouse, or friend in an ongoing fashion, as judged by conditions at the time. These documents, in general, are legally binding and obligate the treating physicians to honor the requests contained therein.

In situations in which honoring patient autonomy would create a moral dilemma for the treating physician, if no acceptable compromise position can be reached with reasoned discussion (not coercion), then the physician's only options are either to honor the patient's requests or to withdraw from the care of that patient. The physician who, in such a circumstance, chooses to simply impose his or her values on a patient does so at the potential risk of both civil and criminal penalties. The American Society of Anesthesiologists has available on its website ethical guidelines for the anesthesia care of patients with do-not-resuscitate orders or other directives that limit treatment.

Other potential ethical conflicts encountered by anesthesia providers concern the permissibility of organ donation that is carefully timed to the withdrawal of life support and the issues raised by requests for anesthesia care providers to participate in capital punishment executions.

The study of ethics allows the physician to better recognize that not all people share common beliefs and values and to accept that a well-informed patient with decision-making capacity is the person most capable of determining the "right" course of action for him or her.

Suggested Readings

American Society of Anesthesiologists. *Ethical guidelines for the anesthesia care of patients with do-not-resuscitate orders or other directives that limit treatment.* 2008. Available at: http://www.asahq.org/publicationsAndServices/standards/09.pdf. Accessed May 1, 2010.

Beauchamp T, Childress J. *Principles of Biomedical Ethics.* 5th ed. New York: Oxford University Press; 2001.

Benson KT. The Jehovah's Witness patient: Considerations for the anesthesiologist. *Anesth Analg.* 1989;69:647-656.

Jonsen A, Siegler M, Winslad W. *Clinical Ethics: A Practical Approach to Ethical Decisions in Clinical Medicine.* 6th ed. New York: McGraw-Hill; 2006.

Lanier WL, Berge KH. Physician involvement in capital punishment: Simplifying a complex calculus. *Mayo Clin Proc.* 2007;82:1043-1046.

Miller F, Truog RD. Rethinking the ethics of vital organ donations. *Hastings Cent Rep.* 2008;38:38-46.

Truog RD. "Do-not-resuscitate" orders during anesthesia and surgery. *Anesthesiology.* 1991;74:606-608.

Truog RD, Waisel DB, Burns JP. DNR in the OR: A goal-directed approach. *Anesthesiology.* 1999;90:289-295.

Waisel D. Physician participation in capital punishment. *Mayo Clin Proc.* 2007;82:1073-1082.

CHAPTER 236

Medicolegal Principles: Informed Consent

J. Robert Sonne, JD

Informed consent is the process of providing sufficient information to the patient or surrogate decision maker to allow that patient or surrogate decision maker to fully participate in respective decisions regarding medical care. This process includes securing authorization from the patient or surrogate decision maker for any proposed surgical or significant diagnostic treatment or procedure.

Along with the moral and ethical obligations that are involved in obtaining informed consent, there are also associated legal requirements. Various state, federal, and accreditation (e.g., Joint Commission) statutes, regulations, and guidelines govern and address the legal parameters of the informed consent process. In addition to general process requirements, legal proscriptions often dictate specific informed-consent provisions for certain treatment or diagnostic procedures (for example, HIV/AIDS testing). Investigation into specific state and federal law on informed consent is encouraged.

In situations in which patients have filed lawsuits, central questions often arise as to whether the anesthesia provider acted within the limits of the patient's consent and whether the patient was given sufficient information to adequately consent to the proposed treatment or diagnostic procedure. Such lawsuits are generally brought under negligence or battery theories.

The Informed-Consent Process

Informed consent for anesthesia often occurs when the patient and anesthesia provider meet moments before the surgical procedure is scheduled to begin. For anesthesia providers, the informed consent process should occur before administration of preprocedure sedation and generally should include a discussion of the elements outlined in Box 236-1. It is largely impractical to discuss all associated risks related to a specific anesthesia treatment or procedure. Thus, in determining what relevant risks to discuss, the physician should consider discussing those procedure or treatment risks that are most common and most severe. In defining how much information a physician should disclose, there are two dominant standards. The "professional" standard holds that the anesthesia provider must disclose information that other anesthesia providers possessing the same skills and practicing in the same or similar community would disclose in a similar situation. The "materiality" standard considers what a reasonable patient would have considered important in making a decision.

During the informed-consent discussion, the anesthesia provider is encouraged to ask patients if they have questions or other concerns about the proposed treatment or procedure. Good communication is often an effective deterrent against future patient complaints and legal claims. During this process, the patient also is generally asked to review and sign a written informed-consent form before the proposed surgical or significant diagnostic treatment or procedure. Whether a signed written informed-consent form is warranted may vary based on applicable state, federal, and accreditation statutes, regulations, or guidelines (e.g., see Center for Medicaid Services Conditions of Participation guidelines). Informed-consent forms generally list the specific procedure or treatment to be performed and may include specific risks, complications, or alternatives. Such forms also may include language indicating that not all discussed risks, complications, or alternatives are expressly listed in the form. Overall, the informed-consent form serves as valuable evidence that the informed process occurred and that the patient consented to the recommended treatment or procedure.

As noted previously, good documentation is effective in preventing and defending complaints and legal claims. Consequently, anesthesia providers are additionally encouraged to timely dictate or otherwise enter a note into the medical record (independent of the signed informed-consent form) that substantiates that the informed-consent discussion occurred. In preparing this note, the anesthesia provider should consider listing the most significant discussed risks and alternatives and should expressly note the patient's consent and election to proceed.

Box 236-1 Elements to Be Discussed by the Patient and Anesthesia Provider During the Preoperative Visit

The patient's diagnosis
The nature and purpose of the proposed anesthesia treatment or procedure
The relevant risks and benefits of the proposed anesthesia treatment or procedure
The relevant risks and benefits of reasonable alternatives (including no treatment) to the proposed anesthesia treatment or procedure

Obtaining Informed Consent When Treating the Incompetent or Minor Patient

If the patient is unable to make his or her own health care decisions or is a minor (under age), an appropriate surrogate decision maker most likely needs to be consulted to make decisions and consent to the patient's care and treatment.

If the patient is an incompetent adult, informed consent is generally obtained from the patient's legal guardian or health care power of attorney. If the patient does not have either a legal guardian or a health care power of attorney, state laws often provide a priority list of surrogate decision makers. These state statutes usually provide highest priority to spouses and then proceed to other family members (e.g., adult children, parents, siblings, grandchildren) and individuals (e.g., domestic partners, close friends). If no surrogate decision maker is available or willing to provide informed consent, some state statutes allow attending physicians to make and consent to health care decisions. This form of consent, however, is typically only permitted after additional approval is obtained from a hospital ethics committee or a second physician.

If the patient is a minor, informed consent is usually obtained from the patient's parents or legal guardian, with assent obtained from the minor, if possible. In certain circumstances, however, a minor may consent without approval from a parent or legal guardian. For example, some states may allow a minor to independently consent to his or her own care if the minor is emancipated, married, in the United States military service, or homeless. In addition, states may allow a minor to independently consent to care related to sexually transmitted diseases, substance abuse treatment, HIV testing, contraception, abortion, or sexual assault. Anesthesia providers are encouraged to review applicable state law for consent exceptions for minors.

Obtaining Informed Consent in Emergent Circumstances

If the anesthesia provider determines that an emergency exists, informed consent is not required to undertake surgical or significant procedures that are necessary to treat or diagnose the patient's emergent condition. When informed consent is not obtained because the circumstances are emergent, the physician should document the circumstances that support the emergency.

Suggested Reading

Paterick TJ, Carson GV, Allen MC, Paterick TE. Medical informed consent: General considerations for physicians. *Mayo Clin Proc*. 2008;83(3):313-319.

CHAPTER 237

Medicolegal Principles: Medical Negligence

J. Robert Sonne, JD

A medical negligence or malpractice lawsuit is a civil action commenced by a patient or an authorized representative of the patient seeking monetary damages for injuries claimed to have resulted from negligent treatment. Medical negligence is the most common threat of liability faced by physicians in the United States.

Elements of Malpractice Actions

A patient is entitled to recover monetary compensation from a physician if the patient can prove that the physician's conduct was below the standard of care and that the conduct caused the patient's injury. It is not enough that the patient suffered a complication or was injured as a result of medical care. The patient must show that the medical care provided by the physician was below the standard of care.

To prevail in a lawsuit, the patient has the burden of proving that a deviation from the standard of care occurred and that the injury was directly caused by that deviation. In most cases, a preponderance of the evidence must support the allegations, and proof must be to a "reasonable degree of medical certainty." To prove deviation from the standard of care, it must be shown that an anesthesiologist failed to use that amount of care and skill commonly exercised by other anesthesiologists with similar training and experience under the same circumstances. Physicians should not be found negligent if they elect to pursue one of several recognized courses of treatment, provided that a respectable number of physicians accept the course of treatment. In addition, reasonable medical judgment, even if in error, should not be considered negligence.

Most often, expert testimony establishes the applicable standard of care. A physician sued for medical malpractice has the right to a jury trial. Because jurors are usually unable to independently evaluate whether medical care is appropriate, physicians and experts explain the medical issues to assist the jury in reaching a conclusion. The expert witness generally has credentials and experience like those of the physician on trial and testifies as to whether the physician acted in accordance with the accepted standards of care. The stringency of the rules on expert qualifications varies by state.

The standard of care may also be established by a variety of other means, including medical treatises or guidelines written by professional organizations, policies of the hospital in which care was provided, and recommendations of drug and device manufacturers. Out-of-court statements by physicians (such as statements to the patient or other colleagues) or documents may constitute admissions against interest and may also be introduced as evidence of a deviation from the standard of care.

If a deviation from the standard of care can be proved, some type of injury must also be proved. Generally, at least some physical injury is necessary. Damages may be awarded to compensate for lost income, past or future medical expenses, and other less tangible elements of an injury, such as pain and suffering and embarrassment.

Finally, a patient must prove that the physician's deviation from the standard of care proximately caused injury and that the injury was not caused by an underlying disease process. A physician's negligent conduct may be a legal cause of harm if it is a substantial factor in bringing about the injury.

Types of Claims Against Anesthesia Personnel

The American Society of Anesthesiologists Closed Claims Project provides important information about the types of claims against anesthesia personnel. The Project, initiated in 1984, collects information from insurance companies about closed claims related to events leading to anesthesia-related injury. Numerous references have been published from the data about specific types of anesthetic injuries and resultant malpractice claims, giving a broad-based rather than an anecdotal picture. In general, the types of injuries that result in malpractice claims against anesthesia personnel include dental injury, nerve injury, and death or brain injury caused by either respiratory or cardiac events.

Lack of Informed Consent

Courts have long recognized that patients have a right to consent to medical treatment. (For more information on informed consent, see Chapter 236.) A patient may allege that no consent was given for a procedure and may seek damages for battery. More often, however, patients allege lack of informed consent or negligent nondisclosure. A physician has a legal obligation to advise the patient of certain risks and benefits associated with medical care, as well as available alternatives. Liability may be based on whether the physician failed to disclose a risk that should have been disclosed and whether that risk occurred.

The Process

Medical malpractice lawsuits are formally commenced by filing or service of a summons and complaint. Notification of the claim may occur before formal commencement of a lawsuit and may come in the form of a letter or formal notice. Individuals as well as corporations may be named as defendants. The lawsuit must be commenced within the statute of limitations, a time period that varies by state. If the lawsuit continues, pretrial discovery occurs in the form of either depositions or written documentation. A relatively small percentage of cases are tried; most are either settled or dismissed. If a trial occurs, a jury is generally charged with determining the facts, and the presiding judge is responsible for determining the applicable law.

Managing Legal Risk

Practicing within accepted standards is the best defense against malpractice liability. Good communication among health care providers and with the patient is critical. Documentation is an essential part of a risk-management strategy and should be comprehensive, accurate, objective, and timely. Inadvertent admissions against interest should be avoided. The most common forms of admissions against interest are self-criticism or criticism of colleagues after an adverse outcome and speculation about the cause of an event before all of the facts are known. Guidelines and policies should be realistic and written to allow for emergencies and physician discretion.

Acknowledgment

The author and editors would like to thank Ann E. Decker, JD for her work on this chapter in previous editions.

Suggested Readings

Cheney FW, Posner KL, Lee LA, et al. Trends in anesthesia-related death and brain damage: A closed claims analysis. *Anesthesiology*. 2006;105:1081-1086.

Choctaw W. *Avoiding Medical Malpractice: A Physician's Guide to the Law*. New York: Springer; 2008.

Sandnes DL, Stephens LS, Posner KL, et al. Liability associated with medication errors in anesthesia: A closed claims analysis. *Anesthesiology*. 2008;109:A770.

CHAPTER 238

The American Society of Anesthesiologists Closed Claims Project

Julia I. Metzner, MD, and Karen B. Domino, MD, MPH

The Impact of Closed Claims Analysis in Anesthesiology

The Closed Claims Project was started in 1985 by the American Society of Anesthesiologists (ASA) as part of a series of initiatives directed at improving the safety of patients undergoing anesthesia and surgery. The specific idea was that rising malpractice insurance costs could be reduced, first, by identifying the scope and causes of significant anesthesia-related patient injuries and, second, by making changes in practice. Over the past 30 years, the Project has successfully contributed to improvements in anesthesia patient safety, and malpractice insurance premiums for anesthesiologists have been substantially reduced. Detailed analysis of adverse outcomes with common patterns has provided valuable insights into important patient risk and safety problems. Discovery of recurrent trends has generated safety and education programs aimed to improve patient safety and the quality of anesthetic care.

Data Collection and Limitations

The database is a structured collection of adverse anesthetic outcomes from the closed claims files of medical liability insurance companies, which insure more than one third of anesthesiologists in the United States. Volunteer ASA members travel to participating medical liability insurance companies to review medical records, depositions, and analyses of closed malpractice claims against anesthesiologists. Clinical data (e.g., patient demographics, procedure, anesthetic technique, type and severity of injury, sequence of events leading to injury, and a detailed summary) as well as liability data (e.g., standard of care, claim resolution, and claim settlement) are collected. Claims for dental injury, the most common claim against anesthesiologists, are not included in the database.

It is important to remember that data concerning how many and what types of anesthetic agents and techniques have been administered by anesthesiologists insured by the companies are not known. Hence, relative risks of a particular anesthetic technique cannot be determined by the Closed Claims Project. The database consists of only claims against anesthesiologists, not other anesthesia providers or medical specialists, unless the provider or specialist worked with the anesthesiologist. In addition, malpractice claims are estimated to represent only 3% to 4% of all patient injuries due to negligence. Because the U.S. medical liability system is a tort-based system with plaintiff payment contingent upon a successful lawsuit, the database is biased for severe injuries that occurred in patients who received substandard care. However, the database does contain a wealth of clinical details of rare, severe, adverse outcomes, and it provides a snapshot of liability in the United States.

Overview of Adverse Outcomes and Their Causes

The database currently contains almost 10,000 claims. The three major adverse outcomes in the database are death (29%); nerve damage (peripheral nerve or spinal cord, 19%) or brain damage (10%); and all other complications (e.g., airway trauma, stroke, myocardial infarction), account for the remaining 42% of claims (Figure 238-1). Although various media outlets have given extensive coverage to the topic of awareness during anesthesia, awareness represents only 2% of the claims in the database and, hence, is not currently a major medicolegal risk in the United States.

The types of complications that are listed in the database vary with the type of anesthesia used (Figure 238-2). A greater proportion of claims for death involve death occurring during monitored anesthesia care, as compared with during general or regional anesthesia. Permanent

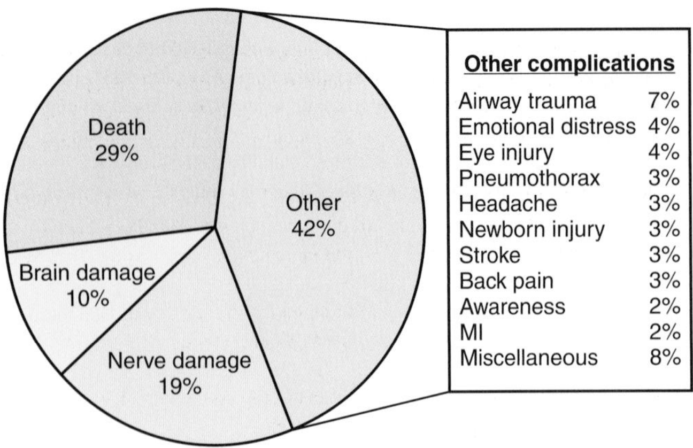

Figure 238-1 The percentage of complications among 7740 claims included in the American Society of Anesthesiologists Closed Claims database. MI, Myocardial infarction.

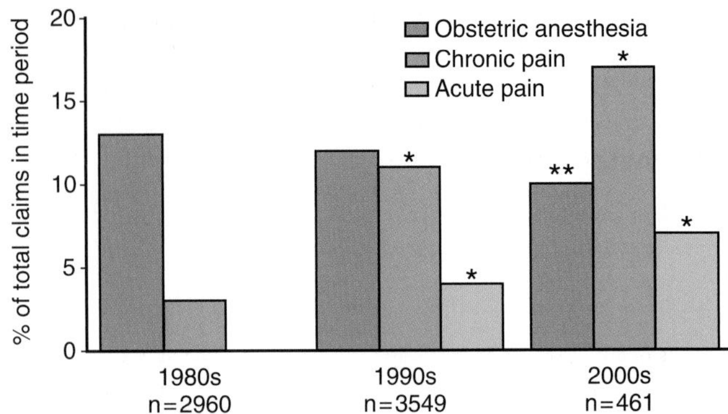

Figure 238-3 Proportion of claims related to obstetric anesthesia, chronic pain, and acute pain by decade among 7740 claims included in the American Society of Anesthesiologists Closed Claims database. $*p < 0.01$; $**p < 0.05$ compared with the 1980s.

nerve injury is more often associated with the use of regional anesthesia (see Figure 238-2).

Four categories of damaging events (i.e., events that caused the injury) account for almost two thirds of all claims: respiratory events (25%), regional nerve block–related events (19%), cardiac events (14%), and equipment-related events (11%). The causes of respiratory events include difficult intubation, inadequate oxygenation/ventilation, esophageal intubation, aspiration of gastric contents, and bronchospasm. Cardiovascular events include excessive blood loss, inadequate fluid replacement, embolism of a variety of causes, and myocardial infarction, among others. Equipment-related events are associated with the use of peripheral and central catheters, electrocautery, infusion pumps, and heating devices, as well as anesthesia ventilators and delivery systems.

Claims associated with acute or chronic pain management have increased since the 1980s and represent more than 15% of all claims collected against anesthesiologists (Figure 238-3). The marked escalation in pain-related claims corresponds with the increasing use of acute and chronic pain therapy over the past decade. Claims associated with obstetric anesthesia make up approximately 10% of current claims (see Figure 238-3).

Trends in Injury

Respiratory Monitoring

An initial finding of the Closed Claims Project was that respiratory-associated adverse events (e.g., inadequate ventilation, esophageal intubation, and difficult intubation) accounted for most claims for death or brain damage in the 1970s and early 1980s. Review of these claims found that the use of pulse oximetry and capnography (or both) would have prevented most of these adverse outcomes. These findings contributed to the ASA adopting pulse oximetry and end-tidal capnography as standards for intraoperative monitoring during general anesthesia in the early 1990s.

A recent review of claims related to monitored anesthesia care found that oversedation, with respiratory depression from sedative or analgesic drugs, was the most important cause of injury during monitored anesthesia care. More than half of claims were judged to have been preventable with the use of better monitoring, including pulse oximetry, capnography, or both. Similarly, monitored anesthesia care was associated with half of the 87 claims for injuries that occurred with anesthesia taking place in remote locations. Respiratory depression secondary to oversedation during monitored anesthesia care accounted for more than a third of remote-location claims. Substandard care, preventable by better monitoring, was implicated in the majority of claims associated with death. These findings contributed to the ASA adding end-tidal capnography as standard for intraoperative monitoring during monitored anesthesia care in 2011.

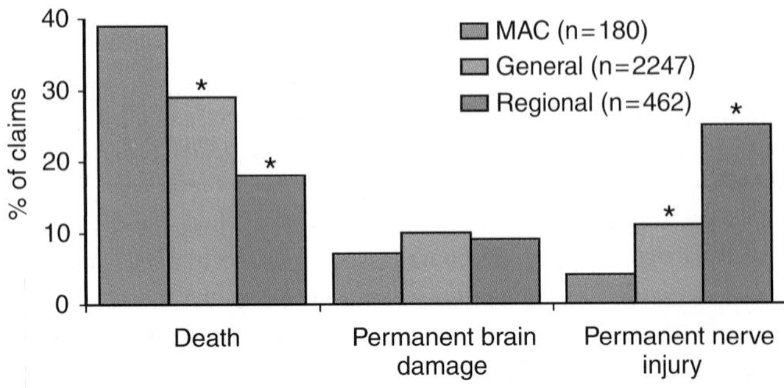

Figure 238-2 Percentages of injuries and type of anesthesia in surgical claims among 7740 claims included in the American Society of Anesthesiologists Closed Claims database. $*p < 0.01$ versus claims associated with monitored anesthesia care (MAC).

Difficult Intubation

The analysis of closed claims for injuries caused by difficult tracheal intubation led to the organization of an ASA Taskforce (1993) that established practice guidelines for management of the difficult airway. A 2005 review of closed claims found that, after implementation of the guidelines, difficult-airway claims associated with death or permanent brain damage during induction decreased from 62% to 35%. In contrast, death or brain damage associated with management of the difficult airway during other phases of the anesthesia did not significantly change after the guidelines were implemented. These results suggest that development of additional strategies for management of the difficult airway encountered during emergence and recovery from anesthesia may improve patient safety. Persistent attempts to intubate were associated with death or brain damage. The 2013 update of the difficult airway practice guideline incorporated additional recommendations for extubation of the difficult airway and the enhanced use of the laryngeal mask airway in difficult intubation.

Obstetric Anesthesia

The practice of obstetrics carries a high medicolegal risk, particularly due to claims related to newborn injury, primarily cerebral palsy. A 2009 review of obstetric anesthesia claims found that claims against anesthesiologists related to newborn death or brain damage represented only 20% of all obstetric claims, with payments made in only a fifth of these claims. Payments were made when anesthesia contributed to the newborn injury, such as a delay from decision to incision of an emergent cesarean section, poor communication with the obstetrician regarding the urgency of delivery, or substandard care in response to an anesthetic catastrophe, such as a difficult intubation or hypotension due to neuraxial anesthesia. Delays in the diagnosis and resuscitation of patients who had received a high neuraxial block were preventable causes of maternal death and brain damage. However, the most commonly occurring claims in obstetric anesthesia are for maternal nerve injury; differentiating between causes related to the block and those related to labor and delivery may be difficult.

Lessons Learned from the ASA Closed Claims Project

Analysis of the Closed Claims Project database has contributed to the use of pulse oximetry and capnography as standards during general anesthesia. Consequently, anesthesia mishaps, particularly those related to inadequate ventilation and esophageal intubation, have decreased since the early 1990s. Recent claims have demonstrated the advantages to using capnography to monitor ventilation during monitored anesthesia care.

Injuries for difficult tracheal intubation motivated the ASA to develop practice guidelines for the management of the difficult airway. As a result, rates of death and permanent brain damage have decreased during the induction of anesthesia. However, claims related to the management of difficult airways, particularly during emergence and recovery from anesthesia, continue to occur.

Suggested Readings

American Society of Anesthesiologists. *Standards for basic anesthetic monitoring* (Approved by the ASA House of Delegates on October 21, 1986, and last amended on October 20, 2010 with an effective date of July 1, 2011). Available at: http://www.asahq.org/For-Members/Standards-Guidelines-and-Statements.aspx.

Apfelbaum JL, Hagberg CA, Caplan RA, et al. Practice guidelines for management of the difficult airway. An updated report by the American Society of Anesthesiologists Task Force on Management of the Difficult Airway. *Anesthesiology*. 2013;118(2):251-270.

Bhananker SM, Posner KL, Cheney FW, et al. Injury and liability associated with monitored anesthesia care: A closed claims analysis. *Anesthesiology*. 2006;104:228-234.

Cheney FW, Posner KL, Lee LA, et al. Trends in anesthesia-related death and brain damage. *Anesthesiology*. 2006;105:1081-1086.

Davies JM, Posner KL, Lee LA, et al. Liability associated with obstetric anesthesia: A closed claims analysis. *Anesthesiology*. 2009;110:8-9.

Domino KB. Medical liability insurance: The calm before the storm? *American Society of Anesthesiologists Newsletter*. 2013;77(10):54-56.

Metzner J, Posner KL, Domino KB. The risk and safety of anesthesia at remote locations: The US closed claims analysis. *Curr Opin Anaesthesiol*. 2009;22:502-508.

Peterson GN, Domino KB, Caplan RA, et al. Management of the difficult airway. *Anesthesiology*. 2005;103:33-39.

CHAPTER 239

Patient Safety and Quality Improvement

Karl A. Poterack, MD

Although patient safety and quality improvement (QI) have been priorities for health care institutions for some time, it was the 2006 report of the Institute of Medicine highlighting the morbidity and mortality risks associated with iatrogenic injury in hospitals that captured the public's interest. Although the report has many problems, the chief executive officers of Fortune 500 companies and third-party payers found the report to be in keeping with their thoughts on the health care industry: reimbursement for health care was increasing at double-digit rates every year, but outcomes were no better, and days of work lost due to illness were not decreasing. Accordingly, over the last several years, QI and the safety of patients in health care institutions has garnered more publicity and increased emphasis on safety.

Quality Improvement

QI is a strategy to guide individual and group decision making. It has its roots in engineering and manufacturing, where systems theory and statistical process control were combined with general management methods. It is variously defined as the reduction of variability in products and processes and as an organized process that assesses and evaluates health services to improve practice or quality of care. International Organization for Standardization (ISO) standard 8402-1986 defines quality as "the totality of features and characteristics of a product or service that bears its ability to satisfy stated or implied needs." The Institute of Medicine defines health care quality as "the extent to which health services provided to individuals and patient populations improve desired health outcomes." W. Edwards Deming defined quality as "meeting customer requirements at a price they are willing to pay."

QI programs in anesthesiology are guided by requirements of regulatory bodies, such as state law, Center for Medicare Services, and The Joint Commission. Unfortunately, many clinicians view QI programs as being driven solely by mandates of these external regulatory groups, which results in the whole system being perceived as "red tape" and "overhead" that add cost but no real value. Such an approach can easily become a self-fulfilling prophecy by consuming resources through the production of unread reports and paperwork, thus diverting resources that could be devoted to actually increasing quality.

Different elements of a QI program may focus on the structure, process, and outcome of health care delivery programs. Structure refers to the setting in which care is provided, (e.g., personnel, facilities, and how they are organized); process, to the patient care activities that are performed; and outcome, to any changes in the patient's health after the care was performed. QI programs, therefore, address all areas of hospital operations. An *adverse event* then, is an untoward, undesirable, and usually unanticipated event, such as the death of a patient, but also of an employee or a visitor in a health care organization. Incidents such as patient falls or improper administration of medications are also considered to be adverse events even if the event has no permanent effect on the patient. A *medical error* is an adverse event or near miss that is preventable with the current state of medical knowledge, and a *sentinel event* is a single isolated event that may indicate a systems problem.

The Joint Commission defines a sentinel event as "an unexpected occurrence involving death or serious physical or psychological injury, or the risk thereof. Serious injury specifically includes loss of limb or function. The phrase 'or the risk thereof' includes any process variation for which a recurrence would carry a significant chance of a serious adverse outcome." The Joint Commission requires all sentinel events to undergo root-cause analysis. In this analysis, the stakeholders who were involved in the care of the affected patient at the hospital in which the sentinel event occurred analyze the events to identify flaws in the system process.

Continuous QI views patient care as a complex system in which undesired results occur because of either a random or a system error. The default assumption is that errors are systems-based until proved otherwise. System errors should be controllable through changing the system. These systems problems ("opportunities for improvement") are identified on an ongoing basis, and strategies are implemented to prevent their occurrence.

Identifying these opportunities for improvement may occur in one of several ways. A common method of identification, mandated by regulatory bodies and with a long history of use in medicine, is to focus on undesirable outcomes—the mortality and morbidity method. In contrast with the shame, blame, and scapegoating of many traditional mortality and morbidity processes, continuous QI focuses not on blame, but, rather, on identification of the system causes of undesirable outcomes. A second way of identifying areas of improvement is the suggestion box method—giving the opportunity to those actually involved in the process to identify problems and suggest solutions. This method may range from planned gatherings at various intervals to specifically gather input, to a very informal open-door policy that fosters and encourages input from those on the front line. A third category is through the systematic measurement of predefined indicators of quality, such as wait times, turnover times, materials waste, and rates of adverse outcomes.

Once specific opportunities for improvement are identified, their current status is measured. The process of care leading to these problems is analyzed. Although the proper way to perform this analysis varies widely, several key points apply to all of them: (1) all areas involved in the actual process (the stakeholders) need to be involved in the analysis, (2) the analysis must be as detailed as possible, (3) the temptation to jump to conclusions must be resisted ("if only the residents would correctly fill out the paperwork, we wouldn't have a problem"), and (4) the goal is to change the system to facilitate the desired outcome.

If change is identified that should lead to improvement, it is implemented. After an appropriate time period, the status is measured again to determine whether improvement actually occurred. Attention may then be directed to continuing to improve this process or turning to a different process to target for improvement.

Medication Errors, Assessment, and Prevention

A common focus of QI programs is the prevention of medication errors. An *adverse drug event* refers to any incident in which the use of a medication (drug or biologic) at any dose, a medical device, or a special nutritional product (e.g., dietary supplement, infant formula, medical food) may have resulted in an adverse outcome in a patient. An *adverse drug reaction*, on the other hand, is an undesirable response associated with use of a drug that compromises therapeutic efficacy, enhances toxicity, or both. The aforementioned Institute of Medicine report identified medication errors as the most common type of error in health care and attributed several thousand deaths to medication-related events.

Numerous organizations have published recommendations for the prevention of medication errors, including, for example, the Agency for Healthcare Research and Quality, the Institute for Healthcare Improvement, the Institute for Safe Medication Practices, The Joint Commission, and the National Quality Forum. These recommendations include implementing computerized provider order entry, using barcoding technology at the point of care, ensuring availability of pharmaceutical decision support, having a central pharmacist supply high-risk intravenously administered medications and pharmacy-based admixture systems, standardizing prescription writing and prescription rules, and eliminating certain abbreviations and dose expressions.

Programs to Improve Outcome

Medication errors can occur anywhere in the hospital. QI efforts that are focused on the operating room, in which anesthesia providers are very involved, include efforts to decrease surgical wound infections and bloodstream infections. For the former, the administration of prophylactic antibiotics, maintenance of normothermia, and more judicious use of fluids and of vasoactive agents are becoming increasingly regulated and monitored. Both the Centers for Disease Control and Prevention and the American Society of Anesthesiologists have promulgated clinical practice guidelines for the placement of central venous catheters. The administration of β-adrenergic receptor blocking agents on the day of surgery to patients who have been taking them is also the focus of many QI programs, and monitored by The Joint Commission. These programs are not static. As part of the QI initiative, the processes are monitored; compliance with the recommendations, systems' problems in implementing the recommendations, and the outcomes themselves must be monitored and assessed, and changes to the recommendations must be implemented when necessary.

Disclosure of Errors to Patients

Not necessarily part of the QI process, one of the areas that has come under increased scrutiny in the last several years concerns how and what to reveal to patients and their family members when errors are discovered. Fear of malpractice action has traditionally made physicians hesitant to disclose medical errors to patients. However, regulatory bodies now encourage, and in some cases state law may require, the disclosure of "serious unanticipated outcomes" to patients. Such disclosure is frequently not protected from admissibility in a legal action. Surveys suggest that most patients want disclosure of errors, an explanation of how the error occurred and how the effects of the error will be minimized, and what actions will be taken to prevent the error from occurring to other patients. Most hospitals and medical staffs, with input from their legal departments, have developed guidelines on how errors and adverse events are disclosed to patients and their families.

Suggested Readings

Agency for Healthcare Research and Quality. *Patient Safety Network*. Available at: http://www.psnet.ahrq.gov/primer.aspx?primerID=2. Accessed October 3, 2012.

Department of Community and Family Medicine. Duke University Medical Center. Patient Safety. *Quality Improvement. A Comparison of the Models*. Available at: http://patientsafetyed.duhs.duke.edu/module_a/methods/comparison_model.html. Published 2005. Accessed October 3, 2012.

Institute of Medicine. *Preventing Medication Errors: Quality Chasm Series*. Available at: http://www.iom.edu/Reports/2006/Preventing-Medication-Errors-Quality-Chasm-Series.aspx. Published July 20, 2006. Accessed October 3, 2012.

The Joint Commission. *Sentinel Event*. Available at: http://www.jointcommission.org/sentinel_event.aspx. Accessed October 3, 2012.

CHAPTER 240

Management of the Difficult Airway

David R. Danielson, MD

Successfully managing difficult airways requires a combination of forethought, proper equipment, and decisiveness. Concentrating on the first two factors makes the third less stressful. Obtaining a thorough patient history and performing a physical examination with particular emphasis on the airway will not reveal every difficult airway but can often avert a crisis and prompt the anesthesia provider to take an alternate approach to managing the airway.

Preoperative Evaluation

The anesthesia provider should preoperatively interview the patient and review the medical record to determine whether the patient has had any previous difficulty while being intubated. Three classic bedside measurements should be obtained: the size of the tongue, as compared with the pharynx; the extension of the atlanto-occipital joint; and the size of the anterior mandibular space. Although none of these parameters is a definitive predictor of airway ease or difficulty, evaluation of as many bedside measures as possible is recommended to increase the predictive power of the preoperative examination. In addition to obtaining the three classic measures, incisor prominence, interincisor distance, width of the palate, temporomandibular joint mobility, and length and thickness of the neck should also be evaluated.

Tongue Versus Pharyngeal Size

Preinduction visualization of the faucial pillars, soft palate, and base of the uvula, with the patient in a sitting position, is used to classify patients according to how well pharyngeal structures can be seen (Table 240-1 and Figure 240-1). Mallampati and colleagues' original recommendation was to examine these structures without the patient phonating and to assign a class level—I through III (see Table 240-1)—to the results. Class II was later subdivided based on whether all of the uvula or only its base can be visualized.

Atlanto-occipital Extension

Mobility of the atlanto-occipital joint enables alignment of the oral, pharyngeal, and laryngeal axes, facilitating mask ventilation and tracheal intubation. Extension of the atlanto-occipital joint can be quantified by observing the angle of the occlusal surface of the upper teeth with respect to horizontal when the patient is upright and extending his or her neck; 35 degrees of extension is a normal value.

Table 240-1 Mallampati Classification of the Upper Airway

Class	Visible Structures
I	Palate, faucial pillars, entire uvula
II	Palate, faucial pillars, base of uvula
III	Palate, some of the faucial pillars
IV	Palate

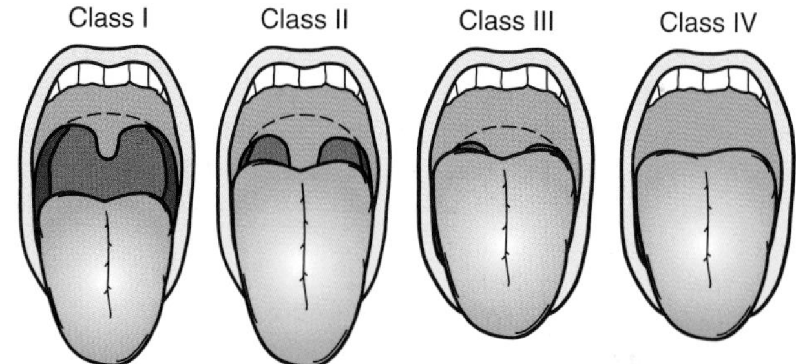

Figure 240-1 Mallampati classification of the upper airway. See Table 240-1 for explanation of each class. (Modified from Mallampati SR, Gatt SP, Gugino LD, et al. A clinical sign to predict difficult tracheal intubation: A prospective study. Can Anaesth Soc J. 1985;32:429-434.)

Anterior Mandibular Space

The anterior mandibular space refers to the thyromental distance, the distance from the thyroid notch to the mental prominence, when the neck is fully extended. A distance of 6 cm in an adult predicts ease of intubation.

Defining the Difficult Airway

By definition, a difficult airway is a clinical situation in which an anesthesia provider experiences difficulty with facemask ventilation of the upper airway, with direct laryngoscopy, or with tracheal intubation. In the 1990s, the American Society of Anesthesiologists (ASA) developed the first practice guidelines and an algorithm for managing the difficult airway and began emphasizing that anesthesia providers needed to learn multiple airway management techniques. This instruction led to anesthesia providers' increased familiarity with multiple airway instruments and a willingness to switch techniques sooner, rather than later, when encountering a difficult airway. The 2013 update of the ASA Difficult Airway Algorithm (Figure 240-2) mentions the use of video laryngoscopy as another useful approach. This mirrors the widespread adoption of video laryngoscopy techniques by most anesthesia providers as their favored approach to anticipated difficult airways.

Management of the Difficult Airway

The anesthesia provider may have more difficulty mask ventilating a morbidly obese patient (i.e., body mass index > 40 kg/m^2), but morbid obesity does not, per se, lead to difficulty in intubating the airway unless

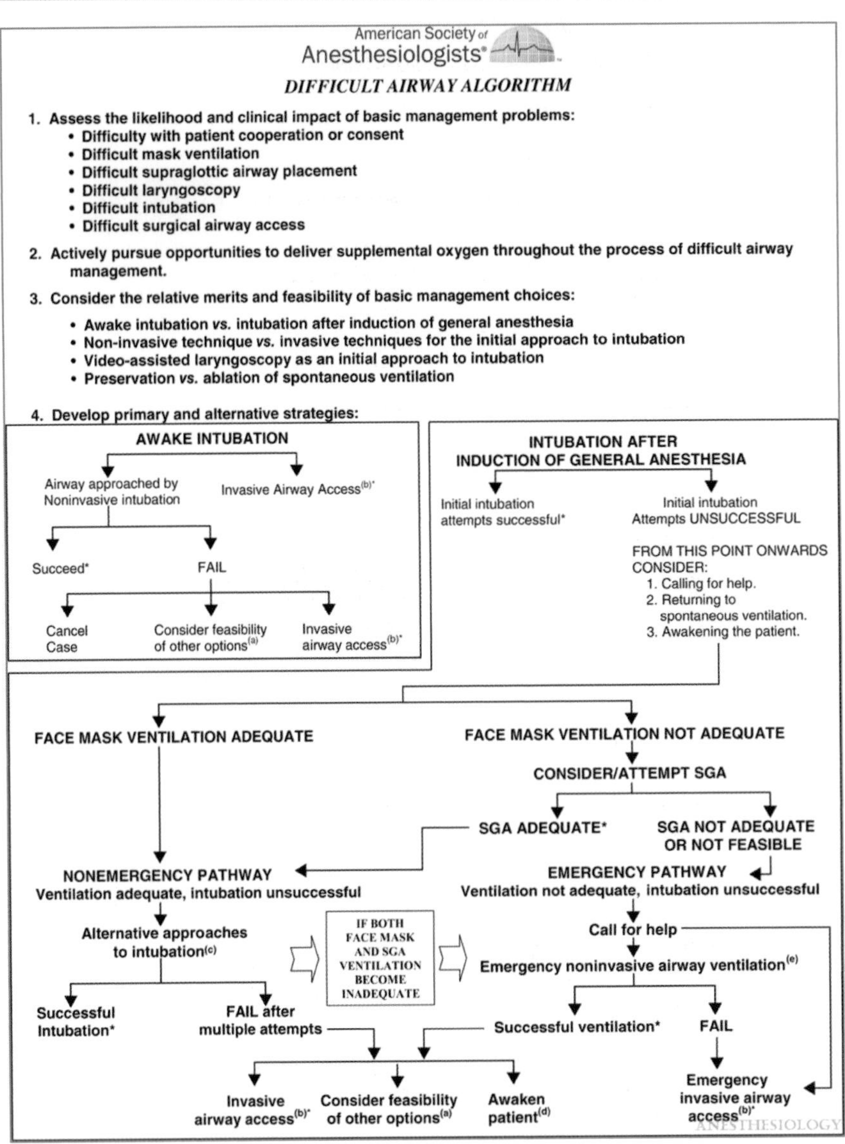

Figure 240-2 ASA Difficult Airway Algorithm. (From Anesthesiology. 2013;118(2):251-270. Difficult Airway Algorithm. Reprinted with permission of the American Society of Anesthesiologists, 520 N. Northwest Highway, Park Ridge, Illinois 60068-2573.)

the patient has increased periglottic tissue or limited neck mobility or if problems are encountered in positioning the patient. Additionally, obese patients develop rapid O_2 desaturation during apnea. These factors can be ameliorated by placing the patient in a "ramped up" position (see Chapter 163).

Only rarely is a surgical airway the first choice for securing an airway. The most common reasons include trauma to the face or cervical spine or a neoplastic disease involving the airway or neck. Because of the differences in managing the airway of patients with trauma, the ASA modified the Difficult Airway Algorithm for use in trauma patients (Figure 240-3).

Identification of a difficult airway after the induction of general anesthesia and administration of neuromuscular blocking drugs leads to the arm of the algorithm that is most stressful for the anesthesia provider. In this circumstance, rapid decisions must be made, and both equipment and knowledge must be immediately available. The anesthesia provider must always be prepared to manage the airway with transoral supraglottic techniques (e.g., laryngeal mask airway, Combitube) as well as with techniques involving emergency invasive airway access (surgical or percutaneous cricothyrotomy plus transtracheal jet ventilation) while moving toward achieving a more definitive airway. Patient safety depends on planning ahead and progressing rapidly down the appropriate arms of the algorithm. Studying the algorithm and being aware of the potential pathways before encountering airway difficulties is likely to result in the best outcome.

Suggested Readings

Apfelbaum JL, Hagberg CA, Caplan RA, et al. Practice guidelines for management of the difficult airway: An updated report by the American Society of Anesthesiologists Task Force on Management of the Difficult Airway. *Anesthesiology*. 2013;118:251-270.

Mallampati SR, Gatt SP, Gugino LD, et al. A clinical sign to predict difficult tracheal intubation: A prospective study. *Can Anaesth Soc J*. 1985;32:429-434.

Wilson WC. Trauma: airway management. *American Society of Anesthesiologists Newsletter* 2005;69(11):10.

AMERICAN SOCIETY OF ANESTHESIOLOGISTS

2003 DIFFICULT AIRWAY ALGORITHM (MODIFIED FOR TRAUMA)

1. Assess the likelihood and clinical impact of basic management problems.
   - A. Difficult Ventilation
   - B. Difficult Intubation
   - C. Difficulty with Patient Cooperation or Consent
   - D. Difficult Tracheostomy
2. Actively pursue opportunities to deliver supplemental oxygen throughout the process of difficult airway management.
3. Consider the relative merits and feasibility of basic management choices:

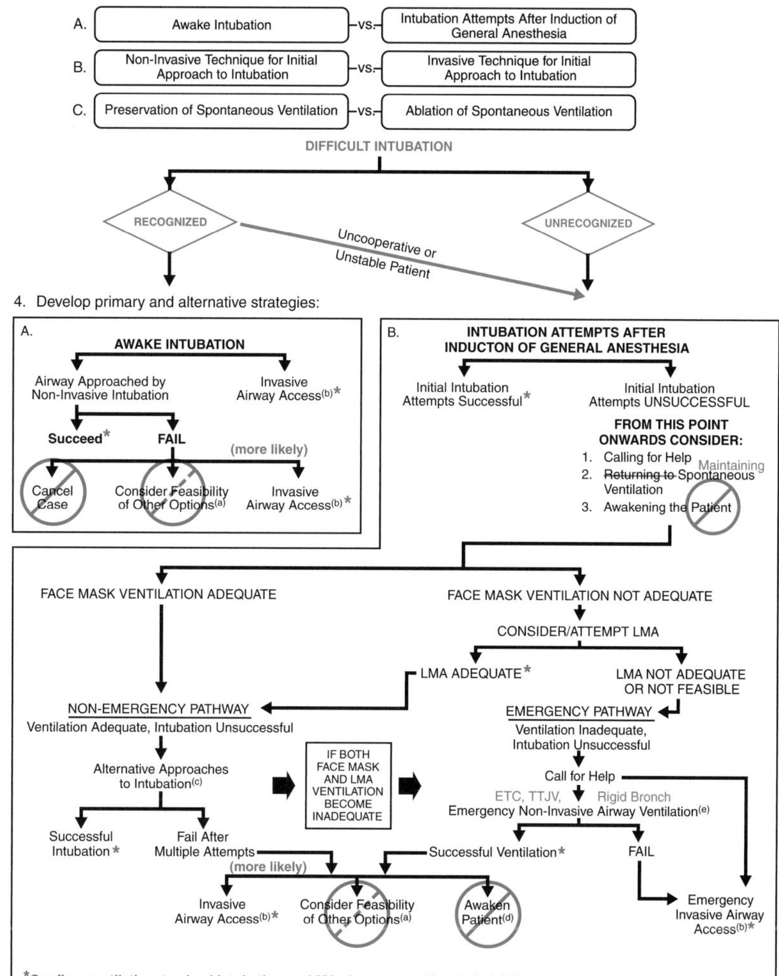

a. Other options include (but are not limited to): surgery utilizing face mask or LMA anesthesia, local anesthesia infiltration or regional nerve blockade. Pursuit of these options usually implies that mask ventilation will not be problematic. Therefore, these options may be of limited value if this step in the algorithm has been reached via the Emergency Pathway. Judgment required. Rarely appropriate for trauma patients.

b. Invasive airway access includes surgical or percutaneous tracheostomy or cricothyrotomy.

c. Alternative non-invasive approaches to difficult intubation include (but are not limited to): use of different laryngoscope blades, LMA as an intubation conduit (with or without fiberoptic guidance), fiberoptic intubation (FOB), intubation stylet or tube changer (airway exchange catheter, (AEC) light wand, retrograde intubation, and blind oral or nasal intubation.

d. Consider re-preparation of the patient for awake intubation or canceling surgery. Rarely applicable in the trauma patient.

e. Options for emergency non-invasive airway ventilation include (but are not limited to): rigid bronchoscope (Rigid Bronch), esophageal-tracheal combitube ventilation (ETC), or transtracheal jet ventilation (TTJV).

f. Extubation strategies include: evaluation of the airway with FOB and extubation over an airway exchange catheter (AEC).

Figure 240-3 2003 American Society of Anesthesiologists Difficult Airway Algorithm Modified for Trauma. LMA, Laryngeal mask airway. (From Wilson WC. Trauma: airway management. American Society of Anesthesiologists Newsletter 2005;69(11):10. Reprinted with permission of the American Society of Anesthesiologists, Park Ridge, IL.)

CHAPTER 241

Perioperative Pulmonary Aspiration

Allen Brian Shoham, MD, and Michael J. Murray, MD, PhD

Perioperative pulmonary aspiration occurs infrequently, but its impact on individual patients can be devastating. Patients who appear to have the greatest risk of aspirating are those who have recently eaten and are undergoing an emergency procedure, those with small bowel obstruction, and those with comorbid conditions such as diabetes or gastroesophageal reflux disease. For patients who do aspirate, the risk of severe pulmonary morbidity or death after aspiration is greatest for those who are sick (American Society of Anesthesiologists physical classification 3 or greater) and elderly. As a general rule, children have less morbidity from pulmonary aspiration.

Importance of Pulmonary Aspiration

Five large studies from 1970 to 2000 documented the overall frequency of perioperative pulmonary aspiration to be approximately 1:3000; the mortality rate is 5% in patients who have a witnessed aspiration. Fortunately, not all patients who aspirate develop respiratory sequelae. The frequency of pulmonary complications and fatality as a consequence of aspiration are shown in Table 241-1.

Based on the information in Table 241-1, if similar mortality rates were to be found within the United States in general, approximately 200 deaths from perioperative pulmonary aspiration would be expected each year. In our largest institutions (i.e., those that perform as many as 50,000 general anesthetics annually), only 1 death from pulmonary aspiration would occur every 18 months. By applying the numbers (1 death per 75,000 general anesthetics) to individual practice settings, an idea of the anticipated frequency of this event can be derived.

Table 241-1 Risk of Aspiration-Associated Pulmonary Complications and Death after General Anesthesia by American Society of Anesthesiologists Physical Status Classification

ASA Physical Status Classification	Frequency	
	Pulmonary Complications*	Deaths†
I	1/39,865 (1:39,865)	0
II	2/87,471 (1:43,735)	0
III	7/78,714 (1:11,245)	1/78,714 (1:78,714)
IV and V	3/9438 (1:3146)	2/9438 (1:4719)
Total	13/215,488 (1:16,576)	3/215,488 (1:71,829)

ASA, American Society of Anesthesiologists.

*Pulmonary complications include acute respiratory distress syndrome, pneumonitis, and pneumonia (with or without positive viral or bacterial identification).

†Death from aspiration-associated pulmonary complications within 6 months of aspiration.

From Warner MA, Warner ME, Weber JG. Clinical significance of pulmonary aspiration during the perioperative period. Anesthesiology. 1993;78:56-62.

Serious morbidity and considerable costs are associated with aspiration of gastric contents that results in an aspiration pneumonitis, acute lung injury, or acute respiratory distress syndrome. Approximately 25% of patients who perioperatively aspirate gastric contents require intensive care support. About 10% of these patients need mechanical ventilation support for more than 24 h, and, as mentioned previously, half of them will die.

Pulmonary Aspiration in Children

The rate of perioperative pulmonary aspiration in children is similar to that in adults, but children rarely die from aspiration. Their outcomes after aspiration tend to be better, and their recoveries seem to be quicker. The children at highest risk for aspiration and serious morbidity are those who are younger than 1 year and who have gastrointestinal ileus.

Use of Medications and Preoperative Fasting

Medications used to decrease gastric contents, acidity, or both clearly work. However, no data suggest that the use of these medications decreases the risk of pulmonary aspiration. Many anesthesia organizations have developed guidelines to decrease the risk of perioperative aspiration, and all guidelines make similar recommendations. The recommendations of the American Society of Anesthesiologists for medications and fasting are given in Tables 241-2 and 241-3, respectively. Routine use of these medications is NOT recommended, and yet many anesthesia providers feel compelled to administer these medications to their patients, despite an adverse risk-benefit ratio. Evidence is lacking, but the only patients who might benefit are those in whom the anticipated risk of pulmonary aspiration is high.

Occurrence of Aspiration in the Perioperative Period

Although aspiration may occur at any time (including immediately before anesthesia induction), it is most common during tracheal intubation and extubation, though a small percentage of those patients who aspirate do so during the intraoperative period. A common factor found in patients who aspirate when a tracheal tube is being used is inadequate muscle relaxation. Laryngoscopy in an inadequately paralyzed patient may cause the patient to gag and vomit. The same sequence occurs during extubation in a patient who is either weak or not alert and nonresponsive. There is insufficient information on the effectiveness of laryngeal mask airways to prevent aspiration, but there are case reports of aspiration with their use in both high-risk and low-risk patients. Patients who have had a previous esophagectomy will regurgitate gastric contents into their pharynx when supine and anesthetized; a tracheal

Table 241-2 Summary of 1999 American Society of Anesthesiologists Task Force Pharmacologic Recommendations to Reduce the Risk of Pulmonary Aspiration*

Drug Type and Common Examples	Recommendation
Gastrointestinal stimulants	
Metoclopramide	No routine use
Gastric acid secretion blockers	
Cimetidine	No routine use
Famotidine	No routine use
Lansoprazole	No routine use
Omeprazole	No routine use
Ranitidine	No routine use
Antacids	
Sodium citrate	No routine use
Sodium bicarbonate	No routine use
Magnesium trisilicate	No routine use
Antiemetic agents	
Droperidol	No routine use
Ondansetron	No routine use
Anticholinergic agents	
Atropine	No use
Scopolamine	No use
Glycopyrrolate	No use
Combinations of the medications above	No routine use

ASA, American Society of Anesthesiologists.
*A 2011 update of these guidelines states that, in patients who have no apparent risk of pulmonary aspiration, the routine preoperative use of gastrointestinal stimulants, antacids, gastric acid blockers, antiemetics, anticholinergics, or combinations thereof is not recommended.

Table 241-3 Summary of 2011 Updated American Society of Anesthesiologists Committee on Standards and Practice Parameters' Recommendations on Preoperative Fasting and the Use of Pharmacologic Agents to Reduce the Risk of Pulmonary Aspiration*

Ingested Material	Minimum Fasting Period (h)†
Clear liquids‡	2
Breast milk	4
Infant formula	6
Nonhuman milk§	6
Light meal¶	6

*These recommendations apply to healthy patients who are undergoing elective procedures. They are not intended for women in labor. Following the guidelines does not guarantee complete gastric emptying.
†The recommended fasting periods apply to all ages.
‡Examples of clear liquids are water, fruit juices without pulp, carbonated beverages, clear tea, and black coffee.
§Because nonhuman milk is similar to solids in gastric emptying time, the amount ingested must be considered in determining an appropriate fasting period.
¶A light meal typically consists of toast and clear liquids. Meals that include fried or fatty foods or meat may prolong gastric emptying time. Both the amount and type of foods ingested must be considered when determining an appropriate fasting period.

tube is probably a better choice than a laryngeal mask airway to secure the airway for general anesthesia in these patients.

Management of Perioperative Pulmonary Aspiration

Patients who aspirate require supportive care. Careful suctioning of aspirated material is useful to decrease the volume remaining in the lungs, but lavage with saline should not be performed because it may increase the spread of aspirate and has not been associated with improved outcomes. If particulate material is present, bronchoscopy should be performed to remove material that might obstruct bronchi. Prophylactic use of antibiotics or steroids has been ineffective in decreasing the frequency of pneumonia and of lung inflammation and has not been associated with improved outcomes. Respiratory care is provided as needed.

The severity of pulmonary aspiration and its consequences vary widely. Scant amounts of aspirated gastric contents may have little impact on the lungs, whereas large volumes of aspirate with a low pH (< 3) may immediately impair oxygenation and lead to the development of severe acute respiratory distress syndrome. Patients who aspirate small volumes perioperatively and who are asymptomatic during the first 2 postoperative hours are unlikely to develop respiratory sequelae. Therefore, it is reasonable to discharge asymptomatic patients to regular postoperative nursing units or even home with little risk of delayed development of respiratory symptoms.

Conclusion

Pulmonary aspiration is an infrequent perioperative event, occurring at a rate of approximately 1 per 3000 children and adult patients undergoing general anesthesia. This rate varies dramatically among patients, with those who are sicker and undergoing emergency procedures, especially if they have recently eaten or have an ileus or small bowel obstruction, are at greatest risk for regurgitation of gastric contents and have the highest rate of aspiration. Approximately 25% of patients who aspirate gastric contents during the perioperative period develop significant respiratory complications. The overall mortality rate from pulmonary aspiration is 5%, and death occurs primarily in adults; children rarely die after perioperative aspiration. The routine use of preoperative medications to reduce the risk of pulmonary aspiration is NOT warranted. Preoperative fasting guidelines suggest shortening fasting periods, especially for clear liquids.

Suggested Readings

American Society of Anesthesiologists Committee. Practice guidelines for preoperative fasting and the use of pharmacologic agents to reduce the risk of pulmonary aspiration: Application to healthy patients undergoing elective procedures: An updated report by the American Society of Anesthesiologists Committee on Standards and Practice Parameters. *Anesthesiology.* 2011; 114:495-511.

Warner MA. Is pulmonary aspiration still an important problem in anesthesia? *Curr Opin Anesthesiol.* 2000;13:215-218.

CHAPTER 242

Eye and Dental Complications

Robert G. Hale, DDS, and Michael J. Murray, MD, PhD

Eye Injury

Anesthesia-related eye injuries are relatively uncommon, but anesthesia providers focus a great deal of attention on avoiding injury to the eye because the eye is one of the major sense organs. An analysis of eye injury claims against anesthesiologists published in 1992 as part of the American Society of Anesthesiologists (ASA) Closed Claims Project found that 3% of all claims in the database were for eye injury. The frequency of payment for eye injury claims was significantly higher than that for claims not related to eye injuries (70% vs. 56%); however, the median cost of eye injury claims was significantly less than that for other claims ($24,000 vs. $95,000).

Corneal Injury

The most often reported eye complications following general anesthesia are corneal abrasion and corneal exposure, both of which are very painful and blur vision. An abrasion is caused by trauma, with complete loss of corneal epithelium, whereas corneal exposure is caused by damage to (but not loss of) the corneal epithelium due to exposure and secondary loss of tear film protection, which is necessary for protecting the integrity of corneal epithelium. Most injuries are thought to be secondary to lagophthalmos, an incomplete closure of the eyelid, with an abrasion being the result of direct trauma to the cornea from facemasks, surgical drapes, fingers, or other foreign objects that inadvertently contact the cornea.

The prevalence of corneal injuries varies depending on the methods used to detect them, but the incidence—as defined by clinical symptoms in patients whose eyes were taped closed during a surgical procedure—ranges from 0.05% to 0.15%. A specific cause of injury can be determined in only approximately 20% of the cases. Because the mechanisms of corneal injury are poorly understood, it is difficult to formulate preventive strategies that will completely eliminate the risk of injury. However, a review of the literature reveals several recurring themes. The pulse oximeter probe should be placed on patients' fourth or fifth finger because patients are less likely to rub their eyes with these fingers. Patients' eyes should be taped closed immediately after induction of anesthesia (do not wait until after intubation). Studies show that, if patients' eyes are taped closed, no extra protection is achieved by using eye ointment unless the surgical procedure is prolonged or if patients are placed in other than the supine position. Even when patients' eyes are taped shut, the anesthesia provider must use caution to prevent foreign objects from coming into contact with the patients' eyes during intubation (e.g., stethoscope draped around the clinician's neck, identification badge clipped to the chest pocket, a loose watchband or bracelet). The patient should be checked periodically, particularly following repositioning, to ensure that movement, moisture, or tears have not loosened or repositioned the tape.

In patients with proptosis, in patients undergoing head and neck procedures, for procedures performed with the patient prone or in the lateral position, and for procedures that are going to last for more than 90 min, the use of ointment on the eyes in addition to taping should be considered. Ointment provides good protection if there is concern that the eyelid tape may come off, but patients who have ointment on their eyes may have some blurred vision at the end of the procedure. The use of petroleum-based ointment is recommended for longer procedures but, because it is flammable, petroleum-based ointment should not be used if electrocautery or electrosurgery is used around the patient's head and neck. Methylcellulose ointment is also an option; because it dissipates more quickly than petroleum-based ointment, it can be used for shorter procedures, and its use is associated with less blurring of vision postoperatively, as compared with petroleum-based products.

Corneal injury should be suspected postoperatively if the patient has pain, photophobia, blurred vision, or the sensation of having a foreign body in the eye. All but the most serious injuries can be managed conservatively. Ophthalmic antibiotic ointment should be administered to the eye, and the patient should be reassured that the injury will resolve within 24 to 48 h without permanent sequelae. An eye patch can be taped in place, but, because it is so often done incorrectly, the use of an eye patch is associated with additional problems.

Postoperative Visual Loss

Postoperative visual loss (POVL) is a rare but devastating complication seen most commonly following spine, cardiac, and head and neck surgical procedures (Figure 242-1). During the 1990s, the incidence of POVL seemed to be increasing, so in 1999 the ASA Committee on Professional Liability established the ASA POVL Registry to tabulate data on POVL following nonocular operations. Seven years later, a review of the registry identified

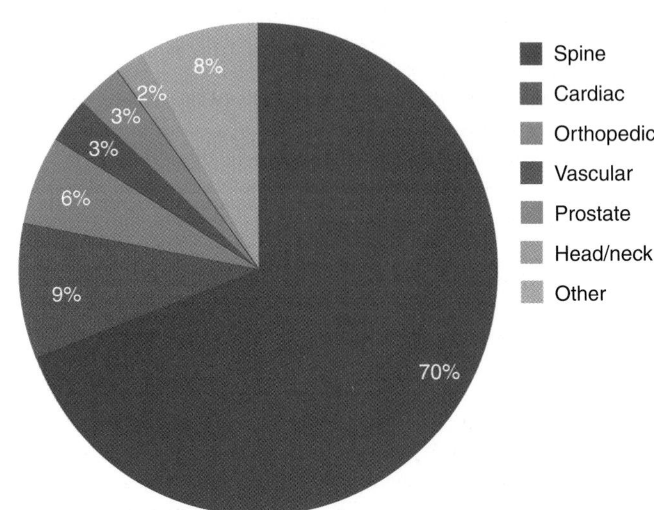

Figure 242-1 Surgical procedures performed in 175 cases from the American Society of Anesthesiologists Postoperative Visual Loss Registry database.

93 cases of POVL associated with spine operations; most were caused by ischemic optic neuropathy (ION)—either anterior or posterior—and not by compression of the globe. Only 10 of the patients had a central retinal artery occlusion, whereas the remainder had ION. Patients with ION, as compared with those without ION, were relatively healthy, were more likely to have an associated blood loss of 1000 mL or greater, or were more likely to have had an anesthetic duration of 6 h or longer; such conditions were found in 96% of the patients.

More recently, the ASA released a Practice Advisory for POVL associated with spine operations. The recommendations are based on observational studies; because the incidence of POVL is so low, prospective randomized studies would be impossible to perform. Among the factors that might increase the incidence of POVL are preexisting vascular disease (e.g., hypertension, diabetes, peripheral vascular disease, coronary artery disease), obesity, tobacco use, and anemia. As reported previously, the advisory commented that POVL is more likely to occur during prolonged procedures ($>$ 6.5 h), during procedures in which substantial blood loss occurs, and during prolonged procedures combined with substantial blood loss.

Reducing the Risk of Postoperative Visual Loss

Of more importance to clinicians were the recommendations of the panel on the intraoperative management of patients as to what might be done to decrease the likelihood of POVL. The panel recommended that special attention be given to the management of blood pressure, intraoperative fluids, and anemia; the use of vasopressors; patient positioning; and staging of surgical procedures.

Blood Pressure Management Many preoperative factors—including the presence of chronic hypertension, cardiac dysfunction, and renal and vascular disease—need to be taken into account in terms of intraoperative blood pressure goals and management for patients undergoing prolonged spine operations in the prone position. In addition, many intraoperative factors must also be taken into account—such as the amount of fluid administered, rate of blood loss, degree of hypotension, and requirement for vasopressors to maintain blood pressure—when making decisions regarding intraoperative blood pressure goals. The use of deliberate hypotension is not contraindicated for these patients but should be determined on a case-by-case basis.

Management of Intraoperative Fluids Monitoring of central venous pressure in patients at high risk of developing POVL should be considered, with administration of both crystalloids and colloids to maintain central venous pressure in patients who have significant blood loss.

Management of Anemia Hemoglobin levels should be monitored periodically during surgery in at-risk patients if sustained or significant blood loss occurs. A hemoglobin target that would eliminate the possibility of POVL has not been established.

Use of Vasopressors Because there have been no controlled trials evaluating the use of α-adrenergic agonists to maintain blood pressure in patients at risk for developing POVL, the decision to use α-adrenergic agonists should be made on a case-by-case basis.

Patient Positioning Other than recognizing that the risk of POVL is increased in patients undergoing procedures in the prone position, the only other recommendation of the ASA task force was to avoid direct pressure on the ophthalmic globe and to periodically check to ensure that nothing impinges or presses on the eye during the surgical procedure.

Recognizing and Treating Postoperative Visual Loss

As soon as at-risk patients are alert following surgery, their visual acuity should be assessed. If they have any evidence of having experienced visual loss, an ophthalmologist should be consulted immediately and asked to examine the patient to document the degree of impairment and to advise as to possible cause. Hemoglobin values, O_2 saturation, and hemodynamics should be optimized, and consideration should be given to ordering a magnetic resonance imaging study to rule out intracranial causes of POVL. There is no evidence to support the administration of diuretics, corticosteroids, anticoagulants, antiplatelet drugs, or drugs that decrease intraocular pressure.

Dental Injury

Damage to the oropharynx is one of the most common, if not the most common, iatrogenic injuries that patients experience while under general anesthesia, occurring in up to 5% of general anesthetics. Injury to the hypopharynx (sore throat) is the most common; in one survey, injury occurred in 45% of patients. One fifth of oral injuries (1% of all general anesthetics) are the result of trauma to teeth, usually to the upper incisors in patients older than 50 years of age. Surprisingly few of these injuries to the teeth require dental or oral surgical intervention, and yet, dental injury is the most frequent cause of complaints and litigation against anesthesia providers.

Fractures of tooth enamel or of crowns account for approximately 40% of cases of dental injury, loosening or frank avulsion of teeth occurs in another 40% of reported cases (in one fourth of those or 10% of the time, a tooth or teeth are found to be missing), and the remaining 20% of cases are due to damage to veneers, dental restorations, prosthetic crowns, and fixed partial dentures.

Etiology

Patient Factors

Children aged 5 to 12 years (who have a mixture of primary and permanent teeth) and adults with carious teeth, gum disease, protruding or loose upper incisors, and difficult airways are at highest risk of experiencing dental injury.

Anesthetic Factors

Dental injury occurs most commonly during induction and emergence from anesthesia. Patients with difficult airways, as mentioned previously, are as much as 20 times more likely to be injured during tracheal intubation, as compared with patients without a difficult airway. The anesthesia provider's skill is also a factor; less experienced providers are more likely to inflict dental injury, as evidenced by one study in which these providers were more likely to contact the laryngoscope with the left upper incisor during intubation. During emergence (or during induction of anesthesia if the depth of anesthesia is not sufficient or if the patient is not adequately relaxed), patients commonly bite, which can generate considerable force concentrated on the incisors and on an oropharyngeal airway, if an oropharyngeal airway is used as a bite block.

Prevention

A thorough preoperative evaluation and examination of the oropharynx should be performed, not only to document whether the patient has a difficult airway, but also to identify those patients with loose or carious teeth. In patients with poor dentition, consideration should be given to postponing the procedure if time permits to allow patients to see their dentists prior to the planned surgical procedure to attend to the dental problem (Figure 242-2). Because two thirds of injuries in one review were due to preexisting conditions (e.g., caries, prostheses, loose or damaged teeth, a single isolated tooth, or functional limitations), the anesthesia provider should document these in the medical record. If the patient requests to proceed after the risks of dental injury have been explained, documentation of the examination and of the counseling should be included in the consent form that the patient signs. Relying on a preprinted standardized "Consent for Anesthesia" that includes "dental injury" as one of the complications of anesthesia provides little protection from a medicolegal perspective.

If removal of a partial denture or bridge leaves an isolated tooth, some experts advise that the benefits of leaving the appliance in place outweigh the benefit of removing it. The use of devices to optimize intubation in

Identify patient factors that increase the risk of dental injury

- Primary teeth
- Loose tooth
- Cavities
- Gum disease
- Mallampati score > 2
- Limited mouth opening
- Partial bridge
- Age > 50 y

Perform a preoperative examination

- Obtain history
- Examine the airway and teeth
- Thoroughly explain findings/risks of proceeding to patient
- Document results

Develop the anesthetic plan

- Assess or plan for removable bridges or partial dentures
- Provide adequate depth of anesthesia and relaxation prior to instrumentation
- Use a bite block between solid molars in high-risk patients
- Ensure additional safeguards for patients with difficult airways and poor dentition

Refer high-risk patients to a dentist or oral surgeon

Figure 242-2 Strategies for decreasing the incidence of intraoperative dental injury.

Avulsed tooth

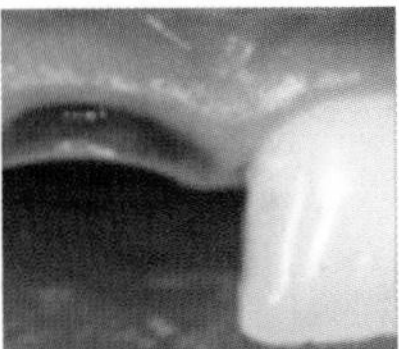

- Act quickly.
- Do not touch the root surfaces.
- Place the tooth in sterile saline.
- Assess whether the tooth can be replaced.
- Consult with a dentist.
- If dentist agrees to see the patient in follow-up, place the tooth back into the socket and hold for several minutes.

Subluxated or chipped tooth

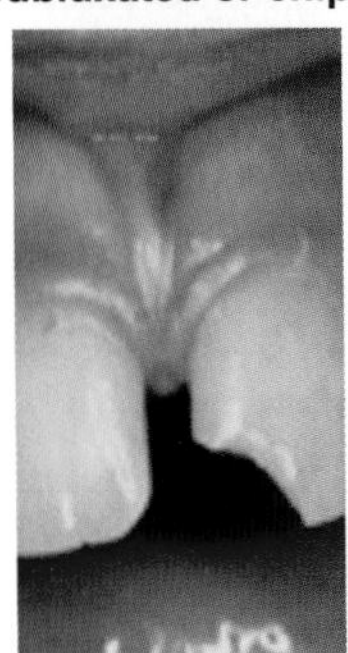

- Find missing teeth, tooth, or fragments.
- Perform imaging studies if unable to account for all fragments.
- Apologize and explain to patient in the presence of her or his responsible companion.
- Document findings and explanation in the medical record.
- Provide the patient with a written follow-up plan.

Figure 242-3 Managing avulsed or subluxated or chipped tooth. Avulsed teeth that are more likely to be able to be replaced include permanent teeth in patients with otherwise good dental health and no evidence of being immunocompromised.

patients with difficult airways and the use of certain dental guards can decrease the incidence of damage to the teeth but do not eliminate the potential for damage and should not be relied on exclusively. Clearly, in these situations, it is incumbent on the anesthesia provider to have a plan for how to protect the airway during induction and intubation and to minimize direct contact with and trauma to the teeth.

Treatment and Management of Dental Injury

Despite our best efforts, injury to teeth can and will occur. Anesthesia departments should have a protocol in place to guide the management and care of dental injuries (Figure 242-3). This protocol should include, at a minimum, the following items:

- Any missing teeth or fragments must be found. If the teeth or fragments are not identified, the patient should have a chest radiograph and an abdominal radiograph, if necessary, to identify fragments that may have been aspirated or swallowed.
- In children, the loss of a primary tooth does not require treatment. However, if a permanent tooth is avulsed, it should be stored in cool sterile saline until placed back in the socket from which it came.
- Once the patient has recovered from anesthesia, she or he should be offered an explanation and an apology. A plan for postoperative care should be documented in the patient's medical record. If indicated, an oral surgical consultation should be obtained while the patient is still in the postanesthesia care unit, or, if treatment is not urgent, arrangements should be made, with a written plan given to the patient, for the patient to see his or her personal dentist.

Suggested Readings

American Society of Anesthesiologists Task Force on Perioperative Visual Loss. Practice advisory for perioperative visual loss associated with spine surgery: An updated report by the American Society of Anesthesiologists Task Force on Perioperative Visual Loss. *Anesthesiology*. 2012;116:274-285.

Contractor S, Hardman JG. Injury during anaesthesia. *Contin Educ Anaesth Crit Care Pain*. 2006;6:67-70.

Gaudio RM, Barbieri S, Feltracco P, et al. Traumatic dental injuries during anaesthesia. Part II: medico-legal evaluation and liability. *Dent Traumatol*. 2011; 27:40-45.

Lee LA. ASA postoperative visual loss registry: Preliminary analysis of factors associated with spine operations. *American Society of Anesthesiologists Newsletter*. 2003;67:7-8.

Lee LA. Postoperative visual loss data gathered and analyzed. *American Society of Anesthesiologists Newsletter*. 2000;64:25-27.

Lee LA, Roth S, Posner KL, et al. The American Society of Anesthesiologists Postoperative Visual Loss Registry: Analysis of 93 spine surgery cases with postoperative visual loss. *Anesthesiology*. 2006;105:652-659.

Windsor J, Lockie J. Anaesthesia and dental trauma. *Anaesth Intensive Care*. 2008; 9:355-357.

CHAPTER 243

Intraoperative Patient Positioning

Roy F. Cucchiara, MD

The art and science of surgical positioning continue to evolve, but the goal remains constant: ensuring optimal surgical access to the operative site while providing a safe environment for the patient. Compromises may have to be made to surgical access so that the anesthesia provider can safely care for the patient no matter what may occur during the operation. Even more compromises may have to be made to protect the patient from injury secondary to prolonged positioning.

Both the surgeon and the anesthesia provider share responsibility for the patient's safety with regard to the surgical position. Few data guide this principle; experience is probably an important factor, but there are no studies to support this claim. In the end, the safety of the position must be balanced against the risk of performing the operation in a position that compromises the surgeon's access.

Commonly Used Positions

The basic patient positions for surgery are supine, prone, and lateral, with the head down (Trendelenburg position) (Figure 243-1) or head up (reverse Trendelenburg). Most other positions are variations on these basic ones. Lithotomy (supine) with the legs elevated and flexed (Figure 243-2), jackknife (prone and flexed), lateral decubitus (Figure 243-3), beach chair, and sitting are commonly used positioning terms.

Complications Resulting from Incorrect Positioning

The most common serious complication of poor positioning is peripheral nerve injury. Common but usually less serious complications relate to the skin. Tape "burns," skin blisters from pressure on surfaces, and skin breakdown from the edges of an unpadded strap are common. A blister forms from abrasion of the skin or from ischemia of the skin area. Abrasions that occur in the operating room are usually shallow enough to heal over without an ulcer. The greatest care must be taken around the patient's face and ears. Although the skin of the face is very vascular and usually heals well, an ischemic area at a fold in the facial tissue can be a serious problem, with poor healing, scarring, and possibly even the need for skin grafting. Particular care must be taken with tube tapes and tapes across the head or face to hold the tracheal tube in position.

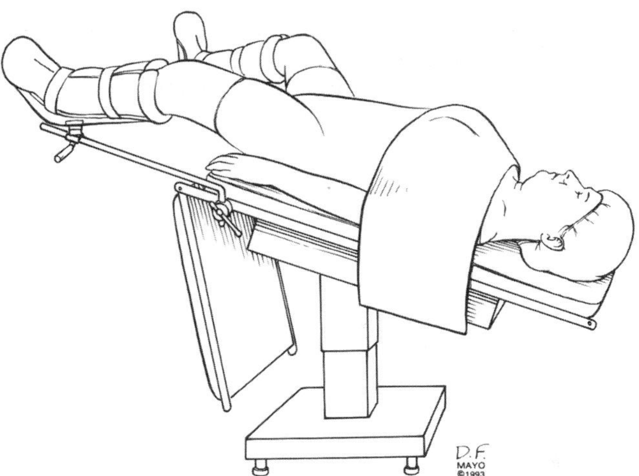

Figure 243-1 The Trendelenburg position. (By permission of Mayo Foundation for Medical Research and Education. All rights reserved.)

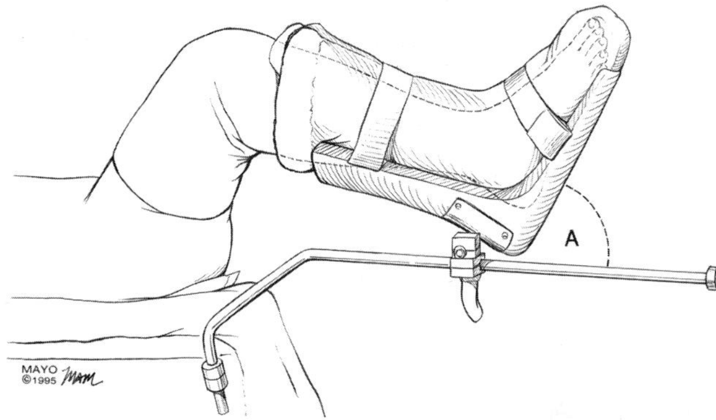

Correct position – Lower leg weight distributed to foot of stirrup by increasing angle A of stirrup to support bar.

Figure 243-2 Correct lower limb positioning in a patient in the lithotomy position. The weight of the lower leg can be distributed to the foot of the stirrup by increasing angle A between the stirrup and the support bar. (By permission of Mayo Foundation for Medical Research and Education. All rights reserved.)

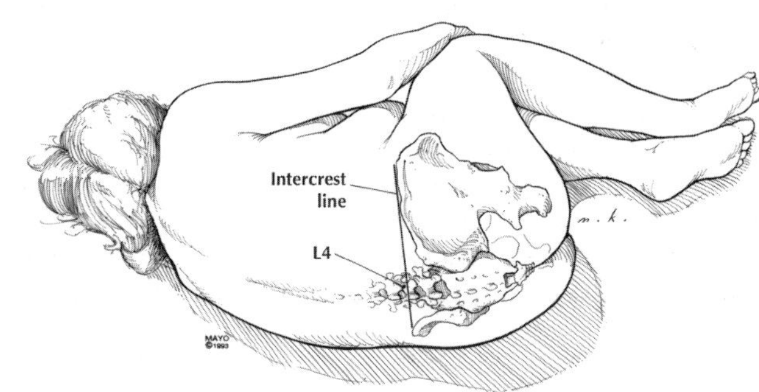

Figure 243-3 The lateral decubitus position for a patient undergoing placement of an epidural catheter. (By permission of Mayo Foundation for Medical Research and Education. All rights reserved.)

Problems Related to the Trendelenburg Position

A steep Trendelenburg position is increasingly being used for laparoscopic procedures, especially for urologic and gynecologic procedures, and can cause occasional difficulties (Figure 243-4). Venous engorgement of the face can be impressive, sometimes resulting in marked conjunctival edema. Airway edema can also result, although this is rarely a problem that delays extubation.

Pulmonary compliance is reduced when the contents of the abdomen press on the diaphragm, which may occur when the patient is in the steep Trendelenburg position. Reduced pulmonary compliance appears to be a transient problem that can be corrected by returning the patient to the supine position. It is reasonable to assume that these patients may have an increase in interstitial lung water that could impair diffusion. An unexplained decrease in O_2 saturation is not uncommon in patients experiencing reduced pulmonary compliance. Applying positive-pressure ventilation when the patient resumes the supine position should correct this phenomenon fairly quickly.

A case report has identified a patient in steep Trendelenburg position who failed to awaken at the end of the case and was found to have had an intracerebral bleed. There are also reports of patients sliding off the operating room table and of extremity compartment syndromes with the weight of the patient pressing against arm straps, with the straps occluding venous return.

Problems Related to the Sitting Position

The sitting position also has associated risks but also many unique benefits. The primary risks are of venous air embolism (Chapter 137) and cerebral ischemia. When intraarterial cannulas are placed to measure blood pressure when the patient is in the sitting position, placing the transducer at the level of the external auditory meatus is considered the gold standard by many to measure cerebral perfusion pressure.

Problems Related to Head Positioning

For many operations involving the cranial nerve or ear, nose, or throat, the patient's head is turned to the side to some degree. Degenerative disease of the cerebral vertebrae or vascular impingement when the head is turned may limit the degree to which the patient's head can be turned. Only rarely will such a patient have somatosensory evoked potentials monitored to detect spinal cord compromise. The best way to determine the degree of cervical movement that the patient can tolerate is to place the patient in the desired position while awake and check the range of motion carefully before inducing anesthesia. The head should not be flexed to the point where there is less than 2 fingerbreadths of space between the bone of the chin and the sternal notch; quadriplegia may result (Figure 243-5). Age should be considered when positioning the patient with the head turned, flexed, or extended. The cervical and vascular degeneration that contribute to problems can begin in middle age and are nearly always present by the seventh decade of life.

Some have suggested that prolonged prone cases should be performed with the patient's head pinned in a headrest to remove the risk of pressure on the eye (Figure 243-6) and to attenuate the possibility of injury. To decrease the risk of blindness in patients in the prone position, some have suggested that, in addition to avoiding pressure on the eyes, a mean arterial pressure of at least 65 mm Hg and a hemoglobin concentration of at least 9 g/dL should be maintained. Other risks in this position include corneal abrasion and injury to the lips, nose, and ears. Flexion of the neck in patients with severe rheumatoid arthritis may sublux the odontoid process, which can narrow the cervical spinal canal.

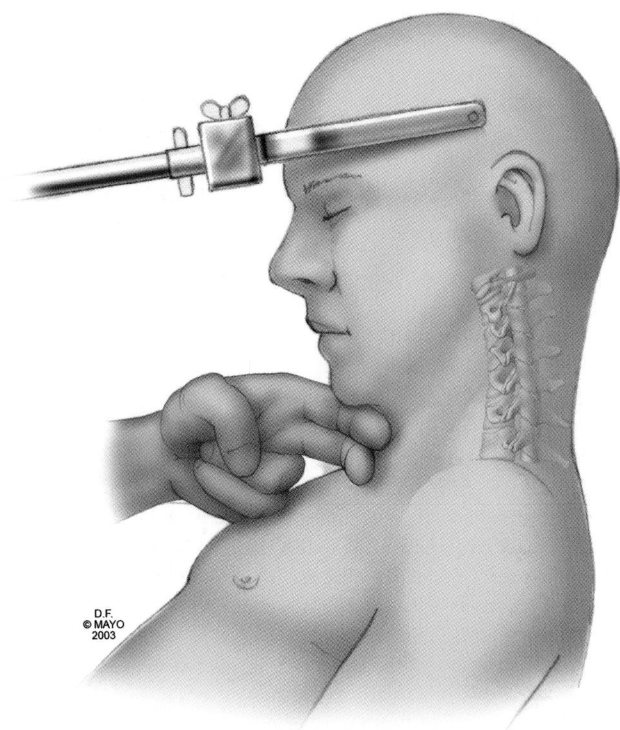

Figure 243-5 Two-finger technique for preventing cervical compression, and therefore quadriplegia, during anesthesia. (By permission of Mayo Foundation for Medical Research and Education. All rights reserved.)

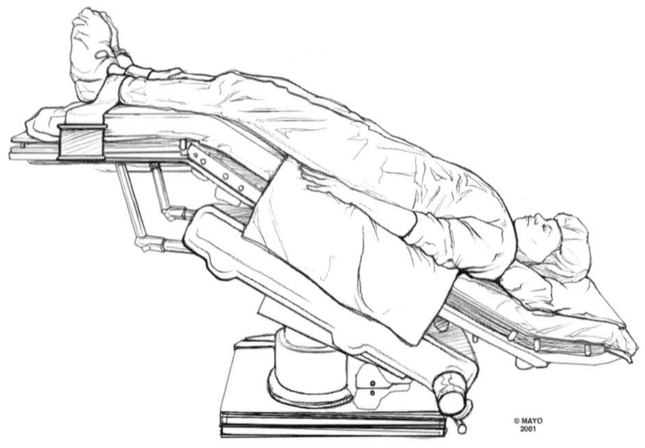

Figure 243-4 The steep Trendelenburg position. (By permission of Mayo Foundation for Medical Research and Education. All rights reserved.)

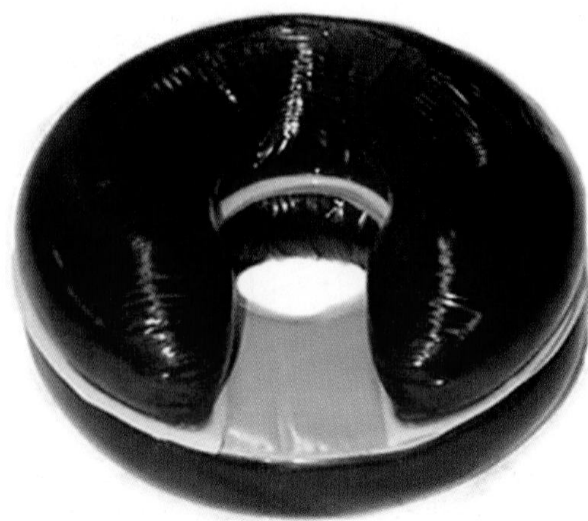

Figure 243-6 Example of a viscoelastic polymer gel headrest. (Used with permission of the David Scott Company. Blue Diamond, David Scott Company, Framingham, MA.)

Correct Positioning

Upper Extremity Positioning

When patients are in the prone position, one or both arms are placed on arm boards in the "surrender" position. In some cases, the arms are tucked beneath the arched frame; in others, both arms are placed at the patient's sides. Risks to the arms include pressure on or stretching of the brachial plexus and pressure on the ulnar nerve. The brachial plexus can often be palpated at the axilla, and the shoulder can be maneuvered so as to ensure that the plexus is not under tension or pressure. For the lateral position, the use of an axillary roll is important to protect the brachial plexus (Figure 243-7).

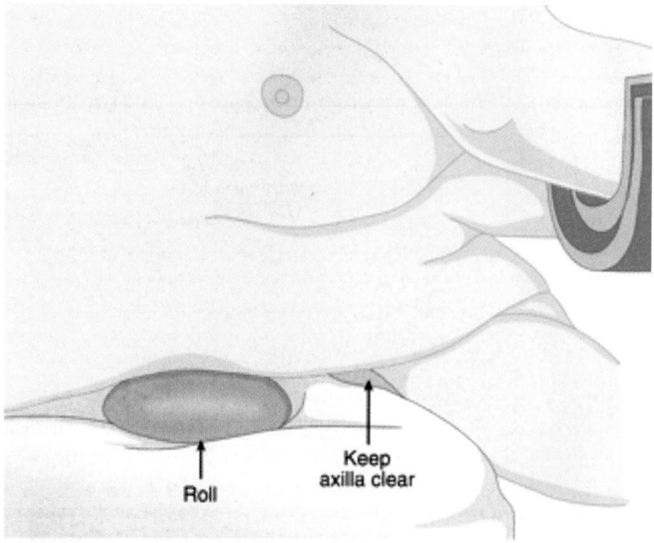

Figure 243-7 Axillary roll. Note that the axillary roll is positioned to protect the brachial plexus, not actually in the axilla. (By permission of Mayo Foundation for Medical Research and Education. All rights reserved.)

Lower Extremity Positioning

The anterior iliac crest must be well padded to avoid pressure injury on the lateral femoral cutaneous nerve with subsequent paresthesias of the side of the thigh. If the patient's legs are large, the knees must be padded or even suspended to prevent pressure blisters. The feet should be free so that the toes are not subjected to supporting the weight of the legs. In older patients, care must be taken to avoid over flexing the hips, which can cause sciatic nerve injury.

Suggested Readings

Akhaddar A, Boucetta M. Subconjunctival hemorrhage as a complication of intraoperative positioning for lumbar spinal surgery. *Spine J*. 2012;12:274.

Apostle KL, Lefaivre KA, Guy P, et al. The effects of intraoperative positioning on patients undergoing early definitive care for femoral shaft fractures. *J Orthop Trauma*. 2009;23:615-621.

Engelhardt M, Folkers W, Brenke C, et al. Neurosurgical operations with the patient in sitting position: Analysis of risk factors using transcranial Doppler sonography. *Br J Anaesth*. 2006;96:467-472.

McEwen DR. Intraoperative positioning of surgical patients. *AORN J*. 1996; 63:1059-1063.

Pannucci CJ, Henke PK, Cederna PS, et al. The effect of increased hip flexion using stirrups on lower-extremity venous flow: A prospective observational study. *Am J Surg*. 2011;202:427-432.

Singh VK, Singh PK, Azam A. Intraoperative positioning related injury of superficial radial nerve after shoulder arthroscopy—A rare iatrogenic injury: A case report. *Cases J*. 2008;1:47.

Warner MA. Perioperative neuropathies. *Mayo Clin Proc*. 1998;73:567-574.

Winfree CJ, Kline DG. Intraoperative positioning nerve injuries. *Surg Neurol*. 2005;63:5-18.

CHAPTER 244

Patient Positioning: Common Pitfalls, Neuropathies, and Other Problems

Mary Ellen Warner, MD

Perioperative neuropathies, vision loss, and positioning-related problems have received increasing attention from the lay press, plaintiffs' lawyers, the anesthesiology community, and clinical researchers in recent years. This chapter will provide an update of current findings and discuss possible mechanisms of injury for these potentially devastating problems.

Upper-Extremity Neuropathies

Ulnar Neuropathy

Ulnar neuropathy is the most common perioperative neuropathy.

Timing of Symptoms

Most symptoms of ulnar neuropathy develop during the postoperative, not the intraoperative, period. Data support the finding that most surgical patients who develop ulnar neuropathy experience their first symptoms at least 48 h postoperatively, suggesting that the mechanism of acute injury occurs primarily outside the operating room. Nonsurgical medical patients also develop ulnar neuropathies during hospitalization.

Impact of Elbow Flexion

The ulnar nerve is the only major peripheral nerve in the body that always passes on the extensor side of a joint, in this case, the elbow. All other major peripheral nerves primarily pass on the flexion side of joints (e.g., median and femoral nerves). This difference in anatomy may play a role in some perioperative ulnar neuropathies. In general, peripheral nerves begin to lose function and develop foci of ischemia when they are stretched by 5% or more of their resting lengths. Elbow flexion, particularly more than 90 degrees, stretches the ulnar nerve. Prolonged elbow flexion and stretch of the ulnar nerve can result in sufficient ischemia to cause symptoms in awake and sedated patients and potential long-lasting damage in all patients.

Anatomy and Elbow Flexion

Prolonged elbow flexion of more than 90 degrees increases intrinsic pressure on the nerve and may be as important an etiologic factor as is prolonged extrinsic pressure. The ulnar nerve passes behind the medial epicondyle and then runs under the aponeurosis that holds the two muscle bodies of the *flexor carpi ulnaris* together. The proximal edge of this aponeurosis is sufficiently thick, especially in men, to be separately named the *cubital tunnel retinaculum*. This retinaculum stretches from the medial epicondyle to the olecranon. Flexion of the elbow stretches the retinaculum and generates high pressures intrinsically on the nerve as it passes underneath the retinaculum (Figure 244-1).

Forearm Supination and Ulnar Neuropathy

Supination of the forearm and hand does not, by itself, reduce the risk of ulnar neuropathy. The action of forearm supination occurs distal to the elbow. Supination is typically used when positioning the patient's arms on armboards or at the patient's sides because of the impact it has on humerus rotation. That is, supination is uncomfortable for most patients, and they will externally rotate their humerus to increase comfort. It is this external rotation of the humerus that lifts the medial aspect of the elbow, including the ulnar nerve, and prevents it from directly resting on the surface of the table or armboard. This rotation helps reduce extrinsic pressure on the ulnar nerve.

Outcomes of Ulnar Neuropathy

Approximately 40% of sensory-only ulnar neuropathies resolve within 5 days; 80% resolve within 6 months. Few combined sensorimotor ulnar neuropathies resolve within 5 days; only 20% resolve within 6 months, and most result in permanent motor dysfunction and pain. The motor fibers in the ulnar nerve are primarily located in the middle of the nerve. Injury to these fibers is likely associated with more significant ischemia or pressure insult to all of the ulnar nerve fibers, and recovery may be prolonged or not possible.

Brachial Plexopathies

Brachial plexopathies occur most often in patients undergoing sternotomies. The risk for this plexopathy in patients undergoing sternotomy is particularly high in those who undergo mobilization of the internal mammary artery, which is presumed to be associated with excessive concentric retraction on the chest wall and potential compression of the plexus between the clavicle and rib cage or stretch of the plexus. In general, patients in prone and lateral positions have a higher risk of developing this problem than do those in supine positions, except in patients having a sternotomy, as mentioned previously.

Brachial Plexus Entrapment

Many insults to the plexus can occur in prone and laterally positioned patients. For example, the brachial plexus can become entrapped between compressed clavicles and the rib cage. Special attention should be given to altering any patient positions that might exacerbate this potential problem.

Prone Positioning

In prone-positioned patients, it is prudent to tuck their arms at their sides if at all possible; many patients have changes in somatosensory evoked potentials when their arms are abducted (e.g., a "surrender" position).

Anatomy of Shoulder Abduction

Abduction of a shoulder of 90 degrees or more places the distal plexus on the extensor side of the joint and potentially stretches the plexus

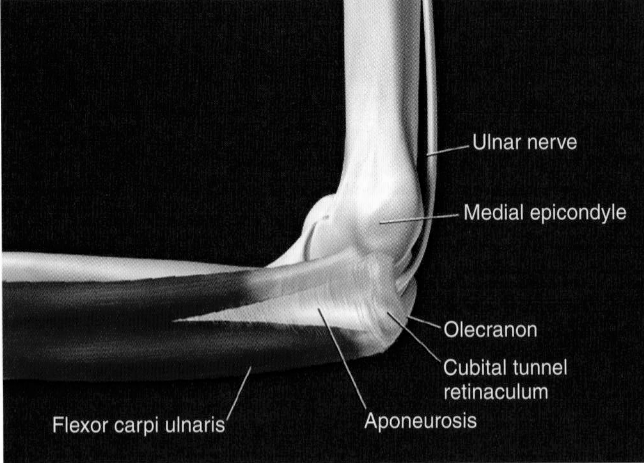

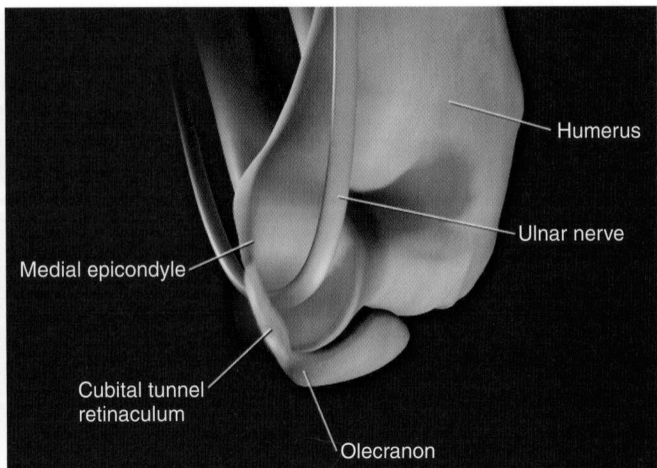

Figure 244-1 **A,** The ulnar nerve of the right arm passes distally behind the medial epicondyle and underneath the aponeurosis that holds the two heads of the *flexor carpi ulnaris* together. The proximal edge of the aponeurosis is sufficiently thick in 80% of men and 20% of women to be distinct anatomically from the remainder of the tissue. It is commonly called the *cubital tunnel retinaculum*. **B,** Viewed from behind, the ulnar nerve is intrinsically compressed by the *cubital tunnel retinaculum* when the elbow is progressively flexed beyond 90 degrees and the distance between the olecranon and the medial epicondyle increases.

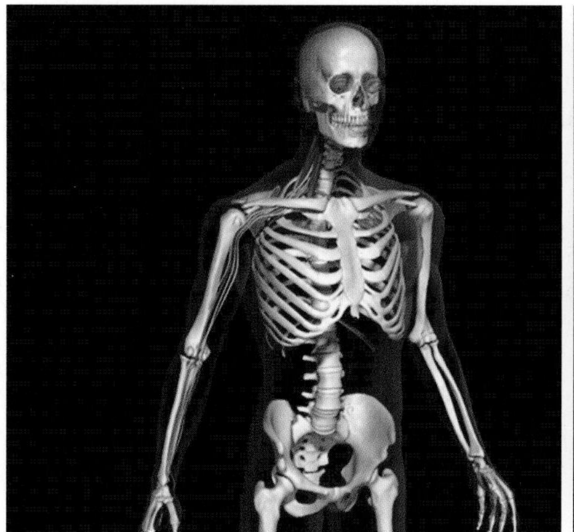

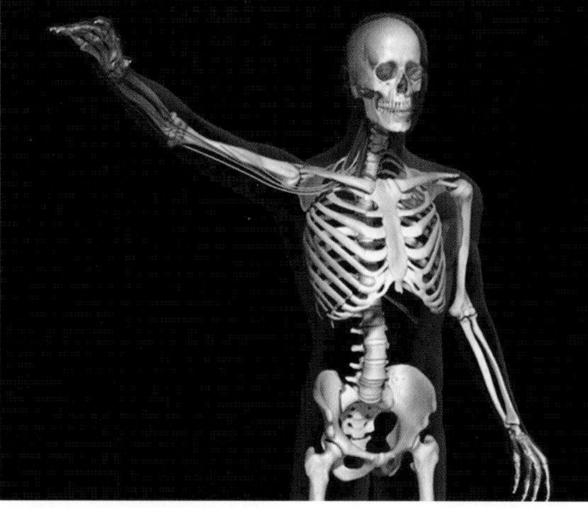

Figure 244-2 A, The neurovascular bundle to the upper extremity passes on the flexion side of the shoulder joint when the arm is at the side or abducted less than 90 degrees. B, Abduction of the arm beyond 90 degrees transitions the neurovascular bundle to where it now lies on the extension side of the shoulder joint. Progressive abduction greater than 90 degrees increases stretch on the nerves at the shoulder joint.

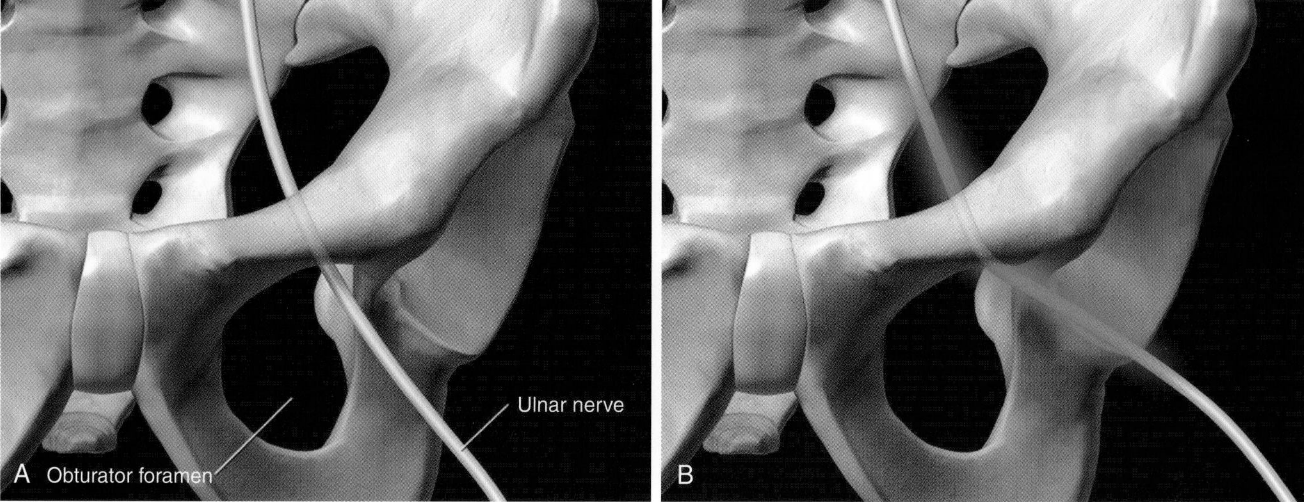

Figure 244-3 A, The obturator nerve passes through the pelvis and exits out the superior and lateral corner of the obturator foramen as it continues distally down the inner thigh. B, Abduction of the hip stretches the obturator nerve and can provoke ischemia, especially at the exit point of the obturator foramen. The point serves as a fulcrum for the nerve during hip abduction.

(Figure 244-2). Therefore, it is prudent to avoid abduction of more than 90 degrees, especially for extended periods of time.

Inflammatory Plexopathy

More than any other nerve or plexus, the brachial plexus is reported to develop perioperative inflammation or idiopathic inflammatory plexopathy. The cause of this problem is unknown, although an increasing amount of information indicates that immunosuppression during the perioperative period might increase the possibility of viral or autoimmune activity in this plexus.

Lower-Extremity Neuropathies

Although peroneal and sciatic neuropathies have the most impact on ambulation, the most common perioperative neuropathies in the lower extremities involve the obturator and lateral femoral cutaneous nerves.

Impact of Hip Abduction on the Obturator Nerve

Hip abduction of more than 30 degrees results in significant strain on the obturator nerve. The nerve passes through the pelvis and out the obturator foramen. With hip abduction, the superior and lateral rim of the foramen serves as a fulcrum (Figure 244-3). The nerve stretches along its full length and is also compressed at this fulcrum point. Thus, excessive hip abduction should be avoided whenever possible. With obturator neuropathy, motor dysfunction is common, and approximately 50% of patients who have motor dysfunction in the perioperative period will continue to have it 2 years later. The dysfunction is usually not painful, but it can be debilitating.

Impact of Hip Flexion on the Lateral Femoral Cutaneous Nerve

Prolonged hip flexion of more than 90 degrees increases ischemia on fibers of the lateral femoral cutaneous nerve. One third of the fibers of this nerve pass through the inguinal ligament as the fibers pass into the thigh (Figure 244-4). Hip flexion of more than 90 degrees results in lateral displacement of the anterior superior iliac spine and in stretch of the inguinal ligament. The lateral femoral cutaneous nerve is compressed by the stretched inguinal ligament and, with time, becomes ischemic and dysfunctional. The lateral femoral cutaneous nerve carries only sensory fibers, so no motor disability occurs when this nerve is injured.

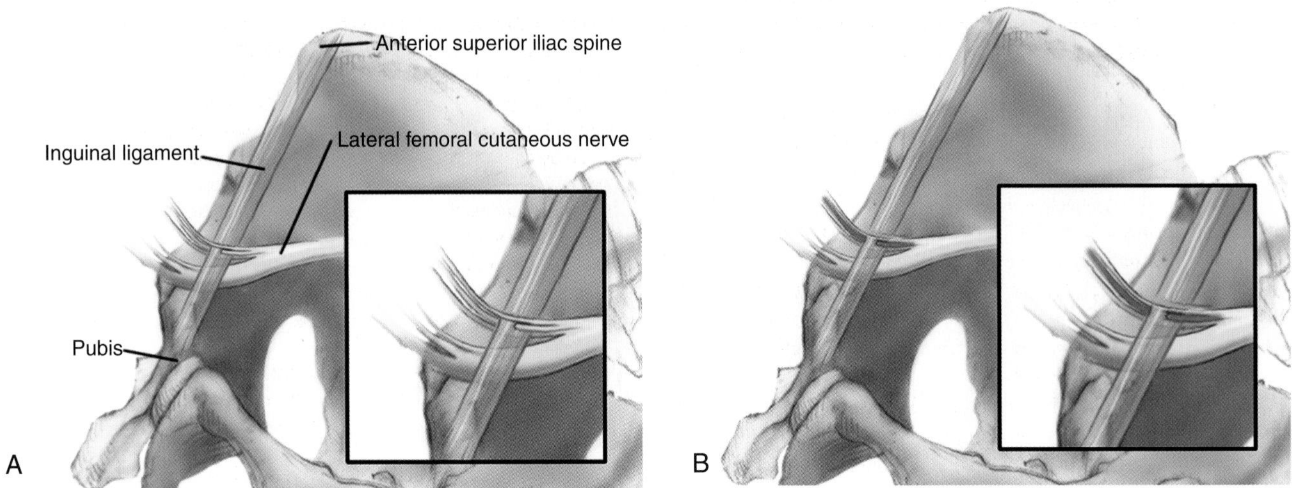

Figure 244-4 **A,** Approximately one third of the lateral femoral cutaneous nerve fibers penetrate the inguinal ligament as the nerve passes out of the pelvis and distally into the lateral thigh. **B,** Hip flexion, especially when greater than 90 degrees, leads to stretch of the inguinal ligament as the ilium is displaced laterally. This stretch causes the intraligament pressure to increase and compresses the nerve fibers as they pass through the ligament.

However, patients with this perioperative neuropathy can have disabling pain and dysesthesias of the lateral thigh. Approximately 40% of these patients have dysesthesias that last for more than a year.

Practical Considerations for Perioperative Peripheral Neuropathies

Prevention

Use padding to distribute compressive forces. Although few studies have been conducted to demonstrate that padding has any impact on the frequency or severity of perioperative neuropathies, it makes sense to distribute point pressure. The use of padding may be viewed favorably by juries in medicolegal actions.

Position joints to avoid excessive stretching. Recognize that stretching any nerve more than 5% beyond its resting length over a prolonged period of time results in varying degrees of ischemia and dysfunction.

Follow-up Care

If your patient develops a peripheral neuropathy and the neural loss is only sensory, it is reasonable to follow the patient's condition daily for up to 5 days. Many sensory deficits in the immediate postoperative period will resolve during this time. If the deficit persists longer than 5 days, it is likely that the neuropathy will have an extended impact. It is appropriate if the sensory deficit lasts longer than 5 days to request that a neurologist become involved to provide an evaluation and long-term care.

If the loss is only motor or combined sensory and motor, it would be prudent to request that a neurologist become involved earlier. Patients with motor or combined sensory and motor loss likely have a significant neuropathy and will need prolonged postoperative care.

Unique Positioning Problems with Catastrophic Results

Spinal Cord Ischemia

Spinal cord ischemia is a rare event that occurs when patients undergoing pelvic procedures (e.g., prostatectomy) are placed in a hyperlordotic position, with more than 15 degrees of hyperflexion at the L2 to L3 interspace. This position results in spinal cord ischemia and infarction. It is best detected with magnetic resonance imaging. Operating room tables made in the United States are designed to limit hyperlordosis in supine patients, even when the table is maximally retroflexed with the kidney rest elevated. In almost all reported cases of spinal cord ischemia, the table had been maximally retroflexed, the kidney rest had been elevated, AND towels or blankets had been placed under the patient's lower back to promote further anterior or forward tilt of the pelvis (to improve the surgeon's vision of deep pelvic structures). In general, anesthesia providers should not allow anyone to place materials under the patient's lower back for this purpose.

Thoracic Outlet Obstruction

Thoracic outlet obstruction, a rare event, occurs when patients with this syndrome are positioned prone or, less commonly, laterally. In almost all reported cases, the shoulder had been abducted more than 90 degrees. In that position, the vasculature to the upper extremity is compressed either between the clavicle and rib cage or between the two heads of the sternocleidomastoid muscle. This entrapment of the vasculature leads to upper-extremity ischemia. When ischemia is prolonged, the results range from minor disability to severe tissue ischemia or infarction that requires forequarter amputation. A simple preoperative question, such as "Can you use your arms to work above your head for more than a minute?" can elicit a history of thoracic outlet obstruction and reduce the risk of this potentially devastating complication occurring.

Steep Trendelenburg Position

As surgeons gain experience with new technologies (e.g., robotics for use in pelvic procedures), they often request that the patient be placed in a steep Trendelenburg position. These positions can be associated with cephalad shifting of anesthetized patients on operating room tables. Patients often are fixed to the table with draw sheets and other retaining devices (e.g., shoulder braces). Cephalad shifting can lead to cervical plexopathies from stretch and to subclavian vessel obstruction from compression. Although intracranial pressure also increases, it rarely results in a negative outcome. However, if orofacial edema occurs, careful attention to the airway is required.

Postoperative Visual Loss

Loss of vision when the patient emerges from an anesthetic following a cardiac or spinal surgical procedure is a devastating event for both the patient and the anesthesia provider. Because postoperative vision loss (POVL) occurs infrequently, it has not been possible to identify the cause, which most authorities agree is multifactorial. Review of the POVL registry of the American Society of Anesthesiologists demonstrates that 67% of patients who developed POVL had undergone a surgical procedure on the spine when they were in the prone position, so it is safe to say that positioning definitely plays a role. In those patients who did develop POVL, the majority had spine procedures that lasted between 5 and 9 h. Many authorities assume that, when the patient is in the prone position, edema in the retina and optic head leads to ischemia. POVL occurs in all age groups but appears to be more common in older patients; however, this may be a reflection more on the number of older patients who have cardiac and spinal surgical procedures or this may also be due to the fact that older patients are more likely to have peripheral vascular disease. Atherosclerosis, then, along with hypotension and anemia, may also play an important role in the development of POVL in these patients.

For patients having spinal surgical procedures that will be performed when the patient is in the prone position, the neck should be maintained in the neutral position with the forehead resting on a pad without any pressure whatsoever on the orbits. Though there is no evidence of benefit to this recommendation, many authorities endorse maintaining a mean arterial blood pressure of greater than 70 mm Hg and a perioperative hemoglobin level of 8 g/dL or higher. Attention to detail in this respect may be beneficial both in terms of patient outcome and, if medical negligence is claimed, if there is an adverse outcome.

Suggested Readings

Beckett AE. Are we doing enough to prevent patient injury caused by positioning for surgery? *J Perioper Pract*. 2010;20:26-29.

Bradshaw AD, Advincula AP. Postoperative neuropathy in gynecologic surgery. *Obstet Gynecol Clin North Am*. 2010;37:451-459.

Fritzlen T, Kremer M, Biddle C. The AANA Foundation Closed Malpractice Claims Study on nerve injuries during anesthesia care. *AANA J*. 2003;71:347-352.

Jones SC, Fernau R, Woeltjen BL. Use of somatosensory evoked potentials to detect peripheral ischemia and potential injury resulting from positioning of the surgical patient: Case reports and discussion. *Spine J*. 2004;4:360-362.

Kamel IR, Drum ET, Koch SA, et al. The use of somatosensory evoked potentials to determine the relationship between patient positioning and impending upper extremity nerve injury during spine surgery: A retrospective analysis. *Anesth Analg*. 2006;102:1538-1542.

Litwiller JP, Wells RE, Halliwill JR, et al. Effect of lithotomy positions on strain of the obturator and lateral femoral cutaneous nerves. *Clin Anat*. 2004;17:45-49.

Pierce V, Kendrick P. Ischemic optic neuropathy after spine surgery. *AANA J*. 2010; 78:141-145.

Practice Advisory for the Prevention of Perioperative Peripheral Neuropathies. A Report by the American Society of Anesthesiologists Task Force on the Prevention of Perioperative Neuropathies. *Anesthesiology*. 2000;92:1168-1182.

Tuncali BE, Tuncali B, Kuvaki B, et al. Radial nerve injury after general anaesthesia in the lateral decubitus position. *Anaesthesia*. 2005;60:602-604.

Winfree CJ, Kline DG. Intraoperative positioning nerve injuries. *Surg Neurol*. 2005;63:5-18.

CHAPTER 245

Malignant Hyperthermia

Denise J. Wedel, MD

History

In 1960, Denborough and Lovell reported the first case of anesthesia-induced hypermetabolism in a patient with a familial history of multiple anesthetic deaths during ether administration. The patient survived a halothane-induced malignant hyperthermia (MH) episode. In 1969, Kalow and Britt described a metabolic error of skeletal muscle metabolism in patients who had recovered from MH episodes. This finding formed the scientific basis for modern diagnostic contracture testing. In 1975, Harrison reported the efficacy of dantrolene in treating porcine MH, a treatment that, used in humans, has lowered the mortality rate associated with this rare problem from as high as 80% to below 10%.

Incidence and Mortality

The incidence of MH reportedly ranges from 1:4500 to 1:60,000 general anesthetics (geographic variation is related to the gene prevalence). Approximately 50% of MH-susceptible (MHS) individuals have had a previous triggering anesthetic without developing MH symptoms. MH is rare in infants, and the incidence decreases after age 50 years, with the highest prevalence of clinical symptoms in males. The reasons for these variations are not understood.

MH has been clearly associated with central core and multi-minicore disease. MH-like symptoms have been associated with other neuromuscular disorders, such as Duchenne muscular dystrophy, although morbidity and mortality are likely to be related to rhabdomyolysis after receiving succinylcholine rather than true MH. The use of nontriggering anesthesia is recommended for these patients. Association with other conditions such as myotonia, sudden infant death syndrome, neuroleptic malignant syndrome, and exercise-induced death in adults is controversial.

Genetics

MH has an autosomal dominant pattern of inheritance, with clinical heterogeneity and variable expression. A single-gene mutation responsible for MH has been identified in a swine model of MH (ryanodine receptor).

The ryanodine receptor is a protein that comprises the calcium-release channel in the skeletal muscle sarcoplasmic reticulum, a site shown to be defective in MHS swine.

Unfortunately, human MH is far more complicated genetically. The ryanodine gene (*RYR1*) (MHS1 locus) encodes the type 1 ryanodine receptor. Mutations in this gene can be identified in 70% to 80% of MHS individuals or people with central core disease. More than 90 mutations have been identified, with more than half of the mutations having been identified in only one family or a few families. The other known MH gene is the *CACMA1S* (MHS5 locus), which encodes the subunit of the dihydropyridine receptor L-type calcium channel. The two identified mutations in this gene account for only about 1% of all MHS. Three additional loci have been mapped (MHS2, MHS4, and MHS6), but the genes have not been identified. The rate of spontaneous mutation is unknown but is probably less than 10% of all cases of MH.

Appropriate patient selection for genetic testing is very important. In a patient with a positive caffeine-halothane muscle biopsy or very strong family history of unequivocal MH, complete sequence analysis of *RYR1* coding results in a 70% to 80% rate of detection. In the case of a multigenerational family (two or more) with unequivocal MH in at least 10 members, linkage analysis for all MHS loci can be performed, and new sites can be detected. However, screening of a single individual with a new diagnosis of clinical MH against the common *RYR1* sites will be positive in only 20% to 30% of cases. Thus, a single preoperative genetic screening test in humans is unlikely to be available in the near future.

Clinical Presentation

The onset of clinical signs can be acute and fulminant or delayed. MH can occur at any time during the anesthetic administration and has been reported to occur as late as 24 h postoperatively.

Trismus (masseter muscle spasm) following inhalation induction and administration of succinylcholine is associated with an approximately 50% incidence of MH diagnosed by contracture testing. Trismus, rarely seen now due to the avoidance of succinylcholine in children undergoing anesthesia, is often not associated with signs of a fulminant MH episode; however, patients must be closely observed for evidence of hypermetabolism as well as rhabdomyolysis. The presence of whole-body rigidity or signs of hypermetabolism following trismus increases the risk of MH susceptibility as a cause, as does a peak creatine phosphokinase level exceeding 25,000 IU/L postoperatively.

Clinical signs and symptoms reflect a state of highly increased metabolism. The onset of hyperthermia is often delayed (Table 245-1). The earliest signs of MH include increased end-tidal CO_2 levels, tachycardia, and tachypnea (in an unparalyzed patient). The results of laboratory tests can be used to support a diagnosis of MH (Table 245-2).

Succinylcholine and all inhalation anesthetic agents are triggers for MH, with the newer short-acting inhalation agents being less likely to trigger MH, as compared with halothane and other longer-acting agents. Potassium is unlikely to cause MH; however, the administration of potassium has been reported to have caused retriggering in a patient treated for MH. Safe anesthetic agents include nitrous oxide, etomidate, ketamine, propofol, all opioids, all local anesthetics, all barbiturates, and all nondepolarizing neuromuscular blocking agents. Drugs used for reversal of neuromuscular blockade are also safe.

Table 245-1 Clinical Signs of Malignant Hyperthermia

↑ Temperature	↑ Sympathetic Activity
Tachypnea	Tachycardia
Rhabdomyolysis	Arrhythmia
Metabolic/respiratory acidosis	Sweating
Rigidity*	Hypertension

*Seventy-five percent of humans will develop rigidity.

Table 245-2 Laboratory Test Findings That Support a Diagnosis of Malignant Hyperthermia (MH)

Laboratory Test	Results in Patients with MH
End-tidal CO_2 concentration	↑
Blood gas analysis*	Metabolic acidosis
Serum CK†	↑
Serum and urine myoglobin	Positive
Serum K^+, Ca^{2+}, and lactate	↑

*Mixed venous, arterial, or venous sample.

†Creatine kinase (CK) levels should be measured every 6 hours for 24 hours.

Mechanism

Exposure to triggering anesthetic agents causes decreased control of intracellular calcium, resulting in release of free unbound ionized Ca^{2+} from storage sites. The calcium pumps attempt to restore homeostasis, which results in adenosine triphosphate (ATP) utilization, increased aerobic and anaerobic metabolism, and a runaway metabolic state. Rigidity occurs when unbound myofibrillar Ca^{2+} approaches the contractile threshold.

Treatment of Malignant Hyperthermia Crisis

The treatment of MH begins with immediate discontinuation of triggering agents and hyperventilation of the patient with 100% O_2. Dantrolene (2 mg/kg) should be intravenously administered early and rapidly when MH is suspected; the dose should be repeated every 5 min to effect or to a maximum of 10 mg/kg (this limit may be exceeded if necessary). After the initial signs of MH have been successfully treated, dantrolene should continue to be intravenously administered at a rate of 1 mg/kg every 6 h for 24 to 48 h to prevent recrudescence of symptoms. Calcium channel blockers should not be concomitantly administered with dantrolene because myocardial depression has been demonstrated with this combination in swine. Treatment efficacy is monitored with arterial blood gases, serum creatine phosphokinase concentrations, and vital signs. Dantrolene has unpleasant side effects (nausea, malaise, muscle weakness) but is generally well tolerated and has minimal toxicity in intravenously administered doses for the treatment of MH.

Symptomatic treatment includes, as appropriate, cooling (taking care to avoid hypothermia); the use of antiarrhythmic agents, diuretics such as mannitol and furosemide (although these drugs are rarely needed because of the mannitol in dantrolene), and sodium bicarbonate; and the management of hyperkalemia with insulin and glucose.

Anesthesia for Patients with Malignant Hyperthermia Susceptibility

Pretreatment with dantrolene is not recommended who have MHS. Nontriggering anesthetic agents should be used, and the anesthesia machine should be prepared by removing vaporizers (if possible), replacing hoses, and flushing the system with high-flow air or O_2 (10 L/min). The Malignant Hyperthermia Association of the United States (MHAUS) recommends that older anesthesia machines be flushed for a minimum of 20 min and no longer recommends that the soda lime canister be

Box 245-1 Indications for Evaluation of a Patient for Malignant Hyperthermia Susceptibility

Unexplained intraoperative death in family members
History of adverse anesthetic event*
Perioperative fever
Idiopathic elevated creatine phosphokinase levels
History of rhabdomyolysis
Presence of associated myopathies†

*For example, trismus.
†For example, central core disease or King-Denborough syndrome.

changed. For some newer anesthesia machines (e.g., Dräger Fabius), MHAUS recommends flushing for a minimum of 60 min. This time can be decreased if the integrated breathing system and diaphragm are replaced with autoclaved components. Because of the large number of newer anesthesia delivery systems on the market, MHAUS recommends following the manufacturer's guidelines to determine the appropriate washout procedure.

Monitoring should include all standard monitors with an emphasis on monitoring end-tidal CO_2, O_2 saturation by pulse oximetry, and core temperature (skin monitors may not reflect core changes). Arterial and central venous pressures should be monitored only if indicated by the surgical procedure or the patient's medical condition.

Evaluation of the Patient with Malignant Hyperthermia Susceptibility

Patients are referred for evaluation of MH susceptibility for a number of reasons (Box 245-1). A serum creatine phosphokinase level is often obtained in patients who are thought to be MHS. This value is elevated in approximately 70% of affected individuals; therefore, the results may be inconclusive.

The muscle biopsy contracture test is the only reliable diagnostic test for MH. Muscle is tested with caffeine and halothane alone, or in combination, and contracture responses are measured. This test has been standardized in European and North American laboratories. Genetic testing is helpful in an unequivocal case of clinical MH, in biopsy-proven cases, and in families in which a genetic mutation has been identified.

Source for Further Assistance

MHAUS is a lay organization with a medical MH expert advisory group that provides support for patients and anesthesia providers. It publishes books, pamphlets, and a quarterly newsletter at nominal costs; sponsors a website (mhaus.org); and manages a 24-h hotline (1-800-MHHYPER) to provide assistance to anesthesia providers managing MHS patients or treating patients with acute MH episodes.

Suggested Readings

Glahn KP, Ellis FR, Halsall PJ, et al, European Malignant Hyperthermia Group. Recognizing and managing a malignant hyperthermia crisis: Guidelines from the European Malignant Hyperthermia Group. *Br J Anaesth*. 2010;105: 417-420.

Gunter JB, Ball J, Than-Win S. Preparation of the Dräger Fabius anesthesia machine for the malignant-hyperthermia susceptible patient. *Anesth Analg*. 2008;107:1936-1945.

Hogan K, Couch F, Powers PA, Gregg RG. A cysteine-for-arginine substitution (R614C) in the human skeletal muscle calcium release channel cosegregates with malignant hyperthermia. *Anesth Analg*. 1992;75:441-448.

Kim TW, Nemergut ME. Preparation of modern anesthesia workstations for malignant hyperthermia-susceptible patients: A review of past and present practice. *Anesthesiology*. 2011;114:205-212.

Klingler W, Rueffert H, Lehmann-Horn F, et al. Core myopathies and risk of malignant hyperthermia. *Anesth Analg*. 2009;109:1167-1173.

Kolb ME, Horne ML, Martz R. Dantrolene in human malignant hyperthermia. *Anesthesiology*. 1982;56:254-262.

Larach MG, Gronert GA, Allen GC, et al. Clinical presentation, treatment, and complications of malignant hyperthermia in North America from 1987 to 2006. *Anesth Analg*. 2010;110(2):498-507.

Malignant Hyperthermia Association of the United States. *Medical Professionals' FAQ: Dantrolene*. Available at: http://medical.mhaus.org/index.cfm/fuseaction/Content.Display/PagePK/MedicalFAQs.cfm. Accessed October 25, 2010.

Prinzhausen H, Crawford MW, O'Rourke J, Petroz GC. Preparation of the Dräger Primus anesthetic machine for malignant hyperthermia-susceptible patients. *Can J Anaesth*. 2006;53:885-890.

Whitty RJ, Wong JK, Petroz GC, et al. Preparation of the Drager Fabius GS workstation for malignant hyperthermia-susceptible patients. *Can J Anaesth*. 2009;56:497-501.

CHAPTER 246

Anaphylactic and Anaphylactoid Reactions

Cornelius B. Groenewald, MB, ChB

Anaphylactic and anaphylactoid reactions, which produce an identical spectrum of clinical signs and symptoms, are acute, potentially life-threatening syndromes that occur in 1 out of every 10,000 to 20,000 anesthetics given. Anaphylactic reactions, which are associated with higher morbidity and mortality rates than anaphylactoid reactions, are type 1, typically IgE-mediated, immune reactions that result in mast cell and basophil degranulation and release of pharmacologically active mediators that affect almost all organ systems. Anaphylactoid reactions reflect nonimmune release of histamine from mast cells and basophils.

Pathophysiology

Prior sensitization or cross-sensitization to similar antigens is necessary to activate an anaphylactic reaction. Antigen-antibody interaction links two IgE molecules that, in turn, bind to and initiate mast cell and basophil degranulation and release of vasoactive mediators, including histamine, serum proteases (such as tryptase), proteoglycans, prostaglandins, and leukotrienes (Figure 246-1).

During anaphylactoid reactions, administered medications may cause nonimmunologic mast cell and basophil degranulation by activation of the complement cascade, of the coagulation system, of the kinin-generating system, or of the fibrinolytic system or by direct nonspecific mechanisms (Figure 246-1).

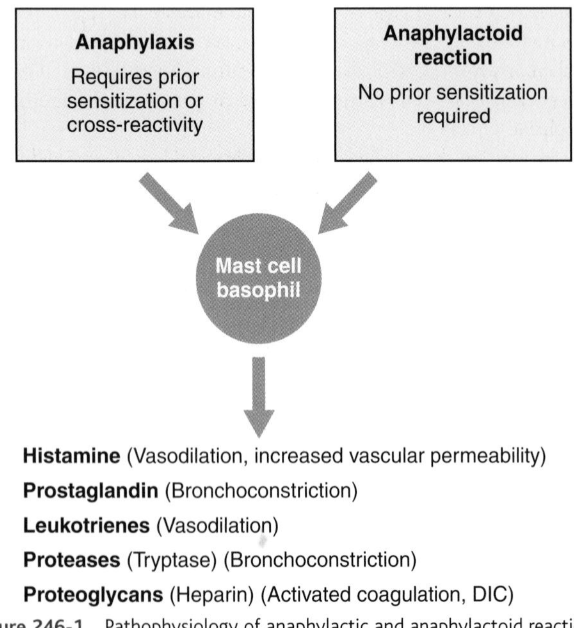

Figure 246-1 Pathophysiology of anaphylactic and anaphylactoid reactions. DIC, Disseminated intravascular coagulation.

Clinical Presentation

Target organs include the skin, upper and lower respiratory tracts, cardiovascular system, hematologic system, and the gastrointestinal tract (Box 246-1); mental status may also be altered. The signs and symptoms of anaphylaxis and anaphylactoid reactions that occur during the perioperative period depend on the types of anesthesia and monitors used. For example, early skin changes may not be appreciated in a covered patient, whereas abdominal and neurologic signs may be apparent only in awake patients.

The clinical presentation is not uniform and depends on the patient's sensitivity and the concentration and route of administration of the antigen. For example, intravenous administration of penicillin may trigger acute cardiovascular collapse, whereas cutaneous exposure to latex may result in only urticaria.

Diagnosis

The occurrence of an anaphylactic or anaphylactoid reaction is suggested by the development of signs and symptoms soon after administration of a potential agent. To distinguish between the reactions, obtaining a serum tryptase concentration may be useful. Tryptase, a serine protease, is released from mast cells during anaphylactic reactions and may correlate with the severity of the reaction. In contrast, anaphylactoid reactions are associated with normal or only slightly elevated tryptase levels. Serum levels rise within 15 min to 2 h and return to baseline levels within 24 h after the reaction, so tryptase concentration should be tested within this time period.

Box 246-1 Signs and Symptoms of Anaphylaxis and Anaphylactoid Reactions

Cardiac	Respiratory
Arterial hypotension	Rhinorrhea
Bradycardia	Angioedema
Tachycardia	↑ Mucous production
Arrhythmia	Bronchospasm
Cardiac arrest	↓ $ETCO_2$
Gastrointestinal	↑ Peak inspiratory pressure
	↓ SaO_2
Nausea	**Cutaneous**
Vomiting	
Hematologic	Angioedema
	Erythema
Coagulopathy*	Flushing
Renal	Urticaria
↓ Urine output†	

*Due to disseminated intravascular coagulopathy.
†Due to acute tubular necrosis.
$ETCO_2$, End-tidal CO_2 concentration; SaO_2, O_2 saturation.

Histamine levels rise early during both anaphylactic and anaphylactoid reactions but return to normal within 30 min; therefore, obtaining histamine levels is rarely useful in assisting with the diagnosis. Sensitivity to a specific medication is diagnosed by skin prick, intradermal testing, and, occasionally, serologic testing.

Substances Commonly Implicated In Anaphylactic and Anaphylactoid Reactions

Neuromuscular Blocking Agents

Neuromuscular blocking agents (NMBAs) are the most common medications involved in perioperative anaphylactic and anaphylactoid reactions, accounting for 50% to 70% of reported cases. The incidence of anaphylaxis is estimated at 1 in 6500 administrations of an NMBA. Cross-reactivity between the NMBAs may approach 60% to 70%. Succinylcholine and rocuronium account for most of the reported cases. The increased incidence of anaphylaxis occurring with the use of these drugs may be due to reporting bias; no epidemiologic studies have shown rocuronium to be more allergenic than other NMBAs. Atracurium, mivacurium, and doxacurium are the NMBAs most likely to cause anaphylactoid reactions that potentially lead to hypotension and tachycardia. However, these effects may be mitigated by slow intravenous administration of the drugs and pretreatment with antihistamines.

Latex

Latex allergy accounts for 20% of perioperative allergic reactions. High-risk groups include health care workers, patients undergoing multiple surgical procedures (such as patients with spina bifida), atopic individuals, and patients with allergies to mango, kiwi, bananas, and other fruits.

Antibiotics

Allergic reactions to the β-lactam ring antibiotics, penicillin, and cephalosporin are the third most common cause of perioperative anaphylaxis. Cross-reactivity between penicillin and the first-generation cephalosporins may approach 10%. The red man syndrome, associated with rapid administration of vancomycin, is caused by nonspecific histamine release.

Other Substances

Anaphylactic reactions to propofol have been reported and occur in 1 in 30,000 to 60,000 administrations. Current evidence suggests that patients who are allergic to egg lecithin (present in the yolk) are perhaps more likely to experience anaphylaxis during propofol administration, as compared with patients without egg-lecithin allergies.

Anaphylactic reactions to opioids are rare but have been reported with the use of fentanyl. Morphine and meperidine cause anaphylactoid reactions rather than anaphylaxis.

Anaphylactic reactions to methylene blue are very rare; however, the incidence approaches 1% to 2% following injection of isosulfan blue or patent blue dye.

The paraaminobenzoic acid preservative in the ester class of local anesthetic agents (procaine, chloroprocaine, tetracaine, and cocaine), rather than the local anesthetic agent itself, is the cause of most anaphylactic reactions with this type of drug; because drugs in this class are not often used, anaphylactic reactions in patients receiving local anesthetic solutions is rare. Drugs in the amide class of local anesthetics (lidocaine, bupivacaine, mepivacaine, prilocaine, and ropivacaine) are not allergenic; however, some individuals are allergic to the sodium bisulfite or metabisulfite used to stabilize epinephrine, and, for these individuals, a local anesthetic without epinephrine should be used.

Reports have implicated colloid volume expanders in 2.3% of perioperative allergic reactions; dextrans have the highest risk, and hetastarch seems to be safest. There is no cross-reactivity between different colloids.

Treatment

The first step in treating an anaphylactic reaction is to discontinue possible causative drugs, thereby decreasing the antigen load. Consideration should be given to switching to a latex-free environment. Supportive treatment is initiated with maintenance of the airway and administration of 100 % O_2. All anesthetic medications should be discontinued. Inhaled anesthetics may produce myocardial depression and worsen hypotension and are not the treatment of choice for bronchospasm in this situation. Increased vascular permeability may result in rapid transit of fluid from the intravascular to the interstitial compartment and, along with vasodilation, could result in hypotension that, if severe enough, could cause hypovolemic shock. Immediate blood volume expansion with 2 to 4 L of crystalloid or colloid solution is indicated. The drug of choice for treating systemic effects is epinephrine, which increases intracellular concentrations of cyclic adenosine monophosphate and thereby stabilizes membrane permeability, resulting in decreased release of pharmacologically active mediators. Vasodilation responds to the α_1-agonist effects of epinephrine on vascular smooth muscle; in addition, epinephrine, with its β_2-agonist activity on bronchial smooth muscle, is the bronchodilator of choice when cardiac collapse is associated with bronchospasm. The route and dose of administration depend on the patient's clinical condition. For reactions that are not severe, a 1:1000 solution of epinephrine may be given subcutaneously at a dose of 0.3 to 0.5 mg. Patients with hypotension should receive 0.5 to 1 mL of double dilute (1:100,000) epinephrine intravenously every 1 to 3 min until they are hemodynamically stable. In cases of life-threatening cardiac collapse, increased doses will be needed. In settings in which intravenous access has not been established, epinephrine may be given via the tracheal tube. It is important to note that epinephrine should not be given intravenously to normotensive patients.

Bronchospasm is treated with inhaled β_2-agonists (such as albuterol or terbutaline).

Antihistamines and corticosteroids are often administered. However, their benefit is less clear. H_1-receptor antagonists, such as diphenhydramine, may competitively bind to histamine receptors and ameliorate some of the signs and symptoms, but there is no evidence to support this use. Corticosteroids (methylprednisolone) are given to prevent delayed release of inflammatory mediators. The use of sodium bicarbonate and arginin vasopressin therapy should be considered in patients not responsive to epinephrine.

Every reaction that occurs perioperatively should be investigated immediately as well as with skin testing 6 weeks postoperatively.

Suggested Readings

Dewachter P, Mouton-Faivre C, Emala CW. Anaphylaxis and anesthesia: Controversies and new insights. *Anesthesiology*. 2009;111:1141-1150.

Hepner DL, Castells MC. Anaphylaxis during the perioperative period. *Anesth Analg*. 2003;97:1381-1395.

Levy JH, Yegin A. Anaphylaxis. What is monitored to make a diagnosis? How is therapy monitored? *Anesthesiol Clin North Am*. 2001;19:705-715.

Mertes PM, Lexenaire MC. Allergy and anaphylaxis in anaesthesia. *Minerva Anesthesiol*. 2004;70:285-291.

SECTION XIII Practice Management

CHAPTER 247

Licensure, Credentialing, and Privileging

R. Scott Gorman, MD, and Carol B. Garrison, CPMSM

Health care organizations—such as hospitals, health plans, and provider networks—must be certain that individuals who provide health care services for their respective organizations are fully qualified, competent, and able to perform those services. This process includes not only evaluating an applicant's licensure and reviewing credentials, but also granting specific privileges to that provider. The determination of both provider qualifications and competency is essential if a health care organization is to provide safe competent care while avoiding lawsuits, bad publicity, and financial loss.

Licensure is the process whereby a government board or agency reviews a provider's education, training, background, and any ethical concerns and, if the standards are adequately met, thereafter grants the provider the right to provide health care services within its jurisdiction. The government views licensure as its primary mechanism of protecting the public from substandard care. The requirements for licensure vary from state to state and sometimes include specific education requirements. Additionally, some states require supplemental competency testing if the provider is several years past formal medical training, received his or her medical training outside the United States, or is not board certified.

Credentialing is the process of assessing and verifying the qualifications of a health care provider to obtain appointment to a medical staff or to be approved as a provider in a health plan or health care network. Although many of the requirements for credentialing are similar to those for licensure, each health care organization determines its own criteria and processes. The health care organization may therefore set standards and expectations for quality, safety, and other performance measures that go beyond licensure standards.

Privileging is the process of evaluating the training, experience, and current competency of an individual to perform specific medical services as a part of a medical staff. Privileges are detailed and specific, and providers may only offer medical services in those areas in which they hold privileges. For most requested privileges, the designated individuals within the health care organization will review the provider's education and training, past clinical performance, malpractice history, and the number of cases performed. An organization's decision to limit a provider's privileges can be grounds for legal action by the applicant or require the organization to submit a report to the applicable state or federal regulatory agency and, therefore, must be done with great care and consistency. Today, most health care organizations also employ a process of ongoing concurrent review after the granting of privileges to ensure that competency is maintained.

How Health Care Organizations Credential and Privilege Providers

The specific processes for credentialing and privileging are delineated in a combination of the health care organization's medical staff bylaws, rules and regulations, and policies and procedures. For legal and regulatory reasons, it is essential that the processes are clearly outlined and precisely followed. Otherwise, the health care organization may have a limited ability to correct or dismiss providers due to inadequate performance.

In most health care organizations, the data collection involved with credentialing and privileging is performed by individuals specifically designated by the organization. These individuals may function solely as credentialing/privileging personnel, or this function may be part of the broader services provided by medical staff services. Following the collection of data, a credentialing or personnel committee or designee reviews the data and makes recommendations to the governing body. In acute care hospitals, the medical executive committee is responsible for forwarding recommendations to the governing body of the health care organization, which is ultimately responsible for the decisions concerning staff membership and clinical privileges.

The information used in licensure, credentialing, and privileging comes from a variety of sources. To decrease the risk that an individual will submit falsified documents for review, licensing boards and health care organizations check information through a process known as primary source verification. This means that verification of an applicant's education, training, experience, work history, board certification, licensure, malpractice history, and legal background check must be obtained directly from the originating source. Although this process can be time consuming, much of the information is now available on secure Internet sites.

At times questions, concerns, or issues (i.e., "red flags," such as incomplete or inconsistent information found on the application form) confront those who are reviewing an application. Among the red flags that cause the greatest concern for reviewers are the following:

- Conflicting information between the information provided on the application and the information received in the verification process.
- Unexplained gaps in time. Organizations may determine what time period is considered an acceptable time gap between transitions (e.g., a time gap between training programs or when relocating). Unexplained or extended time gaps are considered a red flag and require additional information.
- Frequent moves from location to location or practice to practice. This situation not only can make competency evaluation for privileging difficult, but may also suggest problems in other areas, such as poor interpersonal skills, health problems, issues with a state licensing board or agency, or excessive malpractice claims.
- Negative references or reference requests that are not returned. References can be a powerful source of information, but because applicants have a tendency to select individuals who will give a positive review, a negative response is particularly important.

- Unanswered questions on the application. Although an omission may be a simple error, it can also signal an effort by the applicant to hide something.
- A large number of liability suits. Recently, the number of lawsuits associated with a provider has become linked to his or her ability to communicate with patients as well as competency.

License Renewal, Reappointment, and Continuation of Clinical Privileges

No longer is it acceptable for licensing bodies or health care organizations to simply "rubber stamp" a health care provider's request for licensure renewal, reappointment to a health care organization, or continuation of clinical privileges. Regulators as well as medical staff leaders expect the renewal process to be every bit as rigorous and perhaps more evidence-based than was the initial licensure, appointment, or privileging process. This rigor is supplemented by the data that can be collected on a provider during the previous practice period. Not only can the information collected during initial licensure, appointment, and privileging be reassessed, but new information may now be available. This information may include the following:

- Quality and safety information, including compliance with practice guidelines
- Complication and infection rate data
- Compliance with policies and procedures
- Patient satisfaction, e.g., number of patient complaints
- Continuing medical education hours
- Maintenance of board certification
- Peer references
- Malpractice history
- Current competency
- Utilization management

Gathering this information can be a complex and sometimes difficult task, but it is necessary if a health care organization is to make the reappraisal process meaningful in terms of patient protection and institution liability.

Perhaps of greatest importance during this reassessment is the ability to more reliably assess providers' competency to continue to provide the services specified in their initial privileging. This competency is usually assessed through a review of cases performed and success and complication rates and an assessment of competency by peers or the individual's department chair. To demonstrate an individual's competency, most health care organizations have established criteria, which may include the number and type of procedures performed. When possible, objective data should be used in this evaluation process because any limitation of privileging may greatly affect the applicant provider's ability to continue her or his practice of medicine.

Delegated Credentialing

Delegated credentialing is the process used when a health care organization outsources or delegates the credentialing responsibility to an outside vendor or credentialing verification organization (CVO) or another health care organization. Often this involves a health insurer or health care network delegating the credentialing to a participating provider group within the health plan or network. The participating provider group or CVO, rather than the health insurer, performs the credentialing process. This process assumes that the participating provider group or CVO is capable of performing the credentialing process and meets the standards set by the delegating organization. Not only does this arrangement obviate the need for the outsourcing organization to perform the detailed work already being done by the provider group or CVO, but it also means less work for the practitioners who would otherwise be burdened with additional, often duplicative, paperwork.

If health care organizations that delegate credentialing are serious about protecting their patients and decreasing their own liability, they must include oversight of the provider group or CVO. The health care organization that delegates credentialing must set standards for the delegated credentialing process that includes a periodic audit of the credentials files and policies and procedures of the provider group or CVO. Review of quality, safety, patient satisfaction or complaints, liability, and other specific data should be included. Only those outsourced provider groups or CVOs that meet these standards are allowed to continue with delegated credentialing status. In most circumstances, the final decision about whether a provider is credentialed by a delegating health care organization rests not with the outsourced group or CVO, but with the health care organization itself.

Suggested Readings

Centers for Medicare & Medicaid Services (CMS). http://www.cms.gov/

Credentials review and the initial appointment process. In: *The Medical Staff Handbook: A Guide to Joint Commission Standards*. 2nd ed. Oak Brook Terrace, IL: Joint Commission Resources; 2004:19-62.

Matzka K. Credentialing, recredentialing, privileging, and appointment. In: *The Compliance Guide to the Joint Commission Medical Staff Standards*. 6th ed. Marblehead, MA: HCPro, Inc; 2008.

National Association Medical Staff Services (NAMSS). http://www.namss.org/

National Committee on Quality Assurance (NCQA). http://www.ncqa.org/

Reappraisal, reappointment, and renewal of clinical privileges. In: *The Medical Staff Handbook: A Guide to Joint Commission Standards*. 2nd ed. Oak Brook Terrace, IL: Joint Commission Resources; 2004:121-160.

The Joint Commission (TJC). http://www.jointcommission.org/

URAC. https://www.urac.org/

Utilization Review Accreditation Commission. Delegated credentialing and physician performance reporting. *URAC Issue Brief*. Washington, DC: Health2 Resources; June 2008.

CHAPTER 248

Board Certification and Maintenance of Certification

Timothy R. Long, MD, and Steven H. Rose, MD

Although participation in the American Board of Anesthesiology (ABA) certification process is voluntary, achieving and maintaining certification are increasingly important to secure and maintain medical licensure and hospital privileges. Board certification (and maintenance of certification) may also be a requirement for membership in a private group practice or academic anesthesiology department. Achieving certification at the first opportunity and maintaining certification are thus important goals for anesthesiologists.

Primary Certification

The ABA, a member board of the American Board of Medical Specialties (ABMS), has established threshold criteria and the training and education requirements, as well as the knowledge and skills, that anesthesiologists must have so that the ABA can certify (and recertify) an anesthesiologist as meeting these criteria. Certification by an ABMS-member board, such as the ABA, has been shown to correlate with medical school evaluations and grades, the duration and type of residency training, and faculty assessment of procedural skills. Interestingly, personal characteristics such as trait-anxiety (the tendency to respond to a wide range of situations as dangerous or threatening) and the ability to maintain focused attention (vigilance) and process information quickly are also associated with clinical competence, but certification by an ABMS-member board is more widely and readily accepted by the public.

Because the knowledge and skill sets that a physician has decline over time, and because of the continuing advances in technology and science, ABMS-member boards are increasingly recertifying physicians. The results of these recertification processes correlate positively with the number of patients anesthetized and with the severity of illness that these patients have; certification correlates with better clinical outcomes.

Physicians who successfully complete the requirements for residency training (the Continuum of Education) in an Accreditation Council for Graduate Medical Education (ACGME)-accredited anesthesiology residency program may qualify to enter the examination process for primary certification by the ABA if they meet the threshold requirements for primary certification in anesthesiology (Box 248-1).

The duration of candidate status to be eligible for the Part 1 examination is limited to one opportunity per calendar year for 3 years. Candidates completing residency training after January 1, 2012, must complete all certification requirements within 7 years of the last day of the year in which residency training was completed. All candidates must complete the Part 2 examination within 3 years of the date of the first Part 2 examination for which they become eligible.

Trainees beginning the clinical base year (CBY) in 2012 or later will be required to complete three stages of ABA examinations. The first stage (Basic examination) is administered following successful completion of the first clinical anesthesia (CA) year. The second stage (Advanced examination) is administered following successful completion of residency training. The oral examination (Applied examination) may be taken following successful completion of both Basic and Advanced written examinations.

Continuum of Education in Anesthesiology

The ABA Continuum of Education in Anesthesiology consists of 4 years of full-time training after a medical or osteopathic degree has been conferred. This continuum includes 1 year of clinical base training and 3 years of training in clinical anesthesiology (CA-1, CA-2, and CA-3 years). The CBY must be completed in a transitional year or primary specialty training program that is accredited by the ACGME or the American Osteopathic Association. Training outside the United States and its territories must be conducted in a program affiliated with a medical school that is approved by the Liaison Committee on Medical Education.

The 3-year clinical anesthesia curriculum includes basic anesthesia training, subspecialty anesthesia training, and advanced anesthesia training during which residents provide care for progressively more complex patients and progressively more difficult procedures. Basic anesthesia training focuses on fundamental aspects of anesthesia. Subspecialty anesthesia training is focused on the subdisciplines of anesthesiology, such as obstetric anesthesia, pediatric anesthesia, cardiothoracic anesthesia, neuroanesthesia, anesthesia for outpatient surgery, the postanesthesia care unit, perioperative evaluation, regional anesthesia, critical care medicine, and

Box 248-1 Threshold Requirements for Primary Certification in Anesthesiology

- A permanent, unconditional, and unrestricted, unexpired medical license to practice medicine or osteopathy in one or more states or jurisdictions of the United States or province of Canada
- Completion of the requirements of the Continuum of Education in anesthesiology
- An ABA Certificate of Clinical Competence with an overall satisfactory rating covering the final 6-month period of clinical anesthesia training in each anesthesiology residency program on file with the ABA
- Documentation of professional standing that is satisfactory to the ABA
- Capability to perform independently the entire scope of anesthesiology practice without restriction, or with reasonable accommodation
- Successful completion of a written (Part 1) and an oral (Part 2) examination. Although many decry the oral examination process, there is evidence that the examination system established by the ABA many years ago also correlates with clinical competence.

ABA, American Board of Anesthesiology.

pain medicine. Advanced anesthesia training occurs in the CA-3 year. Training in the CA-3 year must be distinctly different from that obtained during the CA-1 and CA-2 years and is characterized by increasing independence to prepare residents for the unsupervised practice of anesthesiology after residency completion. Additional details about the specific requirements for completion of the Continuum of Education in Anesthesiology is available in the ABA Booklet of Information accessible on the ABA website.

Clinical anesthesia training (CA-1 through CA-3 years) must be conducted in no more than two ACGME-accredited programs with at least 3 months of uninterrupted training in each. The 6-month period of clinical anesthesia training in any one program must end with receipt of a satisfactory Certificate of Clinical Competence for this training to receive credit toward requirements to complete the Continuum. Part-time training is assessed on an individual basis by the ABA Credentials Committee and must be approved prospectively. Total absence from training must not exceed 60 working days during the CA-1 through CA-3 years. Absences beyond this limit require extension of total training time based on the duration of the absence. After a prolonged absence from training (>6 months), the ABA Credentials Committee will determine the number of months of training after the absence that are required.

Subspecialty Certification

The ABA also offers subspecialty certification in critical care medicine, pain medicine, hospice and palliative care medicine, sleep medicine, and pediatric anesthesiology (Box 248-2). Subspecialty recertification is offered through successful completion of a written examination. A transition from subspecialty recertification examination programs to Maintenance of Certification in Anesthesiology for Subspecialties (MOCA-SUBS) began January 1, 2010. The last subspecialty recertification examinations will be conducted in 2016 and the first MOCA-SUBS examinations will be conducted in 2017. The MOCA-SUBS program is the only option for holders of ABA subspecialty certification or recertification awarded after January 1, 2010. After 2016, the MOCA-SUBS program is the only option to maintain subspecialty certification.

Maintenance of Certification

Maintenance of Certification in Anesthesiology (MOCA) is required for ongoing certification of anesthesiologists who achieved primary certification in anesthesiology during or after 2000. The MOCA process is completed in 10-year cycles intended to assure the public of a diplomate's continuing competence in the practice of anesthesiology. MOCA requirements are divided into four parts: professional standing, lifelong learning and self-assessment, cognitive examination, and practice performance assessment and improvement. MOCA requirements are summarized in Table 248-1.

Box 248-2 Requirements for Subspecialty Certification

Status as a diplomate of the ABA
Fulfillment of the licensure requirement for certification
Fulfillment of the specialty training requirements as determined by the ABA
Satisfactory completion of the subspecialty certification examination requirements as determined by the ABA
Professional standing satisfactory to the ABA
Capability of performing independently the entire scope of subspecialty practice without or with reasonable accommodations
For subspecialty certification in sleep medicine and pediatric anesthesiology, enrollment in the MOCA process

ABA, American Board of Anesthesiologists; MOCA, Maintenance of Certification in Anesthesiology.

Table 248-1 Maintenance of Certification in Anesthesiology Requirements

Part	Requirement(s)
1	Continual assessment of professional standing through maintenance of valid medical licensure
2	Lifelong learning and self-assessment Current knowledge through CME and other forms of learning 350 CME credits • 250 must be category 1 • Limited to ≤70 per year • ≥90 must be ASA CE or Self-Education and Evaluation Programs or ABA-approved equivalent evaluative CME program • >20 must be patient safety through HealthStream's ABMS PSIP or the ASA's FPS
3	Cognitive examination during years 7-10 of the 10-year accreditation cycle: 200 multiple-choice questions, 50 of which address anesthesiology subspecialties
4	During the 10-year cycle, participate in two evaluations—one during years 1-5 and one in years 6-10 *Case* A four-step process to assess practice and implement changes that improve outcomes *Simulation* A contextual learning opportunity to assess and improve practice conducted in an ASA-endorsed center Confirmation of a diplomate's clinical practice and ongoing practice assessment and performance improvement activities through attestations

ABA, American Board of Anesthesiologists; ABMS, American Board of Medical Specialties; ASA, American Society of Anesthesiologists; CE, continuing education; CME, continuing medical education; FPS, Fundamentals of Patient Safety; MOCA, Maintenance of Certification in Anesthesiology; PSIP, Patient Safety Improvement Program.

Summary

Board certification and MOCA are critical achievements that may impact medical licensure (and maintenance of licensure), hospital privileges, and employment. The requirements for certification and MOCA are detailed and numerous. This chapter provides an overview of current primary certification, subspecialty certification, and MOCA requirements. However, it is important for candidates and diplomates to periodically review current requirements on the ABA website to be aware of the specific requirements.

Suggested Readings

Brennan TA, Horwitz RI, Duffy FD, et al. The role of physician specialty board certification status in the quality movement. *JAMA*. 2004;292:1038-1043.

Lowy J. Board certification as prerequisite for hospital staff privileges. *Virtual Mentor*. 2005;7(4). Available at: http://virtualmentor.ama-assn.org/2005/04/pdf/ccas4-0504.pdf. Accessed November 25, 2012.

Reich DL, Uysal S, Bodian CA, et al. The relationship of cognitive, personality, and academic measures to anesthesiology resident clinical performance. *Anesth Analg*. 1999;88:1092-1100.

Rose SH, Burkle CM. Accreditation Council for Graduate Medical Education competencies and the American Board of Anesthesiology Clinical Competence Committee: A comparison. *Anesth Analg*. 2006;102:212-216.

The American Board of Anesthesiology. *The ABA Booklet of Information*. Available at: http://theaba.org/pdf/BOI.pdf. Accessed September 21, 2012.

CHAPTER 249

Principles of Medical Professional Liability Insurance

Brian J. Thomas, JD

Medical professional liability insurance is provided by third-party liability insurance companies and is purchased by an insured to protect against potential tort liability, a civil wrong, to others. When civil wrong occurs, it creates liability against the wrongdoer (tortfeasor) in favor of the injured party. The civil wrong in a medical malpractice case typically involves an alleged breach of the standard of care by a physician or other health care provider in the form of a negligent act or omission that substantially leads to the patient's injury or death. In the case of a physician, the physician-patient relationship gives rise to the "duty" owed by the physician to the patient. A patient can recover money from a physician if the patient can prove that the physician's conduct both fell below the accepted standard of care and caused the patient's injury or death. Most physicians purchase medical professional liability insurance to defend and pay claims resulting from medical negligence or malpractice lawsuits.

Scope of Coverage—What Is Covered?

The purpose of medical professional liability insurance is to protect the insured physician's personal assets. Medical professional liability insurance generally provides coverage for a physician's legal liability for "injury" that results from professional services provided or that should have been provided by the physician. "Injury" might include bodily injury and intangible injury such as pain, mental suffering, and loss of consortium (conjugal fellowship of husband and wife including not only material services, but also such intangibles as society, guidance, companionship, and sexual relations). "Injury" might also include purely economic losses, such as lost past and future wages, past and future medical expenses, and funeral expenses, as long as the loss derives from an act or omission of a professional nature. The protection provided by medical professional liability insurance varies and is typically defined by a policy's "scope of coverage" provision.

Exclusions—What Is Not Covered?

Medical professional liability insurance policies generally contain exclusionary language expressly limiting coverage in specifically defined situations. Although the exclusionary language varies among different policies, most medical professional liability policies routinely exclude coverage for specific situations (Box 249-1).

Limits of Liability—How Much Is Covered?

A medical professional liability insurance policy limits the amount of damages the insurance company will pay under the policy. Most medical professional liability insurance policies contain two limits—a "per claim" limit and an aggregate limit. The per claim limit is the maximum amount of damages the insurance company will pay for each claim. The aggregate limit is the total amount of damages the insurance company will pay for all claims within in a specified period of time—typically 1 year. Physicians may purchase different limits of liability coverage, typically ranging from $200,000 to $1 million per claim and with an annual aggregate that is typically three times the per claim limit. The amount of professional liability coverage purchased depends on the individual physician's needs. Additionally, some states and health care facilities may require physicians to carry a minimum amount of professional liability coverage.

In addition to the limits of liability, most medical professional liability insurance policies provide coverage for the costs of defending a covered claim. The costs of defending a medical negligence lawsuit typically include attorney fees, expert fees, deposition fees, textbooks, and trial exhibits. The costs of defending a medical negligence lawsuit are most typically provided in addition to the limits of liability; however, under some policies, the limits of liability are reduced by defense expenditures.

Occurrence Versus Claims-Made Coverage

Medical professional liability insurance was traditionally written on an occurrence form. Under an occurrence form, the injury that precipitates a claim for damages simply must occur during the policy period to trigger coverage. Owing to the fact that many claims are not recognized, reported, or filed until years after the alleged negligent professional act occurred, insurance companies experience difficulty calculating how much premium should be collected today to cover claims that might not be reported for years.

To address this problem, many medical professional liability insurance companies now use a claims-made form instead of the occurrence form. Under a claims-made medical professional liability insurance policy, coverage is not triggered by the event giving rise to the injury (the occurrence) but, instead, by when the claim is first made. The term *claims made* refers to the notification that an injured third party is seeking redress from the insured. Typically, coverage is triggered when a physician receives a demand for money from an injured patient or receives a notice or summons from the

Box 249-1 Typical Exclusions by Medical Professional Liability Insurance Policies

- Any intentional, willful, wanton, fraudulent, or malicious acts or omissions
- Liability arising from substance abuse
- Liability arising from the alteration, falsification, or destruction of medical records with fraudulent intent
- Liability assumed under a written or oral contract or agreement
- Punitive or exemplary damages

patient's legal representative and gives notice to the insurance company. Frequently, the meaning of *claims made* includes allowing coverage to be triggered by a precautionary reporting of adverse outcomes or incident report to the insurance company within the policy period regardless of third-party involvement.

Another feature of claims-made policies is the extended reporting period, which guarantees the insured an extended period in which claims may be reported if the policy is canceled or not renewed. The extended reporting period—also known as tail coverage—applies only to claims made after the policy expires or is canceled and arising from events that occur after the date the policy was issued but before the expiration of the policy. These provisions vary substantially among insurance companies.

Consent-to-Settle Clauses

The relationship between a physician and his or her medical professional liability insurance company is also defined by the extent to which the physician can influence the settlement of claims. Some medical professional liability insurance policies contain consent-to-settle clauses that require the insurance company to obtain the insured physician's permission before settling a claim. Because many physicians view an out-of-court settlement as an admission of guilt or feel strongly that their care and treatment were appropriate, a consent-to-settle clause might be an important policy provision for those physicians. Some insurance policies do not include consent-to-settle clauses and allow the insurance company the right to settle claims—even those without merit—without the insured physician's consent.

Suggested Readings

Dobbyn JF. *Insurance Law in a Nutshell*. 3rd St. Paul, MN: West Publishing; 1996:43.

Jerry RH. *Understanding Insurance Law*. 3rd ed. Newark, NJ: Matthew Bender & Co.; 2002:409-410.

Mangan JF, Mangan CM. *Underwriting Commercial Liability*. 2nd ed. Malvern, PA: Insurance Institute of America; 2000;7:288-293.

Pegalis SE, Wachsman HF. *American Law of Medical Malpractice*. 2nd ed. New York: Clark Boardman Callaghan;1992:3-6.

CHAPTER 250

Medicolegal Principles: The Anesthesia Record

Nancy J. Cummings, Esq

The anesthesia record is a part of the complete patient medical record. As such, the anesthesia record is reviewed for the same purposes as the general medical record. The record is for (1) immediate or ongoing care of the patient, (2) communication and coordination among health care professionals treating the patient, (3) claims submission for payment, (4) utilization review and quality-of-care review, (5) accreditation surveys, (6) medical research and education, and (7) evidence in lawsuits.

Physicians should understand the importance of proper record documentation. Government payers, such as the Centers for Medicare and Medicaid Services; private payers, such as Blue Cross/Blue Shield; and accrediting entities, such as The Joint Commission have developed formal minimum requirements or "standards" regarding medical records that must be followed for payment and accreditation. Hospitals and health care professionals typically adopt these requirements to ensure efficient payment of claims and to maintain industry-recognized standards of practice.

Utilization reviews and quality-of-care reviews are routinely performed by hospitals and large payers using medical record documentation as the primary source of information. Physicians who do not comply with hospital standards put themselves and the hospital at risk; therefore, most hospitals will resort to discipline and eventual privilege loss if a physician is seriously and chronically noncompliant with medical record policies.

Medical records are also reviewed for medical research and medical education; for these purposes, specific federal rules also apply. For example, to bill Medicare for a service rendered in a teaching setting, surgical and invasive medical procedures must be documented in a way that demonstrates the direct involvement of the teaching physician in the critical portion of a procedure. Graduate medical education has accrediting standards that include medical documentation requirements. Research grants may also be contingent upon proper record documentation.

In certain types of legal proceedings, the medical chart is highly scrutinized and used as important evidence to prove an element of the case. Lawsuits that often involve medical-record documentation include medical malpractice, workers compensation, job-related injuries, guardianships, and competency determinations. At trial, it is common for copies of or verbatim excerpts from the medical record to be presented for the judge or jury to review in deciding the case. Depending on the nature of the case, the physicians who authored the medical record documentation may also be deposed and questioned on the witness stand regarding their patient care and their record documentation. In such circumstances, the record typically provides significant help for the authoring physician trying to recall details of the care that was provided to the patient.

The quality of the documentation in a medical record reflects on the quality of the care and services rendered to the patient. Incomplete or inadequate documentation may be due to poor care or poor documentation habits, but either casts a poor light on the physician/documenter and the facility that maintains the record. It is in the best interest of the patient, the attending physician, and the health care facility to have accurate and complete documentation in the medical record. For additional information see Chapter 251, Anesthesia Information Management Systems.

Suggested Readings

Centers for Medicare and Medicaid Services. *1997 documentation guidelines for evaluation and management services*. Available at: https://www.cms.gov/MLNProducts/Downloads/MASTER1.pdf. Accessed May 28, 2010.

National Committee for Quality Assurance. *Guidelines for medical record documentation*. Available at: Guidelines_Medical_Record_Review.pdf. Accessed May 28, 2010.

Wood DL. Documentation guidelines: Evolution, future direction and compliance. *Am J Med*. 2001;110:332-334.

World Health Organization. *Guidelines for medical record and clinical documentation; 2007*. Available at: http://www.searo.who.int/LinkFiles/2007_Guidelines_for_Clinical_Doc.pdf. Accessed May 28, 2010.

CHAPTER 251

Anesthesia Information Management Systems

Daniel V. Simula, MD, and Jeff T. Mueller, MD

An anesthesia information management system (AIMS) is the anesthesia component of an electronic medical record (EMR). This data acquisition system collects and displays real-time perioperative data from anesthesia machines, patient monitors, and other medical devices. An advanced AIMS also provides decision support capability for clinicians and facilitates information management and quality improvement functions. Much like the flight deck management and flight control systems found in modern aircraft, an AIMS can minimize manual clinical documentation duties and facilitate increased situational awareness and attention to critical tasks.

Anesthesiologists have long been at the forefront of improving monitoring capabilities and enhancing patient safety. With advances in minicomputers in the 1970s and the advent of desktop computing in the early 1980s, anesthesiologists began to explore the viability of an automated anesthesia record. Given that a single anesthetic can create millions of bits of information and that up to 40% of an anesthesia provider's time is spent as an information scribe, computer automation was seen as a natural way to create a higher quality record that required less manual documentation. Early designs consisted primarily of homegrown proprietary designs that did not benefit from standardization or integration with other systems. Over the past 30 years, established medical device and information technology companies have entered the AIMS market. Even today, this market is continuing to mature, and AIMS vendors currently provide products with wide variations in functionality and integration.

Architecture and Configuration

Conceptually, an AIMS is simply the clinical information system that supports perioperative care. An AIMS can be a stand-alone system or can be integrated within a larger medical records system. In integrated environments, an AIMS might interface with clinical systems, such as an EMR or a CPOE (computerized physician order entry) system, or with practice management systems focused on surgical scheduling, supply management, quality improvement, or coding and billing.

A proper AIMS requires high-reliability hardware, software, and networks. Special attention to human factors engineering and user interface technologies has been shown to be extremely important for the successful design, deployment, and, perhaps most important, user acceptance of any AIMS installation. An AIMS presents all of the attendant requirements of a mission critical system. Dedicated support from the organization's information technology department is an essential ingredient of a successful AIMS.

Prevalence and Utilization

It is widely believed that AIMS utilization lags behind that of many other EMR components. A 2008 study demonstrated that only 14% of U.S. academic anesthesiology departments had fully operational systems.

Even today, the majority of AIMS implementations are stand-alone systems focused primarily on producing an automated anesthesia record. They tend to be poorly integrated with hospital EMRs, operating room management systems (e.g., surgical scheduling, patient tracking, supply management), and other operational systems (e.g., pharmacy, blood banking, physician orders, accounting, billing, quality reporting). However, evolving requirements created by pay-for-performance, quality, and safety initiatives and other administrative expectations are increasing the demand for integration and advanced AIMS. In response to these demands, a number of AIMS vendors are broadening their product offerings to include support for a wide variety of capabilities, such as preanesthesia evaluations, barcode-enabled drug and blood product administration and charting, drug-conflict checking, and user-accessible databases for outcomes research and quality reporting. Even with these attempts to offer more advanced functionality, there are significant downsides if these capabilities are poorly integrated with EMRs and hospital-wide information systems.

As with any evolving technology, early implementations deliver value primarily through singular feature–specific capabilities. Only later in the technology lifecycle does higher-order value from integration begin to overtake the more discrete functions of the system. The current literature on EMRs and medical informatics rarely mentions the use of AIMS. These omissions highlight just how different AIMS requirements are when compared with more general EMR functions and hospital information systems and how little actual integration currently exists. Given that the operating room is arguably one of the most fast-paced, resource-intensive, and high-risk environments in all of health care, it is surprising that anesthesiology is still faced with large "information gaps" and a general lack of advanced information technology.

Benefits

At first glance, the most obvious benefit of an AIMS is the elimination of manual charting on a paper anesthesia record, which not only reduces the need for mundane recordkeeping, but also provides real-time display of higher-order, clinically relevant information. Although they were viewed as significant progress at the time they were implemented, first-generation systems provided little more than the convenience of automatic charting and a legible record. As AIMS technology has progressed, additional benefits have been realized. A well-designed AIMS can add value to an anesthesia practice and the associated facility that is not attainable with paper anesthesia records. Benefits in quality improvement, safety, cost management, revenue capture, and medical liability have all been demonstrated. However, deploying any new and evolving technology introduces risks, and many of these risks and pitfalls have also been noted in the literature. Institutions without the necessary financial and technical resources or the full commitment of senior leadership should consider AIMS implementation cautiously. Making an informed decision includes consulting the literature and specialty organizations for guidelines, policies, technical recommendations, and best practices.

Although an increasing array of benefits have been attributed to AIMS technologies, the question of whether these systems broadly and consistently produce a positive financial return remains hotly debated. One significant confounding factor regarding return-on-investment discussions is determining who receives the benefit and who pays the cost. Although both anesthesia groups and facilities may realize significant benefit from an AIMS, the acquisition and support costs are frequently provided by hospitals or academic institutions. For the limited number of organizations that have deployed an AIMS, survey findings show that return-on-investment expectations have "generally been met," with specific benefits attributed to improved clinical documentation, data collection for clinical research, enhancement of quality improvement programs, and improved regulatory compliance. Despite these benefits, the adoption of EMRs, and AIMS, has not yet occurred in many smaller health care facilities, where the majority of Americans receive their care. To provide the health care community with incentives to overcome the obstacles to EMRs, in 2009 the U.S. Congress passed the Health Information Technology for Economic and Clinical Health Act (HITECH). Through Medicare and Medicaid, the U.S. government will make available $27 billion over a 10-year period to facilitate the transformation to EMRs and, by extension, AIMS.

Summary

In their most basic stand-alone form, AIMS do little more than collect intraoperative anesthesia data and automate the recordkeeping for anesthesia care providers. More advanced AIMS include interfaces with other systems and decision support and information management functions. These advanced capabilities can directly facilitate improvements in billing, quality improvement, safety, regulatory compliance, and research. An integrated AIMS, by interfacing directly with the EMR and other hospital information systems, can facilitate improved and more efficient care far beyond the operating room. Generally, health care lags behind other industries in the utilization of integrated information technology. With fewer AIMS installations relative to other EMR components, this is particularly true for anesthesiology. However, AIMS implementation and use should increase significantly as the technology matures and its value becomes increasingly demonstrated and understood.

Suggested Readings

Balust J. Can anesthesia information management systems improve quality in the surgical suite? *Curr Opin Anaesthesiol*. 2009;22:1-8.

Egger Halbeis CB, Epstein RH, Macario A, et al. Adoption of anesthesia information management systems by academic departments in the United States. *Anesth Analg*. 2008;107:1323-1329.

Epstein RH, Vigoda MM, Feinstein DM. Anesthesia information management systems: A survey of current implementation policies and practices. *Anesth Analg*. 2007;105:405-411.

Stonemetz J. *Anesthesia Informatics*. London: Springer Verlag: 2009:508.

CHAPTER 252

Medical Coding and Payment Systems

Norman A. Cohen, MD, and Sharon K. Merrick, MS, CCS-P

Coding and billing are important elements of every medical practice. Failure to understand coding and payment systems can harm the cash flow of an anesthesia practice. Contracts with payers, as well as a complex web of laws and regulations, govern correct coding. Compliance with these rules, laws, and contractual terms protects against allegations of fraudulent or abusive practices and the potentially severe legal consequences that may occur. In this chapter, we will provide a top-down review starting with issues that are relevant to all medical specialties and then drill down to those that are unique to anesthesia.

Medical Diagnosis and Procedure Codes

Medical codes provide a convenient shorthand way to tell payers and others what you did and why you did it. The Health Insurance Portability and Accountability Act of 1996 (HIPAA) standardized the code sets to be used on claims submitted to Medicare, Medicaid, and most third-party payers. CPT (Current Procedural Terminology) codes describe professional services. The American Medical Association (AMA) owns and maintains this code set. Professional medical services include patient visits with a physician or other qualified health care professional; therapeutic procedures, including major and minor operations; anesthesia care; certain diagnostic tests; and many other categories.

Physicians use ICD-9-CM codes to explain the reason or reasons behind the need for a medical service. *ICD* stands for *International Classification of Diseases*, and *CM* means that the code set has been *clinically modified* to be relevant for use in the United States. The World Health Organization created and maintains the ICD, and the United States government, through the National Center for Health Statistics and the Centers for Medicare and Medicaid Services (CMS) maintains the ICD-9-CM, including instructions for proper use. ICD-9-CM includes three volumes. When reporting professional services, only volumes 1 and 2 are applicable. These volumes contain a listing of diagnoses or conditions. Hospitals use volume 3 codes to describe and get paid for the inpatient facility costs associated with a service.

At the time of this writing, the United States is transitioning to version 10 of the ICD, known as ICD-10, with implementation expected in late 2014. ICD-10 has been adopted in many other countries, beginning in the early 1990s. Both diagnosis and procedure codes will increase in number and change substantially in form with this new version. Because implementation details currently are ill defined, the ICD-10 will not be discussed further in this chapter.

CPT Code Development and Valuation Process

CPT codes describe a medical service; payment systems link these codes to a defined value. This section will describe the method in which CPT codes are created and the most common systems of payment important to anesthesia providers.

When a specialty society, physician, or any interested stakeholder identifies a need for a new procedure code, that individual or group submits a formal proposal to the AMA, which has established a well-defined process that must be followed. Representatives from all specialties seated in the AMA House of Delegates have the opportunity to review all proposals and offer comments or suggestions. The members of the CPT Editorial Panel make decisions on acceptance, rejection, final wording, and guidelines for use. The 2013 Panel consisted of 17 members, including its chair and co-chair. The AMA Board of Trustees selects 11 members from a pool of physicians nominated by the participating specialty societies. Two members represent nonphysician health care professionals nominated by the AMA Health Care Professionals Advisory Committee (HCPAC). The remaining members are representatives from CMS, America's Health Insurance Plans (AHIP), the American Hospital Association (AHA), and the Blue Cross Blue Shield Association (BCBSA).

In 1992, the U.S. government introduced a payment system for the Medicare program to value medical procedures based on the resources used, rather than using the local usual and customary fee. Each service paid under this resource-based relative value system (RBRVS) scale has associated relative value units (RVUs) to account for work, practice expense, and professional liability insurance. Long before the introduction of RBRVS, the American Society of Anesthesiologists (ASA) developed a relative value system for anesthesia services. This system uses a different scale in which each code has an associated base unit value assigned, recognizing the complexity of the case. Time units reflect the time taken to perform the anesthetic service, and modifier units reflect patient condition, emergency status, and several other situations that impact anesthesia care. Medicare uses a modification of the ASA system to pay for anesthesia care in the RBRVS. At this time, nearly all payers use the anesthesia payment system and well over 70% use RBRVS.

Once the CPT Editorial Panel approves a new code or revises an existing code, the next step is to assign or update the value of the code in the RBRVS. In the early 1990s, the AMA and many medical specialty societies jointly created a committee to provide comments to CMS on the value of services covered by this new system. This AMA Specialty Societies Relative Value Scale Update Committee, known as the RUC, has played a very important role in the ongoing refinement of the RBRVS over the ensuing years. The composition of the RUC includes representatives from the AMA, the American Osteopathic Association, a representative of HCPAC, permanent seats for the large medical specialties (including the ASA), and rotating seats for smaller specialties. Representatives from CMS attend the meetings as well. For new and revised codes, specialty societies conduct surveys of physicians who are knowledgeable about the service under review, comparing the work associated with this service with that of a service with an established and accepted valuation. Specialty societies analyze the data and present the results, along with their recommendations as to the value of the service, to the RUC. The specialty societies also submit information on clinical staff, equipment, and supply expenses associated with the service that CMS uses in creating practice expense relative values. The RUC reviews all of the materials and listens to the specialty societies' arguments. The RUC then forwards its own recommendations to CMS. These recommendations requires a two-thirds vote to approve, helping to ensure that the RUC's submissions reflect the consensus opinion of organized medicine. Although CMS accepts the RUC's recommendations more than 90% of the time, specialty societies typically do not enjoy that same success in persuading the RUC to agree with their proposed values.

Anesthesia Coding

Anesthesia services are described by CPT codes 00100 through 01999. This section of CPT is subdivided into body regions. For example, anesthesia for procedures on the shoulder is grouped into codes 01610 to 01682. Codes 01710 to 01782 are used to report anesthesia for procedures on the upper arm and elbow. When coding for anesthesia care, modifiers are used to provide additional information about the patient or to provide additional information about the circumstances in which the care was provided, or both. The former is accomplished via a Physical Status (PS) modifier and the latter with a Qualifying Circumstance code. The ASA physical status assessment, which ranges from 1 for healthy patients through 5 for moribund patients and 6 for an organ donor, has corresponding modifiers (P1 to P6). Depending on the payer, these modifiers can yield higher payments.

A number of practice models exist for delivering anesthesia care in the United States. Sometimes, anesthesiologists work alone. Sometimes, resident physicians or nonphysician anesthesia providers (anesthesiologist assistants or certified registered nurse anesthetists) work with an anesthesiologist on the anesthesia care team; sometimes the anesthesia provider may work under the supervision of a surgeon or, depending on state law, independently. Medicare and some private payers have specific payment rules that impact payment depending on the mode of anesthesia practice. Medicare has created certain payment modifiers to report these various circumstances, which some private payers use as well.

The ASA publishes two very important resources to aid practices in coding for the anesthesia services they provide. The Relative Value Guide (RVG) provides a basic overview of anesthesia coding, along with a list of all of the anesthesia CPT codes with the associated base unit value. The CROSSWALK offers assistance in selecting the exact code that best describes the anesthesia service provided, based on the surgical service or services performed. All of the coding resources cited in this chapter (CPT, ICD-9-CM, RVG, and CROSSWALK) are reviewed and updated each year. For this reason, use of outdated editions is pennywise and dollar foolish, as it will eventually lead to incorrect codes being submitted, may be seen as fraudulent or abusive practice, and could lead to civil or criminal prosecution.

Payment Methodology Illustrations—Anesthesia

The following formula is used to determine payment for an anesthesia service:

Allowed amount = (Base units + Time units + Modifying factors)
× Conversion factor

where the *allowed amount* is the total payment for the service received from the insurer and the patient.

The *base unit* is a measure of the work involved in providing the anesthesia care. The higher the base unit value, the more complex the care. The work covered by the base unit value includes all of the typical preanesthesia and postanesthesia work and excludes only the time spent directly delivering anesthesia and any modifying factors.

The *time unit*, according to the ASA RVG, is determined as follows: "Anesthesia time begins when the anesthesiologist begins to prepare the patient for anesthesia care in the operating room or in an equivalent area and ends when the anesthesiologist is no longer in personal attendance, that is, when the patient is safely placed under post-anesthesia supervision."

Medicare requires that anesthesia time be reported in minutes, with 15 min equal to 1 time unit.. The *modifying factor* is a modifier based on the physical status or qualifying circumstance code. The *conversion factor* is the number of dollars paid per unit.

Illustration 1

An anesthesiologist provided anesthesia care for a patient undergoing a cholecystectomy. Anesthesia time was 60 min, and the patient had severe systemic disease, classifying him as a P3, worth 1 unit. According to the group's contract with the patient's insurer, the conversion factor is $55 per unit, and the anesthesia time of 60 min is reported. Per the ASA CROSSWALK, the proper anesthesia code associated with a cholecystectomy is 00790. Code 00790 has 7 base units. Assuming the payer uses a 15-min time unit, calculation is as follows:

Allowed amount = (Base units + Time units + Modifying factors)
× Conversion factor

= (7 + 4 + 1) × $55

= $660.00

Illustration 2

The anesthesiologist provided anesthesia care for a female patient undergoing drainage of a deep periurethral abscess. In this instance, the CROSSWALK offers two potential anesthesia codes. The primary selection is code 00920—Anesthesia for procedures on male genitalia (including open urethral procedures); not otherwise specified. The alternate code is code 00942—Anesthesia for vaginal procedures (including biopsy of labia, vagina, cervix or endometrium); colpotomy, vaginectomy, colporrhaphy, and open urethral procedures. The patient's sex directs you to select the alternate offering. The RVG tells you that code 00942 has 4 base units. The anesthesia time is 45 min (3 units), there are no modifying factors, and the conversion factor is $62 per unit:

Allowed amount = (Base units + Time units + Modifying factors)
× Conversion factor

= (4 + 3 + 0) × $62

= $434.00

Medicare payments adjust to account for economic differences based on geography. Each Medicare billing area applies slightly different adjustments to the national anesthesia conversion factor, which was $21.92 in 2013. For example, the 2013 conversion factor as $21.87 in Arizona and $20.70 in South Carolina.

Payment Methodology Illustrations—Resource-Based Relative Value System

A different formula is used to determine payment for nonanesthesia services. Medicare and many private payers use the RBRVS. Under RBRVS, RVUs are assigned to the work, practice expense, and professional liability insurance components of each service. These RVUs are added together, and the resulting sum is multiplied by a conversion factor. The formula is as follows:

Allowed amount = (Work RVU + PE RVU + PLI RVU)
× Conversion factor

where PE refers to practice expense, and PLI, to professional liability insurance.

Illustration 3

An anesthesiologist provides anesthesia care for a patient, and the patient requires placement of an arterial line to provide a more detailed level of monitoring. We will use the 2013 Medicare RBRVS conversion factor of $ 34.0230 per unit. Placement of an arterial line is reported with CPT code 36620. The RVUs assigned to this code in 2013 are shown in Table 252-1. Multiplying the total RVUs by the conversion factor results in an allowed amount of $50.69.

The RBRVS method accounts for geographic differences by making adjustments to the RVUs assigned to each component (work, practice expense, and professional liability insurance) of each service, leaving the conversion factor constant across the country.

Table 252-1 Relative Value Units Assigned to Placement and Monitoring of an Arterial Catheter in 2013

Category	RVU
Work	1.15
Practice expense	0.24
Professional liability insurance	0.10
TOTAL	1.49

RVU, Relative value unit.

Conclusion

Anesthesiologists perform some services paid under the anesthesia methodology and others that are paid under the RBRVS method. As such, they need to understand both systems. They also need to have a broad-based understanding of the CPT coding system because the anesthesia codes they report depend upon the more than 5000 diagnostic and therapeutic CPT-described services that may require anesthesia care. Finally, anesthesiologists must understand how to code for line placement, image guidance, pain procedures, transesophageal echocardiography, critical care, inpatient and outpatient evaluation and management visits, and other services related to anesthesia care.

Suggested Readings

American Medical Association. *CPT 2014*. Available at: https://catalog.ama-assn.org/Catalog/cpt/cpt_home.jsp. Accessed November 10, 2013.

American Medical Association. *2014 ICD-9-CM Vol. 1*. Available at: https://catalog.ama-assn.org/Catalog/cpt/cpt_home.jsp. Accessed November 10, 2013.

2014 CROSSWALK Book. A Guide for Surgery/Anesthesia CPT Codes. Park Ridge, IL: American Society of Anesthesiolgists; 2013.

2014 Relative Value Guide Book. A Guide for Anesthesia Values. Park Ridge, IL: American Society of Anesthesiolgists; 2013.

CHAPTER 253

Professional Citizenship and Medical Advocacy

Jeff T. Mueller, MD, and Daniel J. Cole, MD

Advocacy, defined as "the act or process of advocating or supporting a cause or proposal," is an important component of professionalism. Anesthesiologists engage in advocacy to promote patient safety and the highest standards of anesthesia care.

Opportunities to advocate for our profession occur on many levels and in a variety of clinical and nonclinical settings, the most basic of which is the opportunity afforded to us daily in our interactions with patients, their families, and other members of the health care team. Conducting thorough preoperative interviews, performing physical examinations, reviewing laboratory and imaging studies, and involving patients in developing anesthetic plans that address their concerns and comorbid conditions provide patients with insights into the complexity of the comprehensive medical care provided by anesthesiologists. Anesthesiologists must remember that many physicians, hospital administrators, nurses, and patients view anesthesiology as a "black box"—a portion of overall health care that is frequently taken for granted and therefore devalued. We must capitalize upon the many teachable moments that occur during each day, explaining the "why" in addition to the "what" that is involved with anesthesia care with the hope that other health care providers will obtain a more accurate view of our profession.

Anesthesiologists who accept positions of institutional leadership (e.g., facility medical director, chief of staff, or member of hospital committees such as those involved in credentialing and privileging or in quality improvement) have additional opportunities for professional advocacy. In academic medical centers, anesthesiologists must accept leadership positions to promote anesthesiologists' education and research. Our knowledge and expertise are essential to developing and maintaining efficient systems of care associated with the best patient outcomes.

Unfortunately, many anesthesiologists avoid participating in leadership activities of their hospitals and academic medical institutions, which in and of itself is a failure in our obligations to our profession and, therefore, to our patients. Being involved in organized medicine and regulatory bodies that oversee health care delivery, such as state medical licensing boards, The Joint Commission, and Medicare Contractor Advisory Committees, provides other opportunities to support our profession. Other venues for anesthesiologists to represent patients and the specialty are through the provision of testimony at public hearings and during comment periods for rules and legislative actions. Anesthesiologists must respond to requests to participate in such venues to help create regulations and rules that promote patient safety and the delivery of the highest standards of anesthesia care. If we do not participate in regulatory decision making, regulatory bodies may create rules and policies that are based more on opinion than on science and that do not improve outcome but, rather, are impractical and expensive to implement.

City and county boards and state and federal legislatures provide outstanding opportunities to advocate for our profession. Legislative advocacy consists of three components: representation by lobbyists and other advocacy professionals, political campaign activity by political action committees (PACs), and direct grassroots activity by individual physicians. Many medical organizations provide professional representation; the American Society of Anesthesiologists maintains an office in Washington, DC, devoted to that purpose. In many states, the state medical association or anesthesiology specialty society provides professional representation to the state legislature.

Participating in PACs presents a second means for an effective legislative advocacy effort. A specialty society PAC provides an opportunity to directly support legislators who value and promote high-quality anesthesia care. PACs collect and pool financial contributions from members of a medical association or a specialty society and then distribute campaign contributions to selected candidates. In a democracy all interest groups work to support legislators who share their priorities and goals. Anesthesiologists, individually and through PACs, must support legislators who take the time to understand and promote patient safety. Health insurance companies, third-party payers, trial lawyers, hospital associations, pharmaceutical companies, and other groups all work vigorously to support candidates who represent their views, and so must we. PACs are a transparent, ethical, and necessary way for groups of professionals to collectively participate in democracy and its inherent political campaigns.

Both professional representation and PACs are requirements for effective legislative advocacy, but direct grassroots activity by anesthesiologists is the most important component of an effective legislative program. Elected officials are most in tune with the views and interests of the individuals whom they represent. Many groups that oppose the patient-centered priorities of anesthesiologists have capable lobbyists and substantial PACs, but they cannot duplicate our credibility when we directly advocate on behalf of our patients, who are also constituents of the same elected officials. Our personal advocacy should be targeted to grassroots networks and cultivating key contacts. Grassroots networks provide anesthesiologists a medium to send messages to legislators on a specific issue. Equally, if not more, important is developing relationships with key legislators. Building a relationship can take a few years, but the occasional phone call, email, or face-to-face discussion does not require a large amount of time and will cumulatively lead to a relationship with an elected official or appointed civil servant. The American Society of Anesthesiologists offers advice and support to physicians who make this important contribution to the profession.

Who of us believes that patient care simply takes place at the bedside? Unfortunately, regulation and legislation have eroded the doctor-patient relationship and affect virtually all aspects of patient care. If we care about our specialty and the patients for whom we provide care, we must be willing to give of ourselves and go beyond our everyday practice and advocate for our specialty. If we do not provide the anecdotes that guide legislative and regulatory action, others who do not share our interests will be more than happy to do so. If our stories are silenced, our issues become invisible, and we can only blame ourselves for the devaluation of our specialty, the erosion of our autonomy, and the lack of choice that our patients have in selecting who will provide their care and where that care will be delivered.

Suggested Readings

ASA Grassroots Network. *Washington Advocacy Guide*. American Society of Anesthesiologists, 2009. Available at: http://www.asahq.org/Washington/2009ASAGrassrootsNetworkDCAdvocacyGuide.pdf. Accessed October 8, 2012.

Gruen RL, Campbell EG, Blumenthal D. Public roles of US physicians: Community participation, political involvement, and collective advocacy. *JAMA*. 2006;296:2467-2475.

Landers SH, Sehgal AR. Health care lobbying in the United States. *Am J Med*. 2004;116:474-477.

Spivey BE, Dyer ER. Managing medicine: Health care politics and policy. In: Albert DM, ed. *A Physician's Guide to Health Care Management*. Malden, MA: Blackwell Science; 2002:14-20.

CHAPTER 254
Chemical Dependency in Anesthesia Personnel

Keith H. Berge, MD

Chemical dependence is a devastating disease that must be recognized before it can be treated. In most cases, the addict is the last to acknowledge the problem. Thus, it is imperative that we—the friends, colleagues, and relatives of the addict—gain a clear understanding of the disease before we are confronted with it.

Chemical dependency, especially opioid addiction, is an occupational hazard for anesthesia providers. We have access to highly potent synthetic opiates in anesthesia practice and work in a stressful environment. Opioid abuse in anesthesia personnel typically occurs in the workplace; independent of the geographic location in which the abuse takes place, there are many tragic reports of anesthesia providers suffering severe illness (e.g., anoxic encephalopathy) or even fatality from an overdose of self-administered opioids.

Although anesthesia providers are at risk of becoming addicted to the same licit (e.g., ethanol) and illicit drugs (e.g., cocaine) as society at large, the "drug of choice" for anesthesia providers undergoing rehabilitation for chemical abuse is typically fentanyl or sufentanil, although ethanol, propofol, marijuana, and cocaine remain common drugs of abuse. Of 45,581 residents entering the American Board of Anesthesiologists certification process in the years 1975-2009, 384 were confirmed to have developed a substance use disorder (SUD) while in residency, for an overall rate of 2.16 per 1000 resident years. Of those, 26 died in training and 2 died shortly after completing residency, all of SUD-related causes. Despite efforts to educate residents on the dangers posed by SUD, the incidence is increasing.

Fentanyl, available as a street drug, is considered by addiction medicine specialists to have an addictive potential similar to that of "crack" cocaine. It carries the risk of extremely rapid addiction (Figure 254-1). This rapid effect is in contrast with that of ethanol or even other opioids, such as morphine or meperidine, for which a longer period of abuse is typically required before psychological and physical addiction occur.

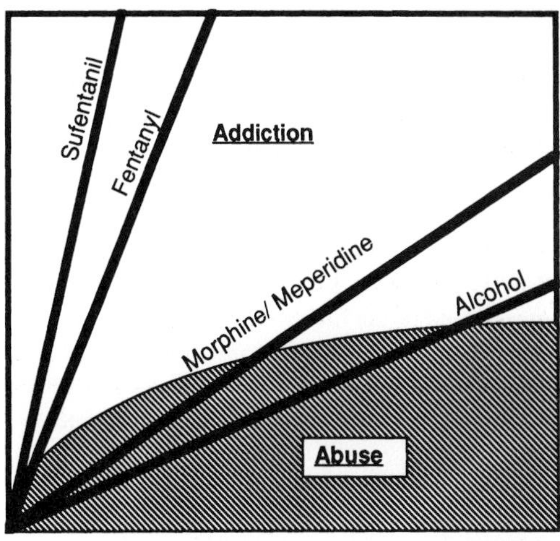

Figure 254-1 Time course of addiction. Dependence on alcohol develops over years, whereas sufentanil or fentanyl addiction develops quickly after a very short period of abuse. (From Arnold WP III. Environmental safety including chemical dependency. In: Miller RD, ed. Anesthesia. 5th ed. Philadelphia, Churchill Livingstone, 2000:2701-2717.)

Recognizing Impairment in a Colleague

Chemical dependency threatens the career and, possibly, the life of an impaired colleague and the lives of patients under his or her care. Therefore, it is imperative that telltale signs of addiction be recognized and treated, not ignored (Box 254-1). These signs, typically subtle, may not be apparent in the workplace until the addictive illness is relatively far advanced. Instead, the afflicted individual may appear to function well in the workplace while his or her family life and social functioning may be in a state of chaos. In the case of opioid addiction, this behavior may be an attempt to preserve both career and access to the needed drug. It is interesting to note that, although the incidence of opioid abuse by anesthesia providers, even while on duty, is known to occur with distressing frequency, documented harm to patients by impaired caregivers is rare.

Box 254-1 Signs of Chemical Abuse in an Anesthesia Colleague

- Exhibiting unusual behavior; mood swings; or periods of depression, anger, and irritability, alternating with periods of euphoria
- "Signing out" unusual and increasing quantities of opioids
- Exhibiting reclusive behavior
- Taking frequent bathroom breaks
- Frequently relieving others
- Volunteering to clean rooms, volunteering for extra call, or spending off-duty hours at the hospital
- Wearing long sleeves to hide needle marks
- Providing operative care for patients arriving in recovery room with pain out of proportion to the amount of opioid charted as having been given during their case
- Exhibiting evidence of withdrawal, including agitation, tremors, and diaphoresis

Intervention

Confronting an impaired colleague is extremely stressful and unpleasant. The intervention process is greatly facilitated if a departmental policy is in place outlining procedures to follow regarding intervention, evaluation, and the option of reentry into the workplace after treatment. If sufficient evidence exists to suggest that a colleague is indeed chemically impaired or addicted, it is imperative that a qualified addiction medicine specialist evaluate this physician. Because denial is a hallmark of addiction, those responsible for the intervention should not attempt to judge the presence or absence of addiction by the response of the colleague suspected of having the addiction. Rather, the purpose of the session should simply be to notify the colleague that she or he must submit to an evaluation by a qualified specialist. Prior arrangements should be made to facilitate immediate evaluation, and the colleague should be physically escorted to the evaluation, with the escort recognizing the potential for the colleague to harm herself or himself. If reasonable suspicion exists that a person is chemically dependent, then an evaluation can be demanded. It is not necessary to achieve the higher legal standard of clear and convincing evidence.

Risk of Relapse

Although the potential for long-term recovery from addiction to ethanol or benzodiazepines has been reported to be good, the risk of relapse into abuse is high for the opioid-addicted physician in recovery. The rate of relapse into opioid abuse has been reported to be between 14% and 70%. In the most recent study, there was an estimated 43% relapse rate predicted over the span of a 30-year career. Relapse rates remain high despite improved treatment, aftercare, and monitoring. Of those who relapsed, death was their initial manifestation of relapse in 13%. Unfortunately, no similar published data exist defining the incidence of SUD or the relapse rate in nurse anesthesia personnel. Due to the high risk of relapse, and the severe consequences that may result, reentry of an anesthesiologist in recovery from opioid abuse into the clinical practice of anesthesiology is controversial. If reentry is undertaken, it is typically associated with an intensive aftercare program mandated by each state. Components of this program usually include random drug screening; active participation in support groups, such as Alcoholics Anonymous or NarcAnon; and prolonged witnessed use of antagonists, such as naltrexone, for those with a history of opioid abuse, or disulfiram, for those with a history of ethanol abuse.

Suggested Readings

Berge KH, Seppala MD, Schipper AM. Chemical dependency and the physician. *Mayo Clin Proc*. 2009;84:625-631.

Booth JV, Grossman D, Moore J, et al. Substance abuse among physicians: A survey of academic anesthesiology programs. *Anesth Analg*. 2002;95:1024-1030.

Bryson EO. Should anesthesia residents with a history of substance abuse be allowed to continue training in clinical anesthesia? The results of a survey of anesthesia residency program directors. *J Clin Anesth*. 2009;21:508-513.

Bryson EO, Levine A. One approach to the return to residency for anesthesia residents recovering from opioid addiction. *J Clin Anesth*. 2008;20:397-400.

Bryson EO, Silverstein JH. Addiction and substance abuse in anesthesiology. *Anesthesiology*. 2008;109:905-917.

Domino KB, Hornbein TF, Polissar NL, et al. Risk factors for relapse in health care professionals with substance use disorders. *JAMA*. 2005;293:1453-1460.

Lanier WL, Kharasch ED. Contemporary clinical opioid use: Opportunities and challenges. *Mayo Clin Proc*. 2009;84:572-575.

Oreskovich MR, Caldeiro RM. Anesthesiologists recovering from chemical dependency: Can they safely return to the operating room? *Mayo Clin Proc*. 2009;84:576-580.

Tetzlaff J, Collins GB, Brown DL, et al. A strategy to prevent substance abuse in an academic anesthesiology department. *J Clin Anesth*. 2010;22:143-150.

Warner DO, Berge KH, et al. Substance use disorder among anesthesiology residents, 1975-2009. *JAMA* 2013;310:2289-2296.

Index

Note: Pages number followed by "b" indicate boxes; "f" figures; "t" tables.

D

E

G

H

I

O

Q

R

S

U

V